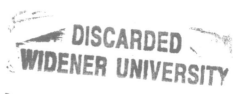

EMERGENCY CARE OF THE WOMAN

NOTICE

Medicine is an ever-changing science. As new research and clinical experience broaden our knowledge, changes in treatment and drug therapy are required. The editors and the publisher of this work have checked with sources believed to be reliable in their efforts to provide information that is complete and generally in accord with the standards accepted at the time of publication. However, in view of the possibility of human error or changes in medical sciences, neither the editors nor the publisher nor any other party who has been involved in the preparation or publication of this work warrants that the information contained herein is in every respect accurate or complete, and they are not responsible for any errors or omissions or for the results obtained from use of such information. Readers are encouraged to confirm the information contained herein with other sources. For example and in particular, readers are advised to check the product information sheet included in the package of each drug they plan to administer to be certain that the information contained in this book is accurate and that changes have not been made in the recommended dose or in the contraindications for administration. This recommendation is of particular importance in connection with new or infrequently used drugs.

EMERGENCY CARE OF THE WOMAN

EDITORS

MARK D. PEARLMAN, M.D.

Associate Professor
Department of Obstetrics and Gynecology
University of Michigan Medical Center
Ann Arbor, Michigan

JUDITH E. TINTINALLI, M.D., M.S.

Professor and Chairman
Steven J. Dresnick, M.D. Distinguished Professor and Chair in Emergency Medicine
Department of Emergency Medicine
University of North Carolina at Chapel Hill
Chapel Hill, North Carolina

Illustrations by Holly R. Fischer, MFA
Ann Arbor, Michigan

McGraw-Hill
Health Professions Division

New York St. Louis San Francisco Auckland Bogotá Caracas Lisbon
London Madrid Mexico City Milan Montreal New Delhi
San Juan Singapore Sydney Tokyo Toronto

McGraw-Hill

A Division of The **McGraw·Hill** *Companies*

EMERGENCY CARE OF THE WOMAN

Copyright © 1998 by The McGraw-Hill Companies, Inc. All rights reserved.
Printed in the United States of America. Except as permitted under the United
States Copyright Act of 1976, no part of this publication may be reproduced or
distributed in any form or by any means, or stored in a data base or retrieval
system, without the prior written permission of the publisher.

234567890 QPKQPK 998

ISBN 0-07-049127-5

This book was set in Times Roman by York Graphic Services, Inc.
The editors were John J. Dolan and Muza Navorozov.
The production supervisor was Richard Ruzycka.
The cover was designed by Marsha Cohen/Paralellogram.
The index was prepared by Irving Tullar.
Quebecor Printing/Kingsport was printer and binder.

This book is printed on recycled, acid-free paper.

Library of Congress Cataloging-in-Publication Data

Emergency care of the woman / editors, Mark D. Pearlman, Judith E. Tintinalli.
    p. cm.
    Includes bibliographical references and index.
    ISBN 0-07-049127-5 (alk. paper)
    1. Obstetrical emergencies.   2. Gynecologic emergencies.
  I. Pearlman, Mark.   II. Tintinalli, Judith E.
    [DNLM: 1. Pregnancy Complications.   2. Emergencies—in pregnancy.
   3. Genital Diseases, Female.   WQ 240 E53 1998]
RG571.E47 1998
618′.0425—dc21   97-36815
                               CIP

To Burt and Dr. Anne
To Susan, Aaron, Allie, Zachary, and Hannah for their love and support.

CONTENTS

PART III
EMERGENCY GYNECOLOGIC DISORDERS IN THE PEDIATRIC PATIENT AND ADOLESCENT / 381

PART IV
EMERGENCY GYNECOLOGIC DISORDERS IN THE REPRODUCTIVE AGE / 433

PART V

EMERGENCY GYNECOLOGIC DISORDERS IN OLDER WOMEN / 621

PART VI

ULTRASONOGRAPHY / 647

PART VII
GYNECOLOGIC ONCOLOGY / 675

APPENDIXES

CONTRIBUTORS

Imran Ali, M.D.
Assistant Professor of Neurology
Medical College of Ohio
Toledo, Ohio

H. Frank Andersen, M.D.
Professor of Obstetrics and Gynecology
Loma Linda University Medical Center
Division of Maternal Fetal Medicine
Loma Linda, California

David A. August, M.D.
Associate Professor of Surgery
Robert Wood Johnson University Medical School
The Cancer Institute of New Jersey
New Brunswick, New Jersey

Mel L. Barclay, M.D.
Associate Professor of Obstetrics and Gynecology
University of Michigan Medical Center
Ann Arbor, Michigan

Steven L. Bloom, M.D.
Assistant Professor of Obstetrics and Gynecology
University of Texas School of Medicine
Dallas, Texas

Brian C. Brost, M.D.
Attending Physician
Department of Obstetrics and Gynecology
Keesler Medical Center
Biloxi, Mississippi

Catherine Christen, Pharm.D.
College of Pharmacy
University of Michigan Medical Center
Ann Arbor, Michigan

Gregory M. Christman, M.D.
Assistant Professor of Obstetrics and Gynecology
University of Michigan Medical Center
Ann Arbor, Michigan

Emmanuel G. Christodoulou, Ph.D.
Research Fellow in Radiological Sciences
University of Michigan Medical Center
Ann Arbor, Michigan

Christine H. Comstock, M.D.
Assistant Professor of Obstetrics and Gynecology
Wayne State University School of Medicine;
Clinical Assistant Professor of Obstetrics and Gynecology
University of Michigan Medical Center;
Director of Fetal Imaging
William Beaumont Hospital
Royal Oak, Michigan

F. Gary Cunningham, M.D.
Jack A. Pritchard Professor and Chair in
Obstetrics and Gynecology
University of Texas Southwestern Medical Center
Dallas Texas

John O. L. DeLancey, M.D.
Associate Professor of Obstetrics and Gynecology
Director, Division of Gynecology
University of Michigan Medical Center
Ann Arbor, Michigan

Diana L. Dell, M.D.
Fellow in Psychiatry
University of North Carolina School of Medicine
Chapel Hill, North Carolina

Gary A. Dildy, M.D.
Associate Professor of Obstetrics and Gynecology
University of Utah Health Science Center;
Director of Perinatology
Utah Valley Regional Medical Center
Provo, Utah

William Patrick Duff, M.D.
Professor of Obstetrics and Gynecology
University of Florida College of Medicine
Gainsville, Florida

Mary Eberst, M.D.
Instructor in Emergency Medicine
University of North Carolina School of Medicine
Chapel Hill, North Carolina

Sebastian Faro, M.D., Ph.D.
John M. Simpson Professor and Chair of
Obstetrics and Gynecology
Rush Medical College and Rush-Presbyterian-St. Luke's
Medical Center
Chicago, Illinois

Larry C. Gilstrap III, M.D.
Professor and Chair of Obstetrics and Gynecology
University of Texas Medical School
Houston, Texas

Mitchell M. Goodsitt, M.S., Ph.D.
Associate Professor of Radiological Sciences
Adjunct Associate Professor of Environmental and Industrial
Health
University of Michigan Medical Center
Ann Arbor, Michigan

Gary D. V. Hankins, M.D.
Professor of Obstetrics and Gynecology
Vice-Chair, Department of Obstetrics and Gynecology
University of Texas Medical Branch
Galveston, Texas

William H. Hurd, M.D.
Associate Professor of Obstetrics and Gynecology
Director of Reproductive Endocrinology
Indiana University School of Medicine
Indianapolis, Indiana

Jean A. Hurteau, M.D.
Associate Professor of Obstetrics and Gynecology
Indiana University School of Medicine
Indianapolis, Indiana

Timothy R. B. Johnson, M.D.
Bates Professor of Diseases of Women and Children
and Chair of Obstetrics and Gynecology
University of Michigan Medical Center
Ann Arbor, Michigan

Kathy Y. Jones, M.D.
Senior Staff Physician in Obstetrics and Gynecology
Henry Ford Hospital
Detroit, Michigan

Vern L. Katz, M.D.
Associate Director of Maternal Fetal Medicine
Sacred Heart Medical Center
Eugene, Oregon

Raymond H. Kaufman, M.D.
Professor of Pathology
Professor of Obstetrics and Gynecology
Baylor College of Medicine
Houston, Texas

Carl B. Lauter, M.D.
Clinical Professor of Medicine
Wayne State University School of Medicine;
Director, Division of Allergy and Clinical Immunology
Member, Division of Infectious Diseases
William Beaumont Hospital
Royal Oak, Michigan

Robert P. Lorenz, M.D.
Associate Professor of Obstetrics and Gynecology
Wayne State University School of Medicine;
Clinical Assistant Professor of Obstetrics and Gynecology
University of Michigan Medical Center;
Vice-Chief of Obstetrics and Director of Maternal Fetal Medicine
William Beaumont Hospital
Royal Oak, Michigan

Mark J. Lowell, M.D.
Associate Medical Director of Survival Flight
Director, Chest Pain Center
University of Michigan Medical Center
Ann Arbor, Michigan

Maurizio L. Maccato, M.D.
Associate Professor of Obstetrics and Gynecology
Baylor College of Medicine
Houston, Texas

Veronica T. Mallett, M.D.
Associate Professor of Obstetrics and Gynecology
Wayne State University School of Medicine and Hutzel Hospital
Detroit, Michigan

Fernando J. Martinez, M.D.
Associate Professor of Internal Medicine
Division of Pulmonary Medicine
University of Michigan Medical Center
Ann Arbor, Michigan

Lisa L. May, M.D.
Associate Professor of Dermatology
University of North Carolina School of Medicine
Chapel Hill, North Carolina

Linda M. Nicholas, M.D., M.S.
Assistant Professor of Psychiatry
University of North Carolina School of Medicine
Chapel Hill, North Carolina

Jennifer R. Niebyl, M.D.
Professor and Head of Obstetrics and Gynecology
University of Iowa College of Medicine
Iowa City, Iowa

Clark E. Nugent, M.D.
Clinical Associate Professor of Obstetrics and Gynecology
University of Michigan Medical Center
Ann Arbor, Michigan

Cheryl J. Paradis, M.D.
Attending Physician
Sherman Hospital
Elgin, Illinois

Mark D. Pearlman, M.D.
Associate Professor of Obstetrics and Gynecology
University of Michigan Medical Center
Ann Arbor, Michigan

Diana O. Perkins, M.D., M.P.H.
Assistant Professor of Psychiatry
University of North Carolina School of Medicine
Chapel Hill, North Carolina

Nancy F. Petit, M.D.
Attending Physician
St. Francis Ob/Gyn and Midwifery Center
Wilmington, Deleware

Carl Pierson, Ph.D.
Director of Clinical Microbiology and Virology
University of Michigan Medical Center
Ann Arbor, Michican

Susan F. Pokorny, M.D.
Associate Professor of Pediatrics
Baylor College of Medicine;
Chair of Obstetrics and Gynecology
Kelsey-Seybold Clinics
Houston, Texas

Margaret R. Punch, M.D.
Clinical Assistant Professor of Obstetrics and Gynecology
University of Michigan Medical Center
Ann Arbor, Michigan

Elisabeth H. Quint, M.D.
Clinical Assistant Professor of Obstetrics and Gynecology
University of Michigan Medical Center
Ann Arbor, Michigan

R. Kevin Reynolds, M.D.
Assistant Professor of Obstetrics and Gynecology
University of Michigan Medical Center
Ann Arbor, Michigan

James A. Roberts, M.D., M.S.
Professor of Gynecologic Oncology
Stanford University School of Medicine
Stanford, California

David S. Rosen, M.D.
Associate Professor of Pediatrics
University of Michigan Medical Center
Ann Arbor, Michigan

Beth S. Rosenberg, M.D., Ed.D.
Clinical Instructor in Internal Medicine
University of North Carolina School of Medicine
Chapel Hill, North Carolina

Thomas F. Rowe, M.D.
Assistant Professor of Obstetrics and Gynecology
Medical Director of Birth Center and Prenatal Diagnostic Center
University of Texas School of Medicine
Galveston, Texas

Andrew J. Satin, M.D.
Associate Professor of Obstetrics and Gynecology
Vice-Chair of Obstetrics and Gynecology
Uniformed Services University of the Health Sciences
Bethesda, Maryland

Elizabeth M. Shadigian, M.D.
Clinical Assistant Professor of Obstetrics and Gynecology
University of Michigan Medical Center
Ann Arbor, Michigan

Monica Sifuentes, M.D.
Assistant Professor of Pediatrics
UCLA School of Medicine
Harbor UCLA Medical Center
Torrance, California

Jack D. Sobel, M.D.
Professor of Medicine
Chief of Infectious Diseases
Wayne State University School of Medicine and Harper Hospital
Detroit, Michigan

Vernon K. Sondak, M.D.
Associate Professor of Surgery
University of Michigan Medical Center
Ann Arbor, Michigan

Rhoda S. Sperling, M.D.
Associate Professor of Obstetrics and Gynecology
Mt. Sinai School of Medicine;
Director of Infectious Diseases
Mt. Sinai Hospital
New York, New York

Kris Strohbehn, M.D.
Assistant Professor of Obstetrics and Gynecology
New England Medical Center
Boston, Massachusetts

Phillip G. Stubblefield, M.D.
Professor and Chair of Obstetrics and Gynecology
Boston University School of Medicine
Brookline, Massachusetts

Judith E. Tintinalli, M.D., M.S.
Steven J. Dresnick, M.D., Distinguished Professor and Chair
in Emergency Medicine
University of North Carolina School of Medicine
Chapel Hill, North Carolina

Marc R. Toglia, M.D.
Attending Physician
Riddle Memorial Hospital
Philadelphia, Pennsylvania

Cosmas J. M. van de Ven, M.D.
Assistant Professor of Obstetrics and Gynecology
University of Michigan Medical Center
Ann Arbor, Michigan

Peter VanDorsten, M.D.
Professor of Obstetrics and Gynecology
Medical University of South Carolina
Charleston, South Carolina

Bradley Vaughn, M.D.
Associate Professor of Neurology
University of North Carolina School of Medicine
Chapel Hill, North Carolina

Ellen C. Wells, M.D.
Associate Professor of Obstetrics and Gynecology
University of North Carolina School of Medicine
Chapel Hill, North Carolina

Catheryn Montgomery Yashar, M.D.
Lecturer in Obstetrics and Gynecology
University of Louisville
Louisville, Kentucky

Kristine M. Zanotti, M.D.
Fellow in Gynecologic Oncology
Cleveland Clinic Foundation
Cleveland, Ohio

Lauren Zoschnick, M.D.
Clinical Assistant Professor of Obstetrics and Gynecology
University of Michigan Medical Center
Ann Arbor, Michigan

PREFACE

Our own practices, in emergency medicine and obstetrics and gynecology, have made us acutely aware of the rapidly changing environment of women's health care. The recent focus on clinical pathways and outcomes makes us ask not only why we do things, but how we do them, and if we all do them in the same way.

We treat more and more complex medical problems, and have learned about the different types and patterns of illnesses in women. We feel stretched to keep ourselves informed about the global objectives of emergency care of women as well as with details of care for specific conditions.

And that is how this book came about.

We hope you will find its organization into clinical presentation by age group helpful. Most chapters are organized by presenting signs and symptoms, allowing problems to be addressed as they present to us. We have tried to provide clinical approaches that best fit the majority of emergency practices or practices where urgent problems are occasionally seen. Most importantly, we have tried to emphasize clinical approaches that best fit our patients and that best instruct our residents and students.

Mark Pearlman, MD
Judith E. Tintinalli, MD, MS

ACKNOWLEDGMENTS

Michelle Burr for her critical role in manuscript management and Rudi Ansbacher, MD, for his careful and thoughtful manuscript reviews.

EMERGENCY CARE OF THE WOMAN

PART I

GENERAL PRINCIPLES

Chapter 1

GENERAL PRINCIPLES OF EMERGENCY MANAGEMENT

Judith E. Tintinalli

All physicians treating women need to be comfortable treating simple obstetric and gynecologic disorders and to be aware of the effect of potential childbearing on diagnostic and treatment plans, socioeconomic circumstances that affect the health care of women, and gender differences in the patterns of acute illness and injury.

EMERGENCY MEDICAL SERVICES

Prehospital evaluation is based upon simple algorithms developed by local medical control. Abdominal or pelvic pain that is severe or unremitting; that is accompanied by other symptoms such as nausea, vomiting, bleeding, distention, or abnormal vital signs; or any pain or bleeding in a woman of childbearing age are general indications for emergency transport.[1] Patients are transported to the nearest appropriate emergency facility in accordance with local, state, or regional planning, and communication is provided to the base hospital by the transporting emergency medical services (EMS) unit. For pregnant women with severe injury, vaginal bleeding, or cardiac arrest or for women of childbearing age in shock, the obstetric consultant should be notified when the EMS call is received, so that he or she can assist in maternal or fetal stabilization as soon as the patient arrives in the emergency department. Transport personnel should provide written documentation of all prehospital care provided, including initial vital signs.[2] This material should be reviewed by the emergency care provider as part of the historical database for clinical evaluation.

TRANSFER

About 40 million Americans lack health insurance.[3] Clarification of a hospital's responsibility to provide emergency health care regardless of the insurance status of the patient was outlined in the Emergency Medical Treatment and Active Labor Act (EMTALA) in 1986. Patients with emergency conditions must be assessed and stabilized before transfer. For appropriate transfer, the transfer must not pose unacceptable risks to the patient, the receiving facility must have the resources to care for the patient, the receiving facility must have accepted the patient, and the transfer itself must be accomplished under conditions appropriate to the patient's medical status.[4]

EMERGENCY DEPARTMENT TRIAGE

There are few studies on the outcomes of emergency department triage and telephone triage and none specifically directed to the triage of chief complaints in women of childbearing potential.[5,6] Injuries and sexual assault and complaints of abdominal pain or vaginal bleeding, especially in a woman of childbearing age, are serious complaints that require emergency evaluation.

EVALUATION

Obtaining the chief complaint is the first step in emergency medical evaluation. After the chief complaint is elaborated, health status information should be recorded. This includes medication allergies, current medications, and tetanus immunization if there is acute injury. Women of childbearing age should be routinely asked if they are pregnant now or trying to become pregnant. These inquiries are necessary no matter what body system is involved in the chief complaint, since the diagnostic tests ordered and the treatment plan will change depending upon the patient's responses. For example, a patient and her physician may decide to forego radiographs or to shield the abdomen if the patient could be pregnant or to obtain a pregnancy test prior to proceeding.

Women of childbearing age who are sexually active should be questioned about contraceptive methods and behaviors. Counseling should be provided for human immunodeficiency virus (HIV), sexually transmitted diseases (STDs), and pregnancy prevention if needed. Patients should be informed about the availability of postcoital contraception in emergencies and how to obtain such treatment.[7] If peri- or postmenopausal women do not report the use of estrogen and progestin or calcium supplementation, the encounter may be used as an opportunity to counsel them on the benefits of such medications for decreasing the risk of cardiovascular disease and osteoporosis.[8]

Depending on the chief complaint, the physical examination may be problem-focused or detailed. Women complaining of upper or lower abdominal pain require a gynecologic and sexual history and pelvic examination in addition to the standard physical examination. Examination for femoral or inguinal hernias should always be performed in women with lower abdominal or groin pain. Direct or indirect inguinal hernias are rare in women. However, femoral hernias are more common in women than in men, possibly because the femoral canal is wider in women. On examination, there is a swelling on the upper part of the thigh, in a location that is lateral to the pubic tubercle and below the inguinal ligament (Fig. 1-1).

Women of childbearing age complaining of acute dysuria and urinary frequency without vaginal discharge probably do not need a pelvic examination and cervical cultures unless there is a reasonable incidence of STDs in the population the physician is treating or the history is otherwise suggestive of STDs. Women of lower socioeconomic status and those who seek treatment at STD clinics are reported to have a high frequency of dysuria and frequency with negative urine cultures but a high incidence of gonorrhea and chlamydial infections.[9] The incidence of urinary tract infection is high in sexually active young women, and the risk is strongest in those with recent sexual intercourse and with the use of a diaphragm and spermicide.[10,11] Thus, a diagnosis of urinary tract infection in a young, sexually active woman should prompt evaluation for possible pregnancy and investigation of coexisting sexually transmitted diseases.

Although women constitute about half of emergency department patients, routine screening for pregnancy is not generally performed unless the chief complaint is gynecologic. In a study of 191 women being treated in an urban emergency department, there was a 6.3 percent prevalence of unrecognized pregnancy, with three historical factors significantly associated with pregnancy: the patient's suspicion of pregnancy, an abnormal last menstrual period, and a chief complaint of abdominal or pelvic pain.[12] When one considers the frequency of radiographic studies ordered and potentially teratogenic drugs prescribed in the emergency department (such as quinolones or tetracyclines), the need to identify unrecognized pregnancy in women of childbearing age becomes obvious.

For women with injury, certain patterns should arouse suspicion of domestic violence. Injuries about the head and neck, such as periorbital hematomas; fractures of the jaw or teeth; injuries to the breasts or genitalia; or wounds with implausible mechanisms of injury suggest domestic violence. Neglect of follow-up—such as suture removal or care of a wound or fracture—also suggests a problematic social situation that could involve domestic violence.[13–15] If domestic violence is suspected, although only one patient (the adult woman) may be present for emergency evaluation, inquiries must also be made about the safety of children in the home. Diseases should not be eliminated from consideration because of a patient's age or assumptions about behaviors. Sexually transmitted diseases and domestic violence can affect older women just as they do younger ones.[15]

Socioeconomic conditions can affect the way in which women seek health care. Immigrant women may be more likely to use the emergency department for pregnancy problems if primary care is unavailable to them. Working women,

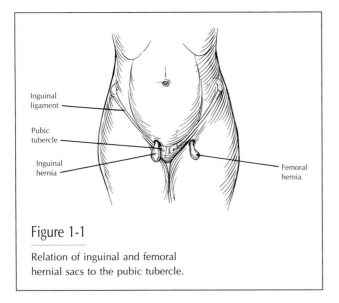

Inguinal ligament

Pubic tubercle

Inguinal hernia

Femoral hernia

Figure 1-1

Relation of inguinal and femoral hernial sacs to the pubic tubercle.

especially from lower socioeconomic classes, may be financially unable to get time off from work for regular medical or dental care and may use the emergency department for after-hours primary care for themselves and their children. Women may escalate or initiate drug or alcohol dependency problems in response to abuse situations that they cannot terminate.[16] Elderly women are reported to account for 25 percent of all U.S. hospitalizations for alcohol-related diagnoses,[17] but failure to consider alcohol dependence as a differential diagnosis in women could be responsible for underreporting bias.

Gender-specific differences in presentation and treatment of acute illness and injury have not been commonly investigated. In epidemiologically important conditions such as coronary artery heart disease, women have often been excluded from clinical trials or results have not been stratified by gender. A body of evidence being developed suggests that there are prominent gender differences in the etiology and expression of chest pain. For example, atypical chest pain appears to be more common in women than in men because diseases associated with atypical chest pain such as vasospasm and mitral-valve prolapse are more common in women. In women with coronary artery disease, chest pain may be present at rest or may be associated with other atypical symptoms during exertion. In addition, some studies have demonstrated that women may receive less aggressive treatment than men for acute myocardial infarction.[18–21]

The passage of Title IX in 1972 has resulted in a marked increase in athletic participation by girls and women and, consequently, the risks of injury in women have increased.[22–25] Cheerleading is reported to result in more deaths and injuries than any women's sport. Among "traditional" sport, girls' cross-country running has a higher injury rate than football or wrestling. Disorders of the knee, leg, ankle, and foot are felt to be more common in women runners because wider hips result in different angular relationships at the knees and ankles. Women athletes have more knee laxity, and women rely more on the quadriceps rather than the hamstrings for knee stabilization, resulting in increased potential for anterior cruciate ligament tears.

RESUSCITATION

Resuscitative techniques are generally no different in women than in men. However, if a woman of childbearing age presents with shock or signs of hypovolemia, ruptured ectopic pregnancy is the first consideration. Resuscitation for critical illness or injury in pregnant women best follows the maxim "Maternal resuscitation is the best fetal resuscitation." Administration of blood or blood products in women should utilize Rh-negative blood. Obstetric consultation should be obtained in tandem with maternal resuscitation to optimize the likelihood of fetal viability.

DISCHARGE INSTRUCTIONS

Follow-up instructions should be clear, explicit, and conveyed in terms the patient can comprehend.[26] The patient should be aware of the expected time course of the condition and should understand why follow-up care may be needed. The physician's concerns about a differential diagnosis should be communicated to the patient so that she will know what symptoms should prompt a return visit. The patient and follow-up provider should be clear about the general and specific reasons for follow-up.

References

1. Grant HD, Murray RH, Bergeron JD, eds: *Brady Emergency Care,* 5th ed. Englewood Cliffs, NJ: Prentice-Hall, 1990.
2. American College of Emergency Physicians: *Position Summaries: V. Principles of Emergency Care.* Dallas: ACEP, 1990.
3. Health Reform: Past and Future. *Health Affairs* 7:225, 1995.
4. Furrow BR: An overview and analysis of the impact of the Emergency Medical Treatment and Active Labor Act. *J Legal Med* 16:325, 1995.
5. Derlet RW, Kinser D, Ray L, et al: Prospective identification and triage of nonemergency patients out of an emergency department: A 5-year study. *Ann Emerg Med* 25:215, 1995.
6. Brillman JC, Doezema D, Tandberg D, et al: Triage: Limitations in predicting need for emergent care and hospital admission. *Ann Emerg Med* 26:493, 1996.
7. Trussell J, Ellertson C, Rodriguez G: The Yuzpe regimen of emergency contraception: How long after the morning after? *Obstet Gynecol* 88:150, 1996.
8. Grodstein F, Stampfer MJ, Manson JE, et al: Postmenopausal estrogen and progestin use and the risk of cardiovascular disease. *N Engl J Med* 335:453, 1996.
9. Chattopadhyay B: Problems with diagnosis and antibiotic treatment of frequency and dysuria syndrome. *J Antimicrob Chemother* 16:680, 1985.
10. Hooton TM, Scholes D, Hughes JP, et al: A prospective study of risk factors for symptomatic urinary infection in young women. *N Engl J Med* 335:468, 1996.
11. Foxman B, Chi JW: Health behavior and urinary tract infection in college aged women. *J Clin Epidemiol* 43:329, 1990.
12. Stengel CL, Seaberg DC, MacLeod BA: Pregnancy in the emergency department: Risk factors and prevalence among all women. *Ann Emerg Med* 24:697, 1994.

13. McCoy M: Domestic violence: Clues to victimization. *Ann Emerg Med* 27:764, 1996.

14. Olson L, Anctil C, Fullerton L: Increasing emergency physician recognition of domestic violence. *Ann Emerg Med* 27:741, 1996.

15. Roberts G, O'Toole B, Raphael B, et al: Prevalence study of domestic violence victims in an emergency department. *Ann Emerg Med* 27:747, 1996.

16. Wailer A, Hohenhaus S, Shah P, et al: Development and validation of an emergency department screening and referral protocol for victims of domestic violence. *Ann Emerg Med* 27:754, 1996.

17. Adams WL, Yuan Z, Barboriak J, et al: Alcohol related hospitalizations of elderly people: Prevalence and geographic variation in the US. *JAMA* 270:1221, 1993.

18. Jackson RE, Anderson W, Peacock WF, et al: Effect of a patient's sex on the timing of thrombolytic therapy. *Ann Emerg Med* 27:815, 1996.

19. Douglas PS, Ginsburg GS: The evaluation of chest pain in women. *N Engl J Med* 334:1311, 1996.

20. Ayanian JZ, Epstein AM: Differences in the use of procedures between women and men hospitalized for coronary heart disease. *N Engl J Med* 325:221, 1991.

21. Weaver WD, White HD, Wilcox RG, et al: Comparisons of characteristics and outcomes among women and men with acute myocardial infarction treated with thrombolytic therapy *JAMA* 275:777, 1996.

22. Kujala UM, Nylund T, Taiamela S: Acute injuries in orienteerers. *Int J Sports Med* 16:1225, 1995.

23. deLoes M: Epidemiology of sports in the Swiss organization Youth and Sports, 1987–1989. *Int J Sports Med* 16:1348, 1995.

24. Bahr R, Karlsen R, Lian O, et al: Incidence and mechanisms of acute ankle inversion injuries in volleyball: A retrospective cohort study. *Am J Sports Med* 22:595, 1994.

25. Tenvergert EM, Ten Duis NJ, Klasen HF: Trends in sports injuries, 1982–88. *J Sports Med Phys Fitness* 32:214, 1992.

26. Morgan D: Emergency room follow-up care and malpractice liability. *J Legal Med* 16:373, 1996.

PART II

THE PREGNANT PATIENT

Chapter 2

CRITICAL PHYSIOLOGIC ALTERATIONS IN PREGNANCY

Mel L. Barclay

According to a recent U.S. Census, approximately 8 percent of American women aged 14 to 44 were pregnant during 1994. Among those women, there were approximately 3.9 million live births.[1] This being the case, the appearance in emergency facilities of pregnant women who are seeking attention for obstetric problems and unrelated medical and surgical care is neither unusual nor unexpected.

As a result of its special physiologic impact on the mother, pregnancy often alters the presentation of a number of disease processes. Elements of physiology that are normal for pregnancy may easily be mistaken for pathophysiology. On the other hand, the appearance of true pathophysiology may be altered or masked by the pregnant state in ways that complicate or delay diagnosis and treatment. Caregivers are in a better position to make an appropriate diagnosis and administer suitable therapy with a more complete understanding of the special physiologic and related anatomic changes produced by pregnancy.

Because a multitude of seemingly unrelated alterations in physiologic processes occur in pregnancy, constructs that permit a unified deductive approach to individual systems are useful. This approach to any problem is referred to as *heuristic*. Heuristic methods permit deduction from simple rules. Using this technique and fundamental changes known to occur in the pregnant state, it is possible to construct models from which one can frequently and logically deduce the important physiologic alterations occurring in pregnancy.

Over the past several decades a number of such models have been suggested by various authors. Each of these models helps to organize what otherwise appear to be diverse alterations into a more manageable set of unified concepts. Armed with tools for assessing how pregnancy alters a given set of circumstances, the emergency medicine physician may be better equipped to make diagnostic and therapeutic decisions.

THREE HEURISTIC MODELS OF HUMAN PREGNANCY

MODEL I: PREGNANCY AS A HYPERPROGESTATIONAL STATE

The first model, and one commonly invoked in discussions of pregnancy, relates to the effect of the enormously increased levels of circulating steroid hormones, particularly progesterone, on maternal systems. Produced mainly by the placenta, progesterone and its metabolic by-products are increased to levels that are more than twenty times normal in the serum of pregnant women.[2]

Progesterone has many effects, but those on smooth muscle are fundamental in producing changes in the normal woman during the course of gestation. Progesterone has the property of hyperpolarizing the cell membranes of smooth muscle, thereby increasing the amount of energy necessary to cause depolarization and the subsequent contraction of the smooth muscle fibers[3–6]; the ultimate effect is to cause smooth muscle relaxation. This has implications for all of the homeostatic mechanisms that depend on the action of smooth muscle for maintenance of the internal milieu. From the uterus, which must be conditioned to contain the rapidly growing fetus, to the most distal peripheral arteriole, the impact of progesterone is at least partly responsible for the multiple changes in the homeostatic mechanisms observed in the pregnant woman.

A large volume of evidence suggests that changes in the responsiveness of the vascular tree to various stressors, decreased peripheral resistance, and changes in circulatory dynamics are due to the relaxing effects of progesterone on smooth muscle. Changes in gastrointestinal motility, compliance of the bronchial tree, and the changes in the urinary collecting system are also attributable, at least in part, to the effects of circulating serum progesterone. These changes are listed in Table 2-1.

Table 2-1

IMPACT OF SMOOTH MUSCLE RELAXATION ON VARIOUS SYSTEMS IN PREGNANCY

System	Effect
Cardiovascular	↑ Mean arterial pressure
	↑ Venous capacitance
	↓ Vascular response to postural change
	↓ Peripheral resistance
Genitourinary	↓ Uterine contractile activity
	↑ Ureteral dilatation
	↑ Renal collecting system volume
Gastrointestinal	↑ Gastric emptying time
	↓ Bowel motility
	↑ Gallbladder emptying time
	↑ Gastroesophageal reflux
Respiratory	↑ Inspiratory capacity

Key: ↓, decreased; ↑, increased.

MODEL II: PREGNANCY AS A STATE OF HOMEOTHERMIC HEAT ADAPTATION

The metabolic activity of the fetus and placenta has the effect of heating the pregnant woman's internal milieu. Abrams and others have documented significant differences between maternal and fetal temperatures during the course of gestation.[7–9] Thermodynamic considerations dictate a net flow of heat energy from the fetus and placenta to the mother. In providing a place for growth and sustenance of the intrauterine fetus and placenta, the pregnant woman houses within her a rapidly metabolizing and heat-producing organism. The total energy output for an average-sized pregnant woman at 36 weeks gestation is approximately 97.72 ± 2.81 W (8443 ± 243 kJ/day). A similarly sized, nonlactating and nonpregnant woman has an energy output of approximately 80.68 ± 1.99 W (6971 ± 172 kJ/day),[10] about 17 percent less.

Homeothermic mammals function within an exceptionally narrow range of temperatures as compared with poikilothermic animals. Being temperature-dependent, the normal function of enzyme systems and the most basic elements of cellular homeostatis require very stable thermal limits. The narrow tolerances of temperature variation permitted in this area of mammalian physiology dictate sometimes profound adjustments in homeostatic mechanisms in order to maintain the constancy of internal temperature.[11] Many of the physiologic adjustments observed in the pregnant state bear a close resemblance to those observed in the heat-adapted homeothermic mammal. Changes observed in heat-adapted humans—such as increased plasma volume, heart rate, respiratory rate, and tidal volume—are similar to physiologic alterations commonly observed in pregnancy. The impressive decrease in peripheral circulatory resistance in pregnancy, manifest as warm skin and fingertips, results from the increased blood flow to the extremities and skin, which is an important aspect of pregnancy physiology.[12]

MODEL III: PREGNANCY AS A STATE OF ADJUSTMENT TO A LARGE ARTERIOVENOUS FISTULA

In 1938, Burwell and others suggested that much of what appears as maternal adaptation in pregnancy could be the result of alterations in maternal circulatory dynamics in response to the large-scale perfusion requirements of the placental and uterine circulation.[13] Particularly in the third trimester, the placental and uterine circulation increases substantially.

Placental and uterine circulation varies linearly with fetal size during the course of gestation. Assali and others have estimated that, at term, the typical flow rate in normal pregnancy is 600 to 800 mL/min. This amounts to approximately 15 to 20 mL/100 g of fetal tissue per min.[14,15] This level of flow is similar to the flow rates in antecubital arteriovenous

(AV) fistulas constructed for purposes of extracorporeal circulation in renal dialysis.[16,17]

Many of the findings associated with AV fistulas of significant size are also seen in pregnancy. These include increased plasma volume, decreased peripheral resistance, increased cardiac output, decreased mean arterial pressure, and Branham's phenomenon (decreased pulse rate and increased blood pressure in response to closure of the fistula; see Table 2-2).

All of these models can be utilized to answer questions regarding how individual systems may be altered in the course of pregnancy. To assume that a pregnant woman's highly adapted physiologic state is identical to that of a nonpregnant woman is potentially dangerous, since what appears normal may not be and what appears to be wildly abnormal may, in fact, be only a result of pregnancy. Interventions made without some attention to the changes described here may be not only unnecessary but also dangerous to mother and baby. From laboratory values to functional measures of organ systems, a surprising variety of changes occur.

IMPORTANT ANATOMIC ALTERATIONS IN PREGNANCY THAT AFFECT DIAGNOSIS AND TREATMENT

Changes in maternal body habitus are among the most obvious alterations in the pregnant state. Some of these changes have significant impact on diagnosis and treatment. Uterine growth, the most obvious anatomic change in pregnancy, has important effects on the location of peritoneal contents. By altering the position and mobility of adjacent structures or by physically impinging on them, the enlarging pregnant uterus has important effects on the presentation of intraab-dominal disease processes as well as on penetrating and blunt abdominal trauma. Women with multiple pregnancies have even greater uterine enlargement and may therefore experience even more profound compression-related physiologic alterations and even disability on the basis of uterine size alone.

During the course of normal gestation, the uterus grows from 50 grams (g) to approximately 1200 g and the fetus from a few grams to 3 to 4 kilograms (kg). Growth of the uterine fundus is approximately linear in the first trimester. Beginning at 20 weeks gestation, the number of weeks of pregnancy approximately equals the straight-line length from the superior margin of the symphysis pubis to the uterine fundus in centimeters. As the uterus emerges from the cavity of the pelvis, changes are produced in the relationships and positions of the movable peritoneal contents. The pattern of uterine growth is depicted in Fig. 2-1. Notably, the uterine fundus becomes a palpable abdominal organ at approximately 10 weeks, when the fundus becomes distinct at the pelvic brim just superior to the upper border of the symphysis pubis. At 16 weeks of gestation, the fundus is palpable approximately halfway between the symphysis and the umbilicus. At 20 weeks, it appears at the umbilicus, and at 38 weeks, it is at the xiphoid. At term, because the fetal presenting part descends into the pelvis, the fundus falls to several centimeters below the level of the xiphoid process (Fig. 2-1).

Bowel is displaced laterally, posteriorly, and upwardly because the anterior surface of the uterus glides along the parietal peritoneum of the anterior abdominal wall with growth. As pregnancy progresses and the uterus enlarges, the uterus becomes the most anterior intraperitoneal organ and is therefore more subject to traumatic injuries than in the first 12 weeks of pregnancy, when it is well protected by the pelvic girdle.

Table 2-2

IMPORTANT CENTRAL HEMODYNAMIC ALTERATIONS IN PREGNANCY[a]

Parameter	Nonpregnant	Pregnant	Units
Cardiac output	4.3 ± 0.9	6.2 ± 1.0	L/min
Heart rate	71 ± 10.0	83 ± 10.0	beats/min
Systemic vascular resistance	1530 ± 520	1210 ± 266	$dyn \cdot s \cdot cm^{-5}$
Pulmonary vascular resistance	119 ± 47.0	78 ± 22.0	$dyn \cdot s \cdot cm^{-5}$
Colloid oncotic pressure	20.8 ± 1.0	10.5 ± 2.7	mmHg
Mean arterial pressure	86.4 ± 7.5	90.3 ± 5.8	mmHg
Pulmonary capillary wedge pressure	6.3 ± 2.1	7.5 ± 1.8	mmHg
Left ventricular stroke work index	41 ± 8	48 ± 6	$g \cdot min \cdot m^{-2}$
Central venous pressure	3.7 ± 2.6	3.6 ± 2.5	mmHg

[a]Measurements between 36 to 38 weeks gestation and 11 to 13 weeks postpartum in ten normal volunteers.
Source: Adapted from Clark et al.,[38] with permission.

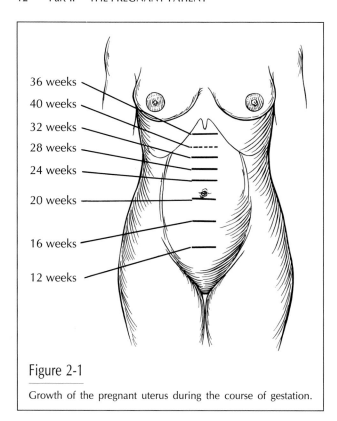

Figure 2-1

Growth of the pregnant uterus during the course of gestation.

36 weeks
40 weeks
32 weeks
28 weeks
24 weeks
20 weeks
16 weeks
12 weeks

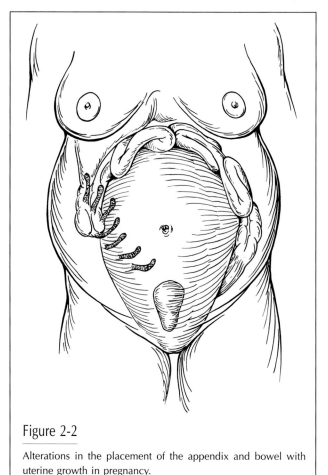

Figure 2-2

Alterations in the placement of the appendix and bowel with uterine growth in pregnancy.

Because of these altered anatomic relationships and the dramatically increased blood supply to the pelvic organs, gunshot wounds with and without fetal injury, abdominal stab wounds, and blunt trauma resulting from vehicular accidents have additional implications[18–22] (see Chap. 8).

Uterine growth and the displacement of peritoneal contents alter the ability of the omentum to wall off subsections of the peritoneal cavity. Infectious processes can become more disseminated than they might in a nonpregnant state. An important aspect of intestinal displacement, which potentially complicates the diagnosis of all intraabdominal problems, is the change in location of the appendix. As the uterus grows, the appendix is displaced laterally and upward. Pictured in Fig. 2-2, this alteration in position can make for more difficult and atypical presentations of appendicitis and make the diagnosis of all causes of abdominal pain in the pregnant woman much more perplexing. For the emergency medicine physician, a strong index of suspicion is necessary when dealing with gravid women, because appendicitis in pregnancy is not unusual on a typical busy obstetric service (see Chap. 19). The presentation of this relatively common process is changed not only by appendiceal location but also by the altered responses that anatomic changes engender. A leaking, partially ruptured appendix elevated out of the pelvis by a pregnant uterus may produce greater peritoneal sepsis because of the inability of the omentum to limit infection. Additionally, measures of intraabdominal infection such as elevations in the neutrophil count, which are normal in the pregnant woman, may confuse the diagnostic picture.

Table 2-3 demonstrates the changes normally observed in the white blood cell count and other laboratory values during the course of pregnancy. Anorexia, common in early pregnancy with appendicitis, is less pronounced later in gestation, as is rectal and rebound tenderness. Delays in diagnosis and treatment of pregnant women occasioned by the effect of the normal physiologic alterations of pregnancy and the varied manner in which they alter the natural history and presentation of disease may increase morbidity and mortality for both mother and baby.[23]

The differential diagnosis of abdominal pain in pregnancy is even more complex than it is in the nonpregnant state and necessarily includes additional diagnoses related to the pregnancy, such as labor, uterine rupture, and placental abruption (see Chap. 19).

Other alterations in the function of the gastrointestinal system in pregnancy include increased gastric emptying time and slowing of peristalsis throughout the entire gut. Common symptoms related to this include constipation and reflux of gastric contents. The major impact of differences in gastrointestinal motility are related clinically to the dangers of aspiration when general anesthesia is needed. In clinical circumstances necessitating the induction of anesthesia

Table 2-3

IMPORTANT LABORATORY VALUES IN PREGNANCY

Test	Nonpregnant Range	Pregnant Effect	Gestational Timing
Serum chemistries			
Albumin	3.5–4.8 g/dL	↓ 1 g/dL	By midpregnancy
Calcium	9.0–10.3 mg/dL	↓ 10%	Falls gradually
Chloride	95–105 meq/L	No change	
Cholesterol	200–240 mg/dL	↑ 50%	Progressive
Creatinine	0.6–1.1 mg/dL	↓ 0.3 g/dL	By midpregnancy
Fibrinogen	200–400 mg/dL	↑ 600 mg/dL	By term
Glucose, fasting	65–105 md/dL	↓ 10%	Gradual fall
Potassium (plasma)	3.5–4.5 meq/L	↓ 0.2–0.3 meq/L	By midpregnancy
Protein (total)	6.5–8.5 g/dL	↓ 1 g/dL	By midpregnancy
Sodium	135–145 meq/L	↓ 2–4 meq/L	By midpregnancy
Urea nitrogen	12–30 mg/dL	↓ 50%	First trimester
Uric acid	3.5–8 mg/dL	↓ 33%	First trimester
Urine chemistries			
Creatinine	15–25 mg/kg per day	No change	
Protein	Up to 150 mg per day	Up to 250–300 mg/day	By midpregnancy
Creatinine clearance	90–130/mL per min per 1.73 m²	↑ 40–50%	By 16 weeks
Serum enzymes			
Alkaline phosphatase	42–98 U/L	↑ 3 to 5-fold increase	By 20 weeks
Amylase	23–84 IU/L	Controversial	
Creatinine phosphokinase	26–140 U/L	↑ 2 to 4-fold increase	After labor (MB bands as well)
Lipase	10–140 U/L	No change	
Transaminase			
Glutamic pyruvic (SGPT)	5–35 mU/mL	No change	
Glutamic oxaloacetic (SGOT)	5–40 mU/mL	No change	
Formed elements of blood			
Hematocrit	36–46%	↓ 4–7%	Nadir at 30–34 weeks
Hemoglobin	12–16 g/dL	↓ 1.4–2.0 g/dL	Nadir at 30–34 weeks
Leukocyte count	4.8–10.8 × 10³/mm³	↑ 3.5 × 10³/mm³	Gradual increase to term, as high as 25 × 10³/mm³ in labor
Platelets	150–400 × 10³/mm³	Slight decrease	

Abbreviations: ↑ = Increased.
↓ = Decreased.

emergently for a nonelective procedure in an unprepared, pregnant patient, the likelihood of aspiration of stomach contents is increased. To minimize the effects of such potential aspiration, many anesthesiologists routinely administer sodium citrate by mouth prior to the induction of any form of anesthesia in pregnant patients to raise gastric pH.

IMPORTANT MILESTONES IN FETAL DEVELOPMENT RELATED TO UTERINE SIZE

Uterine growth is a reflection of fetal growth, and medical and surgical interventions that involve the mother obviously and necessarily involve the fetus. Along with uterine size for estimation of gestational age, a number of fetal parameters are useful. Auscultation of the fetal heart is the most basic means of determining the state of fetal welfare and may also provide a means of assessing gestational age.

Fetal heart tones are typically first audible at 20 weeks of gestation with a Delee auditory-type stethoscope (fetoscope) and at about 10 weeks with a Doppler ultrasound device. The earliest visual confirmation of heart activity is at about 6 weeks with sonographic methods. The detection of heart tones using these various modalities can serve to establish a baseline for estimating fetal age. Quickening, or the occurrence of the first maternally detectable fetal movements, generally occurs at about 17 to 18 weeks in multiparous women and at 19 to 20 weeks in nulliparas. This information can be useful clinically and may be the only data available when rapid decision making regarding gestational age is necessary.

With the most current neonatal intensive care, a majority of infants born before term can survive from about 26 weeks onward and sometimes prior to this. The incidence of serious neurologic problems, such as cerebral palsy, in babies born prematurely is considerable, however; in the face of maternal circumstances that portend serious compromise, the determination of the possibility of fetal viability adds to the burden of those caring for the mother under less than ideal circumstances.

IMPORTANT CARDIOVASCULAR ALTERATIONS IN PREGNANCY

Symptoms such as increasing dyspnea at rest, decreasing exercise tolerance, and light-headedness are common in pregnancy and do not necessarily imply pulmonary or cardiovascular disease. These symptoms are probably produced by the interaction of the pregnancy with the cardiovascular and respiratory adjustments occasioned by fetal needs and the extra demands on the maternal cardiovascular system produced by the need for perfusion of the growth in placental and uterine circulation.

Anatomic alterations produced by uterine and fetal growth have major implications for cardiovascular function in pregnancy and for the emergency treatment of the pregnant woman. From a functional standpoint, pregnancy represents an augmented (yet not hyperdynamic) cardiac state.[24] Many parameters traditionally used to assess the state of the cardiovascular system—including pulse rate, stroke volume, and cardiac output—are increased significantly. All of the changes observed are conditioned by the growth needs of the pregnancy and thus change over the time span of the gestation. Parameter values are often different at different stages of gestation. Typical normal values are listed in Table 2-2 and illustrated in Fig. 2-3 as they relate to maternal position and time in gestation.

During the course of normal pregnancy, a number of

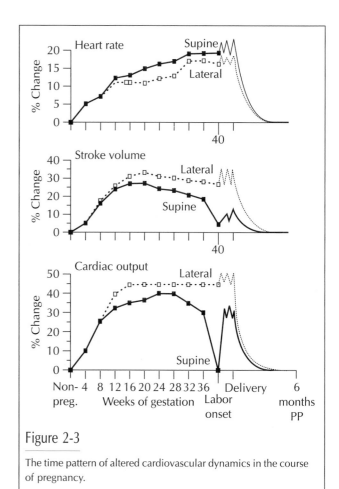

Figure 2-3

The time pattern of altered cardiovascular dynamics in the course of pregnancy.

changes occur in the anatomy of the heart. Both by physical examination and various imaging techniques, the heart is increased in size. Cardiac volume is increased by approximately 12 percent or 70 to 80 mL. Radiologically, images of the pregnant heart show straightening of the upper left cardiac border and simulate left atrial enlargement in right oblique and lateral views. These features, which are normal for pregnancy and the immediate puerperium, can be mistaken for similar radiographic findings associated with mitral stenosis.[25] Recently published ultrasonic measurements of left atrial and left ventricular end-diastolic dimensions as well as cross-sectional measurements of the aortic, pulmonary, and mitral valves have confirmed these well-established observations. Robson and others have reported a 12 to 14 percent increase in the cross-sectional areas of the aortic, pulmonary, and mitral valves during the course of pregnancy, presumably on the basis of increased flow and cardiac output.[26]

Changes in blood flow produce alterations in the auscultative findings on the pregnant heart. The first heart sound is louder and more widely split than in the nonpregnant state. Systolic murmurs, particularly along the lower portion of the left sternal border and over the pulmonary valvular area, are very common in pregnancy. Typically they are most audible at midsystole and have the diamond-shaped characteristics of ejection-type flow murmurs. A continuous cervical venous hum over the supraclavicular fossa just lateral to the insertion of the sternocleidomastoid muscle may be present. When present, this is more prominent on the right side. Mammary artery souffle is occasionally present and may be mistaken for a pathologic diastolic murmur.[27]

The increased dimensions and work of the heart in pregnancy operate to change the position of the heart in the thorax. The cardiac apex is moved upward and laterally. This change in position makes for alterations in normal physical findings, moving the palpable point of maximal cardiac impulse lateral to the midclavicular line and up several intercostal spaces. Electrocardiographic (ECG) findings may suggest left axis deviation. Oram and Holt,[28] among others, have reported ST-segment depression and T-wave changes in approximately 14 percent of normal pregnant women. T-wave inversions are most commonly seen in V_2. These changes are seen in the ECG of a pregnant woman as pictured in Fig. 2-4. Small Q waves can normally be seen in leads II, III, and aVF. These changes, which are apparently innocent, have recently been reported to occur frequently during operative delivery and during exercise. The major importance of these findings relates to the possibility of confusing these nonserious changes with signs of myocardial ischemia.[28,29]

In addition to the changes noted in the ECGs of normal pregnant women, Abramov et al.[30] have stressed the importance of considering the impact of pregnancy and labor on the assessment of laboratory data, with particular regard to the interpretation of results in the area of cardiac diagnosis. In a prospective study, these investigators report a significant elevation of serum creatine phosphokinase and its MB isoenzyme in normal postpartum women without any evidence of myocardial disease.[30]

Among the reported changes in the maternal cardiovascular system, there is a unique and important alteration relating cardiac output to the mother's posture. When the pregnant woman who is near term is in the supine position, the enlarged uterus falls onto the inferior vena cava. The resulting compression produces decreased venous return to the right heart and a decrease in cardiac output of between 25 and 30 percent.[31] The anatomic relationships that produce this phenomenon are pictured in Fig. 2-5. As demonstrated

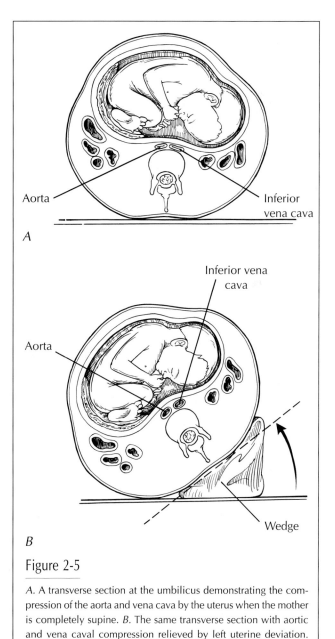

Aorta

Inferior vena cava

A

Inferior vena cava

Aorta

Wedge

B

Figure 2-5

A. A transverse section at the umbilicus demonstrating the compression of the aorta and vena cava by the uterus when the mother is completely supine. *B.* The same transverse section with aortic and vena caval compression relieved by left uterine deviation.

V_1

V_2

V_3

Figure 2-4

An electrocardiogram showing T-wave inversion in lead V_2 in early pregnancy.

in Fig. 2-5*B*, this effect can be minimized by placing the patient in the lateral position or displacing the uterus manually. During spinal or epidural conduction anesthesia, where sympathectomy accompanies the anesthetic effect, this can be very important. Also, when managing the pregnant trauma victim on a backboard, displacing the uterus off the inferior vena cava and aorta can be critically important in maintaining adequate perfusion.

Caval and aortic compression based on this phenomenon may be of critical importance during cardiopulmonary resuscitation of the pregnant patient. Lee and others have written about the special circumstances surrounding cardiopulmonary resuscitation of the pregnant woman and the effect that this particular phenomenon can have.[32] Left uterine deviation of the gravid uterus or placing the woman being resuscitated into some degree of lateral recumbency may make the difference between successful resuscitation and death. The possibility that immediate delivery of the fetus may facilitate both fetal and maternal resuscitation efforts based on these factors is supported by the recent case reports of O'Connor and DePace (see Chap. 29).[33,34]

During the course of normal gestation, the cardiac output is increased by 30 to 50 percent over levels normal for nonpregnant women. The increase in cardiac output begins as early as the tenth week of gestation and increases steadily until the 20th to 24th weeks of pregnancy. This increased level of cardiac output is then sustained at approximately the same level until the time of delivery. Early in the course of pregnancy, this increase in cardiac output seems to be more dependent on increasing stroke volume than on increased heart rate. Later in the course of gestation, the heart rate becomes the more important component of the increase in cardiac output.

In the longitudinal studies done by Mabie and colleagues,[35] total peripheral resistance fell consistently during the course of pregnancy. Duvekot and others have found that most of the fall in total peripheral resistance in pregnancy occurs during the first trimester, at the same time that cardiac output increases most appreciably.[36,37] Systolic blood pressure decreases 10 to 15 mmHg during the middle trimester and gradually increases to prepregnancy levels in the third trimester.

Clark and Cotton have reported a significant fall in pulmonary vascular resistance in normal pregnancy that surpasses the decrease in total peripheral resistance.[38] They found no change in pulmonary capillary wedge pressure or central venous pressure during the course of pregnancy. The implications of these findings are that pregnancy is not normally characterized by hyperdynamic left ventricular function. A tabular summary of central cardiovascular measurements made on normal women is given in Table 2-2.

The expansion of the total blood volume by 45 to 50 percent above nonpregnant levels is probably generated by a number of related factors, including the increase in the size of the vascular tree produced by the addition of the placental circulation, the effects of enormously elevated levels of estrogen and progesterone, and the thermal and metabolic demands of pregnancy.

Changes in total blood volume and red cell mass are illustrated in Fig. 2-6. The clinical impact of expanded blood volume has important ramifications in the dosing of some drugs, as expansion of the intravascular space may effectively dilute the concentration of certain medications, such as anticonvulsants, below therapeutic levels. Expansion of the plasma volume also occurs at a faster rate than the accompanying increase in circulating red cell mass. Early in pregnancy, this produces a dilutional anemia that can be mistaken for an authentic anemia. Serum proteins are also diluted significantly, creating a decrease in plasma colloid osmotic pressure. This change in serum protein is thought to be partially responsible for the dependent edema often seen in later pregnancy. These notable and important changes in plasma and blood volume have major implications for all forms of drug, fluid, and electrolyte therapy. Changes in body fat content are also important for fat-soluble or fat-stored substances, where uptake by fatty tissues is an important factor in the metabolism or excretion of drugs.

Table 2-3 summarizes how a number of important laboratory tests are altered during the course of pregnancy.

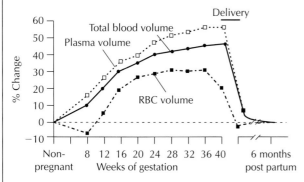

Figure 2-6

Changes in blood volume, plasma volume, and red cell mass during the course of normal gestation. (From Bonica JJ: *Obstetric Analgesia and Anesthesia*, 2d ed. Amsterdam: World Federation of Societies of Anesthesiologists, 1980, p 2, with permission.)

IMPORTANT CHANGES IN THE PULMONARY SYSTEM IN PREGNANCY

Dyspnea occurs during the course of normal, healthy pregnancy in as many as 60 to 70 percent of normal women. This alteration in normal pulmonary function complicates the diagnosis and management of pulmonary difficulties when they do occur. The presence of the pregnant uterus in the abdominal cavity necessitates some changes in pulmonary physiology that are particular to pregnancy. As the uterus grows, the diaphragms are elevated. Compensation for this effect is demonstrated by the resulting increased circumference of the maternal thorax and the increased subcostal angle. Somewhat paradoxically, the tidal volume is increased in pregnancy, as are the alveolar and minute ventilation. Although there are mixed data regarding the issue of respiratory rate, there is general agreement that hyperventilation is the normal state of affairs in pregnancy. This results in a decreased P_{CO_2}, increased pH, and decreased bicarbonate. The pregnant woman is, by most methods of assessment, in a state of partially compensated respiratory alkalosis. The picture can be confusing when one is dealing with other causes of respiratory alkalosis, including altitude sickness, salicylate poisoning, pneumonia, or pulmonary embolism.[39] The functional pulmonary changes seen in pregnancy are depicted in Fig. 2-7.

The changes in pulmonary function that occur in pregnancy, particularly the increase in minute ventilation, promote more efficient transfer of gases from the maternal lung to the blood. This implies that changes in maternal respiratory status occur more rapidly than in the nonpregnant state. Hypoxia as well as hyper- and hypocarbia occur more easily with assisted ventilation. During anesthesia with inhalational agents, the patient gets deeper faster and emerges from anesthesia faster. Because of additional fetal oxygen consumption, hypoxia can become more significant sooner when there is hypoventilation or respiratory obstruction. The greater affinity of fetal hemoglobin for oxygen at a lower partial pressure of oxygen in maternal blood may compound maternal hypoxia.

SUMMARY

A large number of important alterations occur in the special life-adapted state represented by pregnancy. Health care professionals in the emergency care environment who do not consider at least the possibility of specific alterations in the physiology of the maternal organism may either fail to recognize importantly altered presentations of disease processes or may be tempted to apply unnecessary therapeutics. The alterations described here represent many of the clinically relevant changes in major systems. For a more exhaustive discussions of pregnancy-altered physiology, the reader will find extensive references and more complete critical summary information in Hytten and Chamberlain[40] or in the periodical literature, referenced below, dealing with specific issues.

References

1. *Fertility of American Women.* Washington, DC: Fertility Statistics Branch, Bureau of the Census, U.S. Government Printing Office, 1994, pp 20–482.
2. Pearlman WH: Progesterone metabolism in advanced pregnancy and in oophorectomized-hysterectomized women. *Biochem J* 67:1, 1957.
3. Csapo AI: The molecular basis of myometrial function and its disorders, in *La Prophylaxie en Gynecologie et Ostetrique.* Geneva: Georg, 1954, p 693.
4. Calzada L, Bernal A, Loustaunau E: Effect of steroid hormones and capacitation on membrane potential of human spermatazoa. *Arch Androl* 21:121, 1988.
5. Mahesh VB, Brann DW, Hendry LB: Diverse modes of action of progesterone and its metabolites. *J Steroid Biochem Mol Biol* 56(1–6, spec issue):209.
6. Fu X, Ulsten U, Backstrom T: Interaction of sex steroids and oxytocin on term human myometrial contractile activity in vitro. *Obstet Gynecol* 84:272, 1994.
7. Abrams RM, Caton D, Curet LB, et al: Fetal brain: maternal aorta temperature differences in sheep. *Am J Physiol* 217:1619, 1969.
8. Walker DW, Wood C: Temperature relationship of the mother and fetus during labor. *Am J Obstet Gynecol* 107:83, 1970.
9. Macaulay JH, Randall NR, Bond K, Steer PJ: Continuous monitoring of fetal temperature by noninvasive probe and its relationship to maternal temperature, fetal heart rate and cord arterial oxygen and pH. *Obstet Gynecol* 79:469, 1992.
10. Heini A, Shutz Y, Jequier E: Twenty-four-hour energy

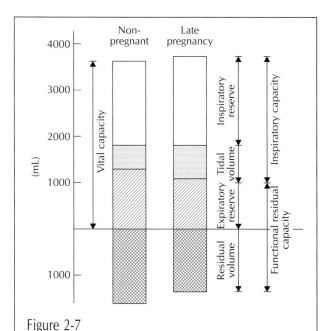

Figure 2-7

Functional changes in measurements of lung volume during the course of pregnancy as compared with the nonpregnant state.

expenditure in pregnant and nonpregnant Gambian women, measured in a whole-body indirect calorimeter. *Am J Clin Nutr* 55:1078, 1992.

11. Kleiber M: Animal temperature regulation, in *The Fire of Life: An Introduction to Animal Energetics.* Huntington, NY: Krieger, 1975, p 150.

12. Nielsen B, Hales JR, Strange S, et al: Human circulatory and thermoregulatory adaptations with heat acclimation and exercise in a hot, dry environment. *J Physiol (Lond)* 460:467, 1993.

13. Burwell CS, Strayhorn WD, Flinkinger D, et al: Circulation during pregnancy. *Arch Intern Med* 62:979, 1938.

14. Assali NS, Rauramo L, Peltonen T: Uterine and fetal blood flow and oxygen consumption in early human pregnancy. *Am J Obstet Gynecol* 79:86, 1960.

15. Romney SL, Reid DE, Metcalfe J, Burwell CS: Oxygen utilization by the human fetus in utero. *Am J Obstet Gynecol* 70:791, 1955.

16. Johnson G, Blythe WB: Hemodynamic effects of arteriovenous shunts used for hemodialysis. *Ann Surg* 171:715, 1970.

17. Oudenhoven LF, Pattynama PM, de Roos A, et al: Magnetic resonance: A new method for measuring blood flow in hemodialysis fistulae. *Kidney Int* 45:884, 1994.

18. Dittrich KC: Rupture of the gravid uterus secondary to motor vehicle trauma. *J Emerg Med* 14:177, 1996.

19. Dahmus MA, Sibai BM: Blunt abdominal trauma: Are there any predictive factors for abruptio placentae or maternal-fetal distress? *Am J Obstet Gynecol* 169:1054, 1993.

20. Neufeld JD: Trauma in pregnancy, what if . . .? *Emerg Med Clin North Am* 11:207, 1993.

21. Awwad JT, Azar GB, Seoud MA, et al: High-velocity penetrating wounds of the gravid uterus: Review of 16 years of civil war. *Obstet Gynecol* 83:259, 1994.

22. Goff BA, Muntz HG: Gunshot wounds to the gravid uterus: A case report. *J Reprod Med* 35:436, 1990.

23. Babaknia A, Parsa H, Woodruff JD: Appendicitis during pregnancy. *Obstet Gynecol* 50:40, 1977.

24. Clark SL, Cotton DB, Lee W, et al: Central hemodynamic assessment of normal term pregnancy. *Am J Obstet Gynecol* 161:1439, 1989.

25. Turner AF: The chest radiograph in pregnancy. *Clin Obstet Gynecol* 18:65, 1975.

26. Robson SC, Dunlop W, Moore M, Hunter S: Combined Doppler and echocardiographic measurement of cardiac output: Theory and application in pregnancy. *Br J Obstet Gynaecol* 94:1014, 1987.

27. Elkayam U, Gleicher N: *Cardiovascular Physiology of Pregnancy in Cardiac Problems in Pregnancy.* New York: Liss, 1982, pp 20–21.

28. Oram S, Holt M: Innocent depression of the ST segment and flattening of the T-wave during pregnancy. *J Obstet Gynaecol Br Commonw* 68:765, 1961.

29. Mathew JP, Fleisher LA, Rinehouse JA, et al: ST segment depression during labor and delivery. *Anesthesiology* 77:635, 1992.

29a. Veille JC, Kitzman DW, Bacevice AE: Effects of pregnancy on the electrocardiogram in healthy subjects during strenuous exercise. *Am J Obstet Gynecol* 175:1360, 1996.

30. Abramov Y, Abramov D, Abrahamov A, et al: Elevation of serum creatine phosphokinase and its MB isoenzyme during normal labor and early puerperium. *Acta Obstet Gynecol Scand* 75:255, 1996.

31. Ueland K, Novy MJ, Petersen EN, Metcalfe J: Maternal cardiovascular dynamics: IV. The influence of gestational age on the maternal cardiovascular response to posture and exercise. *Am J Obstet Gynecol* 104:856. 1969.

32. Lee RV, Rodgers BD, White LM, Harvey RC: Cardiopulmonary resuscitation of pregnant women. *Am J Med* 81:311, 1986.

33. O'Connor RL, Sevarino FB: Cardiopulmonary arrest in the pregnant patient: A report of successful resuscitation. *J Clin Anesthesiol* 6:66, 1994.

34. DePace NL, Betesh JS, Kotler MN: Postmortem cesarean section with recovery of both mother and offspring. *JAMA* 248:971, 1982.

35. Mabie WC, DiSessa TG, Crocker LG, et al: A longitudinal study of the cardiac output in normal human pregnancy. *Am J Obstet Gynecol* 170:849, 1994.

36. Metcalfe J, Ueland K: Maternal cardiovascular adjustments to pregnancy. *Prog Cardiovasc Dis* 16:363, 1974.

37. Duvekot JJ, Cheriex EC, Pieters FA, et al: Early pregnancy changes in hemodynamics and volume homeostasis are consecutive adjustments triggered by a primary fall in systemic vascular tone. 169:1382, 1993.

38. Clark SL, Cotton DB, Lee W, et al: Central hemodynamic assessment of normal term pregnancy. *Am J Obstet Gynecol* 161:1439, 1989.

39. Prowse CM, Gaensler EA: Respiratory and acid-base changes during pregnancy. *Anesthesiology* 26:381, 1965.

40. Hytten F, Chamberlain G (eds): *Clinical Physiology in Obstetrics,* 2d ed. Boston: Blackwell, 1991.

Section I

PROBLEMS OF FIRST-TRIMESTER PREGNANCY

Chapter 3

ECTOPIC PREGNANCY

Veronica T. Mallett

Ectopic pregnancy is defined as *any pregnancy occurring outside the uterine cavity.* It can result from the implantation of a fertilized ovum in the abdomen (abdominal pregnancy), cervix (cervical pregnancy), ovary (ovarian pregnancy), interstitial portion of the uterine wall or tubal cornua (cornual pregnancy), peritoneal surface, or distant sites. Most commonly, ectopic pregnancies are located in the fallopian tube (99 percent). This form of ectopic pregnancy is the focus of this chapter.

A total of 70,000 ectopic pregnancies are reported annually in the United States. The incidence has increased approximately threefold from the 1970s. In the past, the incidence of ectopic pregnancy was reported as 4.5 per 1000 pregnancies.[1] The current incidence is closer to 16 per 1000. Although changing etiologic factors are partly responsible (see Table 3-1), previous inconsistencies in reporting, improved diagnostic tools, and an increase in acquired risks for the disease are some of the factors thought to contribute to the increase. Factors commonly associated with ectopic pregnancy are assisted reproduction, in vitro fertilization, tubal surgery or tubal occlusion, diethylstilbestrol exposure, and tubal sterilization procedures. However, the major predisposing factor for tubal pregnancy is the increasing incidence of pelvic inflammatory disease.

Ectopic pregnancy is the leading cause of maternal mortality in African American women and the second leading cause of maternal mortality among all races.[2] Hemorrhage due to ectopic pregnancy is the leading cause of pregnancy-related death during the first trimester. Annual cost estimates due to ectopic pregnancy in the United States exceed $1 billion. After an ectopic pregnancy, a woman's chance of conception declines from 85 to 60 percent, while her risk for another ectopic pregnancy escalates eightfold from 1.6 to 13.0 percent. This altered reproductive opportunity translates into an increase in the number of infertile women and further increases the risk of future morbidity to those affected.

This chapter provides the clinician with an overview of the pathophysiology, clinical manifestations, differential diagnosis, laboratory and diagnostic evaluation, prognosis, and treatment of this often life-threatening condition.

PATHOPHYSIOLOGY

Ectopic pregnancy results from ovum implantation at an extrauterine location. In the majority of cases, the cause of ectopic pregnancy is mechanical interference with the passage of a fertilized ovum. This delay in ovum transport is most often secondary to a diseased fallopian tube. The most common cause of tubal damage is salpingitis resulting in tubal occlusion or ciliary damage. Less commonly, a congenital malformation of the tube or spasm of the tubal musculature results in obstruction. Extrauterine implantation may be influenced by abnormalities of the fertilized ovum. Also implicated in contributing to abnormal implantation site is the use of ovulation induction agents such as human menopausal gonadotropin. Contraceptive failures in women wearing intrauterine devices (IUDs) are also more likely to be tubal pregnancies, because the IUD preferentially interferes with intrauterine implantation.

Implantation of the embryo in the oviduct is unique to humans; thus no animal model exists for the study of this condition. Much of our knowledge about pathophysiology is thus observational. What has been observed is that implantation occurs on the inner surface of the lumen. Following this, the growing conceptus penetrates the lamina propria and muscularis portions of the tube. Tubal damage is a result of destruction of the tube by the invasive trophoblast. The trophoblast invades blood vessels in the tubal wall, thus obtaining a blood supply for further growth.

Table 3-1

RISK FACTORS FOR ECTOPIC PREGNANCY

Pelvic inflammatory disease
Assisted reproduction
In vitro fertilization
Pelvic or tubal surgery
Tubal occlusion
Sterilization procedures
Diethylstilbestrol exposure

Four different processes may occur when the ectopic tubal embryo outgrows its blood supply. One is formation of a tubal blood mole, a process whereby the blood flows around the chorionic sac, overdistends the tube, and leads to intraluminal rupture of the sac into the tube. Second, there may be a tubal abortion of the tubal blood mole through the fimbriated end (distal end) of the tube, either completely or incompletely into the abdominal cavity. Third, there may be reabsorption of the conceptus as a result of early separation from the tubal blood supply. Last, tubal rupture into the peritoneal cavity may occur as a result of either erosion of chorionic villi or mechanical overdistention of the tube.

The most common site of implantation of an ectopic pregnancy is the ampullary portion of the tube, accounting for over 78 percent of such pregnancies. The isthmic region of the tube is the second most likely, accounting for 12 percent of ectopic pregnancies, followed by fimbrial implantation (5 percent) and cornual (2 percent) or interstitial implantation (Fig. 3-1). The remainder are implanted in cervical, ovarian, abdominal, or distant sites.

DIAGNOSIS

With improved resolution of ultrasound and sensitive quantitative beta human chorionic gonadotropin (β-hCG) assays, the diagnosis of ectopic pregnancy can be made more accurately and earlier in gestation than in the past. As in the past, maternal death is most often due to delay in diagnosis, leading to rupture of the tube and exsanguination. Even with current diagnostic methods available, the diagnosis is missed in 50 percent of cases at the first office visit and in 36 percent at the time of the first emergency department visit.[3]

Any woman of reproductive age presenting with pelvic pain or bleeding should have ectopic pregnancy ruled out. This should begin with a brief but accurate gynecologic and menstrual history including a last menstrual period (LMP). Not only the first day of the LMP but also the timing of two or more immediate past periods should be recorded so as to determine the interval between "normal" menses. Any regularly menstruating woman whose LMP is greater than 4 weeks prior to the current date is likely to be pregnant. If the LMP is determined to be normal and the patient is less than 4 weeks past her menses, the possibility of a pregnancy complication is less likely. If the stated LMP was lighter and shorter than normal, pregnancy must also be considered, since implantation can be associated with normal "menstrual" flow.

The presence of risk factors associated with ectopic pregnancy (Table 3-1) should heighten clinical suspicion. However, ectopic pregnancy frequently occurs without any risk factors.

The clinical presentation of ectopic pregnancy is variable, ranging from the asymptomatic patient to the patient in hy-

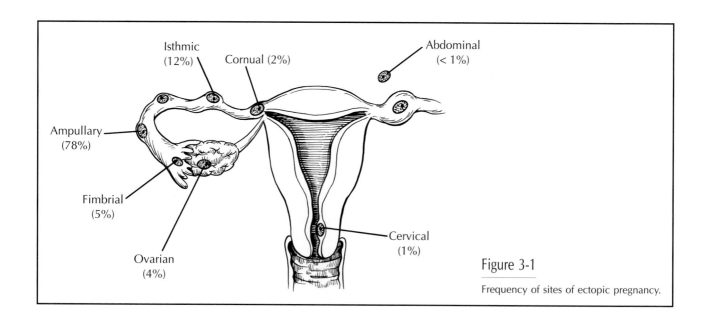

Figure 3-1

Frequency of sites of ectopic pregnancy.

povolemic shock. Symptoms depend on the amount of trophoblastic tissue that has developed, the site of implantation, and whether or not rupture has occurred. History and physical examination can be unreliable, since they are often nonspecific, particularly before bleeding into and distention of the tube have occurred. Menstrual history may also be misleading, but patients with tubal ectopic pregnancies generally present prior to 8 weeks of gestation. Amenorrhea of less than 4 weeks and of more than 12 weeks is seen in 15 percent of cases. Moreover, 15 percent of ectopic pregnancies rupture before the first missed period. Cornual (interstitial) ectopic pregnancies may progress further, manifesting as late as 12 to 14 weeks.

Abdominal pain is the most common symptom of ectopic pregnancy, followed by amenorrhea. After a period of amenorrhea, abnormal vaginal bleeding is frequently present. Pain is characteristically sudden, severe, sharp, and unilateral. The pain may be variable in intensity, quality, location, and duration. Absence of pain is a useful negative predictor of a ruptured ectopic pregnancy. Lack of pain is not, however, useful if the goal is early diagnosis and tubal preservation prior to tubal rupture.

Abnormal bleeding occurs in up to 80 percent of cases. This results from a lack of support of the endometrium by the corpus luteum. The bleeding is generally scant compared to that associated with menses, and it is usually dark in color. A large amount of vaginal bleeding suggests a complication of an intrauterine pregnancy (e.g., threatened abortion). Passage of tissue may represent an incomplete abortion, but a decidual cast of endometrial tissue passed in the presence of an ectopic pregnancy can resemble fetal tissue.

Dizziness or syncope is not a common presentation of ectopic pregnancy. Those patients presenting with such symptoms have most likely experienced rupture of the ectopic pregnancy. Rupture of this magnitude will most likely be accompanied by signs of hemoperitoneum.

Physical examination should begin with hemodynamic assessment. In the past, patients presenting with signs of shock and an adnexal mass were considered to have a "classic presentation." Shock is now the presenting sign in less than 5 percent of ectopic pregnancies. Variation in the degree of hypotension and tachycardia depends on the acuity and degree of hemorrhage. Clinical signs include abdominal tenderness, adnexal tenderness, and an adnexal mass. Over 70 percent of the time, the uterus is normal in size, but one can sometimes be led astray when the uterus is enlarged. Usually the uterus is softened, but not as enlarged as would be expected for gestational age. Irritation of the peritoneum from blood may create abdominal tenderness, involuntary guarding and rebound tenderness. In the obese patient, pelvic examination maybe less reliable. The use of pelvic US and serum β-hCG is particularly useful in this group of patients (see Fig. 3-2).

The presence of a simultaneous intrauterine and ectopic pregnancy is unusual. The incidence of combined gestation (also called *heterotropic pregnancy*) is most often quoted as

1 per 30,000; this number, however, is thought to be increasing because of the increased frequency of assisted reproduction. In fact, recent estimates place the incidence at 1 to 8 per 100 in an in vitro fertilization program as compared with 1 per 6000 in the general population.[4] The classic presentation of combined gestation is abdominal pain, adnexal mass, peritoneal irritation, and enlarged uterus.

Other clinical scenarios in which one might consider a combined gestation are a uterine size compatible with menstrual dates in a person believed to have an ectopic pregnancy; absence of bleeding following removal of an ectopic pregnancy; and hemoperitoneum following termination of a pregnancy. A diagnostic and treatment algorithm is presented in Fig. 3-2.

DIFFERENTIAL DIAGNOSIS

Ectopic pregnancy must be considered in any patient of childbearing potential presenting with abdominal pain, vaginal bleeding, or a missed period. The differential diagnosis of an ectopic gestation includes normal intrauterine pregnancy, acute salpingitis, torsion of an enlarged ovary, ruptured corpus luteum cyst, gastroenteritis, appendicitis, threatened or incomplete abortion, or endometriosis (Table 3-2). Pelvic inflammatory disease (PID) is a common condition confused with ectopic pregnancy, because up to 20 percent of patients with ectopic pregnancy may have temperature elevation as high as 38°C (100.4°F). However, PID is rare in pregnancy, occurring less than 1 percent of the time, and a positive pregnancy significantly lessens the likelihood of PID. Pregnancy protects against bacterial invasion, since the decidua and membranes effectively seal off the uterine cavity preventing organisms from ascending. Patients presenting with low-grade temperature, a positive pregnancy test, and lower abdominal pain are often misdiagnosed as having PID. Consultation with a gynecologist and laparoscopy are often necessary to arrive at the correct diagnosis.

LABORATORY TESTS

HUMAN CHORIONIC GONADATROPIN

All currently used quantitative pregnancy tests are dependent on the ability to detect the beta subunit of human chorionic gonadotropin in serum or urine. This glycoprotein hormone is produced by the trophoblast. The current monoclonal antibody technology allows detection of β-hCG within 2 to 3 days postimplantation. In a normal intrauterine gestation, the β-hCG level increases by at least 66 percent every 2 days until 9 to 10 weeks gestation, at

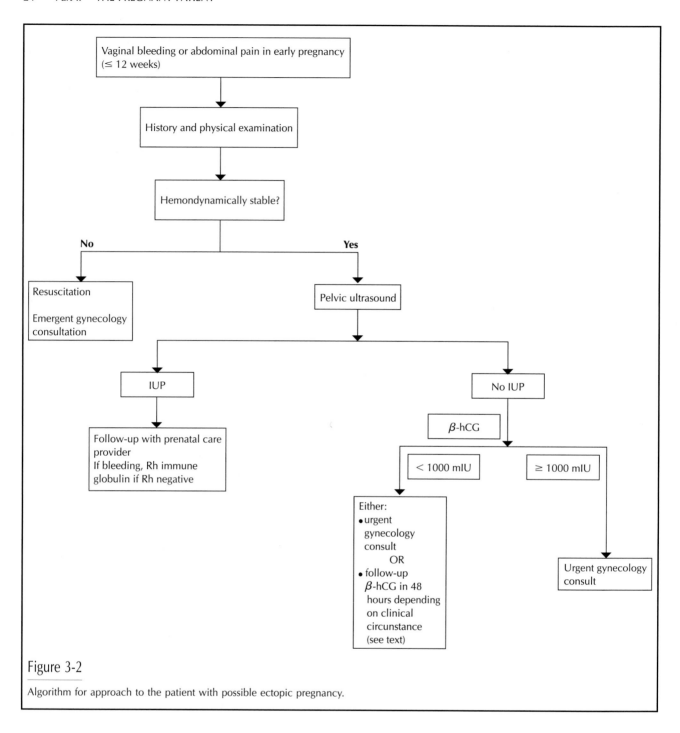

Vaginal bleeding or abdominal pain in early pregnancy (≤ 12 weeks)

History and physical examination

Hemondynamically stable?

No

Yes

Resuscitation

Emergent gynecology consultation

Pelvic ultrasound

IUP

No IUP

Follow-up with prenatal care provider
If bleeding, Rh immune globulin if Rh negative

β-hCG

< 1000 mIU

≥ 1000 mIU

Either:
• urgent gynecology consult
      OR
• follow-up β-hCG in 48 hours depending on clinical circunstance (see text)

Urgent gynecology consult

Figure 3-2

Algorithm for approach to the patient with possible ectopic pregnancy.

which time β-hCG levels decline (Fig. 3-3). A patient in whom β-hCG levels fall, plateau, or fail to reach a predicted slope before 9 to 10 weeks usually has an abnormal pregnancy. The absolute value of a single β-hCG without other testing is not useful during the first nine weeks of pregnancy to determine the location of a pregnancy. Ectopic gestations have a slower increase in β-hCG titer. This fact has led to the frequent clinical use of serial β-hCG measurements (in the stable patient) to assess whether or not there has been at least a 66 percent rise in 48 hours. However, up to 15 percent of ectopic gestations have been reported to have a normal doubling time, and 10 percent of viable pregnancies will have an abnormal doubling time.[5] Serial β-hCG levels can also be used to signal the optimal time for ultrasonography as a gestational sac can be visualized by transvaginal sonography at a level of approximately 1000 mIU/mL. Absence of a sac with a β-hCG level above this increases the likelihood of an abnormal pregnancy, including ectopic pregnancy. In addition, after medical treatment with either an abortifacient or systemic methotrexate, falling β-hCG levels help to determine the effectiveness of treatment.

Table 3-2

DIFFERENTIAL DIAGNOSIS OF ECTOPIC PREGNANCY

Normal intrauterine pregnancy
Threatened or incomplete abortion
Ruptured corpus luteum cyst
Acute salpingitis
Torsion of an enlarged ovary
Gastroenteritis
Appendicitis

ever, is that the lowest progesterone level associated with a normal pregnancy in their series was 5.1 ng/mL.[6,7]

The test is not ideal, as normal intrauterine gestations are reported to exist in the presence of a low progesterone. Moreover, the test is often unavailable on a short-turnaround 24-hour basis, thus limiting its usefulness. If the test is immediately available, a value >25 ng/mL will confirm viability and eliminate the need for further testing, potentially decreasing cost. If the value is <5 ng/mL, the patient can undergo dilatation and curettage. If villi are present, ectopic pregnancy can be ruled out. If no villi are present, the patient should undergo laparoscopy to rule out ectopic pregnancy.[8] Use of a single measurement of progesterone should be considered a potential tool for future use. Its routine use in pregnancy evaluation will need to await further published prospective experience.

PROGESTERONE

Testing of a single serum sample of progesterone has recently emerged as a controversial tool for the evaluation of potential ectopic pregnancy. A serum progesterone greater than 25 ng/mL confirms a viable intrauterine gestation. A progesterone below 5 ng/mL is consistent with a nonviable gestation but is not location-specific. With progesterone values of <25 ng/mL but >5 ng/mL, viability must be established with ultrasound. Use of this diagnostic tool is attractive, as only one measurement need be obtained. Stovall et al. performed receiver-operator characteristics curve analysis on 1120 patients and compared progesterone levels to β-hCG doubling times as predictors of ectopic pregnancy. Their data suggests that serum progesterone is a better predictor of viability than β-hCG doubling time. Of note, how-

ULTRASOUND

The location of the pregnancy can frequently be determined with a real-time ultrasound examination of the pelvis. The findings on ultrasound will be dependent on the gestational age and the type of sonographic approach used. In general, real-time sonography using an abdominal transducer can identify an intrauterine gestational sac by the fifth week, a sac with an embryonic or fetal pole by the sixth week, and an embryonic mass with cardiac motion by the seventh week (see Chap. 52). The use of high-resolution transvaginal ultrasound has improved the accuracy of diagnosis and decreased the gestational age at which an ectopic pregnancy can be diagnosed.

Timor-Tritsch studied 145 patients and found the sensitivity of diagnosing ectopic pregnancy with transvaginal sonography to be 100 percent.[9] The specificity was 98.2 percent, with a positive predictive value of 98 percent. The negative predictive value in this study was 100 percent. With skilled examiners and high-resolution vaginal ultrasound probe, the size and location of an ectopic pregnancy has been detected at as little as 31 to 32 days after LMP. The minimal β-hCG titer at which a sac should always be seen is unclear, but an experienced transvaginal sonographer should be able to visualize a viable intrauterine pregnancy at >1000 mIU/mL (Third international standard). A transabdominal transducer can visualize an intrauterine pregnancy at 6500 mIU/mL. Color Doppler allows even better visualization of an ectopic gestation. Ultrasound is still considered diagnostic of an ectopic pregnancy only when the sac is visible outside the uterus.

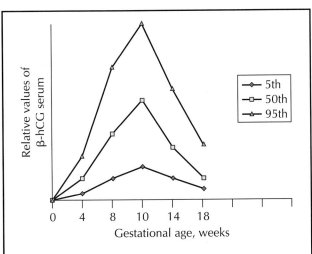

Figure 3-3

Normal rise in β-hCG levels in normal pregnancy through 18 weeks. (From Hay DL: Placental histology and the production of human choriogonadotropin and its subunits in pregnancy. *Br J Obstet Gynaecol* 95:1268, 1988, with permission.)

CULDOCENTESIS

Although the availability of ultrasonography is increasing, there are still areas where radiologic or ultrasound support is not available in a timely fashion. In this case, when ectopic pregnancy is suspected, culdocentesis may be used to

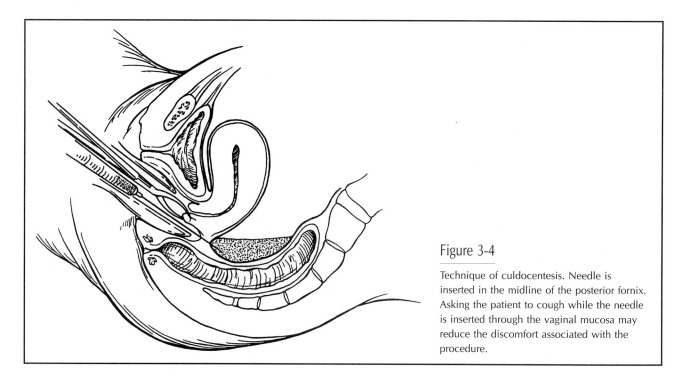

Figure 3-4

Technique of culdocentesis. Needle is inserted in the midline of the posterior fornix. Asking the patient to cough while the needle is inserted through the vaginal mucosa may reduce the discomfort associated with the procedure.

determine whether intraperitoneal hemorrhage is present (Fig. 3-4). If a significant hemorrhage has occurred, cervical motion tenderness may be present, accompanied by cul de sac fullness or bulging. With or without such a finding, however, culdocentesis can be considered in all patients with a suspected ectopic pregnancy. Culdocentesis is negative if serous fluid is aspirated and positive if nonclotting blood is aspirated. Culdocentesis is not used to determine whether or not a tubal pregnancy has ruptured, since culdocentesis is positive in the majority of ruptured or unruptured ectopic pregnancies (85 and 65 percent, respectively). Failure to aspirate blood on culdocentesis is nondiagnostic and may represent difficulty entering the peritoneal cavity. The presence of blood is not always diagnostic of ectopic pregnancy and may represent bleeding from a ruptured corpus luteum in about 5 percent of cases. Use of culdocentesis in the workup of ectopic pregnancy is generally limited to those diagnostic settings where ultrasound is not available.

DILATATION AND CURETTAGE AND LAPAROSCOPY

After identifying an abnormal pregnancy with either a low progesterone (<5 ng/mL), serial β-hCG (<66 percent rise in 48 hours), or ultrasound, curettage can be used to identify villi rendering the diagnosis of ectopic gestation remote. Some treatment algorithms suggest repeating the β-hCG in 24 hours if the β-hCG was less than 2000 mIU/mL and villi were absent. The presence of a rising or plateauing titer would suggest an ectopic gestation, while a falling titer would indicate spontaneous resolution of the ectopic pregnancy. Stovall et al. recommend dilatation and curettage in those whose β-hCG titer rises less than 50 percent in 48 hours.[10] Use of this algo-

rithm is most appropriate for patients who are compliant with follow-up (Fig. 3-2).

SUPPORTIVE TREATMENT

Management of the unstable patient with ectopic pregnancy is initiated with hemodynamic support. Oxygen should be administered and volume resuscitation started immediately. The patient should be given type-specific blood as indicated. Immediate gynecologic consult should be summoned for surgical management.

Management of the stable patient varies depending on the degree of suspicion and the gestational age. Where there is a low degree of suspicion and a menstrual period has just been missed, patients may be followed as outpatients with serial quantitative β-hCG measurements or serum progesterone. Not every patient in this situation needs an ultrasound examination. Even if the diagnosis is delayed 48 to 72 h, little harm is done because rupture of such an early ectopic pregnancy is not usually life-threatening. Once the β-hCG value is >1000 mIU/mL, transvaginal ultrasound should be able to identify an intrauterine sac if the gestation is located in the uterus.

SURGICAL TREATMENT

Operative laparoscopy has largely replaced laparotomy for the first-time treatment of ectopic pregnancy. This has occurred to reduce both morbidity and cost.[11] Tubal conservation procedures, linear salpingectomy, and segmental resection are attempts to preserve fertility. Unfortunately, these conservative treatments have not led to an increase in the intrauterine pregnancy rate.

In addition, persistent ectopic pregnancy or the continued growth of the trophoblast after incomplete removal by conservative surgery complicates 5 to 20 percent of tubal operations. Occasionally this persistent tissue grows and tubal rupture occurs, requiring salpingectomy for hemostasis.

MEDICAL TREATMENT

SYSTEMIC METHOTREXATE

Methotrexate has been used for years in the treatment of gestational trophoblastic disease. Its mechanism of action is through inhibition of spontaneous synthesis of purines and pyrimidines, thus interfering with DNA synthesis and the multiplication of cells.

Stable patients with unruptured ectopic gestation less than 4 cm in diameter by ultrasound are eligible for treatment.

Numerous dosing regimens have been published; however, current practice is to use single-dose treatment of 50 mg/m^2, which is accompanied by fewer side effects. Patients are followed on posttherapy days 4 and 7 with serial quantitative β-hCG titers. If there is a <15 percent decline in β-hCG between days 4 and 7, a second, similar dose is given.[12–14] While high doses of methotrexate can cause bone marrow suppression, acute and chronic hepatotoxicity, stomatitis, pulmonary fibrosis, alopecia, and photosensitivity, these side effects are rarely seen in the dosing schedules used here.

To make sure that the ectopic pregnancy remains unruptured, care should be taken to minimize pelvic exams. Transient pelvic pain or vaginal spotting frequently occurs 3 to 7 days after the start of methotrexate therapy. This pain is presumably due to tubal abortion and normally lasts less than 4 to 12 h in duration. Distinguishing between this pain and that of tubal rupture can be difficult. Observation in the hospital may be required in doubtful cases. Surgical intervention is required when tubal rupture leads to intrabdominal hemorrhage. Rupture remote from administration of methotrexate has been reported but is associated with a plateau or rise in β-hCG titer.

Rarely, following conservative surgical therapy (e.g., laparoscopic salpingostomy), there is persistence of viable trophoblastic tissue. Symptoms can persist in those patients from low-level proliferation of tissue in the tube. After surgery, serial weekly β-hCG levels are followed and should continue to decline until it can no longer be measured (<5 mIU/mL). Persistent or rising β-hCG levels after surgical therapy suggests residual trophoblastic tissue in the fallopian tube, which can cause continued pelvic pain or tubal rupture. This persistent tissue can be successfully treated with methotrexate using the same regimen as described above.[15,16] Gynecologic referral for this treatment is appropriate."

DISCHARGE INSTRUCTION AND FOLLOW-UP

Stable patients in whom the diagnosis of ectopic pregnancy has not been ruled out should be instructed to return for a repeat quantitative measurement of β-hCG in 48 h and every 48 h thereafter until a critical value for ultrasonic scanning has been reached. Warning signs that should prompt immediate return are acute onset lower abdominal pain, dizziness or syncope, shortness of breath, or extreme fatigue. The patient should be warned to refrain from sexual intercourse, as that trauma has been associated with signs of rupture in close proximity to coitus.

Given the differential diagnosis of threatened abortion, acute salpingitis, or corpus luteum cyst, discharge instructions should advise the patient to report fever, passage of clots or tissue, or excessive bleeding. If a lack of understanding or compliance with the follow-up is suspected, admission for observation or laparoscopy should be considered.

References

1. Ory SJ: New options for diagnosis and treatment of ectopic pregnancy. *JAMA* 267:534, 1992.
2. Bernstein J: Ectopic Pregnancy: A nursing approach to excess risk among minority women. *J Ob Gyn & Neo Nurs* 24:803, 1995.
3. Brennan DF: Ectopic pregnancy—Part II: Diagnostic procedures and imaging. *Acta Emerg Med* 2:1090, 1995.
4. Reece EA, Petrie RH, Sirmans MF, Finster M, Todd WD: Combined intrauterine and extrauterine gestations: A review. *Am J Obstet Gynecol* 146:323, 1983.
5. Stovall TG, Ling FW: Some new approaches to ectopic pregnancy. *Cont ObGyn* 5:35, 1992.
6. Cowan BD: Ectopic pregnancy. *Curr Op Ob Gyn* 5:328, 1993.
7. Stovall TG, Ling FW, Cope BJ, et al: Preventing ruptured ectopic pregnancy with a single serum progesterone. *Am J Obstet Gynecol* 160:1425, 1989.
8. Stovall TG, Ling FW, Carson SA, et al: Serum progesterone directed endometrial curettage in the diagnosis of ectopic pregnancy. *Fertil Steril* 57:456, 1992.
9. Timor-Tritsch IE, Yeh MN, Peisner DB, Lesser KB, Slavik TA: The use of transvaginal ultrasonography in the diagnosis of ectopic pregnancy. *Am J Obstet Gynecol* 161:157, 1989.
10. Stovall TG, Ling FW: Some new approaches to ectopic pregnancy. *Cont ObGyn* 5:35, 1992.

11. Silva PD, Schaper AM, Rooney B: Reproductive outcome after 143 laparoscopic procedures for ectopic pregnancy. *Obstet Gynecol* 81:710, 1993.

12. Stovall TG, Ling FW, Buster JE: Reproductive performance after methotrexate treatment of ectopic pregnancy. *Am J Obstet Gynecol* 162:1620, 1990.

13. Stovall TG, Ling FW: Single-dose methotrexate: An expanded clinical trial. *Am J Obstet Gynecol* 168:1759, 1993.

14. Stovall TG, Ling FW, Gray LA: Single-dose methotrexate for treatment of ectopic pregnancy. *Obstet Gynecol* 77:754, 1991.

15. Rose PG, Cohen SM: Methotrexate therapy for persistent ectopic pregnancy after conservative laparoscopic management. *Obstet Gynecol* 76:947, 1990.

16. Dumesic DA, Hafex GR: Delayed hemorrhage of a persistent ectopic pregnancy following laparoscopic salpingostomy and methotexate therapy. *Obstet Gynecol* 78:960, 1991.

Chapter 4

BLEEDING IN THE FIRST TWENTY WEEKS OF PREGNANCY

Catheryn Montgomery Yashar

Vaginal bleeding is a common reason for women to seek care in the emergency department, especially if pregnancy is known or suspected. It complicates up to 40 percent of pregnancies, with approximately half of these ending in abortion. Pregnancies with vaginal bleeding lasting 3 or more days are three times more likely to abort than pregnancies with only 1 or 2 days of bleeding (24 versus 7 percent).[1]

Some 15 to 20 percent of clinically apparent pregnancies abort spontaneously, and 75 percent of the losses occur in the embryonic stage, before 8 weeks of gestation.[2] Some late-onset menses noted by women are, in fact, "chemical pregnancies" only demonstrable by sensitive pregnancy blood tests. On the basis of such tests used as evidence of pregnancy, it is believed that close to 40 percent of conceptions are lost before they become clinically evident. Combining the loss rates of evident and "chemical" pregnancies, the true loss rate may be close to 50 to 60 percent.

DEFINITIONS OF ABORTION

To competently evaluate and manage bleeding in the first 20 weeks, it is important to understand the difference between threatened, inevitable, incomplete, complete, and missed abortion. Table 4-1 lists common causes of first-trimester bleeding. Strictly defined, abortion is loss of pregnancy before 20 weeks or loss of a fetus weighing less than 500 g (World Health Organization). *Threatened abortion* is any amount of uterine bleeding in the first 20 weeks of pregnancy without passage of tissue or cervical dilatation.

Inevitable abortion is a gestation dating less than 20 weeks with bleeding and cervical dilatation but no passage of fetal tissue; it can be associated with profuse bleeding and cramping. *Complete abortion* is passage of all fetal tissue before 20 weeks of gestation and is commonly accompanied by a decrease in cramps and closure of the cervix. *Incomplete abortion* is defined as passage of only part of the products of conception and is more likely to occur between 6 and 14 weeks of pregnancy. Properly differentiating between complete and incomplete abortion is crucial, as only an incomplete abortion requires dilatation and curettage, whereas a completed spontaneous abortion can be managed without surgical intervention. *Missed abortion* is a fetal death at less than 20 weeks without passage of any fetal tissue for 4 weeks after fetal death. Where sensitive pregnancy tests and ultrasound are available, missed abortion is not frequently seen in clinical practice. A *septic abortion* is any stage of abortion accompanied by signs of intrauterine infection, including any combination of elevated temperature, leukocytosis, abdominal tenderness, peritoneal signs, cervical motion tenderness, and foul discharge. Septic abortion complicates 1 to 2 percent of all spontaneous abortions. Induced abortion and its complications are covered in Chap. 5.

RISK FACTORS

There are recognizable factors that predispose a woman to spontaneous abortion. Advanced maternal age,[3] prior poor obstetric history, infertility, concurrent medical disorders (such as diabetes, cystic fibrosis, or systemic lupus erythematosus),

Table 4-1

CAUSES OF VAGINAL BLEEDING BEFORE
THE 20th WEEK OF PREGNANCY

Final Diagnosis	Number of Patients	Percent
Threatened abortion	211	13.6
Inevitable and incomplete abortion	951	61.4
Complete abortion	203	13.1
Septic abortion	67	4.3
Missed abortion	27	1.7
Benign hydatidiform mole	12	0.8
Tubal pregnancy	78	5.1
Total	1549	

Source: Adapted from Herbst et al.,[1] with permission.

abortion even in the presence of vaginal bleeding decreases to around 3 to 5 percent if fetal cardiac activity is seen on ultrasound.[4,5]

The most common cause of fetal wastage is chromosomal abnormalities, accounting for 50 to 60 percent of all losses. As a group, the most common abnormalities are trisomies, though monosomy X is the most common single karyotype in abortuses (15 to 20 percent). If a patient presents with an incomplete abortion and has had one or two prior spontaneous abortions, most clinicians recommend sending the tissue for chromosomal analysis. If possible, fresh tissue should be retrieved and placed in a physiologic solution such as saline or lactated Ringer's. Placement in formalin will destroy the cells, preventing chromosomal evaluation. Because a single spontaneous abortion is so common, chromosomal analysis is generally not recommended after a single abortion in the first or early second trimester, and is generally reserved for women who have had two or three spontaneous abortions.

and exposure to certain agents (Table 4-2) all increase the likelihood of spontaneous abortion. In addition, anatomic abnormalities of the upper genital tract may increase the risk of miscarriage. Agents shown *not* to increase pregnancy loss are birth control pills, video display terminals, diagnostic radiographs (less than 10 rads; see Appendix A-2), or first-trimester minor trauma to the abdomen. After three successive losses, the chance for subsequent pregnancy loss is 30 to 55 percent.[3] Finally, the likelihood of spontaneous

Table 4-2

AGENTS THOUGHT TO BE ASSOCIATED
WITH INCREASED RISK OF ABORTION

Chemical Agents	Infectious Agents
Tobacco	Variola
Anesthetic gases	Vaccinia
Arsenic	*Salmonella typhi*
Aniline	*Vibrio fetus*
Benzene	Malaria (*Plasmodium*)
Ethylene oxide	Cytomegalovirus
Formaldehyde	*Brucella*
Lead	*Toxoplasma*
	Treponema pallidium
	Varicella zoster
	Mycoplasma hominis
	Chlamydia trachomatis
	Ureaplasma urealyticum

Source: Adapted from Gabbe et al.,[12] with permission.

APPROACH TO THE PATIENT

A complete history and physical examination, laboratory testing, and ultrasound will help delineate the cause of bleeding for a majority of women presenting with vaginal bleeding during pregnancy. As a general rule, a reproductive-age woman with abnormal vaginal bleeding should be considered pregnant until a negative pregnancy test is obtained. A careful menstrual history should be obtained, including the first date of the last normal menstrual period (LMP), the previous menstrual period, the usual menstrual interval, and the regularity of menses. It is particularly important to ask specific questions about the character of the LMP. Was it on time? Was it heavier or lighter, longer or shorter than expected? Associated with the usual amount of cramping? Deviations from the normal menstrual period may represent bleeding of implantation of a normal or abnormal pregnancy, which can make accurate dating of the pregnancy difficult. Further important history includes medication use since the LMP; alcohol, tobacco, and recreational drug use; current and past medical problems such as diabetes mellitus, recent infections, bleeding diathesis, thyroid diseases, or systemic lupus erythematosis; surgical history, particularly operations involving the uterus; past obstetric history; and coital frequency and timing. Past obstetric history should at minimum include the number of pregnancies, number of term and preterm deliveries (<37 weeks of gestation), number of abortions (spontaneous and induced), number of living children, and major complications associated with deliveries or abortions (e.g., blood transfusions, perforated uterus, septic abortion). Past gynecologic history should include the most recent Pap smear, history of abnormal Pap smears, history of sexually transmitted diseases or other pelvic infections (e.g., salpingitis), and treatment. Number of sexual partners and contraception use (type and regularity of use) should also be recorded. The volume of bleeding should be recorded, and whether the bleeding is improving or deteriorating. Finally, associated pain or cramping with the location, severity, and duration of the pain should be recorded.

The physical exam begins with attention to vital signs, including orthostatic changes, looking for signs of hypovolemia or sepsis. An abdominal exam should be performed, paying particular attention to tenderness, bloating, or peritoneal signs suggestive of intraperitoneal hemorrhage. If possible, the source of bleeding should be identified by a visual and digital examination of the cervix. Is the bleeding originating from the vaginal walls or the surface of the cervix, or is it coming through the cervical os? If the vaginal or cervical discharge appears abnormal, a wet prep and cervical cultures for gonorrhea and *Chlamydia* should be taken. These should be done before the digital exam to avoid contamination by bacterostatic lubricant. On bimanual exam, note whether a finger can be easily inserted into the cervical os. Ready passage of a digit through the internal cervical os in the bleeding patient is evidence of an inevitable abortion. A finger should never be forcibly placed into the cervix. The size of the uterus should be noted and the adnexa gently palpated for tenderness or a mass. If a mass is suspected, palpation should be gentle, as iatrogenic rupture of an ectopic pregnancy or an ovarian cyst is possible. Further identification of masses in the cul-de-sac are often identified with a careful rectovaginal exam, and this portion of the exam should not be overlooked.

If tissue is extruding from the cervical os, the clinician must be cautious in removing the tissue. Tissue still attached to the endometrium or cervix can result in hemorrhage if separated mechanically. If it is clear that the tissue is completely separated from its uterine/cervical attachments, it is safe to remove it. All other cases should be handled with gynecologic consultation or with immediate dilatation and curettage available. Suction curettage for incomplete abortions can be performed, but only by properly trained personnel.

LABORATORY TESTING

Laboratory tests should include a complete blood count, blood and Rh type, antibody screen, urinalysis, and quantitative beta human chorionic gonadotropin (β-hCG). Recall that acute bleeding may not immediately be reflected in a complete blood count. Any woman with significant bleeding (e.g., brisk bleeding from the cervical os) or in whom intraperitoneal bleeding or a pelvic infection is suspected should have at least one intravenous line placed.

Human chorionic gonadotropin is a hormone that rises rapidly until the 10th week of pregnancy; then, from the 10th

week, it declines until the third trimester, when it again increases gradually (see Fig. 3-3). Human chorionic gonadotropin is composed of an alpha and beta subunit; standard pregnancy tests usually detect the beta subunit (β-hCG). It is first detectable as early as 9 to 11 days following ovulation, which in most women is around 24 days after the LMP; it reaches approximately 100 mIU/mL at the expected time of menses. A single value can be particularly helpful when combined with ultrasound exam, as certain β-hCG values are correlated with specific findings on ultrasound in the normal pregnancy. Even if results are not readily available, a quantitative β-hCG level should generally be determined in first-trimester bleeding, as serial β-hCGs can be helpful for follow-up. The β-hCG should rise by at least 66 percent every 48 h in a viable intrauterine pregnancy.[6] Serial β-hCGs that plateau or fall before the 10th week of gestation usually indicate an abnormal pregnancy. An abnormally high β-hCG may indicate multiple gestation, gestational trophoblastic disease, or, very rarely, an ovarian tumor. In a threatened abortion, the provider should be certain to see a definite, consistent and convincing downward or plateauing trend in the β-hCG, preferably in conjunction with an ultrasound exam, before mention of a nonviable pregnancy is made to the patient. Even mentioning this possibility without adequate cause can create undue anxiety for the patient.

Another potentially useful test in evaluating bleeding during pregnancy is serum progesterone. Progesterone is a hormone that rises after ovulation and continues to rise throughout pregnancy. Women with first-trimester bleeding and serum progesterone of <10 ng/mL will abort approximately 80 percent of the time, and viable pregnancies are generally never seen with a level <5 ng/mL. Only 2 percent of ectopic pregnancies will have a serum progesterone of 25 ng/mL or greater.[6] The test is limited in an emergency department setting because it can take hours to days to return.

ULTRASOUND

Ultrasound (see also Chaps. 52 and 53) has drastically improved the evaluation of bleeding in the first half of pregnancy. In many cases, it can allow a definitive diagnosis and guide treatment (e.g., dilatation and curettage). After a pregnancy is known to be viable by ultrasound (demonstrable fetal heart motion), the average rate of fetal loss is around 3 percent. Mackenzie and colleagues maintain that the spontaneous abortion rate of a sonographically proven live fetus for women with no prior history of miscarriage is 0.6 percent and in women with a history of spontaneous abortion approximately 5 percent.[7] The pregnancy loss rate also varies depending on the gestational age at the time of ultrasound (3.8 percent for those less than 10 weeks and 1.2 percent for those greater than 10 weeks).[5,7] If the ultrasound was performed only for dating purposes, Wilson demonstrated a loss rate of 1.3 percent, which increases to 5.4 percent if the indication for ultrasound was spotting.[5]

As with all diagnostic tests, it is advisable to consult with your radiology department to understand their level of confidence with the equipment and interpretation. Keeping this in mind, abdominal sonography should demonstrate a gestational sac if the quantitative β-hCG is greater than 6000 mIU/mL or greater than 1000 mIU/mL by vaginal ultrasound (corresponding to about 40 days of pregnancy from last menstrual period).[8-10] At 30 to 40 days of gestation, a gestational sac of 1 to 3 mm can be seen eccentrically located inside the uterus (Fig. 52-2). A midline uterine fluid collection may be a decidual sac associated with ectopic pregnancy (Fig. 52-6). A yolk sac is seen around 36 days, and a fetal heartbeat is noted at 41 to 47 days from the LMP.[8,11] At 8 weeks gestational age, the sac is generally 25 mm in size and an embryo should easily be seen (crown-rump length about 14 mm at this age).[8] Gestational sacs with a mean diameter greater than 25 mm without an embryo or greater than 20 mm without a yolk sac are definitely abnormal and a woman can be reliably counseled on pregnancy loss.

DIFFERENTIAL DIAGNOSIS

In virtually all cases of bleeding in the first 20 weeks of pregnancy, a careful investigation utilizing history and physical examination, β-hCG levels, and quality-level ultrasound can establish either the correct diagnosis or a logical management plan that will safely lead to a correct diagnosis.

There are other reasons why direct visualization of the cervix and vagina is important; not least among these is that bleeding may be due to lesions entirely unrelated to the pregnancy (e.g., from the urinary or gastrointestinal tract). A carefully collected midstream clean-catch urine specimen or catheterized specimen may demonstrate whether the blood is from a urinary source. In the absence of infection, blood in the urine should raise suspicion of nephrolithiasis, which is more common in the pregnant than in the nonpregnant population. All urinary tract infections and asymptomatic bacteruria should be treated during pregnancy, as they are associated with preterm labor if untreated (see Chap. 24). If the cause of spotting or bleeding is not readily apparent, bleeding from the lower gastrointestinal tract should be evaluated by inspection of the anus for hemorrhoids and palpation of the rectal canal, and evaluation for blood in the stool. Cervical carcinomas can cause watery, foul, or bloody discharge, frequently presenting after intercourse. A recent normal Pap smear does not definitively rule out carcinoma, and any suspicious lesion should be referred to a gynecologist for biopsy. A lesion on the pregnant cervix should not be biopsied in the emergency department, as profuse bleeding can ensue and may be difficult to control. Nonspecific

inflammation or infectious cervicitis from gonorrhea, *Chlamydia, Trichomonas,* or bacterial vaginosis can lead to a spectrum of symptoms ranging from no symptoms to abnormal discharge, pain, or vaginal spotting. A wet-prep examination may assist in differentiating these diagnoses (see Table 43-2). Cervical cultures for chlamydia and gonorrhea should be performed.

Other cervical findings, such as ectropion or polyps, can cause bleeding as well, especially if the bleeding is consistently postcoital. *Cervical ectropion,* common in pregnancy, is easily recognizable. This is a normal condition, where the more friable columnar epithelium that lines the endocervical canal is present on the portio vaginalis of the cervix. It appears as a smooth, reddened ring of tissue surrounding the cervical os. When touched with a cotton swab, it may start to ooze gently or cause a surprisingly steady stream of bleeding. *Cervical polyps* are pinkish buds that may protrude from the os. Although a polyp can be readily and safely removed in the nonpregnant patient in this setting, it is wise not to attempt removal of a cervical polyp from the pregnant cervix in the emergency department setting, as profuse bleeding may ensue. A cervical polyp is a benign condition and does not require immediate removal. The walls of the vagina should also be inspected, as ulcers, small lacerations, and erosions due to infections, trauma, or neoplasm can cause vaginal bleeding.

If the bleeding is experienced around the time of or just after the expected normal menses, *implantation bleeding* should be considered. This is a fairly common occurrence with a benign physiologic cause. As the embryo burrows into the highly vascular decidual tissue, blood escapes into the uterine cavity and out through the cervix. It ranges from a pinkish discoloration of the vaginal discharge to bleeding equivalent to that of a menstrual period. It can last 1 or 2 days but usually not longer. Most commonly, it occurs in the fifth or sixth week after the LMP and women sometimes mistake this bleeding for a normal menses. Thus, it is a common cause of inaccurate dating as well. *Ectopic pregnancies* occur in 1 to 2 percent of all pregnancies and are covered in detail in Chap. 3.

GESTATIONAL TROPHOBLASTIC DISEASE

Although gestational trophoblastic disease (commonly called *molar pregnancy*) is unusual, it typically presents as bleeding in the first half of pregnancy. It is more commonly seen in those of Asian descent, those who have had prior trophoblastic disease, and first pregnancies in the early or late years of childbearing (<15 or >35 years old). In the general population, the incidence is 1 in 1000, though may be as high as 1 percent in the Asian population. Although usually benign, it does have malignant potential and requires long-term and careful follow-up.

Abnormal proliferation of the trophoblastic cells is the underlying pathophysiology of gestational trophoblastic disease (GTD), which is generally divided into two categories, the complete and the partial mole. In the complete molar pregnancy, fetal tissues are absent and the 46XX karyotype is generally of duplicated paternal origin (that is, both X chromosomes come from the sperm). In the partial mole, fetal tissues are present (there can even be a viable fetus) and, as a result of dispermy, the usual karyotype is triploidy (69 XXY). Complete moles are more likely to lead to persistent or metastatic disease.

At the more serious end of the spectrum of GTD is choriocarcinoma. It usually follows a partial molar pregnancy but may follow a full-term pregnancy or can arise in the ovaries, unassociated with pregnancy. Choriocarcinoma is a frankly malignant lesion that is, fortunately, usually responsive to chemotherapy.

Frequently, GTD presents with abnormal bleeding mimicking an incomplete or threatened abortion. Other signs are passage of hydropic villi (that tend to have a grapelike appearance) through the vagina. Uterine size is larger (50 percent) or smaller (25 percent) than the estimated gestational age or there may be enlarged cystic ovaries resulting from theca-lutein cysts. In addition, common patient complaints include severe nausea or vomiting. Unusually, the patient may have signs of preeclampsia (Chap. 7) or hyperthyroidism.

A characteristic but unusual pattern on ultrasound (*snowstorm pattern*) may accompany a molar pregnancy. The ultrasound appearance of frequent lucent areas interspersed with brighter areas is shown in Fig. 52-10. The β-hCG level is usually higher than expected for gestational age (generally greater than 100,000 mIU/mL). The definitive diagnosis is made by histologic evaluation of the tissue, which is frequently not done until after surgical evacuation. After removal, follow-up measurements of β-hCGs should be done to make sure that there is no persistent or metastatic disease. If GTD is suspected, the uterus should be evacuated as soon as possible, although this is not an emergency unless signs of preeclampsia are present. Nevertheless, the patient should be seen by an obstetrician-gynecologist within the next 24 h so that definitive therapy can be arranged. Prior to discharge from the emergency department, her thyroid status should be evaluated, because some moles produce thyroid hormone and any hyperthyroidism should be treated prior to operative intervention. Further discussion of the neoplastic nature of GTD is covered in Chap. 55.

SEPTIC ABORTION

Fortunately, the estimated fatality rate from septic abortion (see also Chaps. 7 and 18) is very low, ranging from 0.4 to 0.6 per 100,000 spontaneous abortions. Septic abortion is a polymicrobial infection and should be treated by prompt admission, broad-spectrum intravenous antibiotics, and evacuation of the uterus. In addition, blood and cervical discharge should be obtained for culture. Disseminated intravascular coagulation is sometimes seen in this setting, either from prolonged retention of fetal tissue due to release of necrotic tissue into the bloodstream or in women who have developed frank septic shock. See Chap. 5 for further discussion of septic abortion.

RHESUS FACTOR

In all pregnant women who present with bleeding—whether it is due to ectopic pregnancy or threatened, complete, incomplete, missed, or septic abortion—a blood-type and antibody screen should be performed. Fifteen percent of women are negative for the rhesus (Rh) D antigen and are therefore at risk to become Rh-sensitized if they are carrying an Rh-positive fetus. The maternal immune system, recognizing any fetal blood in the maternal circulation as foreign, will make antibodies against the D antigen. In subsequent pregnancies with an Rh-positive fetus, these antibodies may cross the placenta and cause fetal hemolysis and hemolytic disease of the fetus or newborn. Although this disease is sometimes treatable, it can be fatal for all subsequent Rh-positive fetuses.

Sensitization can occur as early as 8 weeks of gestation, and although the frequency of sensitization is not known precisely, it is estimated to be about 9 percent with an abortion at 12 weeks. Therefore, it is recommended that all unsensitized Rh-negative women with bleeding during pregnancy receive Rh immune globulin (Rhogam) if unsensitized. If the gestation is less than 12 weeks, a dose of 50 μg is sufficient; but because gestational age testing can be inaccurate, we recommend administering 300 μg of Rh immune globulin to all unsensitized Rh-negative women with bleeding in the first or second trimester. Many hospitals, for simplicity's sake, carry only the 300-μg dose. Ideally, Rh immune globulin is given before the woman leaves the emergency department, but protection occurs if it is administered within 72 h of the bleed and perhaps as late as 2 to 4 weeks after bleeding.

TREATMENT

If fetal cardiac activity is detected either by ultrasound or Doppler, the stable patient should be followed expectantly. A proven nonviable intrauterine pregnancy in the stable patient without heavy bleeding can be managed, depending on the comfort level of the physician and patient, with close follow-up and warnings to return immediately with excessive bleeding (more than a pad per hour), pain, or fever. Short-term follow-up (within a week) with a prenatal care provider is recommended. Warnings that the uterus may evacuate its contents spontaneously and thereby obviate the need for surgical management should be discussed with the patient. Another appropriate alternative in this scenario is scheduled surgical evacuation, recognizing that at times a family needs to adjust to news of pregnancy loss before they are emotionally ready for surgical intervention. Excessive pain or cramping, bleeding, signs of sepsis, or suspicion of an ectopic pregnancy will make expectant management imprudent, and a gynecologic consultation is indicated. Management of septic abortion is covered in Chaps. 5 and 15. Some emergency departments are able to accommodate these women with suction evacuation equipment and anesthetic capabilities on site. This has the advantage of allowing immediate evacuation, which is simpler for the physician and family.

Incomplete abortions typically occur between 8 and 14 weeks of gestation and require surgical evacuation of the uterus. As bleeding may be profuse, it is appropriate to manage these patients in a hospital setting, though usually on an outpatient basis. If the emergency department is equipped with a suction curettage machine, these cases can be handled in the emergency department if there are trained personnel in suction curettage. The physical examination should demonstrate that the cervical os is open as manual dilation of the cervix is generally too uncomfortable to allow the procedure to be performed in this setting. An intravenous line with lactated Ringers containing 20 U of oxytocin per liter should be begun. IV sedation or IM administration of meperidine, 75 mg, and diazepam, 5 mg, can be administered. A paracervical block can be used by injecting 0.5% lidocaine at the 3 and 9 o'clock positions at the junction of the cervix and vagina in the submucosal tissues, The total dose of lidocaine should not exceed 2 mg/lb of lean body weight. In general, approximately 10 mL is utilized. A 21 gauge spinal needle is useful to perform this. Two or 3 mL can be placed at the 12 o'clock position of the cervix to make placement of the single tooth tenaculum more comfortable. The choice in suction curettes should be based on the size of the uterus and weeks gestation. In general, the diameter of the curette in millimeters should be one less than the gestational age in weeks, calculated from the last menstrual period. The curette should carefully be placed through the cervix, not exerting excessive pressure to avoid perforating the fundus of the uterus. The pregnant uterus is remarkably soft and excessive force must be avoided. The suction machine is turned on and the cannula is rotated, evacuating the uterine contents. This should be continued until bubbles are seen in the tubing. Gentle, sharp curettage follows to be certain all pregnancy tissue is removed. Contraindications to suction curettage in the emergency department include: untrained personnel, suspected ectopic pregnancy, a uterus ≥ 12 weeks gestation, closed cervical os, inability to perform adequate bimanual exam, an allergy to anesthetic or sedative agents without acceptable alternatives, and pain or anxiety which in the clinician's judgment would interfere with the successful completion of the procedure.

Any patient sent home for expectant management should be advised to bring passed tissue with her on return to the hospital. A simple description of the difference between blood clots and tissue is sometimes helpful for the patient.

There is no evidence that reduction of activity or medical therapy will affect the outcome of threatened abortion. Although there is no evidentiary support that rest will affect outcome, it is often prescribed for social and psychological reasons. It is important to emphasize to a patient diagnosed with threatened abortion that normal pregnancies tolerate normal physical activity. The possibility of losing a pregnancy is distressing to a family and should be approached sensitively. It is also crucial to emphasize that there is nothing a woman can do to prevent aborting an abnormal pregnancy. Many women harbor secret feelings of guilt when they face a threatened abortion. These may include guilt over drinking excessively prior to knowing about the pregnancy, arguments between the woman and the baby's father, or unresolved issues surrounding prior elective terminations. If this is suspected, exploration of these feelings and reassurance are warranted. Progestational agents, although advocated by some authors, have not been proved to affect outcome in threatened abortion.

If a woman with a threatened abortion continues her pregnancy, there may be a slightly increased risk of preterm labor and of fetal anomalies. It is judicious to allow the prenatal care provider to discuss these risks in detail with her rather than counseling her in an emergency department setting.

COUNSELING

The emotional response to a spontaneous pregnancy loss is variable, from relief (if the pregnancy was not desired) to overwhelming grief. A sensitive approach to these families is a critical part of treatment and is often the most significant effect that a clinician can have in the setting of pregnancy loss. Offering referral to professional counseling or support groups should be a routine part of the management of these women, and policy should be developed to make the necessary phone numbers available to these families. Occasionally, social work or psychiatry consultation is helpful prior to discharge.

References

1. Herbst A, Mishell D Jr, Stenchever M, Droegemueller W: *Comprehensive Gynecology,* 3d ed. St Louis: Mosby–Year Book, 1996.
2. Harlap S, Shiono PH, Ramcharam S: A life table of spontaneous abortions and the effects of age, parity, and other variables, in Porter IH and Hook EB (eds): *Human Embryonic and Fetal Death,* New York: Academic Press, 1980.

3. Knudson UB, Hansen V, Juul S, Secher NJ: Prognosis of a new pregnancy following previous spontaneous abortions. *Eur J Obstet Gynecol* 39:31, 1991.

4. Simpson JL, Mills JL, Holmes LB, et al: Low fetal loss rates after ultrasound-proved viability in early pregnancy. *JAMA* 258:2555, 1987.

5. Wilson RD, Kendrick V, Wittmann BK, McGillivray B: Spontaneous abortion and pregnancy outcome after normal first-trimester ultrasound examination. *Obstet Gynecol* 67:353, 1986.

6. Stovall TG, Ling FW, Carson SA, Buster JE: Serum progesterone and uterine curettage in differential diagnosis of ectopic pregnancy. *Fertil Steril* 57:456, 1992.

7. Mackenzie WE, Holmes DS, Newton JR: Spontaneous abortion rate in ultrasonographically viable pregnancies. *Obstet Gynecol* 71:81, 1988.

8. Chervenak F, Isaacson G, Campbell S: *Ultrasound in Obstetrics and Gynecology.* Boston: Little, Brown, 1993.

9. Callen P: *Ultrasonography in Obstetrics and Gynecology.* Philadelphia: Saunders, 1988.

10. Cacciatore B, Tiitinen A, Stenman U, Ylostalo P: Normal early pregnancy: Serum hCG levels and vaginal ultrasonography findings. *Br J Obstet Gynaecol* 97:899, 1990.

11. Fossum G, Davajan V, Kletzky O: Early detection of pregnancy with transvaginal ultrasound. *Fertil Steril* 49:788, 1988.

12. Gabbe S, Niebyl J, Simpson J: *Obstetrics: Normal and Problem Pregnancies,* 2d ed. New York: Churchill Livingstone, 1991.

Chapter 5

COMPLICATIONS OF INDUCED ABORTION

Phillip G. Stubblefield

BACKGROUND

Induced abortion as practiced in the United States is generally safe and only infrequently associated with complications.[1] Prior to legalization, induced abortion frequently led to serious complications and death. In the 1940s, more than 1000 women died each year from abortion complications.[2] In recent years, there are fewer than 10 deaths per year from induced abortion in the entire United States. Because most abortions take place in the first trimester, when they are safest, the death-to-case rate for legal abortion is less than 1 per 100,000 abortions. The risk of death from legal abortion induced prior to 16 weeks is five- to tenfold less than that from continuing the pregnancy.[3] Abortion services are generally provided in freestanding specialty clinics. This pattern of care has reduced cost and made abortion services available where they would otherwise not be. However, when complications occur, the fragmentation of care, divided between clinic and emergency department, poses special problems.[4] Providing emergency care is more difficult because essential information from the abortion clinic may not be available after hours, when the patient presents in the emergency department. Emergency physicians and their gynecologic consultants who do not themselves provide abortion services may be insufficiently familiar with the diagnosis and management of abortion complications. Serious complications are rare and are therefore easily mistaken for more common and much less severe problems. In healthy young women, serious injury may not be appreciated until significant complications develop. Often the patient's family does not know that she has obtained an abortion and there is a delay in seeking help because of concern about the abortion being disclosed. Management becomes simpler and more likely correct when the abortion clinic chart can be accessed.

ATTITUDES AND BELIEFS OF HEALTH CARE PROFESSIONALS

Though induced abortion has been legal in the United States since 1973, intense feelings are still aroused by it. Health care professionals must be sure to maintain a nonjudgmental, supportive attitude in dealing with patients who have sought abortion. We have a duty to "put health first" in the care of these women and to deal with the medical issues without burdening the patient with our own emotional responses to abortion.[5] Similarly, it is divisive and harmful and potentially increases medicolegal risk for all involved providers if a presumption of error in management is conveyed to the patient.

METHODS OF INDUCED ABORTION

Some discussion of the technology of legal abortion is necessary to understand the possible complications and their management.

SURGICAL ABORTION IN THE FIRST TRIMESTER

First-trimester abortion is usually performed by some variation of vacuum curettage.[6] Analgesia is usually provided by paracervical block with lidocaine or chloroprocaine. Conscious sedation with intravenous sedatives and analgesics is common. Some clinics offer general anesthesia. After initiation of the selected analgesic, the cervical canal is progressively stretched with dilators, or tapered metal rods of graduated sizes. Then a hollow vacuum curette 6 to 12 mm in diameter is introduced through the cervix, connected to a vacuum source, and the uterine contents evacuated. Some surgeons use a spoon-shaped metal curette following the vacuum to check that the cavity is empty. Afterwards, it is good practice to rinse the aspirated tissue, place it in a glass dish, and examine it over a source of backlighting such as a photographer's light box. This allows immediate confirmation of products of conception, decreasing the likelihood of failure to diagnose ectopic or molar pregnancy. Often, screening for gonorrhea and *Chlamydia* is performed immediately prior to the procedure. Most clinics provide prophylactic antibiotics, usually a short course of tetracycline or doxycycline. Rh-negative patients are given Rh immune globulin prior to discharge to prevent isoimmunization. Patients with a problem requiring extra attention—for example, insufficient tissue aspirated and therefore risk of ectopic pregnancy—should be listed for tracking until the problem is resolved. Clinics often have a 24-h telephone number for emergencies, and the covering physician may have the list of any patients with unresolved problems. Usually the patient is given a single-page summary of her care to take back to her referring physician. This summary will contain essential information such as apparent length of gestation at time of termination, how the procedure is performed, which medications are frequently administered, and types of problems encountered.

MEDICAL ABORTION IN THE FIRST TRIMESTER

The combination of the antiprogesterone, mifepristone (RU486), and misoprostol, a prostaglandin E_1 analogue, has been preliminarily approved by the U.S. Food and Drug Administration.[7] Several centers are currently studying another medical abortifacient regimen, intramuscular methotrexate followed in 5 to 7 days by vaginally administered misoprostol.[8] Either regimen can present problems of incomplete abortion and heavy bleeding after administration of the misoprostol. Failed abortion with continuation of the pregnancy occurs in a small percentage of cases. Sulprostone, the prostaglandin E_2 analogue used in Europe, has led to myocardial ischemia in a small number of older smokers, but this has not been seen with misoprostol.

SURGICAL METHODS FOR MIDTRIMESTER ABORTION

Dilatation and evacuation (D&E) is the most prevalent method for midtrimester abortion in the United States. The cervix is dilated more widely than for first-trimester procedures. This is usually accomplished with hygroscopic dilators, stems of the sea plant *Laminaria,* or rods of synthetic hydrogel. Hygroscopic dilators are placed in the cervical canal; they expand slowly over several hours, producing dilatation. Then, under conscious sedation or general anesthesia, strong ovum forceps are inserted through the cervix to extract the fetus and placenta. Immediate complications of D&E include uterine perforation with potential visceral and vascular injury and embolic phenomena. Later complications include incomplete abortion with bleeding and infection and disseminated intravascular coagulation.

MEDICAL METHODS FOR MIDTRIMESTER ABORTION

A variety of techniques are used to induce labor. Typically combinations are employed, as, for example, *Laminaria* tents to dilate the cervix and prostaglandin E_2 vaginal suppositories to produce uterine contractions. Hypertonic solutions, either saline or urea, may be instilled into the amniotic cavity in combination with prostaglandins. Intravenous oxytocin is often used. The labor induction methods have specific complications depending on the method used: water intoxication with concentrated oxytocin, high fever with prostaglandin E_2, frequent vomiting and diarrhea with either prostaglandin E_2 or methyl $F_{2\alpha}$. Hemolysis, cerebral edema, and renal failure occur if hypertonic saline is inadvertently given intravascularly. Another group of complications are common to all labor induction methods: failure of the primary method, incomplete abortion, sepsis, hemorrhage, uterine rupture, cervical laceration, cervical-vaginal fistula. Disseminated intravascular coagulation (DIC) and embolic phenomena are rare but the risk is greater with labor induction methods than with D&E.

SELECTIVE TERMINATION

Women carrying multifetal gestations may be offered selective termination to reduce the number of gestations usually to two, thus reducing the risk for severely premature birth for the surviving fetuses. This is done by passing a needle through the abdominal and uterine walls and into the heart of an individual fetus under ultrasound guidance. Concentrated potassium chloride is then injected into the fetal heart to produce asystole.[9] Generally the pregnancies treated in this fashion are absorbed without incident, but subsequent spontaneous loss of the remaining gestations can occur and will cause abdominal pain and vaginal bleeding.

ABORTION METHODS USED BY NON-MEDICALLY TRAINED PROVIDERS

A variety of techniques are used in many cultures around the world to induce abortion.[10] Occasionally, U.S. women resort to untrained providers or attempt self-abortion. Complications from these procedures are likely to be more severe and more frequent than with legal abortion induced by a skilled provider. Insertion of a foreign body through the cervix is one such method. Rubber urinary catheters are used in this fashion. Over time, the presence of the foreign body will provide uterine contractions and expulsion of the pregnancy. However, hemorrhage and severe infection are likely. If a rigid foreign body is used, perforation of the uterus and injury to the bladder, bowel, or uterine vessels may occur. In Asia, the "massage technique" is used. The practitioner applies manual or even foot pressure to the gravid uterus through the abdominal wall. This apparently disrupts the placental attachment, leading to placental abruption and labor. Prior to legalization of abortion in the United States, transcervical instillation of chemical pastes and soap solutions into the extraamniotic space was sometimes employed. Entry of soap solutions into the systemic circulation caused intravascular hemolysis and widespread damage to membranes, with resultant pulmonary and renal failure.[11] Sepsis is common with use of unsterile instruments and techniques that do not immediately evacuate the uterus. Clostridial sepsis, a special problem with illegal induced abortion, is much less frequently encountered with legal procedures. Botanical preparations may be ingested as infusions and teas to attempt abortion. In the United States in the nineteenth century, pennyroyal and oil of juniper were commonly taken for this purpose and are still occasionally encountered. Tablets of potassium permanganate are sometimes inserted vaginally to produce abortion. This causes sharply demarcated, deep ulcerations of the vaginal mucosa, with resultant bright red vaginal bleeding. The intent of the abortionist was to mislead medical personnel so they would perform a dilatation and curettage evacuation of the uterus for a presumed incomplete spontaneous abortion.

COMPLICATIONS AND MANAGEMENT

COMPLICATIONS ARISING DURING THE ABORTION PROCEDURE

Freestanding abortion facilities rely on a hospital emergency department as backup, but the need will be infrequent; hence, emergency departments must be prepared for uncommonly occurring, unfamiliar situations that may require prompt intervention. One such emergency is the inability of the abortion facility to complete the abortion. The provider will have begun the procedure but is unable to complete evacuation of the pregnancy. This may be because the gestation is too far advanced for the instruments available in the clinic or because of an abnormality of anatomy. Bleeding will likely be present, and unrecognized uterine perforation may have occurred. Initial assessment of the patient includes physical examination and review of information provided by the clinic as to medical history, gestational age, and details of the abortion procedure, whether membranes were ruptured, estimated blood loss, whether fetal parts were extracted, and whether perforation is suspected. Hypovolemia should be expected. Blood is drawn for a complete blood count plus blood type and crossmatch, and serum electrolytes. A large-bore intravenous line is placed for hydration and blood replacement as needed. If there is bleeding, high-dose intravenous oxytocin therapy should be started with 50 U of oxytocin in 500 mL of 5% dextrose and normal saline administered at 125 mL/h. Immediate transfer to the operating room is required if there is known perforation, continuing external bleeding, or signs of peritoneal irritation (e.g., marked tenderness and rebound). Ultrasound examination is important provided that the patient is stable enough to wait until this study can be obtained (Fig. 5-1). The ultrasound should demonstrate the extent of tissue remaining in the uterus; it may show a large amount of fluid in the pelvis, suggesting intraabdominal hemorrhage; and it may allow determination of gestational age if intact fetal tissue remains in the uterine cavity, where it can be visualized and measured. An anatomic abnormality such as uterine duplication, septate uterus, or pregnancy in a blind horn of a double uterus (i.e., bicornuate or didelphic uterus) should be suspected. Uterine perforation can often be confirmed by inserting a sterile blunt instrument into the uterine cavity and visualizing it under ultrasound guidance.[12] This procedure is best performed in the operating room or with immediate availability to perform suction curettage, as heavy bleeding may result. Next, a decision is made as to means for evacuating the uterus. This will depend upon the estimated gestational age of the pregnancy. First-trimester pregnancies will be evacuated with vacuum curettage usually under laparoscopic guidance and general anesthesia. Management of more advanced gestation depends upon the skills of the consulting gynecologist: whether he or she is trained to perform midtrimester D&E at the suspected gestational age. If not, the uterus will be evacuated by a medical means that induces labor, either prostaglandin or high-dose oxytocin (see Table 5-1). Prophylactic antibiotics are indicated (e.g., cefoxitin 2 g IV or ampicillin/sulbactam 1.5 g IV).

COMPLICATIONS PRESENTING AFTER THE ABORTION PROCEDURE

POSTABORTAL TRIAD

Mild to moderate lower abdominal cramping, vaginal bleeding of moderate amount (similar to a menstrual period), and

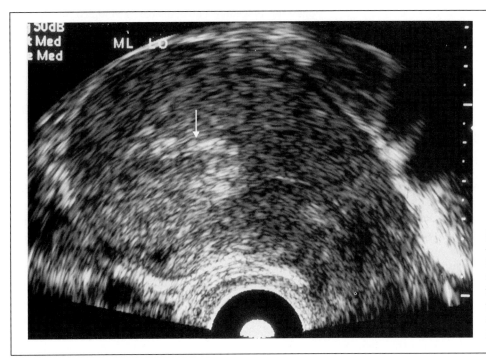

Figure 5-1

Heterogeneous echoes in midposition of uterus representing retained products of conception after pregnancy termination. (Photo courtesy of Robert Bree M.D., University of Michigan.)

low-grade fever (38°C or less) has been described as the "postabortal triad" and is the most common complaint after an abortion procedure. These symptoms usually indicate some amount of retained tissue or blood clot within the uterus and in some cases an associated mild endometritis. Unfortunately, these symptoms can also indicate the early phase of septic incomplete abortion or other serious problems such as those listed in Table 5-2. After an initial assessment, a decision is made as to whether there is retained tissue in the uterus. When retained tissue or clot is present, in most cases, an enlarged, soft, tender uterus is found or there is ultrasound demonstration of intrauterine echoes (see Fig. 5-1), and prompt uterine evacuation is required.

If abdominal tenderness is limited to the lower abdomen and uterus, the uterus feels firm and only minimally enlarged, and transvaginal ultrasound shows no intrauterine tissue, the patient can be treated for presumed early endometritis with

Table 5-1
MEDICAL REGIMENS FOR UTERINE EVACUATION IN THE MIDTRIMESTER

Dinoprostone vaginal suppositories 20 mg q3h
Carboprost 250 μg IM q2h
Misoprostol 800 μg (four 200-μg tablets) administered vaginally or rectally every 12 h
High-dose oxytocin[a]
  Add 50 U of oxytocin to 500 mL of 5% dextrose and normal saline. Administer over a 3-h period. Rest patient 1 h off oxytocin. Repeat, adding 100 U of oxytocin to 500 mL of dextrose/saline solution; administer over 3 h. Rest 1 h. Repeat, adding another 50 U of oxytocin to each 500-mL infusion over 3 h, alternating with 1 h of rest until the patient aborts or a final solution of 300 U of oxytocin in 500 mL is reached.

[a]Adapted from Winkler et al.,[24] with permission.

Table 5-2
CONDITIONS THAT MAY PRESENT AS POSTABORTAL TRIAD[a]

Retained pregnancy tissue (incomplete abortion) without sepsis
Failed abortion (continued intact gestation)
Hematometra
Uterine perforation
Ectopic pregnancy
Early stages of septic incomplete abortion

[a]Lower abdominal pain, bleeding, and fever.

appropriate antibiotics. Because of the multiple possible pathogens, no one antibiotic is ideal. Ofloxacin (400 mg PO b.i.d.) plus either clindamycin (450 mg PO q.i.d.) or metronidazole (500 mg PO b.i.d.) for 14 days, as in the management of early pelvic inflammatory disease, is one acceptable regimen. Oral ergot (methyl ergonovine or ergotamine, 0.2 mg PO t.i.d. for 3 days) is prescribed to minimize bleeding. If the patient is hemodynamically stable without active bleeding, she may be discharged home with follow-up planned in 48 h.

HEMORRHAGE

Possible causes of post-procedure excessive bleeding include uterine atony, cervical laceration, uterine perforation, hematometra, a cervical pregnancy, or retained products of conception (e.g., a gestation too far advanced for completion of abortion by the means available in the clinic). With midtrimester abortion, DIC must also be considered. Management requires rapid action to stabilize the patient, as described in Table 5-3, and immediate communication with the abortion provider to determine what has been done thus far. Gynecologic consultation is frequently necessary. Temporizing measures to control bleeding include insertion of a Foley catheter into the uterine cavity and inflating the 30-mL balloon. As an additional emergency measure to control bleeding, intramuscular carboprost (0.250 mg) or rectal misoprostol (0.800 mg) is given. With the bleeding temporarily controlled, a complete history of the events is obtained and abdominal and pelvic examination and ultrasound examination are performed if this can be done promptly. If perforation is suggested by the history or the findings of abdominal tenderness, guarding, and rebound, the patient is prepared for immediate laparoscopy. An incomplete abortion will require uterine evacuation.

CERVICAL LACERATIONS

Typically, cervical lacerations are on the anterior lip of the cervix, a result of tears from the tenaculum, the instrument placed on the cervix to steady it and provide countertraction during the procedure. If the laceration is deep enough to cause persistent bleeding, it should be repaired with absorbable sutures. The upper extent of the laceration must be visualized prior to repair. If the laceration extends to the internal cervical os, perforation must be considered and ruled out by probing the laceration with a uterine sound or other small blunt instrument, preferably under ultrasound guidance (see "Uterine Perforation," below). As the bladder and ureters lie on the anterior wall of the vagina, lacerations extending to the anterior vaginal wall require an evaluation of the integrity of these structures. Gynecologic or urologic consultation may be helpful in this setting.

UTERINE ATONY

Increased bleeding during or immediately after the abortion procedure may indicate uterine atony, or failure of the uterus to contract normally. This will respond to uteronic agents—intravenous oxytocin—or, if this fails, prostaglandin (see Table 5-1). Failure to respond to these methods may indicate cervical laceration, uterine perforation, retained tissue in the uterus, or DIC.

HEMATOMETRA

Hematometra or "postabortal syndrome" is a type of uterine atony.[13] It may present immediately after the abortion as increasing lower abdominal pain, tachycardia, and prostration, but it may also be more subtle, evolving slowly over several days before reaching sufficient intensity to bring the patient to the emergency department. Differential diagnosis includes the conditions listed in Table 5-2, especially perforation with formation of a broad ligament hematoma. Diagnosis is made on physical exam by demonstration of a tense, tender midline mass arising from the cervix and absence of a tender mass lateral to the uterus. Ultrasound is

---

Table 5-3

GENERAL APPROACH TO MANAGEMENT OF POSTABORTAL COMPLICATIONS

1. Rapid initial assessment including history from patient and written material from abortion facility if available (preoperative ultrasound findings; details of procedure—type, suspected complications or problems encountered, whether tissue was removed, and pathologic analysis of tissue if done).
2. Vital signs and focused physical exam (especially abdomen and pelvic exam).
3. Begin large-bore intravenous line (16 gauge or larger) with lactated Ringers or 0.9% saline.
4. Lab studies: CBC, type and cross-match, blood cultures if febrile or septic abortion suspected.
5. Begin antibiotics if fever or septic abortion suspected (e.g., cefotetan 2 g every 12 h or cefoxitin 2 g every 6 h, or ampicillin/sulbactam 1.5 g every 8 h, or clindamycin 900 mg every 8 h plus gentamicin 2 mg/kg loading followed by 1.5 mg/kg every 8 h IV).
6. If significant bleeding present, administer high-dose oxytocin (see Table 5-1), carboprost 0.25 mg IM, or ergotamine 0.2 mg IM.
7. Rh immune globulin administration (300 μg) if not performed already.
8. Treat specific complications with gynecologic consultation as needed (see text).
9. Arrange aftercare and follow-up.

not essential if the physical findings are clear-cut, but it is helpful to demonstrate the enlarged uterine cavity distended with multiechoic material. Treatment is immediate reevacuation of the uterine contents and intravenous oxytocin. The diagnosis is confirmed by the aspiration of clotted blood from the uterus, its prompt contraction, and resolution of the midline mass. The patient is discharged on an oral ergot regimen (methyl ergotamine or ergonovine, 0.2 mg PO t.i.d. for 3 days).

DISSEMINATED INTRAVASCULAR COAGULATION

Disseminated intravascular coagulation (DIC) must be considered with persistent unexplained bleeding, especially after midtrimester abortion. Passage of blood that does not clot, or persistent hemorrhage after uterine massage and oxytocin therapy, are indications for measurement of platelets, fibrinogen, and fibrin split products. Quick confirmation of the diagnosis is provided by a bedside clotting time, observing the length of time to formation of clot in a glass tube of blood. Firm clot should be present by 5 to 7 min. A longer interval and incomplete coagulation in the tube strongly suggest DIC. In most cases, postabortal DIC can be treated successfully with intramuscular carboprost. This usually produces sufficient contraction of the uterus to stop the bleeding within several minutes of administration, avoiding the need for blood products and transfusion. If hemorrhage persists, then treatment of the DIC with fresh frozen plasma and cryoprecipitate is indicated.

ECTOPIC PREGNANCY

With the exception of the rare heterotopic pregnancy (pregnancy in both uterus and tube at the same time), risk for ectopic pregnancy should be recognized at the time of induced abortion when the surgeon's fresh examination of the tissue fails to reveal chorionic villi. When this is not performed or recognized, the patient leaves the facility thinking that her problem is solved. When, later on, pain from the ectopic pregnancy begins, the patient may initially attribute this to expected postabortal discomfort and may delay seeking help. Unfortunately, emergency department staff can easily make the same mistake. Women with ectopic pregnancies who seek abortion are much more likely to die than are women who do not seek termination.

Ruling out an ectopic pregnancy after an abortion is complex, because modern beta human chorionic gonadotropin (β-hCG) assays will detect hCG for several days after an induced abortion. The problem is much more easily solved when the abortion facility can be contacted and the results of pathologic examination of the aborted tissue determined. Ultrasound may show an adnexal mass with cardiac echoes, pathognomonic for a tubal pregnancy, or an empty uterus and abundant fluid in the pelvic cavity, suggestive of hemoperitoneum. More common is the finding of any empty uterus in the face of persistent β-hCG on serial assays, suggesting the diagnosis of ectopic pregnancy. If the patient has severe abdominal pain and peritoneal signs, then surgical intervention, laparoscopy, or laparotomy is required without delay. It is the less acute situations that present diagnostic and management dilemmas. Most patients who present with mild to moderate pain and minimal to moderate bleeding will not have an ectopic pregnancy but rather a low-grade endometritis with some amount of retained tissue or clot and will respond to uterine evacuation. However, unless the symptoms and findings can be explained by one of these other diagnoses, the patient must be considered at risk for ectopic pregnancy. If she is clinically stable with minimal findings, she may need to be followed as an outpatient with serial quantitative assays of β-hCG until it is clear that the levels are falling rapidly, consistent with a complete induced abortion. Follow-up within 48 to 72 h must be assured. The patient must be instructed about the risk that the ectopic pregnancy may rupture during this waiting period. If the levels plateau or start to rise, the patient should be treated as having an ectopic pregnancy. Therapeutic alternatives include surgery or intramuscular methotrexate. Unruptured ectopic pregnancies with an adnexal mass size by ultrasound of less than 3.5 cm and no fetal heartbeat detectable by transvaginal ultrasound can be treated with intramuscular methotrexate, 50 mg/m^2, with a high probability of success (see Chap. 3).[14]

PAIN

Patients presenting with a primary complaint of lower abdominal pain but with little bleeding and no fever may still have any of the conditions listed in Table 5-2, but hematometra or perforation are the most likely explanations.

A less common cause of pain is a degenerating leiomyoma. An enlarged uterus with point tenderness over a mass in the uterine wall plus ultrasound demonstration of an empty uterine cavity with some degree of uterine enlargement or an actual fibroid is consistent with this diagnosis. Consideration must still be given to the other possibilities—perforation and endomyometritis—but absent adnexal tenderness and fever, with the physical findings as described, suggest that a degenerating fibroid is likely. The treatment is a short course of nonsteroidal anti-inflammatory medication with follow-up in 48 h.

UTERINE PERFORATION

Uterine perforation is part of the differential diagnosis in any patient presenting with the postabortal triad (i.e., bleeding, cramping, and fever) or any of its individual complaints. In a study of U.S. national data of 67,175 abortions, perforation occurred at a rate of 0.9 per 1000 abortions, but it is more likely with procedures performed at a later gestational age: each 2-week increase in gestational age was associated with a 1.4-fold increase in risk.[15] The anatomy of uterine perforation is shown in Fig. 5-2. Perforation markedly increases risk for serious bleeding, infection, and death. Perforations range from a simple puncture of the uterine wall with no other injury to arterial laceration, avulsion, or laceration of the small and large intestine or the urinary bladder. A simple puncture with no visceral or vascular injury will require only evacuation of any retained pregnancy tissue under laparoscopic guidance. More extensive injury will require major surgery, potentially hysterectomy, bowel resection, and colostomy. The clinical challenge is to efficiently determine the extent of injury and manage the injury appropriately.

When the diagnosis of perforation is unclear and physical findings are minimal, ultrasound may be of help. The uterine cavity is visualized, and a uterine sound or small blunt dilator is used to gently explore the cavity under ultrasound guidance. A defect in the uterine wall permitting passage of the sound into the abdomen confirms the diagnosis.

Suspected perforations are best managed by immediate laparoscopy to assess the extent of injury and plan repair and complete the abortion under laparoscopic guidance.[16] The urinary bladder is catheterized to look for grossly bloody urine that would indicate a bladder laceration. Pelvic portions of the large and small intestine are carefully inspected. If any injury is seen, it must be completely visualized. An experienced operator may accomplish this with the laparoscope, but laparotomy is indicated if the site of injury cannot be completely visualized. Perforations occurring at second trimester D&E procedures will usually require laparotomy for adequate evaluation and management.

BOWEL INJURY

If perforation was not immediately recognized by the operator, the bowel may have been grasped with the vacuum cannula or forceps and lacerated or stripped of its mesentery. This can present as fever and increasing abdominal pain 24 to 48 h after the procedure. Small areas of injury can be managed by oversewing the lesion, irrigating thoroughly, and leaving a large intraabdominal drain. Full-thickness injury or stripping of the mesentery will require segmental resection and anastomosis. Larger injuries to the colon will require the creation of a diverting colostomy after repair. Antibiotics are given prophylactically or as treatment, depending on the extent of injury.

BLADDER INJURY

Bladder injury during an abortion is likely to be in the region of the trigone. Suprapubic pain, anuria, bloody urine, or pain on urination are all suggestive of bladder injury. For safe repair, a cystotomy incision is made on the dome of the bladder to provide good visualization. The ureters are

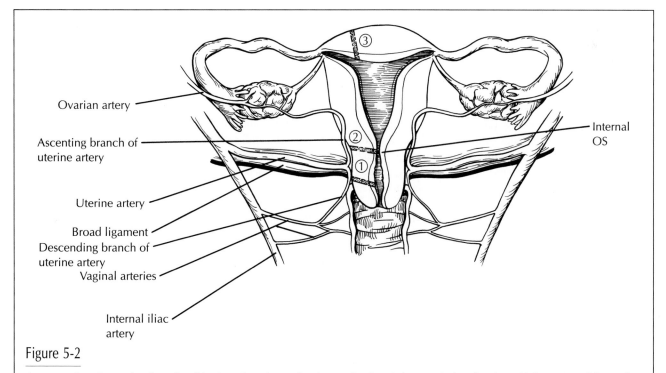

Figure 5-2

Anatomy of uterine perforations. Possible sites of uterine perforation at abortion. 1, low cervical perforation with laceration of descending branches of uterine artery; 2, perforation at junction of cervix and lower uterine segment with laceration of ascending branch of uterine artery; 3, fundal perforation (most common site). (After Berek and Stubblefield,[17] with permission.)

catheterized and the laceration is then repaired in two layers; a urinary catheter is left in place for 5 to 7 days.

The best possible operative consultation with an experienced surgical specialist is advised for management of these more extensive injuries. Inadequate initial management of major injury adds great risk and may jeopardize the patient's survival.

LATERAL UTERINE PERFORATION

Lateral uterine perforations present special problems, as they may cause extensive vascular injury that is unrecognized initially. The operator may perforate laterally with initial dilatation, note a spurt of bright blood that is not appreciated as abnormal, and then find the correct channel through the internal os, complete the dilatation, and successfully evacuate the pregnancy. The injured vessels constrict and bleeding stops, but it later recurs. Perforations at the junction of the cervix and lower uterine segment can lacerate the ascending branch of the uterine artery, giving rise to severe pain, a broad ligament hematoma, and intraabdominal bleeding (Fig. 5-2).[17] These perforations are usually recognized at the time they occur. They are managed by laparoscopy to confirm the injury and then by laparotomy to ligate the severed vessels and repair the uterine injury. Hysterectomy should not be required to manage such an injury; indeed, hysterectomy may not solve the problem. Uterine artery branches may be lacerated lateral to the usual site of their ligation in standard hysterectomy techniques. If this is not appreciated, the patient will rebleed after hysterectomy and must be subjected to a second laparotomy, at considerable risk to her survival.

Low cervical perforation injures the descending branch of the uterine artery, within the dense collagenous tissue of the cardinal ligaments. In this case there is no intraabdominal bleeding. The bleeding is only outward, through the cervical canal, and may subside temporarily as the artery goes into spasm. These vascular injuries produce recurrent episodes of hemorrhage that appear to respond to repeated uterine evacuation and therapy with uterotonic agents and have led to deaths when this phenomenon was not recognized.

Lateral perforations into the cervix or into the broad ligament may escape diagnosis at laparoscopy, as the injury can be retroperitoneal. A perforation at the junction of cervix and lower uterine segment into the broad ligament can be demonstrated in the operating room by carefully passing a uterine sound or other instrument up through the cervix from the vagina. It likely will follow the same course as the perforating instrument did initially and will be seen to tent the broad ligament when observed through the laparoscope. Low cervical perforations cannot be diagnosed even with laparoscopy and will not be appreciated until hysterectomy is begun, the peritoneum between the uterus and bladder is incised, and the bladder is pushed down to expose the perfo-

ration near the cardinal ligaments immediately adjacent to the cervix.

Treatment by selective embolization during arteriography is becoming an increasingly utilized method for controlling pelvic hemorrhage. If low cervical perforation is suspected because of recurrent postabortal hemorrhage, arteriography of the internal iliac arteries should be considered. If a bleeding vessel is identified, it can be selectively embolized via the arterial catheter.

SEPTIC INCOMPLETE ABORTION

If retained pregnancy tissue is not evacuated promptly, septic incomplete abortion may develop. Septic shock and adult respiratory distress syndrome (ARDS) can rapidly ensue.[18] This condition should be suspected when a woman of childbearing age presents with unexplained fever, vaginal bleeding, and amenorrhea, even if there is no history of attempted abortion. The diagnosis can be made with a sensitive pregnancy test and pelvic examination.

To eradicate the infection, blood cultures and cultures from the cervix and endometrial cavity should be obtained and high-dose broad-spectrum antibiotics begun. A variety of infecting organisms are possible: vaginal and bowel flora plus *Neisseria gonorrhoeae* and *Chlamydia*. Any of the Centers for Disease Control regimens for severe pelvic inflammatory disease can be used (see Table 44–6). For these very seriously ill patients we favor triple therapy: ampicillin 2 to 3 g IV q4h, clindamycin 900 mg IV q8h or metronidazole 7.5 mg/kg q6h (usual adult dose, 500 mg), and either gentamicin or tobramycin (loading dose of 2 mg/kg of body weight, followed by 1.5 to 1.7 mg/kg q8h, depending upon blood levels and renal status).

The uterus must be emptied. In the first trimester, this can be accomplished with vacuum curettage under conscious sedation. A retained fetus in the midtrimester creates special problems. If a physician skilled in D&E is available, D&E under ultrasound guidance may be performed; otherwise, labor can be induced with carboprost, misoprostol, or high-dose oxytocin (Table 5-1). Prostaglandin E_2 should probably be avoided in septic abortion, because it elevates body temperature.

Expert support in an intensive care unit is essential, as with septic shock from other causes. Cuff blood pressures are not reliable in septic shock. An arterial line should be placed for blood pressure monitoring, and a balloon flotation right heart catheter inserted so that pulmonary artery wedge pressure (PAWP), cardiac output, and systemic vascular resistance can be monitored. Urinary output is monitored via an indwelling catheter. Intravenous fluids are given in large volume until a target mean arterial pressure (MAP) is achieved of ≥ 60 mmHg without exceeding a target PAWP of 12 to 15 mmHg. If the PAWP reaches 15 mmHg before the target MAP is achieved, vasopressors are added. Dopamine is commonly used: 1 to 3 μg/kg per minute initially, with gradual increases as needed. Dopamine increases heart rate, myocardial contractility, and MAP while maintaining perfusion at lower doses. As the dose is increased, alpha-adrenergic effects occur with vasoconstriction. If target MAP is not reached by 20 μg/kg per minute, norepinephrine is added at 2 to 10 μg/kg per minute. Dopamine is continued at 2 to 5 μg/kg per minute to enhance renal perfusion.

Tissue oxygenation is monitored with pulse oximetry and arterial blood gases. Adult respiratory distress syndrome occurs in 25 to 50 percent of patients with septic shock; it should be treated early with intubation and mechanical ventilation if O_2 saturation falls below 90% or pulmonary compliance begins to decrease.

If after a few hours there is no response to uterine evacuation and medical therapy, laparotomy is indicated. Other indications are suspected uterine perforation, bowel injury, pelvic abscess, and clostridial myometritis. Hysterectomy is frequently necessary in addition to drainage of any abscess. In severely ill patients with septic abortion, early hysterectomy may improve survival. The abdominal cavity should be thoroughly irrigated free of all purulent material and the peritoneum drained with a closed suction system. Bowel injury will require a diverting enterostomy. Abdominal closure should be with internal stay sutures (Smead-Jones or similar) or a running mass ligature including peritoneum, rectus muscle, and rectus fascia. The skin and subcutaneum are left open with sutures placed for a delayed primary closure, and the wound is packed.

Clostridial sepsis should be suspected from the presence of large gram-positive rods on Gram stain from the endometrial cavity or curetted tissue. Other signs of clostridial sepsis are tachycardia that seems out of proportion to the fever and hematuria and shock that develop rapidly. Severe ARDS develops rapidly in these patients. Initial treatment is as described above, but with high-dose penicillin G (4 million units IV q4h) instead of ampicillin. A superficial clostridial infection will respond to these measures. If hemolysis is present, this indicates systemic release of clostridial toxins; prompt hysterectomy and bilateral salpingoophorectomy will probably be necessary.[19] Hyperbaric oxygenation may play a role in treatment, in addition to effective surgical and medical management of clostridial sepsis.[20]

SEIZURE

Patients with epilepsy have occasionally seized during or after abortion procedures. They are managed in the conventional fashion with maintenance of the airway. Vasovagal syncope may occur during cervical dilatation under paracervical block, especially in the unsedated patient. This has been termed *cervical shock*. The patient may have brief tonic-clonic activity and will exhibit bradycardia but quickly recovers when the painful stimulation ceases. This phenomenon is differentiated from true seizure by its brevity, associated cardiovascular changes, and complete absence of a postictal state. After the patient has recovered, atropine (0.4 to 1.0 mg IV) can be administered and the abortion procedure completed. Generalized convulsions followed by cardiorespiratory arrest may follow inadvertent intravascular injection or overdose of local anesthetic for paracervical block.[21] Management requires endotracheal intubation with ventilatory support plus anticonvulsant therapy.

PULMONARY COMPLICATIONS

Anaphylaxis

Fatal anaphylaxis has been reported in asthmatic patients from allergy to the preservative sodium metabisulfite[22] and can also be provoked by preservatives found in oxytocin. These patients develop severe bronchospasm immediately following an otherwise uncomplicated abortion procedure. Treatment is with oxygen, intubation, and agents to relieve bronchospasm, but caution must be used to avoid giving the patient more metabisulfite, so epinephrine containing this preservative, routinely used in these circumstances, is absolutely contraindicated. Terbutaline, the selective beta$_2$ agonist, contains no preservative; it or other similar preservative-free compounds should be used.

Amniotic Fluid Embolism

Amniotic fluid embolism (AFE) or thrombotic pulmonary embolism will present as sudden cardiorespiratory collapse during the performance of a D&E, or during labor in midtrimester abortion induced with hypertonic saline or prostaglandins. Initial therapy is cardiopulmonary resuscitation, oxygen, and intubation. Differentiating between AFE and thrombosis may be difficult, but severe respiratory difficulty leading to cardiac arrest during the abortion procedure will more likely be AFE. Patients who survive the initial episode develop DIC, usually severe, which will require therapy with fresh frozen plasma and possibly cryoprecipitate. Fortunately, AFE during abortion is very rare, because most reported cases are fatal.[23] However, milder forms may occur more frequently, because it is not uncommon, during the performance of a midtrimester D&E, to have a transient, sudden drop in oxygen saturation, which returns to normal in a few minutes without therapy and with no sequelae. The awake patient will report sudden dyspnea and air hunger, which immediately resolves.

Adult Respiratory Distress Syndrome

Adult respiratory distress syndrome (ARDS) occurs with septic abortion and is occasionally seen in the context of a uterine perforation with major hemorrhage. Management in an intensive care unit is required in order to have expert ventilatory support (see Chap. 18). Mortality is high even in previously healthy young women.

CERVICAL AGGLUTINATION SYNDROME

Occasionally postabortal women will present months following the procedure with pelvic pain recurring monthly and no menstrual bleeding. On examination, the uterus is somewhat tender. The ultrasound appearance of this phenomenon has not been described, but ultrasound would be expected to show a distended uterine cavity filled with echogenic material. Treatment is gentle passage of a small blunt cervical dilator through the cervical canal. This is followed by extrusion of mucoid old blood from the cervical canal. This condition is distinct from Asherman's syndrome, where there are intrauterine adhesions and no or minimal collections of blood within the uterus.

SURGICAL EVACUATION OF THE UTERUS IN THE EMERGENCY DEPARTMENT

Key to adequate treatment of most postabortal complications is prompt evacuation of any retained pregnancy tissue. Most patients with postabortal pain, bleeding, or fever will require uterine evacuation. Stable patients with these complications of first-trimester abortion and no evidence of perforation can be safely treated in an emergency department or office setting without the delay or exposure of transportation to the operating room. Many institutions now provide uterine evacuation using suction curettage under conscious sedation in the emergency department. Vacuum curettage can be performed with conventional rigid plastic vacurettes and an electric vacuum pump or with manual vacuum systems, such as the hand-held double-valve syringe used with flexible vacuum cannula (International Projects Assistance, Chapel Hill, NC). Instruments for surgical evacuation are pictured in Fig. 5-3. Paracervical block with 1% lidocaine augmented with conscious sedation allows the procedure to be done without discomfort. One such regimen is midazolam 2 mg IV, followed with one to two doses of 50 μg of fentanyl. The patient is monitored with frequent pulse blood pressure and pulse oximetry until recovery from sedation.

COMPLETING CARE

Prior to discharge, unsensitized Rh-negative patients should be given Rh immune globulin (300 μg IM) if they have not al-

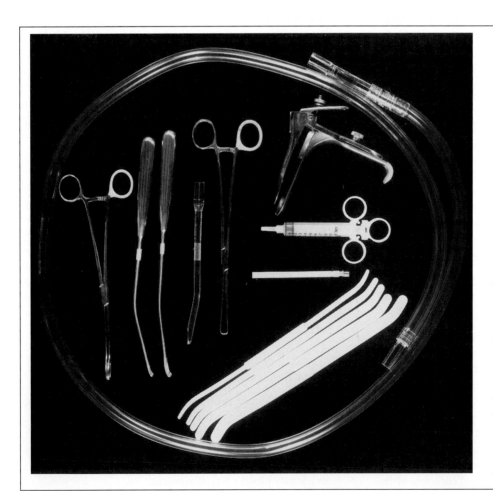

Figure 5-3

Instruments for vacuum extraction in the emergency department. From upper right corner, clockwise: Graves vaginal speculum, "control top" syringe—10 mL, 22 gauge spinal needle 3½", Deniston uterine dilators, Forester ovum forceps, #1 curette, #3 curette, 9-mm vacuum cannula, and single tooth tenaculum. Surrounding the instruments is disposable vacuum tubing. (Photo courtesy P. G. Stubblefield, M.D.)

ready been treated at the abortion facility. Plans for contraception should be discussed and a method prescribed. Follow-up should be arranged. Patients treated on an ambulatory basis for presumed early infection should be evaluated at 48 h to be certain of the adequacy of clinical response to initial therapy. Other patients should be seen in a week. Postoperative instructions include monitoring temperature morning and evening for several days and attention to the amount of pain and vaginal bleeding. The patient should be given a 24-h telephone contact for questions and instructed to call or return if temperature exceeds 38°C or there is persistent abdominal pain or vaginal bleeding sufficient to require changing a pad every hour.

References

1. Hakim-Elahi E, Tovell HMM, Burnhill MS: Complications of first trimester abortion: A report of 170,000 cases. *Obstet Gynecol* 76:129, 1990.
2. Cates W Jr, Rochat RW: Illegal abortions in the United States: 1972–1974. *Fam Plan Perspect* 8:86, 1976.
3. Lawson HW, Frye A, Atrash HK, et al: Abortion mortality: United States, 1972–1987. *Am J Obstet Gynecol* 171:1365, 1994.
4. Hodgson JE: Major complications of 20,248 consecutive induced abortions: Problems of fragmented care. *Adv Planned Parenthood* 9:52, 1975.
5. Susser M: Induced abortion and health as a value. *Am J Public Health* 82:1323, 1992.
6. Stubblefield PG: Pregnancy termination, in Gabbe SG, Niebyl JR, Simpson JL (eds): *Obstetrics: Normal and Problem Pregnancies,* 2d ed. New York: Churchill Livingstone, 1991, p 1303.
7. Peyron R, Aubeny E, Targosz V, et al: Early termination of pregnancy with mifepristone (RU486) and the orally active prostaglandin misoprostol. *N Engl J Med* 328:1509, 1993.
8. Hausknecht RU: Methotrexate and misoprostol to terminate early pregnancy. *N Engl J Med* 333:537, 1995.
9. Evans MI, Dommergues M, Wapner RJ, et al: Efficacy of transabdominal multifetal pregnancy reduction: Collaborative experience among the world's largest centers. *Obstet Gynecol* 170:874, 1993.
10. Potts M, Diggory P, Peel J: *Abortion.* Cambridge, England: Cambridge University Press, 1977.
11. Burnhill MS: Treatment of women who have undergone chemically induced abortions. *J Reprod Med* 30:610, 1985.
12. Darney PD, Horbach NS, Korn AP: *Protocols for Office Gynecologic Surgery.* Cambridge, MA: Blackwell, 1996, p 178.
13. Sands RX, Burnhill MS, Hakim-Elahi E: Post-abortal uterine atony. *Obstet Gynecol* 43:595, 1974.
14. Stovall TG, Ling FW: Single dose methotrexate for ectopic pregnancy: An expanded clinical trial. *Am J Obstet Gynecol* 168:1759, 1993.
15. Grimes DA, Schulz KF, Cates WJ: Prevention of uterine perforation during curettage abortion. *JAMA* 251:2108, 1984.
16. Lauersen NJ, Birnbaum S: Laparoscopy as a diagnostic and therapeutic technique in uterine perforations during first-trimester abortions. *Am J Obstet Gynecol* 135:181, 1979.
17. Berek JS, Stubblefield PG: Anatomical and clinical correlations of uterine perforation. *Am J Obstet Gynecol* 117:522, 1973.
18. Stubblefield PG, Grimes DA: Septic abortion. *N Engl J Med* 331:310, 1994.
19. Faro S, Pearlman M: *Infections and Abortion.* New York: Elsevier, 1992.
20. Grimm PS, Gottlieb LJ, Bodie A, et al: Hyperbaric oxygen therapy. *JAMA* 263:2216, 1990.
21. Grimes DA, Cates W: Deaths from paracervical anesthesia used for first trimester abortion, 1972–1975. *N Engl J Med* 295:1397, 1976.
22. U.S. Food and Drug Administration: Warning for prescription drugs containing sulfite. *Drug Bull* 17:2, 1987.
23. Cates W Jr, Boyd C, Halvorson-Boyd G, et al: Death from amniotic fluid embolism and disseminated intravascular coagulation after a curettage abortion. *Am J Obstet Gynecol* 141:346, 1981.
24. Winkler CL, Gray SE, Hauth JC, et al: Mid second trimester labor induction: Concentrated oxytocin compared with prostaglandin E₂ vaginal suppositories. *Obstet Gynecol* 77:297, 1991.

Chapter 6

NAUSEA AND VOMITING IN EARLY PREGNANCY

Cosmas J. M. van de Ven

Nausea is the feeling of an imminent desire to vomit, whereas *vomiting* is the forceful oral expulsion of gastric contents. *Retching* refers to the physical sensation of vomiting without expulsion of gastric contents, and *regurgitation* is a more gentle return of esophageal contents into the hypopharynx. Two separate entities are discussed in this chapter: nausea and vomiting of pregnancy and hyperemesis gravidarum. *Hyperemesis gravidarum* is a prolonged course of intractable nausea and vomiting associated with weight loss, dehydration, ketonemia, and electrolyte imbalance.

EPIDEMIOLOGY

Nausea and vomiting of pregnancy and hyperemesis gravidarum are most commonly seen in the first 12 weeks (first trimester) of the pregnancy. The incidence of nausea during pregnancy is estimated to be 70 percent[1] and the incidence of vomiting is estimated to be at least 50 percent.[2] In three separate studies, the overall incidence of nausea alone was 23 to 28 percent and of nausea with vomiting 46 to 52 percent. The median day of onset is day 39 after the last normal menstrual period; the average time of onset is in the weeks 4 through 6. The worst symptomatology occurs in weeks 8 through 12. The median day of resolution is day 84 and complete resolution occurs by 20 weeks.[2–4]

More than 50 percent of pregnant women with nausea and vomiting of pregnancy experience their symptoms mainly in the morning, one-third experience them throughout the day, and the remainder have symptoms mainly at night.[1] The re-

currence rate in future pregnancies is 60 percent.[2] Most pregnant women, however, will never become sick enough to present to the emergency department, and only 1 to 2 percent will require admission.[5]

ETIOLOGY/RISK FACTORS

The etiology of nausea and vomiting of pregnancy and hyperemesis gravidarum is still unknown. Hormonal, neurologic, metabolic, toxic, and psychosomatic factors are all described. Increased maternal age was found to be associated with a decrease and younger maternal age with an increase in both incidence and severity of nausea and vomiting.[5,6] Nulliparous women (no prior deliveries >20 weeks gestation), either primigravidae (no prior pregnancies) or patients with previous early pregnancy losses, experienced more nausea and vomiting.[7] However, other investigators reported an increase in nausea and vomiting in multiparous patients. [5–7] Women working outside the home experience more nausea,[7] while women who smoke reported a decreased incidence of both nausea and vomiting.[1,5] Ninety-eight percent of women who have demonstrated an intolerance to oral contraceptives experience nausea and vomiting in early pregnancy. In addition, 90 percent of patients with preexisting gastritis and 100 percent of women with preexisting gallbladder disease experience nausea and vomiting in pregnancy.[1]

Some investigators have implicated human chorionic gonadotropin (hCG) as a causative factor,[8] whereas others provide evidence that there is no such association.[9,10] Goodwin and associates described higher total as well as free beta subunits of hCG concentrations in women with hyperemesis as compared with asymptomatic controls.[11] There is a significant difference in the incidence of nausea and vomiting in patients with spontaneous abortions (50 percent) as compared with those having induced abortions (80 percent), suggesting an inverse association with inadequate production of placental hormone.[12]

Fifty to 70 percent of patients with hyperemesis gravidarum have elevated levels of free T_4 and T_3, which return to normal as soon as the hyperemesis improves.[13] Goodwin and colleagues evaluated biochemical parameters in 57 patients with hyperemesis gravidarum,[14] of whom 60 percent had suppressed thyroid stimulating hormone (TSH). Serum β-hCG levels correlated negatively with TSH and positively with free T_4 levels. Multiple studies suggest that the transient changes in free T_4 and TSH are due to the bioactivity of hCG and not secondary to a primary altered thyroid function.[15,16]

Investigators have suggested a psychological basis for nausea and vomiting in pregnancy.[17] Reported psychological factors associated with hyperemesis gravidarum include immaturity, dependency, hysteria, depression, and anxiety.[18] However, Wolkind et al.[19] found a higher incidence of psychiatric disease in women who did *not* experience nausea and vomiting, and Fitzgerald was unable to show any association at all.[20] Psychological and sociologic factors probably play a role in the patient's experience of nausea and vomiting during pregnancy.[21] However, there is no evidence that these psychological factors play a causative role.

PREGNANCY OUTCOME

A decreased risk of miscarriage,[1,3,4] fetal mortality,[5,22] and perinatal mortality[4] has been noted for women with nausea and vomiting during pregnancy. In their metaanalysis, Weigel and Weigel concluded that the association between nausea and vomiting of pregnancy and pregnancy outcome is limited to a decrease in fetal mortality in the first 20 weeks of gestation.[4] In their study, there were no associations with length of gestation, birth weight, placental weight, fetal body length, fetal head circumference, or Apgar scores or in perinatal or neonatal mortality. In a retrospective study by Chin, no increase in neonatal morbidity or mortality was reported and no increase in medical diseases complicating the pregnancy occurred as compared with women without vomiting.[23]

The degree of maternal weight loss may be more specific in predicting fetal outcome. Gross demonstrated an increased risk of intrauterine growth restriction and low birth weight in those patients who lost more than 5 percent of their prepregnancy body weight.[24]

PATHOPHYSIOLOGY

Gastric peristaltic waves normally occur at three contractions per minute; they originate in the pacemaker area on the greater curvature of the stomach and travel toward the pylorus. Electrical pacemaker cell and contractile–smooth muscle cell activity are controlled by the autonomic nervous system and a variety of hormones.

Nausea is almost always associated with an increase in gastric wave frequency from four to nine contractions per minute, decreased vagal tone, increased sympathetic tone, and increased vasopressin and epinephrine levels. On the other hand, delayed gastric emptying due to antral hypomotility or gastric dysrhythmia provokes symptoms of nausea and vomiting of undigested food. Gastric dysrhythmias have been described in patients with nausea and vomiting of pregnancy by several investigators.[25–27] High levels of β-hCG may play a role in nausea and vomiting of pregnancy, as women with gestational trophoblastic disease (molar pregnancy) or multiple gestations frequently experience excessive nausea and vomiting.

DIAGNOSIS

HISTORY

The usual sequence of events of nausea and vomiting of pregnancy includes loss of appetite or anorexia at 5 to 6 weeks of gestation, followed by nausea and subsequently vomiting. The history should determine the duration and types of symptoms. Pregnancy causes a gradual onset of anorexia, nausea, and vomiting. Other entities with a long course of nausea and vomiting include peptic ulcerative disease, hepatitis, malignancies, metabolic derangements like diabetes, and psychiatric disease. Acute presentations are more commonly due to inflammatory processes such as appendicitis, gastroenteritis, pancreatitis, and cholecystitis. Other acute presentations of nausea and vomiting include recreational drug use and central nervous system events (e.g., meningitis). Pregnancy-induced nausea and vomiting is usually accompanied by anorexia, and eating or drinking quickly makes the symptoms worse. Similarly, in obstructive disease or with gastroparesis, gallbladder or pancreas pathology, the nausea and vomiting will worsen soon after a meal or other oral intake. By contrast, nausea and vomiting associated with mucosal disorders, like peptic ulcer disease, may be relieved by food.

The presence or absence of abdominal pain should be assessed, including the quality of the pain, radiation, severity, and factors that either exacerbate or relieve the pain. Pain is uncommon in pregnancy-induced nausea and vomiting and should alert the care provider to another etiology. Appendicitis is not more common in pregnancy but is prevalent in the reproductive age group. Cholelithiasis and cholecystitis occur more frequently in pregnancy. Both acute and chronic gastroenteritis, pancreatitis, severe constipation, irritable bowel syndrome, and inflammatory bowel disease are other causes of abdominal pain that may be associated with nausea and vomiting. The presence of blood in the contents of the vomitus may reflect mucosal injury or a tear in the esophagus (Mallory-Weiss tear). Undigested food usually indicates gastric obstruction or delayed emptying. Bilious or fecal material suggests a more distal small intestinal or colonic obstruction. Finally, a medication history is necessary to identify prescription, over-the-counter, or other drugs that can cause nausea and vomiting.

PHYSICAL EXAM AND LABORATORY TESTING

Pregnancy-induced nausea and vomiting presents with few physical signs other than those of dehydration. Check orthostatic vital signs and assess dehydration status. Dry mucosa, poor skin turgor, and concentrated urine are present with dehydration. Assess for icteric sclerae or jaundice. Check for costovertebral tenderness. The presence of abdominal tenderness or distention must lead to assessments for gynecologic, surgical, or infectious disorders. Rectal examination is necessary to identify stool impaction and should include testing for occult blood. Pelvic examination is necessary in the presence of abdominal, or pelvic pain, or vaginal bleeding, or discharge.

Lab testing includes a complete blood count, serum electrolytes and ketones, BUN and creatinine, and urinalysis. Elevated hematocrit and BUN may be present due to hemoconcentration. Hyper- or hyponatremia, or hypokalemia may be evident. Urinalysis is important to determine the specific gravity and for evidence of infection.

In patients with hyperemesis gravidarum, vaginal ultrasonography may be helpful to assure the presence of fetal cardiac activity, to identify multiple gestations, or to diagnose molar pregnancies. An upper abdominal ultrasound should be ordered if the exam suggests gallbladder disease, pancreatitis, or liver disease. A plain abdominal flat plate is helpful to rule out bowel obstruction or renal calculus.

DIFFERENTIAL DIAGNOSIS

A multitude of other conditions can induce nausea and vomiting aside from delayed gastric emptying due to pregnancy, including gastric mucosal irritation from nonsteroidal antiinflammatory agents or alcohol, appendicitis, cholelithiasis, pancreatitis, hepatitis, thyrotoxicosis, gastrointestinal dis-

tention secondary to bowel obstruction, vestibular nerve stimulation, increased cranial pressure, meningeal irritation, cerebrovascular dilation, and seizure activity.

Other causes of chronic nausea and vomiting, usually without abdominal pain, include metabolic disorders like thyrotoxicosis, endocrine disorders including diabetic ketoacidosis, hypo- or hyperparathyroidism, and adrenal insufficiency. Toxicity from medications, although rare, includes antiepileptic agents, theophyllines, digitalis glycosides, and salicylates.

Reflux esophagitis may induce or worsen recurrent nausea and vomiting. Relaxation of the lower esophageal sphincter leads to esophagitis with a retrosternal burning sensation. Raising the head of the bed (placing 3- to 4-in. wood blocks under the bedposts) and the use of oral antacids may be helpful. If symptoms persist, H_2-receptor antagonists may be used, including cimetidine, ranitidine, or famotidine in their usual doses.

Preexisting peptic ulcer disease usually improves during pregnancy. Clark studied 313 pregnancies in 118 women and reported a clear remission in 90 percent.[28] However, within 3 months of delivery, symptoms recurred in over half the patients. Medical therapy consisting of antacids and H_2 receptor antagonists is helpful.

Less common causes of nausea and vomiting in pregnancy are diaphragmatic hernia and achalasia. The diagnosis is established by a barium esophagogram or endoscopy. Kurzel and associates reported 18 cases of symptomatic diaphragmatic hernia complicating pregnancy. Those patients presenting with acute obstruction had a maternal mortality of 45 percent. Based on their experience, these authors recommend repair during pregnancy even in asymptomatic patients.[29] Mayberry and Atkinson described the clinical course of 16 women with achalasia who became pregnant; 11 had no change in symptomatology, 2 improved, and 3 worsened. Management consists of giving soft foods and anticholinergic drugs.[30] Successful pneumatic dilatation for severe achalasia during pregnancy has been reported by Fiest et al.[31]

Additional laboratory tests should be ordered based on clinical presentation. Liver function test results may be slightly elevated [aspartate transaminase (AST) and alanine aminotransferase (ALT) two times normal values] in hyperemesis gravidarum, but they are significantly more elevated with hepatitis. Lactate dehydrogenase is normally up to 1.5 times higher during pregnancy as a result of placental production but is significantly elevated in obstructive gallbladder disease (cholelithiasis or cholecystitis). Amylase and lipase are usually normal or minimally elevated in hyperemesis gravidarum but substantially elevated in pancreatitis. Blood urea nitrogen (BUN) is elevated due to dehydration, and creatinine may also be slightly above normal for pregnancy (see Table 2-3 for normal lab values in pregnancy). Thyroid-stimulating hormone may be quite suppressed in hyperemesis gravidarum. Thyrotoxicosis is suggested by an elevated free T_4 and a resin T_3 uptake in the normal range.

Additional diagnostic tests may be indicated, but usually only after expert consultation. These tests may include endoscopy, gallbladder emptying studies, endoscopic retrograde cholangiopancreatography (ERCP), small bowel series, barium enema, computed tomography, magnetic resonance imaging, or colonoscopy.

TREATMENT

This section is limited to the management of nausea and vomiting of pregnancy and hyperemesis gravidarum (Fig. 6-1). Management of specific intraabdominal disease states is covered elsewhere (see Chap. 19). When another etiology for the nausea and vomiting is established, management guidelines should follow a similar pattern as if the patient were not pregnant. In those cases, consultation with the antenatal care provider is recommended to coordinate the patient's care.

NAUSEA AND VOMITING OF PREGNANCY

If the patient appears clinically dehydrated or when ketonuria is present, infusion of 20 mL/kg (usually 1 to 2 L) of D5-lactated Ringers or D5-normal saline should be performed. If laboratory studies are within normal limits, the goal is to correct the dehydration and teach the patient about nausea and vomiting in pregnancy. Counseling may include the following: nausea and vomiting of pregnancy carries minimal fetal risk and is transient in nature; avoid strong odors like cigarette smoke, cooking odors and fumes; helpful dietary advice includes, decreasing the size and increasing the frequency of meals; discontinue prenatal vitamins and iron supplements during this time; avoid mixing solids and liquids; avoid fat-containing foods; maintain oral hydration if possible with electrolyte rich drinks (e.g., Gatorade or bouillon, 2 to 3 oz/h); avoid sweet drinks; start oral intake with soups, followed by complex starches like noodles, pastas, potatoes and rice, and adding chicken or turkey for protein.

The following additional recommendations that have been shown to be safe to treat mild to moderate nausea and vomiting during pregnancy with some established efficacy include: accupressure, for patients with mainly nausea and little vomiting[32] (wrist or "sea bands" are available in boating stores, sutomobile clubs and some drug stores); ginger ale or ginger root containing capsules of 250 mg four times a day[33]; dextrose, levulose, and phosphoric acid (Emetrol), 1 to 2 tablespoons upon awakening and every 3 h thereafter; and, Vitamin B_6, 25 mg three times a day.[34]

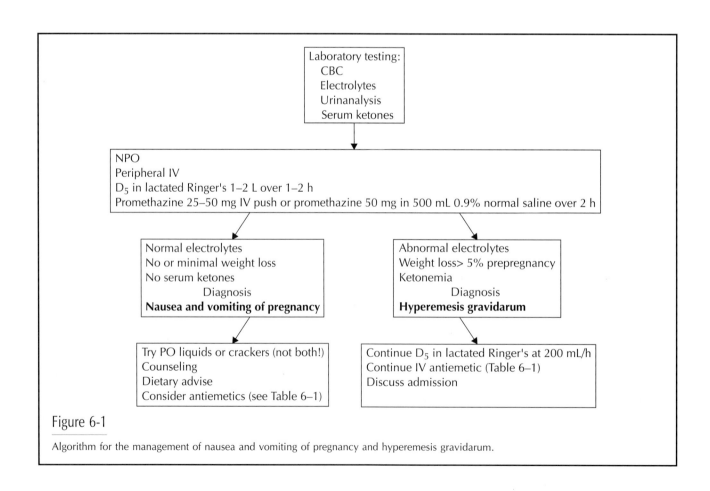

Figure 6-1

Algorithm for the management of nausea and vomiting of pregnancy and hyperemesis gravidarum.

Bendectin® (doxylamine 10 mg, dicyclomine 10 mg and pyridoxine 10 mg) was once the only drug approved by the Food and Drug Administration for the treatment of nausea and vomiting in pregnancy. Unfortunately, it was voluntarily withdrawn from the market in 1983 because of the costs of numerous lawsuits blaming Bendectin as a cause for congenital malformations, including cardiac defects[35] and pyloric stenosis.[36] A causative association has never been established[30,43] and the Center for Disease Control (CDC) eventually concluded that there was no evidence for teratogenicity of Bendectin.[37] Patients may benefit from doxylamine 25 mg at nighttime in combination with pyridoxine (Vitamin B$_6$) 25 mg t.i.d. Doxylamine is sold over the counter as Unisom; however the package insert lists pregnancy as a contraindication.

HYPEREMESIS GRAVIDARUM

When a patient presents to the emergency department with intractable vomiting and weight loss, and laboratory studies reveal hypokalemia or ketonemia, the criteria are met for the diagnosis of hyperemesis gravidarum. Frequently, this will not be the first time the patient has presented with nausea and vomiting. As solid food or liquid usually aggravates the vomiting, the patient should initially take nothing by mouth. Intravenous rehydration is started with 5% dextrose in lactated Ringer's or 5% dextrose in normal saline at 30 to 40 mL/kg. For initial rehydration, 3 to 5 L of crystalloid are commonly necessary. Urine ketones and specific gravity should be followed during rehydration until they improve. Antiemetics are often necessary in this circumstance and should be administered either intravenously or rectally (Table 6-1). Phenothiazines, (Phenergan, Compazine), diphenhydramine (Benadryl), dimenhydrinate (Dramamine), and trimethobenzamide (Tigan) are commonly used in this setting with no apparent risk to the fetus (see below).

Phenothiazines are dopamine receptor antagonists acting in the area postrema and, in addition, have a histamine blocking effect. Benzamides (e.g., Reglan) stimulate motility of the upper intestinal tract without stimulating gastric, biliary, or pancreatic secretions. The antiemetic properties of these drugs may result from their central antidopaminergic effects. Cisapride (Propulsid) is a cholinomimetic that increases gastric contractility. The use of

Table 6-1

ANTIEMETICS

Antiemetic	Brand Name	FDA Category	Oral	Rectal	Intravenous
Acute intervention for both N/V and HG					
Promethazine	Phenergan	C	25 mg q4h	25 mg q4h	25–50 mg IV push
					50 mg in 500 mL 0.9% normal saline over 2 h
Prochlorperazine	Compazine		10 mg q6–8h	25 mg q12h	10 mg over 2 min
					Maximum of 40 mg q24h
Chlorpromazine	Thorazine	C	10–25 mg q4–6h	100 mg q6–8h	25 mg in 500 mL 0.9% normal saline at 250 mL/h
Maintenance therapy for N/V					
Doxylamine with	Unisom		25 mg every evening		
pyridoxine	Vitamin B$_6$		25 mg q8h		
Diphenhydramine	Benadryl	B	25–50 mg q6h		
Cisapride	Propulsid	C	10 mg q6h		
Maintenance therapy for HG					
Metoclopramide	Reglan	B			10 mg over 1–2 min q4–6h or 1 mg/kg in 50 mL D$_5$ in 0.45% normal saline over 30 min
Trimethobenzamide	Tigan	C	250 mg q6–8h	200 mg q6–8h	Should not be given IV
					May be given 200 mg IM q6–8h

N/V=nausea and vomiting of pregnancy; HG=hyperemesis gravidarum.

H2 blockers may also be considered (e.g., ranitidine). Use of a serotonin antagonists (e.g., ondansetron) has been reported in a recent case report,[38] but are prohibitively expensive and are generally not used. Finally, some form of psychotherapeutic counseling has been proven useful in selected cases.[21]

Diphenhydramine (Benadryl), dimenhydrinate (Dramamine), and doxylamine have been studied extensively without evidence of a causative association between the use of these antihistamines and fetal malformations.[24,39] In the Collaborative Perinatal Project 340 patients took trimethobenzamide (Tigan) and no increase in congenital malformations were seen.[40] In 1309 children followed after *in utero* exposure to phenothiazines during the first 16 weeks, no increase in congenital malformations was found.[41] No statistical increase in congenital malformations have been described with promethazine (Phenergan), prochlorperazine (Compazine) or metoclopramide (Reglan).[34] Brompheniramine (Dimetane) should not be used because of potential teratogenicity. Meclizine (Antivert) and cyclizine (Marizene) have also been avoided after reports of teratogenicity, however several studies demonstrated no evidence of teratogenicity in humans.[40,43]

There are circumstances under which outpatient treatment is not advisable, and admission is warranted. Suggested admission guidelines include: uncertain cause of nausea and vomiting; an inability to reverse electrolyte imbalance or ketosis; persistent vomiting in spite of being NPO; and weight loss greater than 10 percent. If the patient requires admission, several steps are useful: continue intravenous infusion using D5/LR at a rate that will maintain adequate hydration (2.5 to 3.5 mL/kg/h); assess and replace electrolytes as necessary; add multivitamins to the intravenous fluids once a day; keep patient NPO; use antiemetics initially around the clock until the patient's symptoms improve; limit physical activity and visitors.

When patients have lost more than 5 to 10 percent of their prepregnancy body weight and oral feeding is not tolerated, placement of a Dobhoff feeding tube should be considered. The successful use of enteral feeding has been reported by several investigators.[44,45] Levine and Esser reported on the use of parenteral nutrition in women with persistent and severe disease.[46] For total parenteral nutrition, central venous access is necessary because the hyperosmolarity of total parenteral nutrition (TPN) requires rapid dilution. This allows the daily delivery of 40 kcal/kg of body weight. Some insurance plans have mandated that some of these women be discharged from the hospital for continued parenteral home care with central lines in place. Therefore, presentation to the emergency department with a number of complications associated with parenteral nutrition and central line problems may be seen. Catheter induced sepsis can be an important source of morbidity in these women. Major mechanical complications include pneumothorax, hematothorax, brachial plexus injury and catheter malpositions. Greenspoon described a maternal death from cardiac tam-

ponade 7 days after successful placement of a subclavian venous catheter for hyperalimentation in a pregnant patient with hyperemesis gravidarum.[47]

Other complications of hyperemesis gravidarum are uncommon but can be severe, including renal and hepatic damage, neurologic syndromes, retinal hemorrhage, hematemesis, and acid aspiration syndrome. Hematemesis, hematochezia, melena, or occult blood in the stool requires further investigation. Causes of significant hematemesis includes gastritis, bleeding ulcers and Mallory-Weiss tear. If persistent or severe, endoscopy is necessary to establish the diagnosis. Acute chest or epigastric pain in the setting of persistent nausea and vomiting may be due to esophageal rupture. Although a rare condition, it is a surgical emergency. Wernicke's encephalopathy due to thiamine deficiency, has been described in association with hyperemesis gravidarum. Once body stores are depleted, Wernicke's encephalopathy can be hastened by ingestion of carbohydrate-rich food or dextrose in intravenous fluids.[48] Therefore, in these rare cases, thiamine must be replaced (1.5 mg/day during pregnancy) and care used in reestablishing the patient's glucose balance.

Readmission for relapse of hyperemesis gravidarum is very common. Godsey and Newman studied 140 women admitted to the Medical University of South Carolina.[49] For 27 percent of these women, multiple admissions were necessary. In women who improve while hospitalized but relapse quickly once discharged, psychiatric consultation is strongly recommended.[21] Psychotherapy, hypnotherapy, and behavior modification have been reported to contribute positively to the management of patients with hyperemesis gravidarum.

References

1. Jarnfelt A, Samsioe G, Velinder GM: Nausea and vomiting in pregnancy: A contribution to its epidemiology. *Gynecol Obstet Invest* 16:221, 1983.
2. Gadsby R, Barnie-Adshead AM, Jagger C: A prospective study of nausea and vomiting during pregnancy. *Br J Gen Pract* 43:245, 1993.
3. Weigel MM, Weigel RM: Nausea and vomiting of early pregnancy and pregnancy outcome: An epidemiological study. *Br J Obstet Gynecol* 96:1304, 1989.
4. Weigel MM, Weigel RM: Nausea and vomiting of early pregnancy and pregnancy outcome: A meta-analytical review. *Br J Obstet Gynecol* 96:1312, 1989.
5. Klebanoff M, Koslowe P, Kaslow R, et al: Epidemiology of vomiting in early pregnancy. *Obstet Gynecol* 66:612, 1985.
6. Depue R, Bernstein L, Ross R, Judd H, Henderson B: Hyperemesis gravidarum in relation to estradiol levels, pregnancy outcome, and other maternal factors: A seroepidemiologic study. *Am J Obstet Gynecol* 156:1137, 1987.

7. O'Brien B, Qiuping Z: Variables related to nausea and vomiting during pregnancy. *Birth* 22(2):93, 1995.

8. Kauppila A, Huhtaniemi I, Ylikorkala O: Raised serum human chorionic gonadotropin concentrations in hyperemesis gravidarum. *Br Med J* 1:1670, 1979.

9. Soules MR, Hughes CL, Garcia JA, et al: Nausea and vomiting in pregnancy: Role of human chorionic gonadotropin and 17-hydroxyprogesterone. *Obstet Gynecol* 55:696, 1980.

10. Swaminathan R, Chin RK, Lao TTH, et al: Thyroid function in hyperemesis gravidarum. *Acta Endocrinol* 120:155, 1989.

11. Goodwin TM, Hersham JM, Cole L: Increased concentration of the free beta subunit of human chorionic gonadotropin in hyperemesis gravidarum. *Acta Obstet Gynecol Scand* 73:770, 1994.

12. Jarnfelt-Samsioe A, Eriksson B, Waldenstrom J, Samsioe G: Some new aspects on hyperemesis gravidarum: Relations to clinical data, serum electrolytes, total protein and creatinine. *Gynecol Obstet Invest* 19:174, 1985.

13. Becks GP, Burrow G: Thyroid disease and pregnancy. *Med Clin North Am* 75:121, 1991.

14. Goodwin TM, Montoro M, Mestman JH: Transient hyperthyroidism and hyperemesis gravidarum: Clinical aspects. *Am J Obstet Gynecol* 167:648, 1992.

15. Kimura M, Amino N, Tamaki H, et al: Gestational thyrotoxicosis and hyperemesis gravidarum: Possible role of hCG with higher stimulating activity. *Clin Endocrinol* 38:345, 1993.

16. Goodwin TM, Montoro M, Mestman JH, et al: The role of chorionic gonadotropin in transient hyperthyroidism of hyperemesis gravidarum. *Endocrinol Metab* 75:1333, 1992.

17. Iatrakis GM, Sakellaropoulos GG, Kourkoubas AH, Kabounia SE: Vomiting and nausea in the first 12 weeks of pregnancy. *Psychother Psychosom* 49:22, 1988.

18. Iancu I, Kottler M, Spivak B, Radwan M: Psychiatric aspects of hyperemesis gravidarum. *Psychother Psychosom* 61:143, 1994.

19. Wolkind S, Zajicek E: Psycho-social correlates of nausea and vomiting in pregnancy. *J Psychosom Res* 22:1, 1978.

20. Fitzgerald C: Nausea and vomiting in pregnancy. *Br J Med Psychol* 57:159, 1984.

21. Deuchar N: Nausea and vomiting in pregnancy: A review of the problem with particular regard to psychosocial and social aspects. *Br J Obstet Gynaecol* 102:6, 1995.

22. Tierson F, Olsen C, Hook EB: Nausea and vomiting of pregnancy and association with pregnancy outcome. *Am J Obstet Gynecol* 155:1017, 1986.

23. Chin RKH: Antenatal complications and perinatal outcome in patients with nausea and vomiting-complicated pregnancy. *Eur J Obstet Gynecol Reprod Biol* 33:215, 1989.

24. Gross S, Librach C, Cecutti A: Maternal weight loss associated with hyperemesis gravidarum: A predictor of fetal outcome. *Am J Obstet Gynecol* 160:906, 1989.

25. Riezzo G, Pezzolla F, Darconza G, Giorgio I: Gastric myoelectrical activity in the first trimester of pregnancy: A cutaneous electrogastrographic study. *Am J Gastroenterol* 87:702, 1992.

26. Koch KL, Stern R, Vasey M, et al: Gastric dysrhythmias and nausea of pregnancy. *Dig Dis Sci* 35:961, 1990.

27. Walsh JW, Hasler WL, Nugent CE, Owyang C: Progesterone and estrogen are potential mediators of gastric slow-wave dysrhythmias in nausea of pregnancy. *Am J Physiol* 270:G506, 1996.

28. Clark DH: Peptic ulcer in women. *Br Med J* 2:1254, 1953.

29. Kurzel RB, Naunheim KS, Schwartz RA: Repair of symptomatic diaphragmatic hernia during pregnancy. *Obstet Gynecol* 71:869, 1988.

30. Mayberry JF, Atkinson M: Achalasia and pregnancy. *Br J Obstet Gynaecol* 94:855, 1987.

31. Fiest TC, Foong A, Chokhavatia S: Successful balloon dilation of achalasia during pregnancy. *Gastrointest Endosc* 39:810, 1993.

32. Belluomini J, Litt RC, Lee KA, Katz M: Acupressure for nausea and vomiting of pregnancy: A randomized blinded study. *Obstet Gynecol* 84:245, 1994.

33. Fischer-Rasmussen W, Kjaer SK, Dahl C, et al: Ginger treatment of hyperemesis gravidarum. *Eur J Obstet Gynecol Reprod Biol* 38:19, 1990.

34. Vutyavanich T, Wongtra-Rjan S, Ruansri R: Pyridoxine for nausea and vomiting of pregnancy: A randomized double blind placebo controlled trial. *Am J Obstet Gynecol* 173:881, 1995.

35. Zierler S, Rothman KJ: Congenital heart disease in relation to maternal use of Bendectin and other drugs in early pregnancy. *N Engl J Med* 313:347, 1985.

36. Eskenazi B, Bracken MB: Bendectin (debendox) as a risk factor for pyloric stenosis. *Am J Obstet Gynecol* 144:919, 1982.

37. Check W: CDC study: No evidence for teratogenicity of Bendectin. *JAMA* 242:2518, 1979.

38. Guikontes E, Spantideas A, Diakakis J: Ondansetron and hyperemesis gravidarum. *Lancet* 340:1223, 1992.

39. Aselton P, Jick H, Milunsky A, et al: First-trimester drug use and congenital disorders. *Obstet Gynecol* 65:451, 1985.

40. Milkovich L, van den Berg BJ: An evaluation of the teratogenicity of certain antinauseant drugs. *Am J Obstet Gynecol* 125:244, 1976.

41. Slone D, Siskind V, Heinonen OP, et al: Antenatal exposure to the phenothiazines in relation to congenital malformations, perinatal mortality rate, birth weight, and intelligence quotient score. *Am J Obstet Gynecol* 128:486, 1977.

42. Kousen M: Treatment of nausea and vomiting in pregnancy. *Am Fam Phys* 48:1279, 1993.

43. Shapiro S, Kaufman DW, Rosenberg L, et al: Meclizine in pregnancy in relation to congenital malformations. *Br Med J* 1:483, 1978.

44. Boyce RA: Enteral nutrition: I. Hyperemesis gravidarum—A new development. *J Am Diet Assoc* 92:733, 1992.

45. Hsu JJ, Clark-Glena R, Nelson DK, Kim CH: Nasogastric enteral feeding in the management of hyperemesis gravidarum. *Obstet Gynecol* 88:343, 1996.

46. Levine MG, Esser D: Total parentenal nutrition for the treatment of severe hyperemesis gravidarum: Marginal nutritional effects and fetal outcome. *Obstet Gynecol* 72:102, 1988.

47. Greenspoon JS, Masaki DI, Uurz CR: Cardiac tamponade in pregnancy during central hyperalimentation. *Obstet Gynecol* 73:465, 1989.

48. Bergin PS, Harvey P: Wernicke's encephalopathy and central pontine myelinolysis associated with hyperemesis gravidarum. *BMJ* 305:517, 1992.

49. Godsey RK, Newman RB: Hyperemesis gravidarum: A comparison of single and multiple admissions. *J Reprod Med* 36:287, 1991.

PROBLEMS OF PREGNANCY IN THE SECOND AND THIRD TRIMESTERS

Chapter 7

PREECLAMPSIA/ ECLAMPSIA

Gary Dildy

The nomenclature system for hypertensive diseases of pregnancy is often confusing. A recent system proposed by the National High Blood Pressure Education Program Working Group[1] is listed in Table 7-1. Preeclampsia is diagnosed when pregnancy-induced hypertension is accompanied by proteinuria or generalized edema. In the United States, preeclampsia complicates approximately 5 to 10 percent of pregnancies[2] and is the second most common cause of maternal mortality in pregnancies beyond 20 weeks.[3] Pathophysiologic changes may adversely affect the maternal cardiovascular, renal, neurologic, hepatic, and hematologic systems.[4] Uteroplacental blood flow may also be affected, resulting in fetal and neonatal complications including death. The presence of a seizure differentiates eclampsia from preeclampsia.

PATHOPHYSIOLOGY OF PREECLAMPSIA

Preeclampsia has been recognized since ancient times; however, the primary inciting factor still remains unknown. A significant amount of clinical and basic science investigation has been undertaken during this century to elucidate the cause of preeclampsia and to improve management, but this problem still remains a considerable contributor to maternal and neonatal morbidity and mortality.

There are numerous theoretical pathophysiologic mechanisms for the development of preeclampsia: an imbalance in prostacyclin and thromboxane, immunologic abnormalities, increased vascular reactivity to vasoactive agents, hyperdynamic increase in cardiac output, abnormal placentation, genetic variations of the angiotensinogen gene, and numerous others have been proposed. However, none are proven and the exact etiology remains unknown.

Risk factors for preeclampsia[5] have been identified (Table 7-2). However, these do not allow accurate prediction of who will develop preeclampsia; therefore, an ideal screening test is not currently available. Risk factors cannot distinguish those who will develop mild disease from those who will develop severe manifestations and multiorgan dysfunction.

From a pathophysiologic standpoint, preeclampsia can be thought of as a process that develops because of generalized systemic vasospasm. Vasospasm leads to tissue ischemia and the various multisystem effects associated with the disease (Table 7-3).

DIAGNOSIS AND DIFFERENTIAL DIAGNOSIS

Specific diagnostic criteria for preeclampsia have been defined by the American College of Obstetricians and Gynecologists based on the triad of hypertension, proteinuria, and edema (Table 7-4).[5] Recognition of the classical triad of signs and varying symptoms is particularly important for health care providers not primarily involved in the management of pregnant patients. Thus it is important to be aware of the pathophysiology and diagnostic criteria of preeclampsia when one is evaluating pregnant women for various apparently unrelated problems.

Preeclampsia is defined as either mild or severe. Mild preeclampsia is characterized by a systolic blood pressure of at least 140 mmHg or a diastolic blood pressure of at least

Table 7-1

CLASSIFICATION OF HYPERTENSION DURING PREGNANCY

Chronic hypertension: Hypertension (BP ≥ 140/90 mmHg) that is present and observable before pregnancy or that is diagnosed before the 20th week of gestation. Hypertension diagnosed for the first time during pregnancy and persisting beyond the 42nd day postpartum.

Preeclampsia-eclampsia: Increased blood pressure accompanied by proteinuria, edema, or both usually occurring after 20 weeks of gestation (or earlier with trophoblastic diseases such as hydatidiform mole or hydrops).

Preeclampsia superimposed on chronic hypertension: Chronic hypertension (defined above) with increases in blood pressure (30 mmHg systolic, 15 mmHg diastolic, or 20 mmHg mean arterial pressure) together with the appearance of proteinuria or generalized edema.

Transient hypertension: The development of elevated BP during pregnancy or in the first 24 h postpartum without other signs of preeclampsia or preexisting hypertension (a retrospective diagnosis).

Source: National High Blood Pressure Education Program Working Group: Report on high blood pressure in pregnancy. *Am J Obstet Gynecol* 163:1689, 1990.

Table 7-2

RISK FACTORS FOR THE DEVELOPMENT OF PREGNANCY-INDUCED HYPERTENSION

Risk Factor	Risk Ratio
Nulliparity	3:1
Age > 40	3:1
African American race	1.5:1
Family history of pregnancy-induced hypertension	5:1
Chronic hypertension	10:1
Chronic renal disease	20:1
Antiphospholipid syndrome	10:1
Diabetes mellitus	2:1
Twin gestation	4:1
Angiotensinogen gene T235	
Homozygous	20:1
Heterozygous	4:1

Source: Adapted from American College of Obstetricians and Gynecologists: *Hypertension in Pregnancy.* ACOG Technical Bulletin 219. Washington DC: ACOG, 1996.

Table 7-3

COMPLICATIONS OF SEVERE PREGNANCY-INDUCED HYPERTENSION

Cardiovascular	Severe hypertension, pulmonary edema
Renal	Oliguria, renal failure
Hematologic	Hemolysis, thrombocytopenia, disseminated intravascular coagulation
Neurologic	Eclampsia, cerebral edema, cerebral hemorrhage, amaurosis
Hepatic	Hepatocellular dysfunction, hepatic rupture
Uteroplacental	Abruption, intrauterine growth retardation, fetal distress, fetal death

Source: Dildy GA, Cotton DB: Hypertensive disease in pregnancy, in Clark SL, Cotton DB, Hankins GDV, Phelan JP (eds): *Critical Care Obstetrics,* 3d ed. Boston: Blackwell, in press.

90 mmHg obtained on two separate occasions at least 6 hours apart. Some clinicians use a relative rise of systolic and diastolic blood pressure of 30/15 mmHg, respectively, over prepregnancy or first-trimester levels; however, these criteria appear to be less accurate. Hypertension must be associated with either proteinuria or edema to be termed preeclampsia.

Significant proteinuria is defined as at least 300 mg of protein in a 24-hour urine collection or at least 1 g/L con-

Table 7-4

DIAGNOSIS OF PREECLAMPSIA

Elevated blood pressure
  Sustained systolic blood pressure ≥ 140 mmHg or diastolic blood pressure ≥ 90 mmHg measured on two separate occasions ≥ 6 h apart

and

Significant proteinuria
  300 mg/24h or ≥ 1 g/mL measured on two separate occasions 6 h apart

or

Edema
  Generalized edema or weight gain of at least 5 lb in 1 week

Source: Adapted from American College of Obstetricians and Gynecologists: *Hypertension in Pregnancy.* ACOG Technical Bulletin 219. Washington DC: ACOG, 1996.

Table 7-5

DIAGNOSTIC CRITERIA FOR SEVERE PREECLAMPSIA[a]

Blood pressure >160–180 mmHg systolic or >110 mmHg diastolic

Proteinuria >5 g/24 h

Oliguria defined as <500 mL/24 h

Cerebral or visual disturbances

Pulmonary edema

Epigastric or right-upper-quadrant pain

Impaired liver function of unclear etiology

Thrombocytopenia

Fetal intrauterine growth retardation or oligohydramnios

Elevated serum creatinine

Grand mal seizures (eclampsia)

[a]Only one condition need be present.
Source: Adapted from American College of Obstetricians and Gynecologists: *Hypertension in Pregnancy.* ACOG Technical Bulletin 219. Washington DC: ACOG, 1996.

Table 7-6

DIFFERENTIAL DIAGNOSES OF HELLP SYNDROME

Autoimmune thrombocytopenic purpura
Chronic renal disease
Pyelonephritis
Cholecystitis
Gastroenteritis
Hepatitis
Pancreatitis
Thrombotic thrombocytopenic purpura
Hemolytic-uremic syndrome
Acute fatty liver of pregnancy

Abbreviation: HELLP = hemolysis, elevated liver enzymes, and low platelets.

centration on two random urine specimens collected 6 hour apart. While "1+ or 2+" proteinuria is frequently considered significant, the semiquantitative dipstick analysis of urine protein is poorly correlated with the actual degree of proteinurias. Classification of preeclampsia is ideally based upon a 24-hour quantitative collection of urine for protein.

The diagnosis of *edema* may be somewhat difficult, as many normal pregnant women will experience some degree of lower extremity edema. Edema must be generalized or a weight gain of at least 5 lb in 1 week should be confirmed.

Preeclampsia almost always occurs after 20 weeks of gestation. An exception to this is the uncommon clinical circumstance of gestational trophoplastic disease (molar pregnancy) (see Chap. 3). Severe preeclampsia is defined as existing when *any* of the manifestations listed in Table 7-5 are identified in the preeclamptic patient.

HELLP SYNDROME

A diagnosis of severe preeclampsia is usually straightforward following careful observation and monitoring of a woman who develops complaints of severe headache, scotomata, swelling, or upper abdominal pain. However, an unusual manifestation of severe preeclampsia is the development of HELLP syndrome (an acronym standing for hemolysis, elevated liver enzymes, and low platelets). HELLP syndrome is a variant of severe preeclampsia, affecting up to 12 percent of women with preeclampsia-eclampsia syndrome. Whereas preeclampsia is usually a disease of primigravidas, HELLP

syndrome has a predilection for the multigravida population. HELLP syndrome may imitate a variety of nonobstetric medical problems (Table 7-6); serious medical and surgical pathology may be misdiagnosed as preeclampsia or HELLP syndrome, or vice versa.[7,8] In addition to varying degrees of hypertension (although not always severe and sometimes not initially evident), the woman with HELLP syndrome usually presents with a complaint of epigastric or right-upper-quadrant pain. Thrombocytopenia is defined as a platelet count less than 100,000/mm^3, but a count of less than 150,000/mm^3 would be suspicious, particularly in the face of hypertension and elevated liver enzymes. Hepatic transaminase levels (AST and ALT) are not elevated during normal pregnancy and may become elevated in association with worsening preeclampsia (with or without HELLP syndrome) but not usually to the levels seen in acute viral hepatitis (i.e., in HELLP, AST and ALT are usually <500 IU/L). Hemolysis is manifest by microscopic observations consistent with microangiopathic hemolytic anemia on the peripheral blood smear (e.g., the presence of schistocytes). Hemolysis is not usually associated with anemia, since plasma volume is often decreased to a more significant degree than is loss of red cell volume in preeclamptic patients. Thus, the hematocrit may actually increase in the face of red cell destruction.

EVALUATION AND TREATMENT OF PREECLAMPSIA

Initial evaluation of the woman who presents with suspected preeclampsia includes several simultaneously initiated steps.[9] Maternal vital signs are monitored initially every 15

Table 7-7

LABORATORY EVALUATION FOR PREECLAMPSIA

Complete blood count with peripheral blood smear
Platelet count
Liver function tests (AST, ALT)
Renal function tests (creatinine, BUN)
Blood type and antibody screen
Urinalysis and microscopy
24-h urine collection for protein and creatinine clearance

Abbreviations: AST and ALT = hepatic transaminase levels; BUN = blood urea nitrogen.

---

to 30 min. The woman is placed in the left lateral recumbent position so that the gravid uterus does not produce aortocaval compression. A clean-catch specimen of urine is obtained for semiquantitative analysis of protein concentration. Initial blood laboratory evaluation should be done as summarized in Table 7-7. If delivery is not felt to be imminent, a 24-hour urine collection should be initiated for volume, creatinine clearance, and total protein excretion.

If the fetus is previable (for example, less than 24 weeks of gestation), the fetal heart rate should be monitored intermittently and recorded. If the fetus is of a viable estimated gestational age (>24 to 26 weeks), then fetal biophysical assessment should be performed by way of a non-stress test or biophysical profile (Table 7-8). An eval-

---

Table 7-8

TESTS OF FETAL CONDITION

Non-stress test (NST): The pattern of the fetal heart rate is evaluated by external electronic fetal monitoring.
Oxytocin challenge test (OCT): The pattern of the fetal heart rate is evaluated by external electronic fetal monitoring after uterine contractions are elicited by intravenous oxytocin infusion.
Biophysical profile (BPP): The fetal condition is assessed by real-time ultrasound monitoring of fetal tone, movement, breathing motions, and amniotic fluid volume.
Ultrasound (US): Fetal number, fetal anatomy, fetal measurements, placental location, amniotic fluid volume, and other parameters are determined by real-time US.
Amniocentesis: A sample of amniotic fluid is aspirated transabdominally under US guidance for evaluation of fetal lung maturity.

---

uation of fetal condition is indicated because uteroplacental blood flow may be compromised in the preeclamptic woman, potentially producing varying degrees of fetal compromise. Initially, fetal growth may diminish as a result of chronic impairment of placental exchange. Intrauterine growth retardation (fetal weight <10th percentile) and oligohydramnios (decreased amniotic fluid volume) may follow. Chronic severe reduction in oxygenation, uterine contractions that further decrease placental perfusion, or umbilical cord compression resulting from oligohydramnios may further compromise the fetus, leading to asphyxia or death. These fetal complications occur more frequently in pregnancies complicated by hypertension than in normotensive pregnancies.

INDICATIONS FOR DELIVERY

Accurate dating of the pregnancy is of paramount importance because the ultimate management decisions for the preeclamptic woman will be based primarily upon fetal maturity (gestational age), maternal well-being (mild versus severe preeclampsia), and fetal well-being (e.g., biophysical testing). Dating of the pregnancy is performed by calculating the estimated date of confinement and the estimated gestational age from the last normal menstrual period. It is important to obtain any previous data that would substantiate gestational age, such as the date of the first positive pregnancy test, first auscultation of fetal heart tones (at 10 weeks by Doppler or 19 weeks by fetoscope), and particularly early obstetric ultrasound biometric data. The non-stress test remains the standard test of fetal well-being but may not be reassuring (reactive) at very early gestational ages—for example, before 28 weeks of gestation. Thus, the biophysical profile may be performed by trained personnel using real-time ultrasound to determine fetal condition. Amniocentesis for a fetal lung-maturity profile may be helpful in cases where fetal pulmonary maturity is in question but the disease process is not severe enough to warrant delivery.

Delivery of the fetus in the preeclamptic patient is dependent upon several maternal and fetal factors. Delivery generally benefits the preeclamptic woman but may result in serious neonatal problems in the preterm gestation. Table 7-9 outlines, in simplified form, the steps in arriving at a decision regarding delivery. It should be noted that exceptions to these broad recommendations may exist; variations in management may be considered in the face of severe preeclampsia at very early gestational ages in tertiary care centers.[10] Certainly when issues of delivery are at hand, involvement of an obstetrician or a perinatologist is indicated.

Two acute emergencies that may be encountered in the emergency department are severe hypertension and eclamptic seizures.

Table 7-9

MANAGEMENT OF PREECLAMPSIA

	Previable Fetus, <23–24 Weeks	Viable Premature Fetus, 24–34 Weeks	Viable Preterm Fetus, 34–37 Weeks	Viable Term Fetus, >37 Weeks
Mild preeclampsia	Consider delivery	Expectant management	Expectant management[a]	Deliver[b]
Severe preeclampsia	Deliver	Deliver[c]	Deliver	Deliver

[a]Assessment of lung maturity by amniocentesis may be of benefit.
[b]May be observed under certain circumstances (e.g., unfavorable cervix).
[c]Expectant management in a tertiary care center may be reasonable in select cases.

MANAGEMENT OF HYPERTENSION

The treatment of severe hypertension is generally necessary when the diastolic blood pressure exceeds 110 mmHg or if the systolic blood pressure is sustained at a level greater than 160 to 180 mmHg. Mild or moderate degrees of blood pressure elevation are generally not treated because of concern for obscuring worsening disease—an important determinant in management decisions such as need for delivery. In addition, treatment of mild to moderate pregnancy-induced hypertension does not necessarily improve outcome for either mother or baby.

However, when severe hypertension does develop, the risk of maternal intracranial bleeding and placental abruption increases. Although many antihypertensive agents are available, obstetricians have met with great success using hydralazine for primary treatment of severe hypertension during pregnancy. Recognizing that the severely hypertensive preeclamptic woman may be significantly hypovolemic, an intravenous line should be established prior to administering antihypertensive agents. Maternal volume is frequently expanded with 500 to 1000 mL of intravenous fluids before antihypertensive therapy is initiated. Hydralazine is usually administered intravenously, with an initial dose of 2.5 mg. The patient should be observed for 20 min, the usual time to onset of action of this agent. If the blood pressure is not corrected to the desired range (systolic of 130 to 150 mmHg and diastolic of 90 to 105 mmHg), then additional 5- to 10-mg boluses of hydralazine may be administered every 20 min up to a total dose of 40 mg. If hydralazine at this cumulative dosage is not efficacious, then a second agent such as labetalol should be considered (Table 7-10). Care should be taken not to create hypotension or sudden drops in BP, since fetal compromise may result. The use of continuous electronic fetal monitoring can help to detect adverse effects of BP treatment on the fetus. Angiotensin-converting enzyme (ACE) inhibitors should not be used during pregnancy because of potential fetal side effects (anuria or renal failure).

SEIZURE PROPHYLAXIS

If severe preeclampsia is suspected during initial evaluation, magnesium sulfate therapy should be initiated to prevent the development of eclamptic seizures.[11–14] Several different regimens of magnesium sulfate ($MgSO_4$) therapy have been recommended (Table 7-11). We would favor an initial loading dose of 6 g intravenously over 15 min, followed by a maintenance dose of 2 g/h intravenously. Maternal deep tendon reflexes, respiratory rate, and urine output should be monitored to prevent magnesium toxicity. Once a decision to deliver has been made, $MgSO_4$ is administered, whether the disease is mild or severe, for the purpose of seizure prophylaxis.

Normal pretreatment serum magnesium levels during pregnancy range from 1.5 to 2.0 meq/L. The desired therapeutic range is 4 to 7 meq/L. When serum magnesium levels exceed therapeutic ranges, toxicity may develop. Loss of deep tendon reflexes (8 to 10 meq/L) precedes respiratory arrest (13 meq/L), and cardiac arrest may follow. With mild magnesium toxicity, the magnesium infusion is simply discontinued. More significant toxicity resulting in respiratory depression is treated by administration of 1 g of calcium gluconate (10 mL of a 10% solution) intravenously over 2 min. Respiratory support, oxygen saturation monitoring, and electrocardiographic (ECG) monitoring are indicated. Magnesium excretion may be enhanced by loop or osmotic diuretics and impaired in renal insufficiency, commonly present in preeclamptic women.

Table 7-10

PHARMACOLOGIC AGENTS FOR ANTIHYPERTENSIVE THERAPY IN PREECLAMPSIA-ECLAMPSIA

Agent Generic	Trade	Mechanism of Action	Dosage	Comment
Hydralazine hydrochloride	Apresoline	Arterial vasodilator	2.5 mg IV, then 5–10 mg IV/ 20 min, up to total dose of 40 mg; IV infusion of 5–10 mg/h, titrated	Must wait 20 min for response between intravenous doses; possible maternal hypotension
Labetalol	Normodyne Trandate	Selective alpha and nonselective beta antagonist	20 mg IV, then 40–80 mg IV/10 min, to 300 mg total dose; IV infusion 1–2 mg/min, titrated	Less reflex tachycardia and hypotension than with hydralazine
Nitroglycerin	Nitrostat IV Tridil Nitro-Bid IV	Relaxation of venous (and arterial) vascular smooth muscle	$5\mu g$/min infusion; double every 5 min	Requires arterial line for continuous blood pressure monitoring; potential methemoglobinemia
Sodium nitroprusside	Nipride Nitropress	Vasodilator	0.25 μg/kg per min infusion; increase 0.25 μg/kg/min every 5 min	Potential cyanide toxicity

Source: Modified from Dildy GA, Cotton DB: Hemodynamic changes in pregnancy and pregnancy complicated by hypertension. *Acute Care* 14–15:26, 1988–1989.

Table 7-11

MAGNESIUM SULFATE (MgSO₄) PROTOCOLS

Investigator	Loading Dose	Maintenance Dose
Sibai, 1990[14]		
Preeclampsia-eclampsia	6 g IV[a] over 15 min	2 g/h
Pritchard[17]		
Preeclampsia	10 g IM[b]	5 g IM[b] q4h
Eclampsia	4 g IV[c] and 10 g IM[b]	5 g IM[b] q4h
Zuspan, 1966[18]		
Severe preeclampsia	None	1 g/h IV
Eclampsia	4–6 g IV over 5–10 min	1 g/h IV

[a]50% solution MgSO₄ diluted in D₅W.
[b]50% solution MgSO₄.
[c]20% solution MgSO₄.

TREATMENT OF ECLAMPTIC SEIZURES

Eclamptic seizures are defined if they occur from the 20th week of gestation to 7 days after delivery, although they have been reported as late as 26 days after delivery. A pregnant or postpartum woman who develops new-onset seizures should be assumed to be eclamptic until proven otherwise. While most eclamptic women also demonstrate hypertension, proteinuria, and edema, up to 30 percent will not. The pathophysiology of the syndrome is poorly understood, and the occurrence of seizures does not necessarily correlate with the severity of other signs. Sibai[14] has reported that in preeclamptics, the incidence of seizures is 1 out of 300.

Eclamptic seizures may be preceded by headache, blurred vision, or decreased visual acuity. Eclamptic seizures may be focal or generalized tonic-clonic seizures.[15] The typical pattern is a single seizure lasting <1 min which responds to intravenous magnesium sulfate (MgSO₄) administration.[16]

The management of eclampsia includes treatment of seizures, hypertension and its complications, and expeditious delivery of the fetus. Emergency obstetrical consultation should be obtained, and transfer to a center with resources for critical obstetrical care will be necessary after maternal stabilization, if that is not available locally.

The initial management of eclamptic seizures is to insure adequate maternal ventilation and oxygenation. Continuous pulse oximetry should be begun and supplemental oxygen administered to maintain the maternal oxygen saturation above 90%, and if undelivered, above 95% if possible. A secure intravenous line should be established, and 6 g magnesium sulfate should be given IV over 15 min, with monitoring of maternal blood pressure, respirations, and pulse rate every 5 min during this infusion. Other MgSO$_4$ regimens have been used (Table 7-11). An indwelling urinary catheter should be placed to carefully monitor urine output. This should be followed by a maintenance infusion of magnesium sulfate of 2 g/h. Most women should respond to this regimen; but if there is continued seizure activity, another 2 g magnesium sulfate should be given intravenously over 15 min. In Pritchard's series at Parkland Memorial Hospital, 88 percent of women had no further seizures after initial treatment of 4 g intravenous magnesium sulfate, and the seizures of an additional 7 percent were controlled with another 2 g given intravenously. Serum magnesium levels should be monitored, but since values are unlikely to be available within minutes, the patient must be monitored closely for clinical evidence of magnesium toxicity, with frequent blood pressures, evaluation of respiratory rate and deep tendon reflexes. Signs and symptoms of magnesium toxicity include slurred speech, muscle weakness and areflexia, hypotension, and respiratory and cardiac depression. Endotracheal intubation and ventilation are necessary for respiratory depression which impairs adequate oxygenation that cannot be otherwise maintained with supplemental oxygen, and 10 mL of 10% calcium gluconate or calcium chloride should be administered intravenously over 5 min. Calcium competitively inhibits the effect of magnesium, and its effect may be transient, so that measures to increase magnesium excretion must be simultaneously begun. Continuous electrocardiographic monitoring is necessary in this setting.

Fetal monitoring should be established as soon as possible, as fetal bradycardia is a common complication of maternal seizures. Once maternal seizures are stopped, and if maternal oxygenation and circulation are maintained, fetal heart rate should return to normal, and plans for expeditious delivery can be made in consultation with an obstetrician.

Reoccurrence of seizures or status epilepticus after the administration of intravenous magnesium sulfate is uncommon, but it poses grave risks to both mother and fetus. Hypertension must be controlled with an intravenous agent such as hydralazine, nitroprusside, or labetalol. Continued seizure activity raises the possibility of intracranial pathology, such as cerebral hemorrhage. Further treatment of acute seizures should proceed as for any adult (see Chap.

25). If it is felt that the magnesium level is therapeutic (serum levels 5 to 7 meq/L), lorazepam, 1–2 mg intravenously, and phenytoin or phosphenytoin, 20 mg/kg phenytoin equivalent intravenously at 50 to 150 mg/min, respectively, should be given.

Lorazepam and other benzodiazepines can result in neonatal respiratory depression. The use of magnesium sulfate as a standard first-line agent for treatment of eclamptic seizures is nearly universally accepted in obstetrics. Some have argued for the use of phenytoin as a first line agent for eclamptic seizures, recent studies evaluating the efficacy of MgSO$_4$ for seizure prophylaxis or eclamptic demonstrate that MgSO$_4$ is the agent of choice.[12,13]

Significant hemodynamic perturbations are observed in preeclamptic women (Table 7-12). Clinical conditions that may merit central hemodynamic monitoring include complications related to central volume status (pulmonary edema of uncertain etiology, pulmonary edema unresponsive to conventional therapy, and persistent oliguria despite appropriate volume expansion), induction of conduction anesthesia in hemodynamically unstable patients, and medical conditions that would otherwise require invasive monitoring.

OBSTETRIC/GYNECOLOGIC OR MATERNAL FETAL MEDICINE CONSULTATION

Any pregnant woman with signs or symptoms consistent with preeclampsia, whether mild or severe, should have a consultation with an obstetrician or perinatologist. This is especially important for women who present with atypical signs and symptoms of medical or surgical disorders which might be confused with the HELLP syndrome (e.g., upper abdominal pains, unexplained thrombocytopenia, or unexplained elevation of liver enzymes). Another primary reason for obstetric consultation is the ordering and interpretation of tests of fetal well-being, such as the nonstress test and biophysical profile in the preeclamptic woman.

Three possible dispositions can be made for the woman with suspected or diagnosed preeclampsia: (1) discharge home, (2) admission to the hospital for observation, and (3) admission to the hospital for delivery. For the preterm woman who is diagnosed with mild preeclampsia, it may be reasonable, after a period of hospital observation, to discharge her home to bed rest after arranging follow-up evaluation. Consultation with an obstetrician is prudent prior to discharge. If there is any question regarding the degree of severity of preeclampsia based on the presenting symptoms or laboratory evaluations or any concerns regarding fetal well-being, admission to the hospital is warranted so that careful observation over a longer period of time may be performed. As

Table 7-12

HEMODYNAMIC PROFILES OF NONPREGNANT WOMEN, NORMAL WOMEN DURING THE LATE THIRD TRIMESTER, AND SEVERE PREECLAMPTICS

Parameter	Normal Nonpregnant ($n = 10$),[a] Mean ± SD	Normal Late 3d Trimester ($n = 10$),[a] Mean ± SD	Severe Preeclampsia ($n = 45$),[b] Mean ± SEM
Heart rate (beats/min)	71 ± 10	83 ± 10	95 ± 10
Mean arterial BP (mmHg)	86.4 ± 7.5	90.3 ± 5.8	138 ± 3
Central venous pressure (mmHg)	3.7 ± 2.6	3.6 ± 2.5	4 ± 1
Pulmonary capillary wedge pressure (mmHg)	6.3 ± 2.1	7.5 ± 1.8	10 ± 1
Cardiac output (L/min)	4.3 ± 0.9	6.2 ± 1.0	7.5 ± 0.2
Systemic vascular resistance (dynes·s·cm^{-5})	1530 ± 520	1210 ± 266	1496 ± 64
Pulmonary vascular resistance (dynes·s·cm^{-5})	119 ± 47	78 ± 22	70 ± 5
Serum colloid osmotic pressure (mmHg)	20.8 ± 1.0	18.0 ± 1.5	19.0 ± 0.5
Left ventricular stroke work index (g·m·M^{-2})	41 ± 8	48 ± 6	81 ± 2

Sources: [a]Clark SL et al: Central hemodynamic assessment of normal term pregnancy. *Am J Obstet Gynecol* 161:1439, 1989.
[b]Cotton DB et al: Hemodynamic profile of severe pregnancy-induced hypertension. *Am J Obstet Gynecol* 158:523, 1988.

previously noted, the decision for delivery will be dependent upon multiple factors, including the fetal gestational age, fetal maturity, and fetal and maternal well-being.

DISCHARGE INSTRUCTIONS AND FOLLOW-UP

When the woman with suspected preeclampsia is discharged from the hospital, she should be instructed to remain at bed rest and to contact her physician for the development of headaches, scintillating scotomata or other visual changes, abdominal pain, vaginal bleeding, or decreased fetal movement. Follow-up should be arranged with the prenatal care provider within 7 days or less.

If the preeclamptic woman presents to a nontertiary care facility, transport to a tertiary care hospital with perinatology and neonatology services is indicated in certain clinical situations. Considering the complex clinical factors, consultation with a perinatologist should be attempted. In general, the patient is transferred when the fetus is viable but preterm and may need delivery (e.g., severe preeclampsia). Transport is sometimes contraindicated during acute emergencies when maternal problems (severe uncontrolled hypertension, uncontrolled eclamptic seizures, severe hemorrhage) or fetal problems (impending delivery, significant fetal compromise) require immediate stabilization. Although maternal transport is generally preferable, in some cases delivery followed by neonatal transport may be in the patient's best interest.

SUMMARY

As with all complications of pregnancy, the physician is faced with the care of two patients, mother and fetus, whose interests are sometimes conflicting. Preeclampsia is a very common complication of pregnancy and is one of the leading causes of maternal and fetal morbidity and mortality in the United States. Preeclampsia may often be confused with other medical and surgical conditions, especially when HELLP syndrome develops. The emergency department physician may be the first to evaluate the pregnant woman presenting with these complications and should recognize the various signs and symptoms of both common and atypical forms of preeclampsia. In all cases where preeclampsia is diagnosed or suspected, the prenatal care provider should be involved with the patient's medical care if possible.

References

1. National High Blood Pressure Education Program Working Group: Report on high blood pressure in pregnancy. *Am J Obstet Gynecol* 163:1689, 1990.

2. Cunningham FG, MacDonald PC, Gant NF, et al: *Williams Obstetrics,* 19th ed. Norwalk, CT: Appleton-Century-Crofts, 1993.

3. Kaunitz AM, Hughes JM, Grimes DA, et al: Causes of maternal mortality in the United States. *Obstet Gynecol* 65:605, 1985.

4. Dildy GA, Cotton DB: Hemodynamic changes in pregnancy and pregnancy complicated by hypertension. *Acute Care* 14–15:26, 1988–1989.

5. American College of Obstetricians and Gynecologists: *Hypertension in Pregnancy.* ACOG Technical Bulletin 219. Washington DC: ACOG, 1996.

6. Dildy GA, Cotton DB. Hypertensive disease in pregnancy, in Clark SL, Cotton DB, Hankins GDV, Phelan JP (eds): *Critical Care Obstetrics,* 3d ed. Boston: Blackwell, in press.

7. Goodlin RC: Preeclampsia as the great imposter. *Am J Obstet Gynecol* 164:1577, 1991.

8. Sibai BM: Pitfalls in diagnosis and management of preeclampsia. *Am J Obstet Gynecol* 159:1, 1988.

9. Dildy GA, Cotton DB: Management of severe preeclampsia and eclampsia. *Crit Care Clin* 7:829, 1991.

10. Sibai BM, Mercer BM, Schiff E, Friedman SA: Aggressive versus expectant management of severe preeclampsia at 28 to 32 weeks gestation: A randomized controlled trial. *Am J Obstet Gynecol* 171:818, 1994.

11. Pritchard JA, Cunningham FG, Pritchard SA: The Parkland Memorial Hospital protocol for the treatment of eclampsia: Evaluation of 245 cases. *Am J Obstet Gynecol* 148:951, 1984.

12. The Eclampsia Trial Collaborative Group: Which anticonvulsant for women with eclampsia? Evidence from the Collaborative Eclampsia Trial. *Lancet* 345:1455, 1995.

13. Lucas MJ, Leveno KJ, Cunningham FG: A comparison of magnesium sulfate with phenytoin for the prevention of eclampsia. *N Engl J Med* 333:201, 1995.

14. Sibai BM: Magnesium sulfate is the ideal anticonvulsant in preeclampsia-eclampsia. *Am J Obstet Gynecol* 162:1141, 1990.

15. Kaplan, PW, Rjepke JT: Eclampsia. *Neurol Clin North Am* 12:565, 1994.

16. Usta IM, Sibai BM: Emergent management of puerperal eclampsia. *Obstet Gynecol Clin North Am* 22:315, 1995.

17. Pritchard JA, Pritchard SA: Standardized treatment of 154 consecutive cases of eclampsia. *Am J Obstet Gynecol* 123:543, 1975.

18. Zuspan FP: Treatment of severe preeclampsia and eclampsia. *Clin Obstet Gynecol* 9:945, 1966.

19. Cotton DB, Lee W, Huhta JC, Dorman KF: Hemodynamic profile of severe pregnancy-induced hypertension. *Am J Obstet Gynecol* 158:523, 1988.

20. Clark SL, Cotton DB, Lee W, et al: Central hemodynamic assessment of normal term pregnancy. *Am J Obstet Gynecol* 161:1439, 1989.

Chapter 8

TRAUMA IN PREGNANCY

Mark D. Pearlman

Some 6 to 7 percent of pregnant women will suffer some degree of physical trauma during their pregnancy.[1] Because most physical trauma suffered during pregnancy will be relatively minor, many of these women will not present for medical care. A critical factor is that the severity of the trauma does not always accurately predict adverse fetal outcome.[2] Recognizing this, a general recommendation should be made that women who suffer any degree of truncal trauma during pregnancy should be evaluated. This is particularly true once fetal viability has been established (i.e., >24 weeks of gestation). Case series of trauma during pregnancy and subsequent fetal loss bear this out, as 60 to 80 percent of all fetal losses result from relatively minor maternal trauma.[2–5]

Penetrating abdominal trauma during pregnancy is particularly problematic for the fetus, because it typically absorbs the brunt of penetrating energy forces, particularly in the latter half of gestation. Management algorithms for penetrating trauma during pregnancy are dependent on gestational age, the penetrating object, the depth of penetration, and the maternal physical examination. Though the basic approach to the management of the gravida following trauma is largely unchanged by the pregnancy, the fetus must be considered early.

ANATOMIC AND PHYSIOLOGIC CHANGES OF PREGNANCY

While prior chapters have addressed both the anatomic and physiologic changes of pregnancy, those that affect the management of trauma in pregnancy are reviewed here.

CARDIOVASCULAR CHANGES

In order to compensate for the metabolic needs of the growing conceptus, fundamental changes in cardiovascular status occur during pregnancy. Changes in blood pressure, heart rate, and blood volume composition have a significant impact on the evaluation of the multiply injured trauma patient. *Blood pressure typically decreases* on the order of 10 to 15 mmHg systolic and 5 to 10 mmHg diastolic during the midtrimester of pregnancy. This is largely due to a decrease in systemic vascular resistance, allowing increased blood flow to the uterus. Systolic blood pressures in the range of 80 to 90 mmHg are not uncommon in the healthy young pregnant woman and should not be mistaken for an indicator of maternal hypovolemia. This is particularly important when one considers that *heart rate increases by 10 to 15 beats per minute* during pregnancy. Again, the increased heart rate is a result of the need to adequately perfuse the uterus, allowing sufficient oxygen and nutrient delivery to the fetus. *The uterine blood flow increases* from 60 mL/min in the nonpregnant state to over 600 mL/min in the last third of gestation. The distribution of cardiac output to the uterus increases from 2 percent prior to pregnancy to 17 percent during pregnancy. This remarkable volume of blood flow is an important consideration if penetrating trauma transects the uterine vasculature or severe blunt abdominal trauma results in uterine vascular avulsion, because rapid exsanguination may result.

The composition of blood during pregnancy changes dramatically, reaching its maximum volume change at 28 weeks of gestation. It is typical for blood volume to increase by 45 percent overall during pregnancy—even more in twins and higher multiple gestations. Plasma volume increases more than does red blood cell (RBC) mass, resulting in a physiologic decrease in hematocrit during pregnancy. It is not uncommon for the normal hematocrit to vary between 33 to 36 percent during pregnancy.

Taken together, the finding of a relatively low blood pressure, increased heart rate, and low hematocrit in the multiply injured trauma patient would understandably raise concern about potential hypovolemia. When the trauma victim is pregnant, interpretation of these findings must be made within the context of the normal physiologic changes outlined above. Probably the most critical anatomic change during pregnancy that can affect resuscitation of the injured trauma victim is the potential for *supine hypotension.* Beyond 24 weeks of gestation, when the pregnant woman is lying supine, the gravid uterus can compress the inferior vena cava and aorta, impeding the return of blood from the lower extremities and pelvis to the central circulation. Because this is a very common position in which to evaluate and manage trauma victims (e.g., strapped to a long board), it is imperative to avoid this position. In the healthy pregnant woman, cardiac output can decrease as much as 30 percent due to a decrease in venous return. In addition, compression of the aorta may further compromise blood flow to the uterus, potentially exacerbating fetal hypoxia. *No woman beyond 24 weeks of gestation should lie supine. Either the lateral decubitus position or manual displacement of the uterus should be performed* (outlined under "General Principles of Trauma Management," below).

GASTROINTESTINAL CHANGES

Gastric and intestinal motility decrease during pregnancy, presumably as a result of elevated progesterone levels (progesterone is a smooth muscle relaxant). These changes in motility result in an *increased gastric emptying time.* As a result, the pregnant trauma victim with head injury and decreased sensorium is at significant risk for aspiration of gastric contents. Clinically, it is best to assume that the injured pregnant woman's stomach is full.

Progressive cephalad and lateral displacement of the small and large bowel result from the enlarging gravid uterus. Therefore, penetrating trauma to the lower abdomen is less likely to result in penetrating intestinal injury during pregnancy. However, an object penetrating in the most superior or lateral aspect of the abdomen may produce complex intestinal injuries during pregnancy with multiple entry and exit wounds to the bowel. Finally, because of the progressive distention and attenuation of the anterior abdominal wall and separation of the rectus muscles that commonly occurs during pregnancy (*distasis recti*), the physical response to intraperitoneal irritation may be altered. For example, rebound tenderness and involuntary guarding may be much less appreciated on physical examination even in the presence of significant intraperitoneal injury (e.g., hemoperitoneum, ruptured viscus).

PULMONARY CHANGES

While tidal volume increases by 30 to 40 percent, respiratory rate does not change appreciably during pregnancy. Cephalad displacement of the diaphragm due to the enlarged gravid uterus results in a decrease in residual volume and functional residual capacity. This may lead to more rapid deterioration of respiratory status with significant pulmonary injury. When these pulmonary changes are taken together with the risk for aspiration due to gastrointestinal changes, serious consideration should be given to early endotracheal intubation in the pregnant trauma victim with multisystem injuries.

CHANGES IN REGIONAL BLOOD FLOW

The 1000 percent increase in uterine blood flow from 60 to 600 mL/min during pregnancy is an important consideration for two reasons. First, in the presence of maternal hypovolemia, the uterus is considered an "expendable organ." Uterine artery vasoconstriction is an adaptive means to maintain cerebral and cardiac perfusion in the presence of maternal hypovolemia, and aggressive intravascular resuscitation is mandatory to maintain adequate fetal oxygenation. Second, avulsion or laceration of the uterine vessels—either through penetrating trauma to the lateral lower abdomen or severe direct abdominal impact—may result in rapid maternal exsanguination. The retroperitoneal pelvic blood vasculature is also hypertrophied during pregnancy, and maternal pelvic fracture may result in impressive bleeding into the retroperitoneal space over a fairly short time frame.

LABORATORY CHANGES OF PREGNANCY

The most frequent and dramatic changes in maternal laboratory values are those found in the complete blood count. Both plasma volume and RBC mass increase during pregnancy, but plasma volume more than RBC mass. As a result, a physiologic anemia in the range of 30 to 36 percent hematocrit, or 11 to 13 g/dL hemoglobin, is normal. Furthermore, leukocytosis is common beginning in the second trimester, with white blood cell counts normally up to 15,000/mm^3. During labor, white blood cell counts normally in the range of 20,000 to 25,000/mm^3 are not uncommon. The platelet count is typically unchanged or minimally lower in the normal pregnancy. Likewise, prothrombin time and partial thromboplastin time are unchanged in normal pregnancy. Arterial pH is unchanged, though a slight increase in minute ventilation results in a decrease in P_{CO_2} to approximately 35 torr. To compensate for this, there is a slight increase in serum HCO_3^- by decreased excretion of bicarbonate into the urine. Measurements of P_{O_2} are unchanged during pregnancy (see Table 2-3, Chap. 2, for other laboratory values in pregnancy).

INJURY PATTERNS IN PREGNANCY

BLUNT ABDOMINAL TRAUMA

Blunt abdominal trauma is most commonly caused by motor vehicle accidents, accounting for 50 to 65 percent of all cases, followed by falls and direct blows to the abdomen.[2,4,6–8] Domestic violence is remarkably common during pregnancy; rates as high as 20 percent have been reported.[9] The most common adverse event resulting from blunt abdominal trauma is abruptio placentae, complicating 1 to 3 percent of non-life-threatening maternal abdominal trauma and 40 to 50 percent of life-threatening maternal trauma (see Fig. 8-1). Similarly, fetal loss occurs uncommonly following trauma during pregnancy, but because most maternal trauma during pregnancy is minor (more than 90 percent), most fetal losses following trauma result from mi-

nor maternal injuries. The clinical implications of this observation is that policies should be developed to allow careful observation of the fetus following maternal trauma of any severity.[10] This specific evaluation is outlined under "Management," below.

Laboratory work in the case of the patient who has suffered blunt abdominal trauma during pregnancy is similar to that in the nonpregnant patient with two notable exceptions: (1) recognizing the differences in normal labs in the pregnant as compared with the nonpregnant patient; and (2) laboratory evidence of fetomaternal hemorrhage.[2,4,11] It has been recommended that all pregnant women undergo Kleihauer-Betke testing if they suffered trauma during pregnancy.[12] This recommendation was based on the observation that evidence of fetal cells in the maternal circulation was found four times more frequently in women who suffered blunt abdominal trauma, with the presumption that identification of fetomaternal hemorrhage could impact decision making (e.g., more intensive fetal surveillance, early delivery).[2,4,11] However, subsequent experience has demonstrated that the results from a Kleihauer-Betke test rarely affect clinical decision making.[13] For example, a fetus that suffers a massive fetomaternal bleed may exsanguinate, but

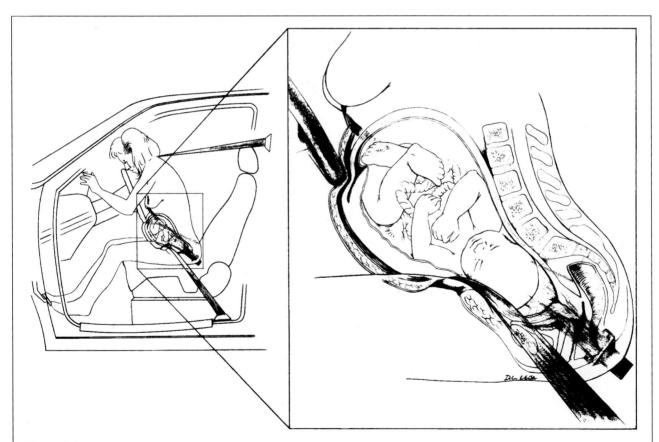

Figure 8-1

Illustration of abruptio placentae resulting from impact with steering wheel. See text for description. (Illustration by Darryl Leja, University of Michigan. From Pearlman and Tintinalli,[10] with permission.)

clinical decision making will be dictated by an abnormal fetal heart tracing rather than Kleihauer-Betke testing, as the latter frequently takes hours to obtain the result.[14] Nonetheless, in the Rh-negative woman, the possibility of isoimmunization due to fetomaternal hemorrhage is real and Rh immune globulin (Rhogam) should be administered to Rh-negative women who have suffered blunt abdominal trauma. A 300-μg dose is sufficient to cover 30 mL of whole blood (equivalent to a 15-mL RBC bleed). Fetomaternal hemorrhage larger than that requires additional Rh immune globulin. Because the Kleihauer-Betke test can identify these occasional large bleeds, its use in the Rh-negative woman may still have utility.

ABRUPTIO PLACENTAE

Abruptio placentae, or separation of the placenta from the decidua basalis of the endometrium, is the most common cause of fetal loss following trauma, accounting for 60 to 70 percent of these losses. The pathophysiology of abruptio placentae is based on the observation that there are fundamental differences in the elastic properties of the uterus and placenta: there are substantial elastic fibers in the uterus, whereas the placenta is relatively devoid of these. When the fluid-filled uterus is struck by a deforming force (e.g., steering wheel), the noncompressible amniotic fluid transmits the force to the entire uterus, causing an outward expansion of the entire uterus except at the point of intrusion by the deforming object. An analogous situation would be attaching a piece of adhesive tape to the inside of a water balloon and squeezing the balloon. The balloon wall is stretched; however, the inelastic tape cannot. If enough stretching occurs, the tape can be sheared off of the balloon. Other mechanisms may be operative in causing placental abruption, e.g., direct placental separation of an anteriorly attached placenta from deformation of the anterior uterine wall.

The signs and symptoms of abruptio placentae vary depending on the severity of separation. Vaginal bleeding is apparent in 80 percent of cases, and abdominal pain is also usually present (Table 8-1). In the most severe cases, there is fetal death associated with a tetanic uterine contraction pattern (less than 15 percent). However, the most sensitive method of diagnosing abruptio placentae following injury is by uterine contraction monitoring using a standard fetal monitor. In several studies, four or more uterine contractions in any 1-h period in the first 4 h of monitoring following trauma identified a group at risk for abruptio placentae.[2,4–6] Women beyond 20 to 24 weeks of gestation should routinely have fetal monitoring, including uterine contraction monitoring, following abdominal trauma of any severity.[12]

UTERINE RUPTURE

Uterine rupture as a result of abdominal trauma is uncommon, complicating only about 0.6 percent of cases of severe

Table 8-1

SIGNS AND SYMPTOMS OF ABRUPTIO PLACENTAE

Finding	Percent
Vaginal bleeding	78
Uterine tenderness or back pain	66
Fetal distress	60
High-frequency uterine contractions	17
Uterine hypertonus	17
Fetal death	15

Source: Adapted from Hurd WW, Miodovnik M, Hertzberg V, Lavin JP: Selective management of abruptio placentae. *Obstet Gynecol* 61:467, 1983.

direct abdominal trauma.[1] The clinical presentation of uterine rupture can vary considerably, from minimal abdominal tenderness in a hemodynamically stable patient to frank peritoneal signs with hypovolemic shock. If there is transmural uterine wall disruption, the fetus may be extruded from the uterus into the peritoneal cavity. Fetal death virtually always occurs in this circumstance. Uterine rupture is nearly always a second- or third-trimester event, as the first-trimester uterus is protected by the bony pelvis. Concomitant visceral injuries including the bladder or gastrointestinal tract can occur.

Uterine rupture should be part of the differential diagnosis of any pregnant woman in the second or third trimester who sustains severe direct abdominal trauma. Findings of abdominal pain and tenderness, signs of hypovolemia (though not always present), and fetal distress or death are clinical clues suggestive of uterine rupture. However, these findings can also be seen in abruptio placentae. More specific findings in uterine rupture include sonographic or x-ray evidence of the fetus outside of the uterine cavity (e.g., extended fetal extremities, oblique fetal lie, or direct visualization of an extrauterine fetus) or a difficult-to-palpate uterine fundus. A history of previous uterine scarring (e.g., cesarean section or myomectomy) increases the risk of uterine rupture, but uterine rupture can occur in the absence of any prior uterine surgery. A positive peritoneal lavage can be suggestive of this diagnosis, but it does not differentiate between uterine rupture and other causes of intraperitoneal bleeding. This can be performed at any gestational age and has been demonstrated to be as accurate as in the nonpregnant patient.[14] However, the hemodynamically unstable patient with signs of peritoneal irritation should be taken directly for exploratory laparotomy while resuscitation efforts are ongoing.

Pelvic fracture during pregnancy poses a significant risk of maternal mortality, because the hypertrophic vasculature can lead to significant retroperitoneal hemorrhage.[15]

Aggressive hemodynamic resuscitation is paramount in the management of these women. Because of the expanded blood volume during pregnancy, blood loss can be underestimated until profound hemodynamic instability ensues. Pelvic fracture in late gestation also places the fetal vertex at risk for skull fracture, because the fetal head engages, or enters the bony pelvis, in late pregnancy. Direct fetal injury (e.g., skull fracture) usually results from severe maternal trauma. In addition to skull fracture, intracranial hemorrhage, fetal splenic rupture, intrathoracic injuries, and extremity fracture have been described. Fortunately, these are rare occurrences.

GENERAL PRINCIPLES OF TRAUMA MANAGEMENT

Because the fetus is wholly dependent on maternal hemodynamic stability for adequate oxygenation, all initial efforts in evaluating and managing the pregnant trauma victim should be concentrated on assessing and resuscitating maternal vital signs (Fig. 8-2). An extensive review of resuscitation of the trauma victim is not offered here because this is discussed in standard trauma texts. However, several anatomic and physiologic changes of pregnancy are discussed because they influence maternal resuscitative efforts. The supine hypotensive syndrome has been described in several chapters in this text (see Fig. 2-5). Beyond approximately 24 weeks of gestation (uterine fundus palpable two finger breadths above the umbilicus), a woman lying in the supine position can develop significant hypotension due to inferior vena caval compression by the uterus, resulting in decreased venous return from the lower extremities. This may lead to a subsequent decrease in cardiac output approaching 25 to 30 percent. In the case of a hypovolemic patient who is marginally compromised, this supine position may cause frank hypovolemic shock. This can be avoided by displacing the uterus to either side by placing a 4- to 6-in. roll underneath the backboard or deflecting the uterus manually. Second, the 50 percent increase in maternal blood volume by 28 weeks of gestation may allow significant blood loss before there is a change in maternal vital signs. Careful attention to the mechanism of injury and the likelihood of significant vascular injury should prompt prophylactic efforts at maternal blood volume expansion and attention to the possible emergent need for blood products.

After assuring adequate ventilation and intravascular volume, efforts should be directed at assessing the extent of maternal injuries, followed by rapid assessment of the fetus. Particular attention should be paid to the maternal abdomen, because the finding of abdominal tenderness may indicate common injuries in accident victims (e.g., laceration of the liver or spleen) or pregnancy-specific injuries (uterine rupture or abruptio placentae). Vaginal bleeding associated with abdominal pain is highly suggestive of abruptio placentae. Beyond 20 to 24 weeks of gestation, a fetal monitor should be placed if available, because it will help to assess fetal

well-being in addition to being the most sensitive test for abruptio placentae. The availability of surgical and obstetric consultation should be anticipated, particularly when the gestational age is such that the fetus is viable outside of the uterus ($\geq$ 24–26 weeks).

Simultaneously with resuscitation efforts, a rapid but complete search for thoracic, intrathoracic, or intraabdominal injury, fractures, or external bleeding sites should ensue. In addition, specific efforts should be made to try to identify uterine or fetal injuries. Examination of the abdomen can be hindered by the recognized fact that findings of peritoneal irritation can be blunted in the pregnant women because of stretching and attenuation of the abdominal musculature.

Fetal monitoring should begin as soon as maternal stabilization has occurred, because abruptio placentae is an event that usually develops early following trauma. Evidence of frequent uterine contractions (four or more in an hour), a nonreassuring fetal heart rate tracing, uterine irritability or tenderness, ruptured amniotic membranes, and vaginal bleeding are all reasons for immediate obstetric consultation. Monitoring of fetal heart rate and uterine contractions should be interpreted by trained personnel. Monitoring is typically continued for a minimum of 4 h.

PENETRATING TRAUMA

Knife and gunshot wounds during pregnancy are not uncommon in urban settings. Understandably, there is considerable concern for fetal well-being when gunshot or knife wounds penetrate the abdomen. Knife and gunshot wounds suffered elsewhere in the body should be managed just as they are in the nonpregnant individual except that the fetus should also be monitored if viable (beyond 24 weeks of gestation) once the woman has been stabilized. However, penetrating wounds to the pregnant abdomen involve different considerations, because fetal or placental injury becomes an important issue.

The proximity of the fetus and placenta to the anterior abdominal wall render them very susceptible to injury or death when there is penetrating abdominal trauma. In fact, there is disparate risk for the woman and her fetus following penetrating trauma. This is because the likelihood of fetal injury is directly related to the size of the uterus in relation to other intraabdominal organs. In this regard, the uterus is dominant in size in the second half of gestation. Furthermore, the anterior abdominal wall, uterine wall, amniotic fluid, and fetus all absorb energy of the penetrating object, protecting other maternal visceral organs. This "shielding effect" is manifest in the most recent series of penetrating abdominal trauma during pregnancy, where there were no maternal mortalities compared with a fetal death rate of nearly two-thirds.[16–18]

With cephalad and lateral displacement of the maternal intraabdominal viscera during pregnancy, penetrating injuries that enter superior or lateral to the uterus are likely to produce complex bowel injuries, resulting in the potential

STABILIZATION

- Maintain airway and oxygenation
- Deflect uterus to left
- Maintain circulatory volume
- Secure cervical spine if head or neck injury suspected

COMPLETE EXAMINATION

- Control external hemorrhage
- Identify/stabilize serious injuries
- Examine uterus
- Pelvic examination to identify ruptured membranes or vaginal bleeding
- Obtain initial blood work

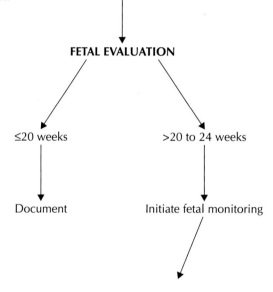

FETAL EVALUATION

≤20 weeks   >20 to 24 weeks

Document   Initiate fetal monitoring

Presence of
- More than four uterine contractions in any 1 h (≥20 weeks)
- Rupture of amnionic membranes
- Vaginal bleeding
- Serious maternal injury
- Fetal tachycardia, late decelerations, nonreactive non–stress test

YES   NO

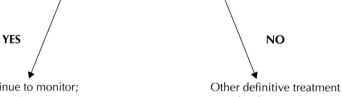

Hospitalize; continue to monitor;   Other definitive treatment
intervene as appropriate   (may be done concomitant with monitoring):
                                             - Suture lacerations
                                             - Necessary x-rays

Discharge with follow-up and instructions

Figure 8-2

Algorithm for management of blunt abdominal trauma during pregnancy. (From Pearlman MD: Motor vehicle crashes, pregnancy loss and preterm labor. *Int J Obstet Gynecol* 57:127, 1997. Used with permission.)

for multiple entrance and exit wounds. Highly projectile objects (e.g., bullets from high-powered rifles) can pass through the uterus, placing the organs posterior to it at risk (e.g., abdominal aorta, inferior vena cava, sigmoid colon).

MANAGEMENT OF PENETRATING TRAUMA

When a pregnant woman presents with penetrating abdominal trauma, three decisions must immediately be made:

1. Whether to perform exploratory laparotomy
2. Whether to deliver the fetus
3. If delivery is planned, what the route of delivery should be

Whether or not to perform exploratory laparotomy will depend on the patient's hemodynamic stability and the presence or absence of hemoperitoneum. It will also depend on the type of penetrating object. Most authors agree that gunshot wounds to the abdomen should be explored in all cases, since the course of the bullet cannot be predicted.[18,19] Furthermore, due to cavitation and shock waves, tissue damage well outside of the projectile's path can be significant. When extrauterine injuries do occur following penetrating abdominal trauma during pregnancy, they typically occur as a result of gunshot wounds. All gunshot wounds to the abdomen should be explored.

Knife wounds to the abdomen are much less likely to cause extrauterine injuries, and these injuries typically have a better prognosis than gunshot wounds. The individual circumstances of knife wounds should be carefully weighed prior to making a decision to perform a laparotomy. Stab wounds to the lower abdomen are much less likely to cause visceral injuries than upper abdominal wounds. However, any midline lower abdominal wound can cause bladder or ureteral injury. Grubb demonstrated that in nonpregnant patients, stab wounds to the abdomen do not penetrate the peritoneum in about one-third of cases.[20] These extraperitoneal wounds generally do not require exploration unless they have injured a large blood vessel in the abdominal wall (e.g., the inferior epigastric artery). However, because of the enlarged gravid uterus, attenuation of the abdominal wall during pregnancy makes it more susceptible to peritoneal penetration. Several invasive tests short of exploratory laparotomy can be utilized to determine if there has been significant intraperitoneal injury. Injection of radiopaque material (e.g., Gastrografin) into the entrance wound followed by a two-view radiograph (e.g., a fistulogram) may demonstrate spillage into the gastrointestinal or genitourinary tract. Such a finding would be an indication for laparotomy. Second, amniocentesis to determine whether the amniotic cavity contains blood or bacteria has been advocated. However, the presence of blood or bacteria does not necessarily mandate delivery, and careful consideration with obstetric consultation should precede this decision.

Injury to the uterine vasculature is uncommon largely because the vessels are located quite lateral and posterior in later gestation. However, because of the tremendous volume of blood flowing through the uterine vessels, injury to these vessels is likely to result in rapid deterioration of vital signs. Unstable vital signs in the presence of a penetrating abdominal wound indicate the need for immediate laparotomy. In the absence of unstable vital signs, peritoneal lavage has been demonstrated to be accurate to diagnose hemoperitoneum during pregnancy and can be helpful in determining whether exploratory laparotomy is necessary.

The decision to deliver depends on (1) gestational age at the time of injury, (2) penetration of the amniotic cavity by the object, (3) evidence of fetal injury or death, and (4) the extent of maternal injuries and the need to empty the uterus to explore the abdomen adequately. These decisions are best made in concert with the obstetrician and trauma surgeon. If exploratory surgery has been performed, incidental cesarean section may be indicated at term if this will improve the ability to explore the abdomen or if there is evidence of fetal distress or injury that would likely be better dealt with in the extrauterine environment. Otherwise, it is acceptable to allow vaginal delivery. The decision to deliver in preterm gestations will depend on several considerations, mainly recognizing that if the pregnancy is allowed to continue in a gestation that is far from term, a better fetal outcome will probably result.

THERMAL AND ELECTRICAL INJURIES

There has been limited published experience with burns and electrical injuries during pregnancy. Matthews and colleagues recommend that severely burned women (more than 50 percent body involvement) should be delivered immediately because maternal death is almost certain otherwise, and fetal survival is not improved by allowing the pregnancy to continue.[21] Their experience was that maternal prognosis with thermal injury is worse as compared with similar injury in nonpregnant women. Other experience has suggested that pregnancy does not affect outcome in patients who have suffered burns.[22,23] More likely, the percentage of body involvement is a reasonably good predictor of maternal survival. In general, fetal prognosis is poor in severely burned women. Typically, these patients will develop spontaneous labor within days to a week postburn. The approach to managing the burn victim in the immediate few hours after injury is similar to that in the nonpregnant woman.

Human experience with electrical injury during pregnancy is limited. Eleven cases of lightning injury during pregnancy were summarized by Pierce and colleagues.[24] In this series, there were no maternal deaths and no long-term sequelae to the fetuses that survived. However, another series of electrical injuries suggests that there may be long-term sequelae in the fetuses who survive the initial insult.[25] In this series of six pregnancies complicated by electrical injury, there was one delayed fetal death complicated by growth retardation and oligohydramnios and two of the three other live births were complicated by oligohydramnios. Because of this, these authors recommend serial ultrasound examinations to follow fetal growth and amniotic fluid volume.

References

1. Pearlman MD, Tintinalli JE, Lorenz RP: Blunt trauma during pregnancy. *N Engl J Med* 323:1609, 1990.

2. Pearlman MD, Tintinalli JE, Lorenz RP: A prospective controlled study of outcome after trauma during pregnancy. *Am J Obstet Gynecol* 162:1502, 1990.

3. Scorpio RJ, Esposito TJ, Smith LG, Gens DR: Blunt trauma during pregnancy. Factors affecting fetal outcome. *J Trauma* 32:213, 1992.

4. Goodwin TM, Breen MT: Pregnancy outcome and fetomaternal hemorrhage after noncatastrophic trauma. *Am J Obstet Gynecol* 162:665, 1990.

5. Williams JK, McClain L, Rosemurgy AS, Colorado NM: Evaluation of blunt abdominal trauma in the third trimester of pregnancy: Maternal and fetal considerations. *Obstet Gynecol* 75:33, 1990.

6. Dahmus MA, Sibai BM: Blunt abdominal trauma: Are there any predictive factors for abruptio placentae or maternal-fetal distress? *Am J Obstet Gynecol* 169:1504, 1993.

7. Esposito JT, Agens DR, Smith LG, Scorpio R: Evaluation of blunt abdominal trauma occurring during pregnancy. *J Trauma* 29:1628, 1989.

8. Kissinger DP, Rozycki GS, Morris JA Jr, et al: Trauma in pregnancy: Predicting pregnancy outcome. *Arch Surg* 126:1079, 1991.

9. Gazmararian JA, Lazorick S, Spitz AM, et al: Prevalence of violence against pregnant women. *JAMA* 275:1915, 1996.

10. Pearlman MD, Tintinalli JE: Evaluation and treatment of the gravida and fetus following trauma during pregnancy. *Obstet Gynecol Clin North Am* 18:371, 1991.

11. Rose PG, Strohm PL, Zuspan FP: Fetomaternal hemorrhage following trauma. *Am J Obstet Gynecol* 153:844, 1985.

12. American College of Obstetricians and Gynecologists: *Trauma during Pregnancy. ACOG Tech Bull* No. 161. Washington, DC: ACOG, 1991.

13. Boyle J, Kim J, Walerius H, Samuels P: The clinical use of the Kleihauer-Betke test in Rh positive patients (abstract). *Am J Obstet Gynecol* 174:343, 1995.

14. Towery R, English TP, Wisner D: Evaluation of the pregnant woman after blunt injury. *J Trauma* 35:731, 1993.

15. Pearlman MD, Tintinalli JE: Trauma in pregnancy (clinical conference). *Ann Emerg Med* 17:829, 1990.

16. Kirshon B, Young R, Gordon AN: Conservative management of abdominal gunshot wound in a pregnant woman. *Am J Perinatol* 5:232, 1988.

17. Awwad JT, Azar GB, Seoud MA, et al: High velocity penetrating wounds of the gravid uterus: Review of 16 years of civil war. *Obstet Gynecol* 83:259, 1994.

18. Buchsbaum HJ: Penetrating injury of the abdomen, in Buchsbaum HJ (ed): *Trauma in Pregnancy*. Philadelphia: Saunders, 1979, p 82.

19. Franger AL, Buchsbaum HJ, Peaceman AM: Abdominal gunshot wounds in pregnancy. *Am J Obstet Gynecol* 160:1124, 1989.

20. Grubb DK: Nonsurgical management of penetrating uterine trauma in pregnancy: A case report. *Am J Obstet Gynecol* 166:583, 1992.

21. Matthews RN: Obstetric implications of burns in pregnancy. *Br J Obstet Gynaecol* 89:603, 1982.

22. Amy BW, McManus WF, Goodwin CW, et al: Thermal injury in the pregnant patient. *Surg Gynecol Obstet* 161:209, 1985.

23. Jain ML, Gary AK: Burns with pregnancy: A review of 25 cases. *Burns* 19:166, 1993.

24. Pierce MR, Henderson RA, Mitchell JM: Cardiopulmonary arrest secondary to lightning injury in a pregnant woman. *Ann Emerg Med* 15:597, 1986.

25. Liberman JR, Mazor M, Molcho J, et al: Electrical burns in pregnancy. *Obstet Gynecol* 67:861, 1986.

Chapter 9

BLEEDING IN THE SECOND HALF OF PREGNANCY; MATERNAL AND FETAL ASSESSMENT

Kristine M. VanDeKerkhove

Timothy R.B. Johnson

Vaginal bleeding after 20 weeks gestation is strongly associated with increased maternal and perinatal morbidity and mortality. Obstetric hemorrhage is also one of the most difficult management problems in medicine, since the well-being of two patients, the fetus and the mother, must be considered and managed simultaneously. Medical decisions in these cases must attempt to optimize the outcome for both patients. At times, however, what is best for the mother is not always best for the fetus. Although the mother seldom benefits from continued pregnancy when significant mid-trimester bleeding occurs, complications of prematurity greatly contributes to the high perinatal morbidity and mortality rates seen in these pregnancies. The decision to deliver or maintain the pregnancy requires a careful assessment of the risks and benefits of all management options for both the mother and the fetus.

The following is a review of causes of vaginal bleeding in the second half of pregnancy and a discussion of the practical aspects of maternal and fetal evaluation and management in the emergency setting.

OVERVIEW OF THE PREGNANT PATIENT WITH BLEEDING AFTER 20 WEEKS GESTATION

The average length of human pregnancy is 40 weeks or 280 days. Pregnancies have, for convenience sake, been broken up into trimesters, each being equal to approximately 13 weeks (i.e., the first trimester lasts until 13 weeks, the second trimester from 14 to 26 weeks, and the third trimester after 26 weeks). The different causes of bleeding during pregnancy are gestational age dependent. For example, the World Health Organization (WHO) has defined abortion as being termination of pregnancy (whether induced or spontaneous) before 20 weeks gestation. Bleeding before 20 weeks gestation is defined therefore as threatened abortion (covered in Chap. 4). This chapter covers bleeding which occurs during the second half of pregnancy. The causes of vaginal bleeding after 20 weeks gestation differ considerably from bleeding prior to that time. The use of both gestational age and the presence (or absence) of abdominal pain are helpful in the initial evaluation of the pregnant woman with bleeding (Table 9-1). The remainder of this chapter deals with the separate causes of vaginal bleeding in the second half of pregnancy and how to approach both diagnosis and management of the pregnant woman and her fetus in that setting.

the placenta has the potential for catastrophic consequences. Bleeding arising from the lower genital tract may be due to cervical changes in labor, ("bloody show"), cervical erosions, cervical polyps, trauma, or cervical cancer. Vulvar varicose veins, common in pregnancy, may also lead to bleeding. Bleeding from the lower genital tract is usually light and, even when heavy, is rarely immediately life-threatening.

THE DIFFERENTIAL DIAGNOSIS

Vaginal bleeding in the second half of pregnancy can arise from either the upper or the lower genital tract. Upper genital tract bleeding may be from the uterus, as with uterine rupture, or from the uteroplacental interface with a placenta previa or abruptio placentae. It may also be from fetal vessels, as in a vasa previa. Bleeding from either the uterus or

BLEEDING ARISING FROM THE UPPER GENITAL TRACT

PLACENTA PREVIA

DEFINITION

Placenta previa occurs when the placenta implants in the lower uterine segment in advance of the fetal presenting part.

Table 9-1

CAUSES OF VAGINAL BLEEDING DURING PREGNANCY

Condition	Weeks of Pregnancy (approx.)	Abdominal Pain or Cramping	Contractions	DIC	Associated Conditions
Abortion	<20	Sometimes	N/A	No	Usually none (see Chap. 4)
Abruptio placentae	>26	Yes	Yes, frequent and intense	Yes	Hypertension, cocaine use, trauma
Placenta previa	>26	No*	No*	No	Multiparity, prior uterine surgery (e.g., cesarean section), multiple gestation
Uterine rupture	Any, usually in labor	Yes	No	+/−	Prior uterine surgery, trauma
Vasa previa	Any, but only with ROM	No*	No*	No	Presents with ROM
Labor ("bloody show")	>20	Yes	Yes	No	
Nonobstetrical causes (e.g., cervicitis, hemorrhoids, postcoital, cervical cancer)	Any	No	No	No	Depends on cause (e.g., cervical cancer, hx of abnormal Pap smear or no recent Pap smear)

ROM=rupture of amniotic membranes.
N/A=not applicable.
*only if in labor.
Hx=history.

RISK FACTORS

Placenta previa occurs in approximately 1 in 200 term births. Multiparity, a history of prior placenta previa, previous cesarean section, and prior abortion with curettage all increase risk for this complication of pregnancy. Pregnancies with a large placenta, as seen in twins gestations, erythroblastosis fetalis, or diabetes also have a higher incidence of placenta previa.

PATHOPHYSIOLOGY

Placenta previa has been subclassified according to the relationship of the placenta to the internal cervical os:

1. Total placenta previa—the placenta completely covers the internal os (Fig. 9-1*A*).
2. Partial placenta previa—the placenta covers part but not all of the internal cervical os (Fig. 9-1*B*).
3. Marginal placenta previa—the placenta approaches but does not cover the internal cervical os (Fig. 9-1*C*).
4. Low-lying placenta—the placenta is implanted in the lower uterine segment within 2 cm of the cervical os.

Bleeding from placenta previa occurs as a result of a marginal separation of the placenta away from the lower uterine segment. The relative lack of myometrial tissue in the lower uterine segment, however, renders it unable to contract effectively for hemostasis when there is separation of the placenta from its implantation site. Bleeding can occur spontaneously or be provoked by physical activity, vaginal examination, or intercourse. Uterine contractions with cervical dilation and effacement at the placental interface may also precipitate bleeding episodes.

CLINICAL PRESENTATION

Placenta previa classically presents with sudden and painless vaginal bleeding in the second or third trimester of pregnancy. Pain, however, may sometimes be present. Clinically, a high fetal presenting part or fetal malpresentation, such as breech or transverse lie, supports the diagnosis. Bleeding is usually from the maternal circulation and, since the functional portion of the placenta is relatively undisturbed, fetal compromise is rare until the development of maternal hemodynamic instability.

IMAGING STUDIES

Digital examination in a patient with placenta previa may precipitate severe hemorrhage. *Ultrasound localization of the placenta is therefore mandatory prior to any vaginal examination* of a patient presenting with obstetric bleeding. Ultrasound studies done earlier in the pregnancy are invaluable. These may be available from the obstetric record at the time of the patient's presentation. If placenta previa was not seen on an earlier examination, then vaginal exam-

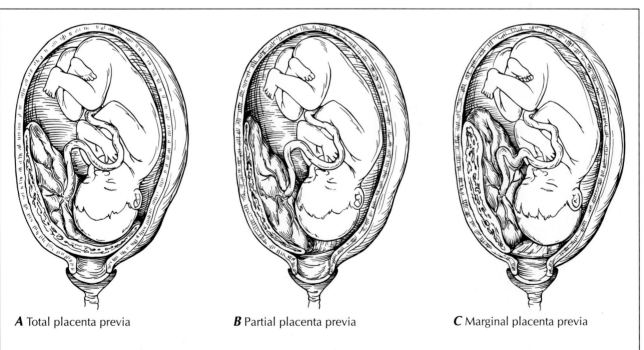

A Total placenta previa   *B* Partial placenta previa   *C* Marginal placenta previa

Figure 9-1

Placenta previa. Placental separation from the lower uterine segment occurs with cervical dilation and formation of the lower uterine segment. Hemorrhage results when the lower uterine segment is unable to contract for hemostasis.

ination may safely be performed. Of note, however, a high percentage of sonographically diagnosed cases of previa encountered early in pregnancy resolve on repeat examination at later gestational ages.[1] This phenomenon may be due to progressive thinning and stretching of the lower uterine segment with differential growth of the placenta away from the cervix. If a previa was seen at an early stage of pregnancy or reports are unavailable at presentation, ultrasound examination for placental location is indicated prior to vaginal examination. Using transabdominal sonography, a midline longitudinal scan is used to evaluate the relationship between the placental structures (Fig. 9-2). Reported false-positive and false-negative rates of 2 to 6 percent and 2 percent, respectively, may be due to shadowing artifact from an ossified fetal presenting part, inability to distinguish a fresh blood clot located in the lower uterine segment from placenta, contractions of the lower uterine segment, maternal obesity, a posterior placenta, or an overdistended maternal bladder.[2,3] With an overdistended bladder, the anterior lower uterine segment is displaced posteriorly and may mimic a cervical os. Ultrasound examinations for the evaluation of placental location should, therefore, include both an initial high-resolution scan performed through a full bladder and a subsequent scan after the bladder is emptied in order to minimize distortion of the lower uterine segment.

Although digital vaginal examination of the cervix is contraindicated until placental location has been determined, translabial or transvaginal sonography may be used if the technical difficulties described above are encountered. A transvaginal probe may be safely introduced into the patient's vagina under direct sonographic visualization (stopping short of the cervix) without causing bleeding.[2] With transvaginal sonography, the shorter distance to the cervix and placenta allows for higher-resolution scans, which are helpful in differentiating the internal cervical os from placental edges. This type of examination, however, should be performed only by persons experienced in the technique and approach.

DOUBLE-SETUP EXAMINATION

If the placenta is not overlying the cervical os, vaginal examination may be safely performed. If, however, ultrasound evaluation is inconclusive, a double-setup examination may be indicated. With this technique, vaginal examination is carefully performed in an operating room setting where cesarean section could be performed emergently should bleeding complications arise. Only an experienced obstetrician should perform this type of examination. In addition, this examination need be performed only if delivery is indicated and a route of delivery remains to be decided—i.e., vaginal versus cesarean section.

ABRUPTIO PLACENTAE

Abruptio placentae is the premature separation of the normally implanted placenta from its uterine implantation site after 20 weeks gestation. Placental separation prior to this time are considered to be part of the process of spontaneous abortion. Severe placental abruption is a leading cause of fetal death and accounts for approximately 14 percent of all

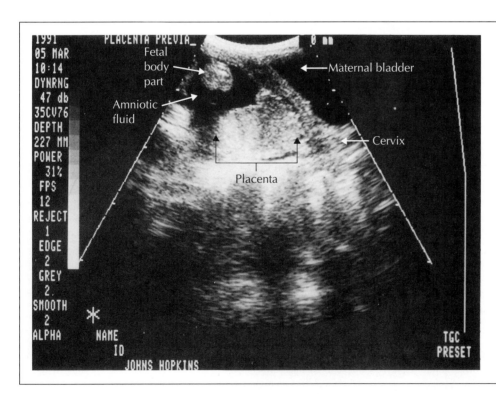

Figure 9-2

Placenta previa—sonographic evaluation.

stillbirths.[4] In addition, the perinatal mortality rate is 25 to 50 percent in these pregnancies, with problems of prematurity such as respiratory distress syndrome, intraventricular hemorrhage, and necrotizing enterocolitis accounting for a high percentage of deaths. Complications of severe hemorrhage, including coagulopathy, emergent surgery, and anesthesia also render abruptio placentae a significant cause of maternal morbidity and mortality in the second and third trimester.

RISK FACTORS

Maternal hypertension is the greatest risk factor for abruptio placentae. In the abruption severe enough to cause fetal death, about 50 percent of cases are associated either with chronic or pregnancy-induced hypertension. In fact, all conditions that predispose to vascular compromise (preeclampsia, chronic hypertension, diabetes mellitus, collagen vascular disease, and chronic renal disease) are associated with an increased risk for premature placental separation.

Blunt abdominal trauma from a direct blow to the abdomen or the shear force created by an acceleration/deceleration event, as in a motor vehicle accident, may also result in abruptio placentae. With severe trauma resulting in major maternal injuries, the reported incidence is as high as 35 percent, while there is a 4 percent risk of abruptio placentae after minor trauma.[5] Other risk factors include placental abruption in a prior pregnancy, advanced maternal age, multiparity, cigarette smoking, and cocaine use.

PATHOPHYSIOLOGY

Abruptio placentae occurs after the spontaneous rupture of blood vessels at the placental bed with hematoma formation. Subsequent bleeding may be external and appear vaginally (Fig. 9-3A), or it may be concealed (about 20 percent) (Fig. 9-3B). In a concealed abruption, blood does not decompress through the vagina and pressure at the placental bed increases. The adjacent myometrium is then unable to contract around the torn vessels to stop them from bleeding. Placental separation is often progressive in these cases. Under pressure, the blood may also rupture through the fetal membranes and into the amniotic fluid (with bleeding evident only with rupture of membranes) or dissect into the myometrium (Couvelaire uterus).

Fetal hypoxia occurs as the placental disruption renders the involved placental surface unable to provide adequate metabolic exchange. Additionally, disrupted maternal and fetal vascular channels may communicate, resulting in a potentially catastrophic fetal blood loss, maternal Rh sensitization, or even a fatal amniotic fluid embolus.

With significant tissue disruption or clot formation, disseminated intravascular coagulation (DIC) may occur. It is believed that the inciting event is tissue thromboplastin release into the maternal circulation and subsequent microvascular coagulation. The maternal fibrinolytic system is then activated, with critical depletion of platelets, fibrinogen, and other clotting factors. Additionally, a true consumptive coagulopathy may occur at the site of a large retroplacental clot. In either case, the final result is inappropriate bleeding and an even greater maternal blood loss.

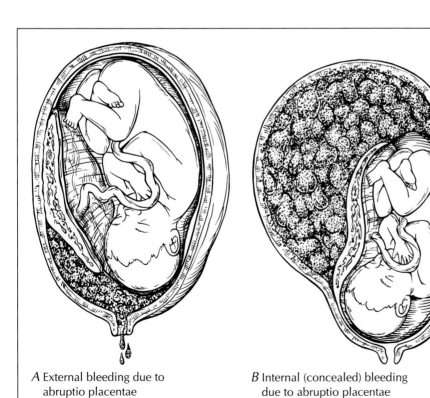

A External bleeding due to abruptio placentae

B Internal (concealed) bleeding due to abruptio placentae

Figure 9-3

Abruptio placentae. Premature separation of the normally implanted placenta after 20 weeks of gestation. *A*. External hemorrhage. *B*. Concealed hemorrhage.

CLINICAL PRESENTATION

Placenta abruption is variable in its presentation, depending on the degree of the placental separation. *Severe abruptio placentae* is placental separation of such magnitude as to cause fetal death. It typically presents with a sudden onset of intense abdominal or back pain. This pain is often focal and constant, and superimposed uterine contractions or even sustained uterine tetany are usually present. Fetal heart sounds are absent and there is no fetal cardiac activity on ultrasound examination. Maternal hemodynamic instability and coagulopathy are common sequelae of severe placental abruption. Clinical signs of DIC, such as mucosal bleeding, excessive bleeding at puncture sites, bruising, or hematuria may be evident. In addition, sequelae of hypotension, such as adult respiratory distress syndrome and acute tubular necrosis, can occur quickly, making aggressive resuscitation and prompt delivery of the fetus and placenta imperative.

Placental separations of smaller magnitude have a subtler and more variable presentation. In these cases, definitive diagnosis of abruptio placentae may be difficult. Focal abdominal or back pain and superimposed uterine contractions or irritability are the commonest findings in these patients. Pain, however, may be absent with small or marginal separations. Placental separations involving a large surface area may result in fetal compromise. The absence of abnormalities in fetal heart rate, however, does not preclude the diagnosis. Maternal hemodynamic instability and coagulopathy are less common with smaller degrees of placental separation.

LABORATORY STUDIES

Although the diagnosis of abruptio placentae is clinical, many of the more readily apparent manifestations of this complication occur late in the disease process. The subtler presentation of mild abruptio placentae often make definitive diagnosis quite difficult. A number of laboratory tests, therefore, have been suggested to assist in the diagnosis. Although positive findings in any of these tests may predict abruptio placentae, how they should guide clinical management remains an area of controversy.

Subclinical coagulopathy seen in mild to moderate abruptio placentae may result in thrombocytopenia and prolongation of the prothrombin and partial thromboplastin times. Fibrinogen will also be consumed, with fibrin degradation products, such as the D-dimer, appearing in the maternal circulation along with a low serum fibrinogen.[6] Also, proteins associated with the fetoplacental unit, such as alpha-fetoprotein (AFP) in amniotic fluid or CA125 from maternal decidua[7,8] can enter the maternal circulation in abruptio placentae, though this latter is not often used clinically in this setting. Finally, disruption of the uteroplacental interface may lead to entry of fetal blood into the maternal circulation.[5] With high-volume fetomaternal hemorrhage, abnormalities in fetal heart rate are seen. Smaller bleeds not resulting in fetal compromise, however, are detectable only by the identification of fetal cells in the maternal circulation such as the Kleihauer-Betke test.

Because of its association with placental abruption, a urine cocaine screen may also lend insight into the mechanism of bleeding. This test, however, is not diagnostic for abruptio placentae.

IMAGING STUDIES

The sensitivity of ultrasound for the diagnosis of abruptio placentae is poor. Although it may sometimes identify a retroplacental clot, this finding is difficult to distinguish from normal placental venous lakes, and is often absent. The sensitivity is greater with severe abruptio, although clinical findings often make the diagnosis straightforward in these cases. The clinical utility of ultrasound in abruptio placentae, therefore, is limited to ruling out placenta previa as a cause of late-trimester vaginal bleeding.

Magnetic resonance imaging (MRI) has a superior ability to differentiate tissue planes and highlight blood. These properties have made it an attractive imaging modality for the diagnosis of abruptio placentae. However, MRI is not mobile; it is also time-consuming and expensive. These impracticalities have limited its usefulness for the evaluation of acute obstetric hemorrhage. Initial studies have shown promise, however, in patients presenting with vaginal bleeding who are clinically stable and whose diagnosis remains uncertain.[9] The use of MRI during pregnancy appears to be safe (see Appendix A-2).

UTERINE RUPTURE

Interruption of the integrity of the uterine cavity in pregnancy has serious consequences. Maternal mortality is 10 to 40 percent in pregnancies complicated by complete uterine rupture and fetal mortality is in excess of 50 percent.

RISK FACTORS

Uterine rupture occurs when there are weaknesses in the uterine wall or excessively high intrauterine pressure forces. The most common predisposing factor for rupture is previous surgery on the uterus, such as cesarean section, fibroid removal (myomectomy), resection of a uterine septum (metroplasty), or uterine cornual resection. Other factors that may predispose to defects in the uterine wall are placental implantation abnormalities (placenta accreta, increta, percreta), invasive mole, or choriocarcinoma. Grand multiparity also increases the risk for this complication. Uterine rupture may also occur after a dramatic increase in intrauterine pressure, as seen with tetanic uterine contractions or in blunt abdominal trauma.

PATHOPHYSIOLOGY

A distinction is made between uterine rupture and dehiscence. Uterine dehiscence is myometrial separation at a site of uterine scar from previous surgery, and the uterine serosa remains intact. The vertical scar from a classical cesarean section, for example, greatly weakens the muscular active segment of the uterus. Increases in uterine pressure may result in tearing at these areas of weakness. Muscle separations may be limited to the relatively avascular scar or may extend into previously uninvolved myometrium. Uterine rupture, on the other hand, involves the entire thickness of the uterine wall, resulting in communication between the uterine and peritoneal cavities (Fig. 9-4). The placenta and fetus may then be extruded into the peritoneal cavities. Bleeding usually occurs from the edges of the defect but may vary from minimal to massive, depending on the size and relative vascularity of the defect and whether the defect involves the placenta or extends into uterine or vaginal blood vessels. In complete uterine rupture, the defect may originate from a previous surgical scar or it may occur spontaneously.

CLINICAL PRESENTATION

In many cases of uterine rupture resulting in fetal or maternal death, the diagnosis is not made until after delivery. Just as the specific anatomic defects in uterine dehiscence and rupture are variable, so is its clinical presentation. Simple uterine dehiscence at the site of a previous low transverse cesarean section may be asymptomatic and discovered only at the time of repeat cesarean section or manual uterine exploration after vaginal delivery. Often, however, local tenderness is reported. A sudden onset of pain may be seen with an increase in uterine irritability in a previously quiescent uterus or, conversely, with cessation of an established contraction pattern in a laboring patient. Fetal heart rate abnormality is often the earliest sign of uterine rupture in the laboring patient. Palpable abnormalities on abdominal examination, recession of the fetal presenting part, and loss of fetal heart tones are seen in massive rupture with extrusion of the fetus and placenta.

Vaginal bleeding is variable and rarely reflects total blood loss. Simultaneous bleeding into the abdominal cavity is common, and signs of fetal distress, maternal hypovolemia, or shock may be seen with only minor vaginal bleeding.

IMAGING STUDIES

In cases of dramatic uterine rupture associated with abnormalities in fetal heart rate and maternal hemorrhage, ultrasound confirmation of clinical suspicions will only serve to delay treatment. Ballooning placental membranes, however, have been described by the use of ultrasound in a case of uterine dehiscence not associated with fetal or maternal compromise.[10]

VASA PREVIA

Bleeding in vasa previa is from fetal vessels as they traverse the placental membranes. The bleeding is purely fetal in origin and therefore is an unusual cause of upper genital tract bleeding in that it poses almost no maternal risk but may rapidly lead to fetal distress and death.

PATHOPHYSIOLOGY

Fetal umbilical vessels usually insert centrally onto the placenta (Fig. 9-5A). Vasa previa occurs with a lateral (velamentous) insertion of the umbilical cord onto the chorionic plate of the placenta or when there is an extra (succencuriate) lobe. With these potentially dangerous variants, fetal vessels traverse within the placental membranes prior to their insertion (Fig. 9-5B and C). If these fetal vessels cross the lower uterine segment and present in advance of the fetus, they are then vulnerable to rupture or laceration with rupture of the placental membranes. Because the circulating blood volume of a fetus is small (approximately 300 to 500 mL), relatively unimpressive amounts of vaginal bleeding may easily lead to severe fetal compromise and rapid fetal exanguination.

Vasa previa is thought to complicate 1 in 2000 to 5000 deliveries, and perinatal mortality due to a ruptured vasa previa is reported to be as high as 50 to 75 percent.[11] This figure, however, is probably an underestimate, as deliveries complicated by vaginal bleeding and fetal distress due to vasa previa are likely to be attributed to much more common causes, such as abruptio placentae.

CLINICAL PRESENTATION

Vaginal bleeding and the rapid occurrence of fetal heart rate abnormalities are the hallmarks of a ruptured vasa previa.

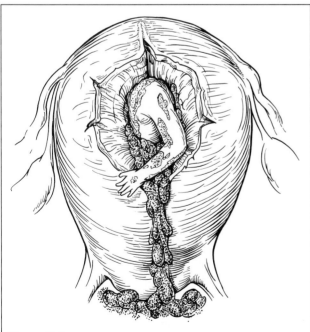

Figure 9-4

Uterine rupture at laparotomy with partial expulsion of the fetus.

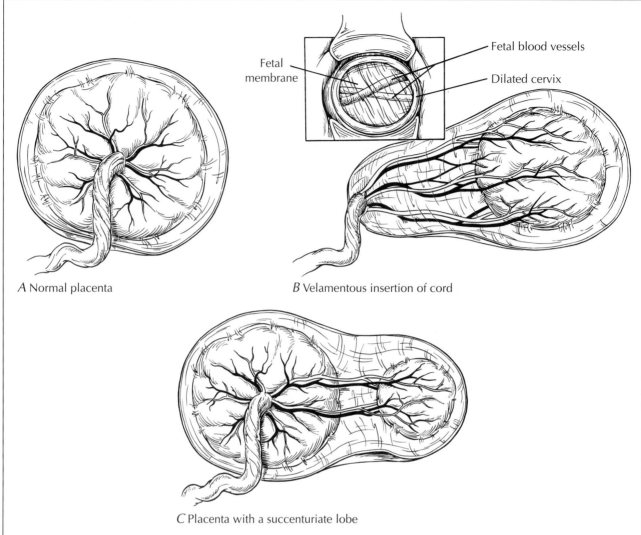

Figure 9-5

Placental variants at risk for vasa previa. *A.* Normal placenta—central attachment of the umbilical vessels to the placenta. *B.* Velamentous insertion of the cord; fetal vessels traverse the placental membranes and divide before they reach the chorionic plate. The inset shows fetal vessels viewed during speculum examination. *C.* Succenturiate placenta: small accessory placental lobules may be joined by fetal vessels traversing the placental membranes.

Occasionally, the aberrant fetal vessels are detected prior to their rupture at the time of elective cesarean section or by palpation of fetal vessels overlying the presenting part during vaginal examination. Unfortunately, however, vasa previa is seldom recognized prior to vessel disruption. Spontaneous or artificial rupture of placental membranes or descent of the fetal presenting part may cause rupture of these vessels. Painless vaginal bleeding as well as the rapid occurrence of fetal compromise occur soon thereafter. Unlike other forms of late-trimester bleeding from the upper genital tract, however, the potential for associated maternal hemodynamic instability is remote.

LABORATORY STUDIES

In cases of vaginal bleeding of uncertain etiology, the Apt test may distinguish fetal from maternal red blood cells in vaginal blood. This test exploits the phenomenon that adult oxyhemoglobin is less resistant to alkali than fetal oxyhemoglobin. It is performed by centrifugation of vaginal blood diluted with five parts water, mixing the supernatant with 0.25 N sodium hydroxide with a second centrifugation and observing the color of this mixture. A pink color indicates fetal origin and a yellow or brown color indicates maternal origin. This test can be time-consuming, however, and is seldom practical in cases of true ruptured vasa previa associated with fetal exanguination.

IMAGING STUDIES

Succenturiate lobes or bilobed placentas may occasionally be seen at ultrasound, identifying patients at risk for this unusual complication. Although direct visualization of aberrant vessels using transvaginal sonography with color-flow Doppler has been described,[12] ultrasound should not be considered a practical or reliable diagnostic tool for an acutely bleeding vasa previa.

BLEEDING ARISING FROM THE LOWER GENITAL TRACT

Vaginal bleeding in the second half of pregnancy may originate from structures in the reproductive tract other than the uterus or placenta. After excluding placenta previa, direct visualization of the vagina and cervix using a bivalve speculum will reveal these sources of bleeding.

OBSTETRIC CAUSES

Progressive cervical dilatation in term or preterm labor may result in the disruption of small blood vessels supplying the cervix. This phenomenon is known as "bloody show." The bleeding is usually relatively minor and signs of labor are often obvious.

NONOBSTETRIC CAUSES

Bleeding arising from the lower genital tract may also be due to visible lesions, such as vulvar varicose veins, cervical eversion, polyps, of carcinoma (Fig. 9-6A–C). Cervical polyps in pregnancy may present with vaginal bleeding and are easily identified on vaginal examination. In addition, metaplastic changes due to the altered hormonal environment in pregnancy result in a cervical ectropion, or an "eversion" of the columnar epithelium of the cervical canal onto the ectocervix. This tissue is relatively friable and may bleed lightly, especially after intercourse or vaginal examination. Similarly, high-grade squamous intraepithelial lesions or carcinoma in situ of the cervix may be more vascular and prone to bleeding in pregnancy. Invasive cervical carcinoma of the cervix, though uncommon, is generally more symptomatic than are in situ lesions. It may present with vaginal bleeding of variable amounts, vaginal discharge, or, in advanced cases, pain.

DIAGNOSIS

History may reveal recent trauma, vaginal examination, or intercourse as precipitating factors. The patient may also report a prior abnormal Pap smear or cervical lesion, possibly noted at initial obstetric evaluation earlier in the pregnancy. Direct visualization using a bivalve speculum may then reveal the source of bleeding. Of note, although cervical carcinoma is an uncommon cause of antepartum bleeding, its consideration in the differential diagnosis is essential. Stander and Lein noted a delay in diagnosis of invasive cervical cancer in 62 percent of their referrals because bleeding was attributed to other complications of pregnancy.[13]

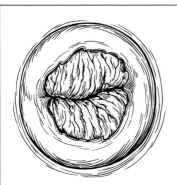
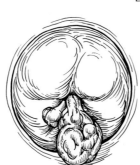
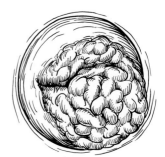

Endocervical origin of polyp

A Portio vaginalis demonstrating cervical eversion

B Large and small cervical polyps

C Advanced carcinoma of the cervix

Figure 9-6

Conditions of the cervix that may lead to bleeding in pregnancy. *A.* Erosion of a cervical ectropion. *B.* Cervical polyp. *C.* Cervical carcinoma.

PRINCIPLES OF CARE FOR VAGINAL BLEEDING IN THE SECOND HALF OF PREGNANCY

The following is a guide for the evaluation and management of the obstetric patient who presents with vaginal bleeding in the second half of pregnancy. Management strategies are based on the etiology of the bleeding, maternal stability, fetal condition and gestational age. Aspects of the guideline may be modified according to the presentation and clinical acuity of each individual patient. The basic principles that apply to the care of *all* obstetric patients who present with vaginal bleeding, however, are listed below.

1. Consultation with an obstetrician is appropriate for *all* cases of bleeding in the second half of pregnancy. If the fetus is potentially viable outside the uterus (≥23 to 24 weeks gestational age), early notification of the pediatrician is also strongly encouraged.
2. Ideally, management should be done at a facility equipped to care for a compromised and possibly premature neonate.
3. Whenever an obstetric patient presents with vaginal bleeding, evaluation and resuscitative efforts should begin immediately. If fetal compromise is present, maternal resuscitation is the first priority and may result in improved fetal status.
4. Remember that there are *two* patients. Evaluation and management must always consider them both.
5. *Never perform a vaginal or rectal examination until placenta previa has been excluded.* These examinations may provoke severe hemorrhage in a patient with placenta previa.
6. Establish gestational age as accurately as possible in all patients. Management decisions are strongly influenced by this information. Previable fetuses (less than 23 to 24 weeks gestational age, incapable of extrauterine existence) are considered very differently from viable fetuses (24 to 25 weeks or greater). Likewise, term or near-term fetuses (36 weeks or greater) are considered differently from preterm fetuses (25 to 35 weeks).

Consultation with an obstetrician is appropriate for all *cases of bleeding in the second half of pregnancy.* At these advanced gestations, many patients will already have initiated prenatal care with an obstetrician. Clinical acuity, however, may require involvement of the most readily available obstetrician. In the vast majority of cases of obstetric bleeding suspected to be from a source in the upper genital tract, hospital admission for either delivery or observation is necessary.

Ideally, management should be done at a facility equipped to care for a compromised and possibly premature neonate. Studies have demonstrated improved outcome for premature fetuses transferred to a regional neonatal intensive care center prior to rather than after delivery.[14,15] Thus, if the initial evaluation of obstetric bleeding occurs at a facility that is not capable of the long-term management of critically ill and possibly premature neonates, then referral to a facility that has these capabilities is desirable. This, however, may not always be feasible if the mother is unstable. If fetal or maternal concerns require immediate delivery or render transport of the pregnant patient unsafe, then delivery, resuscitation, and postpartum neonatal transport are advised. The issues of transport are discussed elsewhere in this book (see Chap. 10).

Whenever an obstetric patient presents with hemorrhage, resuscitative efforts should begin immediately. If fetal distress is present, maternal resuscitation may result in improved fetal status. The position of the gravid patient greatly affects cardiac output and must always be considered. In the supine position, a large uterus may compress the inferior vena cava and compromise venous return. This is relieved by placing the patient on her side or, if that is not possible, by displacing the uterus laterally with a pillow under one side of the maternal pelvis and lumbar spine. If hypotension is present, the Trendelenburg position may also improve venous return. As for all patients, the ABCs (airway, breathing, circulation) of resuscitation are followed. Intravenous access is established with two large-bore intravenous catheters, and crystalloid fluid resuscitation is initiated.

MATERNAL HEMODYNAMIC ASSESSMENT

Visual appraisals of vaginal blood loss are notoriously underestimated. Additionally, maternal hemorrhage may be concealed in abruptio placentae and uterine rupture. Clinical signs of hypovolemia must therefore be used to guide resuscitative efforts. A quick inspection of the patient may reveal obvious hemodynamic compromise. Decreased skin tone, warmth, and delayed capillary refill reflect compromised tissue perfusion. Maternal vital signs may also reflect changes in volume status. During pregnancy, however, compensatory hemodynamic mechanisms (e.g., expanded blood volume) are such that a normal blood pressure and heart rate may be seen in the setting of dangerous hypovolemia. Normal vital signs, therefore, should be interpreted with caution.

Other parameters of organ perfusion, such as urine output via an indwelling catheter, more accurately reflect volume status. A urine flow of at least 30 to 60 mL/h is desirable. Although maintaining a hematocrit above 30 percent is ideal, measurements obtained during resuscitative efforts may be inaccurate. In cases where hemodynamic assessment remains difficult, invasive hemodynamic monitoring is recommended.

Obstetric hemorrhage can also be associated with disseminated intravascular coagulopathy. A coagulopathy should be suspected with abruptio placentae, uterine rupture, or when hemorrhage has been severe. The patient may demonstrate clinical evidence of an evolving coagulopathy with mucosal bleeding, excessive bleeding at puncture sites, bruising, or hematuria. Initial laboratory studies on presentation include a complete blood count and a type and cross-match. A coagulation profile should also be sent, including fibrin split products, D dimers, fibrinogen, and platelet count. A quick bedside assessment of clotting function, however, may be performed with the clot observation test. Blood in a red-topped test tube (without additives) that does not clot within 6 minutes may indicate a coagulopathy with significant fibrinogen depletion.

RESUSCITATION

Normal saline is used for the initial resuscitation. When blood loss is excessive, however, large-volume crystalloid infusion may have deleterious effects on plasma oncotic pressure, oxygen-carrying capacity, and coagulation factor concentration. When blood loss is massive (class III or IV hemorrhage), therefore, blood transfusion is necessary.

Transfusion of whole blood provides both oxygen-carrying capacity and blood-volume expansion. One unit of whole blood contains approximately 450 mL of blood and 63 mL of preservative and anticoagulant and will increase the hematocrit of an adult by about 3 percent. Whole blood stored for over 24 h, however, contains few viable platelets or granulocytes and decreased levels of factors V and VII.

To maximize the benefits of each donated unit, blood banks are now fractionating whole blood into its specific components. Thus, whole blood is almost never available for transfusion. Red blood cells are prepared from whole blood by removing 200 to 250 mL of plasma and stored in preservative and anticoagulant. Packed cells do not contain functional platelets or granulocytes but have the same oxygen-carrying capacity as whole blood; each unit will also increase the hematocrit by about 3 percent.

Ideally, blood should be typed and cross-matched to avoid hemolytic transfusion reactions. With massive obstetric hemorrhage, however, urgent transfusion of O-negative blood may be substituted. Facilities equipped to handle obstetric emergencies should always have O-negative blood available for immediate use.

CORRECTION OF COAGULOPATHY

Massive transfusion and fluid resuscitation lead to dilutional thrombocytopenia and decreased coagulation factor concentration. Additionally, bleeding may initiate a DIC or a dangerous consumptive coagulopathy. When clinical signs of inappropriate bleeding or laboratory confirmation of coagulopathy with continued obstetric hemorrhage are present, intervention is warranted.

Platelet concentrate is administered for thrombocytopenia associated with obstetric hemorrhage and coagulopathy. Each unit increases the platelet count by approximately $10,000/\mu L$. When DIC is present, however, the half-life of each transfused unit is markedly diminished. Fresh frozen plasma, prepared by separating plasma from whole blood,

may be used to correct coagulation factor deficiencies. Clinical improvement or normalization of the prothrombin and partial thromboplastin times is used to guide management.

TRANSFUSION RISKS

Despite blood bank testing, hemolytic transfusion reactions with ABO incompatibility remain a risk of blood transfusion. Rh sensitization may also occur if an Rh-negative recipient receives Rh-positive blood. This, of course, poses a special problem for the obstetric patient with a potentially Rh-positive fetus. Due to small amounts of red blood cells in platelet concentrates. Rh-negative patients should also receive only Rh-negative platelets. If this is unavailable, however, 300 μg of Rh immune globulin may be administered at the time of platelet transfusion to prevent Rh sensitization.

Transmission of viral infections, such as hepatitis, human immunodeficiency virus, and cytomegalovirus (CMV) also remains a risk with blood transfusion. In the adult, transfusion of CMV-containing blood is a concern primarily for the immunocompromised patient. In the pregnant patient who has not been previously exposed to the virus, however, there is potential for transplacental passage to the fetus and possible adverse fetal and neonatal sequelae. Transfusion of CMV-negative or frozen-thawed-deglycerolized red blood cells is ideal, but it is not always practical with acute hemorrhage.

VASOACTIVE DRUGS

With obstetric hemorrhage, hypovolemia may lead to maternal hypotension. Fluid resuscitation and blood component therapy are critical components of resuscitation. Vasopressors, if used in a hypovolemic pregnant patient, may critically compromise blood flow to vital maternal organs and to the fetus. These drugs, therefore, should be used only when hypotension persists despite adequate fluid resuscitation. Invasive hemodynamic monitoring is strongly recommended to guide fluid management when these drugs are necessary.

OTHER ASPECTS OF THE MATERNAL EVALUATION

HISTORY

An accurate history is invaluable to both diagnosis and clinical decision making in obstetric hemorrhage. Questions regarding the acute event are helpful in determining the cause of bleeding. Did activity, such as trauma or intercourse, precede the bleeding? If pain is present, what is its quality and character? Is the pain episodic, like uterine contractions? Did contractions precede the bleeding? Has there been fetal movement since the bleeding episode?

The prenatal history is also important. Has the patient received prenatal care? Have there been prior bleeding episodes? Is the estimated date of delivery known, and if so, how was it determined? Have there been prior ultrasounds that may have evaluated placental location? Are there any other complications, such as high blood pressure or premature contractions? Have any lower genital tract lesions been identified during the course of prenatal care?

The past obstetric history may also be useful to evaluate maternal risk for various complications. What is the patient's gravidity (how many times has she conceived?) and parity (how many times has she given birth after 20 weeks gestational age?). Have there been any abortions requiring uterine curettage? Have there been any cesarean sections or other surgeries on the uterus? Have prior pregnancies been complicated by placental abruption or previa?

Finally, maternal medical and social history may identify risk factors that could guide management of the potentially critically ill patient. Are there maternal vascular disorders, such as hypertension or vasculitis? Is there any history of renal disease? Does the patient have a history of abnormal Pap smears? Does she smoke or use cocaine?

PHYSICAL EXAMINATION

In addition to the hemodynamic assessment outlined above, other aspects of the maternal physical examination are critical for both diagnosis and management of obstetric hemorrhage. Abdominal examination may identify areas of focal tenderness. Additionally, fetal movements, uterine contractions, or frank uterine tetany are identified during palpation of the gravid uterus. To identify fetal lie, Leopold's maneuvers are performed. A fetal malpresentation is diagnosed when the cephalic prominence is not presenting in the pelvis or palpation of the uterine fundus fails to identify a fetal part (transverse lie), as is often seen in placenta previa. With uterine rupture, the fetus may also be noted to be in an abnormal lie or the extruded fetus may be palpated in the maternal abdomen.

TOCODYNAMOMETRY

Evaluation of uterine activity is an important aspect of diagnosis. Uterine activity is usually present with abruptio placentae; it occurs less commonly with placenta previa. Uterine contractions, however, are not always palpable. External tocodynamometry measures the change in shape of the abdominal wall with uterine contractions and is used to provide a graphic display of the frequency and duration of uterine contractions over time. Contraction monitoring should be used in all patients being evaluated for obstetric hemorrhage, if available.

Never perform a vaginal or rectal examination until placenta previa has been ruled out. Vaginal examination is deferred until placenta previa has been ruled out. If a placenta previa was not seen on a prior ultrasound during this pregnancy or one performed at presentation, then vaginal exam-

ination may be safely performed. Speculum examination allows for direct visualization of the site of the bleeding. Blood exiting through the uterine cervix indicates an upper genital tract source. Lesions of the vagina and cervix, on the other hand, may also be identified at this time.

After the speculum is removed, digital vaginal examination is performed to obtain information regarding cervical dilation and effacement. Confirmation of the fetal presenting part and its station in the maternal pelvis is also an important part of this examination.

ASPECTS OF THE FETAL EVALUATION

Clinical decision making in obstetric hemorrhage is profoundly influenced by fetal condition and gestational age.

ASSESSMENT OF GESTATIONAL AGE

Establish gestational age as accurately as possible in all patients. Accurate knowledge of fetal gestational age is critical to rational decision making in obstetrics. Term pregnancies are considered to be those between 38 and 42 weeks gestational age. Continued intrauterine existence in the setting of obstetric bleeding rarely benefits and may even harm these fetuses. The threshold of fetal viability, on the other hand, is approximately 24 weeks (depending on the capabilities of the facility caring for the neonate). Fetuses at less than 24 weeks of gestation are previable; this means that their immaturity renders them incapable of extrauterine existence. Facilitation of delivery is not lifesaving for these fetuses and will only lead to their demise. Finally, fetuses between 25 and 38 weeks of gestation are preterm. These fetuses may benefit from continued intrauterine existence and should be delivered only if the risk of continuation of the pregnancy to both the mother and the fetus outweighs the risk of morbidity and mortality due to complications of prematurity. It is strongly emphasized that within this gestational age range there is dramatic variation in potential for neonatal morbidity and mortality. This must be considered carefully when one is making management decisions in preterm pregnancies (Table 9-2).

There are several methods for estimating fetal gestational age (Table 9-3). Each method has a standard error associated with it; in establishing gestational age, this standard error must be considered. This is especially critical in patients who present at the threshold of fetal viability. For example, if a patient presents with bleeding and is found to be at 22 weeks of gestational age by a method with a standard error of 3 weeks, the fetus may, in fact, be viable. With this uncertainty, decision making can be extremely difficult.

Last menstrual period (LMP), when known with accuracy, is a reliable clinical estimator of gestational age. *Postmenstrual weeks* is an acceptable unit of time for dating pregnancies. A known LMP will be less reliable for dating pregnancies in patients with irregular menstrual cycles or in those who conceived while using hormonal contraceptives.

Table 9-2

PERCENT SURVIVAL BY BIRTH WEIGHT AND GESTATIONAL AGE AMONG NEONATES BORN AT THE UNIVERSITY OF MICHIGAN MEDICAL CENTER, 1991–1994

	Percent Survival	N
Gestational age		
≤24 weeks	31	16
25 weeks	69	26
26 weeks	92	24
27 weeks	89	38
28 weeks	97	38
29 weeks	98	46
30 weeks	100	58
Birth weight		
<500 g	0	2
501–750 g	65	48
751–1000 g	92	64
1001–1250 g	96	74
1251–1500 g	100	107

[a]These data exclude neonates with congenital anomalies; those that lived to be discharged home were considered to be survivors. (Data courtesy of Roger Faix, MD, University of Michigan.)

When an LMP is unknown or unreliable, obstetric ultrasound may be used to establish an estimated date of confinement. Using the crown-rump length in the first trimester, the standard deviation of ultrasound dating is approximately 1 week. Assignments of gestational age using nomograms for biparietal diameter, abdominal circumference, and femur length have a standard deviation of approximately 2 weeks in the second trimester and 3 weeks in the third. Since early ultrasound examinations are more accurate, studies performed earlier in the pregnancy are preferable.

If a patient is unable to provide a history, the prenatal record is unavailable, and the patient's clinical condition precludes a lengthy ultrasound evaluation to estimate gestational age, a fundal height measurement may be used. A simple rule is to consider gestational age in weeks to be grossly equivalent to the height in centimeters from the symphysis to the uterine fundus (Fig. 9-7). This crude method, however, has a standard error that is quite large, and it is particularly inaccurate with maternal obesity or in multiple gestations. Additionally, with obstetric bleeding due to abruptio placentae, concealed uterine hemorrhage may increase the fundal height and render the measurement even less reliable.

ASSESSMENT OF FETAL LUNG MATURITY

Knowledge of gestational age and estimated fetal weight enables prediction of the potential for neonatal morbidity and mortality in fetuses delivered prematurely. Respiratory distress syndrome (RDS) is one of the most common complications of prematurity and the risk for this complication decreases with advancing gestational age. Although lung maturity is generally present by 36 weeks of gestational age, there is considerable variation among individual fetuses.

Since decisions regarding expectant management versus facilitating a delivery in complicated pregnancies are optimized if the risk of an adverse outcome is known with accuracy, laboratory tests for the evaluation of fetal lung maturity in utero have been developed. If the patient and fetus are both clinically stable, amniotic fluid may be obtained by amniocentesis and tested for the presence of phosphotidylglycerol (PG). The presence of PG indicates a low risk for RDS if the fetus is delivered. Tests for the presence of pulmonary surfactant, such as the shake test, the foam stability index, or the lecithin/sphingomyelin (L/S) ratio also provide information regarding risk for RDS.

Because these tests are invasive, they should be performed only if there is a reasonable chance of demonstrating pulmonary maturity. In addition, although the predictive value for RDS can be quite high, other complications of prematurity—such as intraventricular hemorrhage, necrotizing enterocolitis, and patent ductus arteriosus—may still occur in the presence of documented fetal lung maturity.[16]

EVALUATION OF FETAL WELL-BEING

With obstetric bleeding, significant reductions in placental blood flow or direct fetal blood loss may result in fetal distress or even death. Therefore fetal well-being should be evaluated promptly. This is of paramount importance in any patient with a potentially viable fetus.

During the initial evaluation of the obstetric patient, fetal heart tones must be established. A Doppler device is usually readily available in most emergency facilities and may be used to identify fetal heart tones. Alternatively, a fetoscope may be used to auscultate fetal heart tones beyond 19 to 20 weeks of gestational age. Maternal pulse signals are easily obtained in the pelvis; therefore, once a signal is received, fetal and maternal pulsations should be differentiated by simultaneous palpation of maternal peripheral pulses. If Doppler is unable to locate a fetal pulse signal, real-time ultrasound may be used to view fetal cardiac activity directly.

With continued management of the bleeding patient, more sensitive indicators of fetal well-being must be employed. Because the fetus cannot be evaluated directly, indirect methods of evaluation for potential fetal compromise have been developed. Decreased oxygen delivery to the fetus and subsequent fetal hypoxemia and/or acidemia lead to central nervous system (CNS) cellular dysfunction. The resultant decrease in fetal activity and reflex changes in cardiac ac-

Table 9-3

ASSESSMENT OF GESTATIONAL AGE AND FETAL LUNG MATURITY

Test	Interpretation	Reliability/Comments
Last menstrual period	Weeks from last menstrual period	A reliable clinical estimator of gestational age if known with accuracy *Caution:* less reliable in patients with irregular menstrual cycles or when cycles are considered greater or less than 28 days.
Fundal height	Distance between the symphysis pubis and the uterine fundus measured in centimeters approximates gestational age in weeks	Accuracy ± 3 weeks from about 18–35 weeks gestational age *Caution:* less reliable with maternal obesity, extremes of maternal height, transverse fetal lie, or abnormalities of fetal growth (intrauterine growth retardation, or macrosomia). Concealed bleeding from abruptio placentae may also affect this measurement.
Ultrasound	First trimester: crown-rump length	Accuracy within 3–5 days between 6–10 weeks gestational age
	Second trimester: biparietal diameter	Accuracy+/− 2 weeks in the second trimester
	Third trimester: multiple parameters (biparietal diameter, long bone length, abdominal circumference)	Accuracy+/− 2–3 weeks in the third trimester
Amniotic fluid pulmonary maturity studies		
Shake test	An assay of fetal pulmonary surfactant that tests the ability of amniotic fluid to generate foam in the presence of a fixed concentration of ethanol	A positive test is predictive of pulmonary maturity *Caution:* unreliable if specimen contains blood contaminants
Foam stability index	Similar to shake test, using various concentrations of ethanol	A value ≥47 is predictive of pulmonary maturity *Caution:* unreliable if specimen contains blood contaminants
L/S ratio	Ratio of lecithin to sphyngomyelin in amniotic fluid	A ratio ≥2.0 is predictive of pulmonary maturity *Caution:* unreliable if specimen contains blood contaminants or in diabetics
DSPC (disaturated phosphotidylcholine)	Measures a component of pulmonary surfactant	A value>500 μg/dL is predictive of pulmonary maturity Note: reliable in the presence of blood contaminants

tivity are associated with altered fetal heart rate patterns. Fetal heart rate patterns seen with continuous monitoring, therefore, reflect fetal condition and is an effective method to assess fetal well-being in bleeding in the second half of pregnancy. When a woman carrying a potentially viable fetus presents with vaginal bleeding, continuous fetal heart rate monitoring should be employed immediately.

Fetal heart rate signals are obtained using a Doppler ultrasound probe on the maternal abdomen. The fetal cardiac wall motion detected is then electronically transformed into a continuous heart rate tracing for evaluation of temporal patterns (Fig. 9-8). Although the basic components of fetal heart rate monitoring and other tests of fetal well-being are discussed briefly below, the interpretation of these tracings

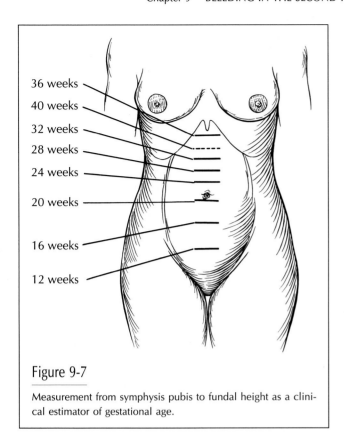

Figure 9-7

Measurement from symphysis pubis to fundal height as a clinical estimator of gestational age.

is often subtle and requires an experienced practitioner. The following discussion, therefore, is intended only to familiarize the emergency physician with the basic elements of the fetal heart tracing.

The *baseline heart rate, short- and long-term heart rate variability,* and the presence of periodic *acceleration* or *decelerations* are significant aspects of the fetal heart rate pattern (Table 9-4).

FETAL HEART RATE

A normal baseline fetal heart rate ranges from 120 to 160 beats per minute. Fetal tachycardia is a sustained elevation of the fetal heart rate above 160 beats per minute. Fetal activity may cause brief elevation in baseline heart rate above 160 beats per minute, or *accelerations.* These, however, are not sustained. Prolonged fetal tachycardia may be associated with maternal fever, intraamniotic infection, fetal anemia, or hypoxia. Administration of certain drugs that increase maternal heart rate, such as beta-sympathomimetic or parasympatholytic drugs, may also result in fetal tachycardia. Rarely, a fetal cardiac tachyarryhthmia may be present.

Fetal bradycardia is a sustained decrease in the fetal heart rate below 120 beats per minute. Decreased fetal heart rates may be associated with fetal hypoxia and acidemia and may potentially require emergent surgical delivery of the fetus. Administration of medications that decrease maternal heart rate, such as beta blockers, may also depress fetal heart rate.

VARIABILITY

Variability in the fetal heart rate baseline represents the normal interplay between cardioinhibitory and cardiostimulatory centers in the fetal brain. It is one of the most sensitive indicators of fetal well-being. Short-term variability represents a beat-to-beat variation of at least 3 beats per minute in fetal heart rate around an overall baseline. Long-term variations in heart rate of about 3 to 5 cycles per minute occur as well (Fig. 9-9A and B). Its absence may indicate fetal compromise. Other causes of decreased variability include evaluation during fetal sleep state, fetal CNS immaturity (fetuses should start to demonstrate variability in heart rate at around 28 weeks), maternal administration of CNS depressants, or fetal CNS anomalies.

FETAL HEART RATE ACCELERATIONS

Accelerations in fetal heart rate typically occur with movement in the healthy fetus. An acceleration is defined as an increase in fetal heart rate of at least 15 beats per minute

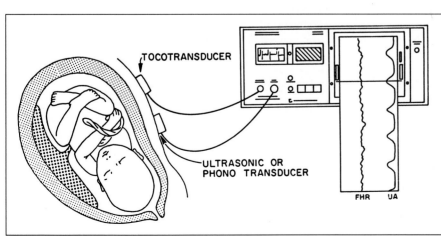

Figure 9-8

Fetal heart rate monitoring and tocodynamometry. Ultrasound Doppler signals are obtained from the moving fetal heart valves and electronically transduced into a fetal heart rate. External uterine contraction monitoring measures uterine displacement for a graphic display of frequency and duration of contractions.

Table 9-4

COMMON PATTERNS OF THE FETAL HEART RATE

FHR Pattern	Characteristic	Cause	Intervention
Normal baseline	Baseline rate 120–160 BPM (Fig. 11-1).	Normal	None
Acceleration	Elevation of fetal heart rate 15 beats per minute above baseline for 15 s (Fig. 11-1).	Normal, reassuring	None
Early deceleration	Shallow, symmetric slowing of the heart rate, which reaches the nadir at the peak of the uterine contraction. Appears as a "mirror image" of the uterine contraction (Fig. 11-2).	Fetal head compression	None
Late deceleration	U-shaped slowing of the fetal heart rate with gradual onsets and returns to baseline that are shallow (10–30 beats per minute). They reach their nadir *after* the peak of the contraction and return to baseline *after* uterine contraction (Fig. 11-3).	Uteroplacental insufficiency; CNS hypoxia; if severe, myocardial depression	1. Consult obstetrician ASAP 2. Start oxygen by mask at 8–10 L/min 3. Begin intravenous lactated Ringer's solution and give 200- to 500-mL bolus of fluid 4. Change position of mother (e.g., left or right lateral decubitus) 5. Avoid supine position
Variable deceleration	Slowing of the fetal heart rate with abrupt onset and return to baseline. Varies in depth, duration and shape, but usually occurs during a uterine contraction (Fig. 11-4).	Cord compression	Consult obstetrician if persistent (occurs with most uterine contractions) or any of the "rule of 60s" are present: more than 60s long, below 60 beats per minute or more than 60 beats per minute below baseline heart rate. Begin in utero resuscitation as in late decelerations.
Beat-to-beat variability (BBV)	The variation of successive beats in the fetal heart rate.	Diminished BBV may be associated with fetal hypoxia; it is also normally seen with fetal sleep cycles or in response to certain medications (e.g., narcotics).	Must be interpreted carefully, paying particular attention to baseline and other periodic changes. Expert consultation should be sought if diminished.
Tachycardia	Sustained fetal heart rate above 160. Mild: 160–180 Severe: >180	Fetal hypoxemia, maternal fever, certain drugs (e.g., beta sympathomimetics) fetal arrhythmias.	Same as with late deceleration.
Bradycardia	Sustained fetal heart rate <120	Fetal hypoxemia, fetal heart block, use of beta blockers.	Same as with late deceleration.

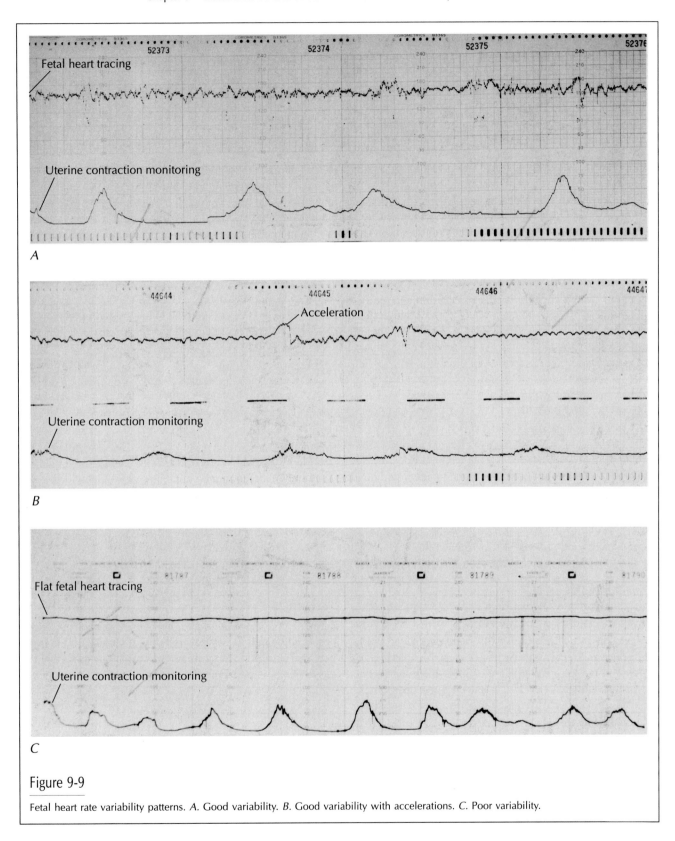

Figure 9-9

Fetal heart rate variability patterns. *A.* Good variability. *B.* Good variability with accelerations. *C.* Poor variability.

over baseline and lasting at least 15 sec. The presence of periodic accelerations is another sensitive indicator of fetal well-being. The differential diagnosis for the absence of periodic accelerations is similar to that for decreased variability.

FETAL HEART RATE DECELERATIONS

Transient slowing of the fetal heart rate is known as a *deceleration.* Decelerations are described as early, variable, or late, depending on their relationship to uterine contractions

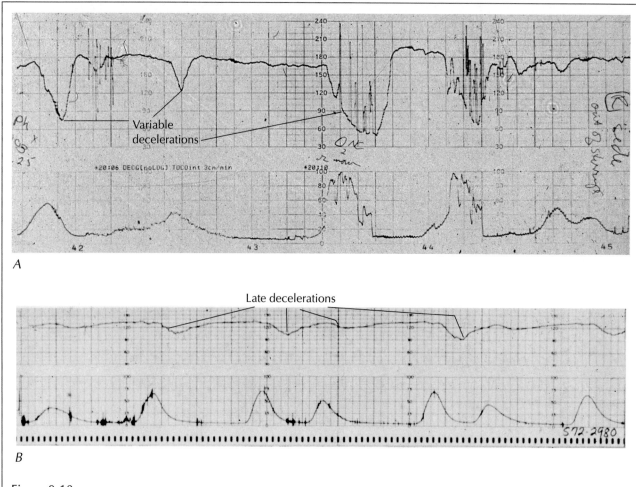

Figure 9-10

Fetal heart rate deceleration patterns. Early decelerations begin with the onset of a contraction and return to baseline at the end of the contraction. *A.* Variable decelerations. There is no consistent relationship with contractions and the pattern is variable in morphology. *B.* Late decelerations. These occur after the onset of a contraction, with a slow return to baseline after completion of the contraction.

and the morphology of the pattern (Fig. 9-10). With early decelerations, mild slowing of the heart rate starts with a contraction and recovers at the end of a contraction. It is often seen in the late, active phase of labor or in the second stage and is thought to represent fetal vagal response to head compression in the birth canal. It is generally not associated with fetal compromise.

Variable decelerations (Fig. 9-10*A*) are not uniform in shape, amplitude, or duration and do not necessarily have a consistent relationship to uterine contractions. They are thought to represent vagal responses to umbilical cord compression. Prolonged, deep, and repetitive variable decelerations may be associated with fetal hypoxemia or acidemia.

Late decelerations (Fig. 9-10*B*) occur after a contraction begins, are uniform in shape, and slowly return to baseline after the completion of a contraction. Pathologic decelerations are repetitive with contractions and usually represent compromised uteroplacental exchange. This pattern is strongly associated with fetal hypoxemia or acidemia and is especially ominous when variability of fetal heart rate is decreased or absent. A summary of various methods used to assess fetal well-being are listed in Table 9-3.

THE KLEIHAUER-BETKE TEST

The Kleihauer-Betke (K-B) test is an acid elution test that identifies the presence of fetal cells in the maternal circulation as evidence of fetomaternal hemorrhage. If nonreassuring fetal heart rate patterns are present, the test evaluates for fetomaternal hemorrhage as a potential cause of fetal distress and can quantitate fetal blood loss if fetal cells are found in the maternal circulation. However, because turn around time is long, clinical decisions are based on the fetal heart tracing, not the K-B result.

In the Rh-negative patient, where fetomaternal hemorrhage of any magnitude may lead to maternal isoimmunization, the test is employed to direct the use of Rh-immune globulin. Rh immune globulin should be administered to D-negative women with bleeding during pregnancy. Generally, 300 μg of Rh immune globulin administered intramuscularly is sufficient to cover a 15-mL packed red blood cell or 30-mL whole blood fetomaternal exchange. If the K-B test indicates a larger bleed, additional Rh immune globulin should be administered.

A few caveats regarding interpretation of the K-B test must be mentioned. First, fetal blood cells last a variable amount of time in the maternal circulation, depending on the maternal-fetal ABO compatibility. When incompatibility exists, fetal cells are quickly lysed in the maternal circulation. Delayed testing must, therefore, be interpreted with caution. Additionally, fetal-type cells may be seen with certain maternal hemoglobinopathies, such as thalassemias, leading to a false-positive K-B test.

SPECIFIC MANAGEMENT PROTOCOLS

MANAGEMENT OF ABRUPTIO PLACENTAE

The approach to managing abruptio placentae depends on three factors: (1) maternal hemodynamic status, (2) fetal condition, and (3) gestational age of the fetus. In general, the management of these cases should be directed by a physician experienced in dealing with bleeding in the second half of pregnancy who can effect immediate operative delivery if necessary.

INTRAUTERINE FETAL DEMISE

With severe abruptio placentae associated with intrauterine fetal demise (IUFD), expeditious delivery is warranted. Hemorrhage and evolution of DIC continues until the fetus and placenta are delivered. Vaginal delivery is the preferred route. Given the high incidence of DIC in severe placental abruption, surgical disruption of maternal tissues by cesarean section may dramatically increase maternal morbidity and should be performed only if absolutely necessary to control hemorrhage. Ongoing blood loss may be rapid and requires aggressive replacement. Central intravenous access should be considered early, since coagulopathy can evolve, resulting in difficulties with central venous cannulation. The volume of ongoing vaginal bleeding is continuously assessed, with an understanding that occult blood loss due to concealed hemorrhage may be present. Since visual estimates of bleeding are unreliable, a disposable pad may be placed beneath the patient. These pads may provide a more objective assessment of blood loss (1 g = 1 mL). To evaluate for possible concealed hemor-

rhage and an enlarging uterus, serial measurements of fundal height are also helpful.

Labor is usually rapid after severe placental abruption. Contractions may be quite strong and are occasionally tetanic. Patients with uterine tetany due to abruptio placentae may also be at risk for rupture of the uterus from the high pressures generated within the cavity. Uterine decompression by artificial rupture of membranes (amniotomy) often improves this contraction pattern. Relief of the excessive intrauterine pressure may also decrease the risk of DIC and amniotic fluid embolus. The progress of labor should be monitored closely, preferably with an intrauterine pressure catheter. If uterine contractions are not adequate in strength, oxytocin should be used to expedite delivery.

In the absence of coexistent maternal medical problems or sequelae of hypovolemia and DIC (adult respiratory distress syndrome, acute tubular necrosis, organ infarction, or hemorrhage), recovery and correction of coagulation defects occur quickly after delivery of the fetus and placenta.

Although cesarean section allows for rapid delivery, the morbidity associated with surgery in this setting makes operative delivery unacceptable as an initial management strategy in most cases. It should be reserved only for failure to progress in labor or excessive maternal hemorrhage with an inability to replace ongoing losses adequately prior to an anticipated vaginal delivery. Hypovolemia and coagulopathy should be aggressively corrected prior to and during the cesarean section.

NONREASSURING FETAL HEART RATE PATTERNS

Lesser degrees of placental separation may not immediately lead to fetal demise but may compromise the fetus and be reflected in abnormal fetal heart rate patterns. In these cases, accurate knowledge of gestational age is critical. If the fetus is viable, urgent delivery by cesarean section is usually warranted. Again, hypovolemia and coagulopathy should be aggressively managed in preparation for surgery. A K-B test in these cases may be helpful to evaluate for potential fetomaternal hemorrhage.

Placental abruption in previable pregnancies is uncommon. If, however, the fetus is not viable (less than 24 weeks gestation and the gestational age is known with certainty), immediate delivery by cesarean section would not be lifesaving for the fetus and management should be based on maternal considerations. If maternal hemorrhage is significant and potentially life-threatening, timely delivery is indicated. Labor is often spontaneous in these cases, but augmentation with pitocin may be necessary. If, however, maternal bleeding is not excessive or potentially life-threatening, expectant management with close observation may be allowed. Maternal resuscitation can sometimes improve fetal condition. Prolonged fetal stress, however, may lead to abnormal fetal growth or eventual demise.

REASSURING FETAL HEART RATE PATTERNS

Frequently, abruptio placentae has a less dramatic presentation, where the fetus is not compromised and reassuring patterns of fetal heart rate are seen. Unfortunately, the natural history and evolution of these nonacute cases is difficult to predict. Marginal sinus separations may lead to transient symptomatology that resolves without recurrence. Cases of minor abruptio placentae that may seem clinically insignificant at initial presentation, however, also have the potential to lead to progressively larger degrees of placental involvement and subsequent fetal distress. The presence of persistent uterine tenderness or uterine activity should increase suspicion of progression. Presently, however, there is no reliable method for distinguishing patients destined for evolution of their placental abruption from those with more benign clinical courses.

If the patient is at term, facilitating a vaginal delivery is appropriate. In equivocal cases, testing of fetal lung maturity may be helpful for decision making. If the patient is not yet at term, expectant management and prolonged observation is the best strategy. Unless the fetus is previable, there must be evidence for ongoing fetal well-being using continuous external fetal monitoring for expectant management to be an option. The risk of recurrent bleeding and premature delivery with poor perinatal outcome, however, remains high with abruptio placentae managed expectantly.[17]

Maternal corticosteroid therapy has been shown to improve neonatal morbidity and mortality with premature delivery.[18,19] Antepartum administration of corticosteroids is therefore recommended in viable pregnancies prior to 34 weeks gestational age being managed expectantly, although the gestational age range in which this therapy is most beneficial is controversial.

MANAGEMENT OF PLACENTA PREVIA

As with abruptio placentae, management approaches depend on maternal hemodynamic status, fetal condition, and gestational age of the fetus. If delivery is elected, cesarean section is indicated with marginal or complete placenta previa. In cases of low-lying placenta, vaginal delivery may be considered provided that there is continued evidence for fetal well-being, the patient is stable, ongoing blood losses are not significant, and personnel and facilities are available should the need for operative delivery arise.

NONREASSURING FETAL HEART RATE PATTERNS

Fetal compromise is seen much less commonly in pregnancies complicated by placenta previa than in abruptio placentae. When fetal compromise is present in viable pregnancies, immediate delivery by cesarean section is indicated.

In the absence of fetal compromise, management is based on maternal hemodynamic stability and fetal maturity.

HEMORRHAGE WITH MATERNAL HEMODYNAMIC INSTABILITY

Potentially life-threatening maternal hemorrhage from placenta previa is an indication for urgent cesarean section. Appropriate fluid and blood component replacement in preparation for surgery is essential. With severe ongoing hemorrhage from placenta previa, maternal blood loss will continue until the fetus is delivered and the placenta is removed. Surgery, therefore, should not be delayed while awaiting crossmatched blood.

HEMORRHAGE WITH MATERNAL HEMODYNAMIC STABILITY

Historically, placenta previa complicated by vaginal bleeding was an indication for urgent delivery, without consideration for fetal maturity. In term patients, the benefits of intrauterine existence have been maximized and timely delivery is warranted. When fetal maturity status is equivocal and delivery is desired, fetal pulmonary maturity studies are helpful.

Complications of prematurity, however, are the major cause of perinatal morbidity and mortality in pregnancies complicated by placenta previa. When the fetus is clearly premature by gestational age or when pulmonary maturity studies reveal an unacceptably high risk of RDS if delivery were to occur, a delay in delivery may result in marked improvement in perinatal outcome.

Because significant maternal bleeding may occur in placenta previa without affecting fetal well-being, protocols for aggressive expectant management of placenta previa—using strict bed rest, volume expansion, and transfusion therapy—have been developed, with positive results. Since bleeding from placenta previa occurs with the development of the lower uterine segment and subsequent disruption of placental vessels, it is reasonable that tocolysis of uterine contractions would result in improved outcome. This, however, remains an area of controversy.[20–23] If expectant management is elected, fetal well-being must be assured with continuous monitoring of the fetal heart rate.

Many episodes of bleeding from placenta previa are self-limited. Recurrences, however, are common and subsequent episodes tend to be more severe. Unfortunately, adverse outcomes—such as premature delivery, intrauterine fetal growth retardation, and perinatal death—remain common despite aggressive expectant management. The severity of these complications tends to correlate with the number of antepartum bleeding episodes.[24] Since these patients have a high likelihood of premature delivery, maternal corticosteroid therapy is indicated in those being managed expectantly.

MANAGEMENT OF UTERINE RUPTURE

Uterine rupture with maternal hemorrhage and fetal distress or demise requires immediate laparotomy. Treatment for hemorrhage, shock, and possible coagulopathy should be instituted without delay in preparation for surgery.

MANAGEMENT OF VASA PREVIA

In vasa previa diagnosed prior to vessel disruption, delivery by cesarean section is indicated. In ruptured vasa previa, if the fetus is viable, delivery should be accomplished by the most expeditious route possible. This usually means cesarean section. The need for intensive neonatal resuscitation, including transfusion therapy, should be anticipated.

MANAGEMENT OF CERVICAL LESIONS

Ordinarily, when a gross cervical lesion is present, diagnosis by removal or biopsy is encouraged. The cervix, however, is a highly vascular organ in pregnancy and removal or biopsy of a lower genital tract lesion may be complicated by profuse bleeding. Specialist consultation prior to tissue sampling, therefore, is recommended when a lesion is seen on speculum examination during pregnancy.

SUMMARY

Vaginal bleeding in the second half of pregnancy is a potential obstetric emergency and always requires prompt evaluation. The principles of emergency care include stabilization of the bleeding patient, evaluation of the status of both mother and fetus, determination of the etiology of the hemorrhage and diagnosis-specific management. Bleeding may be minor and without impact on either maternal hemodynamics or fetal well being, or it may be massive, resulting in both fetal and maternal death. In general, bleeding from the lower genital tract is less immediately life-threatening. On the other hand, bleeding arising from the upper genital tract, regardless of its apparent severity, may be life-threatening. Once evaluation and resuscitative efforts are initiated, management options are ultimately limited to deciding whether the patient should be expectantly managed or delivered. If delivery is indicated, then a route must be selected (vaginal versus cesarean section). These decisions critically depend on an accurate and timely evaluation of maternal hemodynamic status, gestational age of the fetus (term, preterm, or previable), the well-being of the fetus (reassuring heart-rate patterns, nonreassuring heart rate patterns, or IUFD), and the etiology of the hemorrhage.

Although a delay of intervention can have dire consequences for both fetus and mother, unnecessary intervention can be equally devastating. Complications of prematurity are the major cause of perinatal death and lifelong morbidity in these fetuses. Expectant management allows for continued intrauterine fetal development and is, therefore, highly desirable in selected pregnancies at premature gestational ages with demonstrated maternal hemodynamic stability and fetal well-being. Bleeding from abruptio placentae and placenta previa, however, is unpredictable and has the potential to evolve into a severe hemorrhage without warning. Even with demonstrated fetal well-being, therefore, expectant management of these patients has an inherent risk.

It is readily apparent, therefore, that a rational approach to some of the most difficult management dilemmas in medicine requires not only knowledge of the unique aspects of maternal and fetal evaluation but also a thorough understanding of the risks of prematurity coupled with a respect for the catastrophic potential of vaginal bleeding in the second half of pregnancy.

References

1. Langlois SLP, Miller AG: Placenta previa—A review with emphasis on the role of ultrasound. *Aust NZ J Obstet Gynaecol* 29:110, 1989.
2. Farine D, Fox HE, Jakobson S, Timor-Tritsch IE: Vaginal ultrasound for diagnosis of placenta previa. *Am J Obstet Gynecol* 159:566, 1988.
3. Leerentveld RA, Gilberts EC, Arnold M, Wladimiroff JW: Accuracy and safety of transvaginal sonographic placental localization. *Obstet Gynecol* 76:759, 1990.
4. Pritchard JA, Cunningham G, Pritchard SA, Mason RA: On reducing the frequency of severe abruptio placentae. *Am J Obstet Gynecol* 165:1345, 1991.
5. Pearlman MD, Tintinalli JE, Lorenz RP: A prospective controlled study of outcome after trauma during pregnancy. *Am J Obstet Gynecol* 162:1502, 1990.
6. Nolan TE, Simthe RP, Devoe LD: A rapid test for abruptio placentae: Evaluation of a D-dimer latex agglutination slide test. *Am J Obstet Gynecol* 169:265, 1993.
7. Witt BR, Miles R, Wolf GC, et al: Ca125 levels in abruptio placentae. *Am J Obstet Gynecol* 164:1225, 1991.
8. Williams MA, Hickok DE, Zingham RW, Zebelman AM: Maternal serum Ca125 levels in the diagnosis of abruptio placentae. *Obstet Gynecol* 82:808, 1993.
9. Kay HH, Spritzer CE: Preliminary experience with magnetic resonance imaging in patients with third-trimester bleeding. *Obstet Gynecol* 78:424, 1991.
10. Shrout AB, Kopelman JN: Ultrasonographic diagnosis of uterine dehiscence during pregnancy. *J Ultrasound Med* 14:399, 1995.
11. Kouyoumkjian A: Velamentous insertion of the umbilical cord. *Obstet Gynecol* 56:737, 1980.
12. Nelson LH, Melone PJ, King M: Diagnosis of vasa previa with transvaginal and color flow Doppler ultrasound. *Obstet Gynecol* 76:506, 1990.
13. Stander RW, Lein JN: Carcinoma of the cervix and pregnancy. *Am J Obstet Gynecol* 79:164, 1960.
14. Lamont RF, Dunlop PD, Crowley P, et al: Comparative mortality and morbidity of infants transferred in utero or postnatally. *J Perinat Med* 11:200, 1983.

15. Obladen M, Luttkus A, Rey M, et al: Differences in morbidity and mortality according to type of referral of very low birthweight infants. *J Perinat Med* 22:53, 1994.

16. Wigton TR, Tamure RK, Wickstrom E, et al: Neonatal morbidity after preterm delivery in the presence of documented lung maturity. *Am J Obstet Gynecol* 169:951, 1993.

17. Nielson EC, Varner MW, Scott JR: The outcome of pregnancies complicated by bleeding during the second trimester. *Surg Gynecol Obstet* 173:371, 1991.

18. Collaborative Group on Antenatal Steroid Therapy: Effects of antenatal dexamethasone administration on the prevention of respiratory distress syndrome. *Am J Obstet Gynecol* 141:276, 1981.

19. Maher JE, Cliver SP, Goldenberg RL, et al: The effect of corticosteroid therapy in the very premature infant. March of Dimes Multicenter Study Group. *Am J Obstet Gynecol* 170:869, 1994.

20. Silver R, Depp R, Sabbagha RE, et al: Placenta previa: Aggressive expectant management. *Am J Obstet Gynecol* 150:15, 1984.

21. Magann EF, Johnson CA, Gookin KS, et al: Placenta previa: Does uterine activity cause bleeding? *Aust NZ J Obstet Gynaecol* 33:22, 1993.

22. Watson WJ, Cefalo RC: Magnesium sulfate tocolysis in selected patients with symptomatic placenta previa. *Am J Perinatol* 7:251, 1990.

23. Besinger RE, Moniak CW, Paskiewicz LS, et al: The effect of tocolytic use in the management of symptomatic placenta previa. *Am J Obstet Gynecol* 172:1770, 1995.

24. Gorodeski IG, Neri A, Bahary CM: Placenta previa—The identification of low- and high-risk subgroups. *Eur J Obstet Gynecol Reprod Biol* 20:133, 1985.

Section 3

PROBLEMS IN
LABOR, DELIVERY,
AND THE POSTPARTUM

Chapter 10

TRANSPORT OF THE PREGNANT WOMAN

Mark J. Lowell

The need for interhospital patient transfer has grown over the past several decades. Critically ill or injured patients may require equipment and expertise that is unavailable at a smaller hospital, or deterioration in status of a previously stable patient may require advanced care that exceeds local capabilities. In the case of pregnant women, the limited number of facilities equipped to care for their special needs makes the need for transfer more likely, because illness or injury frequently occurs in areas far away from tertiary care centers. The recent development and proliferation of freestanding "birthing centers" has also contributed to the need for transport. Although many are affiliated with a hospital, they are usually physically separate and sometimes great distances from the main facility. A review of care in birthing centers from 1989 reported an overall transfer rate of 15.8 percent.[1] A more recent descriptive study of a university-based center reported transfer rates of 12 percent for ante-partum patients and 19 percent for intrapartum patients during a 20-month study period.[2] As the number of these centers increases, it is reasonable to assume that the number of transfers will rise as well. Last, the recent growth of health maintenance organizations (HMOs) and their practice of caring for their clients at designated institutions will assure the continued need for critical care transport.

Thus, it is reasonable to assume that the need to transport pregnant women will continue to increase. This chapter focuses on some of the issues involved in the prehospital and interhospital transport of the pregnant patient.

PREHOSPITAL TRANSPORTATION

Prehospital transport refers to transport that originates at a nonmedical facility such as a residence or accident scene. The majority of transports of pregnant patients done by emergency medical technicians and paramedics are routine and uncomplicated. From a prehospital perspective, the management is based upon two principles: (1) that definitive care cannot be provided in the prehospital setting and (2) that appropriate care of the mother is the best treatment for the fetus.[3]

Most emergency medical services (EMS) systems are successful because the prehospital care providers have specific protocols that specify the care to be rendered for various medical conditions. This is known as *off-line medical control.* In the event of an unusual or unclear situation, provisions are made for direct assistance via radio or telephone from a physician or his or her designee. This is known as *on-line medical control.*

It is important for EMS systems to develop protocols that specifically identify those facilities capable of caring for the pregnant woman with a medical or surgical emergency.[3] It may be appropriate in some instances to bypass certain hospitals to get to a more sophisticated facility; for example, a woman with severe preeclampsia at 30 weeks of gestation. Other patients should be transported to the closest facility for initial stabilization. For example, pregnant patients with non-pregnancy-related complaints, patients in need of urgent airway interventions, or a newborn in distress might best be initially cared for at the closest facility. Protocols must take into account differences in transport times and the risk that a potentially longer transport may cause adverse sequelae. Both on-line and off-line medical control should be available to assist in these situations.

Although most deliveries are uncomplicated, patients that deliver in the prehospital environment or in the emergency department do have a higher risk of complications.[4] Therefore, prehospital personnel must consider the likelihood of imminent delivery versus the ability to transport the mother to the hospital safely. If delivery appears imminent, it is usually most prudent to deliver at the scene, because delivery in the close confines of a moving ambulance, especially if there is only one caregiver, can be difficult. The prehospital caregiver should assist the delivery. Only two conditions require insertion of the sterile gloved hand into the vagina by the prehospital provider[3]: (1) In the event of a breech presentation, it may become necessary to insert a hand into the vagina to flex the fetal neck to assist in the delivery of the aftercoming head (see Chap. 12). (2) In the event of a prolapsed umbilical cord, the provider's hand should gently dis-

place the presenting part off the cord to restore normal blood flow. The mother should be placed in the knee-chest position to help decrease cord compression. In both cases, rapid transport to an obstetric facility is required.

INTERHOSPITAL TRANSPORTATION

The most widely recognized system of regional distribution of care designates three different levels of facility and expertise. The capabilities of these different levels are listed in Table 10-1.

Interhospital transports can be classified as one- or two-way. When the patient is transferred using ambulances and personnel based at or near the referring facility, it is classified as a *one-way transport*. When a team is sent from the receiving institution to pick up and return with the patient, it is classified as a *two-way transport*.

One-way transports involve some significant disadvantages, especially for pregnant patients. When a patient is being transferred because of a complication of pregnancy, stan-

Table 10-1

FACILITY DESIGNATION BY LEVEL OF OBSTETRIC NEONATAL SERVICES

	Obstetric Services	Neonatal Services	Example
Level I	1. Ability to provide surveillance and care to all obstetric patients with a triage system to identify high-risk patients for transport to level II or III facility 2. Ability to perform cesarean section within 30 min 3. 24-h laboratory facilities including blood bank facilities	1. Care for healthy neonates 2. Resuscitation and stabilization of near-term neonates 3. Stabilization of unexpectedly small or sick neonates before transfer to a level II or III facility	1. Uncomplicated term or near-term vaginal and cesarean delivery 2. Mild preeclampsia at term
Level II	1. All level I services 2. Management of high-risk mothers and fetuses (generally 1500–2500 g, 32–36 weeks of gestation)	1. All level I services 2. Management of small, sick neonates with a moderate degree of illness, either admitted or transferred	1. Preterm labor at 32–36 weeks
Level III	1. All level II services 2. Comprehensive care for mothers of all risk categories 3. Evaluation of new high-risk technologies	1. All level II services 2. Management of extremely small (<1500 g) or sick neonates	1. Preterm labor <32 weeks 2. Fetal anomalies requiring correction (e.g., diaphragmatic hernia, open neural tube defects) 3. Need for maternal intensive care (e.g., severe cardiac or pulmonary disease)

Source: Modified from Hauth and Dooley,[11] with permission.

dard ambulance crews frequently lack the clinical experience to continue the level of care provided at the hospital. Furthermore, if the patient's condition should worsen en route, appropriate evaluation and intervention is dependent on the skill and expertise of the transport team; these may not be available from EMS personnel. In an effort to overcome this problem, staff members from the referring institution (e.g., a nurse or physician) may accompany the patient with the ambulance crew. However, these personnel are usually unfamiliar with transport medicine. They are not used to working in the unstable environment of a moving ambulance, where noise, vibration, and cramped space place limitations on the ability to identify and manage changes in a patient's condition. Additionally, available equipment and resources may not match those available at the hospital. The nurse or physician who accompanies a patient will be absent from the institution and therefore unable to perform his or her usual hospital duties. Last, since most of these transports originate from small communities, the community will be deprived of an ambulance and its crew for several hours.[5]

Two-way transports overcome many of these problems. Two-way systems usually have dedicated transport teams that are specially trained to function in the transport environment and carry special equipment and devices to allow them to do so quickly and efficiently. Dedicated teams, because of the frequency with which they perform transports, generally develop expertise in all types of transports. The major drawback of the two-way transport system is the delay in the patient's arrival at the receiving institution, since the team must be assembled ("scrambled") and must then travel to the referring institution. The referring physician must consider the risks of sending an unstable (or potentially unstable) patient with an inexperienced crew using a one-way transport system versus waiting for a more experienced crew to arrive who can stabilize and prepare the patient for transport and who are better prepared to care for any problems that may arise en route.

CREW CONFIGURATION

The issue of ideal crew configuration for transport remains controversial. The most important goal is the safe and effective transfer of the patient. Regardless of the level of certification or degrees possessed, the caregiver must have general knowledge of and expertise in critical care. Furthermore, for this patient population, a working knowledge of the physiology of labor and delivery, experience with drugs used during pregnancy and childbirth, familiarity with fetal heart monitors and the ability to interpret them, and competency in newborn resuscitation are important skills to possess.

Suggested crew configuration guidelines are given in Table 10-2. Note that a low-risk patient is one in whom the

---

Table 10-2

GUIDELINES FOR CREW CONFIGURATION

Patient Category	Crew Configuration
Low-risk patient (e.g., patient with controlled diabetes mellitus)	Emergency medical technician (EMT)
Moderate-risk patient (e.g., mild preeclampsia)	Obstetrically trained provider
High-risk patient (e.g., premature labor, any patient with significantly abnormal vital signs, etc.)	Obstetrically trained critical-care transport provider

Source: Adapted from Elliott,[6] with permission.

---

risk of the development of complications or delivery en route is minimal. A moderate-risk patient is one who has been stable for several hours and in whom there is a small chance of complications developing. A high-risk patient is one who is critically ill.

In addition to crew configuration, the mode of transport is an important consideration (Table 10-3). Options may include private automobile, ambulance, helicopter, or fixed-wing aircraft. This decision is frequently not an easy one; the type of vehicle chosen should be agreed to by both the referring and receiving physicians. Several factors must be considered in deciding the most appropriate mode of transfer. These include the severity of the patient's illness, the distance between facilities, options for stopping at other facilities should problems arise during transport, total transport times, personnel availability, vehicle availability, weather limitations, traffic limitations, terrain, safety, and cost. Sometimes a combination of transport modalities may be required. One published review of air transport of pregnant patients (via helicopter and fixed-wing aircraft) demonstrated that appropriately screened patients have an extremely low incidence of in-flight delivery.[7]

Another controversial issue is how much time should be spent at the referring facility. For patients with time-intensive disease processes who are being transferred for specific interventions (for example, the patient with acute trauma or a ruptured abdominal aneurysm), it is usually prudent to spend as little time as possible at the referring institution so that the patient can be brought quickly to the place of definitive care. Conversely, there are transport teams whose philosophy is based on bringing the intensive care and expertise to the bedside, so that, to the extent possible, stabilization takes place at the referring facility prior to initiating the transfer.

A pregnant patient frequently presents an interesting dilemma. As noted above, the interhospital transport envi-

Table 10-3

ADVANTAGES AND DISADVANTAGES OF MODES OF TRANSPORT

Advantages	Disadvantages
Ground ambulance	
Usually readily available	Lengthy travel times over long distances
Only two transfers of the patient required	Limited by geographic, traffic, and weather conditions
Adequate working environment	Variable capacity and capability for additional specialized equipment
Easily diverted and adaptable to destination changes	
Low maintenance costs	
Helicopter	
Rapid transport time	Adequate landing zone required
	Multiple patient transfers may be necessary if landing area is remote from the referring facility
	Prone to weather restrictions
	Limited working space
	Noise and vibration may limit evaluation and monitoring
	High maintenance costs
Fixed-wing aircraft	
Rapid transport time	Multiple patient transfers may be necessary if landing area is remote from the referring facility
Able to fly around or over weather (assuming pressurized cabin)	Requires airport with appropriate service availability at each end
Cabin size usually adequate	High maintenance costs
	May require lengthy "scramble time"

Source: Adapted from Pon and Notterman,[5] with permission.

ronment poses particular challenges; it is not the ideal birthing environment, especially given the restricted confines of a helicopter or airplane. If it appears that despite all interventions delivery is likely to occur during the transport, the best approach is usually to await delivery and then transfer both patients (the newborn and the postpartum woman) if necessary.

LOGISTICS OF TRANSFER

In order for an interhospital transfer to proceed smoothly, adequate communications between parties are essential. This process begins from the time of the initial request, where there should be one central number answered by an appropriately trained communications specialist (dispatcher), through whom all communications should be directed. This person should provide rapid coordination of vehicles and personnel. The communications specialist should also be able to contact the receiving physician in the event that problems arise during the transport. This should include radio communications from the ambulance. It should be noted that cellular phones may cause certain medical devices to malfunction and should be used with extreme caution, if at all, around patients. Additionally, it is against federal regulations to use ordinary cellular phones aboard aircraft.

The transferring team should ensure that copies of all pertinent medical records and x-rays accompany the patient. To help the receiving facility prepare for the patient's arrival, facsimile (fax) machines may be used to send documents prior to the transport.

INDICATIONS FOR TRANSPORT

Maternal transport should be considered if there is a significant chance of maternal or fetal risk that cannot be adequately addressed at the referring institution. There is overwhelming evidence that neonates cared for in a neonatal intensive care unit (ICU) beginning at birth have a greater probability of survival, a lower mortality rate, and a shorter length of hospitalization than those transferred after birth.[8–10] Any insult that occurs during the first 24 h of life can have significant effects on a neonate's outcome. Even the most efficiently organized neonatal transport program is subject to logistical problems or errors that may delay care or result in a medical mishap.

The uterus is the ideal transport incubator and assures immediate access to the modern care of a neonatal ICU. From a logistical standpoint, it is usually easier to transport prior to delivery rather than having to assemble a neonatal team with all of its sophisticated but bulky and cumbersome equipment. In addition, with antepartum transfer, there is less separation of mother and infant, increasing mother-infant bonding.[9]

According to the American Academy of Pediatrics and the American College of Obstetricians and Gynecologists, the goal of interhospital transport should be "to care for high-risk perinatal patients in a facility appropriate to their needs."[11]

The decision as to who is a candidate for transfer and appropriate timing of the transfer should be agreed upon by the transferring and accepting physicians. Transport should be considered "when the resources immediately available to the maternal, fetal, or neonatal patient are not adequate to deal with the patient's actual or anticipated condition."[11] The following conditions, largely adopted from the *Guidelines for Perinatal Care*,[11] list some of the conditions under which transport should be considered. It should be noted that the need for transport should be considered individually, based on patient condition and the capabilities of the sending physician and institution.

The maternal conditions possibly requiring transport are as follows:

Obstetric complications
    Premature rupture of membranes
    Premature labor
    Severe preeclampsia, eclampsia, or other hypertensive complication
    Multiple gestation
    Third-trimester bleeding

Medical complications
    Serious infections
    Severe heart disease
    Poorly controlled diabetes
    Thyrotoxicosis
    Renal disease with deteriorating function or increased hypertension
    Drug overdose/substance abuse
    Other medical conditions such as sickle cell anemia, blood dyscrasias, liver disease, malignancy, etc.[12]

Surgical complications
    Trauma requiring intensive care or surgical correction or requiring a procedure that may result in the premature onset of labor
    Acute abdominal emergencies

The fetal conditions possibly requiring transport are as follows:
    Anomalies that may require surgery
    Rh disease with or without hydrops
    Other conditions[12] such as:
        Congenital malformations potentially requiring special diagnostic procedures or surgical care
        Fetal arrhythmia or bradycardia
        Intrauterine growth restriction
        Abnormal fetal testing
        Severe oligohydramnios
        Vaginal breech delivery

Transport should be arranged as soon as the decision to transfer is made. For example, patients with premature rupture of membranes should be transferred as soon as possible. Unfortunately, this is not always the case, and transport teams are frequently asked to perform rushed transports of women in active labor with advanced cervical dilatation. If labor has progressed to the point where delivery en route is likely, it is usually preferable to delay transport and await the arrival of the neonatal team. It is frequently difficult to predict whether or not the transport can be completed prior to delivery. When the transporting vehicle is a helicopter or airplane, where the space to perform delivery and/or resuscitation is severely limited, the decision becomes even more difficult. Elliott and colleagues retrospectively reviewed 1080 patients who were requested to be transported for preterm labor.[13] Of these, 54 patients were dilated 7 cm or more at time of request for transport and 5 were delivered at the referring hospital, so that 49 were ultimately transported. Forty were transported by helicopter (average transport time, 15 min), 8 by fixed-wing aircraft (average transport time, 90 min), and 1 by ground (transport time, 27 min). Fifteen patients had cervical dilatation of 7 cm, 9 had cervical dilatation of 8 cm, and 5 had cervical dilatation of 10 cm. The station of the presenting part was −2 in 12, −1 in 7, 0 in 10, +1 in 10, and +2 in 10. All transported patients received magnesium sulfate and terbutaline sulfate for tocolysis during transport. All patients who were completely dilated and +2 station delivered within 1 h of arrival at the tertiary hospital. The authors conclude that when confronted with this situation, factors to consider prior to the transfer include the skill and expertise of the transport team, distance between hospitals, facilities at the transferring hospital, gestational age, and cervical exam. The decision to transfer should be based on individual patient assessment and not on protocol. The presence of a team member with extensive labor and delivery experience is encouraged so as to assist in the evaluation and decision (e.g., an obstetrician). It is important that there be ongoing communication between the sending and receiving physicians as these issues arise. These discussions should be carefully documented in the patient's chart.[14]

CARE DURING TRANSPORT

Caregivers who are called upon to transport pregnant patients must consider the physiologic changes that occur during pregnancy. These changes require alteration in the usual transport procedures. There are three interventions that should be performed on almost all pregnant patients during transport. They are (1) transport in the left lateral tilt position, (2) administration of supplemental oxygen, and (3) administration of intravenous fluid.

PATIENT POSITION

Fetal compromise may result when pregnant patients are placed in the supine position. When supine, the gravid uterus (after about 20 to 24 weeks) lies directly against the vena cava and potentially the aorta, compressing both and leading to diminished venous return and decreased blood pressure.[15] Compression of the vena cava can reduce preload significantly, leading to a reduction in cardiac output of up to 25 to 30 percent.[16] Hemodynamically compromised patients (who are usually the ones in need of transport), especially those with reduced circulating volume, will have an even lower tolerance for alterations in hemodynamics. Blood vessels in the pregnant uterus are maximally dilated at rest, and no intrinsic autoregulatory mechanism exists for increasing uterine blood flow. Therefore, any decrease in cardiac output may lead to decreased uterine blood flow and possible uteroplacental insufficiency. In response to decreased cardiac output, hypotension, or hypoxia, the uterine vasculature constricts. This can cause significant fetal compromise without any detectable change in the mother's vital signs.[17] Studies in animals have demonstrated that interruption of inferior vena caval blood flow can produce placental separation.[18] Observations in humans have corroborated these findings.[19] It should also be noted that supine positioning of the pregnant patient may lead to respiratory compromise, as functional residual capacity is reduced by 15 to 20 percent at term.[20,21]

The problems outlined above can be avoided by transporting patients beyond 20 weeks of gestation in the left lateral tilt position (i.e., with the right side of the body higher than the left). This can be accomplished by placing pillows under the mother's right side. If the patient requires spinal immobilization due to traumatic injuries, the backboard should be angled at approximately 15° to the horizontal. This can be accomplished by placing the pillows or an oxygen cylinder under one edge of the backboard. If these options are not available, the uterus can be displaced manually to the left by one of the caregivers.

SUPPLEMENTAL OXYGEN

It seems prudent to administer supplemental oxygen to all pregnant patients being transferred. During pregnancy, increasing maternal oxygen saturation will increase fetal saturation as well.[22] Because the fetal oxygen hemoglobin dissociation curve is shifted to the left, oxygen extraction from the maternal circulation is increased.

Special consideration should be given to supplemental oxygen administration when pregnant patients are transported by air. Most commercial jet aircraft cabins are pressurized to an altitude of 8000 feet. At this altitude in a depressurized chamber, maternal P_{O_2} may decrease from 100 to 55 mmHg, with the fetal arterial cord P_{O_2} decreasing from 32 to 25.6 mmHg. Because of the differences in the fetal oxygen-hemoglobin dissociation curve, the normal fetus is able to maintain a greater degree of oxygen saturation and thus appears to be in no danger from cabin pressures of modern jet aircraft.[23,24] Studies in animals have shown that at altitudes up to 7500 feet, there is no significant effect on oxygen exchange in a normal placenta.[25] It should also be

noted that the altitudes at which most rotor-wing (helicopter) transports take place have no significant effects on maternal or fetal oxygenation. However, because women being transported or their fetuses usually have some degree of compromise, it is prudent to administer supplemental oxygen to all pregnant patients being transported, regardless of altitude.

INTRAVENOUS FLUID THERAPY

All patients being transported should have at least one functioning intravenous line in place. The rate of fluid administration should be appropriate to the clinical condition of the patient and fetus. As noted above, an early maternal compensatory mechanism for hypovolemia is a decrease in uterine blood flow, resulting in potential fetal compromise with little or no change in maternal vital signs. Because maternal blood volume increases up to 45 percent during pregnancy, it is estimated that the mother can lose up to 10 to 20 percent of her circulating blood volume acutely before her vital signs become abnormal.[26] Therefore, volume replacement should be given at a rate that ensures adequate uterine perfusion. Any woman with significant hypovolemia should have at least two large-bore peripheral intravenous lines placed. Significant blood loss may require transfusion of blood in addition to crystalloid therapy.

Special mention should be made of the use of pressor agents in pregnancy. Catecholamines cause decreased uterine blood flow[17] and thus should be used only when all other mechanisms have failed. Additionally, efforts to calm the patient so as to decrease endogenous catecholamine production may be useful as well.

It is important to stabilize the mother and fetus to the extent possible prior to transport. Therapeutic agents that are frequently administered safely en route include glucocorticoids, antihypertensives, anticonvulsants, antibiotics, and tocolytics.[27]

MATERNAL AND FETAL EVALUATION

While in transport, standard nursing evaluation, monitoring, and documentation should be performed, with close monitoring of the mother's cardiopulmonary status (Table 10-4). The mother should also be observed for evidence of uterine contractions. Fetal heart rate should be monitored and documented at 15- to 30-min intervals or more often for more critically ill patients. This can be done using a Doppler device or, if available, continuous electronic fetal monitoring. If a Doppler device is chosen for intermittent monitoring and the patient is contracting regularly, fetal heart tones should be documented after a uterine contraction.[28] These devices have been used successfully both on the ground and in the air.[24]

Table 10-4

KEY FACTORS TO BE MONITORED DURING TRANSPORT[a]

Mother	Neonate
Uterine contractions and fetal heart tones	Temperature
Cardiopulmonary status	Respirations
Deep tendon reflexes	Heart rate
Infusion rates of intravenous lines	Blood pressure
Administration of medications	Color
	Activity
	Oxygen concentration

[a]Frequency of monitoring key factors will depend on patient stability, but at least every 30 min is prudent.

MEDICOLEGAL CONCERNS

The transfer of a patient from one institution to another raises many medicolegal issues. Hospitals must develop policies that comply with all applicable federal and state laws. It is best for institutions to have written letters of agreement that cover these issues.

The transfer of patients was addressed in the Consolidated Omnibus Budget Reconciliation Act of 1986, commonly referred to as the COBRA law. Under terms of this law, the transferring physician must discuss the case with a physician at the receiving institution, who must accept the transfer. A "medical screening examination" must be performed prior to the transfer. Evaluation and stabilization should be performed to ensure that, within reasonable medical probability, no harm will come to the patient and that the medical benefits of transfer will outweigh the risks.[29] A patient may be transferred without being stabilized if the transfer is from a lower level to a higher level of care and necessary interventions are beyond the capability of the sending institution.[30] Failure to comply with COBRA laws can result in fines, loss of Medicare reimbursement, a lawsuit by the patient for injuries suffered, or a suit for damages from the receiving hospital for inappropriate patient transfer.[5,31,32]

Prior to the transfer to a higher level of care, the risk and benefits of the transfer should be documented in the medical record by the sending physician. Documentation should also include the capabilities that the receiving institution has over the sending institution, the options for transfer and the reason for the mode chosen, the name of the receiving physician who accepted the transfer, and how availability of space at the receiving facility was assured.[30]

It should be noted that one-way transport systems are generally not as sophisticated as two-way systems. In the eyes of the law, a patient is the responsibility of the sending physician until such time as the patient arrives at the accepting facility. Thus, the sending physician must understand and accept the risk of sending the patient with a level of care less than that which was provided at the sending facility or make arrangements for a transport with personnel capable of meeting the potential needs of the patient.

When members of a two-way transport service arrive at a referring hospital, questions may also arise as to when the responsibility and liability shifts to the accepting institution. Some hospitals consider a patient their responsibility when the transport team assumes care, even though they are physically outside of the home institution. Other institutions assume liability when the patient enters "their" ambulance. To avoid potential problems, these issues should be addressed formally and prospectively through written letters of agreement between institutions. Institutions should develop written transfer policies and procedures that are in compliance with all applicable state and federal laws.

References

1. Rooks JP, Weatherby NL, Ernst EKM, et al: Outcomes of care in birth centers—The National Birth Center Study. *N Engl J Med* 321:1804, 1989.
2. Garite TJ, Snell BJ, Walker DL, Darrow VC: Development and experience of a university-based, freestanding birthing center. *Obstet Gynecol* 86:411, 1995.
3. Pons PT: Prehospital considerations in the pregnant patient. *Emerg Med Clin North Am* 12:1, 1994.
4. Brunette DD, Sterner SP: Prehospital and emergency department delivery: A review of eight years experience. *Ann Emerg Med* 18:1116, 1989.
5. Pon SP, Notterman DA: The organization of a pediatric critical care transport program. *Pediatr Clin North Am* 40:241, 1993.
6. Elliott JP: *Maternal Air Medical Transport, Air Medical Physician's Handbook.* Salt Lake City: Air Medical Physician Association, 1996.
7. Low RB, Martin D, Brown C: Emergency air transport of pregnant patients: The national experience. *J Emerg Med* 6:41, 1988.
8. Giles HR: Maternal transport. *Clin Obstet Gynecol* 6:203, 1979.
9. Mondanlou HD, Dorchester WL, Thorosian A, et al: Antenatal versus neonatal transport to a regional perinatal center: A comparison between matched pairs. *Obstet Gynecol* 53:725, 1979.
10. Merenstein GB, Pettett G, Woodall J, et al: An analysis of air transport results in the sick newborn: II. Antenatal and neonatal referrals. *Am J Obstet Gynecol* 128:520, 1977.

11. Hauth J, Dooley S. (eds): Inpatient perinatal care services, in *Guidelines for Perinatal Care,* 4th ed. American Academy of Pediatrics and American College of Obstetricians and Gynecologists, 1997, pp 13–63.

12. Garmel SH, D'Alton ME: When maternal transport is necessary. *Contem OB/GYN* 40:94, 1995.

13. Elliott JP, Sipp TL, Balazs KT: Maternal transport of patients with advanced cervical dilatation—To fly or not to fly? *Obstet Gynecol* 79:380, 1992.

14. Bowes WA, Jr: Clinical management of preterm delivery. *Clin Obstet Gynecol* 31:652, 1988.

15. Ueland K, Novy MJ, Peterson EN, et al: Maternal cardiovascular dynamics: IV. The influence of gestational age on the maternal cardiovascular response to posture and exercise. *Am J Obstet Gynecol* 104:856, 1969.

16. Pearlman MD, Tintinalli JE, Lorenz RP: Blunt trauma during pregnancy. *N Engl J Med* 323:1609, 1990.

17. Katz VL, Hansen A: Complications in the emergency transport of pregnant women. *South Med J* 83:7, 1990.

18. Howard BK, Goodson JH: Experimental placental abruption. *Obstet Gynecol* 2:442, 1953.

19. Menger WF, Goodson JH, Campbell RG, et al: Observation on the pathogenesis of premature separation of the normally implanted placenta. *Am J Obstet Gynecol* 66:1104, 1953.

20. Novy MJ, Edwards MJ: Respiratory problems in pregnancy. *Am J Obstet Gynecol* 99:1024, 1967.

21. Cheek TG, Gutsche BB: Maternal physiologic alterations during pregnancy. In Schnider SM, Levinson G (eds): *Anesthesia for Obstetrics.* Baltimore: Williams & Wilkins, 1993.

22. Shaw DB, Wheeler AS: Anesthesia for obstetric emergencies. *Clin Obstet Gynecol* 27:112, 1984.

23. Barry M, Bia F: Pregnancy and travel. *JAMA* 261:728, 1989.

24. Elliott JP, Trujillo R: Fetal monitoring during emergency obstetric transport. *Am J Obstet Gynecol* 157:245, 1987.

25. Parer JT: Effects of hypoxia on the mother and fetus with emphasis on maternal air transport. *Am J Obstet Gynecol* 142:957, 1982.

26. Baker DP: Trauma in the pregnant patient. *Surg Clin North Am* 62:275, 1992.

27. Semonin-Holleran R: *Flight Nursing: Principles and Practice,* 2d ed. St. Louis: Mosby–Year Book, 1996.

28. American College of Obstetricians and Gynecologists: *Fetal Heart Rate Patterns: Monitoring, Interpretation, and Management.* ACOG Technical Bulletin 207. Washington, DC: 1995.

29. ACEP Policy Statement, Appropriate Interhospital Patient Transfer. *Ann Emerg Med* 22:766, 1993.

30. Strobos J: Tightening the screw: Statutory and legal supervision of interhospital patient transfers. *Ann Emerg Med* 20:302, 1991.

31. Frew SA, Roush WR, LaGreca K: COBRA: Implications for emergency medicine. *Ann Emerg Med* 17:835, 1988.

32. Mookini RK: Medical-legal aspects of aeromedical transport of emergency patients. *Leg Med* 1, 1990.

Chapter 11

EMERGENCY MANAGEMENT OF PRETERM LABOR

H. Frank Andersen

SIGNIFICANCE OF PRETERM LABOR

Preterm delivery is the leading cause of perinatal death and morbidity in the United States. Approximately 10 percent of pregnancies end in preterm delivery, defined as delivery before 37 completed weeks of gestation.[1] Despite more than a decade of effort to reduce preterm birth by various means, its incidence is stable or increasing slightly. Recent research has demonstrated that some effects of preterm delivery can be ameliorated by appropriate treatment. Also, new diagnostic modalities may help the physician to determine more accurately which woman with symptoms of preterm labor is likely to progress to preterm delivery. These modalities allow interventions to be directed in a more precise and cost-effective manner for those most likely to benefit.

Causes of preterm labor include infection, premature rupture of membranes, abruption, drug abuse (particularly cocaine and amphetamines), multiple gestation, polyhydramnios, and cervical incompetence. Many instances of preterm labor have no identifiable cause, although there is increasing evidence that low-grade infection plays a large role in many cases previously thought to be idiopathic.[2] For the physician seeing a patient with possible preterm labor, the root causes are often not as important as the necessity to recognize the presenting signs and symptoms of preterm labor and begin initial steps to confirm the diagnosis.

RECOGNIZING PRETERM LABOR

Labor is defined as regular uterine contractions resulting in progressive cervical effacement and dilatation. Although any gestation prior to 37 completed weeks is preterm by definition, many clinicians think that those who experience preterm labor before 34 weeks of gestation represent the group at highest risk for poor infant outcomes. Despite the low morbidity and mortality among infants born between 34 and 37 weeks, the presence of even low levels of morbidity suggests that simple measures to reduce the likelihood of delivery are reasonable. Table 11-1 gives approximate risks of complications of prematurity by gestational age.[3]

The principal signs and symptoms of preterm labor are listed in Table 11-2. Women are commonly instructed, during prenatal care, to be aware of these symptoms and to report them. If a pregnant woman with less than 35 weeks of gestation reports regular uterine contractions four or more times per hour, she should lie down, drink fluids, and continue to monitor her contractions. If four or more contractions occur in the second hour of monitoring, she should be evaluated. Women who report vaginal bleeding or leakage of fluid should be instructed to come immediately for examination. Fluid leakage from preterm rupture of membranes (PROM) may occur as a sudden gush or as a steady trickle of fluid over time. Many women experience occasional urinary incontinence during later pregnancy, which

Table 11-1

OUTCOMES OF PRETERM INFANTS[a]

Gestational Age	26 Weeks, Percent	30 Weeks, Percent	34 Weeks, Percent	Term, Percent
Respiratory distress syndrome	93	55	14	<1
Intraventricular hemorrhage	30	2	<1	<1
Sepsis	33	11	4	<1
Necrotizing enterocolitis	11	15	3	<1
Patent ductus arteriosis	48	23	2	<1
Mortality	30–50	7–10	1	<1

[a]Mortality and morbidity may vary significantly among different institutions and different clinical situations. These data are presented as representative and approximations only. Patients should always be counseled that there is a large degree of variation in outcomes.
Sources: Adapted from Robertson et al.,[3] with permission. Mortality data derived from Cunningham FG, MacDonald PC, Gant NF, et al (eds): *Williams Obstetrics,* 19th ed. East Norwalk, CT: Appleton & Lange, 1993, and data from Loma Linda University Medical Center, with permission.

may be difficult to differentiate from PROM without an examination. Whenever doubt exists about possible PROM or preterm labor, it is advisable to examine and monitor the patient.

INITIAL EVALUATION

HISTORY

Initial evaluation includes a brief but careful history of symptoms of preterm labor, review of obstetric history—particularly the outcomes of prior pregnancies—and a review of medical history. Special note should be made of conditions

Table 11-2

SYMPTOMS OF PRETERM LABOR

Menstrual-like cramps
Low, dull backache
Pelvic pressure
Sudden increase in vaginal discharge
Vaginal spotting or staining
Painful uterine contractions, occurring four or more per hour

that may predispose to preterm labor, such as acute urinary tract infection, and conditions that may contraindicate the use of tocolytic drugs to stop preterm labor (Table 11-3). Particular attention should be given to time of initial onset of contractions and frequency of contractions. The presence of any vaginal bleeding contraindicates vaginal examination until an ultrasound examination or review of prior ultrasound reports can rule out placenta previa. A history of leaking fluid from the vagina suggests possible PROM. Initial history and evaluation are summarized in Table 11-3.

Accurate knowledge of the estimated date of delivery (EDD) is necessary for making informed decisions about treating preterm labor. Unfortunately, prenatal records are often not available in the emergency department setting. In addition, many pregnant women who present to the emergency department have not had prenatal care. Most women who attend prenatal care know their EDD, but in some cases history or clinical examination must suffice until records or ultrasound examination are available.

Gestational age is defined as the number of elapsed weeks from the first day of the last normal menstrual period (LMP). If the exact date of the LMP is known, this is an accurate estimator of current gestational age.[4] If the patient is unsure or gives an approximation (e.g., "I know it was in the first week of July"), it should be treated as unreliable and clinical estimators should be used instead to predict gestational age.[4] Clinical markers of gestational age are listed in Table 11-4. Of note, clinical estimators of gestational age are significantly affected by obesity, twins, and polyhydramnios.

Ultrasound evaluation can be very useful to determine fetal gestational age, estimate fetal weight, evaluate amniotic

Table 11-3

INITIAL EVALUATION OF THE PATIENT WITH SUSPECTED PRETERM LABOR

Review obstetric history and medical history, with special attention to:

Predisposing factors for preterm labor

Multiple gestation

History of preterm birth

Drug use

Symptoms of urinary tract infection

Absolute contraindications to tocolysis

Active vaginal bleeding

Eclampsia or severe preeclampsia

Dead fetus or major fetal malformation incompatible with survival

Intrauterine infection

Maternal cardiac disease

Any obstetric or medical condition that contraindicates prolongation of pregnancy

Maternal hyperthyroidism (contraindicates beta-sympathomimetic therapy)

Conditions that limit chance of success with tocolysis

Ruptured fetal membranes

Advanced labor (cervix >4 cm dilated)

Untreated urinary tract infection

Incompetent cervix

Review gestational age. If necessary, estimate gestational age by physical exam and history (Table 11-4)

Review vital signs and perform physical exam, with special attention to uterine size, uterine tenderness, vaginal bleeding, or fluid leakage

Obtain urinalysis (consider urine drug screen); if urinalysis is abnormal, culture and begin empiric therapy for urinary tract infection

Perform sterile speculum exam; evaluate for possible ruptured membranes (presence of pooling fluid, alkaline pH of fluid, ferning of dried smear); culture the cervix for beta streptococcus, *Neisseria gonorrhea,* and *Chlamydia;* consider fetal fibronectin analysis if available

If membranes are ruptured, evaluate cervical length and approximate dilatation visually; if membranes are intact and there is no bleeding, perform digital vaginal examination to evaluate cervical dilatation and effacement

Initiate (or continue) monitoring for uterine contractions and fetal heart rate

---

fluid volume and fetal movement, and determine if fetal structural anomalies exist[5] (see Chap. 52). Although the accuracy of ultrasound estimation of gestational age is poor in the third trimester (± 3 weeks), it is generally sufficient to make treatment decisions. The clinician must consider the possibility of confounding factors which may affect the ultrasound measurements. In the presence of intrauterine growth restriction, ultrasound may underestimate gestational age. Fetal macrosomia in the pregnant woman with diabetes may cause gestational age to be overestimated. Estimated fetal weight in preterm gestation has an error of approximately ± 10 percent. Figure 11-1 shows average fetal weight for gestational age; large for gestational age and small for gestational age are defined as above the 90th and below the 10th percentiles.[6]

EXAMINATION

The pregnancy-specific portion of the physical examination includes estimation of fundal height measured in centimeters from the symphysis pubis to the uterine fundus, auscultation of fetal heart tones, and, if possible, determination of fetal lie by abdominal palpation (Leopold's maneuvers). Differentiation of cephalic, breech, or transverse lie is important to decision making regarding route of delivery but is often difficult by physical examination alone prior to 34 weeks of gestation. Normal fetal heart rate is between 120 and 160 beats per minute. If available, external fetal monitoring can be instituted to evaluate patterns of fetal heart rate and uterine contractions. If a fetal monitor is not available, abdominal palpation over 10 to 15 min is just as accurate to determine the frequency and quality of uterine contractions.

Before performing a digital vaginal examination of the cervix, vaginal bleeding (possible placenta previa) should be excluded by history and ultrasonography. If there is a history of leaking fluid, a sterile speculum examination should be performed prior to digital cervical exam to diagnose or exclude rupture of membranes. This is advisable in any case to obtain cervical cultures for *Chlamydia* and *Neisseria gonorrhoeae* prior to performing a cervical exam. A sterile speculum is introduced into the vagina and the posterior fornix is observed for pooling of fluid. Vaginal fluid should be swabbed on nitrazine (pH) paper; an alkaline pH (>6.5) indicates likely amniotic fluid leakage. Finally vaginal fluid swabbed on a microscope slide and allowed to dry can be examined for the presence of ferning, which indicates amniotic fluid. If membranes are ruptured, the cervix should be examined visually for approximate dilation and effacement but *not* examined manually (i.e., with the gloved hand), as this increases the risk of infection. If membranes are intact, a manual cervical examination is performed to measure cervical dilation, effacement, position (anterior or posterior), consistency (soft or firm), and station of presenting part (degree of descent into the pelvis).

During the sterile speculum examination, I recommend

Table 11-4

CLINICAL ESTIMATORS OF GESTATIONAL AGE

Clinical Estimator	Gestational Age, Weeks	Error (90% Confidence), Weeks
Quickening (first perception of fetal movement)		
Nulliparous	18	±4
Multiparous	17	±4
Uterus reaches the umbilicus	20	±3
Fundal height measurements		
Top of symphysis to top of fundus in centimeters	Number of centimeters equals number of weeks	±4

that cultures for *Chlamydia* and *Neisseria gonorrhoeae* be performed and that the patient be evaluated for bacterial vaginosis. Bacterial vaginosis is diagnosed by the presence of at least three of four criteria: a homogenous vaginal discharge; vaginal pH >4.7; fishy amine odor when vaginal secretions are mixed with 10% potassium hydroxide ("whiff test"); and presence of clue cells on a wet mount or Gram stain of vaginal secretions. Current evidence suggests that bacterial vaginosis predisposes women to preterm labor.[7] While treatment of presumed vaginal infections has not been shown to be immediately effective in treating preterm labor, this information may be of importance in ongoing prenatal

care if the episode of preterm labor does not progress. Group B streptococcal culture should also be obtained (see below).

LABORATORY STUDIES

The initial laboratory study for evaluation of suspected preterm labor is a urinalysis. Acute cystitis and pyelonephritis are common causes of preterm labor. An abnormal urinalysis should be followed by urine culture and is an indication to begin empiric therapy for a urinary tract infection. Cultures of group B streptococcus should be obtained by

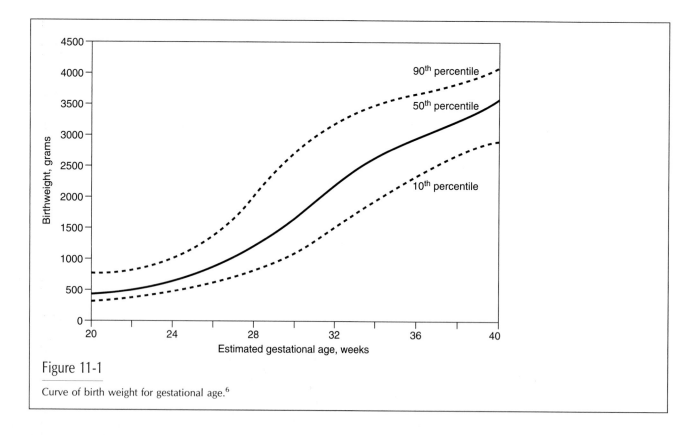

Figure 11-1

Curve of birth weight for gestational age.[6]

swabbing the lower third of the vagina and anorectum with a single cotton swab. The swab should then be placed in an aerobic transport medium or, if available, a selective broth medium (e.g., modified Todd-Hewitt broth) and specifically labeled as group B strep culture. Urine drug screening should be considered in all women with preterm labor, regardless of social class. Cocaine and amphetamine abuse are especially associated with preterm labor. Acute intoxication with either may result in preterm labor, PROM, or placental abruption. A standard prenatal panel may be ordered if it has not already been performed by the prenatal care provider; however, the standard prenatal labs are not of particular value in the immediate evaluation of preterm labor.

Recently, the Food and Drug Administration (FDA) approved an enzyme-linked immunosorbent assay (ELISA) test for the presence of fetal fibronectin in vaginal secretions collected by swabbing the posterior fornix. The presence of fetal fibronectin in cervical secretions (>50 ng/mL) is associated with a 29 percent risk of preterm delivery within the next 7 days. More important, a negative fetal fibronectin is associated with less than 1 percent risk of preterm delivery in the next 7 days.[8] In clinical practice, this test may be useful to identify women with a low risk of preterm delivery in the next week and thus avoid expensive and risky interventions to stop preterm labor. Presently, the ELISA test is time-consuming (a minimum of 6 h turn around), but development of more rapid fetal fibronectin assays is under way. Despite the limitations of the present methodology, fetal fibronectin assay may be an important adjunct to the initial assessment in the future, since the presence or absence of fetal fibronectin may assist decisions about continuing tocolytic therapy.

ULTRASOUND

Ultrasound evaluation may be helpful to determine gestational age, fetal presentation, placental location, and amniotic fluid volume.[5] If vaginal bleeding is present, digital cervical examination should not be performed until ultrasound confirms that there is not a placenta previa. Findings of cervical shortening or funneling of the upper cervical canal by endovaginal or transperineal ultrasound are highly predictive of preterm delivery; however, performing and evaluating cervical ultrasound requires a fairly high degree of experience and is not available in many areas.[9]

Unless physical examination reveals ruptured membranes or advanced cervical dilation (>2 cm), the decision to initiate treatment for preterm labor depends on the presence of continuing uterine contractions and cervical change. Although most monitoring of uterine contractions is done by external electronic monitors, continuous palpation is equally effective. The presence of more than four uterine contractions per hour is abnormal before 34 weeks of gestation. Repeat cervical examination after 1–2 h should be performed if there are frequent uterine contractions to determine if the cervix is progressively effacing or dilating.

INITIAL TREATMENT

Before considering treatment of preterm labor, the physician should evaluate possible contraindications to tocolytic therapy. The most common reasons to withhold tocolytic therapy are situations where tocolysis is unlikely to improve outcome, such as gestational age over 34 weeks or advanced labor (cervix dilated >4 cm), or situations where delivery is indicated, such as abruption, bleeding placenta previa, or preeclampsia (Table 11-3). Another common situation is PROM, in which most clinicians discourage tocolysis. Preterm rupture of the membranes is associated with a high risk of chorioamnionitis, and the onset of uterine contractions is sometimes an early indication of developing infection in PROM.

HYDRATION

Initial treatment of preterm labor is bed rest and hydration. Up to 30 percent of preterm labor resolves with only these measures. It is not clear whether these instances represent preterm labor "treated" by hydration and bed rest alone or whether these are cases of "false" labor. Regardless, in the absence of advanced or changing cervical effacement of dilation, observation is the preferred initial treatment. Observation of patients with uterine contractions and minimal cervical dilatation (<2 cm) does not reduce the effectiveness of tocolysis or increase the chance of preterm delivery.[10]

BETA SYMPATHOMIMETICS

If observation of cervical change and regular contractions confirm the diagnosis of preterm labor and there are no contraindications to tocolytic therapy, further treatment of uterine contractions is warranted. Prospective randomized trials demonstrate that intravenous tocolysis is effective in delaying delivery for at least 48 h. However, mean gestational age at delivery is not substantially changed. The principal advantage of tocolytic therapy is to allow the administration of steroid therapy for fetal lung maturation. The most common choices of tocolytic medications are beta sympathomimetics, magnesium sulfate, or calcium channel blockers. The only drug currently approved by the FDA for the treatment of preterm labor is ritodrine hydrochloride (Yutopar, Astra); however, this drug is now rarely used due to the incidence of side effects and the common use of the less expensive but pharmacologically similar terbutaline.

A common initial tocolytic therapy is 0.25 mg of terbutaline (Brethine, Geigy) given subcutaneously and repeated hourly as needed until contractions stop.[11] Contraction frequency usually decreases within a few minutes. Common side effects of beta sympathomimetics include tachycardia, hypotension, palpitations, headaches, and tremor. Terbutaline therapy should be withheld if the pulse exceeds 140/min. Because of its convenience, terbutaline is often used without an intravenous infusion in place; this may be hazardous if the patient is dehydrated. Despite its ease of use, patients should be carefully monitored for side effects including pulmonary edema, which has been reported with both beta sympathomimetic and magnesium sulfate therapy. If terbutaline is ineffective in controlling uterine contractions, the next step is intravenous tocolytic therapy, usually with magnesium sulfate.

MAGNESIUM

Intravenous magnesium sulfate is initiated with a 4- to 6-g bolus given over 15 to 20 min followed by 2 g/h continuous infusion. The infusion rate may be increased gradually (1 g/h) if uterine contractions are not controlled. Doses above 4 g/h should be used only with extreme caution because of the potential for magnesium toxicity and/or pulmonary edema.[12] Total intravenous fluids should be limited to 125 mL/h.

Normal pretreatment serum magnesium levels during pregnancy range between 1.5 and 2.0 meq/L. When serum magnesium levels exceed therapeutic ranges (4 to 7 meq/L), toxicity may develop. Loss of deep tendon reflexes (8 to 10 meq/L) precedes respiratory arrest (13 meq/L), and cardiac arrest may follow. With mild magnesium toxicity, the magnesium infusion is simply discontinued. More significant toxicity resulting in respiratory depression is treated by administration of 1 g calcium gluconate (10 mL of a 10% solution) intravenously over 2 min. Respiratory support, oxygen saturation monitoring, and ECG monitoring are indicated. Magnesium excretion may be enhanced by loop or osmotic diuretics.

CALCIUM CHANNEL BLOCKERS AND OTHER TOCOLYTICS

Some physicians prefer to use the calcium channel blocker nifedipine (Procardia, Pratt) rather than terbutaline or magnesium sulfate. Similar precautions and contraindications apply to calcium channel blockers used for tocolysis. The initial dose is 10 mg of nifedipine sublingually. If uterine contractions persist after 20 min, repeat the dose at intervals of 20 min up to a maximum of 40 mg during the first hour. If uterine activity is controlled, continue oral therapy with 20 mg of nifedipine every 6 h.[13] Hypotension is a potential complication of nifedipine therapy; for this reason I prefer

repeated 10-mg doses rather than protocols that deliver 20 to 30 mg as an initial bolus.

Indomethacin has been used to stop preterm contractions. This prostaglandin synthetase inhibitor appears to be effective in reducing contractions but has several notable fetal side effects, in particular premature closure of the ductus arteriosus, development of oligohydramnios with prolonged use, and increased risk of necrotizing enterocolitis in the infant after delivery. With few exceptions, I do not recommend its use in most situations of preterm labor.

GLUCOCORTICOIDS

When a suspicion of preterm labor exists between 24 and 34 weeks of gestation, glucocorticoid therapy should be initiated to promote fetal lung maturation unless a clear contraindication exists. A 1994 National Institutes of Health (NIH) Consensus conference strongly encouraged broader use of prenatal glucocorticoid therapy in women at risk of preterm delivery.[14] Women between 24 and 34 weeks of gestation at risk of preterm delivery (24 and 32 weeks in cases of PROM), including all women with suspected preterm labor, should receive glucocorticoids unless contraindicated by maternal disease or the presence of chorioamnionitis. The usual dose is betamethasone acetate (Celestone Soluspan, Schering), 12 mg IM in two doses 24 h apart, or dexamethasone (Decadron, Merck; or Dalalone, Forest Pharmaceuticals), 6 mg IM q6h for four doses. Maximum benefit occurs if delivery is delayed at least 48 h from initial administration. Table 11-5 summarizes tocolytic and glucocorticoid protocols.

Table 11-5

ADMINISTRATION PROTOCOLS FOR COMMONLY USED TOCOLYTIC MEDICATIONS AND GLUCOCORTICOIDS TO PROMOTE FETAL LUNG MATURATION

Terbutaline sulfate (Brethine, Geigy)

Intravenous infusion may not be necessary if patient is well hydrated, but observe closely for hypotension

Monitor maternal heart rate, blood pressure, uterine activity, and fetal heart rate

Initial dose, 0.25 mg terbutaline SC

Repeat dose every hour if contractions recur

Hold dose for tachycardia, chest pain, hypotension

Table 11-5 (*Continued*)
ADMINISTRATION PROTOCOLS FOR COMMONLY USED TOCOLYTIC MEDICATIONS AND GLUCOCORTICOIDS TO PROMOTE FETAL LUNG MATURATION

Magnesium sulfate

Establish intravenous infusion

Monitor maternal heart rate, blood pressure, respiratory rate, deep tendon reflexes, uterine activity, fetal heart rate, and serum magnesium and calcium levels

Calcium gluconate should be available to reverse toxic side effects or to keep serum calcium levels above 7 mg/dL

Initial dose 4–6 g magnesium sulfate over 20 min, then continuous infusion of 2 g/h

Increase infusion rate (to maximum of 4 g/h) if contractions continue; reduce infusion rate if deep tendon reflexes disappear; discontinue infusion if respiratory compromise occurs

If labor is successfully stopped, infusion should be maintained for 12–24h

Discontinue intravenous therapy after 12–24h of successful tocolysis (control of uterine contractions with no further cervical change)

Nifedipine (Procardia, Pratt)

Establish intravenous infusion

Monitor maternal heart rate, blood pressure, respiratory rate, uterine activity, and fetal heart rate

Initial dose: 10 mg sublingual, repeat every 20 min up to four doses or until contractions subside

Maintenance therapy: 20 mg PO q6h

Maintenance therapy may be discontinued after 1–3 days

Oral maintenance tocolytic therapy

Oral maintenance therapy after initial tocolysis of preterm labor is commonplace but of unproved value. Usual oral maintenance therapy is terbutaline sulfate 2.5–5 mg PO q4–6h. Some physicians use nifedipine 20 mg PO q6h for maintenance

Glucocorticoid therapy to promote fetal lung maturation
(24–34 weeks of gestation)

Betamethasone acetate (Celestone Soluspan, Schering) 12 mg IM given twice, 24 h apart, or Dexamethasone (Decadron, Merck, or Dalalone, Forest Pharmaceuticals), 6 mg IM q6h for four doses

Maximum benefit occurs if delivery is delayed at least 48 h from initial administration

ANTIBIOTICS

Infants who deliver preterm are at increased risk from group B beta streptococcus infection; therefore empiric antibiotic therapy with penicillin G (unless the patient is allergic) should be initiated in patients with progressive preterm labor.[15] The reason for presumptive treatment for beta streptococcus is the severity of streptococcal pneumonia, particularly in preterm infants, despite its relative infrequency. The usual dose of penicillin G is 5 million units IV followed by 2.5 million units q4h. Although infection is increasingly thought to play a large role in the genesis of preterm labor, antibiotic therapy in general has not been shown to affect the success of tocolytic therapy in patients with active preterm labor and is not recommended unless there is evidence of a specific infection.[16]

TRANSFER GUIDELINES

Perhaps the most important decision for the emergency department physician treating a patient in preterm labor is the decision on when and where to transfer the patient for continuing care and possibly delivery. Perinatal units are often designated as level I, II, or III based on the ability of the obstetric and neonatal teams to care for preterm infants (see Table 10-1). Although definitions of levels of perinatal care differ widely in different states and among different organizations, in general, level I hospitals are those with the capabilities only to care for full-term, normal infants. Level II facilities include nurseries that can care for infants with moderate complications, sometimes but not always including ventilator care for preterm infants with respiratory distress syndrome. Level III units include teams of perinatologists and neonatologists who can care for the sickest and smallest of neonates, including the use of prolonged ventilator support and the availability of a complete range of neonatal consultation services, such as cardiology, pediatric surgery, and so on. It is important for emergency physicians to be familiar with the capability of their own hospital's perinatal unit and the capabilities of surrounding hospitals to which patients may be transported.

In general, very preterm infants have better outcomes if delivered in a level III perinatal unit than similar infants delivered in a level I or II unit and transported after delivery (neonatal transport) to a level III nursery.[17] Despite the benefit of maternal transport of women in preterm labor, the physician must carefully weigh the risks of transport during pregnancy against the benefits of delivery in the level III unit. The principal risks are maternal or fetal decompensation during transport and delivery en route. Patients should be hemodynamically stable prior to transport and fetal monitoring should show no signs of "fetal distress" (e.g., late decelerations, severe variable decelerations, or tachycardia with loss of baseline variability). If there is evidence of fetal compromise by external fetal monitoring, it is probably preferable to deliver the infant locally, resuscitate and stabilize the infant, and then transport.

Determining the speed of labor progression and exact time of delivery is sometimes difficult. Individual patients may unexpectedly progress very rapidly in labor and deliver precipitously, whereas others may progress slowly despite presenting with advanced cervical dilatation. In general, multiparous women progress more rapidly in labor than nulliparous women. Labor progresses more rapidly in the active phase of labor; however, determination of the active phase of labor can be difficult. Common signs of active-phase labor include cervical dilatation ≥4 cm and complete effacement of the cervix. In nulliparous women, active-phase labor often progresses at about 1 cm/h; however, individuals may exceed this rate of dilatation.

If it is determined to transport the patient prior to delivery, communication with the receiving hospital is important in order to discuss the patient's condition and also to decide on initial therapy during transport. Many of these specific transport issues are covered in Chapter 10. Specifically in regards to preterm labor, the transporting physician may wish to consider initial tocolytic therapy even in patients who are not clearly in preterm labor. For brief transports (≤1 h), subcutaneous terbutaline, 0.25 mg, will usually decrease contraction intensity and frequency. For longer transports, it may be wise to initiate magnesium sulfate therapy, as discussed above.

Transport of women in active labor should include an attendant who is capable of monitoring fetal status by Doppler or external electronic fetal monitor. If evidence of rapidly advancing labor develops during transport, the team must be prepared to perform an emergency delivery en route and initiate infant resuscitation and stabilization until arrival at the receiving hospital.

FOLLOW-UP

Women who present with symptoms of preterm labor appear to be at increased risk for future preterm delivery, even if the current episode is not determined to be true preterm labor. It is important that these women be educated to identify signs and symptoms of preterm labor and to assure good follow-up care. Common symptoms of preterm labor are listed in Table 11-2. The patient who has had an episode of preterm labor should be instructed to watch for these symptoms and report them immediately to her prenatal care provider. A common instruction is that if she experiences four or more contractions per hour she should lie down, drink fluids, and continue to monitor contractions. If contractions

continue at four or more during the second hour, she should immediately call her prenatal care provider or come to the hospital for further evaluation. Fluid leaking from the vagina or bleeding are causes to immediately seek further evaluation.

If the patient has received tocolytic therapy, such as a dose of subcutaneous terbutaline sulfate, some physicians initiate oral treatment with terbutaline 2.5 to 5 mg, q4–6h (daily dose 10 to 30 mg). Oral terbutaline appears to decrease contraction frequency and intensity, according to many patient reports, but is associated with significant side effects, such as headaches, tachycardia, insomnia, and orthostatic hypotension. To date, the evidence suggests that tocolysis with oral terbutaline is not effective in prolonging pregnancy or reducing the incidence of preterm delivery.[18]

Patients who have an episode of preterm labor are usually advised to restrict activity. Activity restrictions and bed rest are among the most commonly prescribed treatments for preterm labor. There is evidence that women who are more active are at increased risk of preterm delivery, but few data demonstrate that activity restriction or bed rest are effective in treating preterm labor.[19] Nonetheless, bed rest in the lateral decubitus position is known to increase uterine perfusion and is often prescribed in the belief that it may be of benefit and does little harm. I suggest a prescription for activity restriction at one of three levels, as outlined in Table 11-6.

SPECIAL CIRCUMSTANCES

Certain special circumstances may necessitate more rapid interventions. Chief among these is fetal distress. While the term *fetal distress* is imprecise, it is typically used in circumstances where fetal heart rate patterns on electronic fetal monitoring suggest a likelihood of fetal hypoxemia or acidosis. Fetal distress is usually suspected by characteristic fetal heart rate (e.g., tachycardia, decreased baseline variability, and recurring late decelerations). Fetal monitoring in preterm infants is somewhat more difficult to interpret. Very preterm fetuses often will be somewhat tachycardic and may have less beat-to-beat variability than more mature fetuses. These fetuses may also show deep decelerations in response to contractions. If fetal distress is suspected, obstetrical consultation should be sought immediately. In some circumstances it is necessary to weigh the advisability of transport to a tertiary institution against immediate delivery if there is suspected fetal distress.

Preterm fetuses are more likely to have an abnormal presentation. Only 60 percent of fetuses at 28 weeks are cephalic, which rises to 98 percent by term. Presentation can usually be determined by abdominal palpation or vaginal examination, but if doubt exists, this should be confirmed by ultrasound examination. Breech presentation does

Table 11-6

SUMMARY OF RECOMMENDATIONS FOR ACTIVITY LIMITATIONS

Patients are instructed to adhere to one of the three levels of activity restriction:

Restricted activity

No heavy lifting (>15 lb), no long walking (>1 block), avoid climbing stairs (>1 flight). Avoid heavy household chores. Take a 1–2 h break at midday and lie down on your side.

Unless instructed otherwise by your prenatal care provider, you may continue to work but should observe the limitations above.

Sexual intercourse is allowable unless your prenatal care provider specifically recommends against it. If you experience contractions during or following intercourse, it is best to abstain from sex until you talk to your prenatal care provider.

Partial bed rest

Lie down on your side for at least 2 h twice daily. No housework other than light cooking. Avoid lifting children. Abstain from sexual intercourse.

Complete bed rest

At complete bed rest, you lie down on your side except to use the bathroom, shower once daily, and sit up for meals. Cooking, housework, and child care must be done by someone else. Abstain from sexual intercourse.

All patients are instructed that if they experience symptoms of preterm labor (four or more uterine cramps or contractions per hour, vaginal spotting, or sudden increase in discharge) during activity to stop that activity and count contractions. If contractions continue at four or more per hour, the hospital or prenatal care provider should be called immediately.

not change the initial management of preterm labor, but if labor progresses, accurate knowledge of presentation is important for deciding on the optimal route of delivery. There is general consensus that in most situations, preterm breech fetuses (less than 34 weeks of gestation but more than 28 weeks) have better outcomes if delivered by cesarean section than if delivered vaginally. Below 28 weeks of gestation, there are no clear data on whether cesarean section offers a distinct benefit.

Prompt recognition of preterm labor is important to give the best possible chance for delaying delivery or at least improving fetal outcome by initiating interventions such as cor-

ticosteroid treatment. The emergency physician plays an important role in this initial evaluation and treatment of the patient in suspected preterm labor.

References

1. Advance report of final natality studies. *Monthly Vital Stat Rep* 40(suppl):8, 1991.
2. Gibbs RS, Romero R, Hillier SL, et al: A review of premature birth and subclinical infection. *Am J Obstet Gynecol* 166:1515, 1992.
3. Robertson PA, Sniderman SH, Laros RK Jr, et al: Neonatal morbidity according to gestational age and birth weight from five tertiary care centers in the United States, 1983 through 1986. *Am J Obstet Gynecol* 166:1629, 1992.
4. Andersen HF, Johnson TRB Jr, Barclay ML, Flora JD: Gestational age assessment: I. Analysis of individual clinical observations. *Am J Obstet Gynecol* 139:173, 1981.
5. Andersen HF: Ultrasonography in labor. *Clin Obstet Gynecol* 34:527, 1992.
6. Alexander GR, Himes JH, Kaufman RJ, et al: A United States national reference for fetal growth. *Obstet Gynecol* 87:163, 1996.
7. Meis PJ, Goldenberg RL, Mercer B, et al: National Institute of Child Health and Human Development Maternal-Fetal Medicine Units Network. The preterm prediction study: Significance of vaginal infections. *Am J Obstet Gynecol* 173:1231, 1995.
8. Iams JD, Casal D, McGregor JA, et al: Fetal fibronectin improves the accuracy of diagnosis of preterm labor. *Am J Obstet Gynecol* 173:141, 1995.
9. Gomez R, Galasso M, Romero R, et al: Ultrasonographic examination of the uterine cervix is better than cervical digital examination as a predictor of the likelihood of premature delivery in patients with preterm labor and intact membranes. *Am J Obstet Gynecol* 171:956, 1994.
10. Utter GO, Dooley SL, Tamura RK, Socol ML: Awaiting cervical change for the diagnosis of preterm labor does not compromise the efficacy of ritodrine tocolysis. *Am J Obstet Gynecol* 163:882, 1990.
11. Stubblefield PG, Heyl PS: Treatment of premature labor with subcutaneous terbutaline. *Obstet Gynecol* 59:457, 1982.
12. Gordon MC, Iams JD. Magnesium sulfate. *Clin Obstet Gynecol* 38:706, 1995.
13. Ferguson JE, II, Dyson DC, Schutz T, Stevenson DK: A comparison of tocolysis with nifedipine or ritodrine: Analysis of efficacy and maternal, fetal, and neonatal outcome. *Am J Obstet Gynecol* 163:105, 1990.
14. National Institutes of Health: Effect of corticosteroids for fetal maturation on perinatal outcomes. *NIH Consensus Statement* 12:1, 1994.
15. Centers for Disease Control and Prevention: Prevention

of perinatal group B streptococcal disease: A public health perspective. *MMWR* 45(RR-7):1, 1996.

16. Lewis R, Mercer BM: Adjunctive care of preterm labor—The use of antibiotics. *Clin Obstet Gynecol* 38:755, 1995.

17. Paneth N, Kiely JL, Wallenstein S, et al: Newborn intensive care and neonatal mortality in low-birth-weight infants: A population study. *N Engl J Med* 307:149, 1982.

18. Boyle JG: Beta-adrenergic agonists. *Clin Obstet Gynecol* 38:688, 1995.

19. Freda MC, Andersen HF, Damus K, et al: Lifestyle modification as an intervention for inner city women at high risk for preterm birth. *J Adv Nurs* 15:364, 1990.

Chapter 12

EMERGENCY VAGINAL DELIVERY

Brian C. Brost

J. Peter VanDorsten

Although many people, including nonobstetric health care providers, view labor and the birth process as mysterious events and situations to be avoided at all costs, deliveries have occurred without assistance throughout history. The most important function in assisting the delivery of a baby is to know when a complication is occurring and methods to improve or correct the situation. This chapter deals with birth as a normal obstetric event, methods to assess maternal and fetal well-being during labor, management of the more common or life-threatening complications, and the care and resuscitation of the newborn infant.

APPROACH TO THE LABORING WOMAN

INITIAL ASSESSMENT OF THE MOTHER AND BABY

On initial evaluation in the emergency department, it is helpful and desirable to obtain and review the patient's prenatal record to look for antepartum complications that may aid in her diagnosis and management. While some obstetricians and family practitioners still use their own forms to record prenatal visits, many providers have switched to a standard obstetric form allowing a quick, systematic review of the patient's antepartum course. Each woman should be evaluated for vaginal bleeding, membrane rupture, preeclampsia, preterm labor, and fetal well-being. Key components of the examination are: maternal vital signs; analysis of fetal heart rate and uterine contractions; assessment of cervical change; and fundal height measurement.

EVALUATION OF THE LABORING PATIENT WITH NO PRIOR OBSTETRIC CARE

For patients without prior obstetrical care, a complete history and physical should be performed to evaluate for possible risk factors that may compromise the maternal or fetal condition during labor. Routine laboratory evaluation should include urinalysis for protein/glucose, urine culture, complete blood count with platelets, maternal blood typing and Rh status, rubella immune status, hepatitis B surface antigen (HBsAg) and possibly human immunodeficiency virus (HIV) status, evaluation for syphilis rapid plasma reagin (RPR) or VDRL, and cervical swabs for *Chlamydia* and gonorrhea. In women with preterm labor, a swab of the lower or "outer third" of the vagina and perianal area for GBS may be helpful to the neonatalogists. Gestational age can be estimated based on LMP, fundal height, and ultrasound (see Table 9-3).

Routine vital signs should include maternal blood pressure and pulse in the sitting position, temperature, and respiratory rate along with documentation of fetal heart tones. Blood pressures during the first and third trimesters are similar to prepregnancy values, while a decrease in both the systolic and diastolic blood pressure is noted in the second trimester. Fetal heart rate can be heard transabdominally using a Doptone by 10 to 12 weeks of gestation or a fetoscope at 18 to 20 weeks estimated gestational age (EGA), and a stethoscope, Doptone, or fetoscope from the later second through the entire third trimester. Figure 12-1 shows typical locations for fundal heights. Normal fetal heart rates are between 120 to 160 beats per minute. Faster (>160 beats per minute, or tachycardia) or slower (<120 beats per minute, or bradycardia) heart rates demand further prolonged evaluation with continuous electronic fetal monitoring while seeking the cause. Obstetric consultation should be obtained to evaluate fetal tachycardia and bradycardia. Causes of fetal tachycardia and bradycardia are listed in Table 12-1. It is important to differentiate the auscultated rate from the maternal pulse to make sure the bradycardia is not maternal pulse. This is done by visualizing fetal cardiac activity by real-time ultrasound or concomitant palpation of the maternal pulse.

Women complaining of cramping, or rhythmic lower abdominal or back pain should be assessed for uterine contractions. This can be done preliminarily by placing a hand lightly over the superior portion of the uterus (fundus). Contractions can be palpated as intermittent tightening of the uterus under the abdominal wall. Important information to obtain includes the frequency, strength, and duration of the contractions. The frequency of contractions is measured from the start of one contraction to the beginning of the next. At the peak of an effective or strong contraction, the uterine fundus cannot be indented with a finger or a thumb.

When uterine contractions occur approximately 10 min or less apart, differentiation between "true" and "false" labor is important. In general, the definition of true labor is

Table 12-1	
CAUSES OF BASELINE FETAL HEART RATE ABNORMALITIES	
Tachycardia (>160 bpm)	**Bradycardia (<120 bpm)**
Fetal hypoxia	Fetal hypoxia
Chorioamnionitis	Congenital heart block
Maternal fever	(more common in women
Maternal hypothyroidism	with SLE)
Fetal tachyarrhythmias	Maternal hypothermia
Fetal anemia	Structural cardiac defects
Fetal heart failure	Prolonged hypoglycemia
Beta sympathomimetic or	Beta blocker drugs
parasympatholytic drugs	
(e.g., terbutaline)	

SLE = systemic lupus erythematosis.

regular contractions increasing in intensity and occurring at progressively closer intervals, leading to gradual cervical dilatation. False labor is defined as contractions without progressive cervical change and is often marked by irregular contractions of steady or irregular intensity that often abate with maternal hydration and sedation.

If it is unclear whether the mother is in labor, particularly if the pregnancy is of less than 37 weeks EGA, it is prudent to observe both the mother and fetus over longer intervals of time to assess for cervical change while continuing to monitor the fetal heart rate. If the patient has no evidence of placenta previa (either documented by ultrasound or in the absence of vaginal bleeding), a sterile vaginal examination will allow assessment of several important factors. The cervix can be evaluated as to its softness, degree of dilation, and effacement (length, measured in centimeters), the status of membranes, and the presenting fetal part. The cervical dilation and effacement are important indicators of imminent delivery. A sterile cervical exam is performed by spreading the labia with the nondominant hand and introducing the first two fingers of the dominant, sterilely gloved hand (palm up) and lubricated with a sterile water-based lubricant. Cervical dilation is measured at the level of the internal os (the cervical portion closest to the presenting fetal part), with the earlier stages of labor (closed to 5 cm) easy to measure. Measurement of more advanced dilation (7 to 10 cm) is obtained by adding together the cervical rim remaining on either side of the fetal head and subtracting this amount from 10 cm. Complete cervical dilation has occurred when the widest portion of the fetal head has passed through the cervical os. The laboring patient is then ready to begin pushing. Preterm pregnancies will reach complete dilation at smaller actual cervical dilation. Cervical examinations in

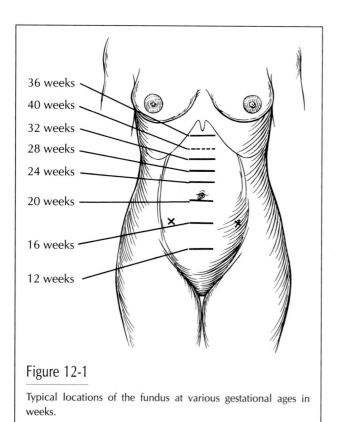

Figure 12-1

Typical locations of the fundus at various gestational ages in weeks.

36 weeks
40 weeks
32 weeks
28 weeks
24 weeks
20 weeks
16 weeks
12 weeks

the low-risk patient should be kept to the minimum needed to evaluate the progression of labor (particularly with evidence of membrane rupture) to lessen the likelihood of infection. If no contractions are noted on monitoring, it becomes important to rule out nonobstetric causes of abdominal or back pain (see Chap. 19).

Women with uterine contractions should be assessed for fetal heart tones during and after the contraction to check for decelerations or transient decreases in the fetal heart rate associated with the contractions. Fetal heart decelerations can be classified as early, variable, or late depending on when they occur in relation to uterine contractions (see Fig. 9-10).

Early decelerations result in fetal heart rate changes that inversely mirror the strength of the uterine contraction. These types of decelerations often occur in the early stages of labor and are not of significant consequence for the fetus. If the nadir fetal heart rate is below 100 beats per minute and repetitive, a vaginal examination for evidence of a prolapsed cord is indicated.

Variable decelerations can be pictured as V- or W-shaped decreases in fetal heart rate (abrupt onset and return to the baseline fetal heart rate) and can occur at the beginning, middle, or end of uterine contractions or even between concentractions. Severe, persistent, variable decelerations (decreases in the fetal heart rate ≥60 beats from the baseline or a nadir of 90 beats per minute), particularly if lasting more than 60 seconds, warrant treatment. Initial management includes sterile vaginal examination, palpating for umbilical cord prolapse, correction of maternal hypotension if present, oxygen by face mask at 10 L/min, and changing the maternal position to lateral decubitus. Amnioinfusion can be performed in labor and delivery units if delivery is not imminent. Amnioinfusion is accomplished by sterile placement of an intrauterine pressure catheter (IUPC), guided through the cervix alongside the fetal head, in a woman with ruptured membranes to allow infusion of fluid into the amniotic cavity. Infusion of 500 to 1000 mL at a rate of 10 to 15 mL/min of body-temperature normal saline solution is thought to relieve compression of the umbilical cord caused by loss of amniotic fluid. Consultation with a practitioner familiar with amnioinfusion should occur prior to its implementation. Tocolysis with terbutaline 0.25 mg subcutaneous injection may allow fetal recovery from severe variable decelerations until obstetric help is available (this should not be used in women with vaginal bleeding or suspected abruption, as it may mask the maternal pulse response). Further discussion of tocolysis can be found in Chapter 11.

Late decelerations occur when the fetal heart rate decreases at the peak of the uterine contraction and returns to baseline after the contraction is completed (see Fig. 9-10). Repetitive late decelerations are usually a result of uteroplacental insufficiency. Repetitive late decelerations indicate possible fetal compromise and require prompt evaluation, continuous fetal monitoring, and/or delivery if not correctable. Administration of oxygen by face mask by 10 L/min, change in maternal position to the lateral decubitus, and administration of intravenous fluids may help to correct the abnormal fetal heart beat.

A prolonged sudden deceleration of the fetal heart rate below 80 beats per minute in a fetus with a prior "normal"-appearing tracing can be related to uterine hyperactivity (contractions closer than every 2 min or lasting >90 s), fetal manipulation on vaginal exam, supine hypotension in the mother, umbilical cord prolapse, or conduction anesthesia. Management includes correction of the cause if possible. When vaginal delivery is not imminent, cesarean section should be performed for a persistent fetal heart rate in the range of 60 to 80 beats per minute for more than 5 minutes in the fetus of viable gestational age, generally above 25 to 26 weeks.

After confirming that the slow fetal heart rate is truly a fetal and not maternal pulse, or in the presence of late decelerations, a series of maneuvers may improve the pattern of the fetal heart rate. It is important to obtain the consultation or services of an obstetrician or surgeon if emergent delivery is indicated. While awaiting their arrival, placing the mother in a left or right lateral tilt or the knee-chest position can improve blood flow to the fetus by increasing blood return back from the lower extremities. Supplemental oxygen can be given via face mask at a rate of 10 L/min. Intravenous access should be obtained with an 18- or preferably 16-gauge catheter to administer a 500- to 1000-mL bolus of normal saline or lactated Ringer's solution. It is important to perform a sterile digital vaginal exam to evaluate for causes of the fetal bradycardia such as cord prolapse, rapid cervical dilatation, or sudden fetal descent. If these maneuvers do not result in an improvement in the fetal heart rate, consider changing the patient's position (e.g. lateral decubitus or knee-chest) every 30 seconds. Continuous fetal monitoring and assessment of uterine contractions are important. Tocolysis or interruption of uterine contractions may be helpful through the use of subcutaneous terbutaline 0.25 mg (if there is no evidence of maternal hemorrhage or abruption).

RUPTURE OF MEMBRANES

Less than 10 percent of women rupture their membranes before spontaneous labor, but confirmation is important because of the increased risk of maternal and fetal infection and risk of cord prolapse if the presenting fetal part is not fixed in the pelvis. Spontaneous rupture of membranes is suspected when a watery discharge is described, whether it presents as a sudden gush or a persistent increase in vaginal moisture. It is important to note the time of rupture of membranes, fetal movement, color (clear versus thin or thick green) and amount of discharge, and continued leakage of fluid. Documentation of membrane rupture can be made and confirmed through a variety of techniques including use of clinical history, nitrazine, ferning, or vaginal pooling (see Table 12-2). The diagnosis of rupture of membranes can never be excluded over the phone.

If the woman's clinical history suggests that membrane rupture has occurred at <37 weeks, digital cervical examination should not be performed until after checking for physical evidence of spontaneous membrane rupture (except in cases of fetal bradycardia to check for cord prolapse or if delivery appears imminent). When membrane rupture is suggested by sterile speculum examination, digital examination should be avoided to decrease the risk of ascending intraamniotic infection. The length and dilation of the cervix can be estimated using a visual estimate during the sterile speculum exam instead of a digital cervical exam.

Visualization of the cervix and posterior fornix allows for assessment for amniotic fluid flow from the cervix or pooling in the posterior fornix. If no fluid is present, having the woman perform the Valsalva maneuver may allow visualization of amniotic fluid flowing from the cervix. Nitrazine paper can be evaluated using a sterile cotton swab of the posterior fornix to document a change in the pH of the vagina from its normal level (pH 4.5 to 5.5, strip remains yellow) in contrast to rupture of membranes (the alkaline amniotic fluid, pH 7.0 to 7.5, turns the pH strip dark blue). False-positive evaluations can be found in the presence of semen, blood, alkaline urine, and bacterial vaginosis. In the presence of one of these substances, the presence of ferning is more reliable. Ferning can be documented by allowing a vaginal pool swab applied to a glass microscope slide to dry and then evaluating it under the microscope. False positives

can be obtained by viewing fingerprints on the slide or collecting a sample of cervical mucus. False-negative tests occur with a dry swab or in the presence of blood.

TECHNIQUES FOR VAGINAL DELIVERY

More than 95 percent of vaginal deliveries at term occur with the fetal head as the presenting part. The goal of the person assisting in vaginal delivery is to decrease the risk of injury or complications for both the mother and the baby during labor and after delivery has occurred. While most women respond to their labor changes instinctively, the assistant can help by optimizing maternal efforts at the appropriate time and monitoring fetal well-being.

STAGES OF LABOR

Although labor is divided into three stages to aid in clinical management, it should be viewed as a continuous process. The first stage of labor typically lasts about 10 hours in nulliparous women and 8 hours in multiparous women; it represents the time from the onset of labor to complete cervical dilation (10 cm). This first stage of labor has been divided into several different phases. The latent phase has a variable duration (averaging 4 to 6 hours up to 13 to 20 hours for nulliparous and multiparous women, respectively) and includes

---

Table 12-2

TESTS TO EVALUATE RUPTURE OF AMNIOTIC MEMBRANES

Test	Findings	Specificity	Causes of False Result
Clinical history of leaking fluid	—	Fair	Urine leakage, vaginitis, normal physiologic discharge of pregnancy
Nitrazine paper	pH > 7.0	Good	Blood, bacterial vaginosis, semen, alkaline urine
Visualization of fluid from os/vaginal pooling	Direct visualization of fluid in vagina or emanating from os	Excellent for direct visualization from cervix	Excellent
Ferning pattern on glass slide	Ferning pattern under microscopy after drying of fluid taken from vaginal pool	Excellent	Cervical secretions will sometime fern
Decreased fluid on ultrasound	Low amniotic fluid index (less than 5 to 10 cm)	Fair to good	Oligohydramnios from other causes (e.g., uteroplacental insufficiency, fetal renal problems)

the time between the onset of labor to the time when an acceleration in the rate of cervical dilatation is noted. The next phase is characterized by maximal cervical dilation with the average rate of cervical dilatation of 3.0 cm/h in nulliparous women and 5 to 6 cm/h in multiparous women.

The second stage of labor begins when the woman reaches complete cervical dilation (10 cm) and ends with delivery of the baby. This stage typically lasts an average of 10 and 35 min in multiparous and nulliparous women, respectively. The fetal head descends an average of 3 to 6 cm/h depending on maternal parity, with descent of less than 1 cm/h in nulliparous women and 2 cm/h in multiparous women being considered abnormal.

The third stage of labor comprises the time from delivery of the baby to delivery of the placenta. The average duration of this stage is about 5 min; it may be longer, though it is not considered abnormally long unless more than 30 min have passed. This stage is similar in both nulliparous and multiparous women. A fourth stage of labor has been described by some authors and is the critical first hour after delivery. During this time, routine evaluation of the placenta and membranes should be performed, looking for vessels at the membrane margins suggesting an accessory lobe or checking for missing segments from the placenta. A thorough examination and repair of any vaginal or cervical lacerations is done during this time. Uterine relaxation, which may lead to increased vaginal bleeding and possibly postpartum hemorrhage, is most likely to occur during this period and should be promptly evaluated and treated, as described in Chap. 13.

FREQUENCY OF MONITORING OF FETAL HEART RATE DURING LABOR

The frequency and type of fetal heart rate monitoring needed depends on the risk classification of the pregnancy. Approximately 20 percent of women have antepartum, surgical, or medical conditions that account for more than half of the poor obstetric outcomes. Another 5 to 10 percent of pregnant women enter this high-risk classification during labor, accounting for an additional 20 to 25 percent of poor obstetric outcomes. The other 20 percent of poor obstetric outcomes occur in pregnancies with no apparent risk factors.

During the first stage of labor in low-risk pregnancies, fetal heart tones should be recorded every 30 min; this should be increased to every 15 min during the second stage of labor. High-risk pregnancies should be evaluated with review of the fetal heart rate every 15 min during the first stage of labor and every 5 min during the second stage, when continuous fetal monitoring or intermittent auscultation is being used. If the intermittent auscultation technique is used, a 1:1 nurse-to-patient ratio is required. If an abnormality of the fetal heart rate is noted (tachycardia, bradycardia, or decelerations), continuous fetal heart rate monitoring is help-

ful in providing a more complete evaluation of fetal well-being. Continuous fetal heart rate monitoring is an alternative and does provide a graphic tracing of the fetal heart rate and uterine activity. This can be helpful for an obstetric care provider who may arrive later.

PROPHYLAXIS FOR GROUP B STREPTOCOCCUS

Neonatal sepsis due to group B streptococcus (GBS) is the leading cause of neonatal sepsis in the United States. With proper intrapartum management, much of the morbidity and mortality associated with this infection can be prevented. Colonization by GBS is present in 15 to 40 percent of all pregnant women. Even if GBS-colonized women are treated during the third trimester of pregnancy, 20 to 70 percent remain colonized at term. While GBS colonization rarely results in maternal morbidity, early-onset GBS sepsis affects 1 to 3 in 1000 live-born infants, resulting in 80 percent of all GBS disease in the newborn. The best technique for prevention appears to be maternal antibiotic prophylaxis during labor, allowing passage of antibiotics to the fetus within 1 to 2 h of maternal administration.

All women delivering preterm (less than 37 weeks gestation) should receive GBS prophylaxis. Current recommendations from the Centers for Disease Control and Prevention (CDC) for the prevention of early-onset GBS disease in term pregnancies includes routine prenatal screening at 35 to 37 weeks of gestation. Women with a positive vaginal or urine culture for GBS at any time during the pregnancy should be given antibiotic prophylaxis during labor. When antepartum cultures are negative or not performed, women are still considered candidates for GBS prophylaxis if they develop an intrapartum fever ≥38.0°C (100.4°F), have rupture of membranes for ≥18 h, or delivered a prior infant with invasive GBS disease.

Recommendations for GBS intrapartum prophylaxis is ampicillin 2 g IV initially, then 1 g IV every 4 h until delivery or an initial dose of penicillin G, 5 million units IV, followed by 2.5 million units IV every 4 h until delivery. In women allergic to penicillin, either clindamycin 900 mg IV every 8 h or erythromycin 500 mg IV every 6 h until delivery may be used.

TECHNIQUE OF DELIVERY

CEPHALIC DELIVERY

The cardinal movements in cephalic delivery are illustrated in Fig. 12-2. After confirming complete dilation and assessing the fetal heart rate, the mother should be encouraged to bear down or push the baby out. Proper maternal positioning can be obtained by having the mother grasp the back

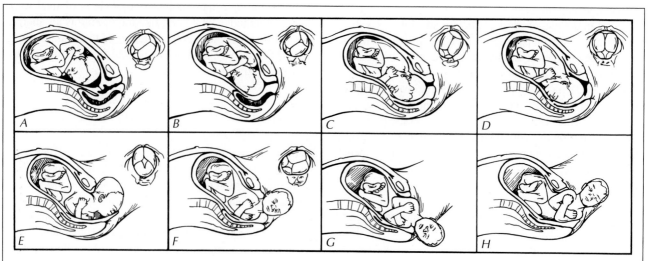

Figure 12-2

Cardinal movements in labor. *A.* Unengaged fetal vertex in the LOA position (inset in upper-right-hand corner). *B.* Descent of the fetal vertex with flexion of the head. *C.* Further flexion and descent of the head with internal rotation of the vertex to near occiput anterior. *D.* Further internal rotation to straight occiput anterior and descent of the fetal vertex. *E.* Fetal head extension underneath the pubic symphysis. *F.* External rotation of the head (restitution). *G.* Downward gentle traction on the fetal vertex allows delivery of the anterior shoulder. *H.* Gentle upward traction on the fetal vertex allows delivery of the posterior shoulder.

of the distal portion of her thighs or assisting her in flexion at the hips and knees by supporting the legs. After the contraction has started, encourage the mother to "bear down" by holding her breath with her chin to her chest while an assistant counts up to 10. The process is repeated two more times during each contraction, with a quick breath in between each pushing effort. An occasional sterile vaginal examination with a gloved finger during the pushing effort is useful to assess fetal descent and providing a focal point for the woman to bear down against through the use of gentle pressure against the posterior vaginal wall toward the rectum. When the fetal head maintains labial separation in between contractions, it is said to be crowning. During this portion of pushing, pressure is maintained on the perineum to decrease the risk of an uncontrolled vaginal delivery and possible extensive perineal laceration.

When the fetal head is crowning, an episiotomy may be performed using a straight Mayo scissors to facilitate delivery of the fetal head. Local anesthesia with several milliliters of 1% lidocaine without epinephrine can be used in the midline of the perineal body and up the vaginal canal. Two fingers are placed inside and along the posterior vagina, to protect the fetal head and the incision is extended twice the distance up into the vaginal canal as is cut posteriorly along the perineal skin with care taken not to extend the incision into the rectum or anal sphincter. If the episiotomy is cut before the fetal head maintains pressure against the perineum, significant bleeding can occur. The routine need for episiotomy is controversial. Most practitioners will utilize episiotomy if forceps are required or a vacuum delivery is used, if it is felt that a significant laceration would otherwise occur, or if more rapid delivery is necessary (e.g., abnormal fetal heart tracing) and an episiotomy would facilitate delivery.

Encourage the mother to continue gradually increasing her bearing down efforts so as to allow the fetal head to dilate the vaginal opening in a controlled fashion while the perineal body is supported with a sterile towel. When the fetal head has been delivered, ask the woman to stop pushing and to breathe, allowing time to suction the oral and nasopharyngeal passages with a bulb suction and to check around the fetal neck for evidence of a nuchal cord. If a nuchal cord is noted, gently reduce it over its head to prevent constriction with delivery of the body. If the cord is too tight to reduce, clamp it with two hemostats and divide between the clamps. Encourage the mother to again bear down gently as you apply gentle posterolateral traction on the side of the head to aid in delivery of the infant's anterior shoulder. To accomplish this, place the palm of each hand over the infant's ears with the fingers pointed to the baby's nose. When the anterior shoulder is evident below the pubic symphysis, redirect the gentle traction in an anterior direction to delivery the baby's posterior shoulder. Support the remainder of the baby's body as it subsequently delivers spontaneously. Hold the back of the infant's head in the palm of your nondominant hand and "trap" the baby's legs and body between your forearm and body. This will enable the birth attendant to hold the baby at the level of the maternal abdomen and repeat bulb suction as needed. Double clamp the fetal cord about 2 to 2½ in. from where the cord enters the body and divide between the clamps. The baby should then be thoroughly dried with clean towels and wrapped in a blanket with coverings around the body and cranium, or it should be placed in a warming unit if available.

BREECH VAGINAL DELIVERY

Breech vaginal presentations occur in 3 to 4 percent of all deliveries. The rate of breech presentation is higher at earlier gestational ages (7 percent at 32 weeks and 25 percent at 28 weeks). Factors associated with breech presentation include polyhydramnios, oligohydramnios, hydrocephalus, previous breech delivery, tumors of the pelvis, and uterine anomalies. Breech presentation is associated with a three to four times greater incidence of perinatal morbidity and mortality, despite the current rate of more than 90 percent cesarean delivery for persistent breech presentation. Morbidity and mortality are related primarily to prematurity, congenital anomalies (two to three times greater), and birth trauma. The major factor contributing to morbidity with vaginal breech delivery is that the smaller fetal feet and abdomen can pass through a partially dilated cervix and the larger fetal head cannot, resulting in head entrapment. Birth injuries can also include brachial plexus or spinal cord injuries, muscular injuries, cephalohematomas or intracranial bleeds, and low Apgar scores.

Fetal position is denoted by the position of the fetal sacrum in relation to the maternal abdomen. Three types of breech presentation can be noted on ultrasound or single-shot flat-plate of the abdomen: frank breech—hips flexed/knees extended; complete breech—hips flexed/knees flexed; and footling breech—one or both hips extended (Fig. 12-3A through C). The risk of cord prolapse increases with inability of the breech to fill the pelvis with rates of 0.5 percent, 4 to 6 percent, and 15 to 18 percent with the above types, respectively. Most obstetricians elect to deliver breech infants by cesarean section because of decreasing experience in breech vaginal delivery and significantly higher risk of fetal and maternal morbidity. External cephalic version may be considered in the term nonlaboring woman (with intact membranes) when the fetus is noted to be presenting breech.

It is important to monitor the fetal heart rate throughout the delivery. As the fetal breech becomes visible through the introitus, maintain pressure on the fetal thighs toward the fetal abdomen to help provide protection for the fetal umbilical cord. Avoid premature outward traction on the fetal feet or lower body until the infant has delivered to the level of the umbilicus. The main goal is to provide encouragement of maternal pushing and support for the delivering fetal body, keeping the sacrum anterior. If the fetus is not footling breech, sweep the medial portion of the fetal thigh laterally and bend the knee by splinting the fetal thigh, using the fingers parallel to the femur (Fig. 12-4A). Grasp and deliver the foot and then repeat the procedure for the other leg (Fig.

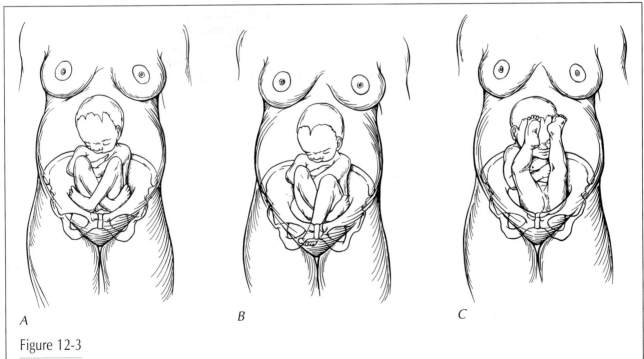

A   B   C

Figure 12-3

Breech variations. A. A complete breech with thighs and knees flexed. B. An incomplete breech with one thigh partially extended and knees flexed (thighs and knees extended results in a footling breech). C. Frank breech with thighs flexed and knees extended.

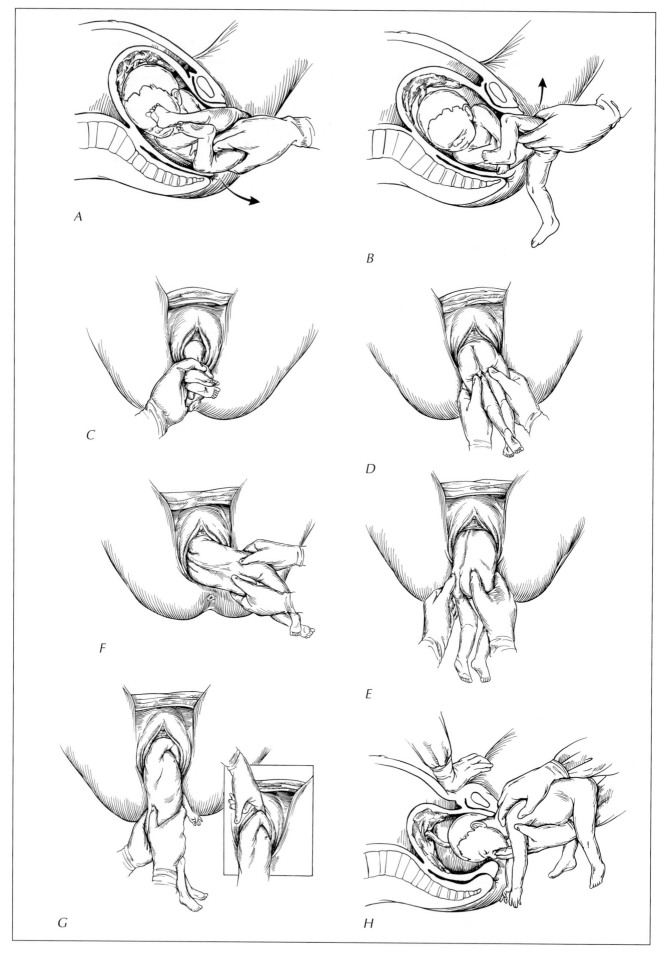

F

G

H

12-4*B*). With a footling breech, grasp both ankles, using three fingers of your hand with the middle finger between the ankles (Fig. 12-4*C*). With thumbs placed over the fetal sacrum and fingers over the anterior iliac crests, allow the delivery of the torso to continue (Fig. 12-4*D*). A moist towel can be used to provide easier handling of the baby's body. Support the infant in a neutral position while encouraging continued maternal pushing until the scapula appears (Fig. 12-4*E*). Then gently rotate the fetal trunk 90° (Fig. 12-4*F*) and deliver the anterior arm by placing your fingers parallel to the humerus at the fetal elbow and sweep the fetal arm downward to deliver the anterior arm (Fig. 12-4*G*). If rotation is difficult, consider delivering of the posterior arm first. Rotate the baby in the reverse direction 180° and repeat the procedure for the other fetal arm. Have an assistant apply abdominal pressure to the fetal head to maintain it in a flexed position with delivery of the fetal body.

The fetus should preferably be delivered in the sacrum-anterior position, maintaining the fetal head in the flexed position by placing the index and middle fingers over the maxilla (Mauriceau-Smellie-Veit maneuver) while applying gentle downward traction by hooking two fingers of the other hand across the fetal shoulders from above (Fig. 12-4*H*). The main force effecting delivery of the fetus should be maternal effort. If the fetus is delivered in the sacrum-posterior position, grasp the fetal feet with one hand and sweep the feet over the maternal abdomen (modified Prague maneuver) while grasping the fetal shoulders to effect delivery of the fetal head. Again, the main force aiding in delivery of the fetus is maternal effort.

Sometimes the cervix is not sufficiently dilated to allow passage of the fetal head after delivery of the fetal body. If the cervix cannot be successfully reduced around the fetal head, cutting Dührssen incisions in the cervix with a long straight mayo scissors at the 2 and 10 o'clock positions can provide release of the fetal head, allowing successful delivery of the infant.

SHOULDER DYSTOCIA

Shoulder dystocia is a peripartum event that is unpredictable and, if not properly managed, can cause serious neonatal morbidity or mortality. It is defined as the inability to deliver the fetal shoulders using normal obstetric maneuvers after delivery of the fetal head.

Shoulder dystocia occurs in 0.13 to 2.0 percent of all vaginal deliveries. Several antepartum and intrapartum risk factors have been noted to increase the risk of shoulder dystocia, including macrosomia (fetal birth weight ≥4000 or 4500 g), maternal obesity, maternal diabetes, postdate pregnancies, pelvic abnormalities, midpelvic delivery, and labor abnormalities including protracted labor or prolonged second stage. Although these factors are present in many cases of shoulder dystocia most shoulder dystocias cannot be predicted prior to delivery.

Maternal morbidity resulting from shoulder dystocia is related to a difficult delivery and maneuvers performed to relieve the dystocia; such complications include lacerations of the birth canal, postpartum hemorrhage, and possible uterine rupture. Fetal complications are more frequent and significant than maternal complications. Brachial plexus injury results from excessive lateral traction on the fetal head in an attempt to dislodge the anterior shoulder. This lateral force stretches the C5 through T1 nerve roots, resulting in a Erb or Klumpke palsy. Brachial plexus injuries occur in about 15 percent of all cases of shoulder dystocia, with one-fifth of these being permanent injuries. Often, brachial plexus injuries noted at birth will resolve over time. Improvement is unlikely if no change in neurologic function has occurred within the first 3 months. Other possible sequelae of shoulder dystocia include an increased incidence of 5-min Apgar scores below 7, neonatal seizures (~13 percent), fractured clavicle or humerus, and spinal cord injury.

Management of shoulder dystocia involves both anticipation and preparation prior to the birth event for this potentially serious obstetric emergency. The key tenet to avoiding fetal injury is to avoid excessive traction on the fetal head during delivery. Typically, shoulder dystocia is evidenced when delivery of the fetal head is followed by a "cranial recoil" or retraction of the head onto the perineum ("turtle sign") during spontaneous or instrumental vaginal delivery. This occurs because the fetal shoulder girdle occupies an anteroposterior position rather than the usual oblique position. When this occurs, the anterior shoulder lodges behind the pubic symphysis, limiting further descent.

Figure 12-4

Management of the vaginal breech delivery. *A.* The Pinard maneuver. The operator's hand is placed behind the fetal thigh, putting gentle pressure at the knee and allowing delivery of the leg. *B.* A similar maneuver of the opposite leg. *C.* The feet are grasped with the thumb and third finger over the lateral malleolus and the second finger is placed between the two ankles. *D.* With maternal expulsive efforts, the breech is delivered to the level of the umbilicus. The sacrum should be kept anterior. *E.* Again, with maternal expulsive efforts, the infant is delivered to the level of the clavicles, keeping the sacrum anterior. Excessive outward traction by the operator will frequently result in nuchal arms. *F.* The fetus is rotated 90° allowing visualization of the now anterior right arm. *G.* The arm is well visualized and a single digit is used to deliver it. Delivery of the opposite arm is accomplished by rotating the fetus 180° in a clockwise direction and repeating the maneuver. *H.* Delivery of the fetal vertex is accomplished by placing the operator's fingers over the maxillary processes of the fetus, keeping the body parallel to the floor. The body should never be lifted above parallel to prevent hyperextension of the neck. An assistant applies suprapubic pressure, aiding flexion of the fetal head and accomplishing delivery.

When a shoulder dystocia has been diagnosed, a deliberate and planned sequence of events should be initiated. Stop the mother from pushing and check for possible obstructive etiologies. Aggressive fundal pressure or further maternal pushing will only impact the anterior shoulder further. Call for help—another physician experienced in the management of shoulder dystocia is very important, if available—and mobilize appropriate nursing staff, anesthesia personnel, and pediatricians. The pH of the fetal blood decreases very slowly at a rate of only 0.04/min, so the worst thing to do in the case of shoulder dystocia is to panic.

Cut a generous episiotomy if it has not already been performed to minimize the effect of maternal soft tissue in obstructing delivery of the fetal shoulders. Have an assistant provide suprapubic pressure by pressing the maternal abdomen just above the pubic bone, in an attempt to dislodge the anterior fetal shoulder under the pubic bone, or directed toward the lateral portion of the maternal pelvis, in an attempt to move the shoulder back into the oblique position (Fig. 12-5). Often this procedure is performed in conjunction with McRobert's maneuver by having two assistants deeply flex the maternal thighs in an attempt to straighten the maternal lumbar and lumbosacral lordosis and displace the anterior fetal shoulder by rotating the pubic symphysis cephalad (Fig. 12-6). These maneuvers reduce the force required to effect delivery of the baby and are sufficient to relieve up to 85 to 90 percent of all cases of shoulder dystocia.

If the infant's shoulders have still not been delivered, a Wood's or "corkscrew" maneuver can be performed by placing a hand behind the posterior shoulder and rotating the baby 180°, so that this shoulder now becomes the "anterior" shoulder (Fig. 12-7). If this is not successful, place a hand

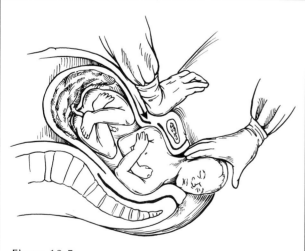

Figure 12-5

Suprapubic pressure is being applied by an assistant while the operator is applying gentle downward traction on the fetal head to disimpact the anterior shoulder.

in the posterior portion of the vagina in an attempt to deliver the posterior arm (Fig. 12-8A and B). Follow the fetal arm to the elbow and apply pressure to the antecubital fossa, causing the forearm to flex. Grasp the fetal arm and sweep it over the fetal chest to deliver the posterior arm. If neither of these maneuvers is successful, a Zavanelli maneuver or "cephalic replacement followed by cesarean delivery" is the last maneuver used to deliver the fetus with extreme shoulder dystocia.

CORD PROLAPSE

If the cord is seen or felt, move the presenting fetal part upward continuously with a gloved hand to prevent compression of the cord. Trying to replace the fetal cord while elevating the presenting fetal part is futile and possibly harmful to the infant, resulting in delay in preparation for an abdominal delivery. Preparations for cesarean delivery include obtaining anesthesia and surgical support, continuous assessment of the fetal heart rate, starting a large-bore intravenous access, placement of a Foley catheter, and clipping the pubic hair above the pubic symphysis. If fetal heart tones are not present, the fetus should be delivered vaginally.

ABNORMAL OR COMPOUND PRESENTATION

The incidence of an infant presenting "face first" (i.e., a hyperextended head) is 1 in 600 to 1200. This presentation is often associated with a contracted maternal pelvis, a large infant, or an anencephalic fetus. Face presentation is distinguished from a breech presentation by the presence of a triangle formed by the fetal mouth and malar prominences. Fetal position in face presentation is denoted by the mentum or chin as anterior or posterior. Infants presenting mentum posterior rarely delivery vaginally unless they spontaneously convert to mentum anterior. It is important not to try to push the fetal head up the birth canal to allow a vertex delivery or to try to rotate the fetal head to mentum anterior, as these maneuvers are frequently associated with significant maternal or fetal morbidity.

Brow presentation is rarer and is usually seen earlier in labor, with later spontaneous conversion to a vertex or face presentation. No attempt should be made to convert a brow presentation. Persistent brow presentation has a poor prognosis for spontaneous vaginal delivery.

Compound presentation is the prolapse of a fetal extremity alongside the presenting fetal part and complicates approximately 1 in 1200 deliveries. Prematurity is a significant factor in more than 50 percent of compound presentations, with 90 percent of these occurring with delivery of a second twin. When a compound presentation is noted, labor should be allowed to progress normally with expectant vaginal delivery. If the fetal limb does not spontaneously retract, a gentle "pinch" to move the extremity up-

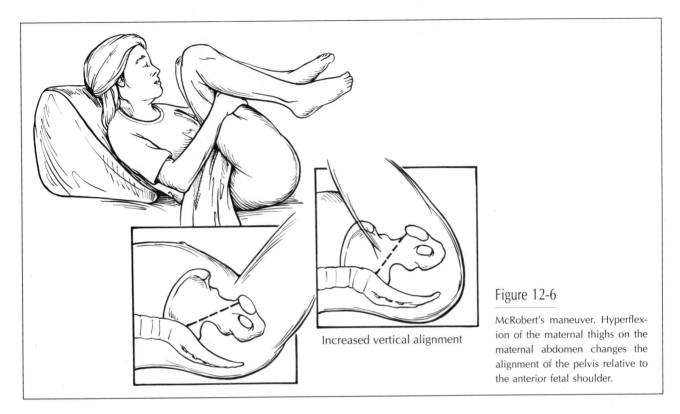

Figure 12-6

Increased vertical alignment

McRobert's maneuver. Hyperflexion of the maternal thighs on the maternal abdomen changes the alignment of the pelvis relative to the anterior fetal shoulder.

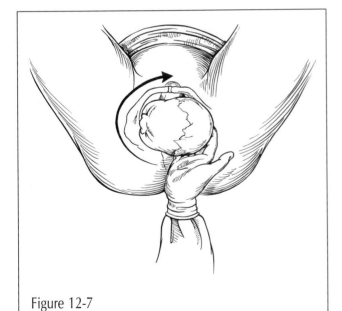

Figure 12-7

Wood's screw maneuver. A hand is placed behind the posterior shoulder and, using firm but gentle pressure, the posterior shoulder is rotated so that it becomes the anterior shoulder. This will usually allow ready delivery of either the anterior or posterior shoulder.

ward with a gloved hand may be sufficient encouragement. Do not lift or move the fetal presenting part in an attempt to reduce or replace the fetal limb.

DELIVERY OF THE PLACENTA

Delivery of the placenta usually occurs within the first 5 min after delivery of the baby, but it can take up to 30 min. If there is no evidence of maternal vaginal hemorrhage, it is useful to await signs of placental separation, including "lengthening" of the umbilical cord, a sudden gush of blood, and a globular appearance of the uterus within the maternal abdomen. Gentle traction on a Kelly clamp placed perpendicular to the umbilical cord can be maintained while pushing against the lower portion of the uterus with the non-dominant hand just above the pubic symphysis toward the upper abdomen. This motion will decrease the risk of uterine inversion, or pulling of the uterus inside-out with the placenta still attached. Excessive traction on the umbilical cord should be avoided to reduce the likelihood of uterine inversion. If the placenta does not freely descend and the patient is not bleeding significantly, it is often prudent to extend the waiting period. After 30 min or with significant bleeding, it may be necessary to separate and remove the placenta from

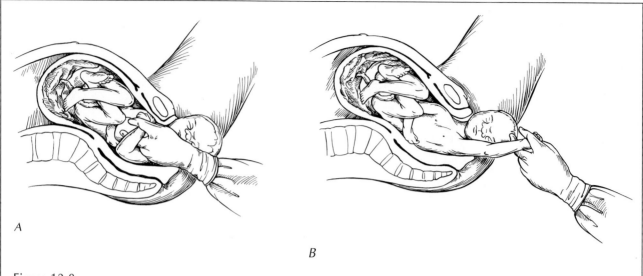

A

B

Figure 12-8

A and *B.* Delivery of the posterior arm. If efforts to disimpact the anterior shoulder have failed to this point, the operator's hand is placed into the vagina, grasping the hand of the posterior arm. The arm is then swept over the fetal thorax and pulled through the maternal vagina. This will result in simultaneous delivery of the posterior shoulder.

the uterus manually. (Fig. 13-15). In most circumstances where the placenta has not delivered in 30 minutes, it is best to await an obstetrician to deliver the placenta because abnormal adherence of the placenta to the uterus (e.g., placenta accreta) is likely. The need for operative intervention (e.g., dilation and curettage) is very possible in this setting.

The following is a description of manual removal of the placenta. This is usually performed by a practitioner familiar with the technique. Coat a sterile gloved hand with iodine solution and introduce the hand into the vagina and through the dilated cervix.

After finding the placental position, gently use the side of the hand to form a cleavage plane between the placenta and the uterus. Grasp the free placenta and remove the hand from within the uterus and vagina. After delivery of the placenta, infusion of 20 U of oxytocin diluted in 1 L of physiologic saline can be infused at rates of 125 mL/h up to 500 mL over 10 to 15 min to maintain uterine tone and decrease the risk of postpartum hemorrhage. Gentle massage of the uterine fundus will also facilitate uterine contractions and lessen bleeding after delivery of the placenta. If a cleavage plane does not easily form, it is best to leave the placenta in place and call an obstetrician, especially if there is no significant maternal bleeding, as this may represent an abnormal placental adherence such as placenta accreta, percreta, or increta.

UTERINE INVERSION

Uterine inversion is a rare (1 in 2000 deliveries) but potentially fatal complication of the third stage of labor. Excessive traction on the umbilical cord in an attempt to expedite delivery of the placenta has been implicated in uterine in-

version, although 15 to 50 percent of inversions occur spontaneously. Diagnosis is made when a pear-shaped, bleeding mass is noted vaginally and abdominal exam confirms that the uterine fundus is not in its usual position.

Treatment involves prompt recognition of the condition, uterine replacement, and correction of shock and hemorrhage, as these clinical conditions are frequently associated with uterine inversions. Do not remove the placenta (if it is still attached) until after replacement of the uterus back to its normal position, as removal may increase the risk of hemorrhage because of the inability of the uterus to contract at the placental insertion site. Manual replacement of the uterus may require the use of halogenated anesthetics to aid in relaxation of the cervix. To replace the uterus, the uterine fundus is grasped in the palm of the operator's hand and manually replaced back through the vagina into the abdominal cavity (Fig. 13-6). Assess for the presence of the fundus above the level of the umbilicus to make sure that all portions of uterus have "unfolded." Once the uterus has been replaced and the placenta removed, oxytocic agents such as oxytocin, methergine (0.2 mg IM—avoid in hypertensive or preeclamptic women), or 15-methyl prostaglandin $F_{2\alpha}$ (0.25 mg IM—avoid in women with asthma or cardiac disease) should be used to promote uterine tone.

EPISIOTOMY AND LACERATION REPAIR

After a vaginal delivery, the vagina and cervix should be examined for evidence of lacerations. Superficial mucosal lacerations involving only the vaginal mucosa may be left "open" to heal by secondary intention if not actively bleeding, or may be reapproximated using 3-0 or 4-0 chromic suture if bleeding. Deeper lacerations should be repaired using a 2-0 chromic suture beginning 1 cm above the laceration to ligate any vaginal veins that may have retracted. If the defect is secured only at the exact ends of the laceration, a hematoma may form. Take care to approximate the entire depth of the laceration using running, locked stitches of the suture and secure the suture with a knot after closing the laceration. Upper vaginal lacerations should be repaired prior to repair of perineal lacerations or the episiotomy site. These may require exposure and lighting only available in an operating room. Lacerations near the clitoris should be carefully repaired with fine suture (e.g., 4-0 chromic) only if there is active bleeding, as scarring or nerve damage may occur. Injuries near the urethra require placement of a Foley catheter prior to repair to make sure that the urethra or bladder is not damaged or inadvertently ligated.

Second-degree perineal lacerations involve the vaginal mucosa and muscles without damage to fascia or muscle of the rectal sphincter. A 2-0 chromic suture is secured about 1 cm above the deepest portion of the incision with closure of the vaginal mucosa to the hymenal ring using a continuous locked stitch (Fig. 12-9*A* through *C*). Without cutting or tying the suture, place the needle through the vaginal mucosa and exit at the deepest point of the muscular defect. Reapproximate the vaginal muscles from the deepest portion out in a continuous unlocked fashion. Bring the needle out at the apex of the perineal defect closest to the rectum and close the perineal skin using a continuous subcuticular stitch to the hymenal ring. Advance the needle under the hymenal ring and secure the suture within the lower vagina.

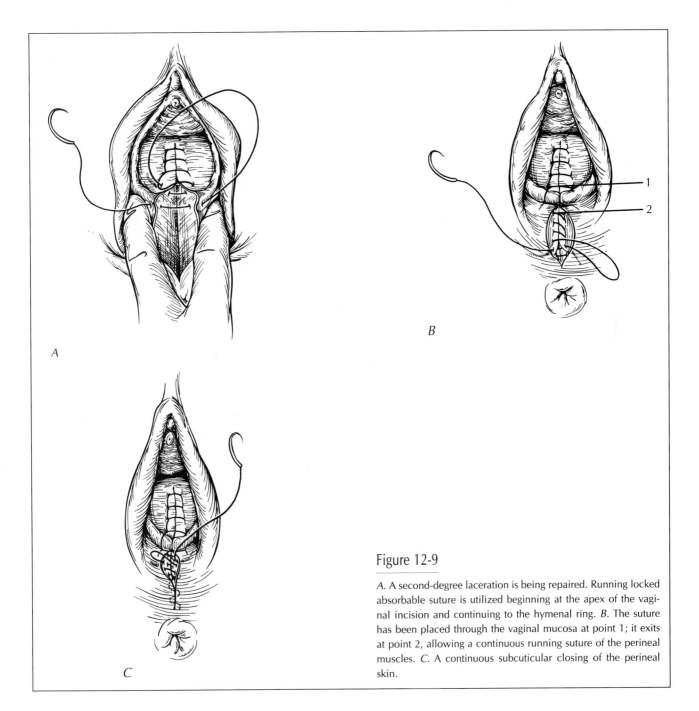

Figure 12-9

A. A second-degree laceration is being repaired. Running locked absorbable suture is utilized beginning at the apex of the vaginal incision and continuing to the hymenal ring. *B.* The suture has been placed through the vaginal mucosa at point 1; it exits at point 2, allowing a continuous running suture of the perineal muscles. *C.* A continuous subcuticular closing of the perineal skin.

Repair of episiotomies or lacerations involving the anal sphincter capsule (third degree) or rectal mucosa (fourth degree) requires careful identification of anatomy (Fig. 12-10*A* through *D*). The rectal mucosa can be closed using a submucosal stitch of 3-0 or 4-0 chromic suture on a small taper needle in a continuous or interrupted fashion. Interrupted stitches of chromic suture may be used to cover the submucosal sutures and avoid direct approximation of the submucosal and upcoming vaginal running locked stitch. Identification of the cut ends of the anal sphincter is essential for successful repair. Grasp the sphincter muscle and capsule with an Allis clamp and suture with 2-0 Vicryl on a taper needle. Closure of this capsule sheath is easiest by first placing two or three interrupted stitches approximating 1 cm of the posterior fascia first, followed by similar approximation of the cephalad, superior, and finally the caudal portions of the sphincter capsule. It is important to reiterate that the strength of this closure is obtained through approximation of the sphincter fascia and not the sphincter muscle. Following reapproximation of the rectal mucosa and anal sphincter, the remainder is closed like a second-degree episiotomy. Consultation with a practitioner skilled in the repair of third- or fourth-degree per-

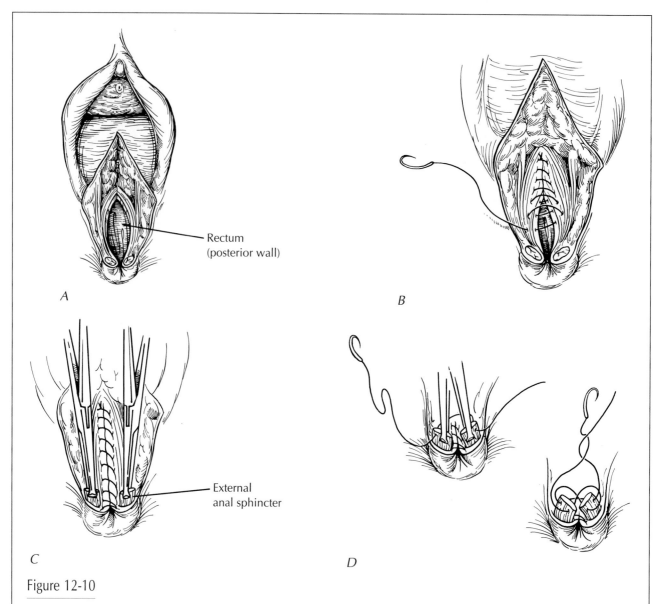

Figure 12-10

A. Appearance of third- and fourth-degree lacerations showing the torn anterior rectal wall and allowing visualization of the intact posterior rectal wall. Interruption in the external anal sphincter is also seen. *B.* Repair of the anterior rectal wall is demonstrated with a continuous running absorbable suture, trying to exclude rectal mucosa. Typically, the perirectal fascia overlying this would be closed separately with interrupted absorbable sutures. *C.* The external anal sphincter is grasped with Alice clamps, as it frequently retracts. *D.* The external anal sphincter is repaired using figure-eight sutures. The remainder of the laceration is repaired as a second-degree laceration (see Fig. 12-7).

ineal lacerations may prevent future problems with fecal or gas incontinence or rectovaginal fistula formation.

MULTIFETAL GESTATION

The perinatal mortality of multifetal gestations is significantly higher than that among their singleton counterparts and is directly related to premature delivery and birth order. These pregnancies also have higher rates of congenital anomalies, malpresentations, cord accidents, placental problems (abruptio placentae or placenta previa), postpartum hemorrhage, and preeclampsia. Important considerations in the management of multifetal gestations include the continuous monitoring of all fetuses during labor and determination of fetal size and presentation.

The recommended route of delivery is dependent on fetal presentation at the time of delivery. Twin pregnancies presenting vertex-vertex will deliver vaginally about 43 percent of the time. No general consensus has been reached on the preferred delivery method for the 38 percent of twins presenting vertex-nonvertex (breech or transverse). Vaginal delivery of the second twin is a reasonable option for clinicians experienced in breech extraction. The relative role of external cephalic version for the second twin is a controversial but reasonable option. Gestations presenting with a nonvertex first twin (19 percent) are routinely delivered by cesarean section because of the increased morbidity and risk of locking of fetal parts.

Higher-order (triplets and above) pregnancies should be delivered at a tertiary care center. No randomized controlled studies exist to support a preference for either vaginal or abdominal delivery of triplets, although most authors believe that delivery by cesarean is preferred. It has been suggested that a low vertical uterine incision is preferable, as fetal malpresentations may make extension of the incision necessary. A reduction in cord gas values and Apgar scores is associated with birth order but tends to be less marked with cesarean delivery.

Preparation of multifetal gestations for vaginal delivery should include evaluation of fetal size and position, continuous monitoring of each infant, availability of an ultrasound in the delivery room, and the presence of a delivery team (anesthesiologist, two obstetricians, and two pediatric care providers for each infant).

MANAGEMENT OF THE NEWBORN INFANT

During the first few minutes of life, the neonate requires assistance to help with the transition from a intrauterine environment to life outside the womb. Preparation is critical to allow rapid resuscitation of the newborn. Basic equipment necessary for neonatal resuscitation is listed in Tables 12-3 and 12-4. Two persons should be assigned to care for the neonate without other responsibilities. Preferably a pediatrician will be in attendance, but this is not always possible in emergent circumstances.

Table 12-3

EQUIPMENT NECESSARY FOR NEONATAL RESUSCITATION

Radiant warmer and blankets
Oxygen with tubing and flowmeter
Suction bulbs and suction source with regulator and DeLee catheters
Stethoscope
Self-inflating bag with infant masks and 100% O_2 adapter
Laryngoscope and #0 and #1 blades with functioning bulbs and batteries
Endotracheal tubes 2.5–4.0 mm internal diameter
Meds: $NaHCO_3$, epinephrine ($1:10,000$), naloxone, dextrose, volume expanders

It is important to dry the infant with warm towels. Then wrap the child in a clean, dry towel or sheet or place it under a radiant heat source to prevent hypothermia. Preterm infants are particularly susceptible to the effects of hypothermia, and their heads should be covered, as heat can be lost rapidly if the head is left uncovered at room temperature. Clearing the infant's oropharynx and nasal passages of mucus or fluid will provide stimulation while assisting its initial breathing efforts. The head should be placed in the "sniff" position. If the fluid is meconium-stained, the delivering physician should suction the mouth, nose, and oropharynx while the head is being delivered. If the resuscitating personnel are trained in neonatal intubation, the trachea should be intubated and suctioned directly with an appropriate-sized endotracheal tube (Table 12-4) and regulated wall suction. If the infant is stable, its stomach contents should be aspirated. Breathing efforts are promoted by the tactile stimulation of drying the amniotic fluid from the baby with towels and one or two slaps to the sole of the baby's

Table 12-4

ENDOTRACHEAL TUBE SIZE BASED ON NEONATAL WEIGHT

Endotracheal Tube Size, (internal diameter) (grams)	Infant Weight
2.5 mm	<1000
3.0 mm	1000–2000
3.5 mm	2000–3000
4.0 mm	>3000

foot or finger flicks to the heel. If there is no response to two to three attempts at stimulation, further attempts are unlikely to be successful.

Evaluation of the infant's heart rate (more or less than 100 beats per minute) is the most reliable indicator of the need for further resuscitation. Evaluation of the newborn includes assignment of an Apgar score at 1 and 5 min of life (Table 12-5). While a low 1-min Apgar score (0 to 3) indicates that the infant requires supportive care, this score does not correlate with subsequent morbidity.

A baby in need of resuscitation can be managed by following the ABC's of neonatal resuscitation, which include assessment of the infant's airway, breathing, and circulation. The mouth and nares should be bulb-suctioned to clear the passages of mucus and fluid while placing the infant at a slight tilt so that the head is lower than the rest of the body. The head should be in a slightly extended or sniffing position so as to maximize airway openings.

A baby with spontaneous respiratory effort and a heart rate above 100 beats per minute should be observed for central cyanosis, which should be treated with a free flow of oxygen while continuing to monitor neonatal respirations and heart rate. If the heart rate falls below 100 beats per minute, begin positive pressure ventilation (PPV), as described below.

Babies making no respiratory effort should receive PPV at a rate of 40 to 60 breaths per minute with >80% oxygen. If a pressure gauge is available, 30 to 40 cm H_2O is required for the initial breath, while subsequent breaths require only 15 to 20 cmH_2O (normal term infants). Repeat assessment for spontaneous breathing should occur

after 20 to 30 seconds of PPV. With spontaneous respirations and a fetal heart rate above 100 beats per minute give free-flow oxygen and continue to monitor the baby. If the heart rate is between 60 to 100 beats per minute, and increasing, continue ventilation; if stable, check adequacy of ventilation; and if below 80 beats per minute, start chest compressions. If the heart rate is less than 60 beats per minute continue ventilation and begin chest compressions. If ventilation continues for more than 2 min place an orogastric tube to relieve abdominal distention.

Chest compressions are performed by placing the thumbs toward the fetal head on the sternum just below an imaginary line connecting the nipples. Compress the sternum (not the infant's ribs) to a depth of $\frac{1}{2}$ to $\frac{3}{4}$ in. using a rate of 90 compressions and 30 PPV per minute. Check the fetal heart rate after 30 seconds of compressions. If the fetal heart rate is less than 80 beats per minute, continue compressions; if greater than 80 beats per minute, use only PPV as above until the heart rate is greater than 100 beats per minute. If the heart rate does not improve, continue the sequence of compressions and PPV until a pediatrician arrives to continue the code. Epinephrine (0.1 to 0.3 mL/kg of 1 : 10,000) should be administered either intravenously or endotracheally if there is no heart rate present. Endotracheal intubation should be conducted only by a provider trained in the technique.

ROUTINE CARE OF THE NEWBORN

The newborn usually makes the transition after delivery without difficulty. Warning signs of potential problems include temperature instability, hypoglycemia, feeding difficulties, rapid respirations, jaundice, cyanosis or pallor of skin, bilious emesis, and prolonged time to first void (>24 h). These infants need more extensive evaluation.

The vernix remaining after immediate delivery care will be readily absorbed by the skin, so there is no urgent need for bathing until the newborn's temperature has stabilized. The infant's umbilical cord should be treated with triple dye, bacitracin ointment, or povidone-iodine to prevent cord infection. It is important to record fetal urination and stool passage after birth (meconium is dark greenish-brown and present for 2 to 3 days). If the infant has not voided by both these routes for the first 24 to 36 hours of life, it should be evaluated for congenital anomalies such as a urethral valve or imperforate anus.

Infants should routinely receive 1 mg of vitamin K IM to prevent hemorrhagic disease of the newborn. Eye care includes drops of silver nitrate 1% solution to the lower eyelid cul-de-sac (this often yields a chemical conjunctivitis) or use of erythromycin ointment to prevent neonatal eye infections such as gonococcal ophthalmia, which can result in neonatal blindness. The American College of Pediatrics and American College of Obstetricians and Gynecologists both recommend that all newborns be routinely immunized against hepatitis B prior to discharge from the hospital. In addition, newborns whose mothers have a positive hepatitis

Table 12-5

APGAR SCORE CRITERIA[a]

Criteria	0	1	2
Heart rate	Absent	<100 bpm	>100 bpm
Respiratory effort	Absent	Slow or irregular	Normal
Muscle tone	Flaccid	Some extremity flexion	Active movement
Reflex irritability	No response	Grimace	Cry
Color	Pale or blue	Body pink and extremities blue	Completely pink

[a]The score is assigned at 1 and 5 min of life.

B surface antigen should be passively immunized using hepatitis B immune globulin.

The mother and infant should not be separated until they have both been properly identified (usually through a combination of arm and leg bracelets or bands). The infant should be footprinted along with a maternal thumbprint to aid in identification. Routine laboratory evaluation should include blood type, hematocrit, serologic test for syphilis, and the state-sponsored screen for inborn errors of metabolism. Infants at risk for hypoglycemia (e.g., maternal diabetes) should have glucose screening. Newborn infants with ABO and Rh incompatibilities (Rh-positive infant and Rh-negative mother) should be observed for at least 48 h postpartum for evidence of jaundice. Jaundice within the first 24 h is never physiologic and warrants further investigation. The daily increase in bilirubin should be <5 mg/dL. Total bilirubin is usually less than 13.0 mg/dL on day 3 to 4 and <15.0 mg/dL on day 5 to 7 in term and premature infants, respectively. Infants with increasing levels of bilirubin should be referred to a pediatrician for care, as they may need phototherapy and/or even exchange transfusion.

POSTPARTUM ISSUES

AMBULATION AND ACTIVITY

Early ambulation after delivery hastens the return of a sense of well-being, providing a more rapid return of strength postpartum. The first attempt at ambulation should be made with assistance during the first hour or two after delivery as the mother is helped to the rest room to void spontaneously. On discharge from the hospital, women who have had uncomplicated vaginal deliveries generally have few limitations on physical activity. They should be counseled to expect greater susceptibility to fatigue and lethargy for a couple of days and to keep their initial activities or chores light. Rest is important and generally hard to come by with a newborn infant to care for. Support from the woman's family and friends can provide her with periods of rest throughout the day by giving her help with housekeeping and infant-care chores.

Return to work depends on the woman's needs and desire. This is an important period during which the maternal-infant attachment established in the hospital is fostered and grows. Also during this time, lacerations and repairs of the genital tract are healing. A rest period of 6 weeks has classically been advised prior to return to work outside the home, although some women elect to return sooner.

BATHING AND EPISIOTOMY CARE

Showering can begin as soon as the woman is able to ambulate without difficulty. Women should be counseled against excessively hot showers in the immediate postpartum period, since these may make them more susceptible to syncopal episodes. Tub baths should be reserved until after the lochia flow has significantly decreased.

A woman with an obstetric laceration or episiotomy may find that a bag of ice wrapped in a towel and applied to the perineum will reduce the incidence of postpartum edema and discomfort. Sitzbaths are also helpful during the postpartum period to reduce discomfort and may be taken as often as desired. Although many proponents advocate the use of warm water, the patient may find that a "cold" sitzbath is more comfortable. A tub is filled with a few inches of water and ice cubes are added after the woman is seated in the tub. Women should be instructed to clean the vulva from front to back. Sanitary napkins should be used during the initial postpartum period. Tampons may be used when their insertion is comfortable, but they should be changed frequently to decrease the risk of toxic shock syndrome.

If the woman complains of increasing perineal pain, it is important to examine her genital tract for evidence of a hematoma, prolapsed hemorrhoids, or infection, such a necrotizing fasciitis, which is a rare but potentially serious complication.

BLADDER FUNCTION

The maternal bladder is subject to potentially significant trauma during delivery, and epidural or spinal analgesia may impair bladder sensation and the ability to void spontaneously. Overdistention of the bladder can also significantly impair bladder function. If a woman is unable to void at 4 h and/or a large suprapubic mass is noted, urinary catheterization may be necessary. Women requiring catheterization are at increased risk of subsequent urinary tract infection and should be counseled as to the warning signs and symptoms of renal infections.

BREAST-FEEDING

The success of postpartum breast-feeding is dependent on the motivation and support of the parturient. The infant should be put to each breast for 5 min every 2 to 3 h the first day. Nursing periods are increased to 10 min on the second day and to 15 min from the third day on. Women should be counseled to increase their dietary intake by an additional 600 kcal/day, drink plenty of liquids, and make sure they get enough calcium to supply 600 to 900 mL of milk per day. Women with inverted nipples require special instructions, and a lactation consultant should be called for prior to delivery if possible.

Breast engorgement occurs on the second to fourth days postpartum as colostrum is replaced with an established milk supply. While this period can be painful, because of markedly distended breasts, it is best managed by giving demand feedings, using warm compresses to encourage milk letdown, and applying cold compresses after feedings for symptomatic relief. It is important to ensure good nipple care by maintaining dry nursing pads between feedings and applying either expressed milk which is allowed to dry or lanolin cream to the areola area after feeding. Nipple soreness can be alleviated by alternating the breasts and fetal position every 5 min if needed.

Several potential problems can be noted while breast-feeding. Vaginal atrophy may lead to vaginal dryness, making intercourse uncomfortable. Breastfeeding women should be counseled as to this expected "side effect" and to the use of vaginal lubricants if desired. Insufficient milk production can be augmented through the use of metoclopramide 10 mg PO three to four times a day for 7 to 10 days or nasal oxytocin (one or two puffs 2 to 3 min prior to breast-feeding).

Women who elect to stop breast-feeding after establishing a milk supply should decrease the frequency of breast-feeding episodes by slowly supplementing with bottle feeds until the infant has been weaned from the breast. To maintain maternal comfort during this period, the women should use bottle supplements so as to maintain approximately equal intervals between breast-feedings. The use of bromocriptine (Parlodel) is no longer recommended for the suppression of lactation.

SEXUAL ACTIVITY

Although sexual activity can be resumed with cessation of bright red bleeding and when the perineum is sufficiently healed to make intercourse comfortable, many women find that they have little or no sexual desire postpartum. Infections are less likely to occur if intercourse is delayed for at least 3 weeks after delivery. While difficulties experienced secondary to lack of adequate lubrication in breast-feeding women can be corrected by using a vaginal lubricant, the tenderness secondary to genital tract trauma and repair requires time to heal adequately. Common sense is the best rule to follow.

DISCHARGE INSTRUCTIONS AND CARE

Prior to discharge after an uncomplicated vaginal delivery, the mother should understand the normal puerperal changes to be expected and indications for return to health care provider. By the third or fourth day postpartum, many women will experience a rapid decrease in their vaginal bleeding to a reddish brown discharge (lochia rubra), which will change and continue as a mucopurulent discharge (lochia serosa) for up to 20 days. The majority of women will then develop a yellowish-white discharge (lochia alba). It is not unusual to have a transient increase in vaginal bleeding 7 to 14 days postpartum, which corresponds to sloughing and regeneration of the placental site eschar. Evaluation for retained placenta or subinvolution of the placental site is necessary if this bleeding persists beyond a few hours.

Return of normal menstrual function is dependent on maternal nutritional status and maternal lactation. Women choosing not to breast-feed have their first menses an average of 7 to 9 weeks after delivery, with a range of 5 to 18 weeks postpartum. Approximately 70 percent of women will have menses by 12 weeks postpartum. Women choosing to breast-feed have a variable return of menses with a risk of ovulation in exclusively breast-feeding women of 1 to 5 percent.

Many providers elect to have a visit 2 to 3 weeks postpartum to detect any postpartum problems and discuss contraceptive options. It is now well understood that many women experience emotional lability during the postpartum period, starting during the first week after delivery. These transient "maternity blues," manifest by tearfulness, irritation, and anxiety, are noted in 50 to 70 percent of all women and can recur for several weeks postpartum. The provider should be alert to more severe psychological reactions such as postpartum depression or psychosis, which requires more intensive support and pharmacologic intervention.

Women who are not immune to rubella should be given a rubella immunization if there are no contraindications. Rh-negative mothers of Rh-positive babies should be given 300 μg of Rhogam. Women should return to their health care provider for increased temperatures ($\geq 38^{\circ}$C or $\geq 100.4^{\circ}$F), abdominal pain, malodorous vaginal discharge, increased vaginal bleeding or clots, increasing episiotomy or laceration repair pain, breast redness, leg pain or swelling—particularly if unilateral, and shortness of breath or chest pain. The postpartum evaluation scheduled can be as a short visit at 2 to 3 weeks for any complications, along with a normally scheduled visit at 6 to 8 weeks postpartum, when the patient's yearly gynecologic examination is performed.

General References

CDC: Prevention of perinatal group B streptococcal disease: A public health perspective. *MMWR* 45(RR-7), 1996.

Creasy RK, Resnik R: *Maternal Fetal Medicine,* 3d ed. Philadelphia: Saunders, 1994.

Cunningham FG, MacDonald PC, Gant NF, et al: *Williams Obstetrics,* 19th ed. Norwalk, CT: Appleton & Lange, 1993.

Gabbe SG, Niebyl JR, Simpson JL: *Obstetrics: Normal and Problem Pregnancies,* 3d ed. New York: Churchill Livingstone, 1996.

Hankins GDV, Clark SL, Cunningham FG, Gilstrap LC: *Operative Obstetrics.* Norwalk, CT: Appleton & Lange, 1995.

Keith LG, Papernik E, Keith DM, Luke B: *Multiple Pregnancy: Epidemiology, Gestation, and Perinatal Outcome.* New York: Parthenon, 1995.

Chapter 13

POSTPARTUM HEMORRHAGE

Clark E. Nugent

Puerperal hemorrhage continues to be a significant cause of maternal morbidity and mortality. Between 1987 and 1990, hemorrhagic complications accounted for 28.7 percent of pregnancy-related deaths.[1] Since most births in the United States take place in a hospital setting, the woman presenting to the emergency department with acute puerperal hemorrhage will usually have either delivered at home, in a freestanding birth center, or in the the emergency department. However, delayed hemorrhage is possible regardless of the delivery setting. This chapter reviews the evaluation and management of common causes of postpartum hemorrhage.

PATHOPHYSIOLOGY

The normal homeostatic mechanisms usually achieve satisfactory hemostasis following delivery. Immediately prior to delivery, the uterus is perfused by up to 750 mL of blood per minute. With separation of the placenta, continued uterine contraction serves to constrict the spiral arteries, which supply the decidua (the lining of the endometrium). Anything that interferes with uterine contraction will result in continued bleeding from the placental attachment site. Persistent uterine bleeding is most commonly caused by uterine atony, although retained placental tissue and uterine rupture must also be considered. Likewise, any traumatic injury that interrupts the integrity of the highly vascular lower genital tract can result in continued brisk bleeding.

Most postpartum hemorrhage takes place within the first 24 h following delivery and is referred to as *immediate hemorrhage*. However, delayed hemorrhage may take place days to weeks following delivery. Delayed hemorrhage is believed to result from either subinvolution of the uterus or placental polyps.

The duration of bleeding following delivery (lochia) has not been extensively studied. In one recent report of 477 lactating women, the median duration of bleeding was 27 days, and 22 percent of these women still reported bleeding five weeks postpartum.[2]

DIAGNOSIS AND DIFFERENTIAL DIAGNOSIS

The initial history should attempt to quantify the amount of bleeding that has taken place. Bleeding patterns may range from sudden, massive hemorrhage to a seemingly harmless, steady flow of blood that ultimately leads to hypovolemia. Details of the delivery should be obtained, especially with regard to delivery of the placenta and whether it was intact.

The initial physical examination should emphasize the vital signs as well as rapid assessment of the magnitude of ongoing vaginal bleeding. Table 13-1 summarizes guidelines from the *Advanced Trauma Life Support Course for Physicians* for estimating blood loss based on the patient's initial presentation.[3] The next step in the evaluation is to determine the etiology of the bleeding. Table 13-2 summarizes the differential diagnosis of postpartum hemorrhage. The commonest etiology is uterine atony, so attention should be directed to palpating the uterine fundus transabdominally. The normal postpartum uterus is firmly contracted, with a globular shape, and is usually palpable at or below the umbilicus. With uterine atony, the uterine fundus will have a

Table 13-1

ESTIMATED FLUID AND BLOOD LOSSES[a] BASED ON PATIENT'S INITIAL PRESENTATION

	Class I	Class II	Class III	Class IV
Blood loss, mL	Up to 750	750–1500	1500–2000	>2000
Blood loss, %BV	Up to 15%	15–30%	30–40%	>40%
Pulse rate	<100	>100	>120	>140
Blood pressure	Normal	Normal	Decreased	Decreased
Pulse pressure, mmHg	Normal or increased	Decreased	Decreased	Decreased
Respiratory rate	14–20	20–30	30–40	>35
Urine output (mL/h)	>30	20–30	5–15	Negligible
CNS/mental status	Slightly anxious	Mildly anxious	Anxious and confused	Confused and lethargic
Fluid replacement, 3:1 rule	Crystalloid	Crystalloid	Crystalloid and blood	Crystalloid and blood

[a]For a 70-kg male.
Source: Committee on Trauma, American College of Surgeons,[3] with permission.

"doughy" consistency; it is readily indented by the palpating hand and frequently palpable above the umbilicus. If the uterus is well contracted, the next step in assessment is to perform a careful visual inspection of the lower genital tract for vaginal or cervical lacerations. Proper lighting in the parallel axis of the vagina and adequate assistance for retraction are essential to carrying out a complete examination. If an adequate examination cannot be accomplished because of patient discomfort, the patient should be moved to the operating room for an examination under anesthesia. It is also possible for there to be continued bleeding from the uterus despite seemingly appropriate uterine tone. This finding should raise the suspicion of either retained placental tissue or uterine rupture. The next step of the physical examination would be to perform a uterine exploration. This is accomplished by gently placing one hand through the dilated cervix and palpating the entire surface of the uterine cavity while the other hand is assisting in positioning the uterus

transabdominally. Again, it may be necessary, for thoroughness, to perform this part of the examination in a setting where adequate anesthesia is available.

The examiner should also consider the location and configuration of the uterine fundus. Inability to palpate the uterine fundus or noting an indentation of the fundus suggests the presence of uterine inversion. This diagnosis can be confirmed by visualization of a red globular mass within the vagina noted on vaginal examination.

Potentially useful laboratory studies include complete blood count with platelet count, type and screen (or crossmatch depending on the magnitude of the bleeding and stability of VS), fibrinogen, prothrombin time, and partial thromboplastin time. Ultrasound has been proposed as a method of determining the presence or absence of retained placental tissue. Although this technology has been successfully used to identify retained placental tissue, its sensitivity and specificity are not currently defined.

Hertzberg and Bowie[4] classified postpartum uterine sonograms into five different categories:

1. Normal uterine "stripe" (Fig. 13-1A): linear pattern of endometrial echoes without endometrial fluid, intensely echogenic foci, or endometrial thickening (thickness of uterine cavity less than 1.5 cm). None of the 18 patients with this pattern had retained placental tissue.
2. Endometrial fluid (Fig. 13-1B): None of the 6 patients with this pattern had retained placental tissue.
3. Echogenic mass (Fig. 13-1C): echogenic material enlarging the uterine cavity [anteroposterior (AP) measurement 1.5 cm or greater], sometimes with a "stippled pattern" of scattered, punctate, intensely echogenic foci. Of 10 patients in this category, 9 had pathologically confirmed retained placental tissue.
4. Hyperechoic foci/no mass (Fig. 13-1D): scattered, in-

Table 13-2

ETIOLOGIES OF POSTPARTUM HEMORRHAGE

Immediate (First 24 h)	Delayed
Uterine atony	Uterine subinvolution
Lower genital tract laceration	Placental polyp
Retained placental tissue or membranes	von Willebrand's disease
Uterine inversion	
Uterine rupture	
Coagulopathy	

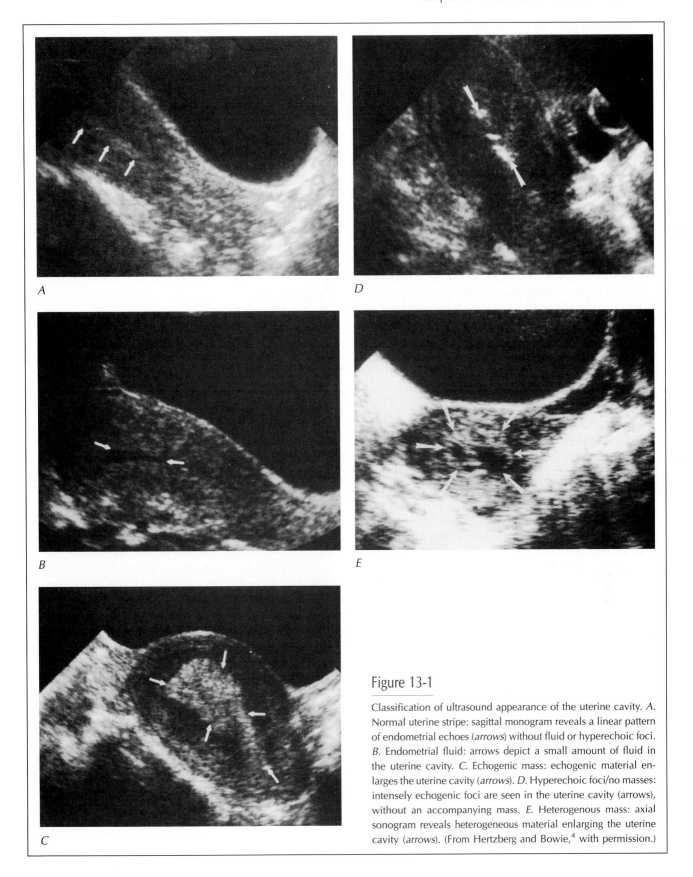

Figure 13-1

Classification of ultrasound appearance of the uterine cavity. *A.* Normal uterine stripe: sagittal monogram reveals a linear pattern of endometrial echoes (*arrows*) without fluid or hyperechoic foci. *B.* Endometrial fluid: arrows depict a small amount of fluid in the uterine cavity. *C.* Echogenic mass: echogenic material enlarges the uterine cavity (*arrows*). *D.* Hyperechoic foci/no masses: intensely echogenic foci are seen in the uterine cavity (arrows), without an accompanying mass. *E.* Heterogenous mass: axial sonogram reveals heterogeneous material enlarging the uterine cavity (*arrows*). (From Hertzberg and Bowie,[4] with permission.)

tensely echogenic foci in the endometrial cavity; no evidence of a uterine cavity mass (cavity less than 1.5 cm in AP diameter). Only 1 of 17 patients with this pattern had pathologically proven retained placental tissue.

5. Heterogeneous mass (Fig. 13-1*E*): endometrial cavity enlarged (1.5 cm or greater) by heterogeneous material exhibiting a mixed pattern of echogenic and echopenic areas. One of two patients had confirmed placental tissue.

TREATMENT OF IMMEDIATE HEMORRHAGE

The initial treatment of postpartum hemorrhage regardless of etiology requires instituting volume resuscitation with isotonic crystalloid through a large-bore intravenous line. Indications for obtaining obstetric consultation are summarized in Table 13-3.

UTERINE ATONY

Uterine atony is treated with bimanual compression and administration of uterotonic agents. Bimanual compression is performed by placing one hand in the vagina against the lower uterine segment while the abdominal hand gently massages the uterine fundus and compresses the uterus against the vaginal hand (Fig. 13-2). When bimanual compression and uterotonic agents are ineffective at controlling hemorrhage, the practitioner should proceed to ruling out other etiologies such as retained placental tissue, undetected lacerations, uterine rupture, or a coagulation disorder.

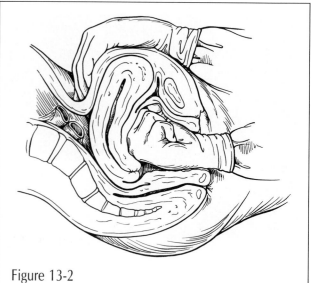

Figure 13-2

Bimanual compression of the uterus for hemorrhage due to uterine atony.

Table 13-3

INDICATIONS FOR OBTAINING OBSTETRIC CONSULTATION

Hemorrhagic shock
Uterine atony refractory to pharmacologic agents
Inability to achieve exposure for adequate vaginal exam
Vaginal or cervical laceration requiring repair in the operating room
Retained placental tissue
Uterine rupture
Coagulation disorder

PHARMACOLOGIC AGENTS FOR TREATING UTERINE ATONY

Oxytocin

Pharmacologic agents useful in the treatment of uterine atony are listed in Table 13-4. Oxytocin is usually the first agent used. It is effective, inexpensive, and has a good safety profile as compared with other uterotonic agents. Oxytocin is an octapeptide that stimulates uterine contraction by binding to specific receptors on the myometrial cells as well as increasing local prostaglandin production. It is administered by diluting 20 to 30 U in 1 L of isotonic crystalloid and infusing at a rate of at least 200 mL/h or by administering 10 U intramuscularly if intravenous access has not been secured. Oxytocin should not be given as an intravenous push because of its ability to relax vascular smooth muscle and cause hypotension. Since oxytocin is structurally similar to vasopressin, there is the potential to produce water intoxication with large doses. However, this can largely be avoided by avoiding administration of free water (e.g., D_5W), which is also ineffective in restoring intravascular volume. The effectiveness of this strategy is demonstrated by a protocol for inducing labor during the second trimester, in which oxytocin rates of up to 100 units/hour diluted in isotonic crystalloid are administered without causing water intoxication.[5] This alternative high-dose strategy is outlined in Chap. 5.

Ergot Alkaloids

Ergot alkaloids have been used in obstetrics since at least the sixteenth century. The most common ergot derivative used for treating postpartum hemorrhage is methyl-

Table 13-4

DRUGS FOR TREATING UTERINE ATONY

Agent	Dosage and Route of Administration	Precautions
Oxytocin	1. 20–30 units in 1 L lactated Ringer's solution or normal saline infused at 200 mL/h 2. 10 units IM	Hypotension with IV push Water intoxication if given with free water
Methylergonovine maleate	0.2 mg IM	Contraindicated with uncontrolled hypertension
15-methyl PGF$_{2\alpha}$ (carboprost tromethamine)	250 μg IM	Arterial desaturation Bronchospasm
PGE$_2$ (Prostaglandin E$_2$)	20-mg suppository per rectum	Hypotension Fever Nausea, vomiting Diarrhea Headache

ergonovine maleate. This agent induces tetanic contraction of the myometrium, thereby effectively compressing the spiral arteries to achieve hemostasis. It is important that methylergonovine maleate be properly stored, since exposure to light and temperatures >30°C (86°F) will lead to loss of activity.[6]

Methylergonovine maleate is usually administered at a dose of 0.2 mg IM. The onset of action is in approximately 7 min with a sustained effect for 2 h. If the patient is hypotensive, the drug will not necessarily reach the target organ. Cautious intravenous administration can be utilized to obtain an immediate effect with a duration of 1 h. The drug should be administered by a slow intravenous push over at least 60 s. Alternatively, 0.2 mg can be placed in 1 L of isotonic crystalloid and infused. A rapid intravenous push should be avoided because of the potential to precipitate a hypertensive crisis. Methylergonovine maleate is contraindicated in the presence of uncontrolled hypertension or preeclampsia. Alternative agents should be utilized in these patients. An oral maintenance dose of 0.2 mg q6h may be administered to maintain increased uterine tone after bleeding has been controlled with parenteral therapy.

Prostaglandins

The prostaglandins stimulate uterine contraction and can be utilized in the treatment of postpartum hemorrhage due to uterine atony. The synthetic 15-methyl analog of prostaglandin F$_{2\alpha}$ (PGF$_{2\alpha}$, carboprost tromethamine) is the most widely used agent, although prostaglandin E$_2$ (PGE$_2$) can also be used. It must be remembered that prostaglandins have systemic effects beyond the myometrium. Their most common side effect is related to the fact that they stimulate gastrointestinal smooth muscle, leading to diarrhea and vomiting. Some patients may experience a marked pyrexia, particularly with the use of PGE$_2$. It usually acts as a bronchodilator whereas 15-methyl PGF$_{2\alpha}$ is a bronchoconstrictor; the latter drug is relatively contraindicated in asthmatic patients. Finally, 15-methyl PGF$_{2\alpha}$ has been associated with arterial desaturation due to increased intrapulmonary shunting.[7]

The usual dosage of 15-methyl PGF$_{2\alpha}$ is 250 μg IM. It can be repeated every 15 to 90 min to a maximal dosage of 2 mg. In actual practice, if satisfactory uterine tonus is not achieved with the first or second dose, it is highly unlikely that repeated doses will accomplish anything beyond accentuating the side effects. Some practitioners advocate injecting the agent directly into the uterus, although there are no trials comparing the efficacy of intramyometrial versus intramuscular injection. The reported success rate of 15-methyl-PGF$_{2\alpha}$ for treatment of postpartum hemorrhage due to atony is approximately 90 percent.[8]

Suppositories of PGE$_2$ have also been used for treating postpartum uterine atony.[9] They should be administered per rectum to avoid being flushed out in the presence of active vaginal bleeding. Hypotension, fever, diarrhea, nausea, and vomiting tend to occur more frequently with PGE$_2$ suppositories than with 15-methyl PGF$_{2\alpha}$.

LACERATIONS OF THE LOWER GENITAL TRACT AND CERVIX

The objective of managing lower genital tract and cervical trauma is to both achieve hemostasis and restore normal anatomy. Adequate lighting and retraction are imperative to be able to delineate the margins of the wound, particularly the superiormost margin of the laceration. If patient discomfort precludes meeting these objectives, obstetric consultation should be obtained and the patient moved to a setting where appropriate anesthesia can be administered for the repair.

Figure 13-3 illustrates the typical repair of a vaginal sulcus laceration. These lacerations can sometimes be quite substantial, extending from the vaginal fornix out into the ischiorectal fossa. The most important aspect of the repair is to include the full thickness of the vaginal wall so that hemostasis is obtained. Incomplete bites of tissue will allow ongoing bleeding into the ischiorectal fossa, with resultant hematoma formation. Care must be exercised if the laceration extends to the anterior aspect of the vagina because of the potential for bladder or ureteral injury. Right-angle or Deaver retractors are often helpful to achieve adequate visualization. A running absorbable suture such as a 3-0 polyglactin is an appropriate choice. The pudendal vessels typically travel along the vaginal walls at 3 to 4 o'clock and 8 to 9 o'clock, care being taken to avoid injuring these vessels during suturing (Fig. 34-3).

Cervical lacerations are especially problematic in that blood loss can be voluminous, but incomplete or over ag-gressive suturing of lacerations can lead to subsequent cervical incompetence or cervical stenosis. Immediately after delivery, the cervix has minimal tone and is redundant. Utilizing a ring forceps to place the cervix on stretch can help avoid the mistake of identifying redundant tissue as a nonexistent laceration and can make suturing easier (Fig. 13-4). If

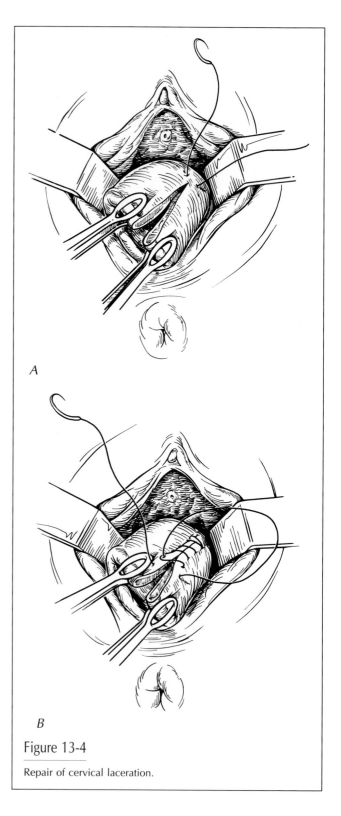

A

B

Figure 13-4

Repair of cervical laceration.

Figure 13-3

Repair of vaginal laceration.

a laceration is identified, its margins should initially be outlined by gently placing ring forceps along the edges, leaving room for subsequent suture placement, taking care not to place a suture through this ring. Once the laceration is clearly demarcated, it can be repaired with a running 3-0 absorbable suture (Fig. 13-4).

Angiographic embolization has been used to control intractable uterine hemorrhaging. Angiographic embolization with absorbable gelatin sponge (Gelfoam, Upjohn) can also be used to control intractable postpartum hemorrhaging.[10] The patient must be sufficiently stable to be transported to the interventional radiology suite. A femoral artery approach is taken. When a specific bleeding vessel is identified, selective embolization of that vessel can be performed. When there is not a specific vessel involved, as with hemorrhage due to uterine atony, hemostasis has been achieved by embolizing the uterine arteries or the anterior branch of the internal iliac arteries. Success rates of approximately 90 percent have been reported.[10]

RETAINED PLACENTAL TISSUE

The approach to the patient with bleeding resulting from retained placental tissue will vary depending on the quantity of tissue retained and the timing of the bleeding episode. If the history indicates that the placenta has not been delivered and more than 30 min have transpired from the time of delivery, manual removal of the placenta is indicated. Bleeding may be precipitated by either partial spontaneous separation of the placenta or by attempts to deliver the placenta by manual traction on the cord, followed by cord avulsion. One should always remember that a potential reason for retained placenta is placenta accreta, where the placenta is abnormally adherent to the uterus and a satisfactory cleavage plain cannot be developed. Attempts at manual removal in the presence of placenta accreta may be associated with catastrophic hemorrhage. It is therefore advisable to perform manual removal of the placenta in a setting where rapid replacement of intravascular volume, uterine curettage, and possible hysterectomy can be performed.

In most instances, manual removal of the placenta will be performed under anesthesia. One hand is used to manipulate the uterus abdominally while the other hand is introduced into the uterus. With the palmar surface of the hand facing the placenta (back of the hand against the uterus), the hand is swept between the placenta and uterine wall to separate the placenta (Fig. 13-5). The placenta can then be grasped and removed from the uterus, taking care to ensure that the fetal membranes are also completely removed. Utilizing ring forceps to grasp and assist with membrane removal is often helpful. On occasion, the cervix and lower uterine segment will be insufficiently dilated, not allowing access to the retained placenta in the uterine fundus. Satisfactory uterine relaxation can be achieved by using either intravenous nitroglycerin or in-

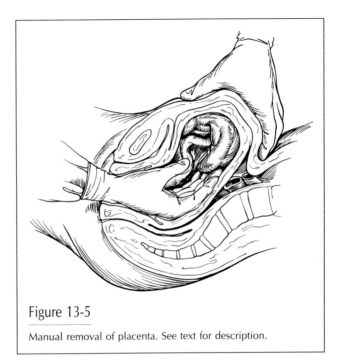

Figure 13-5

Manual removal of placenta. See text for description.

halation anesthesia in the operating room. A uterotonic agent such as oxytocin should be started following delivery of the placenta.

If only placental fragments are retained, they can sometimes be removed at the time of manual exploration of the uterus. However, uterine curettage with a large, sharp curette is often required to achieve complete removal of the retained tissue. An experienced operator is important because the placental implantation site normally has a "shaggy" texture and the temptation to continue scraping until it is smooth should be avoided. Overaggressive curettage for bleeding in the absence of retained tissue should be discouraged because of the potential to cause additional bleeding secondary to trauma as well as leading to intrauterine synechiae, with resultant amenorrhea and infertility.

UTERINE INVERSION

Uterine inversion complicates approximately 1 in 2500 deliveries.[11] Inversion can range in severity from simply the presence of the uterine fundus within the cervix to complete inversion of the uterus and vagina extending beyond the perineum. Most uterine inversions are believed to occur following cord traction with a fundally implanted placenta; however, inversion can follow any delivery, even when the third stage has been managed appropriately. The hemorrhage accompanying uterine inversion can be substantial and life-threatening. The classic teaching is that uterine inversion presents with hypovolemic shock out of proportion to the visualized blood loss, although contemporary series have not substantiated this teaching.[11]

As with all forms of puerperal hemorrhage, obtaining large-bore intravenous access and initiating volume replacement is crucial. Obstetric and anesthesiology consultation should be arranged as soon as possible. When the inversion is acute and the cervix has not contracted around the inverted uterus, it may be possible to reposition the uterus by applying manual pressure to the inverted uterine fundus (Fig. 13-6). Once the uterus has been restored to the proper anatomic location, the operator's hand should remain in the uterus to prevent reinversion while a uterotonic agent (e.g., oxytocin) is administered to obtain normal uterine tone. The blood loss is most severe in cases where the placenta has already separated. If the placenta is still attached when the diagnosis of uterine inversion is made, it should be left in place until repositioning has been accomplished to avoid potentially catastrophic hemorrhage.

Repositioning without uterine relaxation is successful in approximately one-third of cases.[11] If the uterus cannot be replaced due to cervical contraction, a number of strategies are available to achieve uterine relaxation. Traditional methods have included either deep inhalation anesthesia or administration of tocolytic agents such as terbutaline or magnesium sulfate. More recently, intravenous nitroglycerin has been utilized to achieve uterine relaxation. It has the advantage of a very rapid onset of action (30 to 40 s) in conjunction with a short half-life of approximately 1 min.[12] Thus, once uterine repositioning has been accomplished,

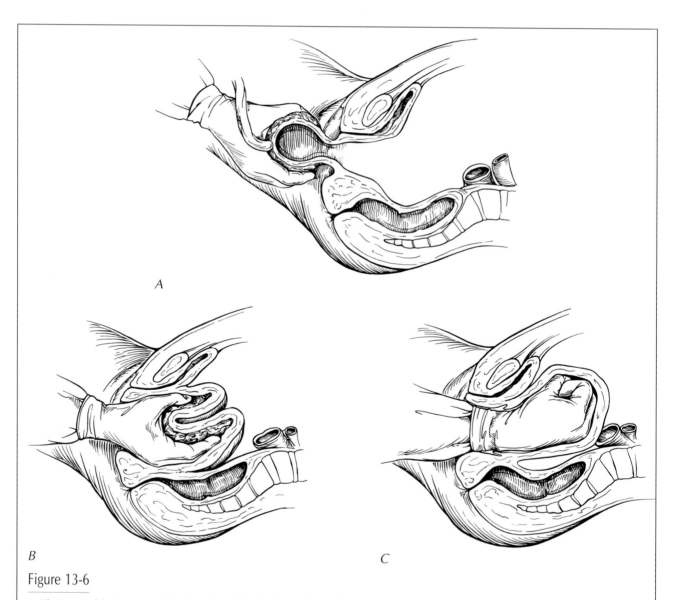

A

B

C

Figure 13-6

A. The inverted fundus grasped in the palm of the hand with fingers directed toward the posterior fornix. The placenta is left attached, if possible. B. The uterus lifted out of the pelvis and directed with steady pressure toward the umbilicus after removal of the placenta. C. The repositioned uterus after removal of the placenta.

uterine tone can be restored very quickly. Doses ranging from 50 to 500 μg have been utilized, with 100 to 200 μg appearing to be a suitable compromise between obtaining acceptable uterine relaxation while avoiding the hypotension possible with larger doses. When hypotension does result, it is transient and can be treated with ephedrine 10 mg given intravenously.[13]

COAGULOPATHY

Coagulopathies that lead to excessive postpartum blood loss may be either hereditary or acquired. Von Willebrand disease is the commonest hereditary blood coagulation disorder affecting women, although occasionally a hemophilia carrier may present with excessive postpartum bleeding. Most reproductive-age women with a coagulation disorder will typically have been previously diagnosed because of excessive menstrual bleeding. These women are at increased risk of either immediate or delayed postpartum hemorrhage as well as hematoma formation.[14] Women with von Willebrand disease are usually treated with either desmopression (DDAVP) or factor VIII concentrate, depending on which of the many von Willebrand variants they may have. The usual dosage of desmopression is 0.3 μg/kg of body weight diluted in normal saline and infused over 15 to 30 min. Human antihemophilic factor (Humate-P) has an advantage over factor VIII concentrate in that there is a decreased risk of transmission of viruses. Humate-P is administered intravenously at an initial dose of 15 to 30 U/kg of body weight followed by 8 to 15 U/kg every 8 h.

Disseminated intravascular coagulation (DIC) is an acquired coagulation disorder characterized by the pathologic generation of thrombin, leading to consumption of clotting factors and platelets. Its presence must trigger a search for the underlying insult (Table 13-5), as treatment will be futile if the primary problem is not corrected. The diagnosis is frequently apparent on the basis of excessive bleeding from lacerations and venipuncture or intravenous sites as well as spontaneous bleeding from mucosal surfaces. Laboratory diagnosis is characterized by decreased fibrinogen and platelets and elevated fibrin degradation products. Given the length of time it may take to perform laboratory studies, many clinicians advocate drawing an extra red-top tube to keep at the bedside. Clot formation within 5 to 7 min usually indicates a fibrinogen level of >100 mg/dL.

The mainstay of treatment of DIC is to correct the underlying problem. Abruptio placentae is associated with DIC only in the most severe cases, which usually involve fetal compromise or even death. Preeclampsia will usually be apparent on the basis of hypertension and proteinuria and is infrequently a cause of DIC. Acute fatty liver disease may present like preeclampsia but is also characterized by nausea and vomiting as well as hepatic dysfunction. Amniotic fluid embolism typically presents with acute cardiovascular collapse. Disseminated intravascular coagulation can occur following fetal demise of any cause, but it is an infrequent event and requires at least 4 weeks to develop.[15] Supportive care measures include adequate volume replacement to minimize the risk of thrombotic complications. Treatment with blood products as summarized below may be necessary as a temporizing measure while the underlying process is being corrected.

VOLUME EXPANSION AND THE USE OF BLOOD PRODUCTS

Restoration of intravascular volume sufficient to maintain perfusion of vital organs and avoid sequelae (e.g., metabolic acidosis, acute tubular necrosis, and pituitary infarction) is the mainstay of therapy for postpartum hemorrhage. Steps to control the ongoing hemorrhage should be initiated simultaneously. The initial volume resuscitation will usually be accomplished with an isotonic crystalloid solution such as lactated Ringer's or normal saline. The use of colloid in this setting appears to offer no survival advantage over crystalloid.[16] Colloidal solutions are also far more expensive and potentially associated with adverse effects. Hydroxethyl starch (Hespan) has been associated with anaphylactoid reactions, allergic reactions, and coagulopathy.[17] Anaphylaxis and interference with platelet function are also concerns with the use of dextran. Although there continue to be recommendations in the obstetric literature for the use of whole blood in treating postpartum hemorrhage, it is not a product that is available in the contemporary blood bank. Attempts to order whole blood will only delay needed therapy and blood products. Contemporary transfusion medicine involves component therapy with the appropriate product to meet the patient's needs.

Table 13-6 summarizes the blood products most commonly used for the obstetric patient. In cases of massive he-

---

Table 13-5

OBSTETRIC ETIOLOGIES OF DISSEMINATED INTRAVASCULAR COAGULATION

Abruptio placentae
Severe preeclampsia
Acute fatty liver
Amniotic fluid embolism
Prolonged retention of dead fetus
Sepsis
Massive hemorrhage
Illegal abortion

Table 13-6

BLOOD PRODUCTS

Product	Indications for Use
Red blood cells	Restore oxygen-carrying capacity
Platelets	Active bleeding with platelet count <50,000 or clinical evidence of microvascular bleeding
Fresh frozen plasma	DIC Emergency reversal of warfarin Antithrombin III deficiency Replacement of isolated factor deficiencies when specific-component therapy is neither available nor appropriate
Cryoprecipitate	Correction of hypofibrinogenemia Von Willebrand disease Hemophilia A (if factor VIII concentrate not available) Fibrin adhesive

Table 13-7

RISK OF TRANSFUSION—TRANSMITTED VIRAL INFECTIONS

	Risk of Infection	95% Confidence Interval
HIV	1:493,000	1:202,000–1:2,778,000
HTLV	1:641,000	1:256,000–1:2,000,000
Hepatitis C	1:103,000	1:28,000–1:288,000
Hepatitis B	1:63,000	1:31,000–1:147,000

Source: Schreiber et al.,[19] with permission.

morrhage, there is no standard formula for blood product administration; rather, the therapy should be tailored to the patient's specific deficiencies. For instance, 35 to 45 percent of platelets usually remain following transfusion of one blood volume.[18] Furthermore, there remains a small but real risk of infectious complication from transfusion, which reinforces the importance of avoiding the unnecessary administration of blood products (Table 13-7).[19]

Regardless of what fluids or blood products are administered to the patient, volume resuscitation will be facilitated by avoiding hypothermia. The infusion of room-temperature fluids and refrigerated blood products can lead to hypothermia, which has a number of deleterious effects.[22] Increased blood viscosity, decreased red cell deformability, and shift of the oxygen-hemoglobin dissociation curve to the left will all serve to impair oxygen delivery to the tissues. Furthermore, hypothermia may interfere with the functioning of coagulation mechanisms.

Red Blood Cells

Packed red blood cells contains the red cells from 1 unit of whole blood, a small amount of plasma, and anticoagulant. A typical volume is 320 to 400 mL with the hematocrit ranging from 70 to 80 percent. A decision to transfuse is not based on a threshold hemoglobin or hematocrit; rather, such a decision is based on the patient's clinical status.[20]

In the event of massive hemorrhage in which immediate improvement of the oxygen-carrying capacity is required, O-negative blood may be administered. Type-specific blood can potentially be available 10 to 15 min after the blood bank receives the patient's specimen. In the absence of unexpected antibodies, an additional 20 min is necessary to provide crossmatched blood. In most instances it should be possible to perform the necessary testing to minimize the risk of transfusion reactions and the formation of alloantibodies that may have significant adverse effects on future pregnancies.

Platelets

One unit of platelets contains the platelets from 1 unit of whole blood suspended in 50 mL of plasma; it also contains coagulation factors. In the absence of accelerated consumptions, 1 unit of platelets will raise the platelet count by 10,000/mm^3. The recommended therapeutic dose of platelets is 1 unit/10 kg of body weight.[18] Platelets are typically transfused as a pool of 6 U. Once the platelets have been pooled, they must be used within 4 h. In the absence of ongoing bleeding, a platelet count above 20,000/mm^3 is a conservative safe value with no need for platelet transfusion.[18] With ongoing bleeding, platelet transfusion should be reserved for instances where the platelet count is documented to be <50,000/mm^3 or if there is evidence of microvascular bleeding. Rh immune globulin should be administered to the Rh-negative woman because of the potential for Rh alloimmunization from Rh-positive red cells that may be contained in the platelets. The dose of Rh immune globulin is 300 μg IM.

FRESH-FROZEN PLASMA

Fresh-frozen plasma is the fluid portion of 1 unit of blood that has been frozen within 6 h of collection to maximize the activity of factors V and VIII. The minimal time for thawing is 45 min. Because of overuse of this scarce resource in the past, specific guidelines for its use have been established[21] (Table 13-6). In the context of postpartum hemorrhage, it will be most frequently indicated in the presence of DIC. The usual starting dose of fresh frozen plasma is 2 bags (400 to 460 mL), although doses as high as 10 to 15 mL/kg may be required for some patients.[21]

CRYOPRECIPITATE

Cryoprecipitate is made from fresh frozen plasma thawed at 1 to 6°C (33.8 to 42.8°F). Fresh frozen plasma provides 80 to 120 units of factor VIII:C, 80 U of von Willebrand factor, 200 to 300 mg fibrinogen, and 40 to 60 units of factor XIII. Clinical indications include correction of hypofibrinogenemia, treatment of von Willebrand disease, treatment of hemophilia A if factor VIII concentrate not available, and as a component of fibrin surgical adhesive.[21] The typical use in obstetrics would be correction of hypofibrinogenemia (<100 mg/dL) due to DIC. The dosage can be calculated using the following formula:

Desired increment in g/L
$$= (0.2 \times \text{number of bags})/\text{plasma volume in liters}$$

Alternatively, 1 bag of cryoprecipiate for every 5 kg of body weight can be administered.[21]

DELAYED HEMORRHAGE

Delayed postpartum hemorrhage is a special circumstance that may present as long as 6 weeks after delivery. Many delayed hemorrhages are thought to be due to placental polyps. A placental polyp is a segment of retained placenta that ultimately undergoes hyalinization. It may represent an area of focal placenta accreta.[23] If ultrasound evaluation indicates retained tissue, uterine curettage is indicated to remove the tissue in the operating room. With either spontaneous passage or removal of placental polyps by curettage, there is often brisk bleeding. With continued hemorrhage after removal of the polyp, hemostasis can be achieved by inflating a Foley catheter with a 30 mL balloon in the uterine cavity.

References

1. Berg CJ, Atrash HK, Koonin LM, Tucker M: Pregnancy-related mortality in the United States, 1987–1990. *Obstet Gynecol* 88:161, 1996.

2. Viness CM, Kennedy KI, Ramos R: The duration and character of postpartum bleeding among breastfeeding women. *Obstet Gynecol* 89:159, 1997.

3. Committee on Trauma, American College of Surgeons: *Advanced Trauma Life Support Course for Physicians.* Chicago: American College of Surgeons, 1993.

4. Hertzberg BS, Bowie JD: Ultrasound of the postpartum uterus: Prediction of retained placental tissue. *J Ultrasound Med* 10:451, 1991.

5. Owen J, Hauth JC, Winkler CL, Gray SE: Midtrimester pregnancy termination: A randomized trial of prostaglandin E_2 versus concentrated oxytocin. *Am J Obstet Gynecol* 167:1112, 1992.

6. Van Dongen PWJ, Van Roosmalen J, De Boer CN, Van Rooij J: Oxytocics for the prevention of post-partum haemorrhages: A review. *Pharm Weekbl [Sci]* 13:238, 1991.

7. Hankins GDV, Berryman GK, Scott RT Jr, Hood D: Maternal arterial desaturation with 15-methyl prostaglandin F_2 alpha for uterine atony. *Obstet Gynecol* 72:367, 1988.

8. Oleen MA, Mariano JP: Controlling refractory atonic postpartum hemorrhage with Hemabate sterile solution. *Am J Obstet Gynecol* 162:205, 1990.

9. Hertz RH, Sokol RJ, Dierker LJ: Treatment of postpartum uterine atony with prostaglandin E_2 vaginal suppositories. *Obstet Gynecol* 56:129, 1980.

10. Mitty HA, Sterling KM, Alvarez M, Gendler R: Obstetric hemorrhage: Prophylactic and emergency arterial catheterization and embolotherapy. *Radiology* 188:183, 1993.

11. Brar HS, Greenspoon JS, Platt LD, Paul RH: Acute puerperal uterine inversion: New approaches to management. *J Reprod Med* 34:173, 1989.

12. Dayan SS, Schwalbe SS: The use of small-dose intravenous nitroglycerine in a case of uterine inversion. *Anesth Analg* 82:1091, 1996.

13. Wessen A, Elowsson P, Axemo P, Lindberg B: The use of intravenous nitroglycerine for emergency cervico-uterine relaxation. *Acta Anaesthiol Scand* 39:847, 1995.

14. Greer IA, Lowe GDO, Walker JJ, Forbes CD: Haemorrhagic problems in obstetrics and gynaecology in patients with congenital coagulopathies. *Br J Obstet Gynaecol* 98:909, 1991.

15. Pritchard JA: Fetal death in utero. *Obstet Gynecol* 14:573, 1959.

16. Peitzman AB, Billiar TR, Harbrecht BG, et al: Hemorrhagic shock. *Curr Probl Surg* 32:925, 1995.

17. Napolitano LM: Resuscitation following trauma and hemorrhagic shock: Is hydroxyethyl starch safe? *Crit Care Med* 23:795, 1995.

18. National Institutes of Health, Consensus Development Conference Statement: Platelet transfusion therapy. *JAMA* 257:1777, 1987.

19. Schreiber GB, Busch MP, Kleinman SH, Korelitz JJ: The risk of transfusion-transmitted viral infections. *N Engl J Med* 334:1685, 1996.

20. Stehling L, Zauder HL: How low can we go? Is there a way to know? *Transfusion* 30:1, 1990.

21. Development Task Force of the College of American Pathologists: Practice parameter for the use of fresh-frozen plasma, cryoprecipitate, and platelets. *JAMA* 271:777, 1994.

22. Nolan TE, Gallup DG: Massive transfusion: A current review. *Obstet Gynecol Surv* 46:289, 1991.

23. Dyer I, Bradburn DM: An inquiry into the etiology of placental polyps. *Am J Obstet Gynecol* 109:858, 1971.

Chapter 14

POSTPARTUM INFECTIONS

Maurizio L. Maccato

Postpartum infections are common obstetric complications. They may involve the soft tissue of the pelvis (e.g., postpartum endometritis), the sites of surgical incisions (e.g., episiotomies or abdominal surgical incision infections), or more distant sites (e.g., urinary tract or breast infections). The potential seriousness of these infections demands accurate, rapid diagnosis, effective antimicrobial therapy, and occasionally surgical therapy. Urinary tract infections (UTI) and mastitis are covered elsewhere (Chaps. 24 and 36). With many third-party payers encouraging early discharge, women will often develop their initial signs and symptoms of postpartum endometritis after discharge, placing an increased burden on emergency departments for their initial evaluation.

POSTPARTUM ENDOMETRITIS

Postpartum endometritis (PPE) involves infection of the endometrium, myometrium, and, frequently, the parametrial tissues. Its incidence varies from 1 to 3 percent following vaginal delivery to as high as 85 percent after high-risk cesarean sections.[1] Several risk factors for PPE have been identified; the most important is delivery by cesarean section. Other major risk factors are chorioamnionitis, the duration of time since rupture of membranes, the presence of labor, many vaginal exams during labor, the presence of high-virulence pathogens, and the use of internal monitoring devices such as intrauterine pressure catheters.

PATHOPHYSIOLOGY

Postpartum endometritis is an ascending infection caused by bacteria that have colonized the vagina and the cervix. It is therefore a polymicrobial infection in the great majority of cases. A large number of aerobes, facultative anaerobes, and obligate anaerobes have been recovered from the endometria of patients with PPE. The most common organisms include group B streptococcus, *Escherichia coli, Prevotella biva,* and *Enterococcus faecalis.* Table 14-1 lists some other common organisms that have been identified.

DIAGNOSIS

The diagnosis of PPE is based primarily on the history and physical exam, with laboratory data and cultures providing supporting evidence. The hallmark of PPE is uterine tenderness and fever. The onset of symptoms may be slow or rapid, depending on the pathogens involved. Pertinent history includes the presence of risk factors (e.g., cesarean section, duration of time since rupture of membranes) and the use of antibiotics during labor and/or delivery. Lower abdominal pain, foul purulent lochia, and rigors are frequently present. Vital signs will usually demonstrate temperature elevation, often >38°C (100.4°F), and tachycardia. Examination of the abdomen may reveal mild to moderate distention and decreased bowel sounds related to an ileus.

Uterine tenderness may involve the fundus of the uterus or be limited to the lower uterine segment. Therefore, palpation of the uterine fundus abdominally may elicit significant

Table 14-1

BACTERIA FREQUENTLY ISOLATED IN
POSTPARTUM ENDOMETRITIS

Gram-negative rods
  Escherichia coli
  Klebsiella-Enterobacter species
  Proteus species
  Serratia species
  Pseudomonas species
  Haemophilus species

Anaerobes
  Clostridium perfringens
  Fusobacterium species
  Bacteroides species
  Peptococcus
  Peptostreptococcus

Gram-positive cocci
  Streptococci, groups A & B
  Pneumococcus
  Staphylococcus aureus
  Enterococcus

Table 14-2

ANTIBIOTICS COMMONLY USED TO TREAT
POSTPARTUM ENDOMETRITIS

Cefoxitin	1–2 g IV q6h
Cefotetan	1–2 g IV q12h
Ampicillin/Sulbactam	1.5–3 g IV q6h
Piperacillin/tazobactam	3.375 g IV q6h
Ticarcillin/clavulanic acid	3.1 g IV q6h
Clindamycin and gentamicin	Clindamycin 900 mg IV q8h + gentamicin 2.0 mg/kg IV bolus, followed by 1.5–1.7 mg/kg q8h (assuming normal renal function)

tenderness. Examination of the abdomen may also identify masses suspicious for abscesses. On pelvic examination, purulent discharge may be present in the vagina. The cervix is frequently softened and dilated. The lower uterine segment is almost invariably tender. If the parametrial tissues are involved, tenderness and induration in the tissue lateral to the uterus will be noted.

Elevation of the white blood cell count is typical, usually in the range of 12,000 to 20,000/mm^3. Ultrasound or computed tomography of the abdomen is usually reserved for the patient who, on physical exam, has evidence of abscess formation or is not responding to appropriate antibiotic therapy. The differential diagnosis of PPE includes UTI with severe cystitis, leading to lower uterine discomfort. A urinalysis generally provides the necessary laboratory support for the diagnosis. Infection of the abdominal wound from a cesarean section may also cause lower abdominal pain and fever. Evaluation of the surgical site is usually sufficient to clarify the diagnosis.

THERAPY

The mainstay of therapy of PPE remains the use of appropriate broad-spectrum antimicrobial agents. Because of the possible severity of the infection, outpatient treatment is usually not indicated. Intravenous broad-spectrum antibiotics will provide the most satisfactory therapy. A number of an-

tibiotics and antibiotic combinations have been utilized in the therapy of PPE with good success (Table 14-2). Broad-spectrum penicillin or a second-generation cephalosporin has most commonly been used. The combination of a penicillin and an aminoglycoside, sometimes with the addition of clindamycin, has also proved satisfactory. Favorable response to antibiotic therapy is expected in 24 to 48 h. If such a response is not present, the development of an abscess, the presence of septic pelvic venous thrombosis, or a wound complication must be ruled out. The therapy of abdominal abscesses usually requires drainage either by interventional radiology or surgically, in combination with effective antimicrobial therapy. In some patients, the presence of a resistant pathogen may be causing the poor response to therapy. Cultures of the endometrium with a protected instrument (i.e., a double-lumen catheter or a disposable endometrial sampling device such as the Pipelle; see Fig. 14-1) may provide important microbial information to help in choosing an antibiotic. It is important to note that enterococci are commonly isolated from the endometria of patients with PPE who have received a cephalosporin as a prophylactic agent at time of delivery. Resistant Enterobacteriaceae have been recovered from patients given penicillin as a prophylactic agent.[2] Because PPE usually requires hospitalization and intravenous therapy, consultation with an obstetrician/gynecologist is appropriate.

An unusual but serious complication of PPE is myometrial necrosis. This infection begins with the development of microabscesses at the site of the uterine surgical incision. These abscesses will progress to a suppurative myometritis with necrosis of the tissue. The syndrome frequently involves the abdominal incision as well. Pain is minimal to mild. The physical examination will disclose a purulent vaginal discharge and a wound abscess at the same time. The cervix is generally open and explorations on a bimanual exam of the lower uterine segment will reveal necrosis of

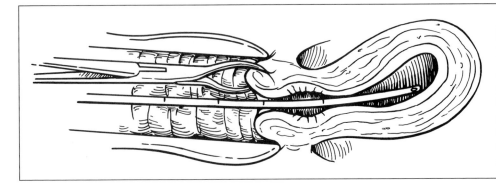

the lower uterine segment, often with fascial dehiscence. X-ray may demonstrate gas within the uterus (Fig. 14-2). Computed tomography or MRI may demonstrate disruption of the uterine wall. Therapy requires emergency surgical exploration and debridement of the uterine wound, which almost invariably leads to hysterectomy. If the abdominal wall is involved, debridement of the abdominal incision is also necessary.

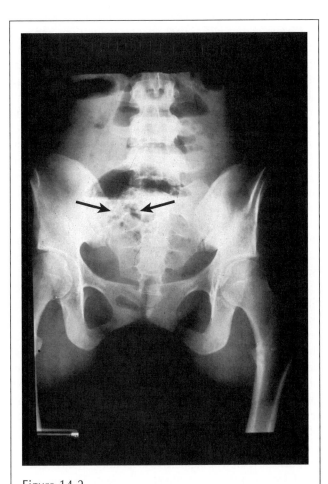

Figure 14-2

Radiograph of abdomen with uterine gas pattern from clostridial myonecrosis. Arrows outline gas within myometrium. (Photograph courtesy of Rudi Ansbacher, M.D., University of Michigan.)

POSTPARTUM ABDOMINAL WOUND INFECTIONS

Infections of the cesarean section abdominal incision occurs after 3 to 16 percent of operations, with an average of 7 percent. Wound infections may be caused either by bacteria present in the lower genital tract, which colonize the incision at time of delivery, or by skin flora. Infections may or may not be associated with PPE. Risk factors for wound infection following cesarean section include obesity, malnutrition, diabetes mellitus, immunosuppression, and circumstances surrounding surgery (e.g., poor hemostasis, breaks in sterile techniques, improper tissue handling, etc.).

Wound infection is suspected when the patient reports symptoms of incisional pain and fever. The physical exam reveals an erythematous and edematous incision, and the wound is usually quite tender to palpation. Frequently, purulent discharge will be noticed at the incision site.

A true wound infection must be differentiated from a seroma or hematoma. As a general rule, hematomas and seromas are not associated with increased temperature or cellulitis. However, the incision may be edematous. In the presence of a wound infection, the white blood cell count is typically elevated. An ultrasound of the incision site may reveal an accumulation of fluid under the subcutaneous or subfascial layers. If the accumulation of fluid is limited to the subcutaneous layer, drainage through the incision site is easily achieved and will provide a specimen for a Gram's stain and culture. This will also help to diagnose uninfected seromas or hematomas. If purulent material is obtained, the incision should be opened, the purulent material evacuated, and the wound debrided. Exploration of the fascia should be performed to ensure that it is intact. Disruption of the fascia requires repair in the operating room.

Therapy is based on the severity of infection. If a cellulitis is noted with no induration, edema, or significant fluid accumulation under the incision, antibiotic therapy alone may be satisfactory. If fluid is noted under the incision line, drainage of the fluid should be performed. Culture and Gram's stain should be obtained. If the stain is positive for organisms and white blood cells, then opening of the incision with drainage of the purulent material and packing of the incision with wet/dry dressing should be initiated. If staining of the aspirated fluid reveals only white blood cells, but no organisms, mycoplasmas and ureaplasmas should be considered possible pathogens. If staining of the fluid reveals no white blood cells and no bacteria, then simple drainage of the pocket of fluid will frequently resolve the problem. The antimicrobial therapy should be directed by the finding on the Gram's stain. The presence of gram-positive cocci suggests staphylococci, streptococci, or enterococci as the primary responsible organisms. The finding of gram-negative bacteria suggests the presence of facultative or obligate anaerobes originating from the lower genital tract. Broad-spectrum antibiotic agents should be used pending the culture results. The patient should be hospitalized if significant temperature elevation is noted (greater than 38°C or 100.4°F orally), if local care of the incision cannot be properly performed on an outpatient basis, or if the patient is unable to tolerate oral antibiotics.

A special circumstance is the rapid development of cellulitis, usually within 24 h of surgery. Unlike typical wound infections, which present 3 to 4 days after surgery along with a fluid collection, women with cellulitis due to group A streptococci do not typically develop an abscess. Rather, they develop a rapidly spreading cellulitis associated with high fever (38 to 40°C or 100.4 to 104°F) tachycardia, and they appear systemically ill. Occasionally, these infections will go on to develop necrotizing fasciitis, an infection requiring surgical intervention (see below).

Rapidly developing cellulitis is typically due to a single organism, but other organisms can coinfect these wounds. Therefore, broad-spectrum antimicrobial therapy is recommended (e.g., ticarcillin/clavulanic acid, ampicillin/sulbactam, or cefotetan). In the absence of a fluid collection, these wounds do not need to be opened. The use of ultrasound or other imaging (e.g., CT) can assist in determining whether a fluid accumulation is present underneath the skin. Because of the potential for significant morbidity (e.g., necrotizing fasciitis), women with rapid development of superficial cellulitis should be hospitalized for parenteral antibiotic therapy and careful observation.

If radiologic evaluation of the incision reveals a collection of fluid below the fascia, drainage of the fluid is necessary. This can be accomplished either by surgical exploration of the incision and subfascial tissues, or by transcutaneous drainage of the fluid under ultrasound or CT guidance. If purulent material is obtained, the patient should be taken to the operating room and the subfascial collection of pus evacuated. At that time, inspection of the uterine incision is recommended. Antimicrobial therapy will be based on culture results. Broad-spectrum antibiotic therapy should be initiated pending culture results. Wound care of the infected postoperative incision is accomplished by a wet/dry dressing changed three to four times daily. The use of 0.25% acetic acid has provided good results in a high-risk population. If a large amount of serous fluid seems to be coming from the incision, it is important to remember the possibility of fascial dehiscence. The fluid volume is frequently increased by a Valsalva maneuver. If a fascial dehiscence is suspected, the patient should be taken to the operating room for exploration of the incision. This will allow for repair of the fascial dehiscence if this is confirmed. If there is no evidence of infection after evacuation of a seroma or a hematoma, the patient's wound can frequently be reapproximated; that is, it does not need to be allowed to heal by a secondary intention. Close follow-up is mandatory. We recommend daily follow-up for approximately a week to make sure that no significant infections develop.

EPISIOTOMY INFECTIONS

The episiotomy is one of the most common surgical procedures performed, and infection of the episiotomy site occurs in less than 1 percent of cases.[3] The severity of infection can be estimated clinically by its depth (Table 14-3 and Fig. 14-3). The infection is usually superficial and accompanied by low-grade fever and pain at the site. Physical examination will reveal edema, induration, and erythema of the perineum and vagina (Fig. 14-4). The therapy of an infected episiotomy site involves debridement of the affected area and the use of a broad-spectrum antibiotic to help speed resolution of the cellulitis. Polymicrobial infection is the rule. Culture of the purulent material may identify resistant organisms. Healing by secondary intention is frequently utilized; however, some centers have used immediate closure of an infected episiotomy site after debridement in the operating room. Satisfactory results in approximately 80 to 90 percent of cases have been reported.[3,4] It is important, therefore, to obtain experienced consultation if surgical closure of the infected episiotomy site is proposed. In the absence of systemic symptoms or extensive cellulitis, outpatient therapy with close follow-up is appropriate.

Necrotizing fasciitis is a rare but frequently fatal infection most often seen in diabetics.[5,6] The hallmark of necrotizing fasciitis associated with the episiotomy site is the presence of severe pain with very mild erythema and edema of the infected area. The pain progresses from very severe to very mild, frequently giving the false impression of an improvement. The skin around the area will then turn bluish and the development of necrosis is apparent toward the latter stage of the infection. Purulence is not a characteristic of this condition. Serous fluid is frequently the only suspicious finding. Soft tissue crepitance due to gas production may also be seen. The supportive laboratory findings include an elevation in the white blood cell count. The microbiology of necrotizing fasciitis involves both aerobic and anaerobic bacteria and frequently includes *Streptococcus pyogenes* or *Clostridium perfringens*. The therapy of necrotizing

Table 14-3

CLASSIFICATION OF SEVERITY OF EPISIOTOMY INFECTION AND TREATMENT RECOMMENDATIONS

Class	Anatomic Borders	Pain	Abscess	Systemic Illness	Fever	Necrosis	Treatment
Simple	Limited to skin and superficial fascia at the incision line	Y	S	N	Y	N	Antibiotics (I) and drainage if abscess present
Superficial fascial infection	Extension to superficial fascia with spreading beyond incision line, *no* necrosis	Y	S	N	Y	N	Antibiotics (I) and drainage if abscess present; may need surgical exploration to rule out necrosis
Superficial fascial necrosis (necrotizing fasciitis)	Extension to and necrosis of the superficial fascia of the perineum (Colk's fascia), spread to the contiguous fascia of the abdominal wall (Scarpa's fascia), or the medial thighs (fascia lata) may be seen; muscle not involved	Y+ (Y−) (late)	N	Y	Y	Y (fascia only, not muscle)	Antibiotics (I + II) plus extensive debridement of fascia
Myonecrosis	Extension to and necrosis of fascia and underlying muscle	Y+	S	Y	Y	Y	Antibiotics (I + II) and extensive debridement of fascia and muscle; hypertonic oxygen therapy sometimes utilized

Key: Y(−) = anesthesia; Y(+) = pain out of proportion to wound appearance; S = sometimes; Y = yes; N = no; I = broad-spectrum therapy (see Table 14-2); II = penicillin G 6–8 million units IV q4h.

---

fasciitis demands wide debridement of the affected area and broad-spectrum antibiotic coverage. Clostridial infections should be treated with high-dose penicillin G (4 to 6 million units IV q4h) in addition to surgical debridement. Immediate obstetric or surgical consultation is imperative.

Myonecrosis is a rare but life-threatening complication. It is caused by *C. perfringens* in 80 percent of cases. The hallmark of the infection is severe pain out of proportion to the wound's appearance, associated with systemic symptoms. *Clostridium perfringens* produces an exotoxin that causes not only necrosis of muscle but also severe systemic symptoms, including hypotension, tachycardia, diaphoresis, and renal tubular necrosis. Ultrasounds and x-rays of the

pelvis will usually reveal gas bubbles at the site of infection (see Fig. 14-2). With *C. perfringens,* surgical debridement is mandatory, along with intravenous antibiotics (e.g., penicillin G 6 to 8 million units q4h).

PERINEAL ABSCESSES

Perineal abscesses will present with development of swelling and tenderness of the perineum, frequently in association with fever and lower abdominal or leg pain.

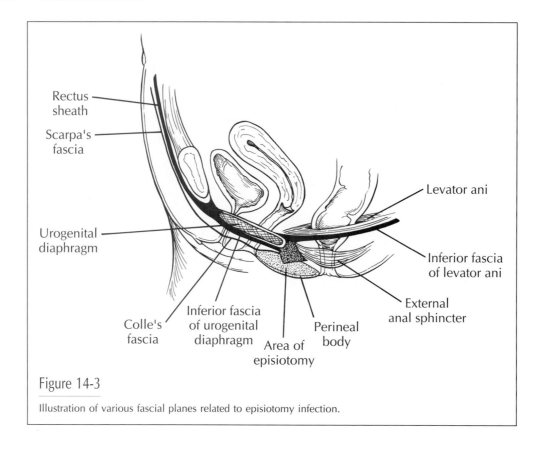

Figure 14-3

Illustration of various fascial planes related to episiotomy infection.

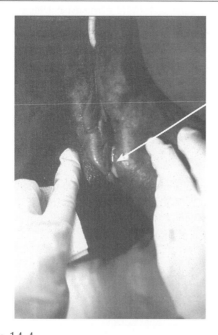

Figure 14-4

Photo of simple episiotomy infection. Arrow points to purulent drainage at episiotomy site.

As in the case of any other abscesses, the hallmark of management is incision and drainage. If the abscess is not surgically drained, it will frequently drain spontaneously, either into the vagina or into the rectum, with the possibility of fistula formation—a significant complication of perineal abscesses. Inpatient therapy and obstetric consultation are necessary for proper care of the condition.

References

1. Casey BM, Cox SM: Chorioamnionitis and endometritis. *Infect Dis Clin North Am* 11:203, 1997.
2. Faro S, Cox SM, Phillips LE: Influence of antibiotic prophylaxis on vaginal microflora. *J Obstet Gynecol* 2(suppl):54, 1986.
3. Arona AJ, al-Marayati L, Grimes DA, Bollard CA. Early secondary repair of third- and fourth-degree perineal lacerations after outpatient wound preparation. *Obstet Gynecol* 86:294, 1995.
4. Ramin SM, Ramus RM, Little BB, Gilstrap LC. Early repair of episiotomy dehiscence associated with infection. *Am J Obstet Gynecol* 167:1104, 1992.
5. Hauster G, Hanzal E, Dadak C, Gruber W. Necrotizing fasciitis arising from episiotomy. *Arch Gynecol Obstet* 255:153, 1994.
6. Goepfert AR, Guinn DA, Andrews WW, Hauth JC. Necrotizing fasciitis after cesarean delivery. *Obstet Gynecol* 89:409, 1997.

Chapter 15

SEPTIC SHOCK IN PREGNANCY

Thomas F. Rowe
Gary D. V. Hankins

Shock describes an acute pathophysiologic state characterized by hypotension despite adequate hydration associated with decreased tissue perfusion, cellular hypoxia, and metabolic acidosis. Shock may result from acute blood loss (hypovolemic shock), cardiac failure (cardiogenic shock), or loss of sympathetic control of resistance vessels (neurogenic shock). *Septic shock* refers to this same pathophysiologic state resulting from an infectious etiology.[1] In an attempt to improve the understanding of sepsis, the American College of Chest Physicians and Society of Critical Care Medicine in 1992 met to develop consensus terms and definitions concerning sepsis and its sequelae (Table 15-1).[2]

The body responds to a wide variety of insults with specific cellular and immunologic mechanisms best described as *systemic inflammatory response syndrome* (SIRS). This is manifested by two or more of the following conditions: temperature >38 or <36°C (>100.4 or <96.8°F), heart rate >90 beats per minute, respiratory rate >20 breaths per minute or Pa_{CO_2} <32 torr (nonpregnant), or white blood cell count (WBC) >12,000 or <4000 cells per cubic millimeter, or >10 percent immature (band) forms. Sepsis is this same systemic response to an active infectious process. Sepsis and its sequelae represent a continuum of clinical and pathophysiologic severity. As such, it has been recommended that the term *severe sepsis* be used if sepsis is associated with organ dysfunction, hypoperfusion, or hypotension. *Hypotension* is defined as a systolic blood pressure (BP) <90 or >40 mmHg reduction from baseline in the absence of other causes for hypotension. *Septic shock* is sepsis complicated by hypotension unresponsive to fluid resuscitation.[2]

Shock is the host's response to an insult (Fig. 15-1); *septic shock* is a pathophysiologic response to a bacterial endotoxin or exotoxin (Fig. 15-2)[3,4] *Sepsis* simply refers to the constellation of clinical signs and symptoms mentioned above associated with the host's response to circulating endotoxins or exotoxins that initiate systemic activation of cytokines, complement, coagulation factors, and immune cellular elements.[4,5] *Sepsis, severe sepsis,* and *septic shock* are progressive states of impaired perfusion of multiple organs resulting in cellular or organ dysfunction or death.[3]

Infections of the pregnant woman are common and primarily involve the genitourinary tract.[4] Listed in Table 15-2 are the most common infections encountered in the obstetric population with shock. Sepsis is most often secondary to gram-negative bacteremia.[1,3–5] Fortunately, when an obstetric patient has clinical evidence of local infection, bacteremia is present only in 8 to 10 percent.[1] The incidence of bacteremia in the general obstetric population is approximately 7.5 per 1000 admissions.[6] Overall, a 0 to 12 percent incidence of septic shock is reported in obstetric and gynecologic patients.[1,5] Ledger and associates identified only a 4 percent rate of shock in obstetric patients with bacteremia.[7] Despite aggressive contemporary medical management, mortality is estimated to occur in 20 to 50 percent of cases of obstetric septic shock.[3] Sepsis is a rare event in obstetrics, but because overall maternal mortality is extremely low, it is a leading cause (10 to 21 percent) of maternal mortality in the United States.[3–6] Multiorgan dysfunction is probably the most important determinant of outcome.[5]

Research in animal models suggests that pregnancy may predispose to septic shock through an increase in sensitiv-

Table 15-1

RECOMMENDED DEFINITIONS OF SEPSIS AND ASSOCIATED TERMS

Infection: Microbial phenomenon characterized by an inflammatory response to the presence of microorganisms or the invasion of normally sterile host tissue by those organisms.

Bacteremia: The presence of viable bacteria in the blood.

Systemic inflammatory response syndrome: The systemic inflammatory response to a variety of severe clinical insults. The response is manifest by two or more of the following conditions:

Temperature >38 or <36°C

Heart rate >90 beats per minute

Respiratory rate >20 breaths per minute or Pa_{CO_2} <32 torr (nonpregnant)

White cell count (WBC) >12,000 or <4000 cells per cubic millimeter or >10% immature (band) forms

Sepsis: The systemic response to infection. Criteria are the same as those above.

Severe sepsis: Sepsis associated with organ dysfunction, hypoperfusion, or hypotension. Hypoperfusion and perfusion abnormalities may include but are not limited to lactic acidosis, oliguria, or an acute alteration in mental status.

Septic shock: Sepsis with hypotension, despite adequate fluid resuscitation, along with the presence of perfusion abnormalities that may include but are not limited to lactic acidosis, oliguria, or an acute alteration in mental status. Patients who are on inotropic or vasopressor agents may not be hypotensive at the time that perfusion abnormalities are measured.

Hypotension: A systolic BP of <90 mmHg or a reduction of >40 mmHg from baseline in the absence of other causes for hypotension.

Multiple organ dysfunction syndrome: Presence of altered organ function in an acutely ill patient such that homeostasis cannot be maintained without intervention.

Source: From Bone et al.,[2] with permission.

ity to circulating endotoxin.[5] Despite this increased sensitivity, mortality from septic shock generally is lower in the obstetric population because of the lack of other medical problems.[1] The emergence of immunocompromised conditions related to the human immunodeficiency virus (HIV) will increase the likelihood of sepsis from microrganisms not typically encountered in immunocompetent hosts. It is therefore critical to recognize patients at greatest risk for septic shock and effect prompt and proper treatment.

MICROBIOLOGY

Gram-negative aerobic bacilli account for approximately two-thirds of confirmed cases of adult sepsis.[3–5] However, gram-positive bacteria, mycoplasmas, fungi, *Rickettsia,* or viruses may also cause sepsis. In the obstetric population, polymicrobial bacteremia accounts for nearly 20 percent of sepsis.[4] Ledger and colleagues reported that *Escherichia coli,* enterococci, and beta-hemolytic streptococci were the most frequently recovered aerobes in a series of 144 bacteremic patients admitted to an obstetrics and gynecology service. Anaerobes accounted for 30 percent of isolates recovered and included streptococci, peptococci, and *Bacteroides* species. *Clostridium perfringens* was found in five patients.[7] Blanco and associates reported that *E. coli* accounted for 57 percent, group B streptococci for 28 percent, and *Bacteroides* for 26 percent of 176 bacteremic obstetric patients.[6] Gram-positive organisms, especially staphylococcal species, may be playing an increasing role in sepsis (Table 15-3).[5]

PATHOPHYSIOLOGY

Septic shock is best understood clinically as an attempt by multiple simultaneously triggered circulating inflammatory mediators to eradicate invading pathogens. The inciting factor is usually an endotoxin from the wall of a gram-negative bacterium or occasionally an exotoxin from gram-positive bacteria (Figure 15-2).[3–5]

Bacterial endotoxin is composed of O-polysaccharide side chains (which are responsible for the O antigenicity), the R core that is shared among these bacteria, and a complex cell-wall lipopolysaccharide that contains a substance known as lipid A or lipopolysaccharide (LPS). Lipid A is the prime mediator of the septic response.[5,8] When the cell wall is disrupted and lipid A is released into circulation, the host responds by producing a number of antibacterial substances, including cytokines such as interleukin 1, 6, 8 (IL-1, IL-6, and IL-8), and tumor necrosis factor-alpha (TNF-α), complement activation and neutrophil activation, which lead to the release of oxygen free radicals.

Lipid A produces most of its deleterious effects through stimulation of monocytes and tissue macrophages, resulting in the production of cytokines, primarily TNF-α. The release

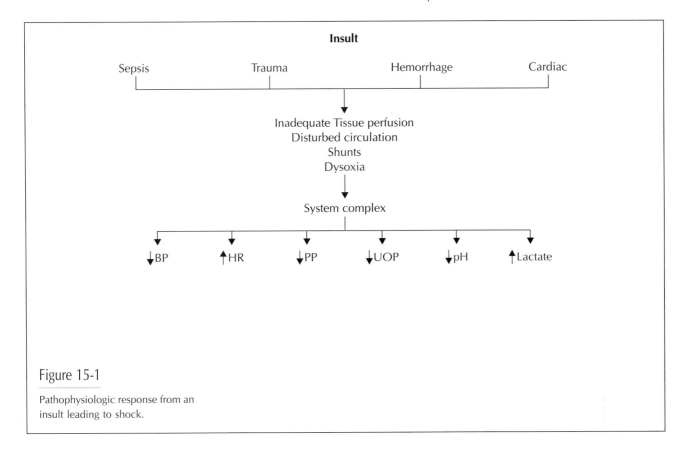

Figure 15-1

Pathophysiologic response from an insult leading to shock.

of cytokines is associated with the formation of fibrin and thrombin and activation of the alternate complement pathway.

This host response is an integral part of the host defense. However, the activation of such mediators can produce adverse host effects and tissue injury. Complement activation leads to bacteriolysis, with subsequent release of histamine and bradykinin. Lipid A directly and synergistically with the above compounds may affect peripheral vasodilatation, promote cell damage, and increase permeability of the endothelial lining. Activated leukocytes also release lysosomal enzymes and produce hydrogen peroxide, superoxide radicals, and hydroxyl radicals, which cause local tissue injury. Fibrin deposition and multiple microthrombi can result in impaired organ perfusion and oxygen delivery. Depletion of coagulation factors occurs because of increased consumption as well as impaired hepatic synthesis, resulting in impaired hemostasis (disseminated intravascular coagulation). Therefore, it is the host response to lipid A that creates the serious clinical sequelae of endotoxin shock.[4,5]

Pathophysiologic vascular alterations that occur in septic shock can result in dysoxygenation. Such derangements in tissue oxygenation result in potential maldistribution of blood flow, so that tissues with low metabolic demands are hyperperfused and those with high metabolic activity are hypoperfused.[4]

STAGES OF SHOCK

Septic shock is clinically divided into three stages: (1) early shock, (2) late shock, and (3) secondary or irreversible shock (Fig. 15-2).[1,4] Clinical features of the stages of shock are described in Table 15-4. Early shock is marked by a hyperdynamic cardiovascular state and peripheral vasodilatation. Clinically, it is characterized at the bedside by fever, tachycardia, tachypnea, and warm extremities. Although the patient may appear ill, the diagnosis of septic shock may be delayed until blood pressure is evaluated. Nonspecific complaints of nausea, vomiting, or diarrhea are frequently present. Despite the hyperdynamic state, patients have decreased tissue oxygen consumption and shunting of blood away from vital organs. Abrupt alterations in behavior may also herald the onset of septic shock and has been attributed to reduced cerebral blood flow.

Laboratory findings are variable in early shock. The white blood cell count may at first be depressed; soon afterwards, a leukocytosis is evident. Hypoglycemia may occur secondarily to hepatic dysfunction. Early evidence of disseminated intravascular coagulation (DIC) may be manifest with thrombocytopenia, decreased fibrinogen, elevated fibrin split products, and an elevation in thrombin time. Early arterial

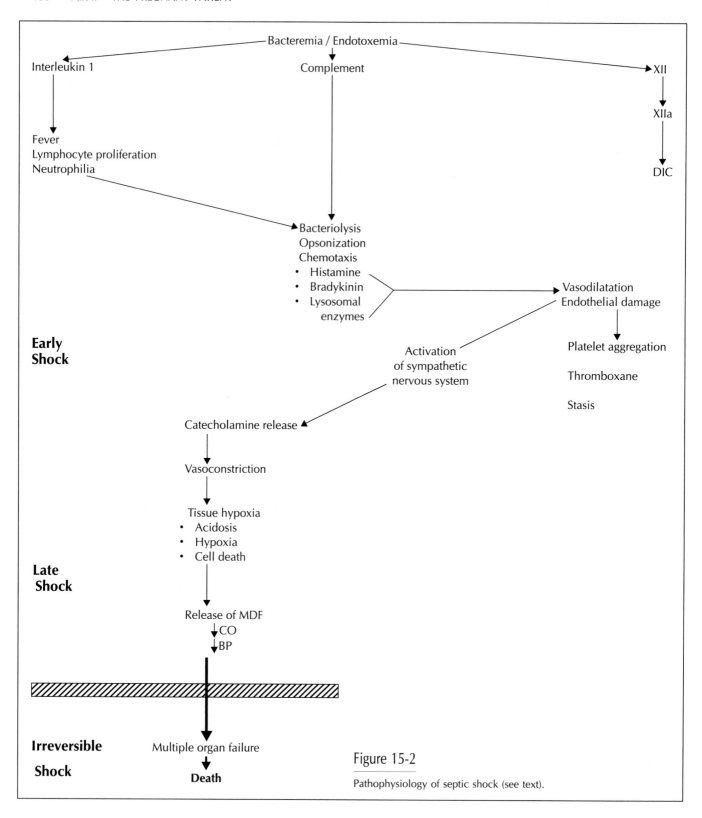

Figure 15-2

Pathophysiology of septic shock (see text).

blood gas analysis may show a transient respiratory alkalosis. Later, metabolic acidosis occurs as tissue hypoxia and lactic acid levels increase.

As the septic process continues, generalized intense vasoconstriction, hypoxia, and decreased cardiac output develop.

Clinically, typical changes of cold shock include cold extremities, oliguria, and peripheral cyanosis. If left untreated, it progresses rapidly to an irreversible state.

The final phase of shock is referred to as *secondary* or *irreversible shock*. Overt signs of prolonged cellular hypoxia

Table 15-2

BACTERIAL INFECTIONS IN OBSTETRIC PATIENTS ASSOCIATED WITH SEPTIC SHOCK

Disorder	Incidence (%)
Chorioamnionitis	0.5–1
Postpartum endometritis	
Cesarean section	15–85
Vaginal delivery	1–4
Urinary tract infections	1–4
Pyelonephritis	1–2
Necrotizing fasciitis (postoperative)	<1
Septic abortion	1–2
Toxic shock syndrome	<1

Source: From Gonik,[1] with permission.

and dysfunction become apparent. Profound alterations in mental status and multiorgan failure are present. Marked metabolic acidosis, electrolyte imbalance, and generalized DIC are common. Hemodynamically, the cardiac output is markedly depressed and generalized peripheral vasodilata-

Table 15-3

PATHOGENS RESPONSIBLE FOR SEVERE INFECTIONS IN OBSTETRIC PATIENTS

Gram-negative rods
  Escherichia coli
  Klebsiella-Enterobacter species
  Proteus species
  Serratia species
  Pseudomonas species
  Haemophilus species

Anaerobes
  Clostridium perfringens
  Fusobacterium species
  Bacteroides species
  Peptococcus
  Peptostreptococcus

Gram-positive cocci
  Streptococci, groups A & B
  Pneumococcus
  Staphylococcus aureus
  Enterococcus

Source: From Fein and Duvivier,[5] with permission.

tion is reflected by a low systemic vascular resistance. Recovery from this phase of shock is difficult and may fail despite aggressive measures.

In treating the gravid patient with sepsis, the normal physiologic adaptations to pregnancy must be recognized, as well as the effects of these changes on presentation and treatment. Critical hemodynamic and ventilatory parameters in pregnancy are listed in Table 15-5. In pregnant experimental animals, Beller and associates demonstrated a more pronounced metabolic acidosis with earlier cardiovascular collapse relative to nonpregnant animals in response to any given dose of lipopolysaccharide.[9] Other investigations have also demonstrated an increased response to endotoxin during pregnancy in several animal species. The reason for such an exaggerated response during pregnancy is unknown. However, the fetus appears more resistant than the mother to the adverse effects of endotoxin, possibly because of the immature status of the fetus's vasoactive response.[1] Conversely, Morishima et al. demonstrated profound asphyxia and rapid deterioration in fetal baboons when the mother was given endotoxin. This response was thought to be due to maternal factors such as hypotension and increased myometrial activity, both of which contribute to reduction in placental perfusion.[10]

MANAGEMENT OF SEPTIC SHOCK IN PREGNANCY

Aggressive therapy of septic shock must achieve a rapid and effective reversal of organ hypoperfusion, improvement of oxygen delivery, and correction of acidosis.[11] Fundamental goals of therapy for the septic pregnant woman are basically the same as those for nonpregnant patients: (1) expanding circulating intravascular volume, (2) securing and maintaining an airway and administering oxygen to improve tissue oxygenation, (3) determining the etiology of sepsis, (4) promptly administering appropriate antibiotic therapy based on likely pathogens, (5) obtaining appropriate laboratory data, and (6) transferring the patient to an appropriate facility or intensive care unit.[1,3] Improvement of the maternal clinical status should positively affect the status of the fetus. Management directed toward maximizing oxygen delivery and extraction and decreasing anaerobic states should improve survival.[4,11]

At times, the source of the infectious process is obvious. At other times, the source is not certain. The combination of ampicillin, gentamicin, and clindamycin or metronidazole covers most of the putative organisms in pelvic infections (Table 15-6). Ampicillin can be withheld with only slightly lower response rates in penicillin-allergic patients. Other acceptable antibiotic regimens include the broad-spectrum penicillins in combination with beta-lactamase inhibitors (e.g., ampicillin/sulbactam or ticarcillin/clavulanic acid).

Table 15-4

CLINICAL FEATURES OF SHOCK

	Early	Late	Irreversible
Cardiovascular system	Hyperdynamic, volume-dependent	Shock Decreased CO	Inotropes required Volume "overload"
Respiratory function	Tachypnea Hypocapnia Hypoxia	Severe hypoxia	Hypercapnia Barotrauma
Renal function	Limited responsiveness Fixed output Minimal azotemia	Azotemia	Oliguria
Metabolism	Severe catabolism Increased insulin requirements	Metabolic acidosis Hyperglycemia	Severe acidosis Increased oxygen consumption
Hepatic function	Normal to chemical jaundice	Clinical jaundice	Encephalopathy
Hematology	Normal to decreased platelets Increased or decreased WBC	Low platelets Low fibrinogen level Increased fibrin split products Prolonged PT, PTT	Immature cells Continued coagulopathy
Central nervous system	Variable	Some response to noxious stimuli	Coma

Table 15-5

HEMODYNAMIC AND VENTILATORY PARAMETERS IN PREGNANCY

	Nonpregnant	Pregnant
Central venous pressure, cmH_2O	1–10	Unchanged
Mean pulmonary artery pressure, mmHg	9–16	Unchanged
Pulmonary capillary wedge pressure, mmHg	3–10	Unchanged
Cardiac output, L/min	4–7	↑ 30–45%
Systemic vascular pressure, dynes/s/cm^{-5}	770–1500	↓ 25%
Pulmonary vascular resistance, dynes/s/cm^{-5}	20–120	↓ 25%
Arterial P_{O_2}, mmHg	90–95	104–108
Arterial P_{CO_2}, mmHg	38–40	27–32
AV oxygen difference, mL/dL	4–5.5	↓ Or normal
Oxygen consumption, mL/min	173–311	249–331

Source: Adapted from Gonik,[1] with permission.

Table 15-6

FREQUENTLY USED ANTIBIOTIC REGIMENS FOR SEPTIC SHOCK DURING PREGNANCY

	Dosage, Intravenous		
	Loading	Maintenance	Frequency
Ampicillin[a] plus	2 g	1–2 g	q4h
gentamicin[a] plus	2 mg/kg	1.5–1.7 mg/kg	q8h
clindamycin or	900 mg	900 mg	q8h
metronidazole	1 g	500 mg	q6h
Ticarcillin/ clavulanic[a] acid	3.1 g	3.1 g	q4h
Imipenem[a]	500 mg	500 mg	q6h

[a]Adjust dose if there is renal failure.

Newer thienamycin antibiotics are also useful in serious pelvic infections (e.g., imipenem or meropenem). Antimicrobial therapy should be based on culture results when available.[1,3–5] In addition, knowledge of the sensitivity patterns of usual organisms at each institution can guide particular antibiotic choices. Common dosage regimens in adults are listed in Table 15-6.

Clinicians should recognize potential adverse fetal effects of some antibiotics (e.g., quinolones, tetracycline).

CARDIOVASCULAR

Maintenance of intravascular volume or volume expansion is critical in the acute management of septic shock. Recalling that the early vascular response to inflammatory mediators is vasodilatation and decreased systemic vascular resistance, the goal of therapy of obstetric septic shock is to achieve rapid reversal of organ hypoperfusion, improvement in oxygen delivery, and correction of metabolic acidosis. Myocardial function may be depressed secondary to myocardial depressant factor (MDF), metabolic acidosis, and increased endogenous endorphin levels, requiring inotropic therapy.[4,11]

Fluid resuscitation should begin with intravenous crystalloids (normal saline or lactated Ringer's solution). A large volume of fluids may be required initially, in part due to extravasation of fluid into extravascular compartments because of increased capillary permeability. If aggressive volume replacement (1 to 2 L of crystalloid administered over 15 to 30 min) is not promptly followed by urinary output of at least 30 mL, further fluid therapy is safest utilizing hemodynamic monitoring with a flow-directed pulmonary artery catheter. Optimal PCWP is usually around 9 to 16 mmHg. Preload optimization is mandatory prior to inotropic therapy. Blood component therapy may also be an important adjunctive measure if significant hemorrhage has occurred or a coagulopathy is present. Diuretic therapy can be administered to correct fluid overload.

If suboptimal or inadequate cardiovascular function continues, vasoactive agents should be added to improve myocardial performance and vascular tone. Dopamine or dobutamine are excellent agents for improving myocardial contractility in an obstetric patient. Dopamine is generally used as the first-line agent, because the effects are dose-dependent. At low doses (1 to 3 μg/kg per minute), dopamine acts primarily on dopaminergic receptors causing vasodilatation and improved perfusion in the renal, mesenteric, coronary, and cerebral vasculature. Higher doses (5 to 10 μg/kg per minute) are associated with predominant beta$_1$ effects, which improve myocardial contractility, stroke volume, and cardiac output. At high doses (>20 μg/kg per minute), alpha-adrenergic effects are noted and generalized vasoconstriction including uterine vasoconstriction occurs.[1,3,4,11]

If the desired hemodynamic state is not achieved, one should try to determine if this is due to persistent vasodilatation or a depressed myocardial function. A vasopressor agent (phenylephrine or norepinephrine) should be added if hypotension is due to vasodilatation. Inotropic therapy (dobutamine, or digoxin) should be used to improve ventricular function.[3]

Later stages of shock are complicated by superimposition of endogenous MDF, which, in the absence of pressor agents, causes further decreased cardiac output and continued low systemic vascular resistance. Hypoxia and lactic acidemia will make it difficult for individual cells to utilize oxygen, with subsequent grave consequences for both mother and fetus.[12]

PULMONARY

Oxygen is administered in an attempt to improve tissue oxygenation. Oxygen consumption is significantly increased following the onset of sepsis. However, in the patient with septic shock, peripheral tissue utilization of oxygen is frequently reduced. This may be due to either cellular dysfunction and underextraction of oxygen or microvascular shunting during later stages of septic shock. Clinical improvement should be reflected in an increase or normalization of peripheral oxygen consumption.[1,5]

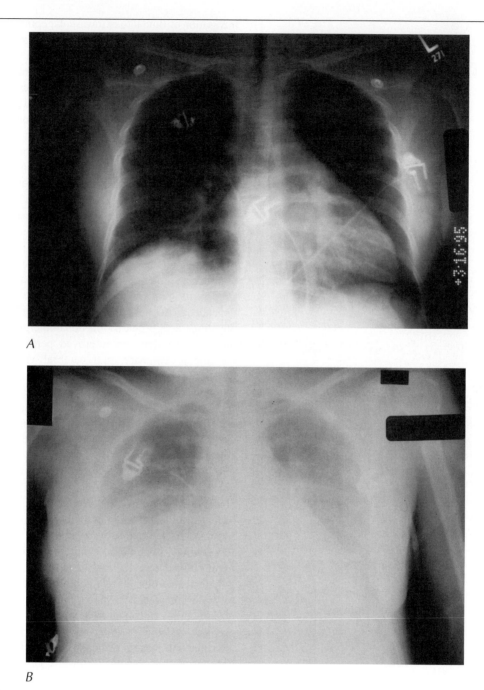

Figure 15-3

A. Chest radiograph upon admission in a pregnant woman with urosepsis *B.* Chest radiograph 36 h later, showing rapid development of adult respiratory distress syndrome.

Pulmonary function early in septic shock is usually remarkable for moderate bronchoconstriction and hyperventilation. Later stages are not uncommonly complicated by the development of adult respiratory distress syndrome (ARDS). This develops in approximately 30 to 40 percent of septic patients and is manifest by tachypnea, dyspnea, stridor, hypoxemia, and cyanosis; it can progress to respiratory failure. Adult respiratory distress syndrome develops following alveolar capillary membrane damage (from the endotoxin) and subsequent accumulation of intraalveolar and interstitial protein and fluid (Fig. 15-3). In addition, surfactant production becomes impaired. Mortality approaches 50 percent in patients with ARDS.

Positive end-expiratory pressure (PEEP) is usually necessary in ARDS to achieve adequate oxygenation at a safe Fi_{O_2}. Airway control is frequently best accomplished by intubation, and mechanical ventilation may be necessary. Although PEEP improves oxygenation by recruiting collapsed alveoli and increasing functional residual capacity, the benefit may be offset by adverse cardiovascular effects if high pressures are used (>10 cmH$_2$O). To that end, use of intravenous fluids and inotropic agents guided by information from the pulmonary artery catheter can assist in "optimizing" ventilatory support. Pulmonary function should be monitored by continuous pulse oximetry, and correlation with intermittent arterial blood gas assessment should be established.[1,3,4]

RENAL

Renal function is best monitored by an indwelling catheter. The kidney can autoregulate perfusion over a moderate range of blood pressures, but as hypoperfusion occurs the glomerular filtration rate decreases and oliguria develops. Poor renal perfusion plus vasoconstriction of afferent arterioles may lead to the development of acute tubular necrosis.[4] Serial creatinine and blood urea nitrogen (BUN) determinations plus hourly urine output determination should be used to evaluate renal function. Correction of hemodynamic and perfusion deficits should result in restoration of renal function.

ANTIMICROBIAL THERAPY

Eradication of the infecting organism(s) is of utmost importance in the management of septic shock. Because the course of septic shock can be short and fulminant, prompt evaluation and administration of appropriate antibiotics is vital to patient survival. In addition, surgical extirpation of infected tissues may be necessary to enhance survival. Expeditious evacuation of the uterus may be required in patients with septic abortion or chorioamnionitis. This is preferably accomplished by the vaginal route, but if the mother's condition is deteriorating, hysterotomy or hysterectomy may be required.

SUMMARY

Septic shock in pregnant patients remains a devastating problem. Early identification, awareness of the state of immunocompromise during pregnancy, and aggressive management based on potential infectious sources may decrease morbidity and mortality for the pregnant patient and her fetus. Appreciation of the systemic inflammatory response and mediators of septic sequelae and their actions should lead to a better understanding of the pathophysiology and therapeutic interventions of septic shock. Optimal therapy includes aggressive volume resuscitation, hemodynamic monitoring and intervention, pulmonary support and oxygen delivery, evaluation of multiorgan failure, and elimination of the infecting organism(s) or tissues. Management is best accomplished in a critical care unit with invasive monitoring capabilities for both the mother and fetus.

References

1. Gonik B: Septic shock in obstetrics, in Clark SL, Cotton DV, Hankins GDV, Phelan JP (eds): *Critical Care Obstetrics*, 2d ed. Boston: Blackwell, 1991, pp 289–306.
2. Bone RC, Balk RA, Cerra FB, et al, Members of the American College of Chest Physicians/Society of Critical Care Medicine Consensus Conference Committee: Definitions for sepsis and organ failure and guidelines for the use of innovative therapies in sepsis. *Crit Care Med* 20:864, 1992.
3. Pearlman M, Faro S: Obstetric septic shock: A pathophysiologic basis for management. *Clin Obstet Gynecol* 33:482, 1990.
4. Yancey MK, Duff P: Acute hypotension related to sepsis in the obstetric patient. *Ob Gyn Clin North Am* 22:91, 1995.
5. Fein AM, Duvivier R: Sepsis in pregnancy. *Clin Chest Med* 13:709, 1992.
6. Blanco JD, Gibbs RS, Castaneda YS: Bacteremia in obstetrics: Clinical course. *Obstet Gynecol* 58:621, 1981.
7. Ledger WJ, Norman M, Gee C, et al: Bacteremia on an obstetric-gynecologic service. *Am J Obstet Gynecol* 121:205, 1975.
8. Wolfe SM: Monoclonal antibodies and the treatment of gram-negative bacteremia and shock. *N Engl J Med* 324:486, 1991.
9. Beller FK, Schmidt EH, Holzgreve W, et al: Septicemia during pregnancy: A study in different species of experimental animals. *Am J Obstet Gynecol* 151:967, 1985.
10. Morishima HO, Niemann WH, James LS: Effects of endotoxin on the pregnant baboon and fetus. *Am J Obstet Gynecol* 131:899, 1978.
11. Lee W, Cotton DB, Hankins GDV, Faro S: Management of septic shock complicating pregnancy. *Ob Gyn Clin North Am* 16:431, 1989.
12. Duff P, Groves AC, McLean LPH, et al: Defective oxygen consumption in septic shock. *Surg Gynecol Obstet* 121:1051, 1969.

Chapter 16

DRUG USE IN PREGNANCY AND LACTATION

Jennifer R. Niebyl

Caution with regard to drug ingestion during pregnancy is usually advised. Until recently, the fetus was thought to rest in a privileged site with little exposure to the mother's environment. The term *placental barrier* has been in widespread use but is truly a contradiction, because the placenta allows the transfer of many drugs and dietary substances. Virtually all drugs cross the placenta to some degree with the exception of large organic ions such as heparin and insulin.

Developmental defects in humans may stem from genetic, environmental, or unknown causes. Approximately 25 percent are known to be genetic in origin; drug exposure accounts for only 2 to 3 percent of birth defects. Approximately 65 percent of defects are of unknown etiology but may be due to combinations of genetic and environmental factors. The incidence of major malformations in the general population is usually quoted at 2 to 3 percent.[1] A major malformation is defined as one that is incompatible with survival, such as anencephaly, one requiring major surgery for correction, such as cleft palate or congenital heart disease, or one producing major dysfunction, such as mental retardation. If minor malformations are also included, such as ear tags or extra digits, the rate may be as high as 7 to 10 percent. The risk of malformation after exposure to a drug must be compared with this background rate.

There is a marked species specificity in drug teratogenesis.[2] For example, thalidomide was not found to be teratogenic in rats and mice but is a potent human teratogen. On the other hand, in certain strains of mice, corticosteroids produce a high percentage of offspring with cleft lip, although no studies have shown these drugs to be teratogenic in humans.

The classic teratogenic period is from day 31 after the last menstrual period (LMP) in a 28-day cycle to 71 days from the LMP. During this critical time, organs are forming, and teratogens may cause malformations that are usually overt at birth. The timing of exposure is important. Administration of drugs early in the period of organogenesis will affect the organs developing then, such as the heart or neural tube. Closer to the end of the classic teratogenic period, the ear and palate are forming and may be affected by a teratogen.

Before day 31, exposure to a teratogen produces an all-or-none effect. With exposure around conception, the conceptus usually either does not survive or survives without anomalies. Because so few cells exist in the early stages, irreparable damage to some may be lethal to the entire organism. If the organism remains viable, however, organ-specific anomalies do not become manifest because either repair or replacement will occur, permitting normal development. A similar insult at a later stage may produce organ-specific defects; after the first trimester, chronic exposure may produce growth restriction.

The Food and Drug Administration (FDA) lists five categories of labeling for drug use in pregnancy:

Category A: Controlled studies in women fail to demonstrate a risk to the fetus in the first trimester, and the possibility of fetal harm appears remote.

Category B: Animal studies do not indicate a risk to the fetus, there are no controlled human studies, or animal studies do show an adverse effect on the fetus, but well-controlled studies in pregnant women have failed to demonstrate a risk to the fetus.

Category C: Studies have shown the drug to have animal teratogenic or embryocidal effects, but no controlled studies in women are available or no studies are available in either animals or women.

Category D: Positive evidence of human fetal risk exists, but benefits in certain situations (e.g., life-threatening situations or serious diseases for which safer drugs cannot be used or are ineffective) may make the use of the drug acceptable despite its risks.

Category X: Studies in animals or humans have demonstrated fetal abnormalities, or evidence demonstrates fetal risk based on human experience, or both, and the risk clearly outweighs any possible benefit.

Patients should be educated about avenues other than the use of drugs to cope with tension, aches and pains, and viral illnesses during pregnancy. Drugs should be used only when necessary. The risk-benefit ratio should justify the use of a particular drug, and the minimum effective dose should be employed. As long-term effects of drug exposure in utero may not be revealed for many years, caution with regard to the use of any drug in pregnancy is warranted.

EFFECTS OF SPECIFIC DRUGS

ANALGESICS

Pregnant patients should be encouraged to use nonpharmacologic remedies, such as local heat and rest, before using analgesics.

ASPIRIN

Aspirin significantly inhibits platelet aggregation, which can increase the risk of bleeding before as well as at delivery. Platelet dysfunction has been described in newborns within 5 days of ingestion of aspirin by the mother.[3] Because aspirin causes permanent inhibition of prostaglandin synthetase in platelets, the only way for adequate clotting to occur is for more platelets to be produced.

There is no evidence of any teratogenic effect of aspirin taken in the first trimester.[4] Aspirin does have significant perinatal effects, however, as uterine contractility is decreased. Patients taking aspirin in analgesic doses have delayed onset of labor, longer duration of labor, and an increased risk of a prolonged pregnancy.[5]

Multiple organs may be affected by chronic aspirin use. Of note, prostaglandins mediate the neonatal closure of the ductus arteriosus. In one case report, maternal ingestion of aspirin close to the time of delivery was related to closure of the ductus arteriosus in utero.[6]

ACETAMINOPHEN

Acetaminophen (Tylenol, Datril) has also shown no evidence of teratogenicity. With acetaminophen, inhibition of prostaglandin synthesis is reversible, so that once the drug has cleared, platelet aggregation returns to normal. The bleeding time is not prolonged with acetaminophen, in contrast to aspirin.[7] Thus, if a mild analgesic or antipyretic is indicated, acetaminophen is preferred over aspirin.

OTHER NONSTEROIDAL ANTI-INFLAMMATORY DRUGS

No evidence of teratogenicity has been reported for other nonsteroidal anti-inflammatory drugs (NSAIDS), such as ibuprofen (Motrin, Advil) or naproxen (Naprosyn). Chronic use may lead to oligohydramnios and constriction of the fetal ductus arteriosus in utero or neonatal pulmonary hypertension, as has been reported with indomethacin. Short courses (less than 48 h) would be expected to be safe.

PROPOXYPHENE

Propoxyphene (Darvon) is an acceptable alternative mild analgesic with no known teratogenicity.[4] However, it should not be used for trivial indications, as it carries potential for narcotic addition.[8]

CODEINE

In the Collaborative Perinatal Project, no increased relative risk of malformations was observed in 563 codeine users.[4] Codeine can cause addiction and newborn withdrawal symptoms if used to excess perinatally.

ANTIASTHMATICS

THEOPHYLLINE AND AMINOPHYLLINE

Both theophylline (Theo-Dur, Slo-Bid) and aminophylline are safe for the treatment of asthma in pregnancy.[4] Because of increased renal clearance in pregnancy, dosages may need to be increased.

EPINEPHRINE

Minor malformations have been reported with sympathomimetic amines, such as epinephrine (Adrenalin), as a group in 3082 exposures in the first trimester, usually from commercial preparations used to treat upper respiratory infections.[4]

TERBUTALINE

Terbutaline (Brethine) has been widely used in the treatment of preterm labor. It is more rapid in onset and has a longer duration of action than epinephrine and is preferred for asthma in the pregnant patient. No risk of birth defects has been reported. Long-term use has been associated with an increased risk of glucose intolerance.[9]

CROMOLYN SODIUM

Cromolyn sodium (Intal) may be administered in pregnancy, and the systemic absorption is minimal. Teratogenicity has not been reported in humans.

ISOPROTERENOL, METAPROTERENOL, ALBUTEROL

When beta-adrenergic agents—isoproterenol (Isuprel), metaproterenol (Alupent), Albuterol (Ventolin)—are given as topical aerosols for the treatment of asthma, the total dose absorbed is usually not significant. With oral or intravenous doses, however, the cardiovascular effects of these agents may result in decreased uterine blood flow. No teratogenicity has been reported.[4]

CORTICOSTEROIDS

All steroids cross the placenta to some degree but prednisone and prednisolone are inactivated by the placenta, and the concentration of active compound in the fetus is less than 10 percent of that in the mother. Therefore, these agents are the drugs of choice for treating medical diseases such as asthma. Inhaled corticosteroids are also effective therapy, and very little drug is absorbed. When corticoid effects are desired in the fetus to accelerate lung maturity, betamethasone and dexamethasone are preferred, as these cross the placenta readily. In several hundred infants exposed to corticosteroids in the first trimester, no increase in abnormalities was noted.[4,10,11]

ANTIBIOTICS AND ANTI-INFECTIVE AGENTS

As pregnant patients are particularly susceptible to vaginal yeast infections, therapy with antifungal agents may be necessary during or after the course of antibiotic therapy.

PENICILLINS

Penicillin, ampicillin, and amoxicillin (Amoxil) are safe in pregnancy, with no increased risk of anomalies.[4] There is little experience in pregnancy with the newer penicillins such as piperacillin (Pipracil) and mezlocillin (Mezlin). These drugs, therefore, should be used in pregnancy only when another, better-studied antibiotic is not effective.

CEPHALOSPORINS

In a study of 5000 Michigan Medicaid recipients, there was a suggestion of possible teratogenicity (25 percent increased birth defects) with cefaclor, cephalexin, and cephradine but not with other cephalosporins.[12] Because other antibiotics that have been used extensively (e.g., penicillin, ampicillin, amoxicillin, erythromycin) have not been associated with an increased risk of congenital defects, they should be first-line therapy when such treatment is needed in the first trimester.

SULFONAMIDES

Among 1455 human infants exposed to sulfonamides during the first trimester, no teratogenic effects were noted.[4] Sulfonamides cause no known damage to the fetus in utero, because the fetus can clear free bilirubin through the placenta. These drugs might theoretically have deleterious effects if present in the blood of the neonate after birth, however. Sulfonamides compete with bilirubin for binding sites on albumin, thus raising the levels of free bilirubin in the serum and increasing the risk of hyperbilirubinemia in the neonate. For that reason, they are not the first choice in the third trimester.

SULFAMETHOXAZOLE WITH TRIMETHOPRIM

Sulfamethoxazole and trimethoprim (Bactrim, Septra) are often given in treating urinary tract infections. Two published trials have failed to show any increased risk of birth defects after first-trimester exposure.[13] However, one unpublished study of 2000 Michigan Medicaid recipients suggested an increased risk of cardiovascular defects after exposure in the first trimester.[14]

SULFASALAZINE

Sulfasalazine (Azulfidine) is used for treatment of ulcerative colitis and Crohn's disease because of its relatively poor oral absorption. However, it does cross the placenta, leading to fetal drug concentrations approximately the same as those of the mother, although both are low. Neither kernicterus nor severe neonatal jaundice have been reported following maternal use of sulfasalizine even when the drug was given up to the time of delivery.[15]

NITROFURANTOIN

Nitrofurantoin (Macrodantin) is used in the treatment of acute uncomplicated lower urinary tract infections as well as for long-term suppression in patients with chronic bacteriuria. Nitrofurantoin is capable of inducing hemolytic anemia in patients deficient in glucose 6 phosphate dehydrogenase (G6PD) and theoretically in infants, whose red blood cells are deficient in glutathione.[16] However, hemolytic anemia in the newborn as a result of in utero exposure to nitrofurantoin has not been reported, and no reports linking the use of nitrofurantoin with congenital defects have been identified.[17]

The microcrystalline form of nitrofurantoin is absorbed more slowly than the crystalline and is associated with less gastrointestinal intolerance. Because of rapid elimination, the serum half-life is 20 to 60 min. Therapeutic serum levels are not achieved; therefore this drug is not indicated when there is a possibility of bacteremia.

TETRACYCLINES

The tetracyclines readily cross the placenta and are firmly bound by chelation to calcium in developing bone and teeth. This produces brown discoloration of the deciduous teeth, hypoplasia of the enamel, and inhibition of bone growth.[18] The staining of the teeth takes place in the second or third trimester of pregnancy, while bone incorporation can occur earlier. Depression of skeletal growth was particularly common among premature infants treated with tetracycline. Alternate antibiotics are currently recommended during pregnancy. Inadvertent first-trimester exposure to tetracyclines has not been found to involve any teratogenic risk.[4,19]

AMINOGLYCOSIDES

Streptomycin and kanamycin have been associated with congenital deafness in the offspring of mothers who took these drugs during pregnancy. Ototoxicity was reported with doses as low as 1 g of streptomycin biweekly for 8 weeks during the first trimester.[20] Among the children of 391 mothers who had received 50 mg/kg of kanamycin for prolonged periods during pregnancy, 9 (2.3 percent) were found to have hearing loss.[21]

Ototoxicity may be increased with simultaneous use of ethacrynic acid (Edecrin),[22] and nephrotoxicity may be greater when aminoglycosides are combined with cephalosporins. Neuromuscular blockade may be potentiated by the combined use of aminoglycosides and curariform drugs; therefore, the dosages should be reduced appropriately. Potentiation of magnesium sulfate–induced neuromuscular weakness has also been reported in a neonate exposed to magnesium sulfate and gentamicin (Garamycin).[23] No known teratogenic effect other than ototoxicity has been associated with the use of aminoglycosides in the first trimester.[24]

ANTITUBERCULOSIS DRUGS

There is no evidence of any teratogenic effect of isoniazid (INH), para-aminosalicylic acid (PAS), rifampin (Rifadin), or ethambutol (Myambutol).

ERYTHROMYCIN

No teratogenic risk of erythromycin has been reported.[19] Erythromycin estolate (Ilosone) has been associated with subclinical reversible hepatotoxicity during pregnancy[25]; thus, other forms are usually recommended.

Erythromycin is not consistently absorbed from the gastrointestinal tract of pregnant women, and the transplacental passage is unpredictable. Both maternal and fetal plasma levels achieved after the administration of the drug in pregnancy are low and vary considerably, with fetal plasma concentrations being 5 to 20 percent of those in maternal plasma.[26] Erythromycin may not be well tolerated in pregnant women who are susceptible to nausea and gastrointestinal symptoms.

CLINDAMYCIN

No increased risk of birth defects was noted among 647 infants exposed to clindamycin in the first trimester.[27] Clindamycin (Cleocin) is nearly completely absorbed after oral administration; a small percentage is absorbed after topical application.

QUINOLONES

The quinolones—e.g., ciprofloxacin (Cipro), norfloxacin (Noroxin)—have a high affinity for bone tissue and cartilage and may cause arthralgia in children. However, no malformations or musculoskeletal problems were noted in 38 infants exposed in utero in the first trimester.[28] Alternative drugs are usually recommended for use in pregnancy.

METRONIDAZOLE

Studies have failed to show any increase in the incidence of congenital defects among the newborns of mothers treated with metronidazole (Flagyl) during early or late gestation.[29,30]

Controversy regarding the use of metronidazole during pregnancy was stirred when metronidazole was shown to be mutagenic in bacteria by the Ames test, which correlates with carcinogenicity in animals. However, the doses used were much higher than those used clinically, and carcinogenicity in humans has not been confirmed.[31] Because some have recommended against its use in pregnancy, metronidazole use should be deferred until after the first trimester if possible.

ACYCLOVIR

The Acyclovir (Zovirax) Registry has recorded 601 exposures during pregnancy, including 425 in the first trimester, with no increased risk of abnormalities in the infants.[32] The Centers for Disease Control recommend that pregnant women with disseminated infection—e.g., herpes encephalitis, hepatitis, or varicella pneumonia—be treated with acyclovir.[33]

Two other agents have been approved for treatment of genital herpes—valacyclovir and famciclovir. Although both are guanosine analogues that require viral thymidine kinase to activate the drug, there is less experience with these drugs during pregnancy.

LINDANE

Toxicity in humans after use of topical 1% lindane (Kwell) has been observed almost exclusively after overexposure to the agent. Although no specific fetal damage is attributable to lindane, it is a potent neurotoxin, and its use during pregnancy should be limited. Pregnant women should be cautioned to wear gloves when shampooing their children's hair, as absorption could easily occur across the skin. An alternate drug for lice is usually recommended, such as pyrethrins with piperonyl butoxide (Rid).

ANTIFUNGAL AGENTS

Nystatin (Mycostatin) is poorly absorbed from intact skin and mucous membranes; its topical use has not been associated with teratogenesis.[19]

The imidazoles are absorbed in only small amounts from the vagina. Clotrimazole (Lotrimin) or miconazole (Monistat) in pregnancy are not known to be associated with congenital malformations. In one study, a statistically significantly increased risk of first-trimester abortion was noted after use of these drugs, but these findings were not considered to be definitive evidence of risk.[34] Nevertheless, for theoretical reasons, use of these drugs should be postponed until after the first trimester if possible.

ANTICOAGULANTS

Warfarin (Coumadin) has been associated with a characteristic embryopathy in about 5 percent of exposed pregnancies. This syndrome includes nasal hypoplasia, bone stippling seen on radiologic examination, bilateral optic atrophy, and mental retardation. The ophthalmologic abnormalities and mental retardation may occur even with use beyond the first trimester.[35] The alternative drug, heparin, does not cross the placenta, as it is a large molecule with a strong negative charge. It should be the drug of choice for patients requiring anticoagulation in pregnancy. Therapy with 20,000 U/day for more than 20 weeks has been associated with bone demineralization.[36] The risk of spinal fractures was 0.7 percent with low-dose heparin and 3 percent with a high-dose regimen.[37] Heparin can also cause thrombocytopenia. Low-molecular-weight heparin is advantageous because it needs to be given only once daily and may reduce the risks of thrombocytopenia and osteoporosis. However, clinical experience with this agent during pregnancy is limited.[38]

The risks of heparin use during pregnancy may not be justified in patients who have had only a single episode of thrombosis.[39,40] Certainly conservative measures should be recommended, such as elastic stockings and avoidance of prolonged sitting or standing.

In patients with cardiac valve prostheses, full anticoagulation is necessary because low-dose heparin has resulted in three valve thromboses (two fatal) in 35 mothers so treated.[41]

ANTICONVULSANTS

Epileptic women taking anticonvulsants during pregnancy have approximately double the general population risk of malformations.[42] Compared to the general risk of 2 to 3 percent, the risk of major malformations in epileptic women on phenytoin (Dilantin) is about 5 percent, especially cleft lip with or without cleft palate and congenital heart disease. Valproic acid (Depakene)[43] and carbamazepine (Tegretol)[44] carry approximately a 1 percent risk of neural tube defects and possibly other anomalies.[45] A combination of more than three drugs or a high daily dose increases the chance of malformations.[46]

Fewer than 10 percent of offspring show the fetal hydantoin syndrome,[47] which consists of microcephaly, growth deficiency, developmental delays, mental retardation, dysmorphic craniofacial features, hypoplasia of the nails and distal phalanges, and hypertelorism. Trimethadione (Tridione) and carbamazepine (Tegretol) are also associated with an increased risk of a dysmorphic syndrome.[48]

Children exposed in utero to phenytoin scored 10 points lower in IQ tests than children exposed to carbamazepine or unexposed controls.[49] A follow-up study of long-term effects of antenatal exposure to phenobarbital and carbamazepine found that anomalies were not related to specific maternal medication exposure. There were no neurologic or behavioral differences between the two groups.[50]

Some women may have taken anticonvulsant drugs for a long period without reevaluation of the need for continuation of the drugs. For patients with idiopathic epilepsy who have been seizure-free for 2 years and who have normal electroencephalograms (EEGs), it may be safe to attempt a trial of withdrawal of the drugs before pregnancy.[51]

Most authorities agree that the benefits of anticonvulsant therapy during pregnancy outweigh the risks of discontinuation of the drugs if the patient is first seen during pregnancy. The blood level of drug should be monitored in order to ensure a therapeutic level but minimize the dosage. Neonatologists must be notified when a patient is on anticonvulsants because this therapy can affect vitamin K–dependent clotting factors in the newborn.

ANTIEMETICS

Remedies suggested to help relieve nausea and vomiting in pregnancy without pharmacologic intervention include taking crackers at the bedside upon first awakening in the morning before getting out of bed, getting up very slowly, omitting the use of iron tablets, consuming frequent small meals, and eating protein snacks at night. Faced with a self-limited condition occurring at the time of organogenesis, the clinician is well advised to avoid the use of medications whenever possible and to encourage these supportive measures initially.

VITAMIN B₆

Vitamin B₆ (pyridoxine) 25 mg t.i.d. has been reported in two randomized, placebo-controlled trials to be effective for treating nausea and vomiting of pregnancy.[52,53] In several other controlled trials there was no evidence of teratogenicity.

DOXYLAMINE

Doxylamine (Unisom) is an effective antihistamine for nausea in pregnancy and can be combined with vitamin B₆ (pyridoxine) to produce a therapy similar to that of the former preparation, Bendectin. Vitamin B₆ (25 mg) and doxylamine (25 mg) at bedtime, and one-half of each in the morning and afternoon, is an effective combination.

GINGER

Ginger has been used with success for treating hyperemesis[54] defined as vomiting during pregnancy severe enough to require hospital admission. A significantly greater relief of symptoms was found after ginger treatment than with placebo. Patients took 250-mg capsules containing ginger as powdered root four times a day.

MECLIZINE

In one randomized, placebo-controlled study, meclizine (Bonine) gave significantly better results than placebo.[55] Prospective clinical studies have provided no evidence that meclizine is teratogenic in humans.[4,56]

DIMENHYDRINATE

No teratogenicity with dimenhydrinate (Dramamine) has been noted, but a 29 percent failure rate and a significant incidence of side effects, especially drowsiness, has been reported.[57]

DIPHENHYDRAMINE

In 595 patients treated with diphenhydramine (Benadryl) in the Collaborative Perinatal Project, no teratogenicity was noted.[4] Drowsiness can be a problem.

TRIMETHOBENZAMIDE

Trimethobenzamide (Tigan), an antinauseant not classified as either an antihistamine or a phenothiazine, has been used for nausea and vomiting in pregnancy. The data collected in a small number of patients are conflicting. In 193 patients in the Kaiser Health Plan study[56] exposed to trimethobenzamide, there was a suggestion of increased congenital anomalies; no clustering of specific anomalies was observed in these children, however, and some of the mothers took other drugs as well. In 340 patients in the Collaborative Peri-

natal Project,[4] no evidence for an association between this drug and malformations was found.

PHENOTHIAZINES

Because of the potential for severe side effects, the phenothiazines have not been used routinely in the treatment of mild or moderate nausea and vomiting but have been reserved for the treatment of hyperemesis gravidarum. Chlorpromazine (Thorazine) has been shown to be effective in hyperemesis gravidarum, and the most important side effect is drowsiness. Teratogenicity does not appear to be a problem with the phenothiazines evaluated as a group.[56,4] In 58 mothers treated with promethazine (Phenergan) and in 48 mothers given prochlorperazine (Compazine), no increased risk of malformations was found.

ONDANSETRON

Ondansetron (Zofran) is no more effective than promethazine and has not been evaluated for teratogenicity.[58]

METOCLOPRAMIDE

Of 192 newborns exposed to metoclopramide (Reglan) during the first trimester, no increased birth defects were observed. The drug can be an effective antinauseant but has not been well studied in human pregnancy.

EMETROL

Emetrol is a phosphorylated carbohydrate solution that acts on the wall of the hyperactive gastrointestinal tract. It reduces smooth muscle contractions in direct proportion to the amount used and is relatively free from toxicity.

ACUPRESSURE

Acupressure is another modality that may be effective in reducing nausea (but not vomiting) in pregnant women.[59]

ANTIHISTAMINES AND DECONGESTANTS

No increased risk of anomalies has been associated with most of the commonly used antihistamines, such as chlorpheniramine (Chlor-Trimeton).[4] Terfenadine (Seldane) has been associated in one study with an increased risk of polydactyly.[60] An association between exposure during the last 2 weeks of pregnancy to antihistamines in general and retrolental fibroplasia in premature infants has been reported.[61]

In the Collaborative Perinatal Project[4] an increased risk of birth defects was noted with exposure to phenylpropanolamine (Entex LA) in the first trimester. In one retrospective study, an increased risk of gastroschisis was associated with first-trimester use of pseudoephedrine (Sudafed).[62] Although these findings have not been confirmed, use of these drugs for trivial indications should be discouraged. If decongestion is necessary, topical nasal sprays will result in a lower dose to the fetus than systemic medication.

Patients should be taught that antihistamines and decongestants are only symptomatic therapy for the common cold and have no influence on the course of the disease. Other remedies should be recommended, such as use of a humidifier, rest, and fluids. If medications are necessary, combinations with two drugs should not be used if only one drug is necessary; e.g., if the situation is truly an allergy, an antihistamine alone will suffice.

ANTIHYPERTENSIVE DRUGS

Methyldopa (Aldomet) has been widely used for the treatment of chronic hypertension in pregnancy. Although postural hypotension may occur, no unusual fetal effects have been noted. Hydralazine (Apresoline) has also had widespread use in pregnancy, and no teratogenic effect has been observed.

SYMPATHETIC BLOCKING AGENTS

Propranolol (Inderal) is a beta-adrenergic blocking agent with no evidence of teratogenicity. Bradycardia has been reported in the newborn as a direct effect of a dose of the drug given to the mother within 2 h before delivery of the infant.[63]

Several studies of propranolol use in pregnancy show an increased risk of intrauterine growth restriction or at least a skewing of the birth-weight distribution toward the lower range.[64] Ultrasound monitoring of patients on this drug is prudent. Studies from Scotland suggest improved outcome with the use of atenolol (Tenormin) to treat chronic hypertension during pregnancy.[65]

ANGIOTENSIN-CONVERTING ENZYME INHIBITORS

Angiotensin-converting enzyme inhibitors [e.g., enalapril (Vasotec) and captopril (Capoten)] can cause fetal renal failure in the second and third trimesters, leading to oligohydramnios, fetal limb contractures, craniofacial deformities, and hypoplastic lung development.[66] Fetal skull ossification defects and hypocalvaria have also been described.[67] For these reasons, pregnant women on these medications should be switched to other agents. Use during the early first trimester has not been reported to be teratogenic.

GASTROINTESTINAL DRUGS

The first step in therapy of heartburn in pregnancy is to avoid both irritating foods and eating foods at bedtime. More frequent, smaller meals may also be helpful.

Antacids taken in the usual therapeutic doses are considered safe, and pregnant women may benefit from the calcium-containing antacids. Liquid antacids have a greater gas acid neutralizing capacity than tablet preparations. The patient should be cautioned not to exceed the recommended daily dosage. Constipation (aluminum) and diarrhea (magnesium) are principal side effects. All, including calcium, may impair absorption of iron and should be taken at a separate time from such supplements.

H$_2$ BLOCKERS

No reports linking the use of cimetidine (Tagamet), ranitidine (Zantac), or famotidine (Pepcid) and birth defects have been located.[68] Cimetidine has been used at term to prevent maternal gastric aspiration pneumonia, with no neonatal adverse effects noted.

There has been some controversy about the antiandrogenic effects of cimetidine in adult humans. Given the possible feminizing effects of cimetidine, ranitidine or famotidine should probably be preferred in pregnancy.[68]

SUCRALFATE

Sucralfate (Carafate) coats the mucosal lesion in an ulcer crater and protects it from gastric acid. It is poorly absorbed from the gastrointestinal tract. Among 183 infants exposed in the first trimester, there was no increased incidence of birth defects.

PSYCHIATRIC DRUGS

There is no clear risk documented for most psychoactive drugs with respect to overt birth defects. However, effects of chronic use of these agents on the developing brain in humans is difficult to study, so a conservative attitude is appropriate. Lack of overt defects does not exclude the possibility of behavioral teratogenesis.

TRANQUILIZERS

Conflicting reports of the possible teratogenicity of the various tranquilizers have appeared, including meprobamate (Miltown) and chlordiazepoxide (Librium), but in prospective studies no risk of anomalies has been confirmed.[69,70] In most clinical situations, the risk-benefit ratio does not justify the use of benzodiazepines in pregnancy.

A fetal benzodiazepine syndrome has been reported in seven infants of 36 mothers who regularly took benzodiazepines during pregnancy.[71] However, the high rate of abnormality occurred with concomitant alcohol and substance abuse and may not be due to the benzodiazepine exposure.[72] Perinatal use of diazepam (Valium) has been associated with hypotonia, hypothermia, and respiratory depression.

LITHIUM

In the International Register of Lithium Babies,[73] 217 infants had been exposed to lithium (Eskalith, Lithobid) at least during the first trimester of pregnancy and 25 (11.5 percent) were malformed. Of these, 18 had cardiovascular anomalies, including 6 with the rare Ebstein anomaly. Of 60 unaffected infants who were followed to age 5, no increased mental or physical abnormalities were noted compared with unexposed siblings.[74]

However, two other reports suggest that there was a bias of ascertainment in the registry and that the risk of anomalies is much lower than previously thought. A case-control study of 59 patients with Ebstein anomaly showed no difference in the rate of lithium exposure in pregnancy from a control group of 168 children with neuroblastoma.[75] A prospective study of 148 women exposed to lithium in the first trimester showed no difference in the incidence of major anomalies as compared with controls.[76] One fetus in the lithium-exposed group had Ebstein anomaly, and one infant in the control group had a ventricular septal defect. The authors concluded that lithium is not a major human teratogen. Nevertheless, we do recommend that women exposed to lithium be offered ultrasound and fetal echocardiography. Also, complications similar to those seen in adults on lithium have been noted in newborns, including goiter and hypothyroidism. Two cases have been reported of polyhydramnios associated with maternal lithium treatment.[77,78] Because nephrogenic diabetes insipidus has been reported in adults taking lithium, the presumed mechanism of this polyhydramnios is fetal diabetes insipidus. Polyhydramnios may be a sign of fetal lithium toxicity. It is usually recommended that drug therapy be changed in pregnant women on lithium to avoid fetal drug exposure. Tapering over 10 days will delay the risk of relapse.[79] However, discontinuing lithium is associated with a 70 percent chance of relapse of the affective disorder in 1 year, as opposed to 20 percent in those who remain on lithium. Discontinuation of lithium may pose an unacceptable risk of increased morbidity in women who have had multiple episodes of affective instability.

ANTIDEPRESSANTS

Imipramine (Tofranil) was the original tricyclic antidepressant claimed to be associated with cardiovascular defects, but the number of patients studied remains small. Among 75 newborns exposed in the first trimester, 6 major defects were observed, 3 being cardiovascular.[80]

Amitriptyline (Elavil) has been more widely used. Although occasional reports have associated the use of this drug and birth defects, the majority of the evidence supports its safety. In the Michigan Medicaid study, 467 newborns had been exposed during the first trimester, with no increased incidence of birth defects.[81]

Fluoxetine (Prozac) is being used with increasing frequency as an antidepressant. In two studies,[82,83] no increased incidence of major malformations was found in 237 infants exposed in utero.

THYROID AND ANTITHYROID DRUGS

Propylthiouracil (PTU) and methimazole (Tapazole) both cross the placenta and may cause some degree of fetal goiter. Thus, the goal of such therapy during pregnancy is to keep the mother slightly hyperthyroid to minimize fetal drug exposure. Because methimazole has been associated with scalp defects in infants,[84] as well as a higher incidence of maternal side effects, PTU is the drug of choice.

Radioactive iodine administered for thyroid ablation or for diagnostic studies is not concentrated by the fetal thyroid until after 12 weeks of pregnancy.[85] Thus, with inadvertent exposure, usually around the time of missed menses, there is no specific risk to the fetal thyroid from radioactive iodine.

The need for thyroxine increases in many women with primary hypothyroidism when they are pregnant, as reflected by an increase in serum thyrotropin (TSH) concentrations.[86] In one study, the mean thyroxine dose before pregnancy was 0.10 mg/day; it was increased to a mean dose of 0.25 mg/day during pregnancy. Although there are no known clinical effects of this modest level of hypothyroidism, it is prudent to monitor thyroid function throughout pregnancy and to adjust the thyroid dose to maintain a normal TSH level.[87]

Topical iodine preparations are readily absorbed through the vagina during pregnancy, and transient hypothyroidism has been demonstrated in the newborn after exposure during labor.[88]

Table 16-1 summarizes drugs with known adverse effects in human pregnancy.

DRUGS IN BREAST MILK

Many drugs can be detected in breast milk at low levels, which are not usually of clinical significance to the infant. If the mother has unusually high blood concentrations, as with increased dosage or decreased renal function, drugs may appear in higher concentrations in the milk.

The amount of drug in breast milk is a variable fraction of the maternal blood level, which itself is proportional to the maternal oral dose. Thus, the dose to the infant is usually subtherapeutic, approximately 1 to 2 percent of the maternal dose on the average. This amount is usually so trivial that no adverse effects are noted. In the case of toxic drugs, however, any exposure may be inappropriate. Long-

Table 16-1

THERAPEUTIC AGENTS COMMONLY USED IN EMERGENCY SETTINGS WITH KNOWN ADVERSE EFFECTS IN HUMAN PREGNANCY

Drug	Effect
ACE inhibitors	Renal failure, oligohydramnios
Aminoglycosides	Ototoxicity
Androgenic steroids	Masculinize female fetus
Anticonvulsants	Dysmorphic syndrome, anomalies
Antithyroid agents	Fetal goiter
Aspirin	Bleeding, antepartum and postpartum
Cytotoxic agents, i.e., methotrexate	Multiple anomalies
Isotretinoin	Hydrocephalus, deafness, anomalies
Lithium	Congenital heart disease (Ebstein anomaly)
Methotrexate	Anomalies
Nonsteroidal anti-inflammatory drugs (prolonged use after 32 weeks)	Oligohydramnios, constriction of fetal ductus arteriosus
Tetracycline (after first trimester)	Discoloration of deciduous teeth, inhibits bone growth
Thalidomide	Phocomelia
Warfarin	Embryopathy—nasal hypoplasia, optic atrophy

Table 16-2

DRUGS CONTRAINDICATED DURING BREAST-FEEDING

Amphetamines
Aspirin (high doses)
Bromocriptine (Parlodel)
Cytotoxic agents
Ergotamine
Lithium
Radiopharmaceuticals

Source: American Academy of Pediatrics,[90] with permission.

DRUGS COMMONLY LISTED AS CONTRAINDICATED DURING BREAST-FEEDING

CYTOTOXIC AGENTS

Cyclosporine (Sandimmune), doxorubicin (Adriamycin), and cyclophosphamide (Cytoxan) might cause immune suppression in the infant, although data are limited with respect to these and other cytotoxic agents. Busulphan (Myleran) has been reported to cause no adverse effect in nursing infants.[91] In general, the potential risks of these drugs, if they were required, would outweigh the benefits of continued nursing.

After oral administration to a lactating patient with choriocarcinoma, methotrexate was found in milk in low levels.[92] Most individuals would elect to avoid any exposure of this drug to the infant. However, in environments in which bottle-feeding is rarely practiced and presents practical and cultural difficulties, therapy with this drug would not in itself appear to constitute a contraindication to breast-feeding.

term effects of even small doses of drugs may yet be discovered. Also, drugs are eliminated more slowly in the infant with immature enzyme systems. As the benefits of breast-feeding are well known, the risk of drug exposure must be weighed against these benefits. However, most maternal medications in breast milk pose little risk to the infants.[89]

For drugs requiring daily dosing during lactation, knowledge of pharmacokinetics in breast milk may minimize the dose to the infant. For example, dosing after nursing will decrease the exposure, as the blood level will be lowest before the next dose.

The American Academy of Pediatrics has reviewed drugs in lactation[90] and categorized the drugs as listed below (Tables 16-2 through 16-5).

Table 16-3

DRUGS WHOSE EFFECTS ON NURSING INFANTS IS UNKNOWN BUT MAY BE OF CONCERN

Metronidazole (Flagyl)
Psychotropic drugs
Antianxiety drugs
Antidepressant drugs
Antipsychotic drugs

Source: American Academy of Pediatrics,[90] with permission.

Table 16-4

DRUGS POTENTIALLY AFFECTING MILK SUPPLY

Decongestants
Diuretics
Combination oral contraceptives

BROMOCRIPTINE

Bromocriptine (Parlodel) is an ergot alkaloid derivative that has an inhibitory effect on lactation. However, in one report, a mother taking 5 mg/day for a pituitary tumor was able to nurse her infant.[93]

ERGOTAMINE

Ergotamine (Ergomar) has been reported to be associated with vomiting, diarrhea, and convulsions in the infant in doses used in migraine medications. However, short-term ergot therapy in the postpartum period for uterine contractility is not a contraindication to lactation.

LITHIUM

Lithium (Eskalith, Lithobid) reaches one-third to one-half the therapeutic blood concentration in infants, who may develop lithium toxicity, with hypotonia and lethargy.[94]

AMPHETAMINES

One report of 103 cases of exposure to amphetamines in breast milk noted no insomnia or stimulation in the infants.[95] However, amphetamines are concentrated in breast milk.

Table 16-5

DRUGS USUALLY CONSIDERED COMPATIBLE WITH BREAST-FEEDING

Analgesics	Antihypertensives
Antiasthmatics	Antithyroid agents
Antibiotics	Corticosteroids
Anticoagulants	Digoxin
Anticonvulsants	Narcotics
Antiemetics	Oral contraceptives
Antihistamines	Sedatives

Source: American Academy of Pediatrics,[90] with permission.

RADIOPHARMACEUTICALS

Radiopharmaceuticals require variable intervals of interruption of nursing to assure that no radioactivity is detectable in the milk. Intervals generally quoted are as follows: 2 weeks for gallium 67, 5 days for iodine 131, 4 days for radioactive sodium, and 24 h for technetium 99. For reassurance, the milk may be counted for radioactivity before nursing is resumed.[96]

DRUGS WHOSE EFFECTS ON NURSING INFANTS IS UNKNOWN BUT MAY BE OF CONCERN

Psychotropic drugs such as antianxiety, antidepressant, and antipsychotic agents are of special concern when given to nursing mothers for long periods. Although there are no data about adverse effects in infants exposed to them via breast milk, psychotropic drugs could theoretically alter central nervous system function.[90] Fluoxetine (Prozac) is excreted in breast milk at low levels.[97]

Temporary cessation of breast-feeding after a single dose of metronidazole (Flagyl) may be considered. Its half-life is such that interruption of lactation for 12 to 24 h after single-dose therapy usually results in negligible exposure to the infant. However, even if a woman continued to nurse, the infant would get a trivial dose.

DRUGS USUALLY COMPATIBLE WITH BREAST-FEEDING

NARCOTICS, SEDATIVES, AND ANTICONVULSANTS

In general, no adverse effects are noted with most of the sedatives, narcotic analgesics, and anticonvulsants. Patients may be reassured that in normal doses, carbamezapine (Tegretol),[98] phenytoin (Dilantin), magnesium sulfate, diazepam (Valium),[99] codeine, morphine, and meperidine (Demerol) do not cause any obvious adverse effects in the infant,[100] since the dose detectable in the breast milk is approximately 1 to 2 percent of the mother's dose, which is sufficiently low to have no significant pharmacologic activity.

The infant eliminates phenobarbital and diazepam (Valium) slowly, however; therefore accumulation may occur. Women consuming barbiturates or benzodiazepines should observe their infants for sedation.

ANALGESICS

Aspirin is transferred into breast milk in small amounts. The risk is related to high dosages, e.g., more than sixteen 300-mg tablets per day in the mother, when the infant may develop sufficiently high serum levels to affect platelet aggregation or even cause metabolic acidosis. No harmful effects of acetaminophen (Tylenol, Datril) have been noted. In one patient taking propoxyphene (Darvon) in a suicide attempt, the level in breast milk was half that of the serum. A breast-feeding infant could theoretically receive up to 1 mg of propoxyphene a day if the mother were to consume the maximum dose continually.[101]

ANTIHISTAMINES AND PHENOTHIAZINES

Although studies are not extensive, no harmful effects have been noted from antihistamines or phenothiazines, and they have not been found to affect milk supply. Decongestants should be avoided by women who are having trouble with milk supply.

AMINOPHYLLINE

Maximum milk concentrations of aminophylline are achieved between 1 and 3 h after an oral dose. The nursing infant has been calculated to receive less than 1 percent of the maternal dose, with no noted adverse effects.[102]

ANTIHYPERTENSIVES

No adverse effects of chlorothiazide (Diuril) have been noted. The drug was not detectable in one nursing infant's serum, and the infant's electrolytes were normal.[103] Thiazide diuretics may decrease milk production in the first month of lactation.[90]

Propranolol (Inderal) is safe in nursing mothers. A nursing infant consumes about 1 percent of a therapeutic dose. This amount of drug is unlikely to cause any adverse effect.[104]

Atenolol (Tenormin) is concentrated in breast milk to about three times the plasma level.[105] One case has been reported in which a 5-day-old term infant had signs of beta-adrenergic blockade with bradycardia, with the breast milk dose calculated to be 9 percent of the maternal dose.[106] Adverse effects in other infants have not been reported.

Neurologic and laboratory parameters in the infants of mothers treated with clonidine (Catapres) are similar to those of controls.[107]

ANTICOAGULANTS

Most mothers requiring anticoagulation may continue to nurse their infants with no problems. Heparin does not cross into milk and is not active orally.

At a maternal dose of warfarin (Coumadin) of 5 to 12 mg/day in seven patients, no warfarin was detected in breast milk or infant plasma. This low concentration is probably due to the fact that warfarin is highly protein-bound. Thus, one liter of milk would contain too small an amount to have an anticoagulant effect.[108,109] The oral anticoagulant bishydroxycoumarin (Dicumarol) has been given to 125 nursing mothers with no effect on the infants' prothrombin times and no

hemorrhages.[110] Thus, warfarin may be safely administered to nursing mothers with careful monitoring of maternal and fetal prothrombin time so that the dosage is minimized.

CORTICOSTEROIDS

Breast-feeding is allowed in mothers requiring corticosteroids. Even at 80 mg/day, the nursing infant would ingest <0.1 percent of the dose, less than 10 percent of its endogenous cortisol.

DIGOXIN

Mothers requiring digoxin (Lanoxin) may continue to nurse. A small amount of the drug enters breast milk due to significant maternal protein binding. The infant receives about 1 percent of the maternal dose,[112] and no adverse effects in nursing infants have been reported.

ANTIBIOTICS

Penicillin derivatives are safe in nursing mothers. In the usual therapeutic doses of penicillin, ampicillin (Amoxil), or dicloxacillin (Pathocil), no adverse effects are noted in infants. In susceptible individuals or with prolonged therapy, diarrhea and candidiasis are theoretical concerns.

Cephalosporins appear in only trace amounts in milk, with the infants exposed to less than 1 percent of the maternal dose.

Tooth staining and delayed bone growth from tetracyclines have not been reported after the drug was taken by a breast-feeding mother. This finding is probably due to the high binding of the drug to calcium and protein, limiting its absorption from the milk. The amount of free tetracycline available in the milk is too small to be significant.

Sulfonamides appear in only small amounts in breast milk and are ordinarily not contraindicated during nursing. However, the drugs are best avoided during the first 5 days of life or in mothers of premature infants when hyperbilirubinemia may be a problem, because the drug may displace bilirubin from binding sites on albumin. In one study of sulfapyridine, the infant received less than 1 percent of the maternal dose. When a mother took sulfasalazine (Azulfidine) 500 mg q6h, the drug was undetectable in all milk samples.

Gentamicin (Garamycin) is transferred into breast milk, and half of nursing newborn infants have the drug detectable in their serum. The low levels detected would not be expected to cause clinical effects.[113]

Nitrofurantoin (Macrodantin) is excreted into breast milk in very low concentrations. In one study, the drug could not be detected in 20 samples from mothers receiving 100 mg q.i.d.[114]

Erythromycin is excreted into breast milk in small amounts, and no reports of adverse effects on infants exposed to erythromycin in breast milk have been noted. Azithromycin (Zithromax) also appears in breast milk in low concentrations.[115] Clindamycin (Cleocin) is excreted into breast milk at low levels, and nursing is usually continued during administration of this drug.

There are no reported adverse effects on the infant of isoniazid (INH) administered to nursing mothers, and its use is considered compatible with breast-feeding. Acyclovir (Zovirax) is excreted in breast milk in low concentrations, with no reported adverse effects.[116]

ORAL CONTRACEPTIVES

Combinations of estrogen and progestin in oral contraceptives can cause a dose-related suppression of the quantity of milk produced. Lactation is inhibited to a lesser degree if the pill is started about 3 weeks postpartum and with doses of estrogen below 50 μg. No consistent long-term adverse effects on children's growth and development have been described.

Evidence indicates that norgestrel (Ovrette) is metabolized rather than accumulated by the infants; to date, no adverse effects have been identified as a result of progestational agents taken by the mother. Progestin-only contraceptives do not cause alteration of breast milk composition or volume,[117] making them ideal for the breast-feeding mother.

PROPYLTHIOURACIL

Propylthiouracil (PTU) is found in breast milk in small amounts.[118] Several infants have been studied up to 5 months of age with no changes in thyroid parameters, including TSH. Lactating mothers on PTU can continue nursing with close supervision of the infant.[118,119] Propylthiouracil is preferred over methimazole (Tapazole) because of its high protein binding (80 percent) and lower breast milk concentrations.

CONCLUSIONS

Many medical conditions during pregnancy and lactation are best treated initially with nonpharmacologic remedies. Before a drug is administered in pregnancy, the indications should be clear and the risk/benefit ratio should justify drug use. If possible, therapy should be postponed until after the first trimester. Most drug therapy does not require cessation of lactation, because the amount excreted into breast milk is so small that it is pharmacologically insignificant.

References

1. Wilson JG, Fraser FC (eds): *Handbook of Teratology.* New York: Plenum Press, 1979.

2. Blake DA, Niebyl JR: Requirements and limitations in reproductive and teratogenic risk assessment, in Niebyl JR (ed): *Drug Use in Pregnancy,* 2d ed. Philadelphia: Lea & Febiger, 1988.

3. Stuart JJ, Gross SJ, Elrad H, et al: Effects of acetylsalicyclic acid ingestion on maternal and neonatal hemostasis. *N Engl J Med* 307:909, 1982.

4. Heinonen OP, Slone S, Shapiro S: *Birth Defects and Drugs in Pregnancy.* Littleton, MA: Publishing Sciences Group, 1977, pp 280–409.

5. Collins E, Turner G: Salicylates and pregnancy. *Lancet* 2:1494, 1973.

6. Areilla RA, Thilenius OB, Ranniger K: Congestive heart failure from suspected ductal closure in utero. *J Pediatr* 75:74, 1969.

7. Waltman TF, Tricomi V, Tavakoli FM: Effect of aspirin on bleeding time during elective abortion. *Obstet Gynecol* 48:108, 1976.

8. Rayburn W, Shukla U, Stetson P, et al: Acetaminophen pharmacokinetics: Comparison between pregnant and nonpregnant women. *Obstet Gynecol* 155:1353, 1986.

9. Main EK, Main DM, Gabbe SG: Chronic oral terbutaline therapy is associated with maternal glucose intolerance. *Obstet Gynecol* 157:644, 1987.

10. Haugen G, Fauchald P, Sodal G, et al: Pregnancy outcome in renal allograft recipients: Influence of cyclosporin A. *Eur J Obstet Gynecol Reprod Biol* 39:25, 1991.

11. Hou S: Pregnancy in organ transplant recipients. *Med Clin North Am* 73:667, 1989.

12. Briggs GG, Freeman RK, Yaffe SJ: *Drugs in Pregnancy and Lactation,* 4th ed. Baltimore: Williams & Wilkins, 1994, pp 148–149.

13. Brumfitt W, Pursell R: Double-blind trial to compare ampicillin, cephalexin, co-trimoxazole, and trimethoprim in treatment of urinary infection. *Br Med J* 2:673, 1972.

14. Briggs GG, Freeman RK, Yaffe SJ: *Drugs in Pregnancy and Lactation,* 4th ed. Baltimore: Williams & Wilkins, 1994, pp 847–848.

15. Jarnerot G, Into-Malmberg MB, Esbjorner E: Placental transfer of sulphasalazine and sulphapyridine and some of its metabolites. *Scand J Gastroenterol* 16:693, 1981.

16. Briggs GG, Freeman RK, Yaffe SJ: *Drugs in Pregnancy and Lactation,* 4th ed. Baltimore: Williams & Wilkins, 1994, p 625.

17. Lenke RR, VanDorsten JP, Schifrin BS: Pyelonephritis in pregnancy: A prospective randomized trial to prevent recurrent disease evaluating suppressive therapy with nitrofurantoin and close surveillance. *Am J Obstet Gynecol* 146:953, 1983.

18. Cohlan SQU, Bevelander G, Tiamsic T: Growth inhibition of prematures receiving tetracycline. *Am J Dis Child* 105:453, 1963.

19. Aselton P, Jick H, Mulnsky A, et al: First-trimester drug use and congenital disorders. *Obstet Gynecol* 65:451, 1985.

20. Robinson GC, Cambon KG: Hearing loss in infants of tuberculous mothers treated with streptomycin during pregnancy. *N Engl J Med* 271:949, 1964.

21. Nishimura H, Tanimura T: *Clinical Aspects of the Teratogenicity of Drugs.* Amsterdam: Excerpta Medica, 1976, p 131.

22. Jones HC: Intrauterine ototoxicity: A case report and review of literature. *J Natl Med Assoc* 65:201, 1973.

23. L'Hommedieu CS, Nicholas D, Armes DA, et al: Potentiation of magnesium sulfate–induced neuromuscular weakness by gentamicin, tobramycin, and amikacin. *J Pediatr* 102:629, 1983.

24. Marynowski A, Sianozecka E: Comparison of the incidence of congenital malformations in neonates from healthy mothers and from patients treated because of tuberculosis. *Ginekol Pol* 43:713, 1972.

25. McCormack WM, George H, Donner A, et al: Hepatotoxicity of erythromycin estolate during pregnancy. *Antimicrob Agents Chemother* 12:630, 1977.

26. Philipson A, Sabath LD, Charles D: Transplacental passage of erythromycin and clindamycin. *N Engl J Med* 288:1219, 1973.

27. Briggs GG, Freeman RK, Jaffe SJ: *Drugs in Pregnancy and Lactation,* 4th ed. Baltimore: Williams & Wilkins, 1994, pp 186–187.

28. Berkovitch M, Pastuszak A, Gazarian M, et al: Safety of the new quinolones in pregnancy. *Obstet Gynecol* 84:535, 1994.

29. Piper JM, Mitchel EF, Ray WA: Prenatal use of metronidazole and birth defects: No association. *Obstet Gynecol* 82:348, 1993.

30. Burtin P, Taddio A, Ariburnu O, et al: Safety of metronidazole in pregnancy: A meta-analysis. *Am J Obstet Gynecol* 172:525, 1995.

31. Beard CM, Noller KL, O'Fallon WM, et al: Lack of evidence for cancer due to use of metronidazole. *N Engl J Med* 301:519, 1979.

32. Centers for Disease Control: Pregnancy outcomes following systemic prenatal acyclovir exposure—June 1, 1984–June 30, 1993. *MMWR* 42:806, 1993.

33. Andrews EB, Yankaskas BC, Cordero JF, et al: Acyclovir in pregnancy registry: Six years' experience. *Obstet Gynecol* 79:7, 1992.

34. Rosa FW, Baum C, Shaw M: Pregnancy outcomes after first trimester vaginitis drug therapy. *Obstet Gynecol* 69:751, 1987.

35. Hill RM, Stern L: Drugs in pregnancy: Effects on the fetus and newborn. *Drugs* 17:182, 1979.

36. deSwiet M, Ward PD, Fidler J, et al: Prolonged heparin therapy in pregnancy causes bone demineralization. *Br J Obstet Gynaecol* 90:1129, 1983.

37. Dahlman TC: Osteoporotic fractures and the recurrence of thromboembolism during pregnancy and the puerperium in 184 women undergoing thromboprophylaxis with heparin. *Am J Obstet Gynecol* 168:1265, 1993.

38. Toglia MR, Weg JG: Venous thromboembolism during pregnancy. *N Engl J Med* 335:108, 1996.

39. Tengborn L, Bergqvist D, Matzsch T, et al: Recurrent thromboembolism in pregnancy and puerperium: Is there a need for thromboprophylaxis? *Am J Obstet Gynecol* 160:90, 1989.

40. Lao TT, deSwiet M, Letsky E, et al: Prophylaxis of thromboembolism in pregnancy: An alternative. *Br J Obstet Gynaecol* 92:202, 1985.

41. Iturbe-Alessio I, del Carmen Fonseca M, Mutchinik O, et al: Risks of anticoagulant therapy in pregnant women with artificial heart valves. *N Engl J Med* 315:1390, 1986.

42. Shapiro S, Hartz SC, Siskind V, et al: Anticonvulsants and parental epilepsy in the development of birth defects. *Lancet* 1:272, 1976.

43. Robert E, Guibaud P: Maternal valproic acid and congenital neural tube defects. *Lancet* 2:937, 1982.

44. Rosa FW: Spina bifida in infants of women treated with carbamazepine during pregnancy. *N Engl J Med* 324:674, 1991.

45. Lindhout D, Schmidt D: In utero exposure to valproate and neural tube defect. *Lancet* 1:1392, 1986.

46. Nakane Y, Okuma T, Takashashi R et al: Multi-institutional study on the teratogenicity and fetal toxicity of antiepileptic drugs: A report of a collaborative study group in Japan. *Epilepsia* 21:663, 1980.

47. Hanson JW, Smith DW: The fetal hydantoin syndrome. *J Pediatr* 87:285, 1975.

48. Jones KL, Lacro RV, Johnson KA, et al: Pattern of malformations in the children of women treated with carbamazepine during pregnancy. *N Engl J Med* 320:1661, 1989.

49. Scolnik D, Nulman I, Rovet J, et al: Neurodevelopment of children exposed in utero to phenytoin and carbamazepine monotherapy. *JAMA* 271:767, 1994.

50. Van der Pol MC, Hadders-Algra M, Huisjes JH, et al: Antiepileptic medication in pregnancy: Late effects on the children's central nervous system development. *Am J Obstet Gynecol* 164:121, 1991.

51. Callaghan N, Garrett A, Goggin T: Withdrawal of anticonvulsant drugs in patients free of seizures for two years. *N Engl J Med* 318:942, 1988.

52. Sahakian V, Rouse D, Sipes S, et al: Vitamin B_6 is effective therapy for nausea and vomiting of pregnancy: A randomized double-blind, placebo-controlled study. *Obstet Gynecol* 78:33, 1991.

53. Vutyavanich T, Wongtrangan S, Ruangsri R: Pyridoxine for nausea and vomiting of pregnancy: A randomized double-blind placebo-controlled trial. *Am J Obstet Gynecol* 173:881, 1995.

54. Fischer-Rasmussen W, Kjaer SK, Dahl C, et al: Ginger treatment of hyperemesis gravidarum. *Eur J Obstet Gynecol Reprod Biol* 38:19, 1990.

55. Diggory PLC, Tomkinson JS: Nausea and vomiting in pregnancy: A trial of meclozine dihydrochloride with and without pyridoxine. *Lancet* 2:370, 1962.

56. Milkovich L, Van Den Berg BJ: An evaluation of the teratogenicity of certain antinauseant drugs. *Am J Obstet Gynecol* 125:244, 1976.

57. Cartwright EW: Dramamine in nausea and vomiting of pregnancy. *West J Surg Obstet Gynecol* 59:216, 1951.

58. Sullivan CA, Johnson CA, Roach H, et al: A pilot study of intravenous ondansetron for hyperemesis gravidarum. *Am J Obstet Gynecol* 174:1565, 1996.

59. Belluomini J, Litt RC, Lee KA, et al: Acupressure for nausea and vomiting of pregnancy: A randomized, blinded study. *Obstet Gynecol* 84:245, 1994.

60. Briggs GG, Freeman RK, Yaffe SJ: *Drugs in Pregnancy and Lactation,* 4th ed. Baltimore: Williams & Wilkins, 1994, p 807.

61. Zierler S, Purohit D: Prenatal antihistamine exposure and retrolental fibroplasia. *Am J Epidemiol* 123:192, 1986.

62. Werler MM, Mitchell AA, Shapiro S: First trimester maternal medication use in relation to gastroschisis. *Teratology* 45:361, 1992.

63. Pruyn SC, Phelan JP, Buchanan GC: Long-term propranolol therapy in pregnancy: Maternal and fetal outcome. *Am J Obstet Gynecol* 135:485, 1979.

64. Redmond GP: Propranolol and fetal growth retardation. *Semin Perinatol* 6:142, 1982.

65. Rubin PC, Clark DM, Sumner DJ: Placebo-controlled trial of atenolol in treatment of pregnancy-associated hypertension. *Lancet* 1:431, 1983.

66. Hanssens M, Keirse MJNC, Vankelecom F, et al: Fetal and neonatal effects of treatment with angiotensin-converting enzyme inhibitors in pregnancy. *Obstet Gynecol* 78:128, 1991.

67. Piper JM, Ray WA, Rosa FW: Pregnancy outcome following exposure to angiotensin-converting enzyme inhibitors. *Obstet Gynecol* 80:429, 1992.

68. Briggs GG, Freeman RK, Jaffe SJ: *Drugs in Pregnancy and Lactation,* 4th ed. Baltimore: Williams & Wilkins, 1994, p 177.

69. Rosenberg L, Mitchell AA, Parsella JL, et al: Lack of relation of oral clefts to diazepam use during pregnancy. *N Engl J Med* 309:1282, 1983.

70. Czeizel A: Lack of evidence of teratogenicity of benzodiazepine drugs in Hungary. *Reprod Toxicol* 3:183, 1988.

71. Laegreid L, Olegard R, Wahlstrom J, et al: Abnormalities in children exposed to benzodiazepines in utero. *Lancet* 1:108, 1987.

72. Bergman V, Rosa F, Baum C, et al: Effects of exposure to benzodiazepine during fetal life. *Lancet* 340:694, 1992.

73. Linden S, Rich CL: The use of lithium during pregnancy and lactation. *J Clin Psychiatry* 44:358, 1983.

74. Weinstein MR, Goldfield MD: Cardiovascular malformations with lithium use during pregnancy. *Am J Psychiatry* 132:529, 1975.

75. Zalzstein E, Koren G, Einarson T, et al: A case-control study on the association between first trimester exposure to lithium and Ebstein's anomaly. *Am J Cardiol* 65:817, 1990.

76. Jacobson SJ, Jones K, Johnson K, et al: Prospective multi-centre study of pregnancy outcome after lithium exposure during first trimester. *Lancet* 339:530, 1992.

77. Krause S, Ebbesen F, Lange AP: Polyhydramnios with maternal lithium treatment. *Obstet Gynecol* 75:504, 1990.

78. Ang MS, Thorp JA, Parisi VM: Maternal lithium therapy and polyhydramnios. *Obstet Gynecol* 76:517, 1990.

79. Cohen LS, Friedman MJ, Jefferson JW: A reevaluation of risk of in utero exposure to lithium. *JAMA* 271:146, 1994.

80. Briggs GG, Freeman RK, Jaffe SJ: *Drugs in Pregnancy and Lactation,* 4th ed. Baltimore: Williams & Wilkins, 1994, pp 435–437.

81. Briggs GG, Freeman RK, Jaffe SJ: *Drugs in Pregnancy and Lactation,* 4th ed. Baltimore: Williams & Wilkins, 1994, pp 38–40.

82. Pastuszak A, Schick-Boschetto B, Zuber C, et al: Pregnancy outcome following first-trimester exposure to fluoxetine (Prozac). *JAMA* 269:2446, 1993.

83. Briggs GG, Freeman RK, Jaffe SJ: *Drugs in Pregnancy and Lactation,* 4th ed. Baltimore: Williams & Wilkins, 1994, pp 374–375.

84. Mujtaba Q, Burrow GN: Treatment of hyperthyroidism in pregnancy with propylthiouracil and methimazole. *Obstet Gynecol* 46:282, 1975.

85. Burrow GN: Thyroid diseases, in Burrow GN, Ferris TF (eds): *Medical Complications during Pregnancy.* Philadelphia: Saunders, 1988, p 229.

86. Mandel SJ, Larsen PR, Seely EW, et al: Increased need for thyroxine during pregnancy in women with primary hypothyroidism. *N Engl J Med* 323:91, 1990.

87. Tamaki H, Amino N, Takeoka K, et al: Thyroxine requirement during pregnancy for replacement therapy of hypothyroidism. *Obstet Gynecol* 76:230, 1990.

88. l'Allemand D, Gruters A, Heidemann P, et al: Iodine-induced alterations of thyroid function in newborn infants after prenatal and perinatal exposure to povidone iodine. *J Pediatr* 102:935, 1983.

89. Ito S, Blajchman A, Stephenson M, et al: Prospective follow-up of adverse reactions in breast-fed infants exposed to maternal medication. *Am J Obstet Gynecol* 168:1393, 1993.

90. American Academy of Pediatrics, Committee on Drugs: The transfer of drugs and other chemicals into human milk. *Pediatrics* 93:137, 1994.

91. Bounaneaux Y, Duren J: Busulphan in nursing infants. *Ann Soc Belg Med Trop* 44:381, 1964.

92. Johns BG, Rutherford CD, Laighton RC, et al: Secretion of methotrexate into human milk. *Am J Obstet Gynecol* 112:978, 1972.

93. Canales ES, Garcia IC, Ruiz JE, et al: Bromocriptine as prophylactic therapy in prolactinoma during pregnancy. *Fertil Steril* 36:524, 1981.

94. Linden S, Rich CL: The use of lithium during pregnancy and lactation. *J Clin Psychiatry* 44:358, 1983.

95. Ayd FJ Jr: Excretion of psychotrophic drugs in human breast milk. *Int Drug Ther News Bull* 8:33, 1973.

96. Berlin CM: The excretion of drugs in human milk, in Schwartz RH, Yaffe SJ (eds): *Drug and Chemical Risks to the Fetus and Newborn.* New York: Liss, 1980, p 125.

97. Burch KJ, Wells BG: Fluoxetine/norfluoxetine concentrations in human milk. *Pediatrics* 91:676, 1992.

98. Niebyl JR, Blake DA, Freeman JM, et al: Carbamazepine levels in pregnancy and lactation. *Obstet Gynecol* 53:139, 1979.

99. Cole AP, Hailey DM: Diazepam and active metabolite in breast milk and their transfer to the neonate. *Arch Dis Child* 50:741, 1975.

100. Briggs GG, Freeman RK, Yaffe SJ: *Drugs in Pregnancy and Lactation,* 4th ed. Baltimore: Williams & Wilkins, 1994, pp 126–692.

101. Ananth J: Side effects in the neonate from psychotrophic agents excreted through breastfeeding. *Am J Psychiatry* 135:801, 1978.

102. Yurchak AM, Jusko NJ: Theophylline secretion into breast milk. *Pediatrics* 57:518, 1976.

103. Miller ME, Cohn RD, Burghart PH: Hydrochlorothiazide disposition in a mother and her breast-fed infant. *J Pediatr* 101:789, 1982.

104. Bauer JH, Pope B, Zajicek J, et al: Propranolol in human plasma and breast milk. *Am J Cardiol* 43:860, 1979.

105. White WB, Andreoli JW, Wong SH, et al: Atenolol in human plasma and breast milk. *Obstet Gynecol* 63:42S1, 1984.

106. Schmimmel MS, Eidelman AJ, Wilschanski MA, et al: Toxic effects of atenolol consumed during breast feeding. *J Pediatr* 114:476, 1989.

107. Hartikainen-Sorri AL, Heikkinen JE, Koivisto M: Pharmacokinetics of clonidine during pregnancy and nursing. *Obstet Gynecol* 69:598, 1987.

108. Orme ME, Lewis PJ, deSwiet M, et al: May mothers given warfarin breastfeed their infants? *Br Med J* 1:1564, 1977.

109. deSwiet M, Lewis PJ: Excretion of anticoagulants in human milk. *N Engl J Med* 297:1471, 1977.

110. Brambel CE, Hunter RE: Effect of Dicumarol on the nursing infant. *Am J Obstet Gynecol* 59:1153, 1950.

111. Ost L, Wettrell G, Bjorkhem I, et al: Prednisolone excretion in human milk. *J Pediatr* 106:1008, 1985.

112. Loughnan PM: Digoxin excretion in human breast milk. *J Pediatr* 92:1019, 1978.

113. Celiloglu M, Celiker S, Guven H, et al: Gentamicin excretion and uptake from breast milk by nursing infants. *Obstet Gynecol* 84:263, 1994.

114. Hosbach RE, Foster RB: Absence of nitrofurantoin from human milk. *JAMA* 202:1057, 1967.

115. Kelsey JJ, Moser LR, Jenning JC, et al: Presence of azithromycin breast milk concentrations: A case report. *Am J Obstet Gynecol* 170:1375, 1994.

116. Meyer LJ, de Miranda P, Sheth N, et al: Acyclovir in human breast milk. *Am J Obstet Gynecol* 158:586, 1988.

117. Committee on Drugs, American Academy of Pediatrics: Breastfeeding and contraception. *Pediatrics* 68:138, 1981.

118. Kampmann JP, Hansen JM, Johansen K, et al: Propylthiouracil in human milk. *Lancet* 1:736, 1980.

119. Cooper DS: Antithyroid drugs: To breast-feed or not to breast-feed. *Am J Obstet Gynecol* 157:234, 1987.

Section 4

MEDICAL DISORDERS IN THE PREGNANT PATIENT

Chapter 17

MANAGEMENT OF VENOUS THROMBOEMBOLISM DURING PREGNANCY

Marc R. Toglia

Venous thromboembolism (VTE) is uncommon but is a leading cause of maternal morbidity.[1] Prompt recognition and treatment of VTE reduces the incidence of fatal pulmonary embolism; however, the diagnosis and management of these conditions during pregnancy remain problematic, in part due to the lack of properly performed clinical trials involving pregnant women. Fortunately, clinicians caring for pregnant women can modify the guidelines established for nonpregnant patients based on an understanding of the physiologic changes that are known to accompany pregnancy.[2] In this chapter, current diagnostic and therapeutic strategies for the evaluation of the acute deep vein thrombosis and pulmonary embolism will be reviewed.

PATHOPHYSIOLOGY

Pregnancy is widely accepted to be a physiologic state with a markedly elevated risk of thromboembolic events, such as deep venous thrombosis (DVT) and pulmonary embolism. It has been estimated that venous thromboembolism is approximately five times more likely to occur during pregnancy than in a nonpregnant woman of a similar age. The reported incidence of venous thromboembolism during pregnancy varies widely and probably reflects the diligence with which the authors sought the diagnosis. Many studies that have used objective criteria for diagnosis suggest that VTE occurs in 1 in 1000 to 1 in 2000 pregnancies.

Physicians have long recognized that each element of Virchow's triad for venous thrombosis—namely, stasis, endothelial damage, and hypercoagulability—is present during pregnancy. Physiologic changes associated with pregnancy result in an increase in venous distensibility and capacitance, which results in an increase in venous stasis. These changes are apparent starting in the first trimester and are thought to be hormonally mediated. As pregnancy progresses, compression of the pelvic vessels by the enlarging uterus further adds to the venous stasis in the lower extremities. Vascular wall injury may occur at the time of delivery, with placental separation or associated with operative delivery.

Pregnancy is also associated with increases in the concentration of coagulation factors, decreases in levels of coagulation inhibitors, and a decrease in the body's fibrinolytic capacity, further contributing to a state of hypercoagulability. The levels of coagulation factors II, VII, X, and fibrin substantially increase by the middle of pregnancy. Protein S, an important coagulation inhibitor, significantly decreases throughout pregnancy, while levels of protein C and antithrombin III remain normal. Inhibition of the fibrinolytic system is also thought to occur and is greatest during the third trimester.

Several independent obstetric risk factors have been associated with an increased risk of venous thromboembolism. These include prolonged bed rest (often prescribed for preterm labor or preeclampsia), hemorrhage, sepsis, instrumental and operative delivery, and multiparity. Traditionally, the risk for venous thromboembolism has been thought to be greatest postpartum and during the late third trimester. However, changes in modern obstetric practices have had a significant impact on the occurrence of venous thromboembolism during pregnancy (e.g., avoiding prolonged bed rest after delivery). Recent investigations, all of which required objective criteria for diagnosis, have suggested that most cases of thromboembolism associated with pregnancy occur prior to delivery. Several studies report that deep venous thrombosis occurs with almost equal frequency in each trimester.[3–6] Though most cases of deep venous thrombosis occur prior to delivery, data suggest that the risk of pulmonary embolism is greatest postpartum, especially following cesarean delivery.

DIAGNOSIS

The signs and symptoms of deep venous thrombosis and pulmonary embolism are nonspecific, and the clinical diagnosis is further hampered by many of the common complaints that occur during pregnancy. For example, leg tenderness, swelling, and shortness of breath occur commonly in the pregnant woman, especially at term. Objective testing should therefore be used liberally if thromboembolic disease is suspected in these patients. Diagnostic algorithms have been well established for the nonpregnant patient.[7] Although these strategies have not been validated in pregnant patients, it is reasonable to adapt them to this population.[2,8]

DEEP VENOUS THROMBOSIS

CLINICAL PRESENTATION

During pregnancy, venous thrombosis most frequently begins in either the calf veins or the iliofemoral portion of the deep venous segment and shows a striking predilection for the left leg.[4,9] The signs and symptoms that accompany deep venous thrombosis vary greatly and depend upon the degree of vascular occlusion, the presence of collateral circulation, and the intensity of the associated inflammatory response. The most commonly recognized symptoms and signs of deep venous thrombosis are leg pain, tenderness, and swelling. Less common physical findings are varicosities, increased temperature, engorged superficial veins, redness, pitting edema, and a palpable cord. Some patients may experience lower abdominal pain. Homans' sign (pain on forced dorsiflexion of the foot) is present in less than one-third of all patients with deep venous thrombosis. The dramatic presentation of classic puerperal thrombophlebitis, phlegmasia alba dolens (or milk leg), with an abrupt onset of severe pain and marked edema of the leg and thigh, is rarely seen in modern-day obstetrics.

Most venous thrombi are clinically silent; among patients with signs or symptoms suspicious for DVT, less than 50 percent will have this diagnosis confirmed by objective testing. Diagnosis based on clinical presentation may be even less accurate during pregnancy, as complaints of leg swelling and discomfort occur commonly in this population. Some investigators believe that if the signs or symptoms are unilateral, if the calf circumference in one extremity is 2 cm or greater than in the other, and if there has been proximal extension of the symptoms or signs, the likelihood of deep venous thrombosis is increased.[2,5] The differential diagnosis of deep venous thrombosis includes many conditions of the thigh and leg that result in a painful, swollen leg, including musculoskeletal causes, superficial thrombophlebitis, impaired venous or lymphatic flow, and popliteal inflammatory cysts (Baker's cyst).

IMAGING STUDIES

Noninvasive imaging studies—including compression ultrasound, impedance plethysmography (IPG), or duplex Doppler scanning—should be used as the initial screening study in both pregnant and nonpregnant patients. These diagnostic studies are highly sensitive (>90 percent) for detecting proximal venous thrombosis (in the popliteal or femoral vein) but significantly less so in detecting calf-vein thrombi. In the nonpregnant patient, compression ultrasonography is currently considered more accurate than IPG.[10] Experience with these modalities during pregnancy is limited, but preliminary studies are promising, suggesting similar accuracy.[9,11] These studies are typically performed with the uterus displaced toward the left side, starting in the late second trimester of pregnancy, to minimize the incidence of false-positive studies due to decreased flow from vena cava compression.

The role of venography in diagnosing DVT during pregnancy remains unresolved. Venography can detect both distal thrombi (in the calf veins) and proximal thrombi (including those in the iliac veins), both of which are common sources of pulmonary emboli during pregnancy. Venography is also more reliable in the diagnosis of recurrent deep venous thrombosis than are noninvasive studies. In nonpregnant patients, a positive noninvasive imaging study is considered sufficient evidence to justify beginning anticoagulant therapy. Pregnant women in whom there is a high clinical suspicion of DVT and who have had positive noninvasive studies can also be treated with this approach. Some clinicians, however, prefer to confirm the diagnosis by performing limited venography prior to exposing the pregnant woman to prolonged anticoagulant therapy. Conversely, many clinicians are reluctant to use venography during pregnancy because of the potential risks of radiation to the fetus. However, exposure data do not support this concern.[12] The estimated fetal radiation exposure with a unilateral procedure is approximately 0.314 rad (0.00314 Gy). Fetal radiation exposure of less than 5 rad has not been associated with adverse fetal outcomes.

Pregnant women with a negative noninvasive study but a strong clinical suspicion of DVT should either undergo venography or be offered serial noninvasive testing. Serial testing is performed on days 2 and 7 following the initial study to evaluate for proximal extension of calf vein thrombi or small, nonocclusive proximal vein thrombi.[10] Hull and colleagues support withholding anticoagulant therapy in pregnant women with a clinical suspicion of deep venous thrombosis and negative results on serial IPG.[9] A diagnostic algorithm for the evaluation of deep venous thrombosis during pregnancy is presented in Fig. 17-1.

PULMONARY EMBOLISM

CLINICAL PRESENTATION

The clinical diagnosis of pulmonary embolism (PE) remains difficult because of the wide spectrum of signs and symptoms, which are often further confounded by the physiologic changes of pregnancy. The most common symptoms of PE are shortness of breath (dyspnea) and pleuritic chest pain. Other symptoms include apprehension and cough, which are present in about half of patients presenting with PE. Hemoptysis occurs in approximately 13 percent of patients. Tachypnea (respiratory rate above 20) is the most common physical finding in patients with PE. Other common signs include pulmonary crackles or rales, tachycardia (>100/min), a pleural friction rub, and an increased pulmonic second heart sound. In one study, dyspnea or tachypnea was found in 90 percent of 383 patients with PE. Dyspnea, tachypnea, or pleuritic pain was present in 97 percent.[13]

Unfortunately, the signs and symptoms associated with PE are not specific for this condition and can be found in a wide variety of other acute pulmonary disease. Asthma is perhaps the most common pulmonary condition encountered in the pregnant woman, followed by pneumonia and pulmonary edema. Pneumonia and asthma can occur at any point during the pregnancy or in the postpartum period. Pulmonary edema is most frequently seen at term, in association with preeclampsia, or as a result of nonjudicious fluid management at the time of labor and delivery. These conditions are usually excluded based on the patient's history and examination and the results of a chest radiograph.

DIAGNOSTIC TESTS

Diagnostic tests such as electrocardiograms, chest roentgenograms, and arterial blood gases may support the diagnosis of PE or identify other etiologies for the patient's complaints. A shielded posterior-anterior chest radiograph (CXR) with lateral views should be obtained to rule out pneumonia or pulmonary edema. A CXR is also necessary for an accurate interpretation of the ventilation-perfusion ($\dot{V}/\dot{Q}$) scan. Nonspecific CXR abnormalities such as atelectasis, unilateral pleural effusions, areas of consolidation, or an elevation of the hemidiaphragm are present in more than 80 percent of patients with PE. Similarly, nonspecific electrocardiographic changes are found in almost 90 percent of individuals with PE. Nonspecific abnormalities of the ST-segment or T-wave inversion are the most common findings. The characteristic $S_1Q_3T_3$ pattern is rarely present.

Most clinically significant pulmonary emboli are associated with hypoxemia (arterial $Pa_{O_2} < 85$ mmHg) and a widened or increased alveolar-to-arterial oxygen gradient ($Da_{O_2} > 20$ mmHg). However, 10 to 15 percent of patients with PE can be expected to have a normal Pa_{O_2}. During the third trimester of pregnancy, the Pa_{O_2} may be as much as 15 mmHg lower in the supine position when compared to the upright condition. Therefore, during the third trimester, arterial blood gases should be measured with the patient sitting upright.

Currently, the radionuclide lung imaging or ventilation-perfusion ($\dot{V}/\dot{Q}$) scan is the primary screening technique used in the evaluation for pulmonary embolism. If the results are interpreted as normal or near normal, the diagnosis of PE is excluded, whereas a high-probability scan is sufficient evidence to begin anticoagulant therapy. Unfortunately, less than one-third of patients with PE can be expected to have a scan with either of these two interpretations. The majority of patients with PE will have a $\dot{V}/\dot{Q}$ scan interpreted as either of low or intermediate (indeterminant) probability and will need to undergo pulmonary angiography. Pregnant patients should be reassured by their physicians that the estimated radiation exposure to the fetus with the combination of chest radiograph, $\dot{V}/\dot{Q}$ scanning, and pulmonary angiography is less than 0.5 rad. A diagnostic algorithm for the evaluation of PE during pregnancy is presented in Fig. 17-2.

MANAGEMENT

All pregnant women with a suspected PE or clinically evident deep venous thrombosis should be promptly hospitalized for anticoagulation and supportive care and managed in consultation with the obstetric team. Patients with large pulmonary emboli and hemodynamic impairment should be monitored in the intensive care unit. In patients with a strong suspicion of PE, anticoagulant therapy may be initiated pending diagnostic studies, such as a $\dot{V}/\dot{Q}$ scan or pulmonary angiography. Acute PE is frequently accompanied by hypoxemia, hypercapnia, right ventricular dysfunction, and elevated pulmonary resistance. Hypoxemia should be aggressively reversed with oxygen therapy, 5 to 10 L/min, by mask to minimize fetal hypoxemia and acidosis. Worsening

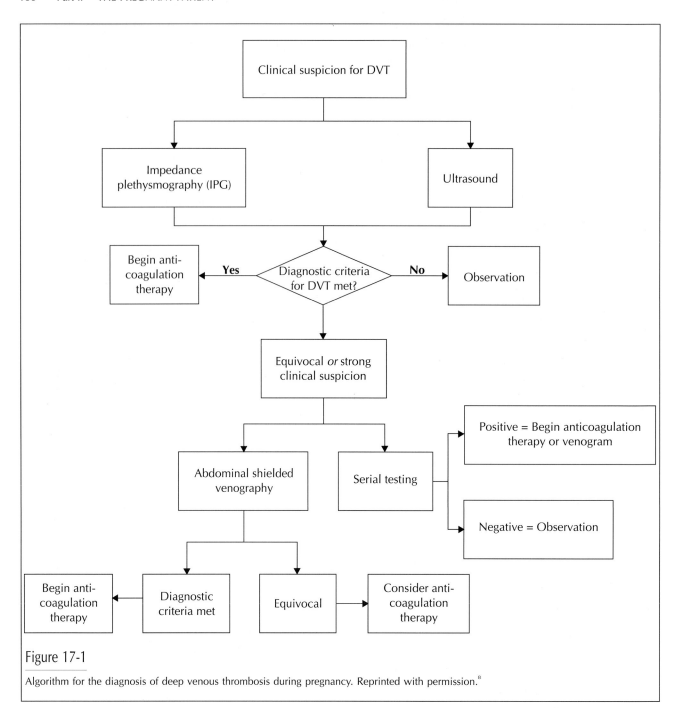

Figure 17-1

Algorithm for the diagnosis of deep venous thrombosis during pregnancy. Reprinted with permission.[8]

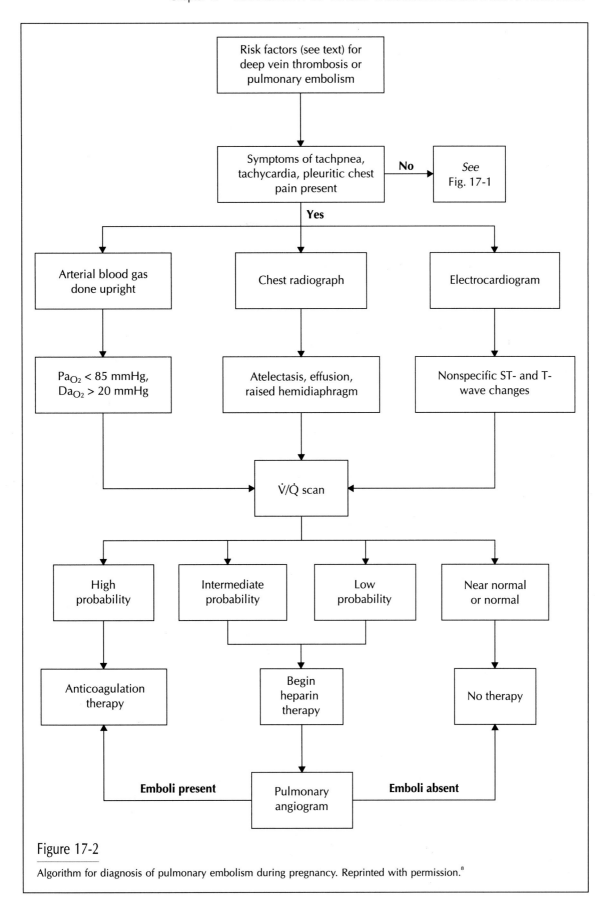

Figure 17-2

Algorithm for diagnosis of pulmonary embolism during pregnancy. Reprinted with permission.[8]

hypercapnia associated with progressive obtundation is an indication for intubation and mechanical ventilation. Intravenous fluids and dopamine should be used in the hypotensive patient to maintain the patient's blood pressure above 80 mmHg, recognizing that the use of pressors may reduce uterine blood flow. Comanagement and monitoring with the obstetric team is highly desirable in this setting. Analgesics such as morphine and meperidine should be used as necessary.

Once diagnosed, venous thromboembolism requires rapid and prolonged anticoagulation to prevent extension of the thrombus, restore venous patency, and limit the risk of PE or its recurrence. Clinical experience and retrospective cohort studies have established heparin as the safest anticoagulant to use during pregnancy because it does not cross the placenta. Cohort studies suggest that the risk of major bleeding in a pregnant patient treated with heparin is 2 percent.[2] Heparin therapy should be instituted for all patients with distal deep venous thrombosis (e.g., in the calf vein), proximal venous thrombosis (e.g., in the iliofemoral or pelvic veins), and PE.

Since therapeutic regimens have not been well established in pregnant patients, heparin therapy should be initiated according to the current recommendations for nonpregnant patients.[2,7] Audits of heparin therapy suggest that heparin administration based on clinical intuition is fraught with difficulty and frequently results in inadequate therapy and prolonged periods of subtherapeutic anticoagulation. The first goal of anticoagulant therapy is to provide sufficiently high starting doses to achieve therapeutic levels quickly in order to minimize the risk of recurrent thromboembolism. Unfractionated heparin should be promptly initiated with an intravenous bolus of 5000 U (or 80 U/kg) followed by a continuous infusion starting at 1300 U/h (Table 17-1). The infusion should then be adjusted on the basis of laboratory tests, such as an activated partial thromboplastin time (aPTT) or heparin level. An aPTT value 1.5 to 2.5 times the patient's baseline value or a heparin concentration of 0.2 to 0.4 U/mL is the recommended target therapeutic range for heparin for both deep venous thrombosis and PE.

Heparin therapy should be monitored every 6 h in the first 24 to 48 h of therapy and the dose adjusted according to one of the standard nomograms for heparin therapy.[7,14] Heparin therapy should be continued for 5 to 7 days, and long-term outpatient anticoagulant therapy using heparin if the patient is still pregnant should be administered for 3 months or longer, depending on when the thromboembolic event occurred during pregnancy.

ANTEPARTUM VENOUS THROMBOSIS

Venous thromboembolism that occurs during pregnancy requires prolonged anticoagulation for the remainder of the pregnancy and for at least 6 weeks postpartum. Conversion to a subcutaneous adjusted-dose heparin protocol is typically the most convenient choice. Subcutaneous adjusted-dose heparin is typically administered either twice to three times daily to maintain a midinterval aPTT within the therapeutic range

---

Table 17-1

GUIDELINES FOR ANTICOAGULATION

Pregnant
- Obtain baseline complete blood count with platelets, aPTT, and PT.
- Give heparin bolus, 5000 U IV or 80 U/kg as a loading dose.
- Start a maintenance heparin infusion of 1300 U/h for DVT and 1500 U/h for PE.
- Check an aPTT at 6 h and adjust the infusion rate to maintain the aPTT between 1.5 and 2.5 times the patient's baseline (or maintain blood heparin level at 0.2 to 0.4 U/mL).
- If aPTT is not prolonged, rebolus with 5000 U, in addition to increasing the rate.
- Repeat the aPTT every 6 h during the first 24 h of therapy. Thereafter, monitor the aPTT daily unless outside of the therapeutic range.
- Monitor the platelet count daily or every other day during the first 10 days of heparin therapy to check for heparin induced thrombocytopenia.

Postpartum
- Begin warfarin therapy on the first day of heparin (in the postpartum patient) at 5–10 mg and administer daily at the estimated maintenance dose.
- Check the PT daily after starting warfarin therapy and adjust therapy to maintain the INR at 2.0 to 3.0.
- Discontinue heparin after an INR of 2.0 to 3.0 has been achieved for 4–7 consecutive days.
- Continue anticoagulation with warfarin for 3 months at an INR of 2.0–3.0.

Abbreviations: aPTT = activated partial thromboplastin time; PT = prothrombin time; DVT = deep venous thrombosis; PE = pulmonary embolism; INR = International Normalized Ratio.
Source: Reprinted with permission from Ref. 8.

(e.g., 1.5 to 2.5 times control). There is very little experience with low molecular weight heparin during pregnancy. Warfarin is uncommonly used during pregnancy because of its adverse effects on fetal development during the first and second trimesters. In addition, warfarin readily crosses the placenta and can result in fetal and neonatal hemorrhage. In general, warfarin should not be used during pregnancy. However, some experts still use warfarin during the second and early third trimesters in women with artificial heart valves because of concern that these patients may be resistant to moderate doses of heparin.

POSTPARTUM VENOUS THROMBOSIS

The postpartum patient is managed in the same way as the nonpregnant patient. Intravenous heparin is initiated as described above, and warfarin may be started on the first day of heparin administration. Warfarin therapy is adjusted according to the prothrombin time (PT), expressed as the International Normalized Ratio (INR). In patients with venous thromboembolism, warfarin therapy should be adjusted to maintain an INR of 2.0 to 3.0. Warfarin therapy produces an early anticoagulant effect (secondary to a rapid fall in factor VII and protein C levels) before it achieves a consistent antithrombotic effect (which lags by at least 24 to 48 h). It is therefore important to continue heparin therapy for at least 4 days and not discontinue it until the INR has been in the therapeutic range for 2 consecutive days after the initiation of warfarin therapy.[15] Warfarin therapy is continued for at least 3 months following the acute event to minimize the risk of recurrence. It is important to inform the patient that neither warfarin nor heparin is secreted in breast milk in significant quantities and that the use of either drug is not a contraindication to breast-feeding. Since warfarin use during pregnancy is associated with the development of birth defects, reliable contraception should be practiced by the nonpregnant sexually active woman while taking this drug.

MANAGEMENT DURING LABOR

Anticoagulant therapy rarely presents a problem at the time of delivery. Heparin has a short, dose-dependent half-life regardless of the route of administration. Women on a subcutaneous adjusted-dose regimen should be instructed to discontinue heparin use with the onset of regular uterine contractions. Upon the woman's presentation to the hospital, an aPTT or heparin level should be measured. The risk of hemorrhage at the time of vaginal delivery or cesarean section has not been reported to be significantly increased when the heparin level is less than 0.4 U/mL. Regional anesthesia is not contraindicated if the aPTT is normal and heparin has not been administered within 4 to 6 h of the delivery. Protamine sulfate can be administered to patients with a heparin level greater than 0.4 U/mL or an aPTT greater than 2.7 times control. One milligram of protamine sulfate will neutralize 100 U of heparin with an almost immediate onset. Protamine sulfate is typically administered in small doses (less than 50 mg given intravenously over 10 min) and titrated against the whole-blood clotting time.

Anticoagulant therapy may be restarted within 4 to 6 h postpartum if the patient is stable and in the absence of heavy uterine bleeding. A continuous heparin infusion should be resumed after a 5000-U loading dose. Warfarin therapy may be initiated on the same day or as soon as the patient can tolerate oral medications, as described above.

Thrombolytic therapy should be avoided in the pregnant patient except in life-threatening situations because of the risk of substantial maternal bleeding, especially at the time of delivery and immediately postpartum. The risk of placental abruption and fetal death due to these agents is currently unknown. Inferior vena caval filters have been used

safely and effectively in pregnant women. Their use is generally restricted to those patients who have recurrent PE despite adequate anticoagulant therapy and those in whom heparin therapy is contraindicated because of a high risk of complications or a history of an adverse reaction to heparin, such as heparin-induced thrombocytopenia. Suprarenal placement has been suggested to avoid injury to the gravid uterus.

SUMMARY

The management of venous thromboembolism during pregnancy continues to present unique and difficult challenges, many of which remain unsolved because of the lack of prospective studies. Pulmonary embolism remains one of the most significant causes of maternal mortality. Because early diagnosis and treatment of these conditions is associated with a marked reduction of serious maternal sequelae, objective testing should be used liberally and aggressively in this population.

References

1. Berg CJ, Atrash HK, Koonin LM, Tucker M: Pregnancy-related morbidity in the United States, 1987–1990. *Obstet Gynecol* 88:161, 1996.
2. Toglia MR, Weg JG: Venous thromboembolism during pregnancy. *N Engl J Med* 335:108, 1996.
3. Bergqvist D, Hedner U: Pregnancy and venous thrombo-embolism. *Acta Obstet Gynecol Scand* 62:449, 1983.
4. Ginsberg JS, Brill-Edwards P, Burrows RF, et al: Venous thrombosis during pregnancy: Leg and trimester of presentation. *Thromb Haemost* 67:519, 1992.
5. Bergqvist A, Bergqvist D, Hallbook T: Deep vein thrombosis during pregnancy: A prospective study. *Acta Obstet Gynecol Scand* 62:443, 1983.
6. Tengborn L, Bergqvist D, Matzsch R, et al: Recurrent thromboembolism in pregnancy and the puerperium. *Am J Obstet Gynecol* 28:107, 1985.
7. Ginsberg JS: Management of venous thromboembolism. *N Engl J Med* 335:1816, 1996.
8. Toglia MR, Nolan TE: Venous thromboembolism during pregnancy: A current review of diagnosis and management. *Obstet Gynecol Survey* 52:1, 1997.
9. Hull RD, Raskob GE, Carter CJ: Serial impedance plethysmography in pregnant patients with clinically suspected deep-vein thrombosis: Clinical validity of negative findings. *Ann Intern Med* 112:663, 1990.
10. Heijboer H, Buller HR, Lensing AWA, et al: A comparison of real-time compression ultrasonography with impedance plethysmography for the diagnosis of deep-vein thrombosis in symptomatic outpatients. *N Engl J Med* 329:1365, 1993.

11. Polak JF, Wilkinson DL: Ultrasonographic diagnosis of symptomatic deep venous thrombosis in pregnancy. *Am J Obstet Gynecol* 165:625, 1991.

12. Ginsberg JS, Hirsh J, Rainbow AJ, Coates G: Risks to the fetus of radiologic procedures used in the diagnosis of maternal venous thromboembolic disease. *Thromb Haemost* 61:189, 1989.

13. Stein PD, Terrin ML, Hales CA, et al: Clinical, laboratory, roentgenographic and electrocardiographic findings in patients with acute pulmonary embolism and no pre-existing cardiac or pulmonary disease. *Chest* 100:598, 1991.

14. Cruickshank MK, Levine MN, Hirsh J, et al: A standard heparin nomogram for the management of heparin therapy. *Arch Intern Med* 151:333, 1991.

15. Gallus AS, Jackaman J, Tillett J, et al: Safety and efficacy of warfarin started early after submassive venous thrombosis or pulmonary embolism. *Lancet* 2:1293, 1986.

Chapter 18

PULMONARY DISORDERS DURING PREGNANCY

Fernando J. Martinez

Pulmonary disorders are frequently noted during the course of pregnancy. To understand the effects of pulmonary disease during pregnancy, one must appreciate the numerous structural and physiologic changes that occur during normal pregnancy.[1]

PHYSIOLOGIC CHANGES DURING PREGNANCY

STRUCTURAL CHANGES WITH PREGNANCY

The structure of the respiratory system changes dramatically during pregnancy. This includes mucosal changes of the respiratory tract—leading to hyperemia, hypersecretion, and mucosal edema—which are most prominent in the third trimester.[1] This is generally attributed to the effects of estrogen and associated with frequent symptoms of rhinitis. The progressive increase in uterine size and maternal weight result in increased circumference of the abdomen and lower chest wall (approximately 5 to 7 cm), elevation of the diaphragm (approximately 4 to 5 cm), and widening of the costal angle (approximately 50 percent).[1] The change in chest wall configuration peaks by 37 weeks of gestation and generally returns to normal within 24 weeks of delivery. Despite this, no change in maximum inspiratory pressure or diaphragmatic pressure has been reported, although diaphragm fatigue has been reported to occur during labor.[2]

CHANGES IN PULMONARY FUNCTION DURING PREGNANCY

The effect of pregnancy on lung function has been well described since the study of Cugell and colleagues.[3] These authors reported changes in lung volumes in women who were 7 to 9 months pregnant compared with nonpregnant individuals (Fig. 18-1). They demonstrated a decrease in expiratory reserve volume (ERV), residual volume (RV), and functional residual capacity (FRC) (approximately 17 to 20 percent). At term there were small declines in total lung capacity (TLC) (approximately 4 percent) but there was no change in vital capacity (VC). Tidal volume (VT) increased significantly (450 to 600 mL).

Lung compliance and routine spirometric indexes change little during pregnancy, although total pulmonary resistance appears to drop. As such, forced VC (FVC), forced expiratory volume in the first second (FEV_1), peak flows, and maximum breathing capacity change little during pregnancy. Data on diffusing capacity (DL_{CO}) are inconsistent, although in general there appears to be no change or a slight increase in DL_{CO} early in pregnancy with a subsequent decrease throughout the remainder of pregnancy to values that are normal or slightly lower than normal.[1]

The respiratory changes in ventilation are illustrated in Fig. 18-2. A dramatic increase in minute ventilation ($\dot{V}E$) occurs, which is predominantly caused by a rise in VT. Respiratory rate changes little throughout pregnancy. Alveolar ventilation rises approximately 50 to 70 percent, as does

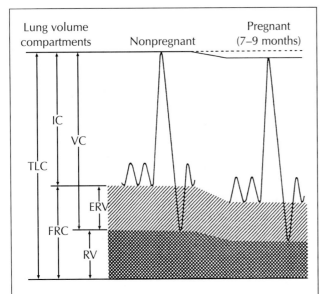

Figure 18-1

Changes in lung volumes in women 7 to 9 months pregnant compared with the lungs of nonpregnant women. TLC = total lung capacity; IC = inspirational capacity; FRC = functional residual capacity; VC = vital capacity; RV = residual volume; ERV = expiratory reserve volume. (Adapted from Elkus R, Popovich J: Respiratory physiology in pregnancy. *Clin Chest Med* 13:555, 1992, with permission.)

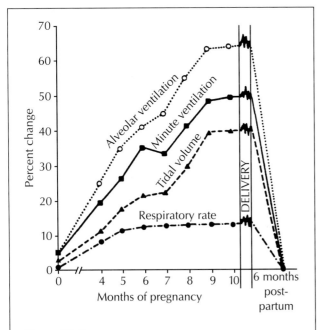

Figure 18-2

Respiratory changes during pregnancy. (Adapted from Elkus R, Popovich J: Respiratory physiology in pregnancy. *Clin Chest Med* 13:555, 1992, with permission.)

metabolic rate. This alveolar hyperventilation is associated with decreases in $P_{A_{CO_2}}$ from 37 to 40 mmHg to 27 to 34 mmHg, which begins by 8 to 12 weeks and plateaus by 20 weeks of gestation. The fall in alveolar P_{CO_2} is associated with an increased alveolar P_{O_2} ($P_{A_{O_2}}$). Moving from a sitting to a supine position is associated with an increased $P(A-a)_{O_2}$ (approximately 6 mmHg) and drop in Pa_{O_2} (approximately 13 mmHg).

During exercise, peak oxygen consumption ($\dot{V}_{O_2}$) does not appear to be significantly different from that of nonpregnant women. For any given work rate, $\dot{V}E$ is increased 20 to 25% in comparison with that of nonpregnant women, such that peak $\dot{V}E$ and $\dot{V}E/\dot{V}_{O_2}$ appear higher in pregnant women.[4] There is a rise in VT with little difference in respiratory rate response during exercise.[4] Lactate threshold also does not appear to change with pregnancy.[4]

EVALUATION OF COMMON RESPIRATORY SYMPTOMS DURING PREGNANCY

DYSPNEA

Dyspnea is one of the more difficult symptoms to evaluate during pregnancy because it occurs frequently during normal pregnancy. Milne and colleagues assessed 62 women eight times during a normal pregnancy.[5] Dyspnea was graded using a three-grade scale. Between 16 and 19 weeks of gestation, the percentage of subjects noting dyspnea rose from 24 to 48 percent. This percentage steadily rose until the 31st week of gestation, when 76 percent of women complained of dyspnea. The severity of dyspnea rose in a similar fashion, such that greater than 30 percent of women experienced moderately severe dyspnea (grade 2 or higher) by the 36th week of gestation. Of interest, no other respiratory symptoms were noted. Determining when dyspnea is pathologic can be quite challenging.

The source of this sensation during pregnancy remains controversial. Most feel that the subjective sensation of hyperventilation during pregnancy plays a large role.[5] The data of Nava and colleagues suggests that the perception of respiratory muscle effort may be important in this sensation.[2]

The evaluation of dyspnea during pregnancy will be guided by the severity of symptoms, the level of work at which symptoms occur, and the time course of symptom development. Studies in nonpregnant adults have examined the etiology of acute dyspnea.[6] A majority of cases are felt to be due to cardiac or pulmonary disease. Similarly, the majority of patients with chronic dyspnea are found to have pulmonary disease or cardiac disease. None of these studies specifically address the pregnant patient, although the type and frequency of diagnoses are likely similar (see Table 18-1). Recent estimates suggest a prevalence of heart dis-

Table 18-1

DISEASE CATEGORIES ASSOCIATED WITH ACUTE OR CHRONIC DYSPNEA DURING PREGNANCY

Disease Category	Acute Dyspnea	Chronic Dyspnea

Cardiovascular	Congestive heart failure
	Ischemic disease
	Infective endocarditis
	Valvular disease
	Pericardial disease
		Valvular disease
		  Mitral stenosis
		  Mitral regurgitation
		  Mitral valve prolapse
		  Aortic stenosis
		  Aortic regurgitation
		  Pulmonic stenosis
		Myocardial disease
		  Dilated cardiomyopathy
		  Hypertrophic cardiomyopathy
		  Restrictive cardiomyopathy
		  Myocarditis
		Ischemic disease
		Congenital heart disease
		Pericardial disease
		Infective endocarditis

Pulmonary disease	Pleural disease
	  Pneumothorax
	  Pleural effusion
	Pulmonary embolism
	Parenchymal infection
	Obstructive lung disease
	  Asthma
	  Upper airway obstruction
	Neuromuscular disease
	Noncardiogenic pulmonary edema
		Obstructive lung disease
		  Asthma
		  Emphysema
		  Cystic fibrosis
		  Upper airway obstruction
		Restrictive lung disease
		  Parenchymal fibrosis
		  Pleural disease
		  Neuromuscular disease
		Pulmonary hypertension

ease in pregnant women ranging from 0.4 to 4.1 percent,[7] although no similar data have been published for pulmonary disease. In the pregnant individual, separating cardiac from pulmonary causes of dyspnea can be difficult.

Table 18-2 compares the features of dyspnea and closely associated symptoms that may be useful in the evaluation of the pregnant, dyspneic patient. Physiologic dyspnea has distinctive chronological features, as it is first noted in the first or second trimester and is most prevalent at term. It is usually described as a sense of difficulty getting a deep breath—as air hunger or increased effort.[7] It is rarely severe and it rarely limits exercise or is noted at rest. In contrast, dyspnea in cardiac or pulmonary disease can occur at rest, may be more severe, and interferes with the ability to exercise. Associated symptoms such as paroxysmal nocturnal dyspnea, orthopnea, and cough should be sought, as they may suggest associated pulmonary or heart disease.

Physical examination should center on the cardiovascular and pulmonary systems. Unfortunately, many of the physi-

ologic changes of pregnancy can limit the value of physical examination in the pregnant, dyspneic patient. The cardiovascular adaptations during pregnancy have been well described previously.[7] These include changes in precordial palpation, heart sounds, jugular venous distention, and murmurs. Chest auscultation can be misleading, as basilar rales may be heard late in pregnancy due to basilar atelectasis. Hyperventilation is frequently seen but is usually due to an increased V_T, as respiratory rate does not change. As such, tachypnea should suggest a pathologic process and lead to further evaluation. Peripheral edema commonly occurs later in pregnancy. The appropriate evaluation of dyspnea during pregnancy will depend on an understanding of these normal physiologic changes.

Diagnostic studies are frequently required if symptoms have features suggestive of a pathologic process. The timing of symptom development (acute versus chronic) will be important in formulating an appropriate diagnostic process.[7] Acute onset of dyspnea is not typical for physiologic dysp-

Table 18-2

SYMPTOMS DURING NORMAL PREGNANCY VERSUS PREGNANCY COMPLICATED BY
CARDIAC OR PULMONARY DISEASE

Symptom	Physiologic Dyspnea of Pregnancy	Dyspnea from Cardiac Disease during Pregnancy	Dyspnea from Pulmonary Disease during Pregnancy
Dyspnea	Occurs frequently First noted in first or second trimester Greatest near term Slowly progressive Does not interfere with activity Rarely noted at rest Rarely severe Associated symptoms less frequent	Occurs occasionally Variable onset Usually begins in second or third trimester May be acute or slowly progressive Worsens with exertion May occur at rest May be severe Associated symptoms frequent	Occurs occasionally Variable onset May occur in all trimesters May be acute or slowly progressive Worsens with exertion May occur at rest May be severe Associated symptoms frequent
Orthopnea	Occurs occasionally Occurs later in pregnancy	Occurs frequently Variable onset	Occurs occasionally Variable onset Frequently associated with cough
Syncope	Occurs uncommonly Occurs later in pregnancy "Supine hypotensive syndrome"	Occurs occasionally Variable onset Occurs while standing or exercising	Occurs occasionally Variable onset Occurs while standing or exercising
Chest pain	Occurs occasionally Occurs later in pregnancy Can be exertional	Occurs frequently Variable onset May be progressive May be exertional	Occurs occasionally Variable onset May be pleuritic Associated symptoms frequent

nea of pregnancy and should lead one to suspect an acute cardiac or pulmonary etiology. Potential causes for acute dyspnea are shown in Table 18-1. A simple algorithm for evaluation is suggested in Fig. 18-3. An abnormality in early studies should lead to appropriate further evaluation. As pulmonary function studies change little during pregnancy, their diagnostic value remains high in the setting of clinical symptoms. Echocardiography must be interpreted with an understanding of the normal physiologic changes expected during pregnancy.[7] It can, however, provide valuable information regarding valvular, myocardial, and pericardial function in the dyspneic individual.[7]

Chronic, progressive dyspnea must be differentiated from physiologic dyspnea as described earlier. Chronic cardiac and pulmonary disease are the most common disease categories leading to pathologic, chronic dyspnea in the pregnant patient. Figure 18-3 illustrates an algorithm that emphasizes simpler studies earlier in the evaluation process. Pulmonary function testing has proven value in the evaluation of the chronically dyspneic patient. As little change occurs in pulmonary function during pregnancy, a similar value for pulmonary function testing should be seen during the evaluation of chronic dyspnea in the pregnant patient.

Echocardiography should be utilized early during the evaluation, as it allows an objective assessment of valvular, myocardial and pericardial function. Bronchoprovocation testing has been reported to be useful in evaluating chronic breathlessness to identify hyperactive airways disease. The safety of this test has not been systemically proven in pregnancy, although limited reports suggest that it is safe.[8] If no obvious etiology is noted during this initial evaluation, a cardiopulmonary exercise test has demonstrated value in evaluating chronic dyspnea in nonpregnant individuals.[9] As noted earlier, pregnancy is associated with elevated resting and peak $\dot{V}_{O_2}$, but measurements during exercise testing can be used to separate cardiac and pulmonary causes for pathologic dyspnea.[4]

COUGH

Cough is a frequent symptom in adults. As with dyspnea, the timing of symptom development is of paramount importance in approaching a differential diagnosis in the pregnant woman. An acute cough is most commonly caused by an infectious pathogen, with viruses most often suspected.

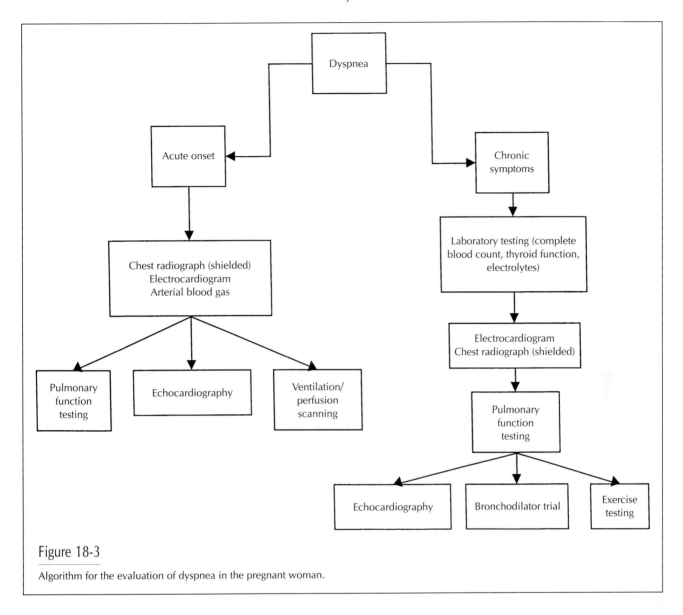

Figure 18-3

Algorithm for the evaluation of dyspnea in the pregnant woman.

This cough is usually self-limited without specific treatment. In women of childbearing age, atypical pathogens such as *Mycoplasma, Chlamydia,* and *Bordetella* (pertussis) have been identified with increasing frequency as the cause of acute cough. Severe cough, sputum production or fever may dictate the need for antibiotic therapy in this setting; erythromycin is particularly well suited for this purpose.

A cough lasting longer than 3 to 4 weeks in a nonsmoker raises a specific differential diagnosis.[10] Most pregnant individuals should present a similar differential. This includes post-nasal drainage, hyperactive airways disease, and gastroesophageal reflux disease (GERD). These processes account for over 90 percent of chronic cough in adults.[10] In the pregnant patient, rhinitis is frequently seen, and as such a cough may be present.[11] Asthma is frequently seen in the childbearing age group. Diagnosis and management are discussed in greater detail subsequently. Gastroesophageal re-

flux is frequent in pregnancy, particularly later in pregnancy, and can certainly be associated with chronic cough.[10] A recent "cost-effective" algorithm for evaluation and treatment of chronic cough has been published,[12] although it was not designed for the evaluation of the pregnant patient. A modified algorithm is suggested in Fig. 18-4.

The safety of many antihistamines in pregnancies has not been established.[13] Schatz and Zeiger recommend tripelennamine first, followed by chlorpheniramine or hydroxyzine if symptoms persist.[14] Because of a risk of adverse reactions in neonates, antihistamines should be avoided in nursing mothers, particularly as many antihistamines are excreted in breast milk.[13] The Food and Drug Administration (FDA) classifies all decongestants as class C, with pseudoephedrine exhibiting a more favorable therapeutic index in pregnancy.[13] Nasal glucocorticoids with the exception of triamcinolone appear to be safe and effective in pregnancy.[13]

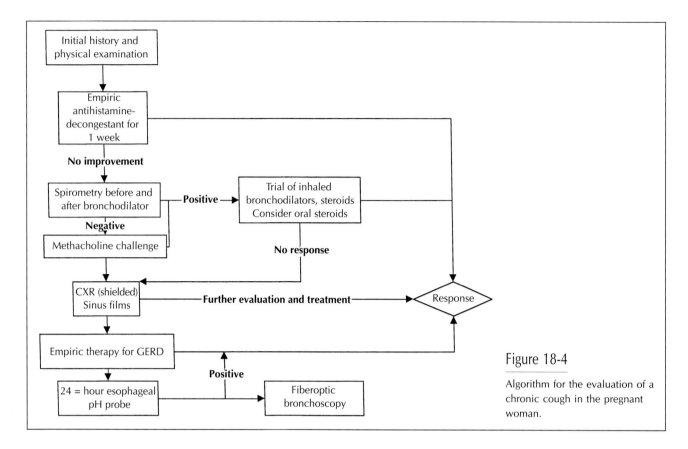

Figure 18-4

Algorithm for the evaluation of a chronic cough in the pregnant woman.

If no response is seen with empiric therapy of rhinitis, hyperactive airways disease should be suspected. An empiric trial of bronchodilators and inhaled steroids should be considered. Bronchoprovocation testing is of unclear safety during pregnancy, although methacholine challenge likely poses little risk.[8] The GERD syndrome is best treated during pregnancy with dietary modification, avoidance of medications that decrease lower esophageal sphincter tone, elevation of the head of the bed, and antacid therapy. Antisecretory agents are generally safe, and ranitidine likely has a favorable safety profile and has been used safely during pregnancy.[15]

HEMOPTYSIS

Hemoptysis, the expectoration of blood from the respiratory tract, is a common sign and symptom of respiratory disease. The evaluation is aimed at quickly establishing an accurate diagnosis and gauging the severity of bleeding. Hemoptysis that is brief in duration and mild in quantity is considered minor. In the ambulatory setting, this is usually caused by bronchitis, pneumonitis, lung carcinoma, or tuberculosis, or it is found to be idiopathic. Hemoptysis of more than 100 mL every 6 hours is considered to be massive, or life-threatening.[16] The cause is usually tuberculosis, bronchiectasis, cystic fibrosis, lung cancer, or a complication of a mycetoma.[16] In the pregnant woman, the etiologies have not been specifically addressed but are likely similar. The increased incidence of venous thromboembolism during pregnancy can present with hemoptysis and must be considered early in the evaluation process. Similarly, the increased size of pulmonary arteriovenous malformations during pregnancy should raise suspicion of this diagnosis in the appropriate clinical setting.

The initial evaluation should aim to confirm a pulmonary source to bleeding. An upper airway source of bleeding is usually evident in the presence of sinusitis, nasal polyps, or neoplasms, recognizing too that epistaxis is more common during pregnancy. A gastrointestinal source of bleeding may be more difficult to identify, although this may be suggested by associated nausea and vomiting or by a dark, acidic color and the presence of food particles. The volume and timing of bleeding should be questioned to allow assessment of bleeding severity.

Physical examination should initially establish stable vital signs and airway protection. Subsequently, one should assess abnormalities of the nose and throat while localizing the site of pulmonary bleeding. The shielded chest radiograph should be considered a basic component of the evaluation, often guiding further evaluation, as shown in Fig. 18-5. Bronchoscopy should be considered when hemoptysis is clinically significant, the initial data base is nondiagnostic, and the results will influence management.[16] Criteria that have been suggested to increase the diagnostic yield

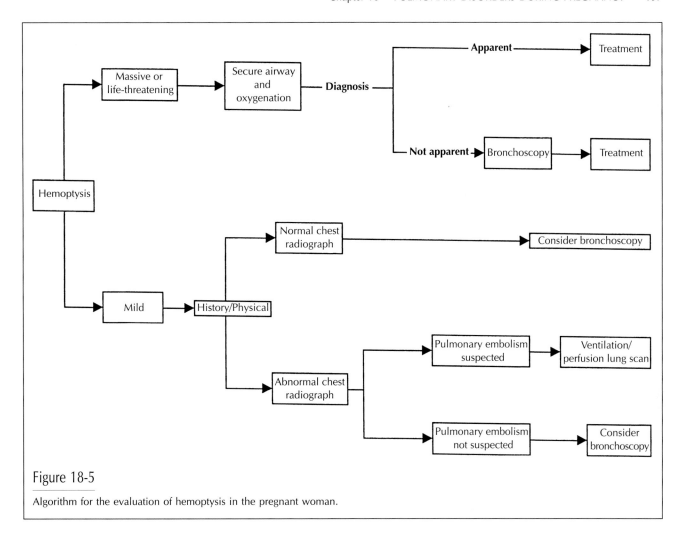

Figure 18-5

Algorithm for the evaluation of hemoptysis in the pregnant woman.

of bronchoscopy include bleeding longer than 1 to 2 weeks, more than 30 mL of bleeding per day, age >40 years, abnormal chest radiograph, smoking history, chronic cough, and worsening anemia.[16] Bronchoscopy during the first 24 hours of presentation increases diagnostic yield, although eventual outcome is not compromised by delaying the procedure.

Therapy of minor hemoptysis is generally supportive. Specific causes such as bronchitis or pneumonitis should be treated with antibiotics, as discussed below. Massive or life-threatening hemoptysis mandates an aggressive evaluation and therapy. A stable airway and oxygenation must be ensured. If the site of bleeding is known, the involved lung should be placed dependent to avoid aspiration of blood into the healthy lung.[17] Mild sedation and cough suppression may be helpful if bleeding slows. If bleeding continues or if the airway is compromised, endotracheal intubation, preferably orally and with a large tube (>8 mm internal diameter) should be considered. Bronchoscopy should be performed in an attempt to localize bleeding. Specific treatment will depend on the known or presumed cause, patient stability, and underlying lung function. Embolization may be used in patients with limited pulmonary reserve, bilateral

parenchymal disease, or multiple arteriovenous malformations.[17] Topical anticoagulants or balloon tamponade may be used in highly selected cases.[17] Multiple authors have suggested better outcome with surgical intervention in patients with adequate respiratory reserve, localized disease, and a stable medical condition.[17]

RESPIRATORY INFECTIONS DURING PREGNANCY

Respiratory infections are very common during the course of pregnancy and should be managed aggressively to minimize maternal and fetal morbidity.

BACTERIAL PNEUMONIA

Bacterial pneumonia represents a very serious infection of the respiratory tract. Although infrequently complicating pregnancy, it can have significant adverse effects on both mother and fetus.

EPIDEMIOLOGY

Pneumonia complicating pregnancy has been reported since the early 1900s. During the preantibiotic era, an incidence of 1 in 158 pregnancies was noted. During the last 20 years, the incidence has varied from 1 in 367 to 1 in 850. More recently, the epidemiology has again changed, with a higher incidence of comorbid illness, particularly human immunodeficiency virus (HIV) infection.[18]

EFFECT OF PNEUMONIA ON PREGNANCY

Maternal Outcome

Aside from the urinary tract, pneumonia is the most frequent cause of nonobstetric infection during pregnancy and the third most frequent cause of indirect obstetric death.[19] Maternal mortality was quite high in the preantibiotic era (12.5 to 32 percent). Oxorn noted a mortality of 20 percent in the preantibiotic era in his series. In the postantibiotic era, he noted a decrease in mortality to 3.5 percent.[20] Subsequent series have confirmed the potential for maternal death from bacterial pneumonia. Recently, reports have pointed to the high incidence of comorbid medical illness (asthma, cystic fibrosis) and HIV infection as a potential cause for this increased mortality. Both of these series reported significant maternal morbidity, particularly in those with comorbid illness. It is important to note that those at risk for complicated pneumonia can successfully complete pregnancy with aggressive management of the respiratory tract infection. Recent experience has demonstrated minimal or no maternal mortality despite a 40 percent incidence of serious, comorbid medical illness.[21]

Obstetric Outcome

The onset of pneumonia can occur at any time during the course of pregnancy, although most cases seem to occur during the second trimester. Premature labor and fetal death can be seen, albeit with a frequency varying from 4 to 44 percent.[19] As with maternal mortality, the majority of variability in poor fetal outcome occurs in women with comorbid, medical illness. It is important to identify those patients with comorbid illness and to manage and monitor them aggressively during the treatment of respiratory tract infection.

BACTERIOLOGY

Extensive literature has been published identifying the most common pathogenic organisms causing community-acquired pneumonia. The majority of authors have noted a high percentage of cases where no pathogen is identified. When a pathogen is recovered, *Streptococcus pneumoniae* is the most common with *Haemophilus* species and atypi-

cal pathogens (*Mycoplasma pneumoniae* and *Legionella* species) seen less frequently. The limited data in pregnant patients with pneumonia suggests that no organism is identified in the majority of the studies. When a pathogen is recovered, the distribution appears similar to that in nonpregnant patients. The incidence of viral infection may be higher in the pregnant individual, as discussed in the subsequent section.

MANAGEMENT

General Aspects

The clinical features of bacterial pneumonia are not dramatically different in the pregnant woman. Cough and fever are the most common symptoms. Dyspnea is less frequently seen than in nonpregnant patients.[22] The recent recommendations of the American Thoracic Society (ATS) are applicable to the pregnant patient with pneumonia.[23] These guidelines, based on simple parameters, group patients into straightforward clinical categories associated with different pathogenic organisms and having varying risk of mortality. These are summarized in Table 18-3.

Features from the history aid in determining comorbid illness and include a history of chronic pulmonary or cardiac disease, diabetes mellitus, hepatic or renal disease, cancer, current or recent smoking, illicit drug use, and, increasingly, HIV infection.[18] Any of these is associated with a higher likelihood of a complicated course and should suggest the possible need for hospitalization. The timing of pneumonia may provide a clue to the cause of pneumonia, as aspiration pneumonia is the most frequent cause of postpartum pneumonia.[22]

Physical findings are useful in judging the severity of pneumonia and the need for hospitalization. As noted earlier, respiratory rate does not usually increase during pregnancy despite the increase in minute ventilation. In the setting of lower respiratory tract infection, a rise in the respiratory rate has clear prognostic significance. Multiple authors have identified an elevated respiratory rate (>20 to 30 breaths per minute) as an independent predictor of complicated community-acquired pneumonia.[23] Hypotension (systolic blood pressure <90 mmHg or diastolic blood pressure <60 mmHg) also serves as a useful predictor of a complicated infection.[23]

Laboratory parameters useful in assessing disease severity include hemoglobin and white blood cell count. Various authors have commented on the lower hemoglobin levels seen in pregnant individuals with pneumonia, some of which may be physiologic.[21] The presence of a markedly elevated or depressed white blood cell count has additional prognostic significance.[23] Azotemia—blood urea nitrogen (BUN) >20 mg/mL—is an additional independent laboratory abnormality predictive of a complicated course.[23] A chest radiograph should be considered in any pregnant patient with upper respiratory tract symptoms lasting more than 2 weeks.[19] It can aid in defining the presence of pneumonia

---

Table 18-3

CATEGORIZATION OF PATIENTS WITH COMMUNITY-ACQUIRED PNEUMONIA

Category	Age	Severity of Illness	Need for Hospitalization	Comorbid Illness	Organisms Likely[a]	Appropriate Antibiotics
1	<60	Mild to moderate	No	No	S. pneumoniae M. pneumoniae Respiratory viruses C. pneumoniae H. influenzae	Erythromycin
2	<60 >60	Mild to moderate	No	Yes	S. pneumoniae Respiratory viruses Aerobic gram-negative bacilli S. aureus	Second-generation cephalosporin or Oral beta-lactam/ beta-lactamase inhibitor ± erythromycin
3	All ages	Moderate to severe	Yes, but not ICU[b]	Maybe	S. pneumoniae H. influenzae Polymicrobial Aerobic gram-negative bacilli Legionella species S. aureus C. pneumoniae Respiratory viruses	Second-generation cephalosporin or Beta-lactam/ beta-lactamase inhibitor ± erythromycin
4	All ages	Severe	Yes, to ICU	Maybe	S. pneumoniae Legionella species Aerobic gram-negative bacilli M. pneumoniae Respiratory viruses	Erythromycin ± third- generation cephalosporin with anti-Pseudomonas activity

[a]Streptococcus pneumoniae, Mycoplasma pneumoniae, Chlamydia pneumoniae, Haemophilus influenzae, Staphylococcus aureus.
[b]ICU = intensive care unit.

---

and also in identifying a high-risk group if multilobar infiltration or pleural effusions are present.

All of these indexes of severity are useful in making decisions regarding the need for hospitalization. Some authors have suggested hospitalization for all pregnant women with radiographically confirmed pneumonia.[24] With appropriate home follow-up, this may not be necessary. However, Table 18-4 demonstrates the published criteria that should be considered in identifying high-risk individuals in whom hospitalization should be strongly considered. In fact, the presence of hypotension, tachypnea, elevated BUN, and confusion are particularly useful in identifying high-risk individuals in whom hospitalization is particularly important.[25]

Antibiotic Therapy

After disease severity is established and a decision to treat the patient is made, the physician must decide on the appropriate antibiotic therapy. The guidelines of the ATS, as illustrated in Table 18-3, are useful in making this decision. Antibiotic therapy in pregnant individuals is complicated by alterations in pharmacokinetics of various antibiotics due to a greater volume of distribution,[13] reduced plasma protein concentration, more rapid clearance, increased hepatic metabolism, and erratic oral absorption of some drugs. Additionally, antibiotics have varying effects on fetal growth and development.[13,26] These effects are listed in Table 18-5 for antibiotics commonly used in the treatment of respiratory tract infections.

Table 18-4

FACTORS SUGGESTING AN INCREASED
MORTALITY IN PATIENTS WITH COMMUNITY-
ACQUIRED PNEUMONIA

Comorbid illness
  Chronic lung disease
  Diabetes
  Renal failure
  Neurologic disease
  Neoplastic disease
  Heart failure
  Chronic liver disease
  Chronic alcohol abuse
  Postsplenectomy state

Clinical data
  Prior hospitalization within 1 year
  Suspicion of aspiration
  Altered mental status

Physical findings
  Respiratory rate >20/min
  Systolic hypotension (<100 mmHg)
  Diastolic hypotension (<60 mmHg)
  Hypothermia (≤37°C)
  Hyperthermia (≥38.3°C)
  Extrapulmonary disease
  Confusion

Laboratory findings
  Leukopenia (<4000/mL)
  Leukocytosis (>30,000/mL)
  Pa_{O_2} <60 mmHg
  BUN >20 mg/dL

Chest radiographic findings
  Multilobar infiltrates
  Bilateral pleural effusions

Sources: Adapted from American Thoracic Society,[23] Farr et al.,[25] Fine et al.,[107] and Hasley et al.[108]

The recommendations of the ATS must be modified in pregnant women. Category 1 individuals are best treated with an appropriate macrolide. Category 2 individuals are best managed with a cephalosporin or penicillin with a macrolide if atypical pathogens are suspected. Category 3 patients are best managed with a second- or third-generation cephalosporin and erythromycin if an atypical pathogen is likely. A category 4 patient is best treated with intravenous erythromycin and an antipseudomonal cephalosporin plus an aminoglycoside.

The duration of intravenous antibiotics remains controversial. Recent investigators have suggested that stability on the third hospital day—as determined by the lack of an obvious reason for continued hospitalization, high-risk pathogen, or life-threatening complication—identified "low-risk" individuals who could be switched to oral antibiotics for approximately 10 days. The length of stay was 4 days with no impact on survival, short- and long-term complications, or patient satisfaction.[27] Clearly, close outpatient follow-up is required to ensure optimal outcome after discharge.

Supportive Therapy

Supportive treatment does not differ in the pregnant patient and must include adequate hydration and antipyretics. Supplemental oxygen is crucial to maintain a maternal Pa_{O_2} greater than 70 mmHg. Close monitoring is required and aggressive respiratory support employed if respiratory failure develops.[28] Tocolysis should be considered if preterm labor complicates pneumonia in pregnancy.

VIRAL RESPIRATORY INFECTIONS

Viral infections are frequently seen in adults and are largely similar between men and women except in the setting of pregnancy. Two common viral infections—influenza and varicella zoster—must be aggressively managed in pregnant women.

INFLUENZA

Influenza is caused by one of the myxoviruses, types A, B, and C. Type A influenza is usually the source of epidemic infection; as such, it is the most problematic. Historical data support a high mortality in pregnant women experiencing influenza pneumonia. In the pandemic of 1918–1919, influenza during pregnancy had a 30 percent maternal mortality—50 percent in the presence of pneumonia. Furthermore, influenza pneumonia in the third trimester was associated with a 61 percent mortality.[22] In the 1957 Asian flu epidemic, 10 percent of all influenza deaths occurred in pregnant women, while almost 50 percent of women of childbearing age who died were pregnant.[19] Pregnant women had twice the mortality of nonpregnant females, with a particular rise in the third trimester. More recent reports have not confirmed such high mortality.

The clinical picture of influenza is typically acute after an incubation period of 1 to 4 days. Fever, malaise, coryza, headache, and cough are frequently seen. Uncomplicated cases usually resolve within 3 days without chest radiographic abnormalities. If symptoms persist longer than 5 days, particularly in a pregnant woman, complications should be suspected. Pneumonia may represent primary progression of viral infection or a complicating secondary bac-

Table 18-5

SAFETY OF ANTIBIOTICS COMMONLY USED TO TREAT BACTERIAL RESPIRATORY TRACT INFECTIONS DURING PREGNANCY

Drug	FDA Category	Effect on Fetus	Effect on Mother
Penicillins	B	None known	Allergic reactions
Cephalosporins	B	None known	Allergic reactions
Macrolides			
Erythromycin	B	None known	Cholestasis with estolate
Azithromycin	B	Limited data	Limited data
Clarithromycin			
Clindamycin	B	None known	Allergic reactions, pseudomembranous colitis
Tetracyclines	D	Discoloration of teeth, inhibition of bone growth	Acute fatty liver, renal failure, pancreatitis
Sulfonamides	B (First and second trimesters)	None known	Allergic reactions, hemolysis (G6PD deficiency)
	D (Third trimester)	Kernicterus, hemolysis (G6PD deficiency)	Allergic reactions, hemolysis (G6PD deficiency)
Aminoglycosides	C	Ototoxicity, nephrotoxicity	Ototoxicity, nephrotoxicity
Quinolones	None	Irreversible arthropathy in animals	Rare pseudomembranous colitis, nephrotoxicity
Chloramphenicol	C	Gray baby syndrome	Bone marrow depression, aplastic anemia

terial infection. These secondary infections are usually caused by *S. pneumoniae, Staphylococcus aureus, H. influenzae,* or enteric gram-negative bacilli.[22] In the 1957–1958 epidemic, pregnant women who died generally expired of fulminant viral pneumonia, while nonpregnant patients died of secondary bacterial pneumonia.[28] Neuzil and colleagues reported results of a large survey and case-control study of pneumonia and/or influenza in pregnancy during epidemics. The risk of acute respiratory illness and hospitalization among women in the third trimester was 4.5 times that of those in the second trimester, which was 2.5 times that of those in the first trimester or nonpregnant women.[29]

Pneumonia complicating influenza must be managed aggressively, especially in pregnant women. Bacterial pneumonia must be treated with appropriate antibiotics using the guidelines described earlier. A picture consistent with primary viral pneumonia must be treated with aggressive oxygen therapy. Occasionally respiratory failure ensues, which

may require mechanical ventilation. Amantadine, an oral antiviral agent that blocks release of nucleic acids, can prevent 70 to 90 percent of infections if used prophylactically.[30] If it is used within 48 hours of symptom onset, the duration of symptoms can be decreased by up to 50 percent and fever can be lowered.[30] Amantadine has been used anecdotally in pregnancy[22,30] and does not appear to be toxic in mice or rabbits.[22] Amantadine and the virustatic agent ribavarin have been successfully used in influenza pneumonia complicating pregnancy.[31]

Pneumonia can be managed during pregnancy without the routine need for induction of labor.[22] Although somewhat controversial, recent reviews have not found convincing data linking maternal influenzal infection with congenital malformation.[19] Because of the potential risks, the Centers for Disease Control (CDC) have recommended that influenza vaccine be considered for pregnant women.[32] This could be of particular value in those women who will be entering the third trimester or early puerperium during the influenza season.

VARICELLA ZOSTER

Varicella zoster is a herpetic DNA virus that generally infects children. Because childhood infection confers immunity, it infects less than 2 percent of adults. But adult cases of chickenpox can be complicated by varicella pneumonia in up to 50 percent of these cases.[19] Multiple reviews of case reports and small series have suggested an increased risk of varicella pneumonia in pregnant women with primary varicella infection.[19,33] In a review of 99 cases of varicella pneumonia, 46 were women, of whom 13 (28 percent) were pregnant.[34] Disease occurred in the third trimester in 21 and in the second trimester in 3 women.[34] Whereas mortality for nonpregnant adults with varicella pneumonia ranges from 11 to 17 percent, it has been reported to be as high as 35 to 40 percent in pregnancy.[22,35]

Varicella pneumonia usually presents 2 to 5 days after the onset of fever, rash, and malaise. Typical symptoms include cough, dyspnea, hemoptysis, and chest pain. In one series, all patients with varicella pneumonia had oral mucosal lesions in addition to the typical skin lesions. The severity of illness can range from asymptomatic to fulminant viral pneumonia with respiratory failure.[22] The chest radiograph typically demonstrates bilateral, peribronchial, nodular infiltrates that are maximal at the height of skin eruption and usually resolve by 14 days. Diffuse pulmonary calcification after clinical resolution is a well-described sequela.[34]

Given the potential for severe, life-threatening disease, aggressive management and observation are required in all patients. Acyclovir, a nucleoside analogue that inhibits herpesvirus DNA synthesis, has been demonstrated to be an effective antiviral agent in herpetic infections.[37] Use within 36 hours of hospitalization has been associated with lower temperature and respiratory rate and improved oxygenation after the fifth hospital day. Retrospective data suggest a decrease in mortality rate from 35 to 17 percent with acyclovir treatment. As such, acyclovir should be used in all patients with varicella pneumonia. The dosage recommendations have varied, although most authorities have suggested at least 7.5 to 10 mg/kg every 8 hours.[36] Acyclovir has been used in more than six hundred pregnancies (more than four hundred in the first trimester) with no increase in the number of birth defects or consistent pattern of congenital malformation. Other aspects of managing varicella during pregnancy are covered in Chap. 23.

Aggressive supportive treatment should be utilized including appropriate hydration to minimize nephrotoxicity with acyclovir. Oxygen supplementation must be optimized and mechanical ventilatory support employed in advanced respiratory failure. Extracorporeal membrane oxygenation has been successfully utilized in at least one pregnant patient with advanced adult respiratory distress syndrome complicating varicella pneumonia.

TUBERCULOSIS IN PREGNANCY

Since the introduction of antituberculosis chemotherapy in the early 1950s, the incidence of tuberculosis (TB) has de-

creased by 5 percent per year.[38] Since the 1980s there has been a clear rise in the incidence of TB. This rise has been felt to be secondary to (1) the increasing incidence of HIV infection, (2) the increase in immigration from countries with a higher prevalence of TB during pregnancy, and (3) the decline in the public health service.[39] The current resurgence has been particularly problematic in urban ethnic minorities, which is the demographic group experiencing the highest rate of HIV infection.[39] In fact, the most populated urban areas account for 18 percent of the population and 42 percent of the TB cases.[38] Although data in pregnant women are limited, there is a potential problem with TB given the recent CDC data confirming that the rate of reported cases increased 44 percent among patients 25 to 44 years of age. Margono and colleagues noted 16 cases of TB at two large community hospitals in New York City between 1985 and 1992.[40] Five of these were noted between 1985 and 1990 (incidence of 12.4 per 100,000 deliveries), while 11 were identified between 1991 and 1992 (94.8 per 100,000 deliveries). Of 11 women, 7 tested positive for HIV.[40] As a result of these data, all physicians caring for pregnant individuals in high-risk groups must be familiar with the care of the pregnant patient with TB. Several excellent reviews of the topic have recently been published.[38,39]

EFFECT OF PREGNANCY ON TUBERCULOSIS

The pathogenesis of TB infection and disease begins with inhalation of tubercle bacilli in 95 percent of patients.[39] The effects of pregnancy on the course of TB have been the source of much controversy dating to antiquity. Hippocrates, Galen, and others felt that pregnancy was beneficial in TB. This opinion drastically changed in the nineteenth century, when it was concluded that pregnancy worsened the course of TB. As a result, abortion was considered a viable therapeutic option for the pregnant woman with TB. The medical opinion again changed in the 1940s and 1950s,[39] when it became evident that TB did not worsen during pregnancy.[38]

Some investigators have suggested that the risk of acquiring TB increases in the first postpartum year,[41] although others have not confirmed this. More importantly, the risk of reactivating quiescent infection during pregnancy remains unclear. Although data are contradictory, the risk of reactivation is likely changed little by pregnancy.[42]

EFFECT OF TUBERCULOSIS ON PREGNANCY

Published reports from the prechemotherapy era suggested a high incidence of impaired fetal outcomes.[39] Some have suggested a higher incidence of pregnancy complications, spontaneous abortion, and labor complications. Jana et al. reported that pulmonary TB was associated with an approximately twofold increase in prematurity and low birthweight, a threefold increase in small size for gestational age, and sixfold increase in perinatal death.[43] These adverse outcomes were more common with late diagnosis, incomplete or irregular treatment, and advanced lesions in the mother.[43] In the postchemotherapy era, most authors feel that appropriately treated TB should have little impact on pregnancy. It is clear that appropriate chemotherapy for TB is crucial during pregnancy and should not be withheld or altered.[44]

CLINICAL MANIFESTATIONS

In general, the clinical manifestations of TB during pregnancy are similar to those in the nonpregnant individual. In the patients described by Good, cough (74 percent), weight loss (41 percent), fever (30 percent), malaise and fatigue (30 percent), and hemoptysis (19 percent) were the most common presenting symptoms, though 19 percent were asymptomatic.[45] This latter point has recently been confirmed by Carter and Mates, who reported that pregnant women were more likely to present without symptoms.[46] Other more unusual presentations include genital TB, which usually involves the fallopian tubes and presents with infertility and menstrual irregularity.[39] Tuberculous mastitis occurs most commonly in women of childbearing age as a single breast mass, with or without drainage. In one report, up to one-third of the cases occurred in lactating women.[39]

Radiographic findings of TB are well described and are generally separated as primary or reactivation disease. In primary disease, involvement of the anterior segment of the upper lobe (50 percent), cavitation (29 percent), pleural effusion (24 percent) and mediastinal adenopathy are noted. In reactivation disease, common changes include exudative or fibroproliferative parenchymal infiltrates (100 percent), apical or posterior segment disease in the upper lobes (51 percent), cavitation (45 percent), and fibrosis (41 percent).

SCREENING AND PROPHYLAXIS OF TUBERCULOSIS DURING PREGNANCY

Given the high frequency of asymptomatic disease and worsened outcome without treatment, early diagnosis is crucial. The most appropriate screening test is the tuberculin skin test, ideally placed using the Mantoux technique.[39] This involves the intradermal injection of 0.1 mL of purified protein derivative (PPD), 5 tuberculin units in strength, which is read as the amount of induration 48 to 72 hours later. This test is safe and is thought to be reliable during pregnancy.[47] Over the last decade the interpretation of the skin test has evolved to more accurately include the purpose of testing and managing false-positive and false-negative interpretation.[48] The American Thoracic Society has formulated guidelines for the evaluation of skin testing in nonpregnant individuals which should be applicable to pregnant women.[48] These recommendations, enumerated in Table 18-6, vary cutoffs for a positive response based on risk factors for disease. It should be noted that approximately 10 percent of individuals with TB have a negative tuberculin skin test.[39] Importantly, a negative test and control skin tests have

---

Table 18-6

CENTERS FOR DISEASE CONTROL RECOMMENDATIONS FOR INTERPRETATION OF THE TUBERCULIN (PPD) SKIN TEST[a]

Lesion Size	Interpreted positive if
>5 mm	Known or suspected HIV infection Recent close contact with active TB Clinical or radiographic evidence of TB
>10 mm	Intravenous drug abuse but HIV-negative Residing in institution, shelter, prison Health care worker Immigrant from country with high prevalence of TB Hispanic, black, Native American Diabetes mellitus Renal failure Postgastrectomy or intestinal bypass Hematologic or reticuloendothelial disease Immunosuppression Silicosis Malnourishment (10% below ideal body weight) Chronic alcoholism
>15 mm	All others

[a]High-risk groups for whom screening should be considered: immigrants from high-risk countries, homeless individuals, known or suspected exposure to high-risk individual, medically indigent urban residents, intravenous drug users, health care workers, nursing home residents, persons confined to prison, persons who are immunosuppressed, individuals with HIV or intercurrent medical illness.

---

been reported in 30 percent of women with HIV infection.[49] As such, a negative test cannot be used to exclude TB, particularly in the setting of appropriate signs and symptoms.

Vaccination with bacille Calmette-Guérin (BCG) is frequently employed in other countries and continues to cause confusion regarding the effect on tuberculin skin testing.[38] In general, a tuberculin skin test is not contraindicated in the face of prior BCG vaccination and should be interpreted as usual if BCG vaccination occurred more than 10 years prior. Previous BCG vaccination should have no impact on the appropriate evaluation and treatment of suspected TB, as the skin test reaction resulting from BCG vaccination is usually less than 10 mm and wanes 3 to 5 years after vaccination.[39]

When a skin test is interpreted as positive, the algorithm illustrated in Fig. 18-6 can be utilized to determine appropriate management in the pregnant woman. Isoniazid (INH) has been shown to be 60 to 90 percent effective in the pro-

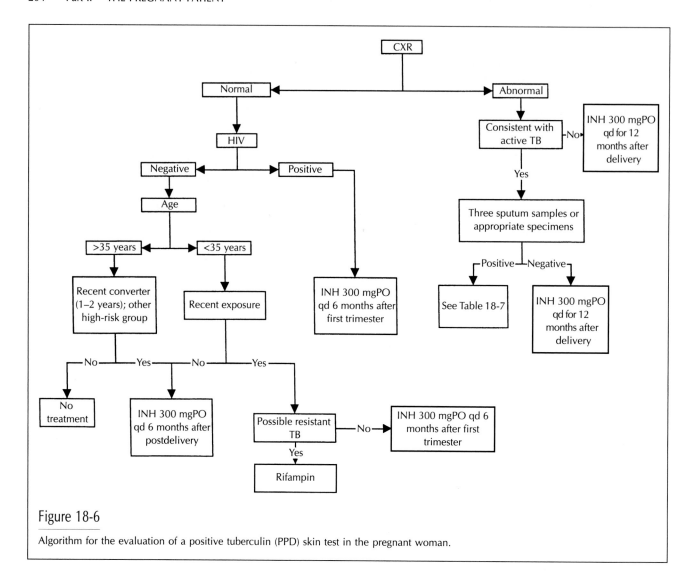

Figure 18-6

Algorithm for the evaluation of a positive tuberculin (PPD) skin test in the pregnant woman.

phylaxis of TB infection.[38] An increased risk of INH hepatitis has been suggested in the perinatal period.[50] As such, INH prophylaxis is best delayed into the postpartum period unless the risk of reactivation is particularly high (a recent PPD conversion or exposure to someone with active TB). In the latter setting, INH prophylaxis can be delayed until the first trimester has passed to minimize risk of teratogenesis. If INH resistance is felt likely because of the presence of appropriate risk factors, rifampin can be used for prophylaxis.

DIAGNOSIS AND MANAGEMENT OF ACTIVE TUBERCULOSIS DISEASE

The diagnosis of TB is best made by identifying *Mycobacterium tuberculosis* in appropriate specimens. These are usually obtained from pulmonary secretions but can include pleural fluid, joint fluid, and cerebrospinal fluid, among others. Occasionally, treatment is provided without microbio-

logic confirmation in the setting of an appropriate clinical and radiographic picture.

Treatment of active TB in the pregnant woman is similar to that of nonpregnant individuals. The potential toxicity to the fetus must be kept in mind. Nevertheless, all authorities agree that the risk of withholding therapy greatly outweighs the risks of treatment.[44] The drugs utilized and their potential toxicity are enumerated in Table 18-7. The current recommendations from the ATS are for a combination of INH, rifampin, and ethambutol.[51] Rifampin and INH for 9 months are appropriate if the risk of INH resistance is small. An abbreviated regimen generally requires pyrazinamide (PZA), which is of uncertain safety in pregnancy.[44] Of interest, others have described anecdotal use of PZA during pregnancy without difficulty.[52] If INH resistance is possible, ethambutol must be added at the outset. It can be deleted from the regimen once microbiologic studies confirm pansensitivity. If multidrug resistance is possible, a regimen of at least four drugs is necessary, ideally under the supervision of a physician familiar with the management of resistant TB. The pres-

Table 18-7

COMMON DRUGS USED TO TREAT TUBERCULOSIS

Drug	Usual Dose	Possible Side Effects
Isoniazid hypersensitivity	300 mg q.d. PO 900 mg twice weekly PO	GI distress, hepatotoxicity, seizures, peripheral neuritis,
Rifampin	600 mg q.d. PO 600 mg twice weekly PO	GI distress, hepatotoxicity, headache, purpura, fever, orange secretions
Ethambutol	2–2.5 g q.d. PO 4 g twice weekly PO	Altered vision, red-green disturbance, optic neuritis, skin rash
Pyrazinamide	2–2.5 g q.d. PO 3 g twice weekly PO	Hepatotoxicity, hyperuricemia, arthralgias, gout
Streptomycin	1 g q.d. IM	Ototoxicity, nephrotoxicity

ence of HIV infection complicates treatment. A detailed discussion is beyond the scope of this chapter; interested readers should consult other sources.[38]

OBSTRUCTIVE DISORDERS

Asthma is one of the most common medical conditions complicating pregnancy; current estimates are that 1 to 7 percent of women of childbearing age manifest asthma. The management of this condition poses unique problems, as both the changing thoracic mechanics of the mother and the effect on the developing fetus of the hypoxia and drugs used for treatment must be considered. Over the past 30 years, multiple attempts have been made to describe the effects of asthma on the mother and fetus. These are summarized in Tables 18-8 and 18-9.

EPIDEMIOLOGY

EFFECT OF ASTHMA ON THE MOTHER AND INFANT

Large retrospective studies published in the 1970s provided a clearer definition of the potential adverse effects of asthma on pregnant women and their infants. Bahna and Bjerkedal[53] demonstrated an increase in preterm births, decreased mean birth weight, increased neonatal mortality, increased neonatal hypoxia, increased hyperemesis gravidarum, vaginal hemorrhage, and increased labor complications. Subsequent studies confirmed increased low birth weight and increased risk of obstetric complications, and recent studies have suggested that a greater prepregnancy severity of asthma is associated with greater pregnancy complications.[54]

In the best-controlled study, Schatz and colleagues reported on 486 pregnant women with asthma compared with 486 pregnant nonasthmatics with normal pulmonary function studied over a 12-year period at the Kaiser-Permanente Medical Center in San Diego.[55] Asthma was managed aggressively with a stepped-care approach (see below) to prevent asthma exacerbations and ensure normal sleep and activity level. Chronic hypertension was significantly more common in the asthmatic subjects (3.7 percent) than in controls (1.0 percent). Trends were observed toward a relation between greater asthma severity (requiring ED therapy) and increased incidence of preeclampsia and low birth weight. There was no difference in perinatal mortality, overall incidence of preeclampsia, preterm births, overall low–birth weight infants, intrauterine growth retardation, or congenital malformations.[55] This suggests that aggressive management of asthma may minimize the risk of asthma for the fetus during pregnancy.

EFFECT OF PREGNANCY ON ASTHMA

Multiple investigators have examined the course of asthma during pregnancy. Gluck and Gluck reviewed studies on 1087 patients reported in the literature from 1946 to 1976. In 36 percent, the asthma improved, while in 23 percent it worsened and in 41 percent it was unchanged.[56] Subsequent studies have in general corroborated these results, albeit with a great degree of variability. Improvement has been reported in 18 to 69 percent, while 6 to 42 percent have experienced

Table 18-8

STUDIES DESCRIBING THE EFFECT OF MATERNAL ASTHMA ON MATERNAL AND PREGNANCY OUTCOME

Reference	Study Type	Number of Subjects	Maternal		
			Preeclampsia	PTD	Asthma Outcomes
Schaefer and Silverman,[100] 1961	R	A: 293 C: 30,000	ND	ND	↔ : 93% ↑ : 3% ↓ : 4%
Gordon et al.,[101] 1970	R	A: 277 C: 30,861	NA	ND	A: 1% death C: NA
Bahna and Bjerkedal,[53] 1972	R	A: 381 C: 112,530	A: 10.5% C: 4.7%	ND	NA
Gluck and Gluck,[56] 1976	P	A: 47	NA	NA	↔ : 43% ↑ : 14% ↓ : 43%
Fitzsimons et al.,[103] 1986	P	A: 56 C: "General population"	NA	A: 12.5% C: 9.6%	NA
Stenius-Aarniala et al.,[104] 1988	P/C	A: 198 C: 198	A: 14.6% C: 4.5%	ND	↔ : 40% ↑ : 42% ↓ : 18%
Shatz et al.,[58] 1988	P	A: 366	NA	NA	↔ : 33% ↑ : 35% ↓ : 28%
Perlow et al.,[106] 1992	R	A: 81 C: 130	ND	A: 14.0% C: 3.9%	NA

Abbreviations: PTD = preterm delivery; R = retrospective; P = prospective; P/C = prospective/controlled; A = study group; C = control group; NA = not available; ND = not described; ↑ = improved; ↓ = worsened; ↔ = unchanged

worsening.[57] The variability noted may reflect different methods of monitoring the years of management and the severity of illness in the population studied.

In the largest series, Schatz and colleagues reported 366 pregnancies in 330 prospectively managed patients with asthma.[58] Asthma worsened during pregnancy in 35 percent, improved in 28 percent, and remained unchanged in 33 percent. Asthma appeared to be less severe with less frequent exacerbation in the last trimester. In those women with worsening asthma, there was an increase in symptoms during weeks 29 to 36 of gestation, which is similar to the data of Gluck and Gluck.[56] Only 10 percent of patients had symptoms during delivery, with only half of these requiring therapy during labor (5 percent). During the 3 months postpartum, the course of asthma tended to revert to the prepregnancy state. In contrast, White and colleagues noted

a worsening of asthma in one-third of patients in the postpartum period.[59] In 34 women prospectively studied during two pregnancies, there was a concordance in asthma course in 58.8 percent.[58]

Upper respiratory tract infections appear to be the most common precipitants of worsening asthma.[60] In adolescents, poor compliance is an additional factor associated with exacerbation of asthma during pregnancy.[60]

MANAGEMENT OF ASTHMA

Goals for the management of asthma in pregnant individuals have been well elaborated in a 1993 report.[61] They include the following:

- Maintain near normal pulmonary function
- Control symptoms

Table 18-9

STUDIES DETAILING THE EFFECT OF MATERNAL ASTHMA ON FETAL OUTCOME

| Reference | Fetal/Neonatal | | | | |
	Low Birth Weight, <2500 g	Perinatal Mortality	Apgar Score	Respiratory Distress	Malformation
Schaefer and Silverman,[100] 1961	A: 8.7% C: 6.3%	ND	ND	ND	ND
Gordon et al.,[101] 1970	ND	A: 5.9% C: 3.2%	ND	NA	Neurologic abnormality, 1 year A: 2.7% C: 1.7% Asthma A: 5.7% C: 0.8%
Bahna and Bjerkedal,[53] 1972	NA	Neonatal: A: 18.5% C: 8.0%	NA	NA	ND
Gluck and Gluck,[56] 1976	NA	NA	NA	NA	NA
Dombrowski et al.,[102] 1986	ND	ND	ND	ND	ND
Fitzsimons et al.,[103] 1986	↑ In those hospitalized with asthma during pregnancy	ND	ND	ND	ND
Lao and Huengsburg,[105] 1990	A: 10.3% C: 1.1%	ND	ND	ND	ND
Perlow et al.,[106] 1992	A: 25.9% C: 4.6%	ND	ND	A: 28.5% C: 4.6%	ND

Abbreviations: A = study group; C = control group; ND = not described; NA = not available.

- Maintain near normal activity levels
- Prevent acute exacerbations
- Avoid adverse effects of medication
- Give birth to a healthy baby.

To achieve these goals, individuals caring for these patients need to understand the role of appropriate monitoring of airway function, the risk-benefit of the various medications available, and the potential role of nonpharmacologic therapy.

Monitoring of Airway Function

The routine monitoring of airway function has been widely accepted as standard care in the management of patients with chronic asthma.[62] The support for this relates in large part to the well-known difficulty by both patients and physicians in predicting severity of airflow obstruction. In an investigation of 22 patients undergoing therapy for an exacerbation of asthma, patients noted resolution of symptoms despite an increase in FEV_1 from 30 percent to only 49 percent of predicted. In the same study, physical signs had resolved when the FEV_1 had risen to 63 percent predicted.[63] Significant airflow obstruction persisted despite improvement in clinical parameters. More recently, emergency physicians estimated pulmonary function in adult asthmatics during an exacerbation prior to spirometry. Pulmonary function was underestimated by an average of 8.1 percent, while knowledge of pulmonary function altered management in 20.4 percent of patients.[64]

Outpatient studies have examined the role of home monitoring of pulmonary function using a simple hand-held peak flow meter. These instruments can reliably estimate pulmonary function during a maximal expiratory maneuver. Beasley and colleagues used such a device to develop a management plan individualized for patients with asthma,[65] improving the outpatient care of these individuals. A larger prospective trial comparing symptom-based self-management plans with a peak expiratory flow–based self-management plan has recently been published.[66] No major difference was noted between the two groups, suggesting that peak flow monitoring may not be routinely needed. Those patients with more severe asthma, however, did appear to fare better with objective measurement of pulmonary function.

Pregnant individuals frequently experience dyspnea during later pregnancy (see above). In these subjects, the routine measurement of pulmonary function could serve to better judge the status of airflow in the face of increasing symptoms. Therefore peak flow monitoring would be expected to improve the management of asthma in such patients. No prospective studies examining this topic are available, however. It has been suggested that 20 to 30 percent of pregnant asthmatics should routinely use peak flow meters throughout pregnancy.[67]

For a typical approach, the patient measures peak expiratory flow rate (PEFR) with a hand-held meter in the morning and evening over a 2-week period and establishes a personal best reading at a time of clinical stability. The level of subsequent peak flows can be used to gauge asthma severity using a zone system.[62,67] In the green zone, there are few asthma symptoms and the peak flows are between 80 and 100 percent of the personal best, with little variation between the morning and evening values (<20 percent). The yellow zone indicates worsening asthma and is associated with 50 to 80 percent of personal best PEFR and a 20 to 30 percent variability between morning and evening values. The red zone is signaled by a PEFR <50 percent of personal best and a >30 percent variability between morning and evening values. This grading of asthma severity has been used to guide a "stepped care" approach to asthma therapy, which is described below.

Fetal Monitoring

Monitoring fetal well-being is as important as monitoring airflow in the mother. This is particularly so in those individuals with greater lability and difficult-to-control symptoms. It is these pregnancies that are most likely to be associated with fetal morbidity. Fetal monitoring should include an accurate determination of gestational age and periodic assessment of fetal growth/activity. It should begin with careful serial measurement of fundal height but should include sonography in poorly controlled asthma or if fetal growth retardation is suspected.[61] If there is an acute exacerbation of asthma, particularly if the condition is poorly responsive to therapy, fetal monitoring should be intensified, including continuous electronic fetal heart monitoring.[61]

Pharmacologic Management

Risk-Benefit Assessment for Commonly Used Drugs

Given the dramatic physiologic changes encountered in pregnancy and the rapid growth and development of the fetus, it is not surprising that much concern is given to possible harmful interactions of agents used to manage asthma. Few controlled studies are available to clearly describe the risk of the many agents available for use in the pregnant mother. Therefore, it is always best to guide pharmacologic therapy by using those agents with documented efficacy and the best safety in animal and human gestational studies. In addition, drugs administered by the inhalational route should achieve lower systemic concentrations in the mother and fetus. Finally, older medications may be safer, as they are more likely to be associated with greater experience for use in pregnancy.[61]

Table 18-10 presents safety data for commonly used drugs in asthma. The FDA uses an alphabetical grading system for drugs based on available animal and human studies as well as an assessment of benefit to risk. In this way category A drugs have negative animal and human studies with a clearly favorable risk-to-benefit ratio. Category B drugs have either negative animal studies and no human studies, or positive animal studies but negative human studies. These drugs also have a favorable risk-to-benefit ratio. Category C drugs have either positive animal studies with little human data or no animal or human data. These agents may have a favorable risk-to-benefit ratio in the appropriate clinical setting. Category D drugs have either positive or negative animal studies but positive human data. These agents may have a role in very select clinical settings. Category X drugs are contraindicated in pregnancy. The FDA categories are not perfect and decisions to use a drug during pregnancy should be based on risk/benefit and not drug category.

It is evident from the review of this table that many medications may have a favorable risk/benefit profile in the appropriate clinical setting. The optimal beta$_2$ agonist would appear to be terbutaline, although the other selective beta$_2$ agonists are probably similar.[68] The optimal inhaled glucocorticoid is clearly beclomethasone. Cromolyn would be an appropriate alternative anti-inflammatory agent in milder disease, while theophylline therapy should be reserved for patients not adequately controlled with beclomethasone, cromolyn, and inhaled beta$_2$ agonists.

Step-Care Approach To Asthma Management

Over the last 15 years, knowledge of the pathogenesis of asthma has grown steadily. Understanding the importance of airway inflammation has revolutionized management, with much greater emphasis on anti-inflammatory therapy earlier in disease. Most experts currently emphasize a stepped-care approach to therapy, which is individualized to disease severity and symptoms.[61,62] Figs. 18-7 through 18-

Table 18-10

RISK-BENEFIT DESCRIPTION OF COMMONLY USED DRUGS IN THE MANAGEMENT OF ASTHMA

Agent	Human Congenital Malformation and Reference Numbers	Additional Data and Reference Numbers	FDA Class
Selective beta$_2$ agonists			
Metaproterenol	—	May inhibit labor[114]	C
Albuterol	—	May inhibit labor[114]	C
Terbutaline	—	May inhibit labor[114] Preserves placental blood flow[114]	B
Pirbuterol	—	—	C
Bitolterol	—	—	C
Nonselective beta$_2$ agonists			
Epinephrine	Positive[110]	Reduced placental blood flow in animals; may inhibit labor[114]	—
Isoproterenol	No association	—	—
Anticholinergic agents			
Ipratropium	None[61,110]	—	—
Nonsteroidal anti-inflammatory agents			
Cromolyn	None[111]	—	B
Nedocromil	—	—	—
Inhaled steroids			
Beclomethasone	None[103,112]	Slight increase in low birth weight and premature delivery[103]	C
Triamcinolone	Fetal growth retardation in one case[113]	Extensive positive animal data[61]	D
Flusinolide	—	—	C
Fluticasone			
Systemic steroids	None[110,114]	Low birth weight in one series[118] but not in another[119]	—
Theophylline	None[110,115–117]	May inhibit labor[114]; theophylline intoxication in newborns particularly with blood levels >12 g/mL[61]	C

11 illustrate an approach to such stepped management based on symptoms and pulmonary function.

In each category, a short-acting beta agonist is available to all patients for use in the setting of acute symptoms. Medications are added as symptoms (particularly nocturnal) increase and as pulmonary function level and/or lability increases. Emphasis is placed on increasing anti-inflammatory medications. In addition, as the patient improves, decreasing use of medication is also encouraged.

Acute exacerbations must be quickly identified and managed. Monitoring remains important to assess severity of illness. Figs. 18-10 and 18-11 illustrate an approach for the management of an acute exacerbation at home (Fig. 18-10) or in the emergency department (Fig. 18-11). The role of rescue beta agonists is clear. Patient education is vital to the appropriate management of individuals during exacerbations.[65] Anti-inflammatory therapy including glucocorticoid therapy should be routinely used as the severity of an exacerbation increases. Aminophylline use remains very controversial, although it is likely that benefits will not outweigh risk.[57] Furthermore, although the loading dose is no different during pregnancy, the maintenance regimen should be more conservative, as clearance may be altered.[57]

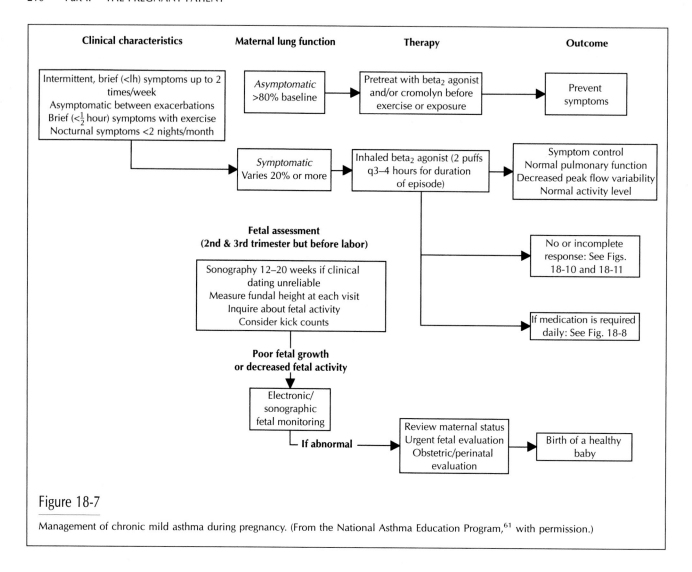

Figure 18-7

Management of chronic mild asthma during pregnancy. (From the National Asthma Education Program,[61] with permission.)

A high index of suspicion must be maintained for the etiology of the exacerbation, including respiratory infections[60] and poor compliance with a chronic medication regimen.[60] Bacterial sinusitis, a well-known cause of asthma exacerbation, has been estimated to be six times more common in pregnant than in nonpregnant patients.

Obstetric Management In The Setting Of Asthma

Most of the principles described for chronic management apply to the pregnant asthmatic during labor. The patient's regularly scheduled medications should be continued during labor and delivery. Figs. 18-12 and 18-13 illustrate the recommended approach to initial assessment and management.[61] Clearly, careful fetal management is crucial to ensure a good outcome. Approximately 10 percent of asthmatics experience an asthma exacerbation during labor.[58]

Oxytocin is the drug of choice for postpartum hemorrhage management in the asthmatic, as both 15-methyl prosta-

glandin $F_{2\alpha}$ and E_2 have been reported to cause bronchoconstriction.[57,67] Recent preliminary data have suggested that prostaglandin E_2 can be used safely in asthmatic women, although more data are required before establishing safety in this setting. During an asthma exacerbation, it is not unusual to experience uterine contractions, although they usually do not progress with successful treatment of the exacerbations.[61] In preterm labor, a beta agonist or magnesium sulfate can be used as a tocolytic agent. In those individuals using systemic beta agonists for preterm labor, the use of two beta agonists should be avoided. In these individuals, magnesium sulfate may be a better choice, possibly adding additional bronchodilation.[69]

For postpartum hemorrhage, oxytocin is the drug of choice, for reasons similar to those stated in the previous paragraph. Methylergonovine and ergonovine may cause bronchospasm and should be avoided.[57] Prostaglandin E_2 may be used with the same caveat discussed earlier. For analgesia, morphine and meperidine should be avoided, as they may potentially cause histamine release, which could precipitate bronchospasm. The preferred agent may be fen-

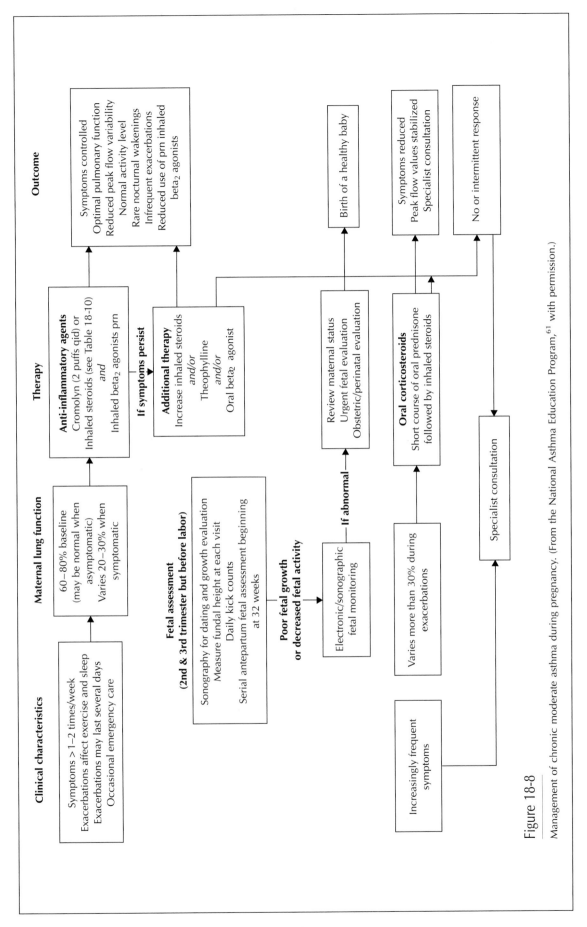

Figure 18-8

Management of chronic moderate asthma during pregnancy. (From the National Asthma Education Program,[61] with permission.)

211

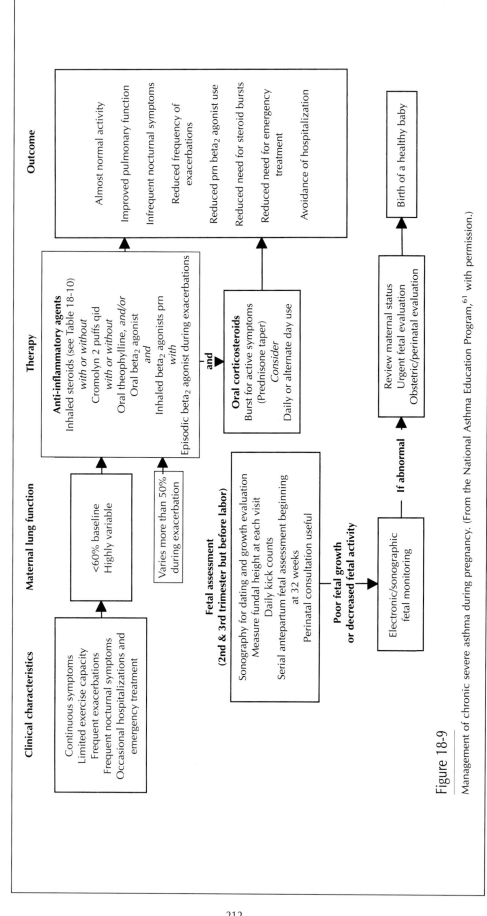

Clinical characteristics

Continuous symptoms
Limited exercise capacity
Frequent exacerbations
Frequent nocturnal symptoms
Occasional hospitalizations and
emergency treatment

Maternal lung function

<60% baseline
Highly variable

Varies more than 50%
during exacerbation

Therapy

Anti-inflammatory agents
Inhaled steroids (see Table 18-10)
with or without
Cromolyn 2 puffs qid
with or without
Oral theophylline, *and/or*
Oral beta$_2$ agonist
and
Inhaled beta$_2$ agonists prn
with
Episodic beta$_2$ agonist during exacerbations

and

Oral corticosteroids
Burst for active symptoms
(Prednisone taper)
Consider
Daily or alternate day use

Fetal assessment
(2nd & 3rd trimester but before labor)

Sonography for dating and growth evaluation
Measure fundal height at each visit
Daily kick counts
Serial antepartum fetal assessment beginning
at 32 weeks
Perinatal consultation useful

**Poor fetal growth
or decreased fetal activity**

Electronic/sonographic
fetal monitoring

If abnormal

Review maternal status
Urgent fetal evaluation
Obstetric/perinatal evaluation

Outcome

Almost normal activity

Improved pulmonary function

Infrequent nocturnal symptoms

Reduced frequency of
exacerbations

Reduced prn beta$_2$ agonist use

Reduced need for steroid bursts

Reduced need for emergency
treatment

Avoidance of hospitalization

Birth of a healthy baby

Figure 18-9

Management of chronic severe asthma during pregnancy. (From the National Asthma Education Program,[61] with permission.)

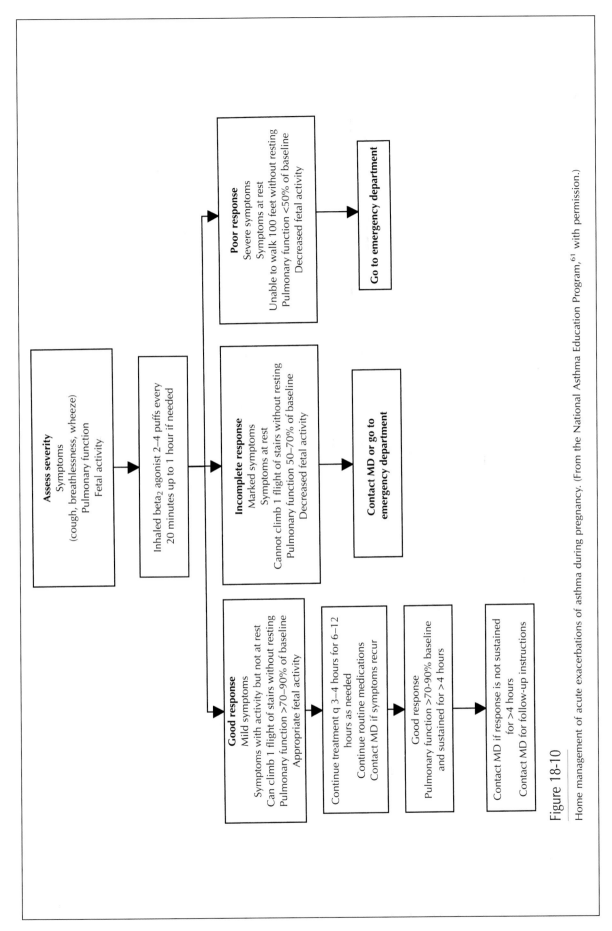

Figure 18-10

Home management of acute exacerbations of asthma during pregnancy. (From the National Asthma Education Program,[61] with permission.)

213

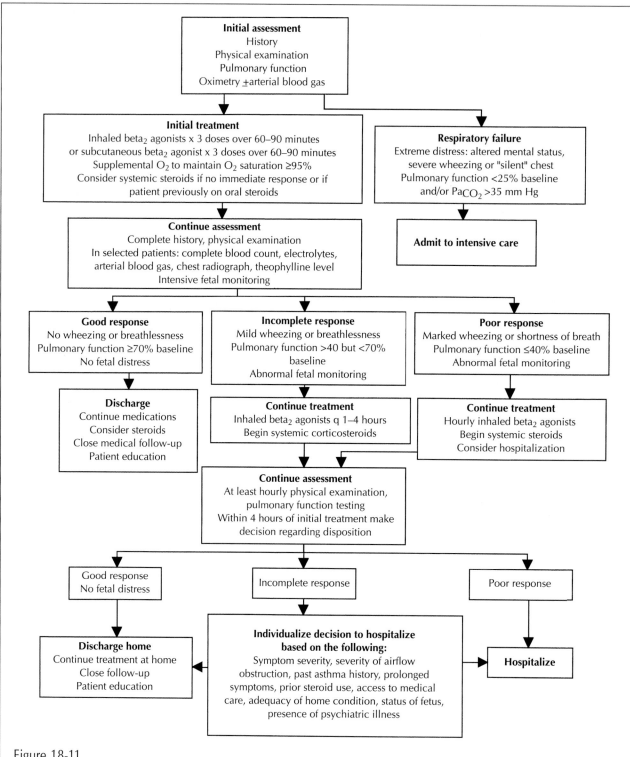

Figure 18-11

Emergency department management of acute exacerbation of asthma during pregnancy. (From the National Asthma Education Program,[61] with permission.)

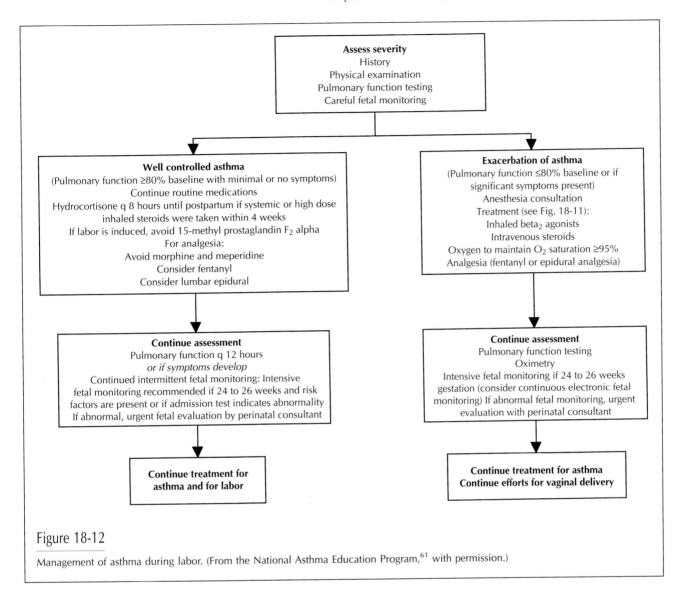

Figure 18-12

Management of asthma during labor. (From the National Asthma Education Program,[61] with permission.)

tanyl.[61] Narcotic analgesics may be associated with respiratory depression and should be avoided if there is a concomitant asthma exacerbation.[61] Lumbar epidural analgesia may be the preferred technique and may enhance the response to bronchodilator therapy. It should be noted, however, that bronchospasm has been reported in 2 percent of patients with asthma receiving regional anesthesia.[70] If general anesthesia is required, ketamine is the preferred agent, while low concentrations of halogenated anesthetics may provide additional bronchodilation but may also increase the risk of postpartum hemorrhage.[61] Preanesthetic use of anticholinergic agents may provide a bronchodilatory effect.

Nonpharmacologic Management

It is vital to identify and avoid potential triggering factors. This would include potential specific allergens or irritants such as cigarette smoke.[57,62] Routine skin testing is not rec-

ommended, as skin testing can be associated with systemic reactions.[57] In fact, abortions have been reported with systemic reactions during allergen immunotherapy. Maintenance immunotherapy has been reported to be safe[71] and can be continued during pregnancy with careful monitoring in those individuals who appear to be deriving benefit and are not prone to systemic reactions.[57] It is probably not wise to begin immunotherapy during pregnancy, in large part due to the risk of systemic reactions.[57]

The most important aspect of nonpharmacologic management is extensive education. Pregnant asthmatics should be instructed that no medicine can be considered *absolutely safe* during pregnancy. On the other hand, the overriding importance of well-controlled asthma must be emphasized; therefore medications (most of which appear to be safe) are preferable to uncontrolled symptoms. The rationale for choosing particular agents must be explained, as well as the development of written treatment plans based on symptoms

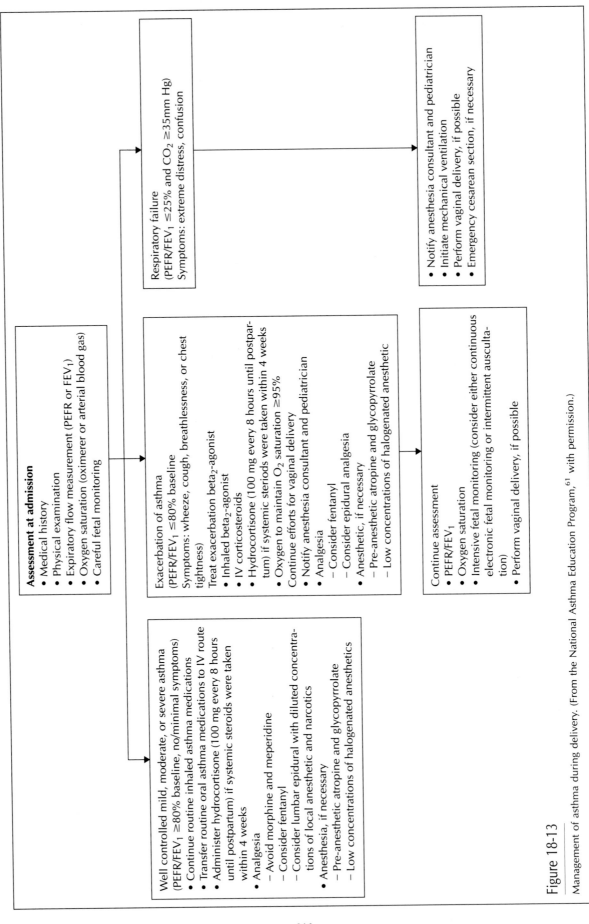

Assessment at admission
• Medical history
• Physical examination
• Expiratory flow measurement (PEFR or FEV_1)
• Oxygen saturation (oximerer or arterial blood gas)
• Careful fetal monitoring

Well controlled mild, moderate, or severe asthma
(PEFR/FEV_1 ≥80% baseline, no/minimal symptoms)
• Continue routine inhaled asthma medications
• Transfer routine oral asthma medications to IV route
• Administer hydrocortisone (100 mg every 8 hours
  until postpartum) if systemic steroids were taken
  within 4 weeks
• Analgesia
  – Avoid morphine and meperidine
  – Consider fentanyl
  – Consider lumbar epidural with diluted concentra-
    tions of local anesthetic and narcotics
• Anesthesia, if necessary
  – Pre-anesthetic atropine and glycopyrrolate
  – Low concentrations of halogenated anesthetics

Exacerbation of asthma
(PEFR/FEV_1 ≤80% baseline
Symptoms: wheeze, cough, breathlessness, or chest
tightness)
Treat exacerbation beta₂-agonist
• Inhaled beta₂-agonist
• IV corticosteroids
• Hydrocortisone (100 mg every 8 hours until postpar-
  tum) if systemic steroids were taken within 4 weeks
• Oxygen to maintain O_2 saturation ≥95%
Continue efforts for vaginal delivery
• Notify anesthesia consultant and pediatrician
• Analgesia
  – Consider fentanyl
  – Consider epidural analgesia
• Anesthetic, if necessary
  – Pre-anesthetic atropine and glycopyrrolate
  – Low concentrations of halogenated anesthetic

Continue assessment
• PEFR/FEV_1
• Oxygen saturation
• Intensive fetal monitoring (consider either continuous
  electronic fetal monitoring or intermittent ausculta-
  tion)
• Perform vaginal delivery, if possible

Respiratory failure
(PEFR/FEV_1 ≤25% and CO_2 ≥35mm Hg)
Symptoms: extreme distress, confusion

• Notify anesthesia consultant and pediatrician
• Initiate mechanical ventilation
• Perform vaginal delivery, if possible
• Emergency cesarean section, if necessary

Figure 18-13

Management of asthma during delivery. (From the National Asthma Education Program,[61] with permission.)

and home pulmonary function in appropriate patients. For medicolegal reasons it is most important to clearly document, in the medical record, that these discussions have taken place and the patient appears to understand the recommendations and home treatment plans. In this way a successful outcome for the management of asthma during pregnancy can be assured.

CYSTIC FIBROSIS

Cystic fibrosis (CF) is an inherited disorder that is transmitted as an autosomal recessive trait and involves epithelial tissues of the pancreas, sweat glands, and mucous glands as well as the exocrine glands. The lung and pancreas are the principal organs affected, with chronic infection of the airways, bronchiectasis, airflow obstruction, and malabsorption, resulting in typical clinical manifestations. Progressive bronchopulmonary disease is the major cause of morbidity and mortality. Approximately 4 percent of the Caucasian population in the United States are heterozygous carriers, with disease occurring in 1 of 3000 live white births.[72]

The severity of clinical disease varies with the extent of organ involvement. Progressive bronchopulmonary involvement is characterized by recurrent infections and increasing chronic airflow obstruction. Cough and dyspnea are commonly seen. Pancreatic involvement is progressive, with resulting exocrine insufficiency and malabsorption. The maldigestion of fats results in major nutritional deficiency. Diabetes mellitus can be seen as a late complication of cystic fibrosis. Several indexes of severity are in clinical use[73,74]; these incorporate general clinical activity (e.g., dyspnea), physical findings, nutritional status, radiographic findings in the grading scheme of Shwachman and Kulczycki,[73] and pulmonary function, chest radiographic abnormality, pulmonary complications, and psychological/behavioral parameters in the Taussig score.[74] The chest radiographic scoring system of Brasfield et al. grades the extent of chest radiographic abnormality.[75]

Improved care and earlier diagnosis over the past decade has progressively improved survival, such that the life expectancy of 1 year in the 1940s has risen to 29 years today. As such, more than one-third of patients are over the age of 16.[72] Because of morphologic abnormalities in the reproductive tract of males with CF, obstructive azoospermia is seen in 95 percent of these patients. On the other hand, women with CF have anatomically normal reproductive tracts. Fertility has not been systematically studied but is probably reduced[72] because of alterations in the properties of cervical mucus in these patients. Despite this, multiple cases and several large series confirm that pregnancy can be seen in a significant proportion of women with CF. Thus patients in their reproductive years need appropriate counseling, and those wishing to avoid pregnancy should use appropriate contraception.

Pregnancy in CF was first documented in the 1960s with 13 pregnancies in 10 patients reported in 1966.[76] Since that time, as the diagnosis has been made earlier and more women have reached reproductive age, the numbers of reported pregnancies has steadily risen. The Cystic Fibrosis Registry reported 32 to 62 pregnancies per year from 1966 to 1988 and 71 to 101 per year from 1990 to 1994.[76] Initial reports suggested marked morbidity associated with pregnancy in CF, although more recent reports suggest improved outcomes.[76]

PHYSIOLOGIC STRESSES OF CYSTIC FIBROSIS

The expected physiologic stress of pregnancy on the pulmonary system was detailed in an earlier section. The stress of these changes in individuals with compromised respiratory status is not surprising. The increased ventilation and widening of the alveolar-arterial Pa_{O_2} gradient would be expected to increased the workload placed on the compromised respiratory system and contribute to respiratory decompensation and hypoxemia.

The increased blood volume and cardiac output usually seen with pregnancy could potentially affect those CF patients with advanced pulmonary disease and limited pulmonary vascular reserve. This would be particularly problematic in patients with clinical pulmonary hypertension. The increased venous return seen during and immediately after delivery would pose particular risk.

With pregnancy there are clear nutritional requirements, estimated at 300 kcal/day, to meet the energy requirement of the fetus and mother.[77] A weight gain of at least 11.5 kg is suggested during pregnancy for normal fetal growth in patients with a normal pregravid weight. In underweight individuals (<90 percent ideal body weight), a weight gain of at least 12.5 kg is recommended.[76] The high frequency of pancreatic exocrine insufficiency and associated malabsorption makes this difficult in CF patients. Furthermore, the excessive energy requirements associated with the increased work of breathing and chronic infection will compound nutritional problems in these patients.

EPIDEMIOLOGY

Effect of Pregnancy on the Course of Cystic Fibrosis

Early reports suggested a high rate of maternal morbidity and mortality associated with pregnancy in CF, including deaths from cor pulmonale in the immediate postpartum period. Early investigators recommend that patients with pulmonary involvement and hypoxemia be advised against pregnancy, while in those with progressive pulmonary deterioration and hypoxemia during pregnancy therapeutic abortion was recommended. Larsen suggested that a vital capacity <50 percent of predicted or the presence of pulmonary hypertension and cor pulmonale should be considered an additional indication for termination of pregnancy.[78]

More recent reports suggest a better outcome for pregnancy in CF,[76] which may represent the higher proportion of patients with milder disease achieving successful pregnancy. In a large survey of CF centers in the United States and Canada, Cohen et al. reported 129 pregnancies in 100 women with CF.[79] Twelve percent died within 6 months of delivery, and these individuals were all noted to have severe pregravid pulmonary disease with further decline during pregnancy. These authors recommended avoiding pregnancy in individuals with a Shwachman or Taussig score <80. Palmer et al. compared the course of eight women during 11 pregnancies.[79a] In five, little change in maternal status occurred (group 1) while in three irreversible deterioration occurred (group 2). Four maternal characteristics distinguished the two groups: Shwachman score, nutritional status, pulmonary function, and chest radiographic score (Brasfield score). Those in group 1 had Shwachman scores above 65 (compared to all <59 in group 2), weight-to-height ratios above 86 percent of normal expected (versus all <74 percent in group 2), much less abnormal chest radiographs (all >14 in group 1 while all <5 in group 2), and better pulmonary function (FVC >78 percent in all of group 1 versus all <37 percent predicted in group 2). Kent and Farquaharson noted a poor outcome associated with a weight gain <4.5 kg and FVC <50 percent predicted.[80] Edenborough et al. retrospectively analyzed 22 pregnancies in 20 patients with CF.[81] Serial pulmonary function testing demonstrated a mean 13 percent drop in FEV_1 and an 11 percent drop in FVC during pregnancy. Much of this was recovered after delivery. Those patients with a pregravid FEV_1 <60 percent predicted more often produced preterm infants and had an increased loss of lung function. The four maternal deaths (0.5 to 3.2 years after pregnancy) occurred in patients with an FEV_1 <50 percent predicted. Of importance, two women with severe pulmonary dysfunction (FEV_1 28 percent and 32 percent predicted) successfully completed pregnancies. Percent of predicted FEV_1 was the single best predictor of maternal and fetal outcome.

Corkey et al. suggested a better outcome during pregnancy in individuals with CF but preserved pancreatic function, although the small number in the series limited the strength of the conclusion.[81a] In conclusion, pulmonary hypertension would serve as an absolute contraindication to pregnancy in women with CF, while an FVC <50 percent predicted identifies a group at particularly high risk. If the patient is otherwise stable, pregnancy may be possible with close observation.

Effect of Cystic Fibrosis on the Course of Pregnancy

Earlier studies suggested a high incidence of premature delivery and perinatal mortality. More recently, data from the CF Foundation Registry have allowed formulation of clearer guidelines. Kotloff et al., in examining the registry database for 1990, confirmed a worse fetal outcome (premature delivery and need for therapeutic abortion) in cases with more severe maternal pulmonary dysfunction.[72] Hilman et al. reported a 17.2 to 34.3 percent rate of abortions and a zero to

10.1 percent incidence of stillbirths during the period of 1990 to 1994.[76] Edenborough et al. confirmed a linear relation between higher pregravid FEV_1 of percent predicted and a higher birth weight ($r = 0.78$, $p < .001$) and longer duration of pregnancy ($r = 0.77$, $p < .001$).[81] Of interest, percent of ideal body weight did not correlate with these outcomes. Clearly fetal outcome is strongly related to the severity of pregravid disease in the mother and the course of pulmonary function during pregnancy.

MANAGEMENT OF THE CYSTIC FIBROSIS PATIENT DURING PREGNANCY

The improving outcome of pregnancy in CF patients likely reflects in part the comprehensive management of these individuals. A coordinated team with knowledge of CF and the stress of pregnancy is necessary to ensure optimal outcomes. As respiratory status is closely related to pregnancy outcome, aggressive follow-up and management of respiratory disease are necessary during pregnancy. Appropriate prepregnancy evaluation is ideal and should include objective measurement of pulmonary function (spirometry and lung volumes) and gas exchange [arterial blood gas (ABG)]. Monitoring of pulmonary function periodically through the course of pregnancy is recommended and should include grading of subjective dyspnea and objective measurement of pulmonary function (spirometry, pulse oximetry, and ABGs if clinically indicated). Routine respiratory management should include postural drainage and exercise to mobilize secretions. Management of bronchospasm shares many similarities to that of asthma during pregnancy (see above). Bronchodilators and anti-inflammatory medications should be utilized as clinically indicated. As in asthmatic patients, optimal airway function should take priority to the theoretical, small risk of these medications. Similarly, oxygen therapy should be utilized freely, as the fetus is intolerant of even minor degrees of maternal hypoxia.

At the first sign of an exacerbation (as signaled by increased cough or dyspnea and worsened pulmonary function or weight loss) aggressive management is mandated. This should include the appropriate use of antibiotics, ideally guided by sputum microbiologic analysis. Antibiotic safety in pregnancy was described in an earlier section, and these principles apply to pregnant CF patients. Several differences must be noted, however. The pharmacokinetics of multiple antibiotics are altered in patients with CF. Beta-lactam antibiotics are cleared more rapidly in patients with CF.[76] The volume of distribution and the rate of clearance of aminoglycosides are also increased in CF patients. As such, higher doses of aminoglycosides and close monitoring of blood drug levels is necessary to assure optimal drug dosing.

Careful attention to nutritional status has been highlighted earlier. At each office visit, the history of caloric intake and symptoms of malabsorption should be sought. Pancreatic enzyme supplementation should be optimized. For those unable to meet nutritional goals, caloric supplementation should be considered. This may include oral supplements or, in more severe cases, nasogastric feedings or parenteral hyperalimentation.[72,76]

Given its cardiovascular stress, close clinical evaluation of hemodynamic status is necessary during the course of pregnancy. This is particularly important in those individuals with more severe pulmonary disease who have a greater limitation in pulmonary vascular reserve. Monitoring of blood pressure, pulse, weight, and edema is mandatory at routine office visits. During delivery and in the immediate postpartum period, additional monitoring is required. The presence of ventricular dysfunction mandates aggressive diuresis and appropriate oxygen administration. A pulmonary artery catheter may aid in optimizing hemodynamics. Inhalational anesthetics that increase pulmonary vascular tone should be avoided in those patients requiring general anesthesia during cesarean section.

COUNSELING OF THE CYSTIC FIBROSIS PATIENT

Counseling of women with CF is an important aspect of their general care. Given the unknown percentage of women with CF who are fertile, it is essential that all patients who wish to avoid pregnancy utilize appropriate contraception. Those wishing to conceive should undergo careful prepregnancy assessment to identify high-risk groups. This evaluation should include Shwachman clinical testing, pulmonary function testing, arterial blood gas measurement, and estimation of nutritional status. Those individuals with pulmonary hypertension, severe hypoxemia, severe airflow obstruction, and marked malnutrition place themselves and the fetus at unacceptable risk and should avoid pregnancy.[72] Patients with severe pulmonary dysfunction (FVC <50 percent predicted) may successfully complete pregnancy if they are otherwise stable. Therapeutic abortion should be considered in the setting of right heart failure, refractory hypoxemia, progressive deterioration in pulmonary function, and progressive hypercapnia with respiratory acidosis.[72]

Genetic counseling should be offered to all women contemplating pregnancy. When the father is a Caucasian who is unaffected, the risk of CF in the offspring is 1 in 50. If the father is a carrier, the risk is 1 in 2. The recent improvements in DNA testing for the chromosomal mutation in CF has improved the ability to provide genetic counseling in this setting. More than 450 mutations of the CF gene have been identified. Current commercial testing is available for up to 90 percent of the reported chromosomal abnormalities.[76] If the DNA screen of the father is negative, the risk of CF in the child is 1 in 492.[82]

CONCLUSION

The accumulated clinical experience suggests that many women with CF can successfully complete pregnancy with few fetal complications. High-risk groups can be identified, improving the ability to counsel women with CF during their childbearing years. Aggressive management during the course of pregnancy can minimize the risk to the mother and ensure optimal fetal outcome.

RESTRICTIVE DISEASES

The physiologic changes noted during pregnancy should exacerbate symptoms in patients with restrictive disease. These disorders are characterized by a decrease in lung volumes (TLC) but preserved airflow (normal or increased FEV_1/FVC) unless superimposed airflow obstruction is present. They include parenchymal inflammatory or fibrotic disorders, pleural diseases, and chest wall or extrathoracic abnormalities. These disorders are unusual and there have been few systematic studies of their effect on or change during pregnancy. Anecdotal reports and small series allow some conclusions and recommendations to be made.

FIBROTIC DISORDERS

SARCOIDOSIS

Sarcoidosis is a multisystem disease of unknown etiology characterized by noncaseating granulomas in a perivascular pattern. The disease affects young adults and involves the lung, peripheral lymph nodes, skin, eyes, and liver most commonly. The clinical manifestations are highly variable, although most commonly an asymptomatic patient presents with an abnormal chest radiograph. The most common clinical symptoms reflect lung involvement and include dyspnea, cough, and chest pain. The classic chest radiographic pattern reveals bilateral hilar adenopathy with or without parenchymal infiltration. The diagnosis is made in the appropriate clinical setting with identification of noncaseating granulomata in tissue samples.

Sarcoidosis does not appear to increase fetal or obstetric complications.[83] The management of pregnancy in patients with sarcoidosis is not generally altered; neither, as a rule, is course of disease,[84] with the majority of patients remaining unchanged or improving. Haynes de Regt described factors that identify "high risk" individuals, including advanced maternal age, parenchymal infiltration/fibrosis on chest radiography, low inflammatory activity, chronic (persistent) sarcoidosis with an insidious onset, and extrapulmonary disease.[85] These individuals should be followed closely through pregnancy and for at least 6 months after delivery, as late-onset disease progression has been reported.[83] The indications for treatment in pregnant women are similar to those in the management of the nonpregnant individual, with prednisone remaining the anti-inflammatory agent of choice.[84]

PULMONARY FIBROSIS

Idiopathic pulmonary fibrosis is a parenchymal lung disease that usually presents in middle age and rarely in women of childbearing age. The clinical manifestations are usually dyspnea on exertion and cough with "Velcro-type" rales on inspiration and digital clubbing. The chest radiograph typically reveals diffuse parenchymal linear infiltrates, while pulmonary function testing confirms restriction and a decreased diffusing capacity. The diagnosis is made by open lung biopsy and disease is treated with prednisone and/or cytotoxic therapy.[84] Few cases of pulmonary fibrosis in pregnancy have been reported, although successful completion of pregnancy has been reported despite severe disease.[84] Close evaluation during and after pregnancy is crucial, as the clinical condition can deteriorate during pregnancy.

EOSINOPHILIC GRANULOMA

Eosinophilic granuloma (EG) or histiocytosis X is an idiopathic granulomatous disease that usually occurs in young adults (ages 20 to 40) who are smokers or former smokers. The disease is more common in men, with the clinical presentation being widely variable.[84] Cough, dyspnea, and chest pain are the most frequent symptoms, while the chest radiograph varies depending on the stage of disease.[84] The typical radiographic presentation includes ill-defined stellate nodules, reticular infiltrates, upper zone predominance, and preservation of lung volumes. Pulmonary fibrosis may document restriction, obstruction, or normal findings. The diagnosis is usually made by examination of involved tissue. Some patients remain asymptomatic or spontaneously improve, although many suffer from persistent or progressive disease.

Many cases of females of childbearing age have been included in series of EG. Some have specifically reported cases of pregnancy in patients with EG, with the course usually remaining unchanged.[84] Most reported cases have complicated systemic histiocytosis X with no apparent effect on pregnancy outcome.[84] In some patients, diabetes insipidus has developed or worsened, requiring specific therapy.[84] Therefore close evaluation and follow-up is required during the course of therapy.

LYMPHANGIOLEIOMYOMATOSIS

Lymphangioleiomyomatosis (LAM) is an idiopathic disorder that classically presents in women of childbearing age.[84,86] It rarely presents after menopause unless estrogen supplementation has been regularly prescribed.[86] Typical symptoms include progressive dyspnea on exertion, cough, chest pain, and hemoptysis. The chest radiograph usually reveals reticulonodular infiltrates with normal or increased lung volumes. Pneumothorax and chylous pleural effusions are frequently noted. Chest computed tomography usually reveals typical changes of multiple thin-walled cysts throughout the lungs. Some consider these changes extremely suggestive. This is one of few pulmonary disorders with interstitial lung disease by chest radiograph but obstruction or mixed obstruction/restriction on pulmonary function testing.[84] As the lung is affected in all cases, biopsy of this organ is the most common method of confirming a histologic diagnosis. The etiology is unclear, although some have suggested a role for estrogen and progesterone stimulation.[84]

Initial reports suggested a dismal prognosis, although more recent reports point to a more favorable outcome. Taylor and colleagues reported that 78 percent of 32 patients were still living a mean of 8.5 years after the onset of disease.[86] Worsening or presentation of disease during pregnancy is well described, although anecdotal reports have described successful pregnancies in patients with LAM.[84] Most women are advised to avoid pregnancy and the use of estrogen in the setting of LAM.[87] Metaanalysis of reported therapy suggests that treatment with progesterone and/or oophorectomy can arrest disease progression in 50 percent of patients.[87] The optimal approach to treatment during pregnancy is unclear.[84]

PLEURAL DISEASE

POSTPARTUM PLEURAL EFFUSION

The physiologic conditions of labor and delivery appear favorable for the development of pleural effusions, including an increased blood volume, decreased plasma colloid osmotic pressure, and increased intrathoracic pressure.[88] Numerous authors have assessed the incidence of pleural fluid in pregnancy. These are summarized in Table 18-11. The techniques utilized to identify pleural fluid have ranged from simple upright radiography[89–91] to thoracic ultrasonography.[92–94] This probably explains much of the variation in incidence. The true incidence is difficult to determine accurately, although the frequency is probably small. El-Naggar and colleagues studied 50 patients weekly during the course of pregnancy with thoracic ultrasonography.[94] Six women had small effusions during pregnancy, which persisted into the postpartum period in three. A moderate-to-large effusion or the presence of signs or symptoms of a complicating illness should prompt further evaluation.[94] In the presence of preeclampsia, the presence of an effusion has been associated with a tenfold higher perinatal fetal mortality, apparently secondary to premature labor and delivery and a shorter gestation.[93]

PNEUMOTHORAX/PNEUMOMEDIASTINUM

Spontaneous pneumothorax is the sudden collapse of a lung in an otherwise healthy person. Although it occurs more frequently in young men, it is occasionally seen in women. It should be suspected in the patient between 20 and 40 years of age with sudden pleuritic chest pain associated with mild to moderate dyspnea.[95] The physiologic alterations of preg-

Table 18-11

STUDIES DESCRIBING PLEURAL EFFUSIONS IN THE PREGNANT WOMAN

Study	Diagnostic Technique	Number of Patients	Route of Delivery		Date Examined Postpartum, Days	Pleural Effusion			
			Cesarean Section	Vaginal		Unilateral	Bilateral	Total (percent)	Volume
El Naggar et al.,[94] 1994	Decubitus CXR	92	—	—	7 to >12	10/92	11/92	21/92 (22.8)	Small 21/21
Wallis et al.,[93] 1989	Upright CXR	142	—	—	≤1	22/142	49/142	71/142 (50.0)	Small 66/142; Moderate 5/142
Udeshi et al.,[92] 1988	Upright CXR	45	35	10	≤2	—	—	44/45 (97.8)	Small 44/45
Stark and Pollack,[91] 1986	Thoracic US	50	21	29	<2	1/50	0/50	1/50 (2.0)	Small 1/50
Hughson et al.,[90] 1982	Thoracic US	34	30	4	<1	—	—	9/34 (26.5)	—
Hessen,[89] 1951	Thoracic US	50	0	50	Weekly during pregnancy and <1	—	—	6/50 (12.0)	Small 6/50

Abbreviations: CXR = chest radiograph; US = ultrasound.

nancy lead to increased minute ventilation and repeated Valsalva maneuvers during labor and delivery, creating an excellent setting for a pneumothorax. Given the frequency of breathlessness during pregnancy, diagnosis can be difficult. A chest radiograph is associated with minimal fetal risk and should be considered when symptoms are acute or moderate in severity.[95]

Van Winter and colleagues recently detailed a literature survey of pneumothorax during pregnancy reported between 1957 and 1996.[96] Twenty-three cases were noted, with 21 occurring in the first (18 of 23) or second (3 of 23) trimesters. Risk factors were seen in 9 of 23 patients, most commonly an acute respiratory infection or a history of chronic lung disease. A prior history of pneumothorax was seen in 12 of 23.

Treatment options are similar for pregnant and for nonpregnant women. Given the sensitivity of the fetus to maternal hypoxia, however, initial observation is required even with a small pneumothorax (<20 percent of the hemithorax).[95,96] Supplemental oxygen during hospitalization may help to accelerate pleural air resorption.[96] If the pneumothorax is large (>20 percent of the hemithorax), aspiration is recommended, with close observation over several hours.[96] If this fails or the pneumothorax recurs, treatment with tube thoracostomy is recommended. Sclerosis with tetracycline, recommended by some for nonpregnant adults, is contraindicated in pregnancy. Patients with continued air leaks, incomplete lung expansion, bilateral pneumothorax, or hemopneumothorax should be treated with surgery.[96] The optimal time for surgical intervention is the second trimester, before the increased risk of premature labor in the third trimester and after organogenesis during the first trimester.[96] With careful technique, the risk of general anesthesia can be minimized during pregnancy.

Spontaneous vaginal delivery with chest tubes in place or after surgery has been well described, with excellent fetal and maternal outcomes.[88,95] A high rate of recurrence (30 to 50 percent) is seen after the first pneumothorax. Therefore a second pneumothorax should lead to consideration of definitive treatment, including surgery.

Pneumomediastinum, the presence of free air in the mediastinum, presents a similar spectrum of management questions in pregnancy. It is a rare phenomenon with an estimated incidence in pregnancy of 1:2000 to 1:100,000. Affected women are typically primigravidas experiencing a prolonged and difficult labor with repeated straining. Pneumomediastinum can occur any time during pregnancy but is most frequently seen during the second stage of labor.

Patients typically complain of acute substernal chest pain, frequently with a tearing sensation and radiation to the neck and arms.[97] Cough and dyspnea may be seen. Tachycardia and subcutaneous emphysema are common physical findings. Pneumomediastinum undergoes spontaneous resolution within 3 to 14 days without sequelae.[88] Treatment in uncomplicated cases includes sedation, analgesics, oxygen supplementation, and elective low forceps delivery to shorten the second stage of labor.[88,97] In cases with severe dyspnea or cyanosis a small incision over the suprasternal notch has been successfully used. In the presence of mechanical ventilation, simultaneous pneumothorax is a distinct possibility.

CHEST WALL DISEASES

Kyphoscoliosis (KS) is a bony deformity of the spine leading to excessive curvature which is usually idiopathic.[84] Patients with untreated scoliosis are at increased risk of respiratory failure, particularly those with a greater degree of curvature and lower vital capacity.

The effects of KS on pregnancy outcome have been minimal except for a possible increase in premature birth.[84] Conflicting reports have been published addressing the risk of progression in spinal curvature during pregnancy.[84] In general, the risk of progression appears to be increased in those with unstable scoliosis or an initial curve greater than 25°. Close observation through pregnancy is required, as major respiratory complications have occurred with KS during pregnancy.[84] Noninvasive ventilatory support using negative-pressure ventilation and nasal positive-pressure ventilation have been successfully utilized during pregnancy.

ACUTE RESPIRATORY FAILURE

Acute respiratory failure in pregnancy remains a major problem, accounting for 30 percent of maternal deaths. The pattern of failure can be characterized as a failure to oxygenate (hypoxic respiratory failure) or to ventilate (hypercapneic respiratory failure), as illustrated in Table 18-12. Thromboembolism, amniotic fluid embolism, and venous air embolism account for 20 percent of maternal deaths, with the other causes in Table 18-12 accounting for an additional 10 percent.

The goals of management include identifying the cause and initiating therapeutic attempts to stabilize maternal physiology. Fetal oxygen delivery must also be preserved. The major determinants of oxygen delivery to fetal tissues include oxygen content of uterine arterial blood (determined by maternal hemoglobin concentration and its saturation), uterine blood flow (determined by maternal cardiac output, blood pressure, and blood pH), placental transfer, and fetal oxygen transport (indirectly measured by fetal heart tracing). Alkalosis causes vasoconstriction of the uterine arteries, with decreased oxygen delivery to the placenta.[98]

Fetal oxygen content is similar to that of the mother despite a fetal umbilical vein P_{O_2} of 28 to 32 mmHg. Compensatory mechanisms include the high-affinity fetal hemoglobin, which is at an elevated concentration and releases oxygen to peripheral tissues more efficiently. Fetal cardiac output is also increased and is optimally distributed to fetal tissues secondary to fetal shunts.

Table 18-12

CAUSES OF RESPIRATORY FAILURE IN THE PREGNANT PATIENT

Hypoxic respiratory failure

Embolic phenomena
    Venous thromboembolism
    Amniotic fluid embolism
    Venous air embolism

Parenchymal disorders
    Adult respiratory distress syndrome
    Aspiration pneumonia
    Bacterial pneumonia
    Viral pneumonia

Cardiogenic pulmonary edema

Atelectasis

Pneumothorax

Hypercapneic respiratory failure

Asthma

Overdose

Neuromuscular disease
    Myasthenia gravis
    Guillain-Barré syndrome

ADULT RESPIRATORY DISTRESS SYNDROME

DEFINITION

Adult respiratory distress syndrome (ARDS) is an acute illness characterized by the physiologic response to an increased pulmonary capillary permeability and resulting increase in lung water. The syndrome is defined by the presence of (1) an appropriate risk factor (see Table 18-13), (2) radiographic infiltrates consistent with pulmonary edema, (3) impaired oxygenation with Pa_{O_2}/Fi_{O_2} ratio ≤ 200, and (4) the absence of heart failure with a pulmonary capillary wedge pressure <18 mmHg or no clinical evidence of elevated left atrial pressure.

Risk factors for ARDS in pregnancy are numerous, as illustrated in Table 18-13. The clinical presentation is non-specific, with dyspnea, tachycardia, and tachypnea being commonly seen. Physical examination may demonstrate diffuse bibasilar rales and cyanosis. Although the chest radiograph may be normal early after the precipitating event, full progression to diffuse bilateral infiltrates typically occurs within 4 to 24 h. Hypoxemia is present, which is relatively resistant to supplemental oxygen.

THERAPEUTIC MEASURES

The overall therapeutic goals in the management of ARDS include optimizing maternal oxygen delivery while mini-

Table 18-13

PREDISPOSING CONDITIONS FOR ADULT RESPIRATORY DISTRESS SYNDROME IN THE PREGNANT WOMAN

Infection
    Bacteremia
    Septic syndrome
    Bacterial pneumonia

Traumatic
    Burns
    Crush injury
    Transfusions
    Fat embolism
    Lung contusion

Inhalation
    Gastric aspiration
    Oxygen toxicity
    Smoke/toxic fume inhalation
    Near drowning

Drugs
    Salicylates
    Opiates
    Diuretic
    Paraquat

Obstetric complications
    Septic abortion
    Eclampsia
    Abruptio placentae
    Dead fetus syndrome
    Retained products of conception
    Amniotic fluid embolism
    Venous air embolism

Pancreatitis

Seizures

mizing oxygen toxicity and iatrogenic complications while also preserving fetal oxygen delivery to tissues. General measures include appropriate oxygen delivery, including mechanical ventilation if necessary. The indications for intubation are similar to those of nonpregnant patients, including (1) inability to maintain Pa_{O_2} >60 to 65 mmHg with oxygen supplementation, (2) uncompensated respiratory acidosis, and/or (3) inability to protect the airway and clear secretions.[98] Intubation may be more difficult because of the hyperemia that can narrow the upper airway of the pregnant woman. Therefore nasotracheal intubation should be avoided.[98] The decrease in functional residual capacity may be exacerbated during intubation; therefore, 100 percent oxygen should be administered before intubation is attempted. In addition, aggressive hyperventilation by hand resuscitation must be tempered by the negative effect of respiratory alkalosis on uterine blood flow.

Mechanical ventilation should be initiated to maintain a relatively normal pH, which usually requires a Pa_{CO_2} of 30 to 32 mmHg. Ventilator settings are similar to those for the nonpregnant patient, with recent literature suggesting that small tidal volumes (6 to 10 mL/kg) are associated with lower airway pressures and potentially lower lung injury. Positive end-expiratory pressure (PEEP) should be utilized to recruit alveoli and allow the minimum $F_{I_{O_2}}$ to be used (ideally <60 percent). It should be applied in increments of 3 to 5 cmH_2O to achieve a satisfactory oxygen saturation (>90 percent) while minimizing potentially harmful peak and plateau pressures (<40 to 45 cmH_2O). Increasing PEEP can depress cardiac output, particularly in those patients with intravascular depletion, and thereby decrease uterine blood flow. The minimum PEEP should therefore be used. When PEEP is raised above 10 cmH_2O or when hypotension and oliguria fail to respond to modest intravenous fluid challenges, a pulmonary artery catheter should be considered. Although cardiac output is usually increased during pregnancy, central pressures (e.g., central venous pressure, pulmonary capillary wedge pressure) should not be significantly different from that in nonpregnant women (see Table 2-2).[99] The data from such a catheter can be used to maximize maternal oxygen delivery during mechanical ventilation.[98]

Fluid management is crucial to optimal outcome in ARDS. Recent data have suggested a better result in patients with a lower pulmonary capillary wedge pressure. When fluid is required to maintain the cardiac output, blood products offer an advantage. Vasopressors may be required to optimize maternal oxygen delivery, with ephedrine providing an optimal degree of alpha and beta stimulation to preserve uterine blood flow.[98] Supine recumbency may cause a marked decrease in venous return during the second and third trimesters because of uterine compression of the inferior vena cava. Similarly, the Trendelenburg position may worsen hypotension. Ideally, the pregnant patient should be positioned with the right hip elevated 10 to 15 cm.[98]

Nutritional support should be ensured, particularly with the elevated requirements of pregnancy and acute respiratory failure. The optimal mode of repletion depends on the clinical setting. A detailed discussion is beyond the scope of this chapter, but the enteral route should be utilized initially if feasible.[98] Specific treatment of ARDS will depend on the underlying cause. Induction of labor is not mandatory, although if the mother is critically ill and the fetus is approaching term, delivery of the fetus may facilitate management.

ASPIRATION PNEUMONIA

The initial description of aspiration pneumonia was given by Mendelson in obstetric patients undergoing labor[98]; this condition has been estimated to cause 2 percent of maternal deaths in the United States. The severity of aspiration depends on the volume, pH, and particulate content of the aspirate. The greater the volume, the lower the pH, and the presence of particulates will worsen the outcome. Generally a pH <2.5 produces a chemical pneumonitis. The clinical presentation includes the development of a fever and cough during labor or the immediate postpartum period. Chest radiography confirms a radiographic infiltrate in a dependent location (basilar segments of the lower lobes or superior segment of the lower lobes). The clinical course generally follows one of three patterns: (1) rapid improvement in 4 to 5 days, (2) initial improvement followed by complicating bacterial pneumonia, and (3) early death from intractable hypoxemia.[98]

If aspiration pneumonia occurs, management generally emphasizes prevention of aspiration and supportive care. Routine antibiotics are not beneficial but may be indicated in the presence of bacterial pneumonia. The bacterial pathogens are usually oropharyngeal anaerobes which may be treated with penicillin therapy.[98] Steroid therapy is not indicated.

References

1. Elkus R, Popovich J: Respiratory physiology in pregnancy. *Clin Chest Med* 13:555, 1992.
2. Nava S, Zanotti E, Ambrosino N, et al: Evidence of acute diaphragmatic fatigue in a "natural" condition. *Am Rev Respir Dis* 146:1226, 1992.
3. Cugell D, Frank N, Gaensler E, Badger T: Pulmonary function in pregnancy: I. Serial observations in normal women. *Am Rev Tuberc* 67:568, 1953.
4. Wolfe L, Mottola M: Aerobic exercise in pregnancy: An update. *Can J Appl Physiol* 18:119, 1993.
5. Milne J, Howie A, Pack A: Dyspnea during normal pregnancy. *Br J Obstet Gynaecol* 85:260, 1978.
6. Mulrow C, Lucey C, Farnett L: Discriminating causes of dyspnea through clinical examination. *J Gen Intern Med* 8:383, 1993.

7. Zeldis S: Dyspnea during pregnancy: Distinguishing cardiac from pulmonary causes. *Clin Chest Med* 13:561, 1992.

8. Juniper E, Daniel E, Roberts R, et al: Improvement in airway responsiveness and asthma severity during pregnancy: A prospective study. *Am Rev Respir Dis* 140:924, 1989.

9. Martinez F, Stanopoulos I, Acero R, et al: Graded comprehensive cardiopulmonary exercise testing in the evaluation of dyspnea unexplained by routine evaluation. *Chest* 105:168, 1994.

10. Irwin R, Curley F, French C: Chronic cough: The spectrum and frequency of causes, key components of the diagnostic evaluation, and outcome of specific therapy. *Am Rev Respir Dis* 141:640, 1990.

11. Schatz M, Zeiger R: Diagnosis and management of rhinitis during pregnancy. *Allergy Proc* 9:545, 1988.

12. Pratter M, Bartter T, Akers S, DuBois J: An algorithm approach to chronic cough. *Ann Intern Med* 119:977, 1993.

13. Hornby P, Abrahams T: Pulmonary pharmacology. *Clin Obstet Gynecol* 39:17, 1996.

14. Schatz M, Zeiger R: The management of asthma during pregnancy. *Curr Obstet Med* 1:65, 1991.

15. Smallwood R, Berlin R, Catagnoli N, et al: Safety of acid-suppressing drugs. *Dig Dis Sci* 40:63S, 1995.

16. Haponik E: Approach to the patient with hemoptysis, in Kelly W (ed): *Textbook of Internal Medicine.* Philadelphia: Lippincott-Raven, 1997, pp 1918–1923.

17. Cahill B, Ingbar D: Managing massive hemoptysis: A rational approach. *J Crit Illness* 11:604, 1996.

18. Richey S, Roberts S, Ramin K, et al: Pneumonia complicating pregnancy. *Obstet Gynecol* 84:525, 1994.

19. Rigby F, Pastorek J II: Pneumonia during pregnancy. *Clin Obstet Gynecol* 39:107, 1996.

20. Oxorn H: The changing aspects of pneumonia complicating pregnancy. *Am J Obstet Gynecol* 70:1057, 1955.

21. Berkowitz K, LaSala A: Risk factors associated with the increasing prevalence during pregnancy. *Am J Obstet Gynecol* 163:981, 1990.

22. Rodrigues J, Niederman M: Pneumonia complicating pregnancy. *Clin Chest Med* 13:679, 1992.

23. American Thoracic Society: Guidelines for the initial management of adults with community-acquired pneumonia: Diagnosis, assessment of severity, and initial antimicrobial therapy. *Am Rev Respir Dis* 148:1418, 1993.

24. Cunningham F: Pulmonary disorders, in Paterson L (ed): *Williams Obstetrics.* Norwalk, CT: Appleton & Lange, 1994, pp 1–14.

25. Farr B, Sloman A, Fisch M: Predicting death in patients hospitalized for community-acquired pneumonia. *Ann Intern Med* 115:428, 1991.

26. Chow A, Jewesson P: Use and safety of antimicrobial agents during pregnancy. *West J Med* 146:761, 1987.

27. Weingarten S, Riedinger M, Hobson P, et al: Evaluation of a pneumonia practice guideline in an intervention trial. *Am J Respir Crit Care Med* 153:1110, 1996.

28. Maccato M: Respiratory insufficiency due to pneumonia in pregnancy. *Obstet Gynecol Clin North Am* 18:289, 1991.

29. Neuzil K, Reed G, Mitchell E Jr, et al: Influenza morbidity increases in late pregnancy. Infectious Disease Society of America 34th Annual Meeting, 1996.

30. Mostow S: Prevention, management, and control of influenza: Role of amantadine. *Am J Med* 82(suppl 6A):35, 1987.

31. Kirshon B, Faro S, Zurawin R, et al: Favorable outcome after treatment with amantadine and ribavirin in a pregnancy complicated by influenza pneumonia. *J Reprod Med* 33:399, 1988.

32. CDC: Prevention and control of influenza: Recommendations of the Advisory Committee on Immunization Practices (ACIP). *MMWR* 45(RR-5):6, 1996.

33. Cox S, Cunningham F, Luby J: Management of varicella pneumonia complicating pregnancy. *Am J Perinatol* 7:300, 1990.

34. Esmonde T, Herman G, Anderson G: Chickenpox pneumonia: An association with pregnancy. *Thorax* 44:812, 1989.

35. Smego R, Asperilla M: Use of acyclovir for *Varicella* pneumonia during pregnancy. *Obstet Gynecol* 78:1112, 1991.

36. Brown Z, Baker D: Acyclovir therapy during pregnancy. *Obstet Gynecol* 73:526, 1989.

37. Andrews E, Yankaskas B, Cordero J, et al: Acyclovir in pregnancy registry: Six years' experience. *Obstet Gynecol* 79:7, 1992.

38. Robinson C, Rose N: Tuberculosis: Current implications and management in obstetrics. *Obstet Gynecol Surv* 51:115, 1996.

39. Vallejos J, Starke J: Tuberculosis and pregnancy. *Clin Chest Med* 13:693, 1992.

40. Margono F, Mroueh J, Garely A, et al: Resurgence of active tuberculosis among pregnant women. *Obstet Gynecol* 83:911, 1994.

41. Hedvall E: Pregnancy and tuberculosis. *Acta Med Scand* 147(suppl 286):1, 1953.

42. Snider D: Pregnancy and tuberculosis. *Chest* 86(suppl):S10, 1984.

43. Jana N, Vasishta K, Jindal et al: Perinatal outcome in pregnancies complicated by pulmonary tuberculosis. *Int J Gynecol Obstet* 44:119, 1994.

44. Snider D, Layde P, Johnson M: Treatment of tuberculosis during pregnancy. *Am Rev Respir Dis* 122:65, 1980.

45. Good J, Iseman M, Davidson P, et al: Tuberculosis in association with pregnancy. *Am J Obstet Gynecol* 140:492, 1981.

46. Carter E, Mates S: Tuberculosis during pregnancy: The Rhode Island experience, 1987 to 1991. 106:1466, 1994.

47. Present P, Comstock G: Tuberculin sensitivity in pregnancy. *Am Rev Respir Dis* 112:413, 1975.

48. American Thoracic Society: Diagnostic standards and classification of tuberculosis. *Am Rev Respir Dis* 142:725, 1990.

49. Mofenson L, Rodriguez E, Hershow R, et al: My-cobacterium tuberculosis infection in pregnant and nonpregnant women infected with HIV in the women and infants transmission study. *Arch Intern Med* 155:1066, 1995.

50. Franks A, Binkin N, Snider D, et al: Isoniazid hepatitis among pregnant and postpartum Hispanic patients. *Public Health Rep* 104:151, 1989.

51. American Thoracic Society: Treatment of tuberculosis and tuberculosis infection in adults and children. *Am J Respir Crit Care Med* 149:1359, 1994.

52. Davidson P: Managing tuberculosis during pregnancy. *Lancet* 346:199, 1995.

53. Bahna S, Bjerkedal T: The course and outcome of pregnancy in women with bronchial asthma. *Acta Allergol* 27:397, 1972.

54. Greenberger P, Patterson R: The outcome of pregnancy complicated by severe asthma. *Allergy Proc* 9:539, 1988.

55. Schatz M, Zeiger R, Hoffman C, et al: Perinatal outcomes in the pregnancies of asthmatic women: A prospective controlled analysis. *Am J Respir Crit Care Med* 151:1170, 1995.

56. Gluck J, Gluck P: The effects of pregnancy on asthma: A prospective study. *Ann Allergy* 37:164, 1976.

57. Schatz M: Asthma during pregnancy: Interrelationships and management. *Ann Allergy* 68:123, 1992.

58. Schatz M, Harden K, Forsythe A, et al: The course of asthma during pregnancy, postpartum, and with successive pregnancies: A prospective analysis. *J Allergy Clin Immunol* 81:509, 1988.

59. White R, Coutts I, Gibbs C, MacIntyre C: A prospective study of asthma during pregnancy and the puerperium. *Respir Med* 83:103, 1989.

60. Apter A, Greenberger P, Patterson R: Outcomes of pregnancy in adolescents with severe asthma. *Arch Intern Med* 149:2571, 1989.

61. National Asthma Education Program, National Heart Lung, and Blood Institute: Executive summary: Management of asthma during pregnancy, in *Report of the Working Group on Asthma and Pregnancy.* NIH publication no. 93-3279A. Washington, DC: NIH, March 1993.

62. Sheffer A: Guidelines for the diagnosis and management of asthma. *J Allergy Clin Immunol* 88:425, 1991.

63. McFadden E, Kiser R, DeGroot W: Acute bronchial asthma: Relations between clinical and physiologic manifestations. *N Engl J Med* 288:221, 1973.

64. Emerman C, Cydulka R: Effect of pulmonary function testing on the management of acute asthma. *Arch Intern Med* 155:2225, 1995.

65. Beasley R, Cushley M, Holgate S: A self-management plan in the treatment of adult asthma. *Thorax* 44:200, 1989.

66. Grampian Asthma Study of Integrated Care (GRASSIC): Effectiveness of routing self monitoring of peak flow in patients with asthma. *Br Med J* 308:564, 1994.

67. Mabie W: Asthma in pregnancy. *Clin Obstet Gynecol* 39:56, 1996.

68. Schatz M, Zeiger R, Harden K, et al: The safety of inhaled beta-agonist bronchodilators during pregnancy. *J Allergy Clin Immunol* 82:686, 1988.

69. Bloch H, Silverman R, Mancherje N, et al: Intravenous magnesium sulfate as an adjunct in the treatment of acute asthma. *Chest* 107:1576, 1995.

70. Fung D: Emergency anesthesia for asthma patients. *Clin Rev Allergy* 3:127, 1985.

71. Metzger W, Turner E, Patterson R: The safety of immunotherapy during pregnancy. *J Allergy Clin Immunol* 61:268, 1978.

72. Kotloff R, FitzSimmons S, Fiel S: Fertility and pregnancy in patients with cystic fibrosis. *Clin Chest Med* 13:623, 1992.

73. Shwachman H, Kulczycki L: Long-term study of one-hundred five patients with cystic fibrosis. *Am J Dis Child* 96:6, 1958.

74. Taussig L, Kattwinkel J, Friedewald W, et al: A new prognostic score and clinical evaluation system for cystic fibrosis. *J Pediatr* 82:380, 1973.

75. Brasfield D, Hicks G, Soong S, et al: The chest roentgenogram in cystic fibrosis: A new scoring system. *Pediatrics* 63:24, 1979.

76. Hilman B, Aitken M, Constantinescu M: Pregnancy in patients with cystic fibrosis. *Clin Obstet Gynecol* 39:70, 1996.

77. Rush D, Johnstone F, King J: Nutrition in pregnancy, in Burrows G, Ferris T (eds): *Medical Complications during Pregnancy.* Philadelphia: Saunders, 1988.

78. Larsen J Jr: Cystic fibrosis and pregnancy. *Obstet Gynecol* 39:880, 1972.

79. Cohen L, di Sant-Agnese P, Friedlander J: Cystic fibrosis and pregnancy: A national survey. *Lancet* 2:842, 1980.

79a. Palmer J, Dillon-Baker C, Tecklin JS, et al: Pregnancy in patients with cystic fibrosis. *Ann Intern Med* 99:596, 1983.

80. Kent N, Farquharson D: Cystic fibrosis in pregnancy. *Can Med Assoc J* 149:809, 1993.

81. Edenborough F, Stableforth D, Webb A, et al: Outcome of pregnancy in women with cystic fibrosis. *Thorax* 50:170, 1995.

81a. Corkey CWB, Newth CJL, Corey M. Levison H. Pregnancy in cystic fibrosis: A better prognosis in patients with pancreatic function? *Am J Obstet Gynecol* 140:737, 1981.

82. Lemna W, Feldman G, Kerem B, et al: Mutation analysis for heterozygote detection and the prenatal diagnosis of cystic fibrosis. *N Engl J Med* 322:8, 1990.

83. Selroos O: Sarcoidosis and pregnancy: A review with results of a retrospective survey. *J Intern Med* 227:221, 1990.

84. King T: Restrictive lung disease in pregnancy. *Clin Chest Med* 13:607, 1992.

85. Haynes de Regt R: Sarcoidosis and pregnancy. *Obstet Gynecol* 70:369, 1987.

86. Taylor J, Ryu J, Colby T: Raffin T: Lymphangioleiomyomatosis: Clinical course in 32 patients. *N Engl J Med* 323:1254, 1990.

87. Eliasson A, Phillips Y, Tenholder M: Treatment of lymphangioleiomyomatosis: A meta-analysis. *Chest* 196:1352, 1989.

88. Heffner J, Sahn S: Pleural disease in pregnancy. *Clin Chest Med* 13:667, 1992.

89. Hessen I: Roentgen examination of pleural fluid: A study of the localization of free effusions, the potentialities of diagnosing minimal quantities of fluid and its existence under physiologic conditions. *Acta Radiol* 86(suppl):1, 1951.

90. Hughson W, Friedman P, Feigin D, et al: Postpartum pleural effusion: A common radiologic finding. *Ann Intern Med* 97:856, 1982.

91. Stark P, Pollack M: Pleural effusions in the post-partum period. *Radiologe* 26:471, 1986.

92. Udeshi U, McHugo J, Crawford J: Postpartum pleural effusion. *Br J Obstet Gynaecol* 95:894, 1988.

93. Wallis M, McHugo J, Carruthers D: The prevalence of pleural effusions in pre-eclampsia: An ultrasound study. *Br J Med* 96:431, 1989.

94. El-Naggar T, Abd-El-Maeboud K, Abdallah M, et al: Peripartum pleural effusion. *Respir Med* 88:541, 1994.

95. Terndrup T, Bosco S, McLean E: Spontaneous pneumothorax complicating pregnancy: Case report and review of the literature. *J Emerg Med* 7:245, 1989.

96. Van Winter J, Nichols F, Pairolero P, et al: Management of spontaneous pneumothorax during pregnancy: Case report and review of the literature. *Mayo Clin Proc* 71:249, 1996.

97. Karson E, Saltzman D, Davis M: Pneumomediastinum in pregnancy: Two case reports and a review of the literature, pathophysiology, and management. *Obstet Gynecol* 64:39S, 1984.

98. Hollingsworth H, Irwin R: Acute respiratory failure in pregnancy. *Clin Chest Med* 13:723, 1992.

99. Cotton D, Beneddti T: Use of the Swan-Ganz catheter in obstetrics and gynecology. *Obstet Gynecol* 56:641, 1980.

100. Schaefer G, Silverman F: Pregnancy complicated by asthma. *Am J Obstet Gynecol* 82:182, 1961.

101. Gordon M, Niswander K, Berendes H, Kantor A: Fetal morbidity following potentially anorexigenic obstetric conditions: VII. Bronchial asthma. *Am J Obstet Gynecol* 106:421, 1970.

102. Dombrowski M, Bottoms S, Boike G, Wald J: Incidence of preeclampsia among asthmatic patients lower with theophylline. *Am J Obstet Gynecol* 155:265, 1986.

103. Fitzsimons R, Greenberger P, Patterson R: Outcome of pregnancy in women requiring corticosteroids for severe asthma. *J Allergy Clin Immunol* 78:349, 1986.

104. Stenius-Aarniala R, Piirila P, Teramo K: Asthma and pregnancy: A prospective study of 198 pregnancies. *Thorax* 43:12, 1988.

105. Lao T, Huengsburg M: Labour and delivery in mothers with asthma. *Eur J Obstet Gynecol Reprod Biol* 35:183, 1990.

106. Perlow J, Montgomery D, Morgan M, et al: Severity of asthma and perinatal outcome. *Am J Obstet Gynecol* 167:963, 1992.

107. Fine M, Smith M, Carson C, et al: Prognosis and outcomes of patients with community-acquired pneumonia: A meta-analysis. *JAMA* 274:134, 1996.

108. Hasley P, Albaum M, Li Y, et al: Do pulmonary radiographic findings at presentation predict mortality in patients with community-acquired pneumonia? *Arch Intern Med* 156:2206, 1996.

109. Turkeltaub P, Gergen P: Prevalence of upper and lower respiratory conditions in the U.S. population by social and environmental factors: Data from the second National Health and Nutrition Examination Survey, 1976 to 1980 (NHANES II). *Ann Allergy* 67:147, 1991.

110. Heinonen O, Slone D, Shapiro S: *Birth Defects and Drugs in Pregnancy.* Littleton, MA: Publishing Sciences Group, 1977.

111. Wilson J: Use of sodium cromoglycate during pregnancy. *J Pharm Med* 8:45, 1982.

112. Greenberger P, Patterson R: Beclomethasone diproprionate for severe asthma during pregnancy. *Ann Intern Med* 98:478, 1983.

113. Katz V, Thorp J, Bowes W: Severe symmetric intrauterine growth retardation associated with the topical use of triamcinolone. *Am J Obstet Gynecol* 162:396, 1990.

114. Schatz M, Hoffman C, Zeiger R, et al: The course and management of asthma and allergic diseases during pregnancy, in Middleton E, Reed C, Ellis E, et al (eds): *Allergy: Principles and Practice.* St Louis: Mosby, 1988, pp 1093–1155.

115. Greenberger P, Patterson R: Safety of therapy for allergic symptoms during pregnancy. *Ann Intern Med* 89:234, 1978.

116. Rubin J, Loffredo C, Correa-Villasenor A, Ferencz C: Prenatal drug use and congenital cardiovascular malformations (abstract). *Teratology* 43(5):423, 1991.

117. Stenius-Aarniala B, Riikonen S, Teramo K: Slow-release theophylline in pregnant asthmatics. *Chest* 107:642, 1995.

118. Reinisch J, Simon N, Karow W, Gandelman R: Prenatal exposure to prednisone in humans and animals retards intrauterine growth. *Science* 202:436, 1978.

119. Smith K, Steinberger E, Rodrigues-Rigav: Prednisone therapy and birthweight. *Science* 206:96, 1979.

Chapter 19

ABDOMINAL PAIN IN PREGNANCY

Steven L. Bloom

Larry C. Gilstrap

Abdominal pain, to one degree or another, is an experience that is shared by virtually all pregnant women. Most abdominal pain is self-limited and has no adverse effect on the pregnancy's outcome. As a result, health care providers are frequently faced with diagnostic challenges in evaluating the etiology and seriousness of abdominal discomfort during pregnancy. In order to address these challenges and to provide optimal care, physicians must integrate their understanding of the normal anatomic and physiologic changes that accompany pregnancy with their clinical findings. They must also recognize common laboratory and diagnostic imaging changes associated with pregnancy, and most importantly, they must avoid placing the gravida in further jeopardy by failing to intervene medically or surgically as they would in facing a similar clinical scenario in a nonpregnant woman. Significant morbidity and even mortality associated with abdominal disease during pregnancy is too frequently the result of such delay.

The diagnosis and management of acute abdominal pain during pregnancy are confounded by many of the physiologic changes that occur throughout gestation. Symptoms classically associated with underlying diseases, such as nausea or urinary frequency, are almost expected to occur during pregnancy. Vital signs such as blood pressure and heart rate, which are fundamental in the evaluation of an ill patient, undergo remarkable changes during pregnancy. The findings noted during the physical exam must be reconciled with the alterations in normal anatomic relationships that occur as the uterus encroaches upon the abdominal organs. Similarly, many of the laboratory studies used in the evaluation of abdominal pain must be interpreted in relation to

the gestational age of the pregnancy. The majority of the anatomic and physiologic changes seen during pregnancy are described in Chap. 2; however, those changes specifically related to the evaluation of abdominal pain are detailed in Table 19-1.

OBSTETRIC CAUSES OF ABDOMINAL PAIN

LABOR

The most common obstetric cause of abdominal pain during pregnancy is labor. Other causes are summarized in Table 19-2. Labor is usually relatively easy to diagnose compared with other causes of abdominal pain. It is characterized by intermittent tightening and relaxation of the uterus and progressive dilatation and effacement of the cervix. Normal labor must be distinguished from uterine irritability or labor associated with other obstetric complications, such as placental abruption and acute chorioamnionitis. It is important to recognize that uterine irritability and labor may be associated with nonobstetric causes of abdominal pain (i.e., appendicitis, acute pyelonephritis, degenerating leiomyoma, etc.). Thus, labor may be either a primary diagnosis or an important sign of other serious conditions.

Women suspected of being in labor should have a digital examination of the cervix to assess for possible dilation and effacement. Such an examination, however, should not be immediately performed if the patient complains of con-

Table 19-1

ANATOMIC AND PHYSIOLOGIC CHANGES OF PREGNANCY THAT MAY ALTER THE EVALUATION OF ABDOMINAL PAIN

Organ	Changes
Abdominal wall	Diastasis recti
	Distention from uterus minimizes pain and rigidity associated with peritonitis
Uterus	Becomes abdominal organ after 12 weeks' gestation
	Growth produces tension upon the broad and round ligaments
Ovaries	Corpus luteum cyst formation
Stomach and intestines	Reduced motility
	Displaced by uterus; appendix may reach right flank
Liver	Does not increase in size
	Spider angiomata and palmar erythema may be present due to elevated estrogen levels
	Decreased serum albumin
	Increased serum cholesterol and alkaline phosphatase

comitant preterm leakage of amniotic fluid or vaginal bleeding. Cervical examination of the woman with preterm rupture of membranes may increase the risk of infection and early delivery. A sterile speculum should be utilized to confirm leakage of amniotic fluid from the cervical os and to gauge the degree of dilation. Women presenting with vagi-

Table 19-2

OBSTETRIC CAUSES OF ABDOMINAL/PELVIC PAIN

Labor
Placental abruption
Uterine rupture/dehiscence
Severe preeclampsia/HELLP syndrome
Acute fatty liver
Incarcerated uterus
Incomplete abortion
Ectopic pregnancy

nal bleeding, moreover, may have a placenta previa. A targeted ultrasound examination for placental location prior to examination should prevent inadvertent injury to the placenta by the examiner.

PLACENTAL ABRUPTION

Placental abruption, or premature separation of the placenta from the uterus, is one of the most serious and potentially life-threatening obstetric causes of abdominal pain encountered in pregnancy. It is characterized by severe abdominal pain, uterine tenderness, tetanic contractions, and varying degrees of bleeding. A significant proportion of the bleeding may be concealed within the uterus and may, therefore, not be readily apparent. As a result, the patient may present with signs of hemodynamic instability or shock which may seem disproportionate to the amount of bleeding observed or reported. Placental abruption severe enough to result in the death of the fetus is usually also associated with a coagulopathy due to the consumption of fibrinogen and other clotting factors. The treatment of placental abruption includes emptying the uterus (usually by cesarean delivery if the fetus is potentially viable) and assuring maternal hemodynamic stability with blood and fluid replacement. The management of placental abruption is further described in Chap. 9.

UTERINE RUPTURE

Placental abruption may occasionally be difficult to distinguish from uterine dehiscence or rupture, especially in women with a previous uterine scar. Many of the signs and symptoms of uterine rupture—such as abdominal pain, bleeding, and ominous fetal heart rate patterns—are also encountered with placental abruption. Unlike the hypertonic contraction pattern seen with placental abruption, however, uterine rupture is classically associated with a loss of intrauterine pressure and an absence of contractions. As in the case of abruption, however, the woman may demonstrate signs and symptoms of hemodynamic instability and shock. Occasionally the diagnosis can be made only at laparotomy. It is important to remember that uterine rupture can occur at any time during pregnancy. In addition, uterine rupture should be strongly considered in the differential diagnosis of women with abdominal pain who have had any prior uterine surgery, including curettage,[1] myomectomy,[2] or cesarean delivery. A prior vertical uterine incision is much more likely to undergo dehiscence than is a low transverse uterine incision. Treatment must be individualized and is dependent upon the size of the laceration, the patient's hemodynamic status, and the surgeon's experience. A small uterine dehiscence can usually be managed by simple repair, especially in the primigravida and in patients for whom preservation of fertility is of utmost importance. Large uterine ruptures in multiparous women are often best managed by hysterectomy.

SEVERE PREECLAMPSIA

The hallmark symptoms associated with severe preeclampsia are headache, scotomata, and right-upper-quadrant pain (see also Chap. 7). The abdominal pain associated with preeclampsia is related to involvement of the liver. While the exact pathogenesis is not completely understood, a combination of hepatic ischemia and edema is theorized to produce the clinical and histologic findings.[3] The most feared complication is the formation of subcapsular hematomas. The rupture of such hematomas is associated with a high mortality rate.

The diagnosis of preeclampsia is based upon an increase in blood pressure accompanied by proteinuria, edema, or both. A blood pressure measurement of 140/90 mmHg during the second half of pregnancy is usually sufficient for the hypertension component of the diagnosis. Women with a history of chronic hypertension are at an increased risk for the development of superimposed preeclampsia; however, the diagnosis of concomitant preeclampsia in these women is more challenging. Increases of 30 mmHg systolic and 15 mmHg diastolic from the usual baseline blood pressure values are suggestive of superimposed preeclampsia. The appearance of proteinuria or nondependent edema (e.g., hand or facial edema) also suggests the possibility of superimposed preeclampsia. For the diagnosis of preeclampsia, proteinuria is defined as at least 300 mg of urinary protein per 24 h or 100 mg/dL or more on two random urinalyses collected 6 h or more apart.[4]

The presence of epigastric pain serves as an important marker to assess the severity of the preeclampsia. When epigastric pain or other signs of severe preeclampsia are present, management of the gravida involves the following:

1. The administration of magnesium sulfate for the prophylaxis of eclampsia
2. The administration of antihypertensive medication (usually hydralazine or labetalol in small incremental doses) for blood pressure measurements of 160/110 mmHg or greater
3. Termination of the pregnancy, which may require transfer to a facility with a nursery capable of caring for a preterm neonate

Of note, it has been observed that the epigastric pain associated with severe preeclampsia may often be temporarily relieved by the intravenous administration of magnesium sulfate.

ACUTE FATTY LIVER OF PREGNANCY

Acute fatty liver of pregnancy, also known as acute yellow atrophy, is relatively uncommon (see also Chap. 7). While the precise incidence is unknown, it has been estimated to occur in approximately 1 in 10,000 deliveries.[5] Acute fatty liver typically occurs in the third trimester and is more common in nulliparous women.[6] The clinical findings, which

---

Table 19-3

SIGNS AND SYMPTOMS ASSOCIATED WITH ACUTE FATTY LIVER OF PREGNANCY

Malaise
Nausea, vomiting, anorexia
Epigastric pain
Hypertension, proteinuria, edema
Jaundice

---

usually present over the course of several days to weeks, are outlined in Tables 19-3 and 19-4.

It may be very difficult to distinguish acute fatty liver from severe preeclampsia, since epigastric pain may be present in both and as many as 50 percent of women with acute fatty liver will have concomitant hypertension and proteinuria.[6] The presence of hypoglycemia, a usually prominent feature presumed to be a result of decreased hepatic glycogenolysis,[5] may serve to help distinguish this entity from severe preeclampsia. Regardless, delivery is the indicated treatment for both these conditions.

The differential diagnosis formulated for women with acute fatty liver may be quite extensive. Pruritus is very uncommon and would suggest cholestasis of pregnancy, a more common pregnancy complication. In addition to preeclamp-

---

Table 19-4

LABORATORY FINDINGS ASSOCIATED WITH ACUTE FATTY LIVER OF PREGNANCY

Test	Result
PT/PTT	Prolonged
Fibrinogen	Decreased
D dimers	Increased
Bilirubin	Usually <10 mg/dL
Transaminases	Usually 300–500 U/L
Alkaline phosphatase	May be 10 times normal
Glucose	Decreased
Platelets	Decreased
Leukocyte count	Increased
Peripheral smear	Features of hemolysis
BUN/creatinine	Increased
Uric acid	Increased
Ammonia	Increased

Abbreviations: PT = prothrombin time; PTT = partial thromboplastin time; BUN = blood urea nitrogen.

sia and cholestasis, the differential diagnosis should include viral hepatitis, gallbladder disease, and Reye syndrome.[5] Correct diagnosis requires a complete history, physical exam, and laboratory profile. Computed tomography (CT) and ultrasound have not been found to be very sensitive for detecting parenchymal liver changes in acute fatty liver unless the fatty changes are severe.[5]

In early accounts of acute fatty liver of pregnancy, maternal and fetal mortality were reported to be as high as 75 percent.[6] More recently, the prognosis has improved, both because of recognition of milder forms of the disease and also because of continuing improvements in supportive care of women with this condition.[6] Acute fatty liver usually resolves following delivery, and recurrence in future pregnancies is rare. This low recurrence may be related to the associated mortality, the reluctance to conceive again, a genuine low recurrence rate, or failure to diagnose the condition correctly.[7]

INCARCERATED UTERUS

Rarely, a retroverted uterus becomes incarcerated in the sacral hollow during the second trimester as it grows from a pelvic organ to an abdominal organ. Although an incarcerated uterus may be associated with severe abdominal pain, the presenting complaints are usually lower abdominal discomfort and difficulty voiding, typically in the early second trimester (14 to 16 weeks of gestation). Less often, affected women will present with "paradoxical" or overflow incontinence due to marked bladder distention resulting from cervical obstruction of the urethra or bladder. The diagnosis is made with a bimanual examination, which reveals a prominent posterior mass in the cul-de-sac and the absence of the uterine fundus rising above the symphysis pubis. Treatment consists of pushing the uterus out of the pelvis with the woman in the knee-chest position. Anesthesia is usually required for this procedure. In addition, an indwelling urinary catheter should be used to drain the bladder until the uterus has grown too large to return into the pelvis.

ECTOPIC PREGNANCY/INCOMPLETE ABORTION

Abdominal pain that occurs during the first trimester is often associated with an ectopic pregnancy or an incomplete abortion (see also Chaps. 3 and 4). Any woman presenting with a complaint of lower abdominal pain and bleeding who is of reproductive age should receive a pregnancy test. In women who have a positive pregnancy test, it must be established that the pregnancy is intrauterine. Findings suggestive of an intrauterine pregnancy include the following:

1. An enlarged uterus that corresponds in size to the estimated weeks of gestation

2. The absence of an adnexal mass or tenderness
3. Auscultation of the fetal heart over the uterus.

When there is doubt about the location of the pregnancy, sonography should be employed. A useful adjuvant to ultrasound is a maternal serum beta human chorionic gonadotropin (β-hCG) level. A normal gestational sac should be consistently demonstrated when the β-hCG level is greater than 1000 mIU/mL (Second International Standard) when using transvaginal sonography.[8] If the location of the pregnancy cannot be established and if the β-hCG level is below 1000 mIU/mL, women without clinical signs of a hemoperitoneum may be followed with serial exams, β-hCG tests, and sonography. Often these women will be admitted to the hospital for observation, especially if they are at increased risk for an ectopic pregnancy. Such risk factors include a prior ectopic pregnancy, previous tubal surgery, or a history of pelvic inflammatory disease.

Women with an incomplete abortion usually present with cramping lower abdominal pain and bleeding. Many times they will report passage of "tissue" prior to presentation. The diagnosis can usually be quickly established by performing a speculum examination. The appearance of a dilated cervical os with visualization of protruding products of conception is diagnostic. Treatment consists of assuring hemodynamic stability and performing a suction and sharp curettage.

GYNECOLOGIC CAUSES OF ABDOMINAL PAIN

Excluding ectopic pregnancy and incomplete or threatened abortion, the most common gynecologic causes of abdominal pain during pregnancy include degeneration of uterine leiomyomata and adnexal masses.

DEGENERATING LEIOMYOMA

Uterine leiomyomata may undergo marked growth during pregnancy, which is thought to be secondary to the hormonal milieu of pregnancy. These enlarging myomas, in turn, may undergo hemorrhagic infarction. The resulting degeneration is associated with pain, fever, and sometimes uterine irritability and premature labor. The differential diagnosis includes placental abruption, appendicitis, and torsion of the adnexa. A history of known leiomyomata or sonographic confirmation of the tumors (Fig. 19-1) is important in establishing the diagnoses. Treatment generally consists of analgesics and nonsteroidal anti-inflammatory drugs such as ibuprofen. Indomethacin has been reported to be effective in the treatment of pain associated with degenerating uterine leiomyomas in pregnancy[9]; however, caution should be used, because indomethacin has been associated with

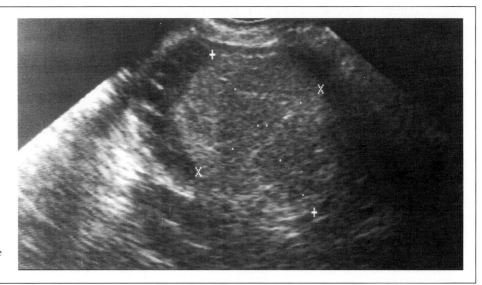

Figure 19-1

Ultrasound image of a uterine leiomyoma.

premature closure of the fetal ductus arteriosus, reduction of fetal urine output, and intraventricular hemorrhage.[10] Surgical intervention is rarely indicated.

ADNEXAL MASSES AND TORSION

The exact incidence of adnexal masses during pregnancy is unknown; with the almost universal use of ultrasound in pregnant women, however, it has been estimated to occur in approximately 1 percent of all pregnancies.[11] The most significant concern regarding adnexal masses is whether or not they are malignant. The rate of malignancy has been reported to vary from less than 1 in 6000 to as high as 1 percent.[12–14] Fortunately, the vast majority of adnexal masses are benign. Simple cysts, theca-lutein cysts, and benign solid tumors (i.e., teratomas) are among the most common masses encountered.

Most adnexal masses are asymptomatic and are discovered at the time of ultrasound examination, cesarean delivery, or tubal ligation. Occasionally such masses may be associated with severe abdominal pain secondary to torsion. The exact incidence of adnexal torsion during pregnancy is unknown. Hogston and Lilford[11] reported an incidence of almost 1 percent for cysts diagnosed in pregnancy by ultrasound. Symptoms of adnexal torsion may range from intermittent lower abdominal pain to those of an acute abdomen, especially if infarction occurs. Most often the pain is intermittent in nature and is associated with an elevated white blood cell count and slight elevation in temperature. Ultrasound is helpful to visualize an adnexal mass, but torsion does not have a characteristic appearance. Treatment consists of surgical exploration with removal of the adnexa if necrosis is suspected or present.

GASTROINTESTINAL CAUSES OF ABDOMINAL PAIN

GASTROESOPHAGEAL REFLUX/PYROSIS

Gastroesophageal reflux or pyrosis is often regarded as a minor malady of pregnancy; however, it may be the cause of significant discomfort. It has been estimated to occur in 30 to 80 percent of all pregnancies and is frequently more troublesome during the third trimester. However, symptoms may occur as early as the first trimester.[15] The signs and symptoms of pyrosis classically involve the sensation of retrosternal burning, or heartburn, and are frequently precipitated by lying supine after the ingestion of a meal. The burning is caused by esophagitis from gastrointestinal reflux. In virtually all women, a history is sufficient to make the diagnosis. In extremely atypical presentations associated with symptoms such as chest pain, cough, or wheezing, further investigation, including endoscopy, may be indicated.[15] Such cases, however, are unusual.

The precise pathogenesis of gastroesophageal reflux during pregnancy is unknown. Most theories involve a combination of hormonal and mechanical factors. Relaxation of the lower esophageal sphincter in combination with increased intragastric pressure produced from the gravid uterus has been thought to contribute to the occurrence of gastroesophageal reflux. Van Thiel and colleagues[16,17] have demonstrated that a progressive increase in plasma progesterone is associated with a lowering of esophageal sphincter pressures. Further investigations[15] involving gastrin and esophageal motility may serve to improve our understanding of the pathogenesis.

The initial treatment of common heartburn should involve elevation of the head while sleeping and avoidance of bending. The woman should be advised to eat frequent smaller meals. Antacids such as sucralfate have been demonstrated to be both safe and efficacious.[15] For more persistent cases, an H_2-receptor antagonist should be considered. Both cimetidine and ranitidine have been used during pregnancy in the usual doses without apparent adverse effects.[10,18]

APPENDICITIS

Appendicitis is one of the most common indications for surgical exploration of the abdomen during pregnancy. The incidence of acute appendicitis has been reported as approximately 1 in 1500 deliveries, a rate comparable to that in a nonpregnant population.[19] Thus, appendicitis does not occur at a greater frequency during pregnancy and appears to represent a purely coincidental event. Similarly, the incidence of appendicitis among pregnant women appears to be evenly divided among the three trimesters.[20] Although appendicitis is not necessarily more severe during pregnancy, physiologic changes associated with pregnancy may make the diagnosis more difficult and exacerbate the pathology. Increased pelvic vascularity may enhance lymphatic drainage, resulting in rapid dissemination of infection.[21] Displacement of the appendix by the enlarging uterus may hamper containment of the infection by the omentum.[21]

The presentation of acute appendicitis during pregnancy is in many ways similar to that in the nonpregnant state. The most common presenting complaint is lower abdominal pain. In the first trimester, the abdominal pain tends to be confined to the right lower quadrant. As the uterus enlarges, however, the appendix is typically displaced more superiorly in the peritoneal cavity. As a result, pain and tenderness due to appendicitis during the last trimesters tend to be located in the right upper quadrant (see Fig. 19-2). It is important to recognize that the physical exam findings of guarding and rebound associated with peritonitis may be less pronounced during later pregnancy and postpartum. The stretching of the peritoneum by the gravid uterus decreases the sensitivity of these signs.

Other signs and symptoms of appendicitis include nausea, vomiting, and diarrhea. Clearly some of these symptoms, such as nausea, are commonly present during normal pregnancies. When a pregnant woman presents with an exacerbation of one or more of these common discomforts, an acute medical or surgical illness such as appendicitis must be excluded. Some of the other signs and symptoms associated with appendicitis in the nonpregnant population occur with less frequency in pregnant women. Fever and anorexia, for example, have been described in less than half of pregnant women with appendicitis.[22]

The diagnosis of appendicitis during pregnancy has long been acknowledged to be a challenge for the practitioner. The diagnostic accuracy has been reported to range between 50 and 80 percent.[20,22] The cardinal signs of appendicitis

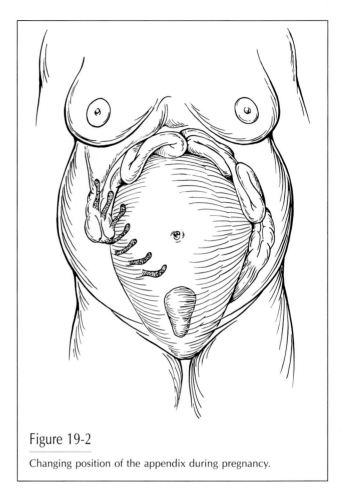

Figure 19-2

Changing position of the appendix during pregnancy.

are considered less reliable because of the frequency with which these symptoms occur in normal pregnancies and in other gastrointestinal illnesses. Two signs, however, which may be helpful in leading to the proper diagnosis of appendicitis during pregnancy are persistent leukocytosis and Bryant's sign. While leukocytosis is common during early pregnancy, labor, and postpartum, its presence in conjunction with the classic findings of appendicitis has been reported to improve diagnostic accuracy.[21] In addition, pain that does not move to the left when a patient turns from a supine to a left lateral decubitus position during pregnancy (Bryant's sign) may be associated with acute appendicitis.[21] Above all, however, a high degree of clinical suspicion is of paramount importance in establishing the diagnosis.

Compression ultrasonography is generally considered to be less reliable for the diagnosis of acute appendicitis in gravid patients due to cecal displacement and uterine interposition.[23] Yet sonography may be useful in ruling out other conditions (e.g., degenerating leiomyoma). If ultrasound is employed, the patient should be examined in the left lateral decubitus position to allow for displacement of the uterus.[24]

The treatment of a suspected acute appendicitis during pregnancy is prompt surgical intervention. Unfortunately, surgery is too often unnecessarily delayed, and as many as 25 percent of pregnant women do not receive treatment until perforation has occurred.[21] Postponement of surgical intervention that leads to perforation and peritonitis greatly increases maternal and fetal morbidity and mortality. It is the delay in diagnosis that appears to contribute most to the maternal (up to 11 percent) and fetal (up to 37 percent) mortality.[22] The risk of misdiagnosis, therefore, appears to be clearly outweighed by the potential complications resulting from delayed intervention.

GALLBLADDER DISEASE

Because gallstones are most commonly encountered in women of reproductive age and because pregnancy is associated with diminished gallbladder motility,[23] pregnant women are at an increased risk for the development of gallstones. Many of these cases are detected at the time of sonography and may be seen in 2.5 to 5 percent of all pregnancies.[23] Asymptomatic gallstones generally do not require therapy during pregnancy. Acute cholecystitis, on the other hand, may be life-threatening and requires prompt recognition and treatment.

As in nonpregnant women, the most common symptom of acute cholecystitis during pregnancy is abdominal pain which is usually abrupt in onset and may vary between severe lancing and cramping sensations. Classically, the pain begins in the midepigastrium and radiates to the right upper quadrant, back, or scapulas.[25] During pregnancy, the gallbladder is rarely palpable. Rebound tenderness, though less common during pregnancy, suggests perforation, abscess formation, or pancreatitis.[25] In women clinically suspected of having symptomatic gallstones during pregnancy, sonography may be useful to help confirm the diagnosis.

There is no unanimity of opinion regarding the optimal management of acute cholecystitis during pregnancy. Medical therapy consisting of the cessation of oral intake, intravenous hydration, and nasogastric suctioning is usually the initial treatment. Women who are conservatively managed during pregnancy should be followed closely for evidence of relapse. Surgery must be considered for women who do not readily respond to such therapy or in whom abscess formation or perforation is suspected. Serious morbidity and mortality may result if surgery is inappropriately delayed.

The treatment of biliary disease during pregnancy was recently reviewed by Swisher and colleagues,[26] who reported the experience in two large urban hospitals over a 6-year period. Seventy-two women were identified with biliary disease out of more than 46,000 pregnancies, for an incidence of 0.16 percent. All women were initially managed medically. Eight women did not respond to such treatment and required surgery, five women who initially responded to medical management later relapsed and required surgery, and three women underwent elective surgery. There was no significant perioperative morbidity resulting from surgery during pregnancy.

Laparoscopic cholecystectomy has gained increasing acceptance as the procedure of choice for gallbladder removal.

In a review of 46 women who underwent laparoscopic cholecystectomy during pregnancy, Lanzafame[27] concluded that the procedure was safe during pregnancy when undertaken by a skilled laparoscopist.

ACUTE PANCREATITIS

Acute pancreatitis is a serious complication during pregnancy that may threaten the lives of both the mother and fetus. The causes during pregnancy are similar to those in the general population with the exception that alcoholism is reported to be less frequent.[28] During pregnancy, cholelithiasis is cited as the most common association.[28,29] Pseudocyst formation is rare.

Recently, Ramin and colleagues reported the results of a large observational study of acute pancreatitis over an 11-year time span at a large urban hospital.[29] Forty-three gravidas were diagnosed among the 147,197 women who were delivered during the study period, for an approximate incidence of one in 3333 pregnancies. Two-thirds of the affected women had associated biliary disease. All had a favorable response to supportive therapy. Cholecystectomy was performed prior to delivery in 8 women and postpartum in another 12. Of 39 women whose pregnancies were followed to delivery, 32 delivered at term and their infants did well. Six infants delivered preterm, two were stillborn, and one died after birth.

During pregnancy, pancreatitis appears to be more common with advancing gestational age.[28,29] The usual presenting symptoms are nausea, vomiting, and abdominal pain, which is classically midepigastric with radiation to the back. As in nonpregnant patients, serial measurements of serum amylase and lipase activity remain the best methods to confirm the clinical diagnosis.[23]

The management of acute pancreatitis during pregnancy includes intravenous hydration and limitation of oral intake in order to decrease enzyme secretion. Other measures include nasogastric suction for severe disease and antimicrobials if infection is suspected. In the report by Ramin and colleagues,[29] all women responded to conservative therapy and they were hospitalized for a mean of 8.5 days. For women with unrelenting disease, intensive supportive therapy and pancreatic debridement and drainage may be lifesaving.[23,30]

INTESTINAL OBSTRUCTION

The incidence of intestinal obstruction during pregnancy has been reported to range between 1 in 1500 and 1 in 66,000 deliveries. This wide variation reflects the general failure to document this complication in the literature.[31] The two most common causes of intestinal obstruction are adhesions from pelvic surgery and volvulus. Adhesions are most likely to precipitate obstruction during pregnancy when the uterus grows from a pelvic to an abdominal organ (12 to 14 weeks of gestation), when the fetal head descends into the pelvis (36 to 40 weeks of gestation), and immediately after delivery, when the uterus undergoes involution.[32] While adhesions are the leading cause of obstruction in both pregnant and nonpregnant women, intestinal volvulus assumes a much greater role in the pregnant woman and may occur in up to 25 percent of women with intestinal obstruction.[31]

The diagnosis of intestinal obstruction during pregnancy can be particularly challenging. The classic signs and symptoms include episodic or continuous abdominal pain, vomiting, and distention. Because this clinical picture can, to a lesser degree, be associated with "normal" pregnancy discomforts as well as other conditions as diverse as labor and acute pyelonephritis, a high degree of clinical suspicion is again required. Severe, persistent emesis, especially after the first trimester, and emesis that is feculent in character should prompt the consideration of intestinal obstruction.[31]

It is important to recognize that women with bowel obstruction during the postpartum period may not manifest peritoneal signs (i.e., rebound and guarding) to the same extent as nonpregnant women since the abdomen has been markedly distended by the uterus and may be "less sensitive." Abdominal x-rays will most often demonstrate the characteristic pattern of small bowel obstruction. In equivocal cases, soluble contrast media can also be utilized safely during pregnancy.

Treatment of suspected bowel obstruction is expedient surgical exploration. A negative laparotomy is associated with very little maternal or fetal morbidity. In contrast, procrastination and delay in diagnosis and treatment are associated with significant morbidity and high mortality.

PEPTIC ULCER DISEASE

Unlike most illnesses that tend to both complicate and be complicated by pregnancy, active peptic ulcer disease usually improves during pregnancy. This is probably a result of decreased gastric acid and increased secretion of mucus.[23] Cunningham reported the occurrence of symptomatic peptic ulcer disease in only one to two out of 200,000 pregnancies.[23] Treatment is similar to that for the nonpregnant patient.

GENITOURINARY CAUSES OF ABDOMINAL PAIN

ACUTE PYELONEPHRITIS

Acute pyelonephritis (see also Chap. 24) occurs in 1 to 2 percent of all pregnant women and is one of the most common serious complications encountered during pregnancy. The presenting symptoms most often seen include fever, chills, nausea, vomiting, and back or flank pain. Gravid women may also experience uterine irritability and contractions. The patient will generally appear ill and is often obviously dehydrated. The most common sign is temperature elevation, often as high as 40°C (104°F). In addition to fever, costovertebral angle tenderness (more common on the right side) and bacteriuria are the key findings. The clinical diagnosis is usually confirmed by a positive urine culture demonstrating more than 100,000 organisms of a single uropathogen per milliliter of urine. The most common organisms are the enteric bacteria, especially *Escherichia coli*. The patient with pyelonephritis will also frequently demonstrate a marked leukocytosis. In addition, a significant number of women will demonstrate a hemolytic anemia. Up to 25 percent of patients will experience a transient decrease in creatinine clearance.

In general, pregnant women with acute pyelonephritis should be admitted to the hospital, as the majority of them are dehydrated and unable to tolerate oral medications. They may have significant complications such as transient renal dysfunction, severe anemia, and adult respiratory distress syndrome. These women should be rehydrated with liberal use of intravenous fluids and started on parenteral antibiotics. In most cases, gravid women will respond well to ampicillin plus an aminoglycoside or to a cephalosporin (see Chap. 24). These women should be observed closely for the onset of preterm labor. Most women will be asymptomatic within 48 to 72 h of initiation of therapy. If after this length of time the patient is still febrile and symptomatic, she should be evaluated for a resistant organism, urinary obstruction, or a perinephric abscess.

Since approximately one-third of pregnant women will experience a recurrence of a urinary tract infection at some time during the pregnancy, it is important either to utilize suppressive antibiotic therapy (such as nitrofurantoin 100 mg given once a day for the remainder of the pregnancy) or to follow the patient with frequent urine cultures during prenatal visits.

URETERAL STONE

Pregnancy is associated with the development of hydroureteronephrosis beginning in the second trimester, a result of both obstructive and hormonal factors.[33] In spite of this predisposition for urinary stasis and infection, urolithiasis is an infrequent complication of pregnancy, with an incidence of about 1 in every 1500 pregnancies.[34] The usual presentation includes abdominal pain, flank pain, and hematuria. During pregnancy, urinary calculi are often diagnosed in association with urinary tract infections.[35] For example, pyelonephritis that does not respond to appropriate antibiotic therapy should increase suspicion for the presence of renal obstruction.

Diagnostic imaging studies are often helpful adjuvants for the evaluation of suspected urinary calculi. Sonography is sensitive for the detection of hydroureteronephrosis but does not readily discriminate between obstruction and physiologic dilatation. The use of Doppler sonography and visualization of ureteral jets have recently been reported to help distinguish ureteral obstruction.[36,37] When sonography is inconclusive, x-ray studies should be considered. The radiation dose to the uterus associated with an intravenous pyelogram has been estimated to be between 686 and 1398 mrad, which is below the threshold associated with fetal risk.[4] The use of a limited intravenous pyelogram consisting of a scout film and a 20-min film will further decrease this exposure (approximately 160 mrad dose to the uterus).

The initial management of urinary calculi during pregnancy consists of hydration and analgesics, which will be sufficient in the majority of women.[34] In approximately one-third of women, further intervention involving stent placement, percutaneous nephrostomy, basket extraction, or surgical exploration is necessary.

References

1. Leibner EC: Delayed presentation of uterine perforation. *Ann Emerg Med* 26:643, 1995.
2. Dubuisson JB, Chavet X, Chapron C, et al: Uterine rupture during pregnancy after laparoscopic myomectomy. *Human Reprod* 10:1475, 1995.
3. Rolfes DB, Ishak KG: Liver disease in toxemia of pregnancy. *Am J Gastroenterol* 81:1138, 1986.
4. Cunningham FG, Gant NF, MacDonald PC, et al: *Williams Obstetrics*, 19th ed. Norwalk, CT: Appleton & Lange, 1993.
5. Watson WJ, Seeds JW: Acute fatty liver of pregnancy. *Obstet Gynecol Surv* 45:585, 1990.
6. Cunningham FG: Liver disease complicating pregnancy, in *Williams Obstetrics*, 19th ed. Norwalk, CT: Appleton & Lange, June/July 1993, suppl 1.
7. MacLean MA, Cameron AD, Cumming GP, et al: Recurrence of acute fatty liver of pregnancy. *Br J Obstet Gynaecol* 101:453, 1994.
8. Callen PW: *Ultrasonography in Obstetrics and Gynecology*, 3d ed. Philadelphia: Saunders, 1994, p 656.
9. Dildy GA III, Moise KJ, Smith LG Jr, et al: Indomethacin for the treatment of symptomatic leiomyoma uteri during pregnancy. *Am J Perinatol* 9:185, 1992.
10. Gilstrap LC, Little BB: *Drugs and Pregnancy*. New York: Elsevier, 1993.
11. Hogston P, Lilford RJ: Ultrasound study of ovarian cysts in pregnancy: Prevalence and significance. *Br J Obstet Gynaecol* 93:625, 1986.
12. Roberts JA: Management of gynecologic tumors during pregnancy. *Clin Perinatol* 10:369, 1983.
13. Thornton JG, Wells M: Ovarian cysts in pregnancy: Does ultrasound make traditional management inappropriate? *Obstet Gynecol* 69:717, 1987.
14. Grant WM: Adnexal masses, in Hankins GDV, Clark SL, Cunningham FG, Gilstrap LC (eds): *Operative Obstetrics*. Norwalk, CT: Appleton & Lange, 1995, pp 405–424.
15. Baron TH, Richter JE: Gastroesophageal reflux disease in pregnancy. *Gastroenterol Clin North Am* 21:777, 1992.
16. Van Thiel DH, Gavaler JS, Joshi SN, et al: Heartburn of pregnancy. *Gastroenterology* 72:666, 1977.
17. Van Thiel DH, Gavaler JS, Stremple J: Lower esophageal spinchter pressure in women using sequential oral contraceptives. *Gastroenterology* 71:232, 1976.
18. Larson JD, Patatanian E, Miner PB Jr, et al: Double-blind, placebo-controlled study of ranitidine for gastroesophageal reflux symptoms during pregnancy. *Obstet Gynecol* 90:83, 1997.
19. Sharp HT: Gastrointestinal surgical conditions during pregnancy. *Clin Obstet Gynecol* 37:306, 1994.
20. Epstein FB: Acute abdominal pain in pregnancy. *Emerg Med Clin North Am* 12:151, 1994.
21. Mahmoodian S: Appendicitis complicating pregnancy. *S Med J* 85:19, 1992.
22. Ellsbury KE: Abdominal pain in pregnancy. *J Fam Pract* 22:365, 1986.
23. Cunningham FG: Gastrointestinal disorders, in *Williams Obstetrics*, 19th ed. Norwalk, CT: Appleton & Lange, June/July 1994, suppl 7.
24. Lim HK, Bae SH, Seo GS: Diagnosis of acute appendicitis in pregnant women: Value of sonography. *AJR* 159:539, 1992.
25. DeVore GR: Acute abdominal pain in the pregnant patient due to pancreatitis, acute appendicitis, cholecystitis, or peptic ulcer disease. *Clin Perinatol* 7:349, 1980.
26. Swisher SG, Schmit PJ, Hunt KK, et al: Biliary disease during pregnancy. *Am J Surg* 168:576, 1994.
27. Lanzafame RJ: Laparoscopic cholecystectomy during pregnancy. *Surgery* 118:627, 1995.
28. Scott LD: Gallstone disease and pancreatitis in pregnancy. *Gastroenterol Clin North Am* 21:803, 1992.
29. Ramin KD, Ramin SM, Richey SD, Cunningham FG: Acute pancreatitis in pregnancy. *Am J Obstet Gynecol* 173:187, 1995.
30. Fernandez-del-Castillo C, Rattner DW, Warshaw AL: Acute pancreatitis. *Lancet* 342:475, 1993.
31. Connolly MM, Unti JA, Nora PF: Bowel obstruction in pregnancy. *Surg Clin North Am* 75:101, 1995.
32. Hill LM, Symmonds RE: Small bowel obstruction in pregnancy—A review and report of four cases. *Obstet Gynecol* 49:170, 1977.
33. Weiss RM: Clinical implications of ureteral physiology. *J Urol* 121:401, 1979.
34. Denstedt JD, Razvi H: Management of urinary calculi during pregnancy. *J Urol* 148:1072, 1992.
35. Lucas MJ, Cunningham FG: Urinary infection in pregnancy. *Clin Obstet Gynecol* 36:855, 1993.
36. Haddad MC, Abomelha MS, Riley PJ: Diagnosis of acute ureteral calculous obstruction in pregnant women using colour and pulsed Doppler sonography. *Clin Radiol* 50:864, 1995.
37. Platt JF, Rubin JM, Ellis JH: Distinction between obstructive and nonobstructive pyelocaliectasis with duplex Doppler sonography. *AJR* 153:997, 1989.

Chapter 20

DIABETES DURING PREGNANCY

Robert P. Lorenz

Every woman of childbearing age seen for emergency care should be evaluated for possible pregnancy. In the diabetic woman, identification of an early pregnancy is critical in providing the best possible chance for a good pregnancy outcome, because spontaneous abortion, birth defects, stillbirth, problems in labor, and illnesses in the newborn and child are inversely related to control of blood sugar during gestation.

Diabetes mellitus (DM) affects 3 to 5 percent of all pregnancies. Types I and II DM complicate approximately 0.5 percent of pregnancies; gestational DM affects 2 to 5 percent, depending on the demographics of the population. Risk factors for gestational DM include maternal age >30 years, obesity, family history of gestational or type II DM, previous large baby, and prior stillbirth.

PATHOPHYSIOLOGY

There is no more sensitive indicator of the metabolic stability of the pregnant diabetic than the condition of the unborn baby. The fetus represents a barometer, with fetal outcome directly dependent on the degree of blood sugar control from the time before conception until delivery. Table 20-1 demonstrates the potential adverse effects of maternal hyperglycemia on the fetus during various stages of gestation.

In normal pregnancy, maternal glucose levels are maintained within a narrow range. Fasting levels are 8 to 10 mg/dL lower during pregnancy, while postprandial levels are slightly higher in pregnancy than otherwise. Glucose is a critical fuel for the fetus and is transported across the placenta by facilitated diffusion. The placenta is an effective barrier to insulin: maternal insulin stays in the mother's circulation for the most part, while fetal insulin remains in the fetal compartment. In most circumstances, the fetal blood glucose level is slightly lower than the maternal level. The fetal pancreas demonstrates islet cells in the first trimester, and insulin is produced at a basal level beginning shortly thereafter. Because of the normal stabilization of blood sugar in a nondiabetic mother, fetal insulin secretion fluctuates very little until birth.

In the diabetic pregnancy complicated by significant hyperglycemia, the fetal environment is disturbed by an excess of glucose transported from the maternal compartment to the fetal circulation. In 1954[1] Pederson proposed a hypothesis for diabetic fetopathy that remains the basis for our understanding. It outlines the following sequence: (1) maternal hyperglycemia, which results in (2) fetal hyperglycemia, which results in (3) early stimulation of excess fetal insulin production as well as hypertrophy and hyperplasia of fetal pancreatic beta cells, which results in (4) increased deposition of fetal fat and protein.

The adverse metabolic conditions involve more than glucose imbalance. There are also alterations in amino acid levels, ketone production, and fatty acid metabolism that can affect the pregnancy. The severity of these other derangements is related to the degree of hyperglycemia.

The mechanisms for pregnancy loss due to poor control of maternal glucose levels are not clearly identified. However, hyperglycemia may be more poorly tolerated by the fetus than by the mother. In the pregnant sheep model, chronic maternal hyperglycemia causes fetal acidemia before maternal acidosis develops.[2] Hyperglycemia can reduce uteroplacental blood flow acutely.[3] Chronic hyperglycemia early in pregnancy may actually cause increased blood flow,

Table 20-1

EFFECTS OF HYPERGLYCEMIA AND/OR KETONEMIA ON PREGNANCY

Stage	Effect: Increased Risk for
Before conception	Infertility
	Spontaneous abortion
	Birth defects
First trimester	Spontaneous abortion
	Birth defects
	Neurologic sequelae
	Fetal growth restriction
Second trimester	Spontaneous abortion
	Fetal death
	Neurologic sequelae
	Excessive size
	Preterm birth
	Birth trauma
Third trimester and labor	Fetal death
	Neurologic sequelae
	Excessive size
	Preterm birth
	Birth trauma
After birth	Metabolic abnormalities in newborn
	Respiratory distress in newborn
	Childhood obesity and related diseases

resulting in macrosomia despite adequate glucose control later in pregnancy.

Maternal diabetic vascular disease is a risk factor for fetal growth retardation due to poor perfusion and inadequate delivery of substrate.

Diabetic ketoacidosis is life-threatening to the fetus. Thirty years ago, the fetal loss rate was 30 percent for maternal acidosis and 64 percent with maternal coma.[4] More recently, Montoro et al. described 20 type I pregnant diabetics in ketoacidosis. Of these, 7 (35 percent) had a dead fetus on admission, but all the fetuses that were alive at presentation survived the acute episode.[5]

Pregnancy does predispose patients with type I DM to ketoacidosis for a number of reasons. When fasting, the pregnant woman's metabolism has been described as a condition of "accelerated starvation," with lower blood sugar and early production of ketones. The normal nausea and vomiting of early pregnancy predisposes the individual to ketosis, and systemic infection—another risk factor for diabetic ketoacidosis—is more frequent during pregnancy.

At birth, infants of diabetic mothers exposed to hyperglycemia are susceptible to hypoglycemia in the newborn period, as their insulin production transiently remains elevated after the maternal glucose overload is removed. Re-

lated metabolic problems in infants of poorly controlled diabetics include hypocalcemia, hyperbilirubinemia, and respiratory distress.

BIRTH DEFECTS

The control of diabetes before conception can lower the risk of birth defects by a factor of 7.[6] The risk of birth defects was 22.4 percent for diabetic women with the highest glycosylated hemoglobin level at the first prenatal visit versus 3.5 percent for those with the lowest level.

Birth defects occur as a result of events before pregnancy and very early in its course. For instance, the neural tube develops at approximately days 23 to 26 after conception, or during weeks 5 to 6 after the first day of the last menstrual period. Most pregnancies in the United States are unplanned and are not diagnosed until 5 to 6 weeks after conception or later. In other words, by the time a woman notices that her period is late, does the home pregnancy test, and calls the doctor, the birth defect "horse" (in the case of neural tube defects, one of the many anomalies that are more common in infants of diabetic mothers) is "out of the barn."

Animal studies have clearly demonstrated the teratogenic effects of hyperglycemia and the associated metabolic derangements in the poorly controlled diabetic pregnancy. Poor control of diabetes results in the following derangements that have been implicated in teratogenesis: elevated beta-hydroxybutyrate, triglycerides, and branched chain amino acid concentrations[7]; myoinositol deficiency[8]; arachidonic acid deficiency; and excess oxygen free radicals.[9]

In contrast to hyperglycemia, hypoglycemia has not been demonstrated to be teratogenic in human pregnancy,[10] although it was found to be teratogenic in some animal studies.[11] However, newborns exposed to elevated levels of maternal serum ketones have lower developmental scores at age 2 than controls.[12]

DIAGNOSIS AND DIFFERENTIAL DIAGNOSIS

From the fetus's standpoint, the impact of DM is related to the degree of hyperglycemia, the stage of gestation, and the attendant metabolic derangements in the mother. However, from the clinician's standpoint, the type of DM present in the mother is very important for an understanding of the pathophysiology and clinical management. The three common types of DM affecting pregnancy are type I, type II, and gestational diabetes mellitus. They are briefly described here; readers are referred to another source for more information.[12]

TYPE I DIABETES MELLITUS

Synonyms include insulin-dependent DM (IDDM), juvenile-onset DM, and ketosis-prone DM. The pathophysiology is a deficiency (early in the disease) or complete lack of production of insulin by the beta cells in the pancreas, often due to an autoimmune process. In the absence of insulin, these patients develop ketoacidosis and die. Often the disease begins before adulthood, but not always. They are at risk of developing vascular complications of all organ systems. Some patients with a long history of type I DM have loss of glucagon production and autonomic dysfunction, placing them at increased risk for severe hypoglycemia.

During pregnancy these patients need frequent meals and snacks, frequent blood sugar monitoring, and close observation for hypoglycemia. Any minor illness can predispose to wide fluctuations in blood sugar and increase the risk for ketoacidosis, which can result in pregnancy loss.

TYPE II DIABETES MELLITUS

Synonyms include non-insulin-dependent DM (NIDDM) and adult-onset DM. The pathophysiology is inappropriate utilization of insulin, usually due to an insulin resistance at the cellular level.[13] Obesity is commonly present in type II diabetics, and in the nonpregnant woman weight loss can cure the disease in some cases. However, weight loss is not recommended during pregnancy. Circulating insulin levels may be normal or actually above normal, but hyperglycemia occurs nevertheless. Ketoacidosis is unusual in the absence of another major illness. Treatment involves diet, exercise, and, in many cases, drug therapy. Oral agents are often effective but not used during pregnancy. Insulin in relatively high doses is effective and is used during pregnancy when diet and exercise are ineffective.

GESTATIONAL DIABETES MELLITUS

This term should *not* be used for patients with type I or II DM who are pregnant. Gestational DM is defined as carbohydrate intolerance of variable severity with onset or first recognition during pregnancy.[14]

The pathophysiology is the same as with type II DM. Normal pregnancy does require increased endogenous insulin production, and this increased demand cannot be met effectively in approximately 2 to 5 percent of women, resulting in gestational DM. Many women given a diagnosis of gestational DM will continue to have carbohydrate intolerance after pregnancy and be shown to be type II diabetics. Within 10 to 20 years of pregnancy, up to 50 percent of women with gestational DM will be identified as type II diabetics. Thus identification of gestational DM is important in the long-term health maintenance of these patients, targeting women who may develop disease later in life. Treatment includes diet, exercise, and insulin. Insulin has been used in some studies for all gestational diabetics and can lower the average birth weight of the newborn, reducing the risk of fetal macrosomia, one of the major problems in these pregnancies.[15] Alternatively, insulin may be used selectively based on past history, maternal weight, risk factors for fetal macrosomia, and/or blood sugars.

MAKING A DIAGNOSIS OF DIABETES DURING PREGNANCY

By definition, a pregnant woman who has DM first diagnosed during pregnancy should be identified as a gestational diabetic. Her treatment should be based on the clinical situation rather than a simple classification.

In the setting of an emergency department, there are a host of possible causes of hyperglycemia in addition to DM: infection, stress, and pharmacologic treatment (e.g., glucocorticoids, intravenously administered glucose, or parenteral nutrition). From a fetal standpoint, both the cause of the hyperglycemia (e.g., overwhelming sepsis from any source, which may cause pregnancy loss) and the elevated blood sugar are threatening. Thus, while identifying the particular type of carbohydrate intolerance in the acute care setting is important (e.g., identifying that a patient has type I DM, took a large dose of insulin 6 h ago, and has not eaten), the immediate need is to treat the underlying condition and stabilize glucose metabolism (see "Management," below).

Although there is no universal agreement regarding the clinical criteria for a diagnosis of gestational DM, a widely

---

Table 20-2

GESTATIONAL DIABETES MELLITUS— TESTING PROTOCOL[a]

I. Screening
   A. Diet: no preparation is necessary; often done as morning fasting
   B. Oral glucose (50 g) ingested quickly
   C. No smoking or vigorous activity
   D. Venous glucose drawn 1 h later
   E. Abnormal: >140 mg/dL if fasted, >130 mg/100 mL if nonfasting test[18]
   F. Abnormal values: do 3 h test with 100 g
II. Diagnosis
   A. Diet: 3-day carbohydrate loading diet
   B. Oral glucose load (100 g) ingested quickly
   C. No smoking or vigorous activity
   D. Abnormal if two or more values meet or exceed:
      1. Fasting—105 mg/dL
      2. One hour—190 mg/dL
      3. Two hours—165 mg/dL
      4. Three hours—145 mg/dL

[a]All glucose measurements performed on venous plasma assayed by glucose oxidase method in a clinical laboratory.[16]

utilized method is the 3-h 100-g oral glucose tolerance test (GTT) administered after a 3-day carbohydrate loading diet[16] (see Table 20-2). There is also no universal agreement regarding which pregnant patients should undergo the diagnostic 3-h GTT. If historic risk factors are used to identify women for laboratory testing, 50 percent of gestational diabetics will be missed.[17] Many clinicians perform laboratory screening of all pregnant women at 24 to 28 weeks of gestation with a 1-h 50-g venous plasma sample. A value of >140 mg/dL is then followed by the diagnostic 3-h test. The screening test has a sensitivity of 90 percent and a specificity of 85 percent.[16]

MANAGEMENT

INSULIN

In order to understand the preexisting treatment program of a pregnant diabetic and the treatment options available in the acute care setting, the many different insulin types are reviewed. During pregnancy, oral hypoglycemic agents are avoided due to adverse fetal effects (see Chap. 16). If a diabetic presents on an oral agent, her treatment plan should include switching to an insulin program as soon as possible.

Over three hundred types of insulin are produced worldwide. They vary based on source, molecular structure, additives to prolong onset and duration of action, buffering agents, and recommended delivery systems. In addition, insulin can be administered intravenously, subcutaneously by single injection or infusion pump, or intramuscularly. Experimental systems include pancreatic cell transplants and other indwelling devices.

Table 20-3

INSULIN TYPES AND ACTION

Type	Method	Time		
		Onset	Peak	Duration
Regular	SQ	15–60 min	2–4 h	5–8 h
	IV	0–5 min	30–60 min	2–4 h
NPH	SQ	2–4 h	6–10 h	12–24 h
Lente	SQ	2–4 h	6–10 h	12–24 h
Ultralente	SQ	4–8 h	10–12 h	24–48 h

Note: The action of insulin given subcutaneously may vary by 25 percent in one person, and by 50 percent among individuals. The action is affected by patient activity, body location of the injection, and local injection site integrity, such as scarring due to long-term use of one site for many injections.

In this country, common types of insulin are "human," beef, and/or pork insulins. Human insulin is produced by bioengineering methods and is identical in molecular structure to endogenous human insulin. Its advantage is that antibodies are produced less often than if beef or pork insulin (each of which varies from human insulin in molecular structure) is used over time. Human insulin tends to be somewhat quicker in onset and shorter in duration than the same type of insulin from animals.

Common formulations of insulin in use include regular, neutral protamine Hagedorn (NPH), Lente, and Ultralente (Table 20-3). The latter three are mixtures of regular insulin with agents that prolong onset, modulate peak action, and extend the duration of a subcutaneous injection. Lente and NPH have a nearly similar pattern of onset, peak, and duration. However, NPH has the advantage of mixing more effectively when a single injection includes a combination of a regular and a longer-acting agent.

During pregnancy, when meticulous control of blood sugar has beneficial effects on pregnancy outcome, many patients are on intensive insulin therapy. Details vary based on the clinical approach in use locally, but certain aspects are uniform. Glucose measurements are frequent (often 6 to 8 times per day), and regular and intermediate insulin are used in combination or singly with scheduled administration 3 to 5 times per day. Continuous subcutaneous infusion pumps using a buffered regular insulin are occasionally utilized.

WORKUP OF PREGNANT DIABETICS PRESENTING FOR ACUTE CARE

HISTORY

The intake history should include the last menstrual period, gestational age, any obstetric problems, past obstetric and medical history, medications, and diet. If the patient is a known diabetic, then the type of diabetes (type I, type II, or gestational), any diabetes-related organic disease, the type of insulin, time and route of last dose of insulin, and diet (daily number of calories, number of meals and snacks per day, time of last meal) should be addressed. Many diabetics will carry a glucometer with them, a written record of their recent blood sugars and insulin doses, and snacks for emergency treatment of hypoglycemia. Many modern glucose reflectance meters have memory storage functions, allowing the clinician to review recent glucose levels quickly. In addition to the chief complaint on presentation for acute care, other recent "minor" illnesses such as a cold, flu, dental problems, or urinary tract infections may identify the cause of worsening carbohydrate intolerance.

PHYSICAL EXAMINATION

The physical examination should include temperature, pulse, respirations, blood pressure, and an estimated or measured weight. Mental status should be assessed, because severe hypoglycemia or hyperglycemia can cause confusion, lethargy, violent behavior, or coma. Examination should concentrate on possible sites of infection if clinically indicated. In patients with long-standing type I DM, the feet can be a source of inflammation or infection due to vascular insufficiency.

A pelvic and abdominal examination should assess the fundal height, cervix, and the presence of fetal heart tones. The fetal heart rate can be auscultated by a nonamplified fetal stethoscope after 20 weeks of gestation in a nonobese patient or after 12 weeks of gestation with Doppler. If the patient is beyond 24 weeks of gestation, fetal assessment for 20 to 40 min by electronic fetal monitoring should be considered.

LABORATORY ASSESSMENT

In a pregnant diabetic presenting for emergency care for any problem, initial blood glucose measurement is advised. A bedside glucose reflectance meter, if properly calibrated, can offer a rapid estimate while the standard laboratory test is under way.

In addition to the laboratory workup of the presenting problem, significant hyperglycemia (e.g., 200 mg/dL in a pregnant woman) in the acute setting should be further assessed for the possibility of diabetic ketoacidosis (DKA). In pregnancy, DKA can occur at glucose levels significantly lower than in the nonpregnant patient.

Diabetic ketoacidosis is defined as hyperglycemia, acidosis, and ketonemia. The laboratory assessment and principles of management of DKA in pregnancy are the same as in the nonpregnant patient.[19,20] Initial laboratory studies include a complete blood count, glucose, electrolytes, blood urea nitrogen, creatinine, venous pH, urinary and serum ketones, arterial blood gases, and urinalysis.

The clinician should be aware that because of the normal physiologic changes of pregnancy, normal ranges of routine laboratory test results may change. By midpregnancy, expanded plasma volume results in a 5 to 10 percent reduction in the hemoglobin and hematocrit and a slight reduction in blood urea nitrogen and serum creatinine. The white blood count is often 10,000 to 15,000 in normal pregnancy and can increase another 50 to 100 percent with labor. Maternal heart rate increases by 5 to 10 beats per minute and midtrimester blood pressures are slightly lower. Increased minute ventilation causes a slight respiratory alkalosis. Small amounts of glucosuria can occur normally in the absence of DM (see also Chap. 2).

Once treatment of DKA is begun, 1- to 2-h assessment of glucose, electrolytes, and pH should follow until stabilization occurs. Other laboratory studies may be repeated as frequently if they remain abnormal. In addition to metabolic therapy, a search for the cause of DKA should be undertaken. Pregnancy per se is not a cause of DKA, but it does predispose a patient to DKA (see "Pathophysiology," above).

If DKA is present, such a patient should be placed in an obstetric intensive care area where both fetal (after about 24 weeks of gestation) and maternal evaluation and treatment can take place.

TREATMENT

HYPOGLYCEMIA

Hypoglycemia may be present on first contact or may be "iatrogenic"—i.e., the result of an extended stay in the acute care setting during which ongoing glucose testing and meals are disrupted. Thus the first aspect of treatment of hypoglycemia in the pregnant diabetic is prevention. Pregnant diabetics who are well controlled by intensive insulin treatment (e.g., six feedings a day and three to five routine insulin injections per day) can quickly develop problems if the routine is disrupted. Such patients may have glucometer values of 50 to 60 mg/100 mL and be comfortable at that level, requiring only their scheduled meal or snack, as opposed to an intravenous bolus of glucose that may disrupt their diabetes for the next 24 h. Patients with a low blood sugar who are symptomatic but are not NPO can be treated orally with crackers or milk. Candy or orange juice often causes an unnecessarily rapid rise in blood sugar, making further treatment more involved.

For severe hypoglycemia associated with obtundation or coma, therapy depends on the setting. Families of type I diabetics (the only group at serious risk of profound hypoglycemia) are often trained and have subcutaneous glucagon available, which they may have given while calling for an ambulance. If intravenous access can be established quickly, then intravenous glucose (e.g., 50 mL of 50% glucose solution) given rapidly can awaken the patient and allow further supportive treatment.

HYPERGLYCEMIA WITHOUT KETOACIDOSIS

Hyperglycemia without ketoacidosis may also be present on initial contact or as the result of management in the emergency department. Prevention of hyperglycemia requires knowledge of the patient's recent diet and insulin treatment and avoidance of large amounts of intravenous fluids containing glucose.

If ketoacidosis is absent, hyperglycemia can be treated on an individualized basis. Often a knowledgeable patient has an understanding of how much subcutaneously administered regular insulin is necessary to normalize her blood level. In some cases, a minor modification of her usual insulin program will suffice. Intravenous insulin has a more rapid onset and shorter duration than subcutaneous insulin and can be used as a bolus or a constant infusion. If the patient is NPO and admission is likely, then an intravenous controlled infusion allows gradual and effective treatment.

DIABETIC KETOACIDOSIS

The principles of metabolic treatment of DKA in pregnancy are the same as in the nonpregnant patient, but attention must be paid to fetal status as well.

Treatment is directed at correcting the multiple abnor-

Table 20-4

TREATMENT OF DIABETIC KETOACIDOSIS IN PREGNANCY

Simultaneously initiate all of the following:

1. Admit to obstetric intensive care area, if available.
2. Insert large-bore intravenous line.
3. Obtain initial laboratory studies (see text).
4. Place patient on her side or in left lateral tilt position to improve venous return.
5. Consider an arterial line for serial blood sampling.
6. Begin a flow sheet including vital signs, glucose, lab values (to be assessed every 1–4 h based on acuity). Glucose and potassium values should be assessed hourly initially.
7. Oxygen by mask (3–6 L/min).
8. Foley catheter, sample to laboratory for urinalysis and culture.
9. Volume replacement (total deficit may be 5–10 L):
   a. 1000 mL normal saline over 1–2 h.
   b. If serum sodium or serum osmolality is elevated, replace with 0.45% NaCl.
   c. After 1–2 h, switch to 0.45% NaCl at 250–500 mL/h; reduce rate as glucose nears 200 mg/dL.
10. Insulin therapy:
    a. Intravenous bolus 0.4 U/kg regular insulin.
    b. Continuous intravenous infusion at 5–10 U/h regular insulin.
    c. Reduce hourly infusion rate as glucose nears 250 mg/dL.
    d. Double infusion rate if no response after first hour.
    e. Continue intravenous infusion for 12–24 h after ketoacidosis clears.
11. Potassium therapy:
    a. Give KCl 40 meq/h if potassium is low.
    b. Give KCl 20 meq/h if potassium is normal.
    c. Withhold KCl if potassium is elevated.
    d. ECG monitoring if KCl is given with oliguria.
12. Etiology:
    Workup for causes of diabetic ketoacidosis.
13. Fetal assessment:
    a. Beyond 12 weeks of gestation, fetal heart rate by Doppler.
    b. Beyond 24 weeks of gestation, continuous electronic fetal monitoring and uterine monitoring.
    c. An abnormal (nonreassuring) fetal heart rate is often present in diabetic ketoacidosis and is usually best treated with intrauterine resuscitation. Maternal oxygen therapy, fluid replacement, and correction of hyperglycemia and ketoacidosis will improve fetal condition. Emergency delivery is rarely necessary and potentially hazardous to the mother.
    d. Uterine contractions are often observed and usually do not result in delivery remote from term. Tocolysis should not be undertaken unless significant cervical dilatation occurs. Beta sympathomimetic agents and maternal administration of glucocorticoids for fetal pulmonary maturity should be avoided during diabetic ketoacidosis.

malities of hyperglycemia, insulin deficiency, ketone excess, acidosis, dehydration, and electrolyte imbalance (see Table 20-4).

DISCHARGE INSTRUCTIONS AND FOLLOW-UP INTERVAL

Any female diabetic of childbearing age should be encouraged to use contraception unless she is enrolled in a program to normalize her blood sugars before conception. All women of childbearing age (pregnant or not) should consume 0.4 mg of folic acid daily to reduce the incidence of neural tube defects. Diabetic women who have a normal pregnancy first identified in the emergency department need urgent follow-up to assure the best possible outcome of the pregnancy. Sometimes admission is appropriate (see below).

DIET

Women of normal weight should consume 36 kcal/kg per day in the first trimester and 40 kcal/kg per day in the last two trimesters.[21] Overweight women (>120 percent of ideal body weight) may benefit from 24 kcal/kg per day, while underweight women (<80 percent of ideal body weight) can consume 40 kcal/kg per day throughout pregnancy.[22] The diet should be divided into three meals and two to three snacks. An American Diabetes Association diet plan provides the appropriate mix of carbohydrate, fat, and protein. Folic acid (0.4 mg/day) and an intake of 1200 mg/day of calcium are advised. Consultation with a nutritionist experienced with pregnant diabetics can be very helpful.

ACTIVITY

Pregnancy does not require special activity restrictions. However, it is ill-advised to institute a vigorous new exercise program in a previously sedentary patient. Because joint laxity increases and weight distribution changes, care should be taken with certain sports. Exercise tolerance in previously fit women will decrease slightly with advancing gestation.

INSULIN

The goal of diet, exercise, and insulin programs is to normalize blood sugars. In the acute care setting, the planning of insulin therapy should be based on prior insulin doses and ideally coordinated with the team who will follow the pregnancy. Insulin resistance due to hormonal changes in pregnancy does not develop until the second half of pregnancy; however, most diabetics who begin pregnancy find that they need more insulin than before because the goals are lower blood sugars. One or two injections a day in a type I or II diabetic who is pregnant will not be adequate to maximize control in most cases.

HOME GLUCOSE MONITORING

Any attempt at normalizing blood sugars has some risk of hypoglycemia and can only be undertaken safely with frequent self-testing. With intensive insulin therapy, measurements may be taken before and 1 or 2 h after each of the three main meals, at bedtime, and at 3 A.M. There is little need for urinary testing at home unless the blood sugar is above 200 mg/dL, in which case urinary ketones indicate a state of increased insulin resistance.

RECORD KEEPING

Frequent measurements are of little benefit without a good record of the dates and times of insulin therapy and blood glucose values.

HYPOGLYCEMIA SAFEGUARDS

Type I diabetics should be advised to keep a glucose meter with them at all times, along with a snack for emergencies. Family members should be instructed in the warning signs of hypoglycemia and equipped with emergency stores of oral glucose treatment and glucagon to be administered subcutaneously.

GUIDELINES

Diabetics under good control with a previously identified pregnancy should keep their regular appointments for follow-up care unless the acute problem dealt with in the emergency department requires otherwise.

Diabetics under less than ideal control who are pregnant and any diabetic with an early pregnancy just identified should be seen quickly, and some may be candidates for admission.

The patient should be instructed that a home blood glucose value of less than 60 mg/dL, an episode of severe hypoglycemia, or a blood sugar that persists above 200 mg/dL is reason to call her doctor immediately.

INDICATIONS FOR ADMISSION AND SPECIALTY CONSULTATION

Indications for admission include moderate or severe hyperemesis gravidarum, persistent ketosis for any reason, diabetic ketoacidosis, and poorly controlled diabetes mellitus (any type) in early pregnancy.

Hyperemesis gravidarum predisposes the diabetic woman to ketoacidosis because of starvation and dehydration. If a patient is unable to eat reliably and drink adequately, the risk of hypoglycemia due to mealtime nausea and vomiting after a premeal insulin dose has been taken is concerning. Hyperemesis gravidarum in a nondiabetic that can be managed on an outpatient basis often requires admission in a type I or II diabetic.

Ketosis without ketoacidosis is concerning because this may adversely affect neurodevelopmental outcome in the offspring. If ketosis can be cleared easily with hydration and the underlying cause addressed, then a trial of outpatient therapy is worthwhile. The most common cause is inadequate oral intake of fluids or calories because of vomiting or poor diet.

If an early pregnancy is first diagnosed in the emergency department and diabetic control is inadequate, admission should be considered. Organogenesis occurs in the first 6 to 8 weeks after the last menstrual period, and persistently elevated blood sugars at this time are a factor in birth defects and pregnancy loss.

If the blood sugars are quite elevated when the diagnosis of gestational DM is first made in the emergency department, admission is appropriate. While there are no strict guidelines, a fasting glucose of above 140 mg/dL or a random glucose of >200 mg/dL would be concerning. Urgent outpatient follow-up as soon as possible is an alternative.

Diabetic ketoacidosis requires emergency admission to an obstetric intensive care area.

Specialty consultation should be used liberally for assistance in the management of DM in pregnancy for any of the above problems. In the metabolically stable patient who is already enrolled in high-risk pregnancy care, the high-risk team involved should be contacted to help plan ongoing care and address the role of admission. In many centers, there is a multidisciplinary team of obstetricians, high-risk pregnancy specialists (maternal-fetal medicine), endocrinologists, diabetes nurse educators, dieticians, and social workers who support these challenging patients. In some settings, an obstetrician along with medical consultants and others care for these patients. If the patient does not have a care team on presentation, arrangements for follow-up with experienced clinicians should ideally be made before discharge.

SUMMARY AND COMMENT

The emergency physician can contribute to improving outcome for pregnancies of diabetics in a number of ways:

1. Regardless of the presenting complaint to the emergency physician, the diabetic woman of childbearing age:
   a. Should be assessed for an early undiagnosed pregnancy. If an early pregnancy is present, then aggressive management to achieve good glucose control should begin immediately, either as an outpatient or an inpatient.
   b. In the absence of pregnancy, the history should address current method of contraception, and patient education should include the importance of preconception glucose control to improve pregnancy outcome.
2. When a pregnant diabetic presents to the emergency physician, regardless of the presenting complaint, assessment of the metabolic condition of the mother and appropriate correction of hyperglycemia and ketosis, if present, should be part of acute care.
3. In the absence of hyperglycemia or ketosis, ongoing care should include a plan for close follow-up to offer the best chance of a good pregnancy outcome.

References

1. Pederson J: Weight and length at birth of infants of diabetic mothers. *Acta Endocrinol* 16:30, 1954.
2. Philipps AF, Porte PJ, Stabinsky S, et al: Effects of chronic fetal hyperglycemia upon oxygen consumption in the ovine uterus and conceptus. *J Clin Invest* 74:279, 1984.
3. Nyland L, Lubell NO: Uteroplacental blood flow in diabetic pregnancy: Measurements with indium 113m and a computer-linked gamma camera. *Am J Obstet Gynecol* 144:298, 1982.
4. Kyle GC: Diabetes and pregnancy. *Ann Intern Med* 59 (suppl 3):1, 1963.
5. Montoro MN, Myers VP, Mestmand JH, et al: Outcome of pregnancy in diabetic ketoacidosis. *Am J Perinatol* 10:17, 1993.
6. Miller E, Hare JW, Cloherty JP, et al: Elevated maternal hemoglobin A1 in early pregnancy and major congenital anomalies in infants of diabetic mothers. *N Engl J Med* 304:1331, 1981.
7. Reece EA, Eriksson UJ: The pathogenesis of diabetes-associated congenital malformations. *Obstet Gynecol Clin North Am* 23(1):29, 1996.
8. Baker L, Piddington R, Goldman AS, et al: Myo-inositol and prostaglandins reverse the glucose inhibition of neural tube fusion in cultured mouse embryos. *Diabetologia* 33:593, 1990.
9. Eriksson UJ, Borg LAH: Diabetes and embryonic malformations: Role of substrate-induced free oxygen radical production for dysmorphogenesis in cultured rat embryos. *Diabetes* 42:411, 1993.
10. Reece KEA, Homko CJJ, Wiznitzer A: Hypoglycemia in pregnancies complicated by diabetes mellitus: Maternal and fetal considerations. *Clin Obstet Gynecol* 37:50, 1994.
11. Sadler TW, Hunter ES III: Hypoglycemia: How little is too much for the embryo? *Am J Obstet Gynecol* 157:190, 1987.
12. Rizzo T, Metzger BE, Burns WJ, et al: Correlation between antepartum maternal metabolism and intelligence of offspring. *N Engl J Med* 325:911, 1991.
13. Pickup J, Williams G: *Textbook of Diabetes.* Boston: Blackwell, 1991.
14. National Diabetes Group: Classification and diagnosis of diabetes mellitus and other categories of glucose tolerance. *Diabetes* 28:1039, 1979.
15. Coustan DR, Lewis SB: Insulin therapy for gestational diabetes. *Obstet Gynecol* 51:306, 1978.
16. American College of Obstetricians and Gynecologists: *Diabetes in Pregnancy.* Technical bulletin #200. Washington, DC: ACOG, 1994.
17. Coustan DR: Screening and diagnosis of gestational diabetes. *Semin Perinatol* 18:407, 1994.
18. Carpenter MW: Testing for gestational diabetes, in Reece EA, Coustan DR (eds.): *Diabetes in Pregnancy.* New York: Churchill Livingstone, 1995, p 267.
19. Ragland G: Diabetic ketoacidosis, in Tintanelli JE, Krome RL, Ruiz E (eds): *Emergency Medicine,* 3d ed. New York: McGraw-Hill, 1992.
20. Chauhan SP, Kerry KG Jr: Management of diabetic ketoacidosis in the obstetric patient. *Obstet Gynecol Clin North Am* 21:143, 1995.
21. National Academy of Sciences: *Recommended Dietary Allowances,* 10th ed. Washington DC: National Academy Press, 1989.
22. Jovanovic-Peterson L, Peterson CM: Dietary manipulation as a primary treatment strategy for pregnancies complicated by diabetes. *J Am Coll Nutr* 9:320, 1990.

Chapter 21

HEMATOLOGIC DISORDERS IN PREGNANCY

Mary E. Eberst

REVIEW OF HEMATOLOGIC CHANGES IN NORMAL PREGNANCY

ANEMIA OF PREGNANCY

Normal pregnancy results in a dilutional anemia with an expected hemoglobin of 11.0 to 12.0 g/dL and a hematocrit of 33 to 34 percent at the time of delivery. During pregnancy, the plasma volume and red blood cell (RBC) mass both increase; however, the increase in plasma volume is proportionately greater, resulting in a decrease in the hemoglobin and hematocrit. Overall, the plasma volume expands 40 to 60 percent, up to 1500 cm^3, most of which occurs during the first and second trimesters. The RBC mass increases 20 to 30 percent beginning in the first trimester and continuing throughout the pregnancy. The expansion of RBCs results from elevated levels of erythropoietin and human placental lactogen and requires adequate levels of iron, folate, and vitamin B$_{12}$. The increased RBC mass can serve as a reservoir to compensate for any blood loss at the time of delivery. The hemodilution serves the metabolic and perfusion needs of the fetal-placental unit. The resultant decrease in blood viscosity may offset the effects of increased levels of fibrinogen and enhanced RBC aggregation in late pregnancy. There is evidence that the failure to develop this expected anemia is associated with an increased risk of low birth weight and preterm delivery. However, anemia that is worsened by iron or folate deficiency is detrimental (see below). Hemoglobin levels below 10.5 g/dL or hematocrit below 32 percent represent anemia beyond that expected. These levels likely represent a true anemia due to a reduction in RBC mass and should be evaluated further.[1]

LEUKOCYTOSIS

During normal pregnancy, leukocytosis is common. Early in pregnancy, the average white blood cell (WBC) count can be at the upper limit of normal for nonpregnant patients. By the third trimester, the WBC may normally rise as high as 15,000 to 18,000/mm^3. During the last month of gestation, the WBC trends downward until the time of delivery, when it may again rise to 15,000 to 20,000/mm^3. White blood cell counts up to 25,000/mm^3 are sometimes seen during normal labor. Elevated levels of plasma cortisol are believed to be responsible for this leukocytosis. The WBC differential may reveal a rare myelocyte or metamyelocyte, and Doehle bodies may be present in the cytoplasm of the WBCs.

PLATELET CHANGES IN PREGNANCY

In conjunction with the increase in plasma volume during normal pregnancy, and perhaps because of compensated low-grade disseminated intravascular coagulation (DIC) within the uteroplacental unit, platelet counts decline during pregnancy as much as 20 percent from baseline values, although usually remaining within the normal limits. This decline in the platelet count is most pronounced after 32 weeks of gestation. In large studies of pregnant women, thrombocytopenia, when diagnosed by conventional criteria, is present in as many as 8 percent at the time of delivery. Most of these women, up to three-fourths, have no identifiable underlying disease state and have what is called "incidental" or "gestational" thrombocytopenia.[2,3] The majority of these women have platelet counts above 80,000/mm^3, although they can be as low as 50,000/mm^3. This "gestational" thrombocytopenia is of no apparent risk to the mother or infant at the time of delivery. Gestational thrombocytopenia can recur in subsequent pregnancies. It rarely predates the development of autoimmune or other underlying disease and is not associated with neonatal thrombocytopenia. Platelet counts should return to normal levels within days of the delivery. Gestational thrombocytopenia is a diagnosis of exclusion; conditions that could have an effect on the neonatal platelet count should be considered. In pregnant women with thrombocytopenia, the clinician should decide the extent of investigation, if any, to evaluate the possibility of underlying disease. An approach to this evaluation is discussed below.

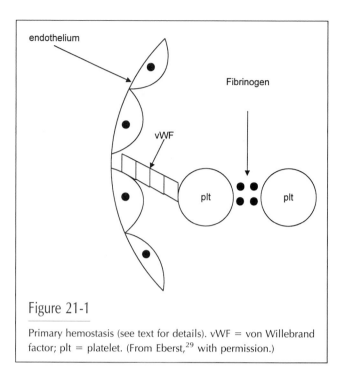

Figure 21-1

Primary hemostasis (see text for details). vWF = von Willebrand factor; plt = platelet. (From Eberst,[29] with permission.)

HEMOSTASIS IN PREGNANCY

REVIEW OF NORMAL COAGULATION

The normal hemostatic system consists of a complex process that limits blood loss by the formation of a platelet plug (primary hemostasis) and the production of cross-linked fibrin (secondary hemostasis), which strengthens the platelet plug. These reactions are counterregulated by the fibrinolytic system, which limits the size of fibrin clot that is formed, thereby preventing excessive clot formation. Congenital and acquired abnormalities occur in both of these systems. The affected patients may have excessive hemorrhage, excessive thrombus formation, or both.

Primary hemostasis is the platelet interaction with the vascular subendothelium that results in the formation of a platelet plug at the site of injury. Required components for this to occur are normal vascular subendothelium (collagen), functional platelets, normal von Willebrand factor (connects the platelet to the endothelium via glycoprotein Ib), and normal fibrinogen (connects the platelets to each other via glycoproteins II$_b$–III$_a$). Figure 21-1 depicts primary hemostasis.

Secondary hemostasis describes the reactions of the plasma coagulation proteins (factors) by a tightly regulated mechanism. The final product is cross-linked fibrin, which is insoluble and strengthens the platelet plug formed in primary hemostasis. Figure 21-2 diagrams the reactions of secondary hemostasis.

The fibrinolytic system is a complex system that regulates the hemostatic mechanism by limiting the size of fibrin clots

that are formed. A simplified schema is depicted in Fig. 21-3. The principal physiologic activator is tissue plasminogen activator (t-PA), which is released from endothelial cells. The t-PA converts plasminogen, which is synthesized in the liver and absorbed in the fibrin clot, to plasmin. Plasmin degrades fibrinogen and fibrin monomer into low-molecular-weight fragments known as *fibrin degradation products* (FDPs) and cross-linked fibrin into D-dimers.

Other physiologic inhibitors of hemostasis with prevalent clinical applicability include antithrombin III and the protein C–protein S system. Antithrombin III is a protein that forms complexes with all the serine protease coagulation factors (factors XII, XI, X, IX, VII, and prothrombin) thereby inhibiting their function. Heparin potentiates this interaction, and this is the basis for its use as an anticoagulant. Protein C, which requires the presence of protein S for activation, is capable of inactivating the two plasma cofactors, factors V and VIII, and inhibiting their participation in the coagulation cascade. Patients with deficiencies of antithrombin III, protein C, or protein S present clinically with abnormal thrombus formation (e.g., pulmonary embolism, deep venous thrombosis).

The screening tests of primary and secondary hemostasis as well as other commonly used coagulation tests are outlined in Table 21-1.

COAGULATION CHANGES IN PREGNANCY

Many dramatic changes in the normal hemostatic mechanism occur during pregnancy, leading to a hypercoagulable state in preparation for the hemostatic challenge that occurs

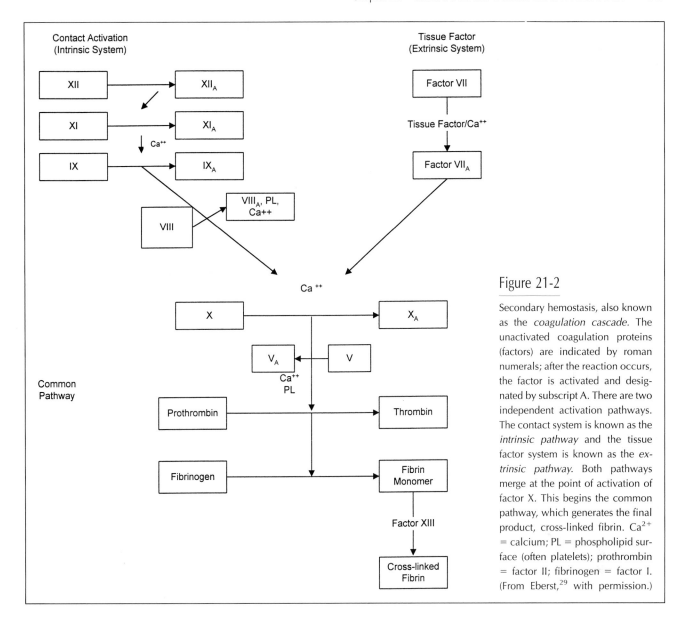

Figure 21-2

Secondary hemostasis, also known as the *coagulation cascade*. The unactivated coagulation proteins (factors) are indicated by roman numerals; after the reaction occurs, the factor is activated and designated by subscript A. There are two independent activation pathways. The contact system is known as the *intrinsic pathway* and the tissue factor system is known as the *extrinsic pathway*. Both pathways merge at the point of activation of factor X. This begins the common pathway, which generates the final product, cross-linked fibrin. Ca^{2+} = calcium; PL = phospholipid surface (often platelets); prothrombin = factor II; fibrinogen = factor I. (From Eberst,[29] with permission.)

at the time of delivery and placental separation.[4,5] These changes lessen the amount of bleeding at the time of delivery but increase the risk of thrombosis throughout the pregnancy and early postpartum period. As a result of these changes, the normal balance between coagulation (clot formation) and fibrinolysis (clot lysis) is tipped in favor of clot formation. The effect of pregnancy on the coagulation factors, naturally occurring anticoagulants, and fibrinolysis is shown in Table 21-1. In general, the factors that promote hemostasis are increased in concentration, while those that

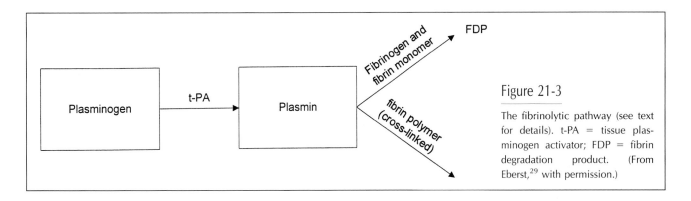

Figure 21-3

The fibrinolytic pathway (see text for details). t-PA = tissue plasminogen activator; FDP = fibrin degradation product. (From Eberst,[29] with permission.)

Table 21-1

TESTS OF HEMOSTASIS

Primary Hemostasis

Screening Tests	Normal Value	Measures	Clinical Correlations
Platelet count	150,000 to 300,000/mm^3	Number of platelets per mm^3	*Decreased platelet count (thrombocytopenia)* Bleeding usually not a problem until platelet count <50,000: high risk of spontaneous bleeding including CNS with count <10,000 per mm^3. Causes: Decreased production—viral infections (measles); marrow infiltration; drugs (thiazides, ETOH, estrogens, alpha-interferon) Increased destruction—viral infections (mumps, varicella, EBV, HIV); ITP, TTP, DIC[a], HUS; drugs (heparin, protamine) Splenic sequestration (hypersplenism, hypothermia) Loss of platelets (hemorrhage, hemodialysis, extracorporeal circulation) Pseudothrombocytopenia—platelets are clumped but not truly decreased in number; examine blood smear to recognize this *Elevated platelet count (thrombocytosis)* Commonly reactive to inflammation or malignancy or in polycythemia vera; can be associated with hemorrhage or thrombosis
Bleeding time (BT)	2.5–10 min (template BT)	Interaction between platelets and the subendothelium	*Prolonged bleeding time caused by:* Thrombocytopenia (platelet count <50,000 per mm^3) Abnormal platelet function (vWD, ASA, NSAIDs, uremia, liver disease) Collagen abnormalities (congenital abnormality, or prolonged use of glucocorticoids)

Secondary Hemostasis

Screening Tests	Normal Value	Measures	Clinical Correlations
Prothrombin time (PT)	10–12 s, but laboratory variation	Extrinsic system and common pathway—factors VII, X, V, prothrombin, and fibrinogen	*Prolonged PT—most commonly caused by:* Use of warfarin (inhibits vitamin K–dependent factors II, VII, IX and X) Advanced liver disease with decreased factor synthesis Antibiotics; some cephalosporins (moxalactam, cefamandole, cefotaxime, cefoperazone) that inhibit vitamin K–dependent factors
Activated partial thromboplastin time (aPTT)	Depends on type of thromboplastin used; "activated" with kaolin	Intrinsic system and common pathway including factors XII, XI, IX, VIII, X, V, prothrombin,	*Prolongation of aPTT most commonly caused by:* Heparin therapy Factor deficiencies; factor levels have to be <30% of normal to cause prolongation "Lupus-type anticoagulant"—can occur in patients with SLE and others; can lead to recurrent pregnancy loss (see text for details) *Note:* high doses of heparin or warfarin can cause prolongation of both the PT and aPTT due to their activity in the common pathway

Table 21-1

TESTS OF HEMOSTASIS (Continued)

Screening Tests	Normal Value	Measures	Clinical Correlations
Secondary Hemostasis (*Continued*)			
Thrombin clotting time (TCT)	10–12 s	Conversion of fibrinogen to fibrin monomer	*Prolonged TCT caused by:* Low fibrinogen level (DIC) Abnormal fibrinogen molecule (liver disease) Presence of heparin, FDPs, or a paraprotein (multiple myeloma); these interfere with the conversion Very high fibrinogen level (acute-phase reactant)
"Mixes"	Variable	Performed when one or more of the above screening tests is prolonged; the patient's plasma ("abnormal") is mixed with "normal" plasma and the screening test is repeated	*If the "mix" corrects the screening test*, one or more factor deficiencies are present *If the "mix" does not correct the screening test*, an inhibitor is present
Other Hemostatic Tests			
Fibrin degradation products (FDP) and D-dimer (evaluate fibrinolysis)	Variable	*FDPs* measure breakdown products from fibrinogen and fibrin monomer; *D-dimer* measures breakdown products of cross-linked fibrin	Levels of these are elevated in DIC, thrombosis, pulmonary embolus, liver disease
Factor level assays	60–130% (0.60–1.30 U/mL)	Measures the percent activity of a specified factor compared to normal	Used to identify specific factor deficiencies and in the therapeutic management of patients with deficiencies
Inhibitor screens	Variable	Verifies the presence or absence of antibodies directed against one or more of the coagulation factors	*Specific inhibitors*—directed against one coagulation factor, most commonly against factor VIII; can be in patients with congenital or acquired deficiency *Nonspecific inhibitors*—directed against more than one of the coagulation factors; an example is the lupus-type anticoagulant

[a]There are many pregnancy-associated causes of DIC (e.g., abruptio placentae, severe preeclampsia, amniotic fluid embolism).
Abbreviations: CNS = central nervous system; ETOH = ethanol; EBV = Epstein Barr virus; HIV = human immunodeficiency virus; ITP = idiopathic thrombocytopenic purpura; TTP = thrombotic thrombocytopenic purpura; DIC = disseminated intravascular coagulation; HUS = hemolytic uremic syndrome; vWD = vonWillebrand disease; ASA = aspirin; NSAIDs = nonsteroidal anti-inflammatory drugs; FDPs = fibrin degradation products.
Source: Adapted from Eberst,[29] with permission.

Table 21-2

HEMOSTATIC CHANGES IN NORMAL PREGNANCY

Effect on Hemostasis		Changes in Concentration (increased plasma volume taken into account)
	Coagulation Factors	
Promote hemostasis	I (fibrinogen)	Increases (2–4 times)
	VII	Increases (up to 10 times)
	VIII	Increases (up to 2 times)
	vWF	Increases (up to 4 times)
	X	Increases
	XII	Increases
	Naturally Occurring Anticoagulants	
Inhibit hemostasis	Antithrombin III	Slight decrease
	Protein C	Slight increase, still in normal range
	Protein S	Slight decrease, still in normal range
	Fibrinolytic System:	
	plasminogen activator inibitor 2 (PAI-2) (inhibits plasminogen)	Increase (derived from placenta)

limit clot formation are unchanged or slightly reduced in concentration. The fibrinolytic system is overall less active during pregnancy, and its response to stimuli is decreased. Most of these changes in hemostasis can be detected by the third month of gestation, and return to normal levels occurs within 4 weeks after delivery. Fibrinolytic activity returns to normal levels within 1 h after delivery of the placenta because the inhibitor of fibrinolysis, placentally derived plasminogen activator inhibitor 2 (PAI-2), is eliminated.

RED BLOOD CELL DISORDERS

CONGENITAL HEMOLYTIC ANEMIAS/HEMOGLOBINOPATHIES

SICKLE CELL DISEASE

Sickle cell disease (SCD) is the most common inherited hemoglobinopathy; 8 percent of African Americans in the United States carry the sickle cell gene. The genetic abnormality that results in sickle cell disease stems from a single amino acid substitution, valine for glutamic acid, at the sixth position on the beta chain of the hemoglobin molecule; the result is hemoglobin S. This genotype can be detected in fetal cells, allowing prenatal diagnosis. The inheritance of one gene for SCD results in the heterozygous carrier state—sickle cell trait. When two genes are inherited, the homozygous state—SCD (SS genotype)—results. Homozygous sickle cell disease occurs in 0.1 to 0.2 percent of the U.S. African American population. Other heterozygous hemoglobinopathies ("major hemoglobinopathies") that are commonly encountered include hemoglobin SC disease and sickle-thalassemia disease.

Most clinicians are familiar with patients with SCD, who commonly present in the emergency setting with "crises." Table 21-3 outlines the acute complications seen in patients with SCD. The reader is referred to standard texts on emergency medicine or hematology for an expanded discussion of the management of these crises. In patients with SCD, the sickled RBCs are rapidly removed from the circulation, resulting in a chronic hemolytic anemia. These patients typically have a hemoglobin of 6 to 9 g/dL. Patients with sickle cell trait are hematologically normal. Crises rarely occur in these patients under conditions of extreme anoxia, dehydration, or acidosis. Sickle cell trait does result in concentrating defects in the kidneys, and papillary necrosis, urinary tract infection, and hematuria can occur. Patients with hemoglobin SC disease usually have a milder hemolytic anemia than those with SCD, and most have fewer clinical complications. Patients with sickle-thalassemia disease have varying degrees of anemia and clinical complications; some are as severely affected as patients with SCD.

The care of pregnant women with sickle cell disease be-

Table 21-3

ACUTE COMPLICATIONS OF SICKLE CELL DISEASE

Vasoocclusive crises
  Musculoskeletal pain
  Cerebrovascular disease
  Pulmonary crisis (acute chest syndrome)
  Abdominal pain
  Renal crisis
  Acute multiorgan failure

Infectious crises
  Sepsis
  Pneumonia
  Urinary tract infection
  Meningitis

Hematologic crises
  Acute splenic sequestration
  Aplastic crisis

Source: Adapted from Eberst,[31] with permission.

gins with the identification of affected patients. Because of the profound clinical consequences, it is unlikely that a patient with a major hemoglobinopathy (SCD, hemoglobin SC disease, or sickle-thalassemia disease) would become pregnant without being aware that she has the disease. Carriers, however, may be unaware of their status. Screening during early pregnancy is desirable in order to identify women who are at high risk of a difficult pregnancy and of giving birth to an affected offspring.[6] Prenatal screening tests, including a complete blood count (CBC), will demonstrate anemia with sickled RBCs and Howell-Jolly bodies on the peripheral smear in patients with major hemoglobinopathies. Carriers of the sickle cell gene, however, who may be unaware of their status, usually have a normal CBC. Hemoglobin electrophoresis is needed to identify the carrier status and is recommended as part of the prenatal screening of all African American patients. Analysis of fetal DNA can be performed as early as 7 to 13 weeks of gestation by amniocentesis or chorionic villus sampling to diagnose hemoglobinopathies in the offspring of affected patients.

Patients with hemoglobinopathies enter pregnancy with an increased risk of morbidity and mortality due to their underlying anemia and chronic organ damage. Many women with sickle cell disease have uncomplicated pregnancies that result in the delivery of full-term infants of normal birth weight. However, compared with hematologically normal women, pregnant women with SCD have an increased risk

of both maternal and fetal complications. With good prenatal care, patients with SCD have a maternal mortality rate of <1 percent, but 30 to 40 percent have complications such as infections (pneumonia and urinary tract infections, including pyelonephritis, as well as skin infections), acute cholecystitis, and increased frequency of crises. Pulmonary complications can occur, including pulmonary emboli. Obstetric complications, which are more frequent in women with hemoglobinopathies, include spontaneous abortion, premature labor, preeclampsia, low-birth-weight infants, and fetal death. One recent study found an incidence of fetal wastage of 32 percent among 270 pregnancies in women with SCD. Vasoocclusion involving the placenta is thought to be responsible for the increased incidence of low birth weight, intrauterine growth retardation, and neonatal death. Thus far, it has been impossible to predict which women will have obstetric complications. One study found that pregnant women with SCD who had higher hemoglobin levels were more likely to have infants with higher percentile birth weights.

Women with sickle cell trait rarely have pregnancy complications as a result of the carrier state. They may have an increased incidence of pyelonephritis, which can precipitate premature labor. There is a case report of maternal death in a patient with sickle cell trait.

Women with hemoglobin SC disease can develop severe anemia during pregnancy and may have severe vasoocclusive events, particularly in the puerperium. When these occur, the course appears to be similar to that of pregnant women with SCD.

During pregnancy, women with SCD require folic acid supplementation (1 mg/day); their levels are often marginal because of chronic accelerated erythropoiesis. Iron supplementation may not be required. Iron deficiency should be documented with serum iron and ferritin levels prior to giving supplements in order to avoid iron overload. The management of crises in pregnant women is the same as for other patients with SCD. An aggressive search for underlying infections should be undertaken and adequate hydration, oxygen supplementation, and analgesia maintained. In the past, pregnant women with SCD were given prophylactic blood transfusions in order to increase the percentage of normal circulating hemoglobin. Theoretically this would lower the incidence of vasoocclusive crises and decrease fetal wastage.[7] This practice has not been validated by controlled studies, and prophylactic transfusions are no longer routinely used. Transfusions have the disadvantages of alloimmunization, potential for viral exposure, and transfusion reactions. In current practice, transfusions are used for obstetric or hematologic complications or severe anemia (hemoglobin below 6 g/dL). Transfusions are indicated for the acute chest syndrome, cerebrovascular events, papillary necrosis, prolonged vasoocclusive crises, multiple-gestation pregnancies, and before general anesthesia or cesarean section delivery.[8] The presence of SCD alone should not affect the type of delivery chosen for a given patient. Prolonged labor, with its risk of acidosis, dehydration, and infection, should be avoided in patients with SCD.

THALASSEMIA

Thalassemia is an inherited hemoglobinopathy that results in reduced formation of the globin chains comprising the hemoglobin molecule. Because the RBCs do not have a normal quantity of hemoglobin, their life span is shortened, resulting in a chronic hemolytic anemia. The genetic abnormality can result in decreased production of the alpha globin chain (α-thalassemia) or in decreased production of the beta chain (β-thalassemia).

Homozygous α-thalassemia is incompatible with life. Patients with heterozygous α-thalassemia have normal or only slightly decreased levels of hemoglobin with microcytic, hypochromic RBC indices [decreased mean corpuscular volume (MCV) and decreased mean corpuscular hemoglobin (MCH)]; β-thalassemia is more common than α-thalassemia. About 10 to 20 percent of patients with the gene for β-thalassemia have a homozygous state; no normal β chains are produced. These patients have a severe hemolytic anemia and are transfusion-dependent; survival past the teenage years is uncommon. Patients with heterozygous β-thalassemia have a mild hemolytic anemia, with microcytic, hypochromic RBC indices. Some patients have a double heterozygous condition with a gene for thalassemia (usually β-thalassemia) and a gene for SCD. Their clinical and hematologic status is variable, depending on the quantity of normal beta-hemoglobin chains produced.

As is the case with other hemoglobinopathies, care of the pregnant patient begins with early screening to identify carriers and offer prenatal diagnosis. The vast majority of pregnant patients encountered with thalassemia will have the heterozygous condition called *thalassemia minor* or *trait*.[9] Less than 20 successful pregnancies have been reported in patients with homozygous β-thalassemia. A screening CBC in patients with heterozygous thalassemia will show a normal to slightly decreased hemoglobin with microcytic, hypochromic indices. Hemoglobin electrophoresis is needed to establish the diagnosis. This anemia can easily be confused with iron-deficiency anemia. Iron studies often show elevated ferritin concentrations prepregnancy in patients with thalassemia trait. The MCV is typically lower in patients with thalassemia than in those with iron-deficiency anemia. During pregnancy, patients with thalassemia trait can become significantly more anemic than hematologically normal women, presumably because of a larger than normal expansion of plasma volume. These patients should receive iron supplementation unless their serum ferritin level is known to be high. They also require folate supplementation; some clinicians recommend 5 mg/day. Red blood cell transfusions are sometimes needed to maintain adequate oxygen-carrying capacity. With good prenatal care, the pregnancy outcome in women with thalassemia trait is no different than that in the general population of women.

NUTRITIONAL ANEMIAS

IRON-DEFICIENCY ANEMIA

Anemia due to iron deficiency is the most common hematologic problem that develops during pregnancy. Among pregnant women not given iron supplementation, up to 55 percent will develop anemia (hemoglobin below 10.5 g/dL) by the end of the third trimester.[10] During pregnancy, iron is used for accelerated erythropoiesis in the mother and for fetal and placental development; iron is preferentially delivered to the fetus. Iron requirements during pregnancy average 800 to 1000 mg, or about 4 mg/day. Most women of reproductive age have 300 mg in iron stores; multiparous women have less. Although iron absorption does increase during pregnancy, typically there are still not adequate supplies without supplementation. Poor appetite, poor nutrition, nausea, vomiting, multiple gestation, and chronic illness can increase the chance of iron depletion. Iron deficiency is also more common in African Americans, Hispanics, and teenagers. Additional iron is also needed to account for blood loss at the time of delivery and that needed during lactation.

The diagnosis of iron deficiency can be difficult to establish during pregnancy. Any woman whose hemoglobin is below 10.5 g/dL should be evaluated. A low hemoglobin level is actually a late manifestation of iron deficiency. The RBC indices are not a reliable indicator of iron deficiency because microcytosis is often a late finding and other deficiencies, such as folate, may be present as well, masking the microcytosis. Iron studies, such as the total iron-binding capacity (TIBC) and serum iron levels, can be artificially increased and decreased, respectively, in normal pregnancy. The serum ferritin level is the most sensitive test for diagnosing iron deficiency in pregnancy. The serum ferritin level reflects the total body iron stores. In general, patients with normal iron stores should have serum ferritin levels above 20 μg/mL. Even the ferritin level is not always reliable, however. Up to 20 percent of pregnant women with normal ferritin levels will be iron-deficient. In addition, after 34 weeks of gestation, ferritin levels as low at 15 mg/mL can be seen and are not indicative of iron deficiency if the serum hemoglobin remains above 11 g/dL. In pregnancy, iron deficiency may be associated with an increased risk of preterm labor and delivery of a low-birth-weight infant. Infants born to iron-deficient mothers usually have significantly decreased iron stores, which may be related to developmental and behavioral abnormalities.

To prevent the development of iron-deficiency anemia during pregnancy, routine prenatal care in the United States typically includes daily supplementation with ferrous sulfate (usually 300 mg/day), which provides 60 mg of elemental iron daily. Some clinicians, however, are more selective regarding which patients are given iron supplementation. Iron supplementation does not always result in an increase in the hemoglobin concentration, but iron stores are repleted.

FOLATE DEFICIENCY

Anemia due to folate deficiency in pregnant women is one of the most common causes of megaloblastic anemia in the world. Megaloblastic anemia in pregnancy is almost always due to folate deficiency; vitamin B_{12} is rarely implicated. Between 10 and 60 percent of pregnant women who do not receive folate supplementation develop megaloblastic changes in their bone marrow. During pregnancy, folate requirements are at least doubled due to accelerated erythropoiesis and growth of the fetus and placenta. Even greater requirements occur in women with a history of poor nutrition; coexistent hemolytic anemias, such as SCD; those taking anticonvulsant medications; those with twin or greater gestations; and during lactation. Total body stores of folate are small. During pregnancy, the daily folate requirement is 300 to 400 μg. Because the placenta has a large number of folate receptors, the fetus preferentially gets any available folate. Nausea and vomiting during pregnancy can lead to increased loss of folate.

Folate deficiency is difficult to establish during pregnancy. Any pregnant woman with a hemoglobin below 10.5 to 11 g/dL should be considered for evaluation. Anemia purely due to folate deficiency is macrocytic; pancytopenia may be present. Many pregnant women have anemia due to a combined deficiency of folate and iron. This combined deficiency gives rise to a dimorphic population of RBCs, and the RBC indices are unreliable. The presence of hypersegmented neutrophils can be a clue to the presence of folate deficiency, but these are not reliably present. Serum folate levels can be decreased in pregnancy when a true deficiency is not present. Determination of the RBC folate level is the most reliable method of diagnosing folate deficiency. In addition to anemia, low folate levels in pregnancy are associated with an increased risk of spontaneous abortion and congenital defects, particularly neural tube defects. Premature infants born with low folate stores can have feeding difficulties and infections.

Routine prenatal vitamins in the United States provide 500 μg to 1 mg of folic acid per day, usually in combination with iron supplementation. Women with hereditary hemolytic anemias, such as sickle cell disease or thalassemia, should receive larger doses of folate, up to 5 to 10 mg daily. Women taking antiseizure medications, particularly phenytoin or phenobarbital, are at increased risk of developing anemia due to folate deficiency. They should be supplemented with 1 mg of folate daily. Recent studies advocate that women contemplating pregnancy begin folate supplements prior to pregnancy of 400 μg/day to prevent neural tube defects in the offspring they may conceive.

ACQUIRED HEMOLYTIC ANEMIAS

In this section, we explore anemias pertinent to pregnancy that result from the hemolysis of the RBCs. These anemias are precipitated by acquired abnormalities, such as antibodies in the case of autoimmune hemolytic anemia, or microvascular changes in the syndromes of disseminated intravascular coagulation (DIC); hemolysis, elevated liver functions, and low platelets (HELLP); and thrombotic thrombocytopenic purpura/hemolytic uremic syndrome (TTP/HUS). Clinically, these patients all have anemia with its inherent signs and symptoms; thrombocytopenia and a coagulopathy may be present, as noted below. Diagnosis of these disorders is based on the history, clinical signs and symptoms, and laboratory evaluation. The general laboratory evaluation of patients with suspected hemolytic anemia is outlined in Table 21-4. More specific tests may be required, and these are discussed below. The acquired hemolytic anemias most commonly encountered in pregnant patients are characterized in Table 21-5.

Table 21-4

LABORATORY EVALUATION OF PATIENTS WITH SUSPECTED HEMOLYTIC ANEMIA

Study	Anticipated Result
CBC	Anemia of a variable degree; verify that WBC and platelet counts are normal
Reticulocyte count	Should be elevated, reflective of a normal bone marrow response; can be as high as 30–40%
Review of peripheral blood smear	*Spherocytes:* Most common RBC morphologic abnormality in hemolytic anemias; most abundant in warm antibody immune hemolysis and hereditary spherocytosis *Schistocytes:* Fragmented RBCs resulting from trauma within the vasculature; markers of nonimmune hemolysis
Unconjugated (indirect) bilirubin	Elevated as a result of heme catabolism
Lactic dehydrogenase (LDH)	Elevated
Haptoglobin	Low or absent in the presence of hemolysis; binds catabolized hemoglobin; is an acute-phase reactant so can be deceptively elevated
Plasma free hemoglobin	Elevated

Abbreviations: CBC = complete blood count; WBC = white blood cells; RBC = red blood cells.

Table 21-5

CHARACTERISTICS OF ACQUIRED HEMOLYTIC ANEMIAS

	AIHA	TTP	HUS	DIC	HELLP
Microangiopathic hemolytic anemia (MAHA)	No	Prominent	Prominent	May have	Present
Coombs test	Positive	Negative	Negative	Negative	Negative
Thrombocytopenia	No	Prominent	Present	Present	Present
Renal abnormalities	No	Present	Prominent	No	No
Neurologic abnormalities	No	Prominent	No or mild	No	No
Hepatic dysfunction	No	May have	May have	May have	Prominent
Fever	No	Present	Present	May have	No
Coagulation studies	Normal	Normal	Normal	Abnormal	Normal
Pregnancy-associated	Can be	Can be	Can be	Can be	Always

Abbreviations: AIHA = autoimmune hemolytic anemia; TTP = thrombotic thrombocytopenic purpura; HUS = hemolytic uremic syndrome; DIC = disseminated intravascular coagulation; HELLP = hemolysis, elevated liver functions, low platelets.

Note: Disease descriptions here are based on the presence of isolated disease without complications; individual patients often have other problems that make syndromes less readily identifiable.

Source: From Eberst,[32] with permission.

AUTOIMMUNE HEMOLYTIC ANEMIA

There are three types of antibody-mediated, "immune" hemolytic anemias:

1. Warm antibody hemolytic anemia. These antibodies react at body temperature.
2. Cold antibody hemolytic anemia. These antibodies react with the RBCs at temperatures below normal body temperatures.
3. Drug-induced immune hemolytic anemia. Certain drugs cause an immune reaction that results in destruction of the RBCs.

The direct Coombs test, also known as the direct antiglobulin test (DAT), is used to specifically identify immune-mediated hemolytic anemias. This test demonstrates the presence of immunoglobulin (IgG) or complement (C_3) on the surface of the RBC. The indirect Coombs test, which identifies free antibodies in the serum, is used primarily for pretransfusion screening of blood. The peripheral blood smear of patients with immune hemolysis often shows abundant spherocytes.

The treatment of autoimmune hemolytic anemias (AIHAs) is primarily immunosuppression, initially with prednisone. Splenectomy and other immunosuppressive drugs (azathioprine or cyclophosphamide) may be required. If AIHA is drug-induced, the offending drug must be stopped. If there is underlying disease, such as malignancy or another immune disorder, that must be treated also.

Autoimmune hemolytic anemia has rarely been reported to occur in pregnancy. Warm antibodies, since they are IgG, can cross the placenta and cause mild hemolysis in the fetus and newborn. When AIHA predates the pregnancy, the mother and fetus will require close monitoring. Ongoing therapy with glucocorticoids should continue. There is limited experience with the use of other immunosuppressives (i.e., azathioprine) in pregnancy. There are rare reports of AIHA developing only during pregnancy, remitting after delivery, and recurring during subsequent pregnancies. This has been successfully controlled with glucocorticoids, although the infant may be affected.

MICROANGIOPATHIC HEMOLYTIC ANEMIAS

Although it is associated with a variety of underlying disorders, the mechanism of hemolysis in microangiopathic hemolytic anemias (MAHA) is consistent: fragmentation of the RBCs resulting from their passage through abnormal arterioles—arterioles that have endothelial damage or fibrin deposited within the arteriole. In pregnancy, MAHA is seen in the syndromes of DIC, HELLP, and TTP/HUS, which are discussed below.

DISSEMINATED INTRAVASCULAR COAGULATION

This syndrome is characterized by activation of the coagulation system. Disseminated intravascular coagulation (DIC) is triggered by the liberation of tissue factor into the vasculature or, alternatively, through endothelial injury. The placenta and uterine contents are rich in procoagulant materials such as tissue factor. In pregnancy, a wide variety of complications can cause DIC through one or both of these trigger mechanisms (Table 21-6). Figure 21-4 outlines the

Table 21-6

OBSTETRIC CAUSES OF DISSEMINATED INTRAVASCULAR COAGULATION

Obstetric Complication	Trigger of DIC	Acuity of Clinical Manifestations
Preeclampsia	Endothelial injury	Low-grade, compensated
Eclampsia	Endothelial injury	Acute, uncompensated
HELLP syndrome	Endothelial injury	Low-grade, compensated (usually)
Septic abortion	Endothelial injury	Acute, uncompensated
Placental abruption	Liberation of tissue factor	Acute uncompensated
Amniotic fluid embolus	Liberation of tissue factor	Acute, uncompensated
Intrauterine fetal death	Liberation of tissue factor	Low-grade, compensated
Uterine rupture	Liberation of tissue factor	Acute, uncompensated
Saline-induced abortion	Liberation of tissue factor	Acute, uncompensated

Abbreviations: DIC = disseminated intravascular coagulation; HELLP = hemolysis, elevated liver functions, low platelets.

pathophysiology of DIC. The resultant bleeding and thrombosis can occur simultaneously, although bleeding manifestations are more common, occurring in up to 75 percent of patients with DIC. In DIC, the usually tightly regulated balance between coagulation/clot formation and fibrinolysis becomes unbalanced. Furthermore, the changes in hemostasis that accompany pregnancy increase the risk of DIC as well as the risk of thromboembolism.

As noted above, bleeding is the most common clinical presentation of DIC. Bleeding from the skin and mucous membranes is common, as well as oozing from venipuncture sites and surgical wounds, petechiae, and ecchymoses. Disseminated intravascular coagulation is one of the more common causes of excessive bleeding in pregnant patients. Placental abruption is the commonest cause of DIC in pregnancy, although only 10 percent of patients with placental abruption develop severe coagulation abnormalities. The effect of microthrombus formation can be seen as hypoperfusion or ischemia involving organs such as the skin, liver, kidneys, central nervous system, gastrointestinal tract, and adrenal gland. There is a spectrum of clinical and laboratory manifestations in DIC, depending on the underlying etiology (Table 21-6). Most often in pregnancy, DIC is acute

in onset and uncompensated, because the liver and bone marrow cannot replace the coagulation factors and platelets as rapidly as they are being consumed. Two complications of pregnancy that are associated with low-grade, compensated DIC are fetal death in utero and preeclampsia. In current medical practice, fetal death in utero is usually detected early and the fetus is removed before fulminant DIC occurs. Preeclampsia causes endothelial injury and usually a chronic, low-grade DIC.

The diagnosis of DIC is based on the patient's clinical signs and symptoms and characteristic laboratory abnormalities, as outlined in Table 21-7. Of note, MAHA occurs in only 25 percent of patients with DIC; the finding of schistocytes on the peripheral smear is helpful, but their absence does not rule out the diagnosis of DIC. There must be evidence of the consumption of platelets and clotting factors.

The management of DIC is reviewed in detail in Chap. 13. In pregnancy, the management of DIC usually involves delivery of the fetus followed by supportive care and replacement blood products.

HELLP SYNDROME

This syndrome, first described in 1982, consists of hemolysis, elevated liver enzymes, and low platelets (HELLP) in patients with preeclampsia. In a recent study,[11] HELLP syndrome was identified in 19 percent of patients with severe preeclampsia or eclampsia. Seventy percent of the cases occur antepartum and 30 percent postpartum, usually within 48 h of delivery. The maternal mortality rate is 1 percent. The pathogenesis of HELLP syndrome is unknown, but there is a microvesicular fatty infiltration of the liver with localized, and possibly systemic, endothelial damage that leads to microangiopathic hemolysis. Some believe that HELLP syndrome is part of the spectrum of disease that includes TTP and HUS (see below). The classic signs of preeclampsia, hypertension, edema, and proteinuria may be absent or minimal in patients with HELLP syndrome. Right-upper-quadrant pain, nausea, and vomiting are frequent presenting complaints at any time after 20 to 24 weeks of gestation. To prevent misdiagnosis, all health care providers should be familiar with this syndrome. There are no standard diagnostic criteria for HELLP. The incidence of concurrent DIC is debated and ranges from 5 to 100 percent. In general, any woman who is pregnant or newly postpartum and who presents with symptoms of upper abdominal pain, severe headache, or visual changes, especially in conjunction with hypertension and/or proteinuria, should be evaluated for thrombocytopenia and liver function test (LFT) abnormalities. HELLP syndrome can lead to hepatic failure or rupture, coma, acute renal failure, severe hyponatremia, cortical blindness, seizures, and congestive heart failure; these sequelae are more likely if the syndrome is left untreated. All patients in whom this diagnosis is established should be referred to a tertiary care center with the capability of caring for high-risk pregnancies for management. The optimal

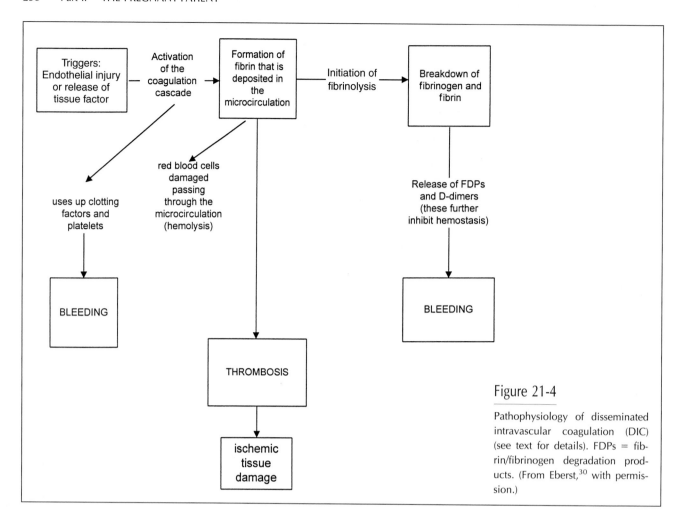

Figure 21-4

Pathophysiology of disseminated intravascular coagulation (DIC) (see text for details). FDPs = fibrin/fibrinogen degradation products. (From Eberst,[30] with permission.)

management of HELLP involves delivery of the fetus. In the setting of extreme fetal immaturity, however, some experts favor a more conservative approach with very careful follow-up in select cases. Experimental treatments that have been used to treat HELLP syndrome include plasmapheresis and prostacyclin.

THROMBOTIC THROMBOCYTOPENIC PURPURA AND HEMOLYTIC UREMIC SYNDROME

Thrombotic thrombocytopenic purpura (TTP) and hemolytic uremic syndrome (HUS) are variant clinical syndromes that reflect a common underlying pathologic process. The first of these, TTP, has been diagnosed in patients of all ages but most commonly in women between ages 10 and 60. Five hundred to a thousand cases are diagnosed per year in the United States. Ninety percent of these patients have no apparent predisposing condition. In others, TTP has been linked to genetic predisposition, immunologic disease (systemic lupus erythematosus, rheumatoid arthritis), infections (viral,

mycoplasmal, human immunodeficiency virus, subacute bacterial endocarditis), or pregnancy. About a hundred cases of TTP occurring in pregnancy and the postpartum period have been reported.[12,13] Hemolytic uremic syndrome is primarily a disease of infancy and early childhood. An adult form also exists, which can be difficult or impossible to distinguish from TTP. Two-thirds of adults with HUS are women. Conditions associated with adult HUS include the use of oral contraceptive agents, preeclampsia, eclampsia, and the postpartum period. In children, HUS is associated with viral and bacterial infections including *Escherichia coli* serotype 0157:H7. In 25 percent of patients, TTP can be recurrent; HUS is rarely recurrent.

Although the precise inciting event is unknown, the pathology in TTP and HUS likely results from the presence of one or more agents that cause platelet aggregation. Abnormalities of endothelial cell function that have been implicated include the release and presence of large von Willebrand factor multimers, deficient production of prostacyclin, and deficient production of tissue plasminogen activator.

Table 21-7

LABORATORY ABNORMALITIES CHARACTERISTIC OF DISSEMINATED INTRAVASCULAR COAGULATION

Studies	Result
Most Useful	
Prothrombin time (PT)	Prolonged
Platelet count[a]	Usually low
Fibrinogen level[b]	Low
Helpful	
Activated partial thromboplastin time (aPTT)	Usually prolonged
Thrombin clot time (TCT)[c]	Prolonged
Fragmented red blood cells[d]	Should be present
FDPs and D-dimer[e]	Elevated
Specific Factor Assays[f]	
Factor II	Low
Factor V	Low
Factor VII[g]	Low
Factor VIII[h]	Low, normal, high
Factor IX	Low (decreases later than other factors)
Factor X	Low

Abbreviation: FDPs = fibrin/fibrinogen degradation products.
[a]Platelet count usually low, most important that it is falling if it started at an elevated level.
[b]Fibrinogen level correlates best with bleeding complications; it is an acute-phase reactant, so it may actually start out at an elevated level; fibrinogen level less than 100 mg/dL correlates with severe DIC.
[c]TCT is not a sensitive test; it is prolonged by many abnormalities.
[d]Fragmented red blood cells and schistocytes are not specific for DIC.
[e]Levels may be chronically elevated in patients with liver or renal disease.
[f]The factors in the extrinsic pathway are most affected (VII, X, V, and II).
[g]Factor VII is usually low early because it has the shortest half-life.
[h]Factor VIII is an acute-phase reactant so its level may be normal, low, or elevated in DIC.
Source: From Eberst,[30] with permission.

Whatever the etiology, the result is the deposition of a hyaline material within the lumina of capillaries and arterioles. The hyaline material is composed of platelets and fibrin-like material that form microthrombi. In TTP, these platelet aggregates are present throughout the microcirculation; in HUS, the renal circulation is primarily affected. The clinical manifestations reflect the thrombocytopenia that is a result of platelet aggregation and the ischemia or infarction of organs resulting from the microthrombi.

The diagnosis of TTP is based on clinical and laboratory findings known as the pentad. This pentad consists of the following:

1. Microangiopathic hemolytic anemia (MAHA) with characteristic schistocytes on the peripheral blood smear and an appropriate reticulocytosis; the degree of anemia is variable, but one-third of patients have a hemoglobin below 6 g/dL.
2. Thrombocytopenia with platelet counts ranging from 5000 to 100,000/mm^3.
3. Renal abnormalities including renal insufficiency, azotemia, proteinuria, or hematuria.
4. Fever.
5. Neurologic abnormalities including headache, confusion, cranial nerve palsies, seizures, or coma.

The presenting complaint is often a neurologic abnormality, although signs and symptoms referable to the anemia or thrombocytopenia are common. Hemolytic uremic syndrome is both a clinical and a laboratory diagnosis. Acute renal failure is the predominant feature. Neurologic abnormalities are seen in one-third of HUS patients. Both MAHA and thrombocytopenia are present in HUS, although the thrombocytopenia is usually not as severe as in TTP. It can be very difficult to distinguish TTP from HUS and other causes of hemolytic anemia. Table 21-5 characterizes this differential diagnosis. Of particular importance, in both TTP and HUS, coagulation studies should be normal.

The diagnosis of TTP or HUS is a medical emergency. Patients suspected of having this diagnosis should have immediate consultation with an experienced specialist (i.e., perinatologist) who can coordinate care. Although the overall survival rate is 80 percent, TTP can be rapidly fatal. The overall survival rate in HUS is 85 to 95 percent; however, older children and adults generally have a worse prognosis. The foundation of therapy of TTP is plasma exchange transfusion (PLEX). Plasma infusion alone may help some patients if PLEX is not readily available. The basis for PLEX is that the exchanged fresh frozen plasma (FFP) or fresh unfrozen plasma (FUP) provides a substance that the patient is lacking or it removes an unknown toxic substance. The use of PLEX therapy may be required daily for weeks to months. Other therapeutic measures for TTP include glucocorticoids and aspirin or dipyridamole. Further immunosuppressive therapy with vincristine, azathioprine, or cyclophosphamide is sometimes used, as is splenectomy. Platelet transfusions should be avoided unless there is uncontrolled hemorrhage because they can aggravate the underlying platelet aggregation problem. The treatment of HUS consists of early dialysis and supportive care. In childhood HUS, up to 90 percent of the renal failure is reversible. Adults with HUS are not as fortunate, but the renal failure may be reversible even after a year or longer.

The relationship between TTP and pregnancy is obscure; some believe it is only coincidental. In early reports, when

TTP occurred in pregnancy, the prognosis was poor for the fetus and the mother. Pregnancy does not appear to influence the course of TTP. As a result of hyaline thrombi affecting the placental vessels and leading to placental insufficiency, intrauterine growth retardation and perinatal death can occur. When TTP is diagnosed in pregnancy, conventional therapy is advocated with delivery of the fetus as soon as possible. The use of PLEX has improved the overall outcome of pregnant women with TTP. Infusions of the high-molecular-weight fraction of plasma have been successfully used in pregnant patients with TTP. In one case, recurrent TTP resolved after delivery of the fetus. When TTP occurs in the third trimester, it must be distinguished from other obstetric complications including severe preeclampsia, eclampsia, and DIC.

OTHER RED CELL DISORDERS

APLASTIC ANEMIA

Aplastic anemia uncommonly complicates pregnancy. Two distinct groups of patients are identified: those with a previous history of idiopathic aplastic anemia who become pregnant and those who develop aplastic anemia during pregnancy. A recent study of pregnancy in patients with idiopathic aplastic anemia reveals that successful pregnancy can occur when these women are in remission, although relapses occurred during nearly one-third of the pregnancies. All of the infants were healthy. Several cases of aplastic anemia that developed during pregnancy have been described. The mechanism is unknown; perhaps it is immunologic, but there is greater than chance occurrence. Of these patients, approximately one-third have spontaneous remission of the aplastic anemia following abortion or delivery of the infant. The aplasia may recur in subsequent pregnancies. When remission does not occur, bone marrow transplantation may be necessary. Maternal outcome is dependent on the severity of the aplasia and any infections that may occur. Treatment is supportive, with transfusions as necessary. The blood counts of the infant are not affected by aplastic anemia in the mother.

POLYCYTHEMIA VERA IN PREGNANCY

Polycythemia vera (PV) is an uncommon myeloproliferative disorder that results in an elevated hematocrit and often elevated WBC and platelet counts. It affects 1 in 50,000 persons, and most patients are middle aged or older; therefore reports of pregnancy in patients with PV are rare. Pregnancy does not seem to change the course of the disease. Hypertension may be associated with PV. While maternal outcome is usually good, fetal outcome is usually poor, with an increased incidence of spontaneous abortion, preterm delivery, and fetal death. During pregnancy, phlebotomy can be used to maintain the hematocrit between 40 and 47 percent.

If thrombocytosis is present, some have suggested the use of low-dose heparin to prevent thrombosis, but this is controversial. After delivery, accelerated erythropoiesis often occurs.

PRIMARY PLATELET DISORDERS

OVERVIEW OF PLATELET DISORDERS

A myriad of platelet disorders can be encountered in the pregnant patient. Quantitative disorders are most common, thrombocytopenia being more common that thrombocytosis. Qualitative platelet abnormalities, characterized by abnormal platelet function, arise in many disease states that can occur in conjunction with pregnancy (Table 21-8). The management of platelet dysfunction is beyond the scope of this text; the reader is referred to standard works on hematology.

Thrombocytopenia can result from several mechanisms as outlined in Table 21-9. In pregnancy, physiologic thrombocytopenia or "gestational" thrombocytopenia is the most commonly encountered cause of thrombocytopenia (discussed earlier). Of those pathologic processes, an increased rate of platelet destruction is the most common mechanism

---

Table 21-8

CLINICAL CONDITIONS ASSOCIATED WITH QUALITATIVE PLATELET ABNORMALITIES

Uremia

Liver disease

Disseminated intravascular coagulation (DIC)

Drugs (aspirin, NSAIDs, tricyclic antidepressants, phenothiazines, nitrofurantion, prostaglandins, antihistamines)

Antiplatelet antibodies (ITP, SLE)

Cardiopulmonary bypass

Myeloproliferative disorders (PCV, CML)

Dysproteinemias (multiple myeloma, Waldenstrom macroglobulinemia)

Preleukemias, AML, ALL

Von Willebrand disease (congenital or acquired)

Abbreviations: ITP = idiopathic thrombocytopenic purpura; SLE = systemic lupus erythematosus; PCV = polycythemia vera; CML = chronic myelogenous leukemia; AML = acute myelogenous leukemia; ALL = acute lymphocytic leukemia.
Source: From Eberst,[30] with permission.

Table 21-9

PATHOPHYSIOLOGIC MECHANISMS OF ACQUIRED THROMBOCYTOPENIA

Mechanism	Associated Clinical Conditions
Decreased platelet production	Marrow infiltration (tumor or infections)
	Aplastic anemia
	Viral infections
	Drugs (thiazides, estrogens, ethanol, alphainterferon, chemotherapeutic agents)
	Radiation
	Vitamin B_{12} and/or *folate deficiency*
Increased platelet destruction	*Preeclampsia/eclampsia*
	Idiopathic thrombocytopenic purpura (ITP)
	Thrombotic thrombocytopenic purpura (TTP)
	Hemolytic uremic syndrome (HUS)
	HELLP syndrome
	Disseminated intravascular coagulation (DIC)
	Viral infections (HIV, mumps, varicella, EBV)
	Drugs (heparin, sulfa-containing antibiotics, ethanol, aspirin, indomethacin, valproic acid, heroin, thiazides, H_2 blockers)
Splenic sequestration	Hypersplenism
	Hypothermia
Platelet loss	Excessive hemorrhage
	Hemodialysis
	Extracorporeal circulation
Multifactorial	*Gestational or incidental thrombocytopenia* in pregnancy
Pseudothrombocytopenia	Not a disease state but a laboratory phenomenon

Abbreviations: HIV = human immunodeficiency virus; EBV = Epstein-Barr virus; HELLP = hemolysis, elevated liver function, low platelets.
Note: Conditions in italic print are exclusively or commonly encountered in pregnancy.
Source: Adapted from Eberst,[29] with permission.

affecting pregnant women. The need for evaluation of thrombocytopenia in pregnant women is controversial. Most clinicians would agree that workup is indicated for a platelet count below 100,000/mm³, though some would initiate this workup for any platelet count below 150,000/mm³. Patients with mild thrombocytopenia (a platelet count of 100,000 to 150,000 mm³) who are without any significant history or signs or symptoms of thrombocytopenia and who do not have a falling platelet count can be managed with monitoring of the platelet count. This degree of thrombocytopenia should not pose a threat to the mother or fetus in an otherwise uncomplicated pregnancy. Platelet counts below 100,000/mm³ are more likely to be due to an etiology that can threaten the mother and the fetus; therefore the patient should be fully studied in order to identify an etiology. There may be important implications for the delivery and postnatal care. Women with a previous history of autoimmune thrombocy-

topenic purpura should be identified early; their management is discussed separately below. Pregnant women with significant thrombocytopenia and no known concomitant disease should be studied as outlined in Table 21-10. Pregnant patients with platelet counts below 50,000/mm³ with an identifiable pregnancy-related cause (e.g., abruptio placentae or DIC) should be referred for hematologic consultation.

The management of bleeding resulting from thrombocytopenia in pregnancy is the same as for any condition with thrombocytopenia.[14] Bleeding complications are usually not seen unless the platelet count is below 50,000/mm³. Spontaneous bleeding, including central nervous system hemorrhage, can occur with platelet levels below 10,000/mm³. The emergency management of patients with thrombocytopenia and bleeding begins with control of the acute hemorrhage and maintenance of an adequate intravascular volume in order to ensure hemodynamic stability. Generally, patients

Table 21-10

EVALUATION OF THROMBOCYTOPENIA IN PREGNANCY

Laboratory and Clinical Setting	Workup
Platelet count 100,000/mm³ to 150,000/mm³ No significant past medical history No clinical signs or symptoms referable to underlying disease or thrombocytopenia Platelet count is stable	Follow serial platelet counts Review of peripheral smear Urinalysis Consider baseline liver function tests and serum creatinine
Platelet count 100,000/mm³ or below May or may not have significant medical history or symptoms referable to thrombocytopenia	Review of peripheral smear Urinalysis Liver function tests, creatinine Coagulation studies Antinuclear antibodies, lupus anticoagulant, anticardiolipin antibodies Antiplatelet antibodies Human immunodeficiency virus antibody Direct Coombs test

with active bleeding and platelet counts below 50,000/mm³ should receive platelet transfusion. Each unit of platelets infused should raise the platelet count by 10,000/mm³. Typically, platelet transfusions are given 6 units at a time. Patients with antiplatelet antibodies, such as those with idiopathic thrombocytopenic purpura (ITP), or patients with hypersplenism are unlikely to respond to platelet transfusion. Some diseases, such as DIC and TTP, may be exacerbated by platelet transfusion. Patients with platelet counts below 10,000/mm³, regardless of the etiology, should receive immediate platelet transfusion because of the high risk of spontaneous hemorrhage. If surgery is necessary, platelet counts below 50,000/mm³ require transfusion so that the platelet count is >50,000/mm³ at the time of surgery if possible.

Thrombocytosis—platelet counts above 400,000/mm³—is discussed below.

IDIOPATHIC THROMBOCYTOPENIC PURPURA

Idiopathic thrombocytopenic purpura (ITP), also called immune thrombocytopenic purpura, is the second most common platelet abnormality encountered in pregnant patients. The incidence is estimated at 1 to 2 per 10,000 pregnancies, although the actual incidence may be higher.[14] Estrogens and other hormones may play a role in the pathogenesis of ITP, which is thought by most to have an immune basis. This is suggested by the increased incidence of ITP in adult female patients and the relapses of previously diagnosed ITP that occur during pregnancy. In ITP, thrombocytopenia is a result of platelet destruction caused by antibodies that are directed against platelet surface antibodies. These antibodies are IgG and can cross the placenta, causing fetal thrombocytopenia.

The diagnosis of ITP is one of exclusion; any pregnant woman with a platelet count below 100,000/mm³ should be evaluated. Drug and chemical exposures should be elicited. The workup of thrombocytopenia (Table 21-10) begins with examination of the peripheral smear to exclude pseudothrombocytopenia (due to clumping of platelets) and to ensure that the WBC and RBC lines appear normal. Other laboratory studies are used to exclude other causes of thrombocytopenia, including anti-DNA and antinuclear antibody (ANA, for systemic lupus erythematosus); direct Coombs test (to exclude autoimmune hemolytic anemia with thrombocytopenia, called Evans syndrome); lupus anticoagulant; anticardiolipin antibodies; thyroid studies; human immunodeficiency virus antibody; and coagulation studies. All of these should be normal in a patient with ITP. A bone marrow examination is usually done and, in the setting of ITP, typically shows normal to increased megakaryocytes and no abnormalities involving the other cell lines. Antiplatelet antibodies can be demonstrated in about 90 percent of patients with ITP. These antibodies are specific for the diagnosis of ITP, but the tests themselves have varying sensitivity. The presence and quantity of maternal antiplatelet antibodies does not correlate with maternal platelet counts. In pregnancy, the presence of antiplatelet antibodies can, according to some, have consequences for the fetus. Some studies show that when maternal antiplatelet antibodies are demonstrable, the fetus is a greater risk for having significant thrombocytopenia at birth.[2] Conversely, when antiplatelet antibodies are not demonstrable in the mother, the fetus is at minimal risk of having significant thrombocytopenia. Women who develop thrombocytopenia for the first time during pregnancy and have a negative workup, including no demonstrable antiplatelet antibodies, may have ITP or "gestational" thrombocytopenia (discussed above). These diagnoses may not be distinguishable without longitudinal follow-up; in either condition, the platelet count may improve after delivery of the fetus.

Most pregnant patients with ITP will have a previously established diagnosis. Recurrent or new-onset ITP during pregnancy may present with easy bruising, petechiae, purpura, or bleeding from the mucous membranes. The presence of lymphadenopathy, splenomegaly, or joint or skin complaints is suspicious for other conditions. Many pregnant patients with ITP are asymptomatic; thrombocytopenia is discovered on routine prenatal screening tests.

The treatment of ITP in the pregnant patient is generally the same as its treatment in nonpregnant patients, keeping in mind potential risks to the fetus and attempting to optimize the platelet count at the time of delivery. Most patients with platelet counts above 50,000/mm^3 who are asymptomatic do not require treatment. When treatment is required, glucocorticoids are the first-line therapy. Care must be used when treating pregnant patients with glucocorticoids; long-term therapy is not advisable. In addition to the usual side effects of glucocorticoids, during pregnancy their use may be associated with an increased risk of preeclampsia, gestational diabetes, and postpartum psychosis. Fetal adrenal suppression is a theoretical hazard. Glucocorticoids are often administered for 3 weeks prior to delivery in order to optimize the maternal and fetal platelet counts. Dexamethasone or beclomethasone are used, because prednisone and hydrocortisone do not cross the placenta well. Glucocorticoid administration to the mother does not prevent all cases of neonatal thrombocytopenia. Intravenous IgG is another commonly used therapy for ITP, in both pregnant and nonpregnant patients. Intravenous IgG is effective in raising the platelet count in up to 80 percent of patients, usually within 48 h; the effect may last for 2 to 3 weeks. Although the mother may have a good response to intravenous IgG, and this does cross the placenta, the response in the fetus is unpredictable. Splenectomy, which removes the major site of platelet destruction in ITP, can produce a cure or long-term remission in 60 to 80 percent of patients with ITP. Splenectomy in pregnancy is not advised unless all other attempts to raise the platelet count are unsuccessful. With modern surgical techniques, splenectomy can be done with minimal risk to the fetus and mother. Other medications that are used to treat ITP with some success are danazol, vincristine, and cyclophosphamide—all of which are contraindicated in pregnancy. There is some experience with the use of azathioprine in pregnancy; fetal morbidity appears to be negligible.

The effect of maternal thrombocytopenia on the fetus and the fetal platelet count has implications for fetal hemorrhage in utero particularly at the time of delivery. While spontaneous fetal hemorrhage in utero due to thrombocytopenia is usually not a problem, there is risk of fetal intracerebral hemorrhage at the time of delivery. Maternal thrombocytopenia at the time of delivery is of little risk to the mother. Platelet transfusions can be given for excessive bleeding (e.g., at the time of delivery) but should not be given prophylactically. The bleeding time can be used to further assess the risk of excessive bleeding in patients with thrombocytopenia. A bleeding time prolonged more than 15 min, although not entirely predictive of surgical bleeding, poses a greater risk of excessive bleeding. In the presence of maternal ITP, the incidence of severe (<50,000/mm^3) thrombocytopenia in the

fetus is 5 to 15 percent.[15,16] Maternal platelet counts do not correlate with fetal platelet counts, and there is no reliable way to predict the latter. Some maternal factors may be associated with an increased risk of fetal thrombocytopenia, such as severe, uncontrolled ITP, the presence of ITP prior to the pregnancy, the presence of antiplatelet antibodies during this or previous pregnancies, and persistent maternal thrombocytopenia in patients with previous splenectomy for ITP. The obstetric management of patients with ITP is beyond the scope of this text; however, in general, fetal platelet counts are used to direct the mode of delivery. The direct measurement of fetal platelet counts can be done by percutaneous umbilical blood sampling (PUBS) usually performed at 37 to 38 weeks of gestation, or fetal scalp sampling during labor. The indications for cesarean section are controversial but are usually considered when the fetal platelet count is below 50,000/mm^3. It is not entirely clear that cesarean section reduces neonatal morbidity and mortality in the setting of severe fetal thrombocytopenia.[17]

ESSENTIAL THROMBOCYTOSIS

Essential thrombocytosis (ET) is a chronic myeloproliferative disorder characterized by persistent elevation of the platelet count above 600,000/mm^3 and other diagnostic criteria as established by the Polycythemia Vera Study Group. Although most common in patients in the sixth and seventh decades of life, ET is increasingly diagnosed in younger patients. ET complicating pregnancy is a rare event; about 40 cases have been described. Clinically, ET is associated with thromboembolic events as a result of thrombocytosis or bleeding complications due to platelet dysfunction. Pregnancy can be successful in patients with ET, but spontaneous abortion, fetal growth retardation, and stillbirth can result from placental thrombosis and infarction. Some studies have found that the platelet counts decline in pregnant women with ET, followed by a rebound in the postpartum period. This, however, is not a consistent finding. Aspirin and dipyridamole have been used in asymptomatic pregnant patients with ET to prevent thrombosis in the placenta, but there are insufficient data to support this as a routine practice. When the platelet count exceeds 1 million/mm^3 or there are symptoms or thromboembolic complications, platelet pheresis can be used. Interferon alpha has been successfully used without apparent effect on the fetus; cytotoxic drugs are avoided in pregnancy.

HEMATOLOGIC MALIGNANCIES

Hematologic malignancies, lymphomas or leukemias, are among the most commonly diagnosed malignancies in pregnant women. Although uncommon, these diseases represent a challenge to the clinician to manage the patient appropriately in order to achieve the best outcome for the patient and fetus.

LYMPHOMA

It is estimated that lymphoma complicates 1 in 1000 to 6000 pregnancies. The vast majority of these patients are diagnosed with Hodgkin disease (HD); non-Hodgkin lymphoma (NHL) is rarely reported during pregnancy. There is no evidence that either type of lymphoma is directly affected by pregnancy, and there is very rarely any direct effect on the fetus. Staging of the extent of disease is essential for proper treatment, although staging during pregnancy can be difficult because extensive radiographs are needed (including computed tomography scan of the abdomen and pelvis). Staging laparotomy may be needed. Some clinicians choose to risk understaging the pregnant patient rather than exposing her to radiation, although consultation with a radiation physicist may demonstrate acceptable risk (see Appendix A.2). Magnetic resonance imaging may be an alternative. Staging laparotomy should be delayed until as late in the pregnancy as possible. Some treatment options can safely be undertaken during pregnancy, including radiotherapy above the diaphragm with abdominal shielding and some chemotherapies after the first trimester.

Women previously treated successfully for lymphoma should avoid pregnancy for 2 years after completing therapy. There is evidence that these women have decreased fertility and may have an increased risk of spontaneous abortion and fetal abnormalities. They do not, however, have a higher rate of disease recurrence in pregnancy.

LEUKEMIA

Leukemias are the second most common fatal malignancy of women in childbearing years and can be expected to occur in about 1 in 75,000 pregnancies. Over 300 pregnancies complicated by leukemia have been reported in the literature. The majority of new leukemias diagnosed in pregnancy, up to 88 percent, are acute leukemias; two-thirds of these are acute myelogenous leukemia (AML). Of the chronic leukemias, chronic myelocytic leukemia (CML) accounts for almost all the cases. The prognosis for the mother and fetus depends on the type of leukemia, stage of pregnancy, clinical effects of the leukemia, and potential toxic effects of the treatment. There is no evidence that the course of leukemia is affected by pregnancy; with aggressive treatment, the prognosis should be the same as for women who are not pregnant. The fetus is at greater risk of poor outcome the earlier during pregnancy the diagnosis is made. Spontaneous abortion is common when leukemia is diagnosed during the first trimester. It is very rare for maternal leukemia cells to be transmitted to the fetus, although leukemic infiltrates are commonly found on the maternal side of the placenta. The infants of women with leukemia are commonly preterm, small for gestational age, and may be transiently cytopenic if the mother is receiving chemotherapy.

Pregnant women diagnosed with AML cannot delay treatment; the median survival of untreated patients is 2 months. Combination chemotherapy is used; it is of minimal risk to the fetus after the first trimester and of limited risk during the first trimester. The goal of aggressive chemotherapy is to attain a remission that optimizes the outcome for the mother and fetus. Some women will relapse and have a rapidly fatal course after delivery.

Chronic myelogenous leukemia typically has a more indolent course, and treatment may be delayed until later in pregnancy or the postpartum period. Alkylating agents are not without risk in the first trimester; leukopheresis may be a treatment option.

Women who have been cured of acute leukemia are usually fertile and have no increased risk of recurrent disease in pregnancy. Chronic myelogenous leukemia is typically cured only with bone marrow transplantation; successful pregnancy can subsequently occur.

HYPERCOAGULABLE STATES

THROMBOEMBOLIC DISEASE

Pregnancy and the postpartum period represent a period of increased risk of thromboembolism in all women. The three components of Virchow's triad—hypercoagulability of blood, trauma to the vessel walls (at delivery), and venous stasis (due to uterine compression of the inferior vena cava and iliac vessels and increased levels of progesterone, leading to decreased peripheral vascular resistance and pooling of blood in veins)—are present. As discussed above, the hemostatic changes that occur in pregnancy are physiologic and intended to limit hemorrhage at the time of placental separation. These changes, however, result in a hypercoaguable state that can be hazardous to both the mother and, in turn, the fetus. The changes in coagulation can be detected by the third month of gestation and return to baseline within 4 weeks of delivery. Deep venous thrombosis and pulmonary embolism are discussed in detail in Chap. 17.

LUPUS ANTICOAGULANT/ ANTIPHOSPHOLIPID SYNDROME

The lupus anticoagulant (LA) is an acquired antibody against phospholipids. The antibody can be IgM or IgG. In vitro, it prolongs the phospholipid-dependent reactions in the coagulation cascade, hence the name *anticoagulant*. In vivo, however, the LA is rarely associated with bleeding complications; it is associated with thromboses and obstetric complications or may be clinically insignificant. First identified in patients with systemic lupus erythematosus (SLE), the LA can be detected in up to 50 percent of these patients when the most sensitive tests are used, although most studies find positivity in 10 to 15 percent of patients with SLE. Several subsets of patients with the LA can be identified. (Fig. 21-5). The presence of the LA has major implications for pregnancy because it is associated with a higher risk of fetal death than any other condition known.

Three groups of women who have the LA can have obstetric complications including recurrent abortions, intrauterine death, intrauterine growth retardation, and premature delivery. These complications result from thrombosis of the placental vessels and placental infarction. The first group of women with the LA and obstetric complications have the primary antiphospholipid syndrome (Table 21-11). This syndrome is characterized by the presence of antiphospholipid antibodies, which includes the LA and/or anticardiolipin antibodies. Clinically, these patients do not have SLE or other identifiable autoimmune disorders. (If they do, it is called "secondary" antiphospholipid syndrome.) They do have venous or arterial thromboses, recurrent fetal loss, and thrombocytopenia.[18,19] It is unclear whether the LA or anticardiolipin antibodies are more specifically associated with fetal loss. Up to 90 percent of pregnancies in patients with the antiphospholipid syndrome who do not receive appropriate treatment have a resultant spontaneous abortion or stillbirth.[20] In this syndrome, fetal death most commonly occurs late in the first trimester or in the second trimester. The second group of women with the LA and fetal loss are those patients with SLE. The last group of women with the LA and recurrent fetal loss have no other medical problems and no other evidence of thromboembolic disease.

The laboratory diagnosis of the LA begins with the finding of mild to moderate prolongation of the activated partial thromboplastin time (aPTT), usually not more than 10 to 15 s above normal, in the presence of a normal or mildly prolonged PT and normal thrombin clot time (TCT). The prolonged aPTT will not correct when "mixed" with normal plasma, indicating the presence of an inhibitor. Specific factor assays will verify that this inhibitor is not specific for any one factor; all will be decreased. Further testing can be done to verify the presence of the lupus anticoagulant. These tests are the dilute Russell viper venom time (dRVVT), Kaolin clot time (KCT), platelet neutralization procedure (PNP), and tissue thromboplastin inhibition (TTI) test. Any one of these tests can verify the presence of the LA. If the PT is prolonged by more than 3 s, the patient should be evaluated for concomitant hypoprothrombinemia (factor II),

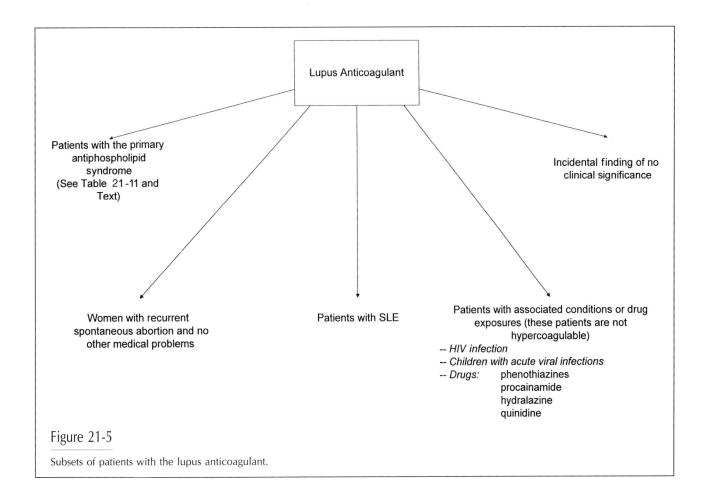

Figure 21-5

Subsets of patients with the lupus anticoagulant.

Table 21-11

PRIMARY ANTIPHOSPHOLIPID SYNDROME

Laboratory Findings	Clinical Findings
1. Presence of antiphospholipid antibodies (one or both) Lupus anticoagulant (up to 70%) Anticardiolipin antibodies (up to 60%)	1. Venous thrombosis (DVT, PE), 34–54%
	2. Arterial thrombosis (CVA, TIA, MI), 24–44%
2. Thrombocytopenia, 30–50%	3. Recurrent fetal loss, 34–90%

Note: These patients do not have SLE or any other autoimmune disorder.

Abbreviations: DVT = deep venous thrombosis; PE = pulmonary embolus; CVA = cerebral vascular accident; TIA = transient ischemic attack; MI = myocardial infarction.

which can occur in patients with SLE and LA. Anticardiolipin antibodies are measured by an enzyme-linked immunosorbent assay (ELISA).

Many women with antiphospholipid antibodies (LA and/or anticardiolipin antibodies) will not have thromboembolic disease or fetal loss. During pregnancy, these women usually do not receive prophylactic therapy. Women with known antiphospholipid antibodies and a history of fetal loss or thromboembolic disease should be considered for prophylactic treatment during pregnancy and the postpartum period. Those women who have experienced fetal loss have a very high risk of subsequent miscarriage, perhaps as high as 60 percent.[21] Pregnant women with a history of thromboembolic disease and antiphospholipid antibodies should be anticoagulated with subcutaneous heparin during the pregnancy and postpartum period (usually 6 weeks). The optimal treatment to prevent fetal loss in women with antiphospholipid antibodies and a previous history of fetal loss is uncertain. Early studies used prednisone (40 to 60 mg daily) and aspirin (75 to 80 mg daily) and had a fetal survival rate of 60 to 80 percent, although preeclampsia and fetal growth retardation were common. Prednisone is used to suppress antibody production and aspirin is used to inhibit thromboxane A_2, which causes vasoconstriction and platelet aggregation. Aspirin alone appears to have no effect on fetal survival, while prednisone alone may actually decrease fetal survival. One small study used subcutaneous heparin in a dose to maintain the aPTT at 1.5 to 2 times control; the pregnancy success rate was 93 percent.

Prior to pregnancy, women with a history of recurrent fetal loss, autoimmune or connective tissue disease, venous or arterial thrombosis, or thrombocytopenia should be screened for the presence of the LA and anticardiolipin antibodies. Women who have had a single spontaneous abortion do not have an increased frequency of antiphospholipid antibodies and do not require screening.

CONGENITAL DEFICIENCY OF NATURALLY OCCURRING ANTICOAGULANTS

Patients with congenital deficiency of the naturally occurring anticoagulants antithrombin III, protein C, and protein S are at increased risk for thromboembolic disease; pregnancy further enhances this hypercoagulable state.

ANTITHROMBIN III DEFICIENCY

Deficiency of antithrombin III (ATIII) is the most common clinically relevant inherited hypercoagulable state, estimated to occur in 1 in 2000 to 5000 in the general population. In women with ATIII deficiency, the risk of thrombotic events during pregnancy and the postpartum period ranges from 45 to 70 percent if they do not receive prophylactic anticoagulant therapy.[22] As discussed above, ATIII levels normally decline during pregnancy. In patients with congenital deficiency, pregnancy can precipitate their first thrombotic episode. There is no way to predict which patients will develop thrombosis, so most clinicians advocate prophylactic anticoagulation for pregnant patients with known congenital ATIII deficiency. Starting early in the pregnancy, most patients are managed with full-dose subcutaneous heparin in order to prolong the aPTT by 5 to 10 s. Anticoagulation is continued for at least 6 weeks postpartum, when the risk of thrombosis may be even higher than during pregnancy. Low-molecular-weight heparin may be a suitable alternative. At the time of delivery, ATIII concentrates are given to raise the ATIII level to 80 to 120 percent of normal. When thrombotic events occur during pregnancy, ATIII concentrates are used; tPA has also been used.[23] If thrombotic events have previously occurred, the patient is usually anticoagulated indefinitely.

PROTEIN C DEFICIENCY

Heterozygous inherited protein C deficiency is estimated to occur in 1 in 300 persons in the general population; however, only a small fraction of these patients have clinical evidence of hypercoagulability. Women with protein C deficiency have a 25 percent incidence of thrombosis during pregnancy and the postpartum period without prophylactic anticoagulation.[22] The risk is greatest during the postpartum period. Based on this, subcutaneous low-dose heparin prophylaxis is used for asymptomatic patients with protein C deficiency during pregnancy and full anticoagulation for 6 weeks postpartum. Placental thrombosis and infarction can cause intrauterine growth retardation. Heterozygous protein C deficiency is associated with the development of warfarin-induced skin necrosis. Homozygous protein C deficiency in newborns is often fatal and is associated with the development of purpura fulminans. A newly developed protein C concentrate has been used to treat these neonates.

PROTEIN S DEFICIENCY

Pregnant patients with protein S deficiency have a risk of developing thrombosis of up to 20 percent when not treated with prophylactic anticoagulation.[22] In normal pregnancies, levels of protein S decrease slightly. Most clinicians treat asymptomatic pregnant patients with protein S deficiency with low-dose subcutaneous heparin throughout the pregnancy and higher doses in the postpartum period. Patients who have had previous thrombotic complications, deep venous thrombosis, or fetal loss due to placental infarction may be managed with full-dose heparin throughout their pregnancies.

PAROXYSMAL NOCTURNAL HEMOGLOBINURIA

Paroxysmal nocturnal hemoglobinuria (PNH) is a rare acquired disorder characterized by RBC hemolysis in conjunction with leukopenia, thrombocytopenia, and thromboses. An abnormal stem cell gives rise to abnormal RBCs, WBCs, and platelets. The RBC membranes have an intrinsic defect that makes them more sensitive to lysis by complement. There is a variable degree of intravascular hemolysis; only 25 percent have hemoglobinuria.

About fifty cases of PNH in pregnant patients are described in the English literature. Complications during pregnancy and the postpartum period include spontaneous abortion, thrombosis (involving the peripheral, hepatic, or cerebral vasculature or pulmonary embolus), and hemolytic crises. Prophylactic low-dose heparin has been used to prevent thrombotic complications, but this is not always effective. In patients with PNH, heparin must be used with caution, because it activates the complement system and can precipitate hemolytic episodes. If thrombotic complications occur during pregnancy, full anticoagulation with heparin is maintained, followed by warfarin in the postpartum period. Transfusions of washed RBCs have been used to maintain the hematocrit between 25 and 30 percent and suppress the production of abnormal cells.

INHERITED COAGULATION: FACTOR DEFICIENCIES

Severe congenital disorders of hemostasis are nearly always diagnosed in infancy or childhood; however, milder forms may not become apparent until adulthood or when there is a significant hemostatic challenge (e.g., at menarche). Preg-

nant patients should be questioned about any personal or familial history of excessive bleeding with surgical procedures, menses, previous pregnancies, or dental extractions. If there has been excessive bleeding in any of these circumstances, further workup should be undertaken. Acquired coagulopathies due to drugs—e.g., nonsteroidal anti-inflammatory drugs (NSAIDs)—or liver disease should also be considered. In this section, we discuss the most common inherited coagulopathies affecting pregnant women—von Willebrand disease (vWD), the hemophilias (factor VIII or IX deficiency), and other coagulation factor deficiencies. The type of bleeding that occurs can give an indication of the abnormality that may be present. For example, mucosal bleeding, epistaxis, gingival bleeding, gastrointestinal bleeding, and menorrhagia occur as a result of problems with primary hemostasis, such as vWD and thrombocytopenia. Bleeding into joints (hemarthroses), fascial planes, and the retroperitoneum is associated with defects in secondary hemostasis, typically coagulation factor deficiencies. Occasionally some patients with noninherited coagulation defects will have more than one type of coagulopathy—for example, DIC, where there is thrombocytopenia along with low coagulation factor levels.

VON WILLEBRAND DISEASE

Von Willebrand disease (vWD), which is caused by a deficiency or abnormality of von Willebrand factor (vWF), is the most common inherited coagulation disorder, with 1 in 100 persons having a defective gene, although only 1 in 10,000 manifests a clinically significant bleeding disorder. Usually inherited in an autosomal dominant pattern, vWD affects men and women equally. One in 1 million patients has type III vWD, with its severe bleeding manifestations, due to an autosomal recessive defect. Von Willebrand factor is a glycoprotein that is synthesized, stored, and secreted by vascular endothelial cells; it has two functions: (1) to participate in primary hemostasis, vWF allows platelets to adhere to damaged endothelium (Fig. 21-1); and (2) vWF carries factor VIII in the plasma.

Clinically, the bleeding manifestations of vWD are highly variable, even among patients with the same type of vWD (Table 21-12, discussed below). Most patients have mild bleeding from mucocutaneous surfaces (such as epistaxis), easy bruising, bleeding after dental extractions, and menorrhagia. Patients with the rare type III vWD have severe, spontaneous life-threatening bleeding comparable with that of severe hemophilia. Patients with vWD should avoid NSAIDs.

A variety of laboratory tests are used to establish the diagnosis of vWD. Coagulation screening tests—the PT, aPTT, and TCT—will usually be normal, although the aPTT may be prolonged in moderate or severe vWD due to the decreased level of factor VIII (vWF is not available in the plasma to carry the factor VIII). The specific tests used to diagnose vWD are outlined in Table 21-13. Often, patients have to be tested on more than one occasion to establish the

Table 21-12

CLASSIFICATION OF VON WILLEBRAND DISEASE

Type	Occurrence	Defect
Type I	70–80% of patients with vWD	All multimers present but in decreased amounts
Type II		
Type IIA	10–15%	Large and intermediate multimers are absent
Type IIB	5%	Large multimers are absent
Type III	<5%	All multimers are absent (virtually no vWF is present)

Abbreviations: vWD = von Willebrand disease; vWF = von Willebrand factor.
Source: Adapted from Eberst,[33] with permission.

diagnosis. The vWF levels can be affected by estrogens, progesterone, thyroid disease, infection, and exercise. Based on multimeric analysis, patients with vWD can be classified into types and subtypes, as outlined in Table 21-12. This can be clinically important in pregnancy, as discussed below.

In nonpregnant patients, the treatment of vWD depends on the type of vWD that is present and the severity of bleeding.[24] Table 21-14 shows the recommended therapy for patients with vWD and bleeding. Desmopressin (DDAVP, or 1-desamino-8-D-arginine-vasopressin) is the treatment of choice for patients with type I vWD. The desmopressin can be administered subcutaneously or intravenously at a dose of 0.3 μg/kg of body weight. This dose can be given every 12 h for three to four doses before tachyphylaxis occurs. Desmopressin causes the release of vWF from endothelial storage sites. Tachyphylaxis occurs when these stores become depleted. Desmopressin is a synthetic product without the risks of blood products; however, it can cause flushing, headache, and hyponatremia. Factor VIII concentrates with high levels of vWF are used to treat patients with types II or III vWD. In an emergency, cryoprecipitate can be used to replace vWF. Each bag of cryoprecipitate contains 100 U of vWF activity but carries a small risk of viral transmission.

VON WILLEBRAND DISEASE IN PREGNANCY

Von Willebrand disease is the most common inherited coagulation abnormality with clinical significance during pregnancy and delivery.[3,25,26] In one 1986 report, 27 percent of women with vWD had abnormal bleeding at the time of abortion, delivery, or in the postpartum period.[25] During pregnancy, under the influence of estrogen, most patients have significant increases in their levels of vWF and factor VIII. These increases begin at about 11 weeks of gestation and often result in normal levels of vWF and factor VIII by the time

Table 21-13

LABORATORY EVALUATION OF PATIENTS WITH VON WILLEBRAND DISEASE

Test	Typical Result	Comments
Bleeding time (BT)	Prolonged	Measures platelet and vessel wall interaction (primary hemostasis); this test has high variability—if prolonged, it represents important data; if normal, it does not rule out vWD
vWF antigen (vWF:Ag)	Low or normal	Is an acute-phase reactant, also increased in stress and pregnancy
vWF activity (vWF:RCo)	Low	Evaluates function by measuring the ability of vWF to agglutinate platelets in the presence of the antibiotic ristocetin
Factor VIII activity	Low or normal	May be normal or slightly decreased in vWD except very low or absent in type III vWD
Multimeric analysis	Variable	Separates the vWF molecule into it subunits (multimers) based on molecular weight; needed to distinguish types of vWD

Abbreviations: vWF = von Willebrand factor; vWD = von Willebrand disease.
Source: From Eberst,[33] with permission.

Table 21-14

RECOMMENDED TREATMENT FOR PATIENTS WITH VON WILLEBRAND DISEASE

Type of vWD	Not Pregnant	Pregnant
Type I	Desmopressin (DDAVP)	*Early:* DDAVP *Delivery:* Intermediate purity factor VIII concentrates (Humate-P, Koate HS)
Type II	Type IIA: Intermediate purity factor VIII concentrate Type IIB: Intermediate purity factor VIII concentrate	*Early, delivery, and postpartum:* Intermediate purity factor VIII concentrate
Type III	Intermediate purity factor VIII concentrates	Intermediate purity factor VIII concentrates

Note: Cryoprecipitate can be used to replace von Willebrand factor and factor VIII in emergencies when these other products are not readily available.

of delivery, although the bleeding time (BT) may remain prolonged. If vWF and factor VIII levels are at least 50 percent of normal at the time of delivery, vaginal delivery can occur without factor replacement and without excessive bleeding. In pregnant women with vWD, excessive bleeding most commonly occurs with first-trimester abortions and in the postpartum period, when vWF and factor VIII levels return to normal. Women with vWD must be closely observed for postpartum hemorrhage, which can be severe.

As noted above, the majority of patients with type I vWD will have factor VIII and vWF levels at least 50 percent of normal at the time of delivery and no bleeding complications. Prior to delivery, a factor VIII level should be determined; this is more readily available than vWF levels and may be more reflective of the risk of excessive bleeding. If the factor VIII level is less than 30 percent of normal, replacement therapy will likely be needed for hemostasis at delivery. Desmopressin will not be effective late in pregnancy because its effect, the release of vWF from endothelial stores, has already been accomplished by the increased estrogen levels. At the time of delivery, intermediate purity factor VIII concentrates rich in vWF are used to replace vWF and factor VIII. Desmopressin can be effective earlier in pregnancy and in the postpartum period (Table 21-14).

Pregnant patients with type IIB vWD can develop severe thrombocytopenia during pregnancy. The abnormal vWF that is present in these patients increases in concentration under the influence of estrogen, and this abnormal vWF binds to platelets, effectively removing them from circulation. This thrombocytopenia is most severe immediately prior to delivery. At the time of delivery, if factor VIII levels are below 30 percent of normal and thrombocytopenia is present, the intermediate purity factor VIII concentrates that are rich in vWF are used for replacement therapy and can correct the

thrombocytopenia. Even in the nonpregnant state, patients with type IIB vWD are usually not treated with desmopressin because of the risk of inducing thrombocytopenia.

Patients with type III vWD have a bleeding diathesis clinically similar to that seen in severe hemophilia A. Circulating levels of factor VIII and vWF are negligible and do not increase significantly during pregnancy. These patients respond poorly to treatment with desmopressin. Intermediate purity factor VIII concentrates are used for replacement therapy to treat bleeding complications and prophylactically prior to delivery. Replacement therapy should be continued several days after cesarean section.

HEMOPHILIAS—DEFICIENCY OF FACTOR VIII OR FACTOR IX

The most common inherited coagulation factor deficiencies, hemophilia A (factor VIII deficiency) and hemophilia B (factor IX deficiency, Christmas disease), are X-linked recessive disorders and therefore rarely of clinical significance in pregnant patients. Female carriers of the gene for hemophilia can have low factor levels and be at risk of symptomatic bleeding if extreme lyonization has occurred, or in phenotypic females with genetic abnormalities such as Turner syndrome (XO). Carriers of hemophilia can usually be identified based on family history. Those with low factor levels may give a history of abnormal or excessive bleeding, especially if they have been hemostatically challenged; menorrhagia is common. Coagulation screening tests, in particular the aPTT when screening for factor VIII or IX deficiency, will be normal unless the factor level is below 25 to 30 percent of normal. Based on history, specific factor VIII or IX levels can be obtained. Pregnant patients with factor levels below 30 percent of normal are at risk of excessive bleeding at the time of delivery and in the postpartum period.[27] Factor levels do not always correlate with bleeding symptoms. Carriers of hemophilia with factor levels below 50 percent of normal should be referred for specialized care by a hematologist or coagulation specialist.

Carriers of hemophilia A should have rising levels of factor VIII during pregnancy, as do other pregnant women. If the factor VIII level remains low (<50 percent) at the time of delivery, replacement therapy, in the form of recombinant factor VIII concentrate, should be given to raise the factor VIII level to at least 50 percent of normal. Levels of 50 percent of normal should be maintained 3 to 4 days postpartum, longer after cesarean section. Desmopressin may be effective in raising the factor VIII level in the postpartum period.

Carriers of hemophilia B reportedly have more clinical problems than carriers of hemophilia A. If factor IX levels are low at the time of delivery, highly purified factor IX concentrates should be used to raise the circulating factor IX level to 50 percent of normal and be continued 3 to 4 days postpartum. Previously, prothrombin complex concentrates were used to replace factor IX. These products can cause thromboembolic phenomena and should be avoided in pregnancy.

It is important to identify carriers of hemophilia early in pregnancy for testing of their factor levels and for genetic counseling. Prenatal diagnosis of hemophilia is possible. Of the offspring of carriers of hemophilia, 50 percent of the males will have hemophilia and 50 percent of the females will be carriers.

OTHER CONGENITAL COAGULATION FACTOR DEFICIENCIES

Although uncommon, congenital deficiency of any coagulation factor can complicate pregnancy. Best described in pregnancy are deficiencies of factors XIII, XII, and XI and fibrinogen abnormalities; these are discussed below. Recently, a patient with congenital factor VII deficiency complicating pregnancy has been described.

FACTOR XIII DEFICIENCY

Congenital deficiency of factor XIII is rare, occurring in one in several million patients. Factor XIII is essential for the cross-linking of fibrin monomers to form a stable clot. An autosomal recessive disorder, factor XIII deficiency typically causes recurrent spontaneous abortions and excessive uterine bleeding. The diagnosis of factor XIII deficiency is established by clot solubility in 5 molar urea. The basic coagulation screening tests will all be normal. Factor XIII is essential for successful pregnancy; it is necessary for normal development of the placenta and fetus. In order to maintain pregnancy, women with factor XIII deficiency must be treated with supplemental factor XIII in the form of fresh

frozen plasma (FFP) or factor XIII concentrates (available only in Europe). This can be accomplished by infusion of FFP, 5mL/kg every 2 to 3 weeks, or factor XIII infusion every 21 days. Factor XIII levels need be only 5 percent of normal to maintain pregnancy.

FACTOR XII DEFICIENCY

Congenital deficiency of factor XII has been identified in several hundred patients. The diagnosis is established by a markedly prolonged aPTT (>100 s) and a very low factor XII level by specific factor assay. Congenital deficiency of factor XII in pregnant women has been associated with spontaneous abortion and premature delivery; however, this relationship is not clear. Factor XII deficiency rarely causes hemorrhage; thromboembolic complications are more common as a result of the involvement of factor XII in fibrinolysis.

FACTOR XI DEFICIENCY

Congenital factor XI deficiency occurs in about one in a million persons in the general population, but in up to three per thousand in the Ashkenazi Jewish population. In factor XI deficiency, clinical bleeding does not always correlate with factor XI levels. Diagnosis is established by the finding of a prolonged aPTT and a low factor XI level on specific factor assay. Postpartum bleeding can be a problem for these women. Factor XI is replaced by FFP. Inhibitors to factor XI rarely occur. A recent report describes a pregnant woman with congenital factor XI deficiency and an inhibitor.

FIBRINOGEN ABNORMALITIES

Abnormalities of fibrinogen, factor I, can be quantitative (low or absent levels) or qualitative (the fibrinogen molecule is structurally abnormal and does not function properly). Both of these fibrinogen abnormalities are associated with obstetric complications such as spontaneous abortion, placental abruption, and postpartum hemorrhage. Patients with fibrinogen abnormalities will usually have prolongation of the coagulation screening tests—the PT, aPTT, and TCT. Fibrinogen levels can be quantitated by specific assay. Abnormal fibrinogen molecules can be demonstrated by functional tests. Successful pregnancy can be achieved with fibrinogen replacement with cryoprecipitate.

ACQUIRED COAGULATION FACTOR DEFICIENCIES

INHIBITORS OF FACTOR VIII

A rare cause of bleeding in previously healthy postpartum women is the development of an inhibitor to a coagulation factor. Inhibitors are circulating antibodies, usually IgG, that are directed most commonly against the factor VIII molecule and less commonly against factor IX. These inhibitors develop in 10 to 15 percent of patients with severe hemophilia A and 10 percent of patients with severe hemophilia B. Occasionally, inhibitors develop in patients who do not have hemophilia. The incidence of inhibitor development in patients who do not have an underlying coagulation disorder is about 1 in 1 million per year. Up to 85 percent of these patients have underlying associated conditions such as autoimmune disorders, lymphoproliferative disorders, or drug reactions. In one series, 7 percent of these inhibitors occurred during pregnancy and the postpartum period.

There are many case reports that document the association of factor VIII inhibitors and pregnancy.[28] Most commonly, the inhibitor develops near term or within several months postpartum; the first pregnancy is typically affected. The patient is usually symptomatic and may present with massive bruising, hemarthroses, ecchymosis, or severe life-threatening bleeding. The diagnosis is established by laboratory findings of a normal PT, greatly prolonged aPTT, and normal TCT. Further studies demonstrate that the aPTT does not "correct" by adding normal plasma (mix); on factor assays, the factor VIII level will be very low or absent and the other factors are normal or only slightly low. When an inhibitor develops during pregnancy, the IgG antibody can cross the placenta and cause a low factor VIII level in the fetus. The etiology of inhibitor development in these patients is unknown; there is a temporary breakdown in the maternal immune tolerance to her own factor VIII. The natural history of these inhibitors is spontaneous resolution over months to 2 years in at least one-half of affected patients. As a rule, inhibitors do not recur in subsequent pregnancies and, in one case, the inhibitor disappeared during a subsequent pregnancy. All patients suspected of having a coagulation factor inhibitor should be referred immediately to an experienced hematologist or coagulation specialist. The bleeding complications in inhibitor patients are managed with high doses of factor VIII concentrates, unactivated or activated prothrombin complex concentrates, and porcine factor VIII. Glucocorticoids, intravenous IgG, and cytotoxic agents can be used to try to suppress the antibody production.

References

1. Williams MD, Wheby MS: Anemia in pregnancy. *Med Clin North Am* 76:631, 1992.
2. Burrows RF, Kelton JG: Fetal thrombocytopenia and its relation to maternal thrombocytopenia. *N Engl J Med* 329:1463, 1993.
3. How HY, Bergmann F, Koshy M, et al: Quantitative and qualitative platelet abnormalities during pregnancy. *Am J Obstet Gynecol* 164:92, 1991.
4. Letsky EA: Mechanisms of coagulation and the changes induced by pregnancy. *Curr Obstet Gynaecol* 1:203, 1991.
5. Walker ID: Management of thrombophilia in pregnancy. *Blood Rev* 5:227, 1991.
6. Perry KG Jr, Morrison JC: The diagnosis and management of hemoglobinopathies during pregnancy. *Semin Perinatol* 14:90, 1990.
7. Koshy M, Burd L: Management of pregnancy in sickle cell syndromes. *Hematol Oncol Clin North Am* 5:585, 1991.
8. Koshy M, Chisum D, Burd L, et al: Management of sickle cell anemia and pregnancy. *J Clin Apheresis* 6:230, 1991.
9. Savana-Ventura C, Bonello F: Beta-thalassemia syndrome and pregnancy. *Obstet Gynecol Surv* 49:129, 1994.
10. Allen LH: Nutritional supplementation for the pregnant woman. *Clin Obstet Gynecol* 37:587, 1994.
11. Sibai BM, Ramadan MK, Usta I, et al: Maternal morbidity and mortality in 442 pregnancies with hemolysis, elevated liver enzymes, and low platelets (HELLP syndrome). *Am J Obstet Gynecol* 169:1000, 1993.
12. Pinette MG, Vintzileos AM, Ingardia CJ: Thrombotic thrombocytopenic purpura as a cause of thrombocytopenia in pregnancy: Literature review. *Am J Perinatol* 6:55, 1989.
13. Miller JM, Pastorek JG: Thrombotic thrombocytopenic purpura and hemolytic uremic syndrome in pregnancy. *Clin Obstet Gynecol* 34:64, 1991.
14. McCrae KR, Samuels P, Schreiber AD: Pregnancy-associated thrombocytopenia: Pathogenesis and management. *Blood* 80:2697, 1992.
15. Burrows RF, Kelton JG: Low fetal risks in pregnancies associated with idiopathic thrombocytopenic purpura. *Am J Obstet Gynecol* 163:1147, 1990.
16. Cook RL, Miller RC, Katz VL, Cephalo RC: Immune thrombocytopenic purpura in pregnancy: A reappraisal of management. *Obstet Gynecol* 78:578, 1991.
17. Burrows RF, Kelton JG: Pregnancy in patients with idiopathic thrombocytopenic purpura: Assessing the risks for the infant delivery. *Obstet Gynecol Surv* 48:781, 1993.
18. Cowchock S: The role of antiphospholipid antibodies in obstetric medicine. *Curr Obstet Med* 1:229, 1991.
19. Infante-Rivard C, David M, Gauthier R, Rivard GE: Lupus anticoagulants, anticardiolipin antibodies, and fetal loss. A case-control study. *N Engl J Med* 325:1063, 1991.
20. Many A, Pauzner R, Carp M: Treatment of patients with antiphospholipid antibodies during pregnancy. *Am J Reprod Immunol* 28:216, 1992.
21. Branch DW, Silver RM, Blackwell JL, et al: Outcome of treated pregnancies in women with antiphospholipid syndrome: An update of the Utah experience. *Obstet Gynecol* 80:614, 1992.
22. Conrad J, Horellou MH, VanDreden P, et al: Thrombosis and pregnancy in congenital deficiencies in AT III, protein C or protein S: Study of 78 women. *Thromb Haemost* 63:319, 1990.
23. Baudo F, Caimi TM, Redaelli R, et al: Emergency treatment with recombinant tissue plasminogen activator of pulmonary embolism in a pregnant woman with antithrombin III deficiency. *Am J Obstet Gynecol* 163:1274, 1990.
24. Aledort LM: Treatment of von Willebrand's disease. *Mayo Clin Proc* 66:841, 1991.
25. Conti M, Mari D, Conti E, et al: Pregnancy in women

with different types of von Willebrand disease. *Obstet Gynecol* 68:282, 1986.

26. Perry KG Jr, Morrison JC: Hematologic disorders in pregnancy. *Obstet Gynecol Clin North Am* 9:783, 1993.

27. Greer IA, Lowe GD, Walker JJ, et al: Hemorrhagic problems in obstetrics and gynecology in patients with congenital coagulopathies. *Br J Obstet Gynaecol* 98:909, 1991.

28. Staikowsky F, Blachin I, Pineat-Vincent F, et al: Inhibitors of factor VIIIc and pregnancy: Review of the literature. *J Gynecol Obstet Biol Reprod* 20:817, 1991.

29. Eberst ME: Evaluation of the bleeding patient, in Tintinalli JE, Ruiz E, Krome RL (eds): *Emergency Medicine*, 4th ed. New York: McGraw-Hill, 1996, pp 973–976.

30. Eberst ME: Acquired bleeding disorders, in Tintinalli JE, Ruiz E, Krome RL (eds): *Emergency Medicine*, 4th ed. New York: McGraw-Hill, 1996, pp 976–982.

31. Eberst ME: Hereditary hemolytic anemias, in Tintinalli JE, Ruiz E, Krome RL (eds): *Emergency Medicine*, 4th ed. New York: McGraw-Hill, 1996, pp 987–991.

32. Eberst ME: Acquired hemolytic anemias, in Tintinalli JE, Ruiz E, Krome RL (eds): *Emergency Medicine*, 4th ed. New York, McGraw-Hill, 1996, pp 991–996.

33. Eberst ME: Hemophilias and von Willebrand disease, in Tintinalli JE, Ruiz E, Krome RL (eds): *Emergency Medicine*, 4th ed. New York: McGraw-Hill, 1996, pp 983–986.

Chapter 22

HUMAN IMMUNODEFICIENCY VIRUS INFECTIONS IN PREGNANCY

Rhoda S. Sperling

EPIDEMIOLOGY AND PATHOPHYSIOLOGY

Infection with human immunodeficiency virus (HIV), the virus that causes acquired immunodeficiency syndrome (AIDS), is pandemic. Worldwide, an estimated 8.8 million women are infected with HIV; most of them reside in sub-Saharan Africa, where identification of infection status and access to treatment are severely limited. Even in the United States, despite the ready availability of antibody screening since 1985, many HIV-infected women remain unaware of their serostatus.[1] Risk factors associated with a woman testing HIV-seropositive include a history of intravenous drug use (IVDU), unprotected intercourse with HIV-infected men or men with high-risk behavior (IVDUs or bisexual men), prostitution or multiple sexual partners, residence in a country with a high prevalence of HIV infection, and blood transfusion between 1978 and 1985. Epidemiologic studies have repeatedly identified a number of cofactors that can facilitate transmission of HIV-1, including genital ulcer disease, anal-receptive intercourse, and severity of HIV-related immunosuppression of a sexual partner.

Perinatal transmission accounts for most HIV-1 infections among children. In the United States, from 1988 to 1993, an estimated 6000 to 7000 children were born each year to HIV-infected women.[1] In 1994, results of a clinical trial of a combined maternal-child zidovudine regimen demonstrated that the risk of perinatal transmission could be dramatically reduced.[2] Utilization of this zidovudine regimen has been credited with the decline in the incidence of perinatally acquired AIDS in this country.[1] Unfortunately, the zidovudine regimen recommended in the United States[3] is not an affordable prevention strategy in most countries.

The etiologic agent of AIDS is a retrovirus designated human immunodeficiency virus type 1 (HIV-1). The T-helper lymphocyte ($CD4^+$ T lymphocyte) is the primary target for HIV infection because of the affinity of the virus for the $CD4^+$ surface marker. The $CD4^+$ T lymphocyte coordinates a number of important immunologic functions, and a loss of these functions results in a progressive impairment of the immune response.

DIAGNOSIS

Because of the long period of clinical latency, most pregnant HIV-infected women will be clinically asymptomatic or have subtle signs/symptoms that may be related to HIV-1. The clinician should be aware of the possible spectrum of illness that may be present.

PRIMARY INFECTION

An acute clinical illness associated with HIV-1 seroconversion occurs in 50 to 70 percent of cases. The incubation period from exposure to time of onset is typically 2 to 4 weeks (average, 21.4 days.) It is generally a self-limiting illness that resolves in 1 to 3 weeks. It can be associated with an appreciable degree of morbidity, and patients may require hospitalization. The main clinical feature of primary HIV-1 infection reflects both the lymphocytopathic and neurologic tropism of HIV-1. Patients typically present with an acute illness characterized by fever, lethargy, malaise, myalgias, headaches, retroorbital pain, photophobia, sore throat, lymphadenopathy, and maculopapular rash. Seroconversion in primary infection is prompt. Second-generation anti–HIV-1 enzyme-linked immunosorbent assays (ELISA, EIA) tend to become positive 14 to 21 days after onset of symptoms. Commercial Western blots demonstrate the presence of specific antiviral antibodies as early as 9 days after the onset of symptoms. The median time from initial infection to the development of detectable anti–HIV-1 antibodies is 2.1 months, with 95 percent of individuals developing antibody within 5.8 months of the initial infection.[4]

CLINICAL LATENCY

During the period of clinical latency there is active viral replication and a progressive decline in CD4$^+$ T lymphocytes. Many conditions, although not pathognomonic for AIDS, may be associated with progressive immunosuppression and are classified by the Centers for Disease Control and Prevention (CDC) as HIV-related (Table 22-1). These conditions include vulvovaginal candidiasis, cervical dysplasia, pelvic inflammatory disease, unexplained fever >30 days, unexplained weight loss, herpes zoster involving two distinct dermatomes, and idiopathic thrombocytopenic purpura. All of these conditions may be seen by the obstetrician/gynecologist or emergency department physician. When these conditions are diagnosed, HIV testing should be encouraged.

ACQUIRED IMMUNODEFICIENCY SYNDROME

Effective January 1, 1993, the CDC expanded the surveillance case definition for AIDS.[5] This new definition now

---

Table 22-1

HIV-RELATED CONDITIONS

Bacillary angiomatosis

Candidiasis, oropharyngeal

Candidiasis, vulvovaginal; persistent, frequent, or poorly responsive to therapy

Cervical dysplasia (moderate or severe)/cervical carcinoma in situ

Constitutional symptoms, such as fever (38.5°C or 101.3°F) or diarrhea lasting ≥ 1 month

Hairy leukoplakia

Herpes zoster (shingles) involving at least two distinct episodes or more than one dermatome

Idiopathic thrombocytopenic purpura

Listeriosis

Pelvic inflammatory disease, particularly if complicated by tuboovarian abscess

Peripheral neuropathy

---

classifies a patient as having AIDS if he or she is an HIV-infected adult with (1) a CD4$^+$ T lymphocyte count of less than 200/mm^3 or less than 14 percent of total lymphocytes; (2) pulmonary tuberculosis; (3) recurrent bacterial pneumonia (more than one episode in a 1-year period); or (4) invasive cervical cancer. These criteria have been added to the 23 other clinical conditions that, under the 1987 CDC guidelines, previously defined patients as having AIDS (Table 22-2). The decision to include cervical cancer as an AIDS-defining condition was controversial; it was based on information from small, uncontrolled case series. The available epidemiologic evidence suggests an increased prevalence of cervical dysplasia, the precursor of cervical cancer, in HIV-infected women, and also an adverse effect of HIV-infection on the progression, clinical course, and treatment of both cervical dysplasia and cancer.

ANTEPARTUM ASSESSMENT

If HIV infection is diagnosed or suspected, symptoms that should be reviewed include weight loss, fever, diarrhea, oral thrush, difficulty swallowing, pulmonary complaints, herpes zoster, genital and extragenital herpes simplex, and central nervous system complaints (Table 22-3).

Table 22-2

CONDITIONS INCLUDED IN THE 1993 AIDS SURVEILLANCE CASE DEFINITION

Candidiasis of bronchi, trachea, or lungs

Candidiasis, esophageal

Cervical cancer, invasive

Coccidioidomycosis, disseminated or extrapulmonary

Cryptococcosis, extrapulmonary

Cryptosporidiosis, chronic intestinal (>1 month's duration)

Cytomegalovirus disease (other than liver, spleen, or nodes)

Cytomegalovirus retinitis (with loss of vision)

Encephalopathy, HIV-related

Herpes simplex, chronic ulcer(s) (>1 month's duration) or bronchitis, pneumonitis, or esophagitis

Histoplasmosis, disseminated or extrapulmonary

Isosporiasis, chronic intestinal (>1 month's duration)

Kaposi's sarcoma

Lymphoma, Burkitt's (or equivalent term)

Lymphoma, immunoblastic (or equivalent term)

Lymphoma, primary, of brain

Mycobacterium avium complex or *M. kansasii,* disseminated or extrapulmonary

Mycobacterium tuberculosis, any site (pulmonary or extrapulmonary)

Mycobacterium, other species or unidentified species, disseminated or extrapulmonary

Pneumocystis carinii pneumonia

Pneumonia, recurrent

Progressive multifocal leukoencephalopathy

Salmonella septicemia, recurrent

Toxoplasmosis of brain

Wasting syndrome due to HIV

Source: Centers for Disease Control and Prevention,[5] with permission.

Table 22-3

COMMON EMERGENCY DEPARTMENT PRESENTATIONS—WHEN TO THINK HIV

Symptoms suggestive of an acute retroviral infection

Upper and lower respiratory tract infections—pneumonia, recurrent bronchitis, recurrent sinusitis

Skin conditions—herpes zoster, nonhealing genital ulcer disease

Unexplained weight loss

Unexplained fever

Oral thrush

Chronic vulvovaginal candidiasis

Abnormal blood count—neutropenia, thrombocytopenia

High-risk behaviors

---

liver function tests, tuberculin skin testing, chest x-ray, testing for sexually transmitted diseases (STDs), serology for toxoplasmosis and cytomegalovirus, and Pap smear.

T cells remain the most commonly used surrogate marker to assess HIV-related disease progression. Those individuals who have absolute T-helper cells counts less than 200 cells/mm^3 are at high risk for the early development of the opportunistic infections that define AIDS. Clinically, T-cell counts are used to determine when prophylactic therapies should be initiated.

An assessment of circulating virus in the plasma should be performed. Studies have demonstrated that plasma viral load can predict progression to AIDS. Combination therapy with antiretrovirals can result in a reduction in plasma HIV RNA and an increase in CD4$^+$ T-cell counts. Most clinicians are now utilizing viral load to determine when therapy should be initiated and to assess adequacy of response to therapy. The most commonly used tests for viral load determinations are the branched deoxyribonucleic acid (bDNA) and the reverse transcriptase polymerase chain reaction (RT-PCR) assay; the results of these tests are reported as plasma RNA copy number per milliliter.

Neutropenia and thrombocytopenia are frequently seen in HIV-1–infected individuals. In addition, many HIV-related therapies are associated with hematologic toxicities; therefore, baseline evaluations are indicated.

Some antiretroviral agents are metabolized by the liver, or they may be associated with hepatotoxicity; therefore, baseline evaluations of liver function are indicated.

The incidence of tuberculosis among HIV-infected patients ranges from 4 to 21 percent, depending on the geo-

Maternal screening tests should be ordered. In the emergency department setting, many of the recommended tests may not be readily available, but they should be obtained as soon as feasible. The following tests are recommended: CD4 count, assays for viral load, complete blood count (CBC),

graphic area. For tuberculin skin testing, the Mantoux skin test (0.1 mL intracutaneous injection into the volar aspect of the forearm) with 5 tuberculin units (5-TU) of purified protein derivative (PPD) is recommended. The only patients who should not be tested are those known to have had a positive PPD previously and/or a history of past treatment for tuberculosis.

The value of anergy testing accompanying PPD testing is debated for individuals who may not have a delayed-type hypersensitivity (DTH) response. Routine evaluation for anergy is no longer recommended by the CDC.

All skin tests should be read in 48 to 72 h. For an HIV-infected adult, a significant PPD skin reaction is ≥ 5 mm of induration. Patients with positive PPD skin tests should be evaluated for preventive treatment with isoniazid (INH) after active tuberculosis has been excluded. A chest x-ray must be obtained; if it is abnormal and/or the patient has unexplained fever or pulmonary symptoms, sputum cultures should be obtained as well.

Pregnancy requires appropriate lead shielding of the abdomen and pelvis in order to reduce the risk of radiation exposure to the embryo or fetus. All patients with a positive PPD and all those with significant pulmonary symptoms or unexplained fevers should be evaluated with a chest x-ray.

The same risk behavior that has led to HIV-seroconversion may have placed a patient at risk for exposure to other sexually transmitted diseases. Screening tests for vaginal trichomoniasis, cervical gonorrhea and chlamydial infection, syphilis, and hepatitis B should be performed.

Reactivation of chronic *Toxoplasma* and cytomegalovirus infections is common in HIV-infected patients as immunosuppression advances. It is unclear whether reactivated maternal disease presents any increased risk for vertical transmission of those pathogens to the fetus. Knowledge of maternal serostatus is helpful in evaluating acute maternal illnesses and also in evaluating the fetus or neonate for evidence of congenital infections.

There is an increased prevalence of cervical dysplasia in patients who are HIV-infected. Studies from the United States have found the prevalence of cervical intraepithelial neoplasia (CIN) in HIV-infected women to be from 15 to 42 percent; in contrast, typical rates of cervical dysplasia in urban populations are 3 to 5 percent. Routine Pap smear evaluations are important and should be in accordance with current clinical guidelines.[6]

ANTEPARTUM TREATMENT

ANTIRETROVIRAL TREATMENT

There is an evolving standard of care based on a better understanding of the pathophysiology of HIV.[7] Guidelines are outdated almost as quickly as they can be published. The number of effective drugs continues to expand rapidly and the use of viral load determinations to govern patient management is quickly becoming standard. Data support the concept that antiretroviral regimens that reduce viral load are associated with better outcome and fewer opportunistic infections or death.[8,9] In nonpregnant adults, agents attacking different aspects of the viral replication cycle are used in combination and are often able to achieve (at least for a short period of time) undetectable levels of virus. Therapies most commonly utilized in clinical practice include three-drug regimens combining nucleoside analogue reverse transcriptase inhibitors with protease inhibitors. Additional therapeutic options currently being studied in clinical trials include combination therapies including nonnucleoside reverse transcriptase inhibitors and integrase inhibitors. In nonpregnant adults, factors to consider in trying to define when early intervention with potent antiretroviral regimens should be initiated include the relative ability of available agents to minimize HIV replication for prolonged periods of time, the relative ability of available agents to delay or prevent the emergence of drug-resistant HIV variants, the relationship between the emergence of drug resistance and treatment failures, and the toxicities associated with prolonged therapy. During pregnancy, additional considerations include the safety (both short- and long-term) of infants following exposure in utero as well as the impact of maternal antiretroviral therapy on mother-to-child HIV-1 transmission. Nucleoside analogues and other antiretroviral agents may be potential human carcinogens or have other unexpected toxicities. As with any therapy that is continued or initiated during pregnancy, the theoretical safety risks must be balanced against the known benefits. It has been demonstrated that zidovudine can dramatically reduce the risk of mother-to-child HIV-1 transmission. The impact on perinatal transmission of other antiretroviral agents, whether used singularly or in combination, remains unknown.

PROPHYLAXIS

There is increasing recognition that bacterial infections, especially those of the upper and lower respiratory tract, occur with greater frequency among HIV-infected individuals and are among the leading causes of HIV-related morbidity and mortality. The rates of these infections increase with decreasing $CD4^+$ T-lymphocyte counts; however, these problems are seen even in patients without advanced immunosuppression. Vaccination, prophylactic antibiotics, and early antimicrobial treatments have all been utilized by clinicians (Table 22-4).

In patients with advanced immunosuppression, chemoprevention has proved to be a successful strategy to reduce the risk for the first occurrence of an AIDS-defining opportunistic infection. Vaccines against pneumococcal disease and influenza are available. Chemopreventive strategies recommended during pregnancy include primary prophylaxis

Table 22-4

RECOMMENDED PROPHYLACTIC THERAPIES DURING PREGNANCY[a]

Disease	Preventive Regimen	Indication
Streptococcus pneumoniae respiratory infections	Pneumococcal vaccine, 0.5 mL IM × 1	First time—all patients; revaccinate if >5 years after first dose
Influenza	Influenza vaccine whole or split virus, 0.5 mL IM × 1	Yearly, all patients
Pneumocystis carinii pneumonia	Trimethoprim/sulfamethoxazole (TMP/SMX), 1 single-strength tablet PO daily	CD4$^+$ T-cell count <200
Mycobacterium avium complex (MAC)	Azithromycin, 1200 mg PO weekly	CD4$^+$ T-cell count <50
Tuberculosis (TB) isoniazid-sensitive	Isoniazid, 300 mg PO daily × 12 months	PPD[b] (≥ 5 mm in duration), radiographic evidence of old TB, exposure to a person with active TB, or prior untreated positive PPD

[a]A comprehensive explanation of currently recommended therapies, including scientific rationale, indications, preventive strategies, dosages, and alternative regimens, is given in the *1997 USPHS/IDSA Guidelines for the Prevention of Opportunistic Infections in Persons Infected with Human Immunodeficiency Virus.*[10]
[b]Purified protein derivative (tuberculin).

against *Pneumocystis carinii* pneumonia (PCP) and disseminated *Mycobacterium avium* complex (MAC).[10] Because of concerns regarding chronic drug exposures during the first trimester, drug therapies should be deferred until after the first trimester whenever possible. Live vaccines (e.g., measles, mumps, rubella, varicella) should not be administered during pregnancy, but inactivated vaccines are safe and effective.

VACCINES

Pneumococcal vaccine efficacy has varied widely, from 60 to 80 percent. Adults with asymptomatic or symptomatic HIV infection should be vaccinated; pregnancy is not a contraindication, as this is not a live vaccine. About half the persons given pneumococcal polysaccharide vaccine may experience mild side effects, such as erythema and pain at the injection site. Fever, myalgias, and severe local reactions have been reported in less than 1 percent. Immunization has been shown to cause a burst of HIV-1 replication; however, there is no evidence that this will have an adverse impact on long-term maternal health. It is unknown whether a burst of HIV-1 replication could be associated with an increased risk of HIV-1 transmission. Because of this concern, many experts recommend, when feasible, that vaccination be deferred until after a zidovudine regimen has been initiated for the prevention of mother-to-child HIV transmission.

Some reports suggest that influenza illnesses may be more prolonged and the risks of complications higher for HIV-infected individuals. Influenza vaccination, an inactivated virus vaccine, may be associated with a transient burst of HIV-1 viral replication.

PREVENTION OF OPPORTUNISTIC INFECTIONS

TUBERCULOSIS

Preventive therapy with 12 months of isoniazid (INH) is recommended for patients who are HIV-seropositive in the following settings: (1) positive tuberculin test of ≥5 mm of induration, (2) history of a previously untreated positive tuberculin skin test, (3) radiographic evidence of old tuberculosis, and (4) history of exposure to active tuberculosis infection.

PNEUMOCYSTIS CARINII PNEUMONIA

The recommended treatment of choice for PCP prophylaxis in nonpregnant adults is trimethoprim sulfamethoxazole, one double-strength (DS) or one single-strength (SS) tablet daily. Metaanalysis suggests that even lower-dose regimens (one DS tablet three times a week) may be as effective but better tolerated. Prophylaxis for PCP is recommended at any time during pregnancy.[10]

DISSEMINATED INFECTION WITH *MYCOBACTERIUM AVIUM* COMPLEX

Controlled trials have demonstrated that chemoprophylaxis for MAC can substantially decrease the incidence of disease and can prolong survival. Primary prophylaxis with either clarithromycin or azithromycin is recommended for non-pregnant adults with CD4$^+$ T-lymphocyte counts <50/mm^3. Prophylaxis for MAC is recommended during pregnancy; however, because of fetal safety considerations, azithromycin is the treatment of choice during pregnancy.[10]

ANTEPARTUM PREVENTION OF PERINATAL HIV-1 TRANSMISSION

Without any treatment, the reported rates of mother-to-child transmission have varied widely in different geographic areas, from 15 to 40 percent.[11–15]

There is scientific evidence to support HIV transmission from mother to infant antepartum (in utero), intrapartum (during labor or delivery), and postpartum (through breast-feeding.) The stage of maternal infection is a significant predictor of the risk of mother-to-infant transmission. Advanced maternal immunosuppression, as judged by a low T-helper cell count,[15–17] more rapid clinical disease progression,[16,18] or increased viral burden as assessed by either p24 antigenemia[16,17] or plasma RNA levels[19–21] have all been associated with an increased risk of perinatal HIV-1 transmission.

In February 1994, the AIDS clinical trial group (ACTG) 076 study was closed to enrollment and unblinded when an interim efficacy analysis demonstrated that a regimen of maternal and newborn zidovudine dramatically reduced the risk of mother-to-child HIV-1 transmission, from 25.5 to 8.3 percent.[2] The details of the ACTG 076 trial have been published.[2] It was a placebo-controlled study that enrolled HIV-infected pregnant women between 14 and 34 weeks of gestation, with CD4$^+$ T-cell counts greater than 200/mm^3 and no maternal indications for antiretroviral therapy. Patients were randomized to either zidovudine (ZDV) or placebo. The active regimen included antepartum ZDV (100 mg PO five times daily) initiated between 14 and 34 weeks of gestation, continued throughout the remainder of pregnancy, followed by intrapartum ZDV (an intravenous loading dose of 2 mg/kg started in labor, followed by a continuous infusion of 1 mg/kg per hour) until delivery. Thereafter oral ZDV (syrup 2 mg/kg every 6 h for 6 weeks beginning 8 to 12 h after birth) was given to the infant.

The availability of a regimen that could prevent the transmission of a fatal pediatric infection led the U.S. Public Health Service to publish guidelines for the use of zidovudine during pregnancy.[3] Other professional groups have published practice guidelines for clinicians as well.

The mechanism by which ZDV reduced the risk of trans-

mission was unknown at the time the ACTG 076 study was stopped. Maternal ZDV may have reduced the circulating viral load and diminished the viral exposure of the fetus in utero and at the time of delivery. Alternatively, or additionally, therapeutic concentrations of the drug in both the fetus and the newborn may have provided protection before and after viral exposure. Stored samples from entry and delivery have been assayed to determine whether maternal plasma viral load predicted either transmission risk or ZDV efficacy. Recently published findings demonstrated that in the 076 population, (1) viral load predicted transmission risk in untreated mother-infant pairs, (2) in both the ZDV and placebo groups transmission occurred across a broad range of entry plasma RNA levels and T-helper cell counts, and (3) a reduction of circulating plasma RNA from entry to delivery explained only part of the ZDV treatment effect.[21] Explanations need to be considered for the apparent lack of association between the observed maternal plasma RNA levels and the effect of ZDV treatment. The possibility of a prophylactic effect both in utero and intrapartum, during and after exposure, has been raised. Until the scientific explanation for the ZDV treatment effect is further elucidated, the current practice of offering a ZDV regimen to all HIV-infected pregnant women and their newborns regardless of their plasma viral burden or CD4$^+$ T-cell counts should continue. In clinical circumstances where alternative therapies are indicated for the treatment of maternal disease, a maternal/infant regimen of ZDV must still be considered.

There are many ongoing clinical trials of both antiretroviral therapies and immune-based therapies to reduce the risk of mother-to-child HIV-1 transmission. In the United States, a phase III trial of a maternal/newborn regimen of hyperimmune HIV immune globulin and a phase I study of maternal nevirapine (a nonnucleoside reverse transcriptase inhibitor) are nearing completion. Internationally, several studies of short-course maternal ZDV and also several studies of maternal ZDV in combination with other antiretroviral agents are under way. The results of all of these trials should add to our understanding of the mechanisms whereby perinatal HIV-1 transmission can be prevented.

INTRAPARTUM MANAGEMENT

Several intrapartum factors have been hypothesized to influence the risk of transmission; these include chorioamnionitis, duration of time since rupture of membranes, and mode of delivery. Theoretically, these factors could alter the duration of exposure of the infant's mucosal surfaces to cell-free and cell-associated virus in either maternal blood and/or cervicovaginal secretions. In a cohort study from Zaire, both chorioamnionitis and funisitis were associated with an increased transmission risk of mother-to-child HIV-1 transmission.[18] Exposure to ruptured membranes may increase the risk of transmission. A recent report from a prospective, longitudinal study in the United States and Puerto Rico found an association with perinatal transmission when the duration of time since rupture of membranes before delivery exceeded 4 h.[22] A similar association between rupture of membranes and mother-to-child transmission has not been reported in other large cohort studies. Definitive data are lacking regarding the role of cesarean delivery and the risk of transmission. Perinatal transmission studies in this country have not reported a significant association between the mode of delivery and the risk of HIV-1 transmission. However, the European Collaborative Study[23] and a meta-analysis of predominantly European studies[24] have reported an association with cesarean delivery and a lower rate of HIV-1 transmission. These data are difficult to interpret and subject to many potential biases, since patients were not randomly assigned to mode of delivery. A randomized trial of the mode of delivery is under way in Italy. Chlorhexidine vaginal cleansing in labor (a low-cost, simple strategy that could be utilized worldwide) was unsuccessful in reducing mother-to-child HIV-1 transmission in a large clinical trial reported from Malawi.[25]

Steps for intrapartum management are listed in Table 22-5.

When the patient presents to either the emergency department or labor and delivery with complaints of labor or rupture of membranes, an appropriate evaluation should include contraction monitoring, speculum examination to exclude spontaneous rupture of membranes (SROM), and a vulvovaginal examination to exclude evidence of genital herpes simplex virus (HSV) infection.

As soon as labor is diagnosed, or SROM is confirmed, maternal ZDV treatment should be initiated.[3] Patients may also be participating in clinical trials to prevent HIV-1 perinatal transmission. This information should be obtained upon admission.

In general, HIV-infected individuals have greater morbidity (and mortality) following common bacterial infections as compared with nonimmunosuppressed individuals. Many experts recommend antibiotic prophylaxis in labor for HIV-infected patients. Theoretically, this may benefit maternal health by reducing the risk for intraamniotic infection (IAI) and its associated sequelae. In addition, if IAI is a risk factor for HIV-1 transmission, it may also reduce the risk of intrapartum HIV-1 vertical transmission.

Obstetric practices that expose the fetus to maternal blood and cervicovaginal secretions should be discouraged. The application of fetal scalp electrodes and fetal scalp sampling should be avoided. Early amniotomy should be discouraged. Induction (or augmentation) of labor should be considered for patients at term with premature rupture of membranes.

POSTPARTUM CARE

Confirmed or suspected maternal endomyometritis, wound infections, and other bacterial infections should be treated aggressively with appropriate antimicrobials. In general, HIV-infected individuals have greater morbidity (and mortality) following common bacterial infections as compared with individuals who are not immunosuppressed.

In the United States, where there is a safe alternative, breast-feeding in HIV-infected women should be actively discouraged, since it may be associated with a 10 to 20 percent incremental increase in perinatal HIV-1 transmission.

Long-term follow-up should be arranged for both mother and child with practitioners who are experienced in managing HIV-1 infections.

Table 22-5

INTRAPARTUM MANAGEMENT OF HIV

1. Assess for:
   Labor
   Spontaneous rupture of membranes
   Vulvovaginal infections
2. Determine if patient is enrolled in clinical trial
3. Administer zidovudine (ZDV) to laboring woman,
   2 mg/kg bolus dose, followed by 1 mg/kg/h
4. Limit fetal exposure to maternal fluids, if possible

References

1. Centers for Disease Control and Prevention: World AIDS day. *MMWR* 45:1005, 1996.
2. Connor EM, Sperling RS, Gelber RD, et al: Reduction of maternal-infant transmission of human immunodeficiency type 1 with zidovudine treatment. *N Engl J Med* 331:1173, 1994.
3. Centers for Disease Control and Prevention: Recommendations for the use of zidovudine to reduce perinatal transmission of human immunodeficiency virus. *MMWR* 43(RR-11):1, 1994.
4. Pantaleo G, Grazios C, Fauci A: The immunopathology of human immunodeficiency virus infection. *N Engl J Med* 320:327, 1993.
5. Centers for Disease Control and Prevention: 1993 Revised classification system for HIV infection and expanded surveillance case definition for AIDS among adolescents and adults. *MMWR* 41(RR-17):1, 1992.

6. Kurman RJ, Henson DE, Herbst ME, et al: Interim guidelines for the management of abnormal cervical cytology. *JAMA* 271:1866, 1994.

7. Carpenter CCJ, Fischl MA, Hammer SM, et al: Antiretroviral therapy for HIV infection in 1996. *JAMA* 276:146, 1996.

8. Hammer SM, Katzenstein DA, Hughes MD, et al: A trial comparing nucleoside monotherapy with combination therapy in HIV-infected adults with CD4 cell counts from 200 to 500 cells per cubic millimeter: AIDS Clinical Trials Group Study 175 Study Team. *N Engl J Med* 375:1081, 1996.

9. Katzenstein DA, Hammer SM, Hughes MD, et al: The relation of virologic and immunologic markers to clinical outcomes after nucleoside therapy in HIV-infected adults with 200 to 500 CD4 cells per cubic millimeter: AIDS Clinical Trials Group Study 175 Virology Study Team. *N Engl J Med* 335:1142, 1996.

10. Centers for Disease Control and Prevention: The 1997 USPHS/IDSA Guidelines for the prevention of opportunistic infections in persons infected with human immunodeficiency virus. *MMWR* 46(RR-12):1, 1997.

11. Ryder RW, Nsa W, Hassig SE, et al: Perinatal transmission of the human immunodeficiency virus type 1 to infants of seropositive women in Zaire. *N Engl J Med* 320:1637, 1989.

12. Hira SK, Kamanga J, Bhat G, et al: Perinatal transmission of HIV-1 in Zambia. *Br Med J* 229:1078, 1987.

13. Hutto C, Parks WP, Lai S, et al: Perinatal transmission of the human immunodeficiency virus type 1. *J Pediatr* 118:347, 1991.

14. Goedert JJ, Mendez H, Drummond JE, et al: Mother-to-infant transmission of human immunodeficiency virus type 1; association with prematurity or low anti-gp 120. *Lancet* 2:1351, 1989.

15. Fischl MA, Richman DD, Grieco MH, et al: The efficacy of azidothymidine (AZT) in the treatment of patients with AIDS and AIDS-related complex: A double blind, placebo-controlled trial. *N Engl J Med* 317;185, 1987.

16. Hague RA, Mok JY, Johnstone FD, et al: Maternal factors in HIV transmission. *Int J STD AIDS* 4:142, 1993.

17. St Louis M, Kamenga M, Brown C, et al: Risk for perinatal HIV-1 transmission according to maternal immunologic, virologic, and placental factors. *JAMA* 269:2853, 1993.

18. Lindgren S, Anzen B, Bohlin AB, Lidman K: HIV and child-bearing: Clinical outcome and aspects of mother-to-infant transmission. *AIDS* 5:1111, 1991.

19. Dickover DE, Garratty EM, Herman SA, et al: Identification of levels of maternal HIV-1 RNA associated with risk of perinatal transmission: Effect of maternal zidovudine treatment on viral load. *JAMA* 275:599, 1996.

20. Fang G, Burger H, Grimson R, et al: Maternal plasma human immunodeficiency virus type 1 RNA level: A determinant and projected threshold for mother-to-child transmission. *Proc Natl Acad Sci USA* 92:12100, 1995.

21. Sperling RS, Shapiro DE, Coombs RW, et al: Maternal viral load, zidovudine treatment, and the risk of transmission of human immunodeficiency virus from mother to infant. *N Engl J Med* 335:1621, 1996.

22. Landesman SH, Kalish LA, Burns DN, et al: Obstetrical factors and the transmission of human immunodeficiency virus type 1 from mother to child. *N Engl J Med* 334:1617, 1996.

23. European Collaborative Study: Cesarean section and the risk of vertical transmission of HIV-1 infection. *Lancet* 343:1463, 1994.

24. Villari P, Spino C, Chalmers TC, et al: Cesarean section to reduce perinatal transmission of human immunodeficiency virus: A metaanalysis. *Online J Curr Clin Trials,* July 8, 1993, document 7410.

25. Biggar RJ, Miotti P, Taha T, et al: Perinatal intervention in Africa: Effect of a birth canal cleansing intervention to prevent HIV transmission. *Lancet* 347:1647, 1996.

Chapter 23

VIRAL INFECTIONS IN PREGNANCY

Patrick Duff

Viral infections occur commonly in pregnancy. Fortunately, the most frequent infections (upper respiratory tract infections, gastroenteritis) usually do not pose a serious risk to either the mother or her fetus. Some infections, however, may cause serious, even life-threatening complications in the pregnant adult and/or may severely injure the developing infant.

This chapter reviews in detail those infections that fall into the latter category: cytomegalovirus, hepatitis, herpes simplex, parvovirus, rubella, rubeola, toxoplasmosis, and varicella. Human immunodeficiency virus is considered in Chap. 22. In each section, attention is directed to the epidemiology and pathophysiology of infection, clinical manifestations, diagnosis, management, and indications for referral for specialty consultation. Table 23-1 provides a concise summary of the key points of this chapter and may be used as a quick reference for patient management. Table 23-2 summarizes the indications and contraindications to the use of viral vaccines in pregnant women.

CYTOMEGALOVIRUS INFECTION

EPIDEMIOLOGY

Cytomegalovirus (CMV) is a double-stranded DNA virus, and humans are its only known host. Like herpes simplex virus, CMV may remain latent in host cells after the initial infection. Recurrent infection is usually due to reactivation of endogenous latent virus rather than reinfection with a new strain of virus. Cell-mediated immunity is more important than humoral immunity in controlling infection.[1]

Cytomegalovirus is not highly contagious; therefore, close personal contact is required for infection to occur. *Horizontal transmission* may result from receipt of an infected organ or blood transfusion, sexual contact, or contact with contaminated saliva or urine. *Vertical transmission* may occur as a result of transplacental (hematogenous) infection, exposure to contaminated genital tract secretions during delivery, or breast-feeding. The incubation period of the virus ranges from 28 to 60 days, with a mean of 40 days.[1-3]

In young children, the most important risk factor for infection is close contact with playmates, particularly in the setting of day care. Infected children, in turn, pose a risk of transmitting virus to adult day care workers and to members of their own families. In addition to acquiring infection from young children, adolescents and adults may develop infection as a result of sexual contact. Cytomegalovirus infection is endemic among homosexual men and heterosexuals with multiple partners.[1-8] Additional risk factors for infection include low socioeconomic status, history of abnormal cervical cytology, birth outside of North America, first pregnancy at less than 15 years, and coinfection with other sexually transmitted diseases (STDs), such as trichomoniasis.[9]

CLINICAL MANIFESTATIONS IN CHILDREN AND ADULTS

Most children who acquire CMV infection are asymptomatic. When clinical manifestations are present, they are

Table 23-1

SERIOUS VIRAL AND PROTOZOAN INFECTIONS IN PREGNANCY

Organism	Risk to Mother	Risk to Fetus/Neonate	Diagnosis		Treatment
			Maternal	Fetal/Neonatal	
CMV	Minimal except in immunocompromised patient	Severe fetal injury with *primary* maternal infection transmitted antepartum	Serology	Amniocentesis—viral culture Ultrasound	Prevention of exposure
Hepatitis A	Minimal	None	Serology	—	Passive immunization with immune globulin after exposure Active immunization with inactivated hepatitis A vaccine prior to exposure (e.g., international traveler and in combination with immune globulin after exposure)
Hepatitis B	Chronically infected patients are at high risk for developing chronic liver disease	Perinatal transmission of infection	Serology	Serology	Passive immunization with hepatitis B immune globulin (HBIG) Active immunization with hepatitis B vaccine (HBV)
Hepatitis C	Chronically infected patients are at high risk for developing chronic liver disease	Perinatal transmission of infection	Serology	Serology	Prevention of exposure Administration of immune globulin exposure
Hepatitis D	Coinfection with hepatitis B increases risk for chronic liver disease	Perinatal transmission of infection	Serology	Serology	Preventive measures for hepatitis B protect against hepatitis D
Hepatitis E	Severe acute infection with 10–20% risk of mortality	Fetal death resulting from maternal death Perinatal transmission of infection rare	Serology	Serology	Prevention of exposure through good sanitation and avoidance of travel to endemic areas

Table 23-1

SERIOUS VIRAL AND PROTOZOAN INFECTIONS IN PREGNANCY *(Continued)*

Organism	Risk to Mother	Risk to Fetus/Neonate	Diagnosis Maternal	Diagnosis Fetal/Neonatal	Treatment
Herpes simplex	Minimal except in immunocompromised patient	Severe neonatal injury when delivered to mother with primary infection	Clinical examination Culture	Same	Cesarean when mother is actively infected at time of delivery Acyclovir for *severe* maternal infection or *any* neonatal infection
Parvovirus	Minimal	Hydrops fetalis Neurologic and hematologic sequelae in neonate are rare	Serology	Ultrasound	Intrauterine transfusion for hydropic fetus
Rubella	Minimal	Congenital rubella syndrome—greatest risk is when maternal infection occurs in first trimester	Clinical examination Serology	Ultrasound	Ensure maternal immunity *prior* to pregnancy by vaccination with live vaccine Pregnancy termination for infected fetus
Rubeola	Serious sequelae, although rare, include pneumonia and encephalitis	Minimal risk of teratogenicity	Clinical examination Serology	—	Ensure maternal immunity *prior* to pregnancy by vaccination with live vaccine Immune globulin for postexposure prophylaxis
Toxoplasmosis	Minimal except in immunocompromised patient	Severe fetal injury with *primary* maternal infection	Serology	Amniocentesis for PCR analysis Ultrasound	Mother—sulfadiazine + spiramycin Neonate—sulfadiazine + pyrimethamine
Varicella	Serious sequelae include pneumonia and encephalitis	Varicella embryopathy affects ≤2% of fetuses exposed prior to 20 weeks of gestation	Clinical examination Serology	Ultrasound	Ensure maternal immunity *prior* to pregnancy by vaccination with live varicella vaccine Administer varicella-zoster immune globulin for postexposure prophylaxis Acyclovir for active maternal or neonatal infection

Table 23-2

GUIDELINES FOR USE OF VIRAL VACCINES IN PREGNANT WOMEN

Vaccine	Type of Vaccine	Indication
Hepatitis A	Inactivated	Pre- and postexposure prophylaxis
Hepatitis B	Inactivated	Pre- and postexposure for mother and neonate
Influenza	Inactivated	Preexposure prophylaxis in pregnant women with chronic cardiopulmonary or renal disease, sickle cell disease, immunodeficiency disorder, or who have had a splenectomy
Mumps	**Live**	**Contraindicated during and within 3 months of anticipated pregnancy**
Rubella	**Live**	
Rubeola	**Live**	
Varicella	**Live**	

usually mild and include malaise, fever, lymphadenopathy, and hepatosplenomegaly. Similarly, most adults with either primary or recurrent CMV are asymptomatic. Symptomatic patients typically have findings suggestive of mononucleosis. Respiratory infection is uncommon in adults with normal immune function, but an increasing number of cases of serious CMV pulmonary infection are likely to occur as a consequence of the rising prevalence of human immunodeficiency virus (HIV) infection in women.

DIAGNOSIS OF INFECTION IN ADULTS AND CHILDREN

The diagnosis of CMV infection can be confirmed by isolation of virus in tissue culture. The highest concentrations of CMV are found in urine, seminal fluid, saliva, and breast milk. Several different cell lines have been used to support viral growth, and techniques such as the viral shell assay, immunofluorescent staining, monoclonal antibody, and polymerase chain reaction permit identification of viral antigen within 24 h.[1,9–11]

Serologic methods also are helpful in establishing the diagnosis of CMV infection provided that the reference laboratory is skilled in performing such tests. In the acute phase of infection, virus-specific IgM antibody is present in serum. IgM titers usually decline rapidly over a period of 30 to 60 days, but in some patients they may remain elevated for 6 to 9 months. There is no absolute IgG titer that will clearly differentiate acute from recurrent infection. However, a fourfold or greater change in the IgG titer is consistent with recent acute infection.[1] Other laboratory tests suggestive of CMV infection include a differential white blood cell count showing atypical lymphocytes, low platelet count, and elevated serum transaminase concentrations.

CONGENITAL AND PERINATAL INFECTION

As a result of exposure to either young children or an infected sexual partner, approximately 50 to 80 percent of adult women in the United States have serologic evidence of past CMV infection. Unfortunately, the presence of antibody is not perfectly protective against vertical transmission; thus pregnant women with both recurrent and primary infection pose a special risk to their fetuses. Fetal and neonatal CMV infection may occur at three distinct times: antepartum, intrapartum, and postpartum. Antepartum or congenital infection poses the greatest risk to the fetus and is perhaps the most difficult to understand because of the confusing array of statistics reported in epidemiologic surveys.

CONGENITAL (ANTEPARTUM) INFECTION

Congenital CMV infection results from hematogenous dissemination of virus across the placenta. Dissemination may occur with both primary and recurrent (reactivated) infection but is much more likely in the former setting. From 1 to 4 percent of uninfected women seroconvert during pregnancy.[12] In women who acquire primary infection, 40 to 50 percent of the fetuses will be infected. The overall risk of congenital infection is greatest when maternal infection occurs in the third trimester—that is, the efficiency of transplacental infection is highest in the third trimester. However, the probability of severe fetal injury is highest when maternal infection occurs in the first trimester.[13]

Of fetuses with congenital infection, 5 to 20 percent are symptomatic at birth. The most common clinical manifestations are hepatosplenomegaly, intracranial calcifications, jaundice, growth restriction, microcephaly, chorioretinitis, and hearing loss. The most frequent laboratory abnormalities in the neonate are thrombocytopenia, hyperbilirubine-mia, and elevated serum transaminase concentrations. Approximately 30 percent of severely infected infants die. Of the survivors, 80 percent have severe neurologic morbidity, ocular abnormalities, or sensorineural hearing loss.[14,15] Approximately 80 to 95 percent of infants delivered to mothers with primary infection will be asymptomatic at birth. Of these infants, 10 to 15 percent subsequently develop hearing loss, chorioretinitis, or dental defects within the first 2 years of life.

Pregnant women who experience recurrent CMV infection are much less likely to transmit infection to their fetuses than women with primary infections. Recurrent infection arises predominantly as a result of reactivation of latent infection rather than reinfection with a new viral strain. The most recent and probably clearest delineation of fetal risk in this situation is the report by Fowler et al.[15] These authors studied 125 women with serologic evidence of primary infection and 64 with recurrent infection. In the former group, 18 percent of infants were symptomatic at birth. An additional 7 percent developed at least one major sequela within 5 years of follow-up. Two percent died, 15 percent had sensorineural hearing loss, and 13 percent had IQs below 70. In contrast, none of the infants delivered to mothers with recurrent infection were symptomatic at birth. During the period of surveillance, 8 percent had at least one sequela, but none had multiple defects. The most common

sequela was hearing loss. The authors concluded that maternal antibody provided substantial but not complete protection against serious fetal infection resulting from recurrent maternal CMV infection.

Overall, approximately 1 percent of infants (40,000) born in the United States each year have congenital CMV infection. Approximately 3000 to 4000 infants are symptomatic at birth, and an additional 4000 to 6000 subsequently have neurologic or developmental problems in the first years of life. Cytomegalovirus infection is now the principal cause of hearing deficits in children. Public health officials estimate that the annual cost of caring for children with congenital CMV is almost $2 billion.[16,17] Figure 23-1 summarizes the sequelae of CMV infection in pregnancy.

PERINATAL (INTRAPARTUM AND POSTPARTUM) INFECTION

Perinatal infection may occur *during delivery* as a result of exposure to infected genital tract secretions. At the time of delivery, up to 10 percent of pregnant women may be shedding CMV in cervical secretions and/or urine. About 20 to 60 percent of exposed fetuses may subsequently shed virus in the pharynx and/or urine. The incubation period for this form of infection ranges from 7 to 12 weeks, with an average of 8 weeks. Fortunately, infected infants rarely have serious sequelae of infection acquired during delivery.[14,17]

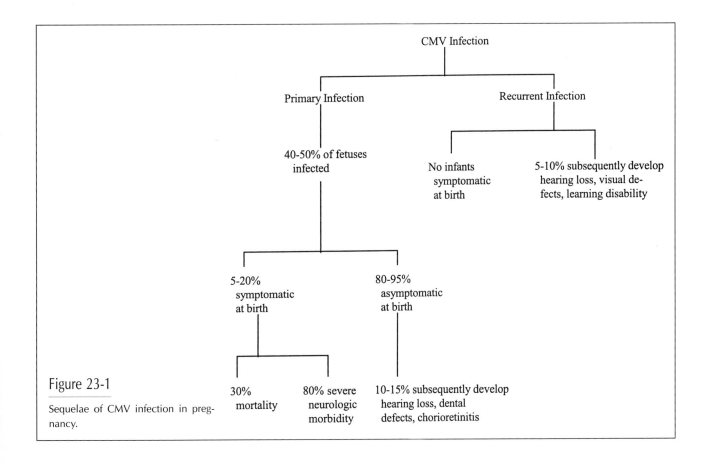

Figure 23-1

Sequelae of CMV infection in pregnancy.

Perinatal infection also may develop *as a result of breast-feeding*. Stagno et al.[18] surveyed 278 women who had recently delivered and who agreed to provide samples of breast milk. Thirty-eight (13 percent) had CMV isolated at least once from colostrum or milk. Twenty-eight of these women were shedding CMV only in breast milk. Nineteen of their neonates were breast-fed, and 11 (58 percent) acquired CMV infection despite the presence of neutralizing antibody in breast milk. Fortunately, serious sequelae did not occur in infected infants.

DIAGNOSIS OF FETAL INFECTION

In recent years, much attention has focused on the analysis of amniotic fluid and fetal serum as a means to diagnose congenital infection. Several authors have compared the relative value of the following diagnostic tests: viral culture of amniotic fluid and fetal serum, determination of total IgM concentration in fetal serum, identification of anti-CMV IgM in fetal serum, and assessment of fetal liver function tests. These reports have uniformly supported the superiority of amniotic fluid culture in confirming the diagnosis of congenital CMV infection and the great value of ultrasound in determining the severity of fetal injury.[10,11]

MANAGEMENT

At the present time, a vaccine for CMV is not available. Antiviral agents such as ganciclovir and foscarnet have moderate activity against CMV, but their use is limited primarily to treatment of severe infections in immunocompromised patients. Their value in preventing severe fetal/neonatal infection has not been demonstrated. Accordingly, physicians should focus their attention on educating patients about preventive measures.

One of the most important interventions is helping patients understand that CMV infection can be a sexually transmitted disease and that sexual promiscuity significantly increases the risk of acquiring infection. Individuals who have multiple sexual partners should be counseled that latex condoms provide an effective barrier to transmission of CMV.[19] Another important intervention is educating health care workers, day care workers, elementary school teachers, and mothers of young children about the importance of simple infection-control measures such as hand-washing and proper cleansing of environmental surfaces. Obstetricians, pediatricians, and emergency medicine physicians must be consistently aware of the importance of transfusing only CMV-free blood products to fetuses, neonates, pregnant women, and immunocompromised patients, and screening potential donors of organs and semen for CMV infection.[2] Finally, health care workers, particularly reproductive-age women, must adhere to the principles of universal precautions when treating patients and handling potentially infected body fluids.[12]

For several reasons, routine prenatal screening for CMV infection is not recommended. First, laboratory resources might be overwhelmed if all pregnant women were screened. Second, if laboratories do not ensure a high level of quality control, the interpretation of serologic tests can be confusing, leading to incorrect and irreversible interventions such as pregnancy termination. Third, neither antiviral chemotherapy nor immunoprophylaxis is available to protect the fetus or neonate. Accordingly, screening should be limited to women who have symptoms suggestive of acute CMV infection, who have had definite occupational exposure to CMV, or who are immunocompromised. Although most immunocompetent adults will not have manifestations of infection, fever (lasting an average of 19 days) and lymph node and spleen enlargement may be seen. Tonsillitis and pharyngitis are rare. Hepatitis (especially biochemical hepatitis) and interstitial pneumonitis can be seen occasionally even in the immunocompetent patient, though they are more commonly seen in transplant and other immunocompromised individuals. Even more uncommon complications of CMV infection are Guillain-Barré syndrome, meningoencephalitis, myocarditis, and thrombocytopenia with hemolytic anemia. A pregnant woman suspected of having primary CMV infection should be referred to an obstetrician-gynecologist or specialist in maternal-fetal medicine for further evaluation and treatment. When a pregnant woman presents to an emergency department or urgent care facility, it is imperative that the prenatal care provider receive results of CMV laboratory testing so that further counseling can be provided in a timely fashion because decisions about test results (e.g., pregnancy termination) are time-dependent.

HEPATITIS

Hepatitis is one of the most common and most highly contagious viral infections. At present, five distinct types of hepatitis virus have been identified: A, B, C, D, and E. Each infection has a slightly different clinical implication for the pregnant woman and her fetus.

HEPATITIS A

EPIDEMIOLOGY

Hepatitis A is responsible for approximately 30 to 35 percent of cases of hepatitis in the United States. It is caused by an RNA virus that is transmitted by person-to-person contact through fecal-oral contamination. Poor hygiene, poor sanitation, and intimate personal or sexual contact facilitate transmission. Epidemics frequently result from common exposure to contaminated food and water. In the United States, individuals at particular risk for hepatitis A are those who have recently immigrated from or traveled to developing na-tions of the world where the disease is endemic.[20] Drug abusers, homosexual men, and children in day care centers also are at increased risk of acquiring hepatitis A.[21-23]

The incubation period of hepatitis A ranges from 15 to 50 days, with a mean of 28 to 30 days. The highest concentration of viral particles is found in fecal material, and the virus is not normally excreted in urine or other body fluids.

CLINICAL MANIFESTATIONS

Some patients with hepatitis A are asymptomatic. Children are more frequently asymptomatic than adults. When symptoms occur, they usually include malaise, fatigue, anorexia, nausea and vomiting, and right-upper-quadrant pain. The characteristic physical findings of acute hepatitis A are jaundice, hepatic tenderness, darkened urine, and acholic stools.

DIAGNOSIS

The most useful diagnostic test for hepatitis A is detection of IgM-specific antibody. This marker can usually be identified 25 to 30 days after the initial exposure, and it persists for up to 6 months. IgG antibody is detectable within 35 to 40 days of exposure and persists indefinitely, thus conferring lifelong immunity. The serum concentration of alanine aminotransferase (ALT), aspartate aminotransferase (AST), and bilirubin is usually moderately to markedly elevated. Liver biopsy is rarely indicated to confirm the diagnosis of viral hepatitis.[23,24] When performed, it characteristically shows extensive hepatocellular injury and a prominent inflammatory infiltrate.

MANAGEMENT

Acute hepatitis A is usually a self-limited illness, and only supportive care is required for the vast majority of patients. Recovery is typically complete within 4 to 6 weeks. Fewer than 0.5 percent of affected patients develop fulminant hepatitis, coagulopathy, or encephalopathy. Infected patients, particularly those who are pregnant, should be advised of the need for sound nutrition. Physical activity should be limited to prevent upper abdominal trauma, and drugs with potential hepatotoxicity should be avoided. Sexual and household contacts should receive immunoprophylaxis with a single intramuscular dose of immune globulin, 0.02 mL/kg, within 2 weeks of exposure. In addition, they also should receive the formalin-inactivated hepatitis A vaccine in a single intramuscular dose of 0.06 mL. The vaccine is highly immunogenic and is safe for use in pregnancy.[24,25]

As a general rule, unless the pregnant mother becomes severely ill, hepatitis A does not pose a serious risk to the fetus. Perinatal transmission of infection does not occur, and a chronic carrier state does not exist. An infant delivered to an acutely infected mother should receive immune globulin to prevent horizontal transmission of infection after delivery. In addition, mothers who develop evidence of en-

cephalopathy, coagulopathy, or severe debilitation should be hospitalized for intensive support.[23,26] An obstetrician-gynecologist should be included in the interdisciplinary team caring for the seriously ill pregnant patient.

HEPATITIS B

EPIDEMIOLOGY

Approximately 40 to 45 percent of all cases of hepatitis in the United States are caused by hepatitis B virus. Over 300,000 new cases occur annually, and about a million Americans are chronic hepatitis B carriers. The frequencies of acute and chronic hepatitis B in pregnancy are 1 to 2 per 1000 and 5 to 15 per 1000 respectively.[26]

Hepatitis B is caused by a DNA virus, and the incubation period is 60 to 110 days. The intact virus is termed the *Dane particle*. The virus has three major structural antigens: surface antigen (HBsAg), core antigen (HBcAg), and e antigen (HBeAg). Transmission of hepatitis B occurs primarily as a result of parenteral injection, sexual contact, and perinatal exposure.[23] Certain population groups have an increased prevalence of hepatitis B: Asians, Eskimos, drug addicts, transfusion recipients, dialysis patients, residents and employees of chronic care facilities, prisoners, and recipients of tattoos.

CLINICAL MANIFESTATIONS

Some patients with acute hepatitis B infection can have a clinically inapparent infection, though most will have elevated transaminases. Symptomatic acute hepatitis B can range from a mild, anicteric course to a considerably more severe, icteric disease. Symptomatic disease is typified by nausea, vomiting, headache, anorexia, malaise, low- to moderate-grade fever (37.5 to 39.0°C or 99.5 to 102.2°F) and right-upper-quadrant discomfort.

Following an acute infection caused by hepatitis B virus, less than 1 percent of patients develop fulminant hepatitis and die. About 85 to 90 percent experience complete resolution of their physical findings and develop protective levels of antibody, while 10 to 15 percent become chronically infected. Of these, 15 to 30 percent subsequently develop chronic active or persistent hepatitis or cirrhosis, and a small percentage develop hepatocellular carcinoma. Chronic liver disease is particularly likely to occur in patients who remain seropositive for HBeAg or who become coinfected with hepatitis C or hepatitis D virus.[23]

DIAGNOSIS

The diagnosis of *acute* hepatitis B is confirmed serologically by detection of the surface antigen and IgM antibody to the core antigen. Identification of HBeAg is indicative of an exceptionally high viral inoculum and active viral replication. Patients who have *chronic* hepatitis B infection have persistence of the surface antigen in the serum and liver tissue. Some individuals, particularly Asians, also remain seropositive for HBeAg.[23,24,27]

Patients with acute and chronic hepatitis B infection pose a major threat of transmission to other household members, especially their sexual partners. Infected women also may transmit infection to their fetuses. Perinatal transmission occurs primarily as a result of the infant's exposure to infected blood and genital secretions during delivery. In the absence of immunoprophylaxis for the neonate, perinatal transmission occurs in 10 to 20 percent of women who are seropositive for HBsAg. The frequency of perinatal transmission increases to almost 90 percent in women who are seropositive for both HBsAg and HBeAg.[23,24,28]

Fortunately, a combination of passive and active immunization is highly effective in preventing both horizontal and vertical transmission of hepatitis B infection. Therefore, it is critically important that pregnant women presenting for care to anyone other than their prenatal care provider have results of hepatitis B serology forwarded to that provider. All individuals who have had household or sexual exposure to another person with hepatitis B infection should be tested to determine if they have antibody to the virus. If they are seronegative, they should immediately receive immunoprophylaxis with hepatitis B immune globulin (HBIG), 0.06 mL/kg intramuscularly. They then should receive the hepatitis B vaccination series. The vaccine is an inactivated agent and is thus safe for use in pregnancy.

Similarly, infants who are delivered to seropositive mothers should immediately receive HBIG, 0.5 mL IM, and then begin the hepatitis B vaccination series within 12 h of birth. At the present time, two recombinant hepatitis B vaccines are available: Recombivax-HB and Engerix-B.[24] Both products are composed of inactivated portions of the surface antigen and are prepared by recombinant DNA technology. Neither poses a risk of transmission of a bloodborne pathogen, and both are safe for administration during pregnancy to patients at risk.

Patients infected with hepatitis B virus also may transmit infection to medical and nursing personnel who care for them. Each year approximately 12,000 American health care workers contract hepatitis B as a result of an occupational injury such as a needle stick or splash to a mucous membrane. Of these, approximately 200 develop fulminant hepatitis and subsequently die.[24,29,30] Health care workers can protect themselves from hepatitis in three principal ways. First, they should be vaccinated for hepatitis B. Second, they should encourage *all* young adults and other individuals who have a specific risk factor to receive the hepatitis B vaccine. Third, they should consistently follow universal precautions to prevent sharp injuries and splashes to exposed mucous membrane or skin surfaces.

Conversely, health care workers who are infected with hepatitis B also pose a risk to others. They, too, must observe safeguards to prevent horizontal transmission of infection to their patients. Infection is most likely to occur as a consequence of direct blood-to-blood exposure during invasive surgical procedures. Unless the patient has documented immunity to hepatitis B, the infected health care worker has an ethical obligation to inform her that some risk of transmission exists. The attendant should then perform the procedure only if the patient explicitly consents. During the actual procedure, the operator must take every precaution to ensure that he or she sustains no sharp injury that would expose the patient to infected blood.

NON-A, NON-B HEPATITIS

Non-A, non-B hepatitis accounts for 10 to 20 percent of cases of hepatitis in the United States. Non-A, non-B hepatitis occurs in two forms: parenterally transmitted hepatitis C and enterically transmitted hepatitis E.

HEPATITIS C

EPIDEMIOLOGY

Hepatitis C is a 30- to 38-nm, single-stranded RNA virus, and its incubation period is 5 to 10 weeks. Approximately 75 percent of patients with hepatitis C are asymptomatic. The remainder have the usual symptoms and physical findings of acute viral hepatitis outlined above (see "Hepatitis B"). The principal risk factors for infection are intravenous drug abuse, transfusion, and sexual intercourse.[31] Approximately 90 percent of all cases of posttransfusion hepatitis are due to hepatitis C, and 2 to 15 percent of patients who receive multiple transfusions become infected with this virus. Hepatitis C is particularly likely to result in chronic liver disease. Approximately 50 percent of infected patients develop biochemical evidence of hepatic dysfunction. Of these, about 20 percent subsequently develop chronic active hepatitis or cirrhosis.[23]

DIAGNOSIS

The diagnosis of hepatitis C infection is confirmed by identification of anti-C antibody. Initial screening for this antibody should be performed with an enzyme immunoassay (EIA). A positive EIA should be followed with a recombinant immunoblot assay (RIBA). The present RIBA is able to detect four specific viral antigens. If at least two antigens are identified, the test is considered positive. If only one antigen is identified, the test is considered indeterminant. The present generation of laboratory assays does not precisely discriminate between IgM and IgG antibody. Moreover, antibody may not be detectable until up to 22 weeks after the onset of clinical illness. Direct detection of antigen also is possible with polymerase chain reaction (PCR) methodology, although this test is not yet widely available.[23]

In a general obstetric population, the prevalence of hepatitis C is 1 to 3 percent. The principal factors that place an obstetric patient at high risk for hepatitis C include concurrent STDs, multiple sexual partners, history of recent multiple transfusions, and history of intravenous drug abuse. Patients with these risk factors should be screened for hepatitis C during pregnancy.[32,33]

MANAGEMENT

In selected series, the frequency of perinatal transmission of hepatitis C infection has ranged from 10 to 44 percent,[31,33] but the epidemiology of perinatal transmission has not been completely delineated. Many of the infected neonates in these series were coinfected with human immunodeficiency virus (HIV).

At the present time, a vaccine for hepatitis C is not available. Passive immunization with immunoglobulin (0.06 mL/kg IM) should be administered following percutaneous exposure to a person with hepatitis C and may be used during pregnancy. The benefit of immunoprophylaxis for the neonate has not been proved in controlled clinical trials. Although alpha interferon has shown some activity against the virus, relapses occur in 44 to 80 percent of patients within 6 to 12 months of discontinuation of therapy.[23]

HEPATITIS D

EPIDEMIOLOGY

Hepatitis D, or delta hepatitis, is caused by an RNA virus that is dependent upon coinfection with the hepatitis B virus for replication. Hepatitis D has an external coat of hepatitis B surface antigen and an internal delta antigen that is encoded by its own genome. The epidemiology of hepatitis D is essentially identical to that of hepatitis B.[41]

CLINICAL MANIFESTATIONS

Acute hepatitis D occurs in two forms: *coinfection* and *superinfection.* Coinfection represents the simultaneous occurrence of acute hepatitis B and D. It is usually a self-limited disorder and rarely leads to chronic liver disease. Superinfection occurs when acute hepatitis D develops in a patient who is a chronic hepatitis B carrier. Approximately 20 to 25 percent of patients with chronic hepatitis B ultimately become superinfected with the delta virus, and about 80 percent of these individuals subsequently develop chronic hepatitis. Of those who have chronic hepatitis, 70 to 80 percent develop cirrhosis and portal hypertension, and, unfortunately, almost 25 percent ultimately die of hepatic failure.[41–43]

DIAGNOSIS

The diagnosis of *acute coinfection* can be confirmed by detection of delta antigen in hepatic tissue or serum and IgM-specific antibody in serum. In addition, the tests for HBsAg and HBcAb-IgM are positive. In patients with *superinfection,* serologic tests reflect acute hepatitis D (positive delta antigen, positive serum IgM antibody) and chronic hepatitis B infection (positive surface antigen, HBcAb-IgG). Patients with chronic hepatitis D usually have detectable serum levels of IgG-specific antibody for the delta virus and are seropositive for HBsAg. Unfortunately, IgG antibody does not eradicate the delta viremia, and the antigen can still be identified in serum and hepatic tissue.[23,41,42]

MANAGEMENT

Patients with acute hepatitis D should receive the general supportive care outlined for hepatitis A. Those with chronic infection should be monitored periodically for worsening hepatic function or coagulopathy. At present, there is no specific antiviral agent or immunotherapy that is curative for either acute or chronic delta infection. Perinatal transmission of hepatitis D virus has been reported. Fortunately, transmission is uncommon because the neonatal immunoprophylaxis for hepatitis B is almost uniformly effective against hepatitis D.[23] Therefore, infants born to these infected women should receive HBIG 0.5 mL IM immediately after birth and then begin the hepatitis B vaccination series within 12 h of birth.

HEPATITIS E

EPIDEMIOLOGY

Hepatitis E is caused by an RNA virus, and the disease may present in either an icteric or anicteric form. The virus is transmitted by the fecal/oral route; therefore the epidemiology of hepatitis E is similar to that of hepatitis A. The incubation period ranges from 2 to 9 weeks, with a mean of 45 days.[34,35] Hepatitis E is rare in the United States but is endemic in developing countries.[36–38] In these countries, maternal mortality has been alarmingly high, ranging from 10 to 20 percent. Extreme poverty, coexisting medical illnesses, malnutrition, and poor prenatal care are at least partially responsible for the poor maternal prognosis. The only cases of hepatitis E in the United States have occurred in patients who traveled to countries where the disease was endemic.[39]

DIAGNOSIS

Three new diagnostic tests are available for confirmation of hepatitis E infection. Viral-like particles can be identified in the stools of infected patients by electron microscopy. These particles will agglutinate when combined with serum from the patient. In addition, a fluorescent antibody blocking assay and Western blot assay are now available for use.[23,40]

MANAGEMENT

Patients with acute hepatitis E should be treated as described previously for patients with hepatitis A. Once a patient has recovered from the acute illness, a chronic carrier state does not develop and perinatal transmission rarely occurs. If the mother survives the acute stage of infection, fetal outcome is usually not adversely affected. Patients with suspected hepatitis E should be managed in consultation with an obstetrician-gynecologist.

HERPES SIMPLEX INFECTION

EPIDEMIOLOGY

Herpes simplex virus (HSV), a double-stranded DNA virus, is transmitted by direct, intimate contact. Following the initial infection, the virus remains dormant in neuronal ganglia and may reactivate at later times. Two strains of the virus have been identified: HSV-1 and HSV-2. The former causes primarily oropharyngeal infection and the latter, genital tract infection. Approximately 0.5 to 1.0 percent of women have an overt herpetic infection during pregnancy. About 400 cases of neonatal herpes occur annually in the United States, and the estimated incidence of neonatal infection ranges from 1 per 7500 to 30,000 live births.[44]

Herpes simplex virus infections are classified as *primary, nonprimary first episode,* and *recurrent* on the basis of historical and clinical findings and serologic testing. Table 23-3 summarizes the criteria for each diagnosis. Approximately 20 to 40 percent of Americans are seropositive for HSV, accounting for approximately 31 million people. Up to 80 percent of these individuals do not have a history of an overt primary infection.[44,45] Stated another way, 60 to 80 percent of individuals who are HSV-2–seropositive are unaware that they are infected.

CLINICAL MANIFESTATIONS

The onset of HSV infection is usually heralded by a prodrome of neuralgias, paresthesias, and hypesthesias, followed by an eruption of painful vesicles on an erythematous base in either the orolabial area or genitalia. The vesicles typically rupture, forming a shallow-based ulcer, and then form a dry crust. Because the infection is limited to the epidermis, some vesicles become secondarily infected and evolve into frank pustules. Ultimately, the vesicles heal without scarring.[44,45]

In patients experiencing a primary HSV infection, vesicles may be present for up to 3 weeks. Systemic symptoms may be moderately severe, and local complications such as urinary retention may occur. In recurrent infections, overt vesicles are fewer in number and less painful and typically persist for ≤14 days. Table 23-4 compares the incubation period and clinical features of primary and recurrent HSV infection.[44]

In some patients, particularly those who are immunocompromised, HSV infection may be widely disseminated, affecting extensive areas of skin, mucosal membranes, and visceral organs. Herpes simplex virus may also cause a severe ocular infection, meningitis, encephalitis, and ascending myelitis.

DIAGNOSIS

Several laboratory tests may be used to confirm the diagnosis of HSV infection. Cytologic preparations may show characteristic multinucleated giant cells and intranuclear inclusions. Polymerase chain reaction assays are extremely sensitive in detecting low concentrations of viral DNA, but such assays are not yet widely available. Serology is especially useful in classifying the initial herpetic episode as *primary* versus *nonprimary first episode.* However, serologic testing is rarely indicated in patients who experience recurrent HSV infection.[44,45]

Table 23-3

CLASSIFICATION OF HERPES SIMPLEX VIRUS INFECTION

Classification	Criteria
Primary	First clinical infection
	No preexisting antibody
Nonprimary first episode	No history of genital tract infection
	Positive antibody for HSV-1 or HSV-2
Recurrent	Prior history of clinical infection
	Positive antibody for HSV-2

Table 23-4

COMPARISON OF PRIMARY VERSUS RECURRENT HERPES SIMPLEX VIRUS INFECTION

Stage of Illness	Type of Infection	
	Primary	Recurrent
Incubation period and/or prodrome (days)	2–10	1–2
Vesicle, pustule (days)	6	2
Wet ulcer (days)	6	3
Dry crust (days)	8	7
Total	**22–30**	**13–14**

Until the advent of PCR, viral isolation in tissue culture has been the standard for confirmation of diagnosis. Viral isolation is usually possible within 72 to 96 h of inoculation of the tissue culture. The highest rate of isolation is achieved when clinical specimens are obtained from fresh vesicles or pustules. Vesicular fluid should be aspirated with a fine needle into a tuberculin syringe. Ulcers should be scraped vigorously with a wooden spatula or cotton-tipped applicator.[44,45] The lowest yield is obtained from the dry, crusted lesion, with viral isolation by culture in only approximately 25 percent. The result of a positive test for HSV must be conveyed to the prenatal care provider.

MANAGEMENT

Severe primary HSV infection has been associated with spontaneous abortion, preterm delivery, and intrauterine growth restriction. Isolated case reports have been published documenting in utero infection even in the presence of intact membranes.[44-46] However, the greatest risk to the fetus occurs when overt HSV infection is present at the time of labor. In this situation, the principal mechanism of infection is direct contact with infected vesicles during the process of vaginal birth. The risk of neonatal infection is clearly dependent upon whether the mother has a primary or recurrent HSV infection. In the setting of a primary infection, the viral inoculum in the genital tract is high, and maternal IgG antibody is not present; together, these factors increase the risk of neonatal infection. Approximately 40 percent of neonates delivered vaginally to such women become infected. In the absence of antiviral chemotherapy, almost half of these infants die, and 35 to 40 percent experience severe neurologic morbidity such as chorioretinitis, microcephaly, mental retardation, seizures, and apnea. In women who have recurrent *symptomatic* HSV infection, the risk of neonatal infection following vaginal delivery is ≤5 percent. In women who have a history of recurrent HSV infection but no prodromal symptoms or overt lesions, the risk of neonatal infection with vaginal delivery is ≤1 per 1000, a result of asymptomatic viral shedding.[44,45,47-49]

Neonatal HSV infection may take many forms. In its simplest manifestation, it may appear as a localized abscess at the site of attachment of a scalp electrode or as isolated mucocutaneous lesions. In its more severe forms, neonatal HSV infection may present as widely disseminated mucocutaneous lesions, visceral infection, meningitis, and encephalitis. In these latter instances, mortality may approach 50 to 60 percent, and up to half of the survivors may have persistent neurologic sequelae.[44,45,47-49]

Clinical management of HSV infection has changed dramatically in recent years. This is true for several reasons. First, surveillance cultures of the genital tract in patients with a history of HSV infection have been ineffective in preventing neonatal HSV infection.[49-51] Second, cultures are not 100 percent sensitive. Third, culture results are not always readily available at the time a patient is admitted for

delivery. Last, about two-thirds of children with neonatal HSV infection are actually born to women who do not have a history of prior infection and who, hence, would not be targeted for surveillance cultures.[48-51]

Accordingly, the following simplified guidelines have now been recommended by the Infectious Diseases Society for Obstetrics and Gynecology and endorsed by the American College of Obstetricians and Gynecologists.[45,48] At the time of the patient's initial prenatal appointment, she should be questioned about a prior history of HSV infection. If her history is positive, she should be screened for other sexually transmitted diseases such as gonorrhea, chlamydial infection, syphilis, hepatitis B, and HIV infection. When the patient ultimately is admitted for delivery, she should be asked about prodromal symptoms and examined thoroughly for cervical, vaginal, and vulvar lesions. If no prodromal symptoms or overt lesions are present, vaginal delivery should be anticipated. If symptoms or lesions are present, cesarean delivery should be performed. Cesarean delivery is indicated even in the presence of ruptured membranes of extended duration, since abdominal delivery significantly decreases the size of the viral inoculum to which the infant is exposed. Laboring patients, particularly those with ruptured membranes, who present to the emergency department should be referred immediately to the labor and delivery ward for management by an obstetrician-gynecologist.

In addition to the guidelines outlined above, clinicians should be aware of possible indications for use of acyclovir during pregnancy. Immunocompromised patients with disseminated infections require hospitalization for treatment with intravenous acyclovir. Oral acyclovir, 200 mg five times daily or 400 mg three times daily for 7 to 10 days, should be considered for immunocompetent patients who have *severe* herpetic infection (e.g., prominent systemic symptoms and urinary retention), especially near term. In addition, prophylactic treatment with acyclovir, 400 mg twice daily, may be appropriate in women with frequent recurrent infections in pregnancy, particularly near term.[52] Acyclovir is classified by the Food and Drug Administration (FDA) as a category C drug. To date, the Acyclovir Registry has reported no increase in the frequency of adverse effects in infants exposed in utero to this antiviral agent.[52-54] Both valacyclovir and famciclovir have recently been approved for treatment of HSV and appear to be as efficacious as acyclovir. The experience with their use during pregnancy, however, is quite limited.

PARVOVIRUS INFECTION

EPIDEMIOLOGY

Human parvovirus B_{19} is a single-stranded DNA virus that can replicate only in cells that are dividing rapidly. The virus is distributed worldwide, and infection may occur in both a sporadic and epidemic form. Humans are the only known host for the B_{19} virus. The organism is transmitted by respiratory droplets and infected blood components, and the incubation period is 4 to 20 days. Serum and respiratory secretions become positive for the virus several days before clinical symptoms develop. Once symptoms or a rash appears in immunocompetent patients, respiratory secretions and serum are usually free of the virus.[55] Prevalence of antibody to parvovirus increases with age. Approximately 2 to 15 percent of children aged 1 to 5 years are seropositive for antibody. In adolescents and adults, the seroprevalence increases to more than 60 percent.[55,56]

CLINICAL MANIFESTATIONS

The most common clinical presentation of parvovirus infection is erythema infectiosum or fifth disease. This illness typically occurs in elementary school and day care populations in the late winter and early spring. Patients may have low-grade fever, malaise, and adenopathy; adults may develop polyarthritis affecting the hands, wrists, and knees. In addition, many children have a characteristic pruritic, erythematous "slapped cheek" rash on the face and a finely reticulated erythematous rash on the trunk and extremities (Fig. 23-2). The rash may wax and wane over a period of several months in response to stress, exercise, sunlight, or bathing. Erythema infectiosum is a self-limited illness. Complete recovery is the norm, and serious long-term sequelae rarely occur.[55,56]

The second major clinical presentation of parvovirus infection is transient aplastic crisis. This disorder occurs almost exclusively in individuals who have an underlying hemoglobinopathy and results from viral infection of the bone marrow, with resultant destruction of red blood cell precursors. Affected patients have prodromal symptoms similar to those of erythema infectiosum. From 1 to 7 days after the onset of the prodrome, signs of anemia develop, such as pallor, weakness, and lethargy. Patients with transient aplastic crisis usually do not have a skin rash. Full recovery without sequelae is the norm provided that the patient receives appropriate supportive care.[55,56]

DIAGNOSIS OF MATERNAL INFECTION

Parvovirus can be grown in tissue culture consisting of fresh bone marrow supplemented with erythropoietin. The virus also can be detected by DNA hybridization assays using serum, leukocytes, respiratory secretions, urine, or tissue. In addition, infection can be documented by characteristic histologic changes in infected cells, such as eosinophilic inclusion bodies, marginated chromatin, and direct detection of viral particles by electron microscopy. However, the clinical mainstay of laboratory diagnosis is serologic testing. Antibody to parvovirus can be measured by enzyme-linked immunosorbent assay (ELISA), radioimmunoassay (RIA),

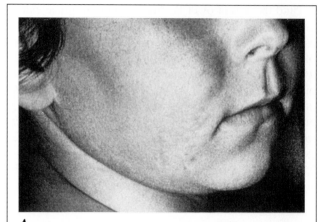

A

B

Figure 23-2

A. Characteristic "slapped cheek" rash of erythema infectiosum. *B.* Lacelike rash on upper extremity. [From Duff P: Maternal and perinatal infection, in Gabbe S, Niebyl J, Simpson JL (eds): *Obstetrics: Normal and Problem Pregnancies.* New York: Churchill Livingstone, 1996, with permission.]

and Western blot; IgM-specific antibody is usually positive by the third day after the onset of symptoms. Typically, IgM disappears within 30 to 60 days, but it may persist for up to 120 days; IgG antibody is detectable by the seventh day of illness and persists for life.[55–57]

FETAL INFECTION

When a pregnant woman develops parvovirus infection, her fetus is at risk for one particularly serious complication: hydrops. This condition results primarily from the propensity of the virus to injure red blood cell precursors in the fetal marrow and, to a lesser extent, from direct viral infection of the fetal myocardium. Either mechanism can result in a picture of high-output cardiac failure with generalized fetal edema and effusions in the pleural space or peritoneal cavity. When maternal infection occurs in the first 12 weeks of pregnancy, the frequency of hydrops ranges as high as 15 to

20 percent. When exposure is in weeks 13 to 20, the risk of hydrops is 10 to 15 percent. When exposure is delayed until >20 weeks, the risk of hydrops is ≤5 percent.[55,56]

Parvovirus does not usually cause a structural defect in the fetus. However, isolated case reports have recently described abnormalities such as hypotonia, arthrogryposis, motor delay, infantile spasms, ventriculomegaly, and prolonged anemia in infants that may be associated with congenital parvovirus infection.[58,59]

DIAGNOSIS OF FETAL INFECTION

The most valuable test for diagnosis of fetal parvovirus infection is ultrasound. Severely affected fetuses typically have evidence of hydrops. Since the incubation period of the virus may be longer in the fetus than in the child or adult, the patient should be followed with serial ultrasound examinations for 6 to 10 weeks after her acute illness. If the fetus shows no signs of hydrops, invasive tests are unnecessary.[55,56]

MATERNAL MANAGEMENT

Following a documented exposure to parvovirus, the mother should immediately have a serologic test to determine if she is immune or susceptible to the virus. If preexisting IgG antibody is present, the patient can be reassured that second infections are extremely unlikely and that her fetus is not at risk. If the patient is susceptible, she should have a repeat serologic test in approximately 3 weeks to determine if she has seroconverted. If seroconversion is detected, the patient should be referred to an obstetrician-gynecologist for further assessment. Hydropic fetuses are candidates for transfusion in utero.[60]

No antiviral agent or vaccine is presently available for treatment of parvovirus infection, but patients with erythema infectiosum rarely need more than simple supportive care. Patients with transient aplastic crisis may require red blood cell transfusion during the acute phase of their illness. As a general rule, isolation of patients with erythema infectiosum is not of value in reducing transmission of infection, since spread by respiratory droplets has already occurred by the time the patient has clear signs of clinical disease. Conversely, if patients with transient aplastic crisis are isolated early in the course of their illness, horizontal transmission to other susceptible individuals may be reduced.[55,56]

RUBELLA

EPIDEMIOLOGY

Rubella is an RNA virus, and only a single serotype is known. Rubella occurs primarily in young children and adolescents, and the disease is most common in the springtime.

Major epidemics of rubella occurred in the United States in 1935 and 1964; minor sporadic epidemics occurred approximately every 7 years until the late 1960s. Following licensure of an effective rubella vaccine in 1969, the frequency of rubella declined by almost 99 percent. The persistence of this infection, albeit at a low level, appears to be due to failure to vaccinate susceptible individuals rather than the lack of immunogenicity of the vaccine.

Rubella virus enters the host through the upper respiratory tract. From this site, the virus travels quickly to the cervical lymph nodes and then is disseminated hematogenously throughout the body. The incubation period of the virus is approximately 2 to 3 weeks. It is present in blood and nasopharyngeal secretions for several days before appearance of the characteristic rash and is shed from the nasopharynx for an equal period of time after appearance of the exanthem.

Antibody against rubella does not normally appear in the serum until after the rash has developed. Acquired immunity to rubella is usually lifelong. Second infections have occurred after both natural primary infections and vaccination. However, recurrent infections generally are not associated with serious illness, viremia, or congenital infection.[61,62]

CLINICAL MANIFESTATIONS

Most children and adults with rubella have mild constitutional symptoms such as malaise, headache, myalgias, and arthralgias. The principal clinical manifestation of this illness is a widely disseminated, nonpruritic, erythematous maculopapular rash (Fig. 23-3). Postauricular adenopathy and mild conjunctivitis are also common. These clinical manifestations are usually short-lived and typically resolve within 3 to 5 days. The differential diagnosis of rubella includes rubeola, roseola, other viral exanthems, and drug reaction.[61,62]

DIAGNOSIS

The diagnosis of rubella is usually based on physical examination. If necessary, serologic tests can be confirmatory. IgM antibody typically reaches a peak 7 to 10 days after the onset of illness and then declines over a period of 4 weeks. The serum concentration of IgG antibody rises more slowly, but protective antibody persists for life. Several types of antibody detection tests are available, including enzyme immunoassay, indirect immunofluorescence, and latex agglutination. The EIA and latex agglutination tests are the most rapid and convenient methodologies.[63]

CONGENITAL RUBELLA SYNDROME

Because of the success of rubella vaccination campaigns, the incidence of congenital rubella syndrome in the United States has declined dramatically over the past 25 years.[64] Unfortunately, however, approximately 10 to 20 percent of

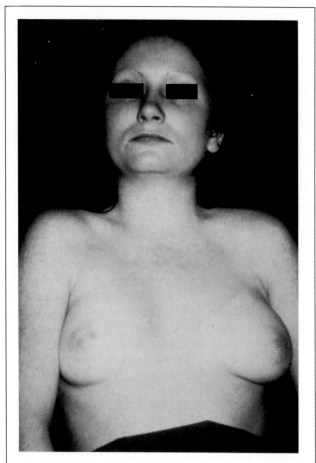

Figure 23-3

Typical disseminated erythematous maculopapular rash of rubella. [From Duff P: Maternal and perinatal infection, in Gabbe S, Niebyl J, Simpson JL (eds): *Obstetrics: Normal and Problem Pregnancies*. New York: Churchill Livingstone, 1996, with permission.]

women in the United States remain susceptible to rubella; hence, their fetuses are at risk for serious injury should they become infected during pregnancy.

The rubella virus crosses the placenta by hematogenous dissemination, and the frequency of congenital infection is critically dependent upon the time of fetal exposure to the virus.[63] Approximately 50 percent of infants exposed to the virus within 4 weeks of conception will manifest signs of congenital infection. When maternal infection occurs in the second 4-week period after conception, approximately 25 percent of fetuses will be infected. When infection develops in the third month, 10 percent of fetuses will be infected. When maternal infection occurs beyond this point in time, less than 1 percent of babies will be infected.[62,65,66]

An entire spectrum of anomalies has been associated with congenital rubella syndrome. The four most common are deafness (affecting 60 to 75 percent of infected fetuses), eye defects (10 to 30 percent), central nervous system defects (10 to 25 percent), and cardiac malformations (10 to 20 percent). The most common cardiac abnormality asso-

ciated with congenital rubella is patent ductus arteriosus, although supravalvular pulmonic stenosis is perhaps the most pathognomonic. Other possible abnormalities include microcephaly, mental retardation, pneumonia, intrauterine growth restriction, hepatosplenomegaly, hemolytic anemia, and thrombocytopenia.[66]

Detailed ultrasound examination is the best test to determine if serious fetal injury has occurred. Abnormalities that can be identified accurately by ultrasound include intrauterine growth restriction, microcephaly, and cardiac malformations. Pregnant women with suspected primary rubella infection in the first 20 weeks of pregnancy should be referred to an obstetrician-gynecologist for further evaluation and treatment.

The prognosis for infants with congenital rubella syndrome is guarded.[65–67] Approximately 50 percent of affected individuals have to attend schools for the hearing-impaired. An additional 25 percent require at least some special schooling because of hearing impairment, and only 25 percent are able to attend regular mainstream schools. Some affected individuals develop insulin-dependent diabetes later in life, presumably secondary to in utero infection of the pancreas. The estimated lifetime cost of caring for a child with congenital rubella syndrome is approximately $200,000 to $300,000.[67]

MANAGEMENT

Ideally, women of reproductive age should have a preconception medical consultation when they are contemplating pregnancy. At this time, they should be evaluated for immunity to rubella. If serologic testing demonstrates that they are susceptible, they should receive rubella vaccine prior to conception and should avoid pregnancy for 3 months.[62] When preconception counseling is not possible, the patient should have a test for rubella at the time of her first prenatal visit. Women who are susceptible to rubella should be counseled to avoid exposure to other individuals who may have viral exanthems.

If a susceptible patient is subsequently exposed to rubella, serologic tests should be obtained to determine whether acute infection has occurred. If acute infection is documented, patients should be counseled about the risk of congenital rubella syndrome. Obviously, specific counseling should be based upon the time during gestation when the maternal infection occurred. The diagnostic tests for detection of infection in utero should be reviewed, and patients should be offered the option of pregnancy termination based upon the assessed risk of serious fetal injury.[68]

Susceptible patients who are fortunate enough to escape infection during pregnancy should be vaccinated immediately postpartum. The present rubella vaccine is the RA 27/3 preparation; it is available in a monovalent form, a bivalent form (measles-rubella, MR) and a trivalent form (measles-mumps-rubella, MMR). Approximately 95 percent of patients who receive rubella vaccine seroconvert. Antibody levels persist for at least 18 years in more than 90 percent of vaccinees.

There are few adverse effects of vaccination, even in adults. Less than 25 percent of patients experience mild constitutional symptoms such as low-grade fever and malaise. Less than 10 percent have arthralgias, and less than 1 percent develop frank arthritis. Women who have received the vaccine cannot transmit infection to susceptible contacts, such as younger children in the home. Breast-feeding is not a contraindication to vaccination. In addition, the vaccine can be administered in conjunction with other immune globulin preparations, such as Rh-immune globulin.

Women who receive rubella vaccine should use contraception for a minimum of 3 months after vaccination. For a number of years, the Centers for Disease Control and Prevention (CDC) maintained a registry of women who received the rubella vaccine within 3 months of conception. That registry included almost 400 patients; fortunately, there were no instances in which congenital rubella syndrome resulted from vaccination.[68] The maximum theoretical risk of congenital rubella resulting from rubella vaccine in early pregnancy is 1 to 2 percent.

RUBEOLA

EPIDEMIOLOGY

The measles virus is a single-stranded RNA virus that is highly contagious and is spread primarily by respiratory droplets. About 75 to 90 percent of susceptible contacts become infected after exposure. The incubation period is 10 to 14 days. Since licensure of the measles vaccine, the reported incidence of measles has decreased by almost 99 percent. In recent years, two major types of measles outbreaks have been reported in the United States. One type has occurred among unvaccinated preschoolers, including children less than 15 months of age. Another has occurred among previously vaccinated school-age children and college students. Approximately one-third of the cases in the latter type of outbreak have been in individuals who were previously vaccinated. Presumably, these cases result from either *primary failure* to respond to the first vaccine or *secondary failure,* a situation where an adequate serologic response develops initially but immunity wanes over time.[69]

CLINICAL MANIFESTATIONS

The clinical manifestations of measles usually appear within 10 to 12 days of exposure. The most common are fever, malaise, coryza, sneezing, conjunctivitis, cough, and photophobia. All patients typically develop a generalized maculopapular rash, and the majority also have Koplik's spots, which are blue-gray specks on a red base that develop on the buccal mucosa opposite the second molars. The skin exanthem typically begins on the face and neck and then spreads to the trunk and extremities. It usually lasts for approximately 5 days and then recedes in the order in which it appeared. The duration of illness is approximately 7 to 10 days. Patients are contagious from 1 to 4 days before the onset of coryza. Immunity to measles should be lifelong following infection by wild virus and is mediated by both humoral and cellular mechanisms.

Although measles is typically a minor illness, some patients develop serious sequelae. Otitis media occurs in 7 to 9 percent of infected patients; bronchiolitis and pneumonia affect 1 to 6 percent. A severe form of hepatitis may also occur. In a recent report by Atmar and associates, 7 of 13 (54 percent) pregnant women with measles developed hepatitis.[70]

Encephalitis occurs in approximately one in a thousand cases of measles. It results from both viral infection of the central nervous system and a hypersensitivity reaction to the systemic viral infection. Measles encephalitis may result in permanent neurologic impairment, including mental retardation; the mortality rate from this complication is approximately 15 to 33 percent.[69,71,72] Another unusual but extremely serious complication of measles is subacute sclerosing panencephalitis (SSPE). This complication occurs in 0.5 to 2 per 1000 cases. The manifestations of SSPE typically develop approximately 7 years after the acute measles infection and the condition is more common in children who had measles before the age of 2. It is characterized by progressive neurologic debilitation and a virtually uniformly fatal outcome.

A final complication is an unusual condition, termed *atypical measles.* This disorder is a severe form of measles reinfection that affects young adults previously vaccinated with the formalin-inactivated killed measles vaccine that was distributed in the United States from 1963 to 1967. Affected patients have extremely high antibody titers to measles. They typically experience high fever, pneumonitis, pleural effusion, and a coarse, maculopapular, hemorrhagic or urticarial rash. Although the disease is usually self-limited, atypical measles can lead to hepatic, cardiac, and renal failure. Interestingly, affected patients are not contagious to others.

DIAGNOSIS

Five clinical criteria should be present to establish the diagnosis of measles: fever $\geq 38.3°C$ (100.9°F), characteristic rash lasting more than 3 days, cough, coryza, and conjunctivitis. Although the virus can be cultured, the mainstay of diagnostic tests is detection of virus-specific antibody.[21,66,69] The confirmation of acute measles virus infection is based upon detection of IgM-specific antibody or a fourfold change in the IgG titer in acute and convalescent sera. The acute titer for IgG antibody should be obtained within 3 days of the onset of the rash and the convalescent titer, 10 to 20 days later.

The differential diagnosis of measles is lengthy. A variety of other infections must be considered, including rubella, scarlet fever, Rocky Mountain spotted fever, toxoplasmosis, enterovirus infection, mononucleosis, meningococcemia, and serum sickness.

COMPLICATIONS OF MEASLES DURING PREGNANCY

Several reports have described an increase in maternal mortality associated with measles infection during pregnancy. Most fatalities have been due to pulmonary complications. In one of the earliest reports, Christensen et al.[73] described a serious epidemic of measles in Greenland in 1951. Of 83 pregnant women, 4 (4.8%) who developed measles died. An unspecified number of these women also had active tuberculosis. In the report by Atmar et al.,[70] 1 of 13 pregnant women (8 percent) with measles died because of severe respiratory infection. In another recent report, Eberhart-Phillips and coworkers[74] evaluated 58 pregnant women with measles: 35 (60 percent) required hospitalization, 15 (26 percent) developed pneumonia, and 2 (3 percent) died.

Measles infection in pregnancy is associated with an increased risk of spontaneous abortion and preterm delivery. The frequency of congenital anomalies is not significantly increased. However, infants of mothers who are acutely infected at the time of delivery are at risk for neonatal measles. This infection typically develops within the first 10 days of life and results from transplacental viral dissemination. In some reports, the mortality in preterm and term infants with neonatal measles has been as high as 60 percent and 20 percent, respectively.[70,74,75] However, these alarmingly high mortality figures were published prior to the era of skilled neonatal intensive care and the availability of broad-spectrum antibiotics for treatment of secondary bacterial infections.

MANAGEMENT

Pregnant women with measles should be referred to an obstetrician-gynecologist and observed carefully for evidence of serious complications such as otitis media, hepatitis, encephalitis, and pneumonia. Secondary bacterial infections should be treated promptly with antibiotics. Administration of aerosolized ribavirin may be of benefit in patients with severe viral pneumonitis.[66] The affected patient should be counseled that the risk of injury to her fetus is very low. The most effective method for evaluating the fetus for infection in utero is detailed ultrasound examination. Findings suggestive of infection in utero include microcephaly, growth restriction, and oligohydramnios. Neonates delivered to a mother who has developed measles within 7 to 10 days of delivery should receive intramuscular immune globulin in a dose of 0.25 mg/kg. These infants should subsequently receive the live measles vaccine when they are 15 months of age.[71]

All children should receive measles vaccine when they are 15 months of age. The immunization should be administered as part of the trivalent measles-mumps-rubella (MMR) vaccine. The appropriate initial dose for young children is 0.5 mL subcutaneously. The original public health recommendations provided for only a single dose of measles vaccine. However, recent outbreaks of measles have occurred in individuals who received only one dose of the vaccine. Accordingly, the CDC now recommends that all individuals who have not been infected with the wild measles virus receive a second dose of vaccine. Children who receive their first dose at age 15 months should receive a second dose at 4 to 6 years of age. Children who are vaccinated with the live vaccine before their first birthday should be considered unvaccinated and should receive the full two-dose series. Individuals who received *further attenuated vaccine,* accompanied by immune globulin or measles immune globulin, should be considered unvaccinated and receive two doses of the vaccine. Individuals who were given the inactivated vaccine during the period 1963–1967 are at risk for developing severe atypical measles syndrome if they are exposed to the natural virus. Accordingly, these individuals also should receive two doses of the live vaccine. Women of reproductive age who have only one documented measles vaccination are also candidates for a second immunization. The seroconversion rate with the new live virus vaccine is ≥95 percent.[69,71]

There are three specific contraindications to vaccination: pregnancy, severe febrile illness, and history of anaphylactic reaction to egg protein or neomycin. The vaccine should not be given for 3 months after a person has received immune globulin, whole blood, or other antibody-containing blood products. However, the vaccine can be administered concurrently with Rh-immune globulin in the immediate postpartum period. Although no cases of congenital infection have been described as a result of treatment with the measles vaccine, patients receiving the vaccine should use effective contraception for 3 months following inoculation.[71]

Few adverse effects are associated with measles vaccination. Approximately 5 to 15 percent of vaccinees develop a low-grade fever; 5 percent or less develop a rash. Less than 1 percent have febrile seizures, and less than one per million develop encephalitis.

When an outbreak of measles occurs, susceptible individuals should be targeted for postexposure prophylaxis. If they are not pregnant, they should receive the live measles vaccine within 72 h of exposure. They also should receive immune globulin within 6 days of exposure. The appropriate dose of immune globulin is 0.25 mL/kg for immunocompetent patients and 0.5 mL/kg for immunocompromised individuals. The maximum dose of the immune globulin preparation is 15 mL. Pregnant patients should receive only immune globulin.[69,71]

TOXOPLASMOSIS

EPIDEMIOLOGY

Although a protozoal rather than a viral infection, toxoplasmosis is usually considered within the category of serious perinatal infections; accordingly, it is reviewed here. *Toxoplasma gondii* has three distinct forms: trophozoite, cyst, and oocyst. The life cycle of *T. gondii* is dependent upon wild and domestic cats, which are the only host for the oocyst. The oocyst is formed in the cat intestine and subsequently excreted in the feces. Mammals, such as cows, then ingest the oocyst, which is disrupted in the animal's intestine, releasing the invasive trophozoite. The trophozoite is then disseminated throughout the body, ultimately forming cysts in the brain and muscle.

Human infection occurs when infected meat is ingested or when food is contaminated by cat feces—e.g., via flies, cockroaches, or fingers. Infection rates are highest in areas of poor sanitation and crowded living conditions. Stray and domestic cats that eat raw meat are most likely to carry the parasite. The cyst is destroyed by heat, and the practice of eating rare or raw meat in France may explain the high prevalence of infection in that country.[76]

Approximately 40 to 50 percent of adults in the United States have antibody to *T. gondii,* and the prevalence of antibody is highest in lower socioeconomic populations. The frequency of seroconversion during pregnancy is ≤5 percent, and approximately 3 in 1000 infants show evidence of congenital infection. Clinically significant congenital toxoplasmosis occurs in approximately 1 in 8000 pregnancies. Toxoplasmosis is more common in western Europe, particularly France.[76,77]

CLINICAL MANIFESTATIONS

The ingested organism invades across the intestinal epithelium and spreads hematogenously throughout the body. Intracellular replication leads to cell destruction. Clinical manifestations of infection are the result of direct organ damage and the subsequent immunologic response to parasitemia and cell death. Host immunity is mediated primarily through T lymphocytes.

Most infections in humans are asymptomatic. Even in the absence of symptoms, however, patients may have evidence of multiorgan involvement, and clinical disease can follow a long period of asymptomatic infection. Symptomatic toxoplasmosis usually presents as an illness similar to mononucleosis.[76,77]

In contrast to infection in the immunocompetent host, toxoplasmosis can be a devastating infection in the immunosuppressed patient. Because immunity to *T. gondii* is cell-mediated, patients with HIV infection and those treated with chronic immunosuppressive therapy after organ transplantation are particularly susceptible to new or reactivated infection. In these patients, central nervous system dysfunction is the most common manifestation of infection. Findings typically include encephalitis, meningoencephalitis, and intracerebral mass lesions. Pneumonitis, myocarditis, and generalized lymphadenopathy also occur commonly.[76,77]

DIAGNOSIS

The diagnosis of toxoplasmosis can be confirmed by serologic and histologic methods. Serologic tests suggestive of an acute infection include detection of IgM-specific antibody, demonstration of an extremely high IgG antibody titer, and documentation of IgG seroconversion from negative to positive.[76,77] Clinicians should be aware that serologic assays for toxoplasmosis are not well standardized. When initial laboratory tests appear to indicate that an acute infection has occurred, repeat serology should be performed in a well-recognized reference laboratory (such as that established by Dr. Jack Remington at Stanford University).

The best tissue for identification of *T. gondii* is a lymph node or brain biopsy specimen. Histologic preparations can be examined by light and electron microscopy. For light microscopy, specimens should be stained with either Giemsa or Wright stain.[76–79]

CONGENITAL INFECTION

Congenital infection can occur if a woman develops *acute* toxoplasmosis during pregnancy. Chronic or latent infection is unlikely to cause fetal injury except perhaps in an immunosuppressed patient. Approximately 40 percent of neonates born to mothers with acute toxoplasmosis show evidence of infection. Congenital infection is most likely to occur when maternal infection develops in the third trimester. Less than half of the affected infants are symptomatic at birth. The clinical manifestations of congenital toxoplasmosis are quite varied and include a maculopapular rash, fever, hepatosplenomegaly, ascites, chorioretinitis, uveitis, seizures, and ventriculomegaly.[70–73]

The most valuable tests for antenatal diagnosis of congenital toxoplasmosis are ultrasound and amniocentesis. Ultrasound findings suggestive of infection include ventriculomegaly, intracranial calcifications, microcephaly, ascites, hepatosplenomegaly, and growth restriction. Hohlfeld et al.[80] have now identified a specific gene of *T. gondii* in amniotic fluid using a PCR test. In their investigation, 34 of 339 infants had congenital toxoplasmosis confirmed by serologic testing or autopsy. All amniotic fluid samples from affected pregnancies were positive by PCR. Test results were available within 1 day of specimen collection.

MANAGEMENT

Toxoplasmosis in the immunocompetent adult is usually an asymptomatic or self-limited illness and does not require treatment. Immunocompromised patients, however, should be treated, and the regimen of choice is a combination of oral sulfadiazine (4-g loading dose, then 1 g four times daily) plus pyrimethamine (50 to 100 mg initially, then 25 mg daily). In such patients, extended courses of treatment may be necessary to cure the infection.

Treatment is also indicated when acute toxoplasmosis occurs during pregnancy. Treatment of the mother reduces the risk of congenital infection and decreases the late sequelae of infection.[72,73] Pyrimethamine is not recommended for use during the first trimester of pregnancy because of possible teratogenicity. Sulfonamides can be used alone, but single-agent therapy appears to be less effective than combination therapy. In Europe, spiramycin has been used extensively in pregnancy with excellent results.[78,79] It is available for treatment in the United States through the CDC.

Aggressive early treatment of infants with congenital toxoplasmosis is indicated and consists of combination therapy with pyrimethamine, sulfadiazine, and leucovorin for 1 year.[81] Early treatment reduces but does not eliminate the late sequelae of toxoplasmosis, such as chorioretinitis.

In the management of the pregnant patient, *prevention* of acute toxoplasmosis is of paramount importance. Pregnant women should be advised to avoid contact with stray cats and cat litter. They should always wash their hands after preparing meat for cooking and should never eat raw or rare meat. Fruits and vegetables should also be washed carefully to remove possible contamination by oocysts. Management of acute toxoplasmosis during pregnancy should occur in consultation with an obstetrician.

VARICELLA

EPIDEMIOLOGY

The varicella zoster (VZ) virus is a DNA herpesvirus. Humans are the only known source of infection. Natural varicella infection occurs primarily during early childhood. Less than 10 percent of cases occur in individuals greater than 10 years of age; however, older patients account for more than 50 percent of all fatalities due to varicella. Varicella is transmitted by direct contact and respiratory droplets. The virus is highly infectious, and approximately 95 percent of susceptible household contacts become infected following exposure. The incubation period is 10 to 14 days. Patients are infectious from 1 day before the outbreak of the rash until all of the cutaneous lesions have dried and crusted over. Immunity to varicella is usually lifelong.[82]

Herpes zoster infection occurs as a result of reactivation of latent virus infection in a patient who has already had varicella. Because of the presence in the host of virus-specific antibody, herpes zoster is usually a much less serious disorder than varicella and rarely poses a major risk to either the mother or her baby unless the former is immunocompromised. However, susceptible patients may develop acute varicella when exposed to individuals with herpes zoster; therefore, they must be counseled appropriately about this risk.[82]

CLINICAL MANIFESTATIONS

The usual clinical manifestations of varicella are fever, malaise, and a skin rash. The characteristic skin lesions usually begin as pruritic macules which appear in crops. The macules progress to papules, then to vesicles, and finally to crusts. The lesions initially appear on the face and trunk and then spread centripetally to the extremities (Fig. 23-4).

In immunocompetent children serious complications of varicella are exceedingly rare. However, in adults, two life-threatening sequelae may develop; encephalitis and pneumonia. The former occurs in ≤ 1 percent of pregnant women; the latter may develop in up to 20% of patients. Prior to the development of acyclovir, the mortality associated with varicella pneumonia in pregnancy approached 40 percent.[82,83]

DIAGNOSIS

The diagnosis of varicella is usually made by clinical examination alone. In problematic cases, the virus can be isolated in tissue culture, and cytologic preparations may show multinucleated giant cells and eosinophilic intranuclear inclusions. Serologic assays are of primary value in assessing a patient's susceptibility to varicella immediately following exposure. The two most useful antibody assays are the fluorescent antimembrane antibody test (FAMA) and ELISA.

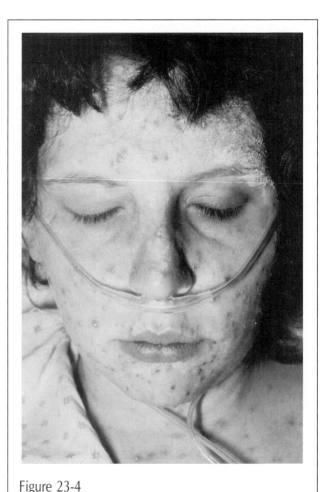

Figure 23-4

Characteristic disseminated vesicular eruption of varicella.

Both assays show sustained elevations, usually lifelong, following natural infection.[82,84]

MANAGEMENT OF MATERNAL INFECTION

The optimal approach to maternal varicella infection is *prevention*. All women of reproductive age should be assessed for immunity to varicella, ideally before they become pregnant. A patient who does not have a clear, positive history of prior infection should have a varicella serology to determine if she is immune or susceptible. Susceptible patients, particularly those who are likely to be exposed to varicella either at home or in the workplace, should be offered the new varicella vaccine. Varivax (Merck) is a live attenuated vaccine, and it is approximately 70 to 80 percent effective in protecting the patient against natural infection. Individuals more than 12 years of age should receive two subcutaneous doses of the vaccine 4 to 8 weeks apart. Vaccine recipients should use effective contraception for 3 months after immunization. The vaccine can be administered simultaneously with the measles-mumps-rubella (MMR) immunization, but it should not be given in conjunction with blood or blood products. In addition, the vaccine is contraindicated in patients who are pregnant, who have immunodeficiency disorders, or who have received high-dose systemic glucocorticoids within 30 days of vaccination.[85]

The most common situation that the clinician encounters is a pregnant patient who has been exposed acutely to an individual who "may have had chickenpox." The first step in the approach to this situation is to verify that the index patient actually has varicella. If infection is confirmed, the pregnant woman should then be questioned about immunity to varicella. If immunity cannot be documented by history, an IgG varicella serology should be obtained and the result reviewed within 24 to 48 h of exposure. If the serology is positive, the patient can be reassured that her fetus is not at risk. If the serology is negative, the patient should receive varicella zoster immune globulin (VZIG). This preparation is 60 to 80 percent effective in preventing infection if given within 96 h of exposure. The dose of VZIG is one vial (125 U) per 10 kg of actual body weight, up to a maximum of five vials. In problematic cases, if waiting for the varicella serology will delay administration of VZIG for more than 96 h after exposure, the immunization should be given without confirmatory serology.[82,86,87]

Patients who receive VZIG, as well as those who present for care too late for passive immunoprophylaxis, should be counseled about the clinical signs and symptoms of varicella. In particular, they must be advised to report immediately if early manifestations of varicella encephalitis or pneumonia develop. If serious sequelae occur, the patient should be referred to an obstetrician-gynecologist and/or infectious diseases specialist and admitted to the hospital for intravenous therapy with acyclovir. The recommended dose of acyclovir is 500 mg/m^2 every 8 h, and treatment should be continued until the patient's systemic symptoms have resolved and the cutaneous lesions have begun to crust. Immunocompromised patients should be treated with acyclovir immediately at the onset of clinical illness because they are at such increased risk for serious complications.[82,83]

CONGENITAL INFECTION

Congenital varicella results primarily from hematogenous dissemination of virus across the placenta. Ascending infection following rupture of membranes is possible but extremely unlikely. Congenital infection may lead to spontaneous abortion, intrauterine fetal demise, and varicella embryopathy. The latter disorder is manifest by multiple abnormalities such as cutaneous scars, limb hypoplasia, muscle atrophy, malformed digits, psychomotor retardation, microcephaly, cortical atrophy, cataracts, chorioretinitis, and microophthalmia.[82]

Fortunately, two recent investigations have demonstrated a relatively low frequency of anomalies even following exposure in the first half of pregnancy. Pastuszak et al.[88] reported a study of 106 women with varicella in the first 20 weeks of gestation. The frequency of varicella embryopathy was 1.2 percent, and the prevalence of preterm birth was 14 percent. Subsequently, Enders and coworkers[89] published the largest prospective study of varicella in pregnancy. They observed a 2 percent incidence of congenital infection when maternal varicella occurred at 13 to 20 weeks' gestation. The frequency of congenital infection was only 0.4 percent when maternal infection occurred before 13 weeks' gestation.

Although varicella virus can be isolated from amniotic fluid and placental tissue, the best test to detect congenital varicella is ultrasound. Sonographic findings suggestive of fetal varicella include polyhydramnios; hydrops; hyperechogenic foci in the abdominal organs, particularly the liver; cardiac malformations; limb deformities; microcephaly; and intrauterine growth restriction.[82]

NEONATAL INFECTION

The final major complication of varicella infection in pregnancy is neonatal varicella. Infection of the neonate occurs in 10 to 20 percent of infants whose mothers have acute varicella within the period from 5 days before to 2 days after delivery.[82] Infection usually results from hematogenous dissemination of virus across the placenta at a time when no maternal antibody is present to provide passive immunity to the fetus. Less commonly, neonatal varicella results from postnatal exposure to the mother or another infected person.

The clinical course of neonatal varicella can be variable in progression and severity. The infant usually becomes symptomatic within 5 to 10 days of delivery. Some neonates have only scattered skin lesions and no systemic signs of illness. Others have a biphasic course, initially presenting with a cluster of skin lesions, followed by more widespread dissemination. Still others have a more severe acute illness associated with extensive cutaneous lesions and visceral infection. The most common life-threatening complication is pneumonia. In reports published before the widespread availability of acyclovir, the mortality associated with neonatal varicella was 20 to 30 percent.[82]

To prevent neonatal varicella, an effort should be made to delay delivery until 5 to 7 days after the onset of maternal illness. If delay is not possible, the neonate should receive VZIG (one vial, 125 U) immediately after birth. An important additional preventive measure is isolation of the infant from the mother until all vesicular lesions likely to come in contact with the infant have crusted over.[82,87]

Occasionally herpes zoster is present in the newborn. This condition is usually a manifestation of intrauterine varicella that occurs in the second half of pregnancy. The clinical course is typically benign, but in rare instances encephalitis has been documented. Intravenous acyclovir is indicated for treatment of severe herpes zoster infection in the neonate.

References

1. Betts RF: Cytomegalovirus infection epidemiology and biology in adults. *Semin Perinatol* 7:22, 1983.
2. Wilhelm JA, Malter L, Schopfer K: The risk of transmitting cytomegalovirus to patients receiving blood transfusions. *J Infect Dis* 154:169, 1986.
3. Stagno S, Pass RF, Dworsky ME, Alford CA: Congenital and perinatal cytomegalovirus infections. *Semin Perinatol* 7:31, 1983.
4. Pass RF, August AM, Dworsky M, Reynolds DW: Cytomegalovirus infection in a day care center. *N Engl J Med* 307:477, 1982.
5. Jones LA, Duke-Duncan PM, Yeager AS: Cytomegalovirus infections in infant-toddler centers: Centers for the developmentally delayed versus regular day care. *J Infect Dis* 151:953, 1985.
6. Hutto C, Little EA, Ricks R, et al: Isolation of cytomegalovirus from toys and hands in a day care center. *J Infect Dis* 154:527, 1986.
7. Adler SP: Cytomegalovirus and child day care. *N Engl J Med* 321:1290, 1989.
8. Demmler GJ, Schydlower M, Lampe RM: Texas, teenagers, and CMV. *J Infect Dis* 152:1350, 1985.
9. Chandler SH, Alexander ER, Holmes KK: Epidemiology of cytomegaloviral infection in a heterogeneous population of pregnant women. *J Infect Dis* 152:249, 1985.
10. Hohlfeld P, Vial Y, Maillard-Brignon C, et al: Cytomegalovirus fetal infection: Prenatal diagnosis. *Obstet Gynecol* 78:615, 1991.
11. Donner C, Liesnard C, Content J, et al: Prenatal diagnosis of 52 pregnancies at risk for congenital cytomegalovirus infection. *Obstet Gynecol* 82:481, 1993.
12. Adler SP: Cytomegalovirus and pregnancy. *Curr Opin Obstet Gynecol* 4:670, 1992.
13. Kumar ML, Prokay SL: Experimental primary cytomegalovirus infection in pregnancy: Timing and fetal outcome. *Am J Obstet Gynecol* 145:56, 1983.
14. Stagno S, Pass RF, Dworsky ME, et al: Congenital cytomegalovirus infection. *N Engl J Med* 306:945, 1982.
15. Fowler KB, Stagno S, Pass RF, et al: The outcome of congenital cytomegalovirus infection in relation to maternal antibody status. *N Engl J Med* 326:663, 1992.
16. Dobbins JG, Stewart JA, Demmler GJ: Surveillance of congenital cytomegalovirus disease, 1990–91. *MMWR* 41:35, 1992.
17. Reynolds DW, Stagno S, Hosty TS, et al: Maternal cytomegalovirus excretion and perinatal infection. *N Engl J Med* 289:1, 1973.
18. Stagno S, Reynolds DW, Huang ES, et al: Congenital cytomegalovirus infection. *N Engl J Med* 296:1254, 1977.
19. Katznelson S, Drew WL, Mintz L: Efficacy of the condom as a barrier to the transmission of cytomegalovirus. *J Infect Dis* 150:155, 1984.
20. Shapiro CN, Coleman PJ, McQuillan GM, et al: Epidemiology of hepatitis A: Seroepidemiology and risk groups in the USA. *Vaccine* 10(suppl 1):S59, 1992.
21. Centers for Disease Control: Hepatitis A among drug abusers. *MMWR* 37:297, 1988.
22. Centers for Disease Control: Hepatitis A among homosexual men—United States, Canada, and Australia. *MMWR* 41:155, 1992.
23. American College of Obstetricians and Gynecologists: *Hepatitis in Pregnancy.* ACOG Technical Bulletin no. 174. Washington, DC: ACOG, 1992, p 1.
24. Centers for Disease Control: Protection against viral hepatitis: Recommendations of the Immunization Practices Advisory Committee. *MMWR* 39(RR-2):1, 1990.
25. Werzberger A, Mensch B, Kuter B, et al: A controlled trial of a formalin-inactivated hepatitis: A vaccine in healthy children. *N Engl J Med* 327:453, 1992.
26. Syndman DR: Hepatitis in pregnancy. *N Engl J Med* 313:1398, 1985.
27. Hoofnagle JH: Chronic hepatitis B. *N Engl J Med* 323:337, 1990.
28. Sweet RL: Hepatitis B infection in pregnancy. *Obstet Gynecol Rep* 2:128, 1990.
29. Centers for Disease Control: Hepatitis B virus: A comprehensive strategy for eliminating transmission in the United States through universal vaccination: Recommendations of the Immunization Practices Advisory Committee (ACIP). *MMWR* 40:1, 1991.
30. Jagger J, Hunt EH, Brand-Elnaggar J, et al: Rates of needle-stick injury caused by various devices in a university hospital. *N Engl J Med* 319:284, 1988.
31. Lynch-Salamon DI, Combs CA: Hepatitis C in obstetrics and gynecology. *Obstet Gynecol* 79:621, 1992.
32. Osmond DH, Padian NS, Sheppard WH, et al: Risk factors for hepatitis C virus positivity in heterosexual couples. *JAMA* 269:361, 1993.

33. Bohman VR, Stettler RW, Little BB, et al: Seroprevalence and risk factors for hepatitis C virus antibody in pregnant women. *Obstet Gynecol* 80:609, 1992.

34. Chauhan A, Jameel S, Chawla YK, et al: Common aetiological agent for epidemic and sporadic non-A, non-B hepatitis. *Lancet* 339:1509, 1992.

35. Bradley DW, Maynard JE: Etiology and natural history of post-transfusion and enterically transmitted non-A, non-B hepatitis. *Semin Liver Dis* 6:56, 1986.

36. Velazquez O, Stetler HC, Avila C, et al: Epidemic transmission of enterically transmitted non-A, non-B hepatitis in Mexico, 1986–1987. *JAMA* 263:3281, 1990.

37. Wong DC, Purcell RH, Sreenivasan MA, et al: Epidemic and endemic hepatitis in India: Evidence for a non-A, non-B hepatitis virus aetiology. *Lancet* 2:876, 1980.

38. Thomas DL, Mahley RW, Badur S, et al: Epidemiology of hepatitis E virus infection in Turkey. *Lancet* 341:1561, 1993.

39. Centers for Disease Control: Hepatitis E among U.S. travelers, 1989–1992. *MMWR* 42:1, 1993.

40. Favorov MO, Fields HA, Purdy MA, et al: Serologic identification of hepatitis E virus infections in epidemic and endemic settings. *J Med Virol* 36:246, 1992.

41. Rizzetto M: The delta agent. *Hepatology* 3:729, 1983.

42. Hoofnagle JH: Type D (delta) hepatitis. *JAMA* 261:1321, 1989. [Erratum to *JAMA* 261:3552, 1989.]

43. Jacobson IM, Dienstag JL, Werner BG, et al: Epidemiology and clinical impact of hepatitis D virus (delta) infection. *Hepatology* 5:188, 1985.

44. Cook CR, Gall SA: Herpes in pregnancy. *Infect Dis Obstet Gynecol* 1:298, 1994.

45. American College of Obstetricians and Gynecologists: *Herpes Simplex Virus Infection.* ACOG Technical Bulletin no. 102. Washington, DC: ACOG, March 1987.

46. Stone KM, Brooks CA, Guinan ME, Alexander ER: National surveillance for neonatal herpes simplex virus infections. *Sex Transm Dis* 16:152, 1989.

47. Prober CG, Sullender WM, Yasukawa LL, et al: Low risk of herpes simplex virus infections in neonates exposed to the virus at the time of vaginal delivery to mothers with recurrent genital herpes simplex virus infections. *N Engl J Med* 316:240, 1987.

48. Gibbs RS, Amstey MS, Sweet RL, et al: Management of genital herpes infection in pregnancy. *Obstet Gynecol* 71:779, 1988.

49. Gibbs RS, Mead PB: Preventing neonatal herpes—Current strategies. *N Engl J Med* 326:946, 1992.

50. Kulhanjian JA, Soroush V, Au DS, et al: Identification of women at unsuspected risk of primary infection with herpes simplex virus type 2 during pregnancy. *N Engl J Med* 326:916, 1992.

51. Arvin AM, Hensleigh PA, Prober CG, et al: Failure of antepartum maternal cultures to predict the infant's risk of exposure to herpes simplex virus at delivery. *N Engl J Med* 315:796, 1986.

52. Brown ZA, Baker DA: Acyclovir therapy during pregnancy. *Obstet Gynecol* 73:526, 1989.

53. Centers for Disease Control: Pregnancy outcomes following systemic prenatal acyclovir exposure—June 1, 1984–June 30, 1993. *MMWR* 42:806, 1993.

54. Whitley RJ, Gramm JW: Acyclovir: A decade later. *N Engl J Med* 327:782, 1992.

55. Kumar ML: Human parvovirus B_{19} and its associated diseases. *Clin Perinatol* 18:209, 1991.

56. Thurn J: Human parvovirus B_{19}: Historical and clinical review. *Rev Infect Dis* 10:1005, 1988.

57. Centers for Disease Control: Risks associated with human parvovirus B_{19} infection. *MMWR* 38:81, 1989.

58. Conry JA, Torok T, Andrews I: Perinatal encephalopathy secondary to in utero human parvovirus B-19 (HPV) infection (abstr). *Neurology* 43:A346, 1993.

59. Brown KE, Green SW, deMayolo JA, et al: Congenital anaemia after transplacental B_{19} parvovirus infection. *Lancet* 343:895, 1994.

60. Sahakian V, Weiner CP, Naides SJ, et al: Intrauterine transfusion treatment of nonimmune hydrops fetalis secondary to human parvovirus B_{19} infection. *Am J Obstet Gynecol* 164:1090, 1991.

61. Centers for Disease Control: Rubella prevention: Recommendations of the immunization practices advisory committee (ACIP). *MMWR* 39:1, 1990.

62. American College of Obstetricians and Gynecologists: *Rubella and Pregnancy.* ACOG Technical Bulletin no. 171. Washington, DC: ACOG, August 1992.

63. Sautter RL, Crist AE, Johnson LM, LeBar WD: Comparison of five methods for the determination of rubella immunity. *Infect Dis Obstet Gynecol* 1:188, 1994.

64. Centers for Disease Control: Rubella and congenital rubella syndrome—United States, January 1, 1991–May 7, 1994. *MMWR* 43:391, 1994.

65. Miller E, Cradock-Watson JE, Pollock TM: Consequences of confirmed maternal rubella at successive stages of pregnancy. *Lancet* 2:781, 1982.

66. Munro ND, Smithells RW, Sheppard S, et al: Temporal relations between maternal rubella and congenital defects. *Lancet* 2:201, 1987.

67. McIntosh EDG, Menser MA: A fifty-year follow-up of congenital rubella. *Lancet* 340:414, 1992.

68. Bart SW, Stetler HC, Preblud SR, et al: Fetal risk associated with rubella vaccine: An update. *Rev Infect Dis* 7:S95, 1985.

69. National Vaccine Advisory Committee: The measles epidemic: The problems, barriers, and recommendations. *JAMA* 266:1547, 1991.

70. Atmar RL, Englund JA, Hammill H: Complications of measles during pregnancy. *Clin Infect Dis* 14:217, 1992.

71. Centers for Disease Control: Measles prevention: Recommendations of the Immunization Practices Advisory Committee (ACIP). *MMWR* 38:1, 1989.

72. Atkinson WL, Hadler SC, Redd SB, Orenstein WA:

Measles surveillance—United States, 1991. *MMWR* 41:1, 1992.

73. Christensen PE, Schmidt H, Bang HO, et al: An epidemic of measles in Southern Greenland, 1951. *Acta Med Scand* 144:430, 1953.

74. Eberhart-Phillips JE, Frederick PD, Baron RC, Mascola L: Measles in pregnancy: A descriptive study of 58 cases. *Obstet Gynecol* 82:797, 1993.

75. Stein SJ, Greenspoon JS: Rubeola during pregnancy. *Obstet Gynecol* 78:925, 1991.

76. Krick JA, Remington JS: Toxoplasmosis in the adult—An overview. *N Engl J Med* 298:550, 1978.

77. Sever J: The dangers of toxoplasmosis in pregnancy. *Contemp Obstet Gynecol* 10:29, 1977.

78. Daffos F: Prenatal management of 746 pregnancies at risk for congenital toxoplasmosis. *N Engl J Med* 318:271, 1988.

79. Desmonts G, Couvreur J: Congenital toxoplasmosis: A prospective study of 378 pregnancies. *N Engl J Med* 290:1110, 1974.

80. Hohlfeld P, Daffos F, Costa JM, et al: Prenatal diagnosis of congenital toxoplasmosis with a polymerase-chain reaction test on amniotic fluid. *N Engl J Med* 331:695, 1994.

81. Guerina NG, Hsu HW, Meissner HC, et al: Neonatal serologic screening and early treatment for congenital *Toxoplasma gondii* infection. *N Engl J Med* 330:1858, 1994.

82. Chapman S, Duff P: Varicella in pregnancy. *Semin Perinatol* 17:403, 1993.

83. Smego R, Asperilla MO: Use of acyclovir for varicella pneumonia during pregnancy. *Obstet Gynecol* 78:1112, 1991.

84. McGregor JA, Mark S, Crawford GP, Levin MJ: Varicella zoster antibody testing in the care of pregnant women exposed to varicella. *Am J Obstet Gynecol* 157:281, 1987.

85. Varicella vaccine. *Med Lett* 37:55, 1995.

86. Duff P: Varicella in pregnancy: Five priorities for clinicians. *Infect Dis Obstet Gynecol* 1:163, 1994.

87. Centers for Disease Control: Varicella-zoster immune globulin for the prevention of chickenpox. *MMWR* 33:83, 1984.

88. Pastuszak AL, Levy M, Schick B, et al: Outcome after maternal varicella infection in the first 20 weeks of pregnancy. *N Engl J Med* 330:901, 1994.

89. Enders G, Miller E, Cradock-Watson J, et al: Consequences of varicella and herpes zoster in pregnancy: Prospective study of 1739 cases. *Lancet* 343:1547, 1994.

Chapter 24

URINARY INFECTIONS DURING PREGNANCY

F. Gary Cunningham

Infections of the urinary tract are the most common bacterial infections encountered during pregnancy. Although *asymptomatic bacteriuria* is more common, symptomatic infection may involve the lower tract to cause *cystitis,* or it may involve the renal calyces, pelvis, and parenchyma to cause *pyelonephritis.* Urinary tract dilation is one of the most significant anatomic alterations induced by pregnancy. It involves dilatation of the renal calyces and pelves as well as the ureters. These changes, which are more prominent on the right side, are secondary to both hormonal and mechanical obstructive factors. The latter create urinary stasis and may lead to serious upper urinary tract infections. Another factor predisposing to infection is increased vesicoureteral reflux. These normal changes associated with pregnancy may also lead to erroneous interpretation of studies done to evaluate suspected pathologic obstruction.

Organisms that cause urinary tract infections are those from the normal perineal flora. There are unique strains of *Escherichia coli* with pili that enhance their virulence.[1] Also called *adhesins* or *P-fimbriae,* these appendages allow bacterial attachment to glycoprotein receptors on uroepithelial cell membranes (Fig. 24-1). Although pregnancy *per se* does not seem to enhance these virulence factors, urinary stasis apparently does; along with vesicoureteral reflux, stasis predisposes to symptomatic upper urinary tract infections. In addition, Hart and colleagues[2] have shown that some strains of uropathogenic *E coli* predominate in causing acute infection in pregnant women. These strains include serotypes O6, O15, and O75.

In the early puerperium, bladder sensitivity to intravesicular fluid tension is often decreased as the consequence of the trauma of labor as well as analgesia, especially epidural or spinal blockade. Sensations of bladder distention are also probably diminished by discomfort caused by a large episiotomy, periurethral lacerations, or vaginal wall hematomas. Following delivery, there is frequently a diuresis with copious urine production and bladder distention. Overdistention, coupled with catheterization to provide relief, commonly leads to urinary infection in the early postpartum period.

ASYMPTOMATIC BACTERIURIA

Asymptomatic or covert bacteriuria involves persistent, actively multiplying bacteria within the urinary tract in the absence of symptoms. The reported prevalence of bacteriuria during pregnancy varies from 2 to 7 percent and depends on parity, race, and socioeconomic status. The highest incidence has been reported in African American multiparas with sickle cell trait, and the lowest incidence has been found in affluent white women of low parity.

Bacteriuria during pregnancy typically is present at the time of the first prenatal visit; after an initial negative urine culture, 1 percent or less of women develop urinary infection.[3] A clean-voided specimen containing more than 100,000 organisms of a single uropathogen per milliliter is considered evidence of infection. Although smaller numbers of bacteria may represent contamination, lower colony counts may sometimes represent active infection, especially in the presence of symptoms. Thus, it seems prudent to treat lower concentrations of known pathogens because pyelonephritis may occur with counts of only 20,000 to 50,000 per milliliter.

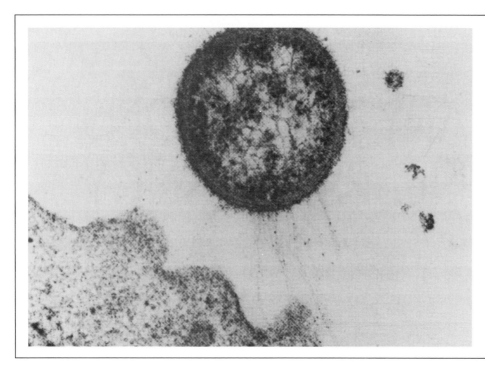

Figure 24-1

Transmission electron microscopy shows fimbriated *E. coli* adhering to transitional cell (original ×180,000). (From Roberts,[37] with permission.)

SIGNIFICANCE

If asymptomatic bacteriuria is not treated, one-fourth of infected women subsequently develop acute symptomatic infection during that pregnancy. Eradication of bacteriuria with antimicrobial agents prevents most of these clinically evident infections. For example, Gratacos and associates[4] reported a decreased incidence of pyelonephritis from 1.8 to 0.6 percent in their population following the introduction of a screening and treatment program for asymptomatic bacteriuria. Although it is reasonable to perform routine screening for bacteriuria in women at high-risk, screening via urine culture may not be cost effective when the population prevalence is low. Less expensive tests such as the leukocyte esterase-nitrite dipstick have been shown to be cost effective with prevalences of 2 percent.[5] Another approach for the low-risk population is to perform screening cultures selected by historical factors.

Although Romero and colleagues[6] concluded from a meta-analysis that covert bacteriuria was associated with preterm delivery and low-birth-weight infants, they were unable to address the effects of prevention of acute pyelonephritis on preterm labor and delivery. From evidence currently available, it seems unlikely that bacteriuria exclusive of pyelonephritis is a prominent factor in the genesis of low-birth-weight or preterm infants. Bacteriuria has been linked to an increased incidence of pregnancy-induced hypertension and anemia. Utilizing a multivariate analysis for a perinatal registry cohort of 25,746 mother-infant pairs, Schieve and colleagues[7] reported increased risks for low-birth-weight, preterm delivery, hypertension or preeclampsia, and maternal anemia. These findings are at variance with those of Gilstrap and colleagues,[8] who compared pregnancy outcomes in 248 pregnant women in whom they localized asymptomatic infection to the bladder or kidney. They found no association of bacteriuria with anemia, pregnancy-induced hypertension, or low-birth-weight infants from growth restriction or preterm delivery.

Bacteriuria persists after delivery in many women, and a significant number of these also have pyelographic evidence of chronic infection, obstructive lesions, or congenital urinary abnormalities.[9,10]

TREATMENT

Any one of several antimicrobial regimens is effective for asymptomatic bacteriuria during pregnancy. Selection can be made on the basis of *in vitro* susceptibilities, but usually empiric treatment suffices. Treatment for 10 days with nitrofurantoin macrocrystals, 100 mg four times daily, is effective in most women. Other regimens include ampicillin, amoxicillin, a first-generation cephalosporin, nitrofurantoin, or a sulfonamide given four times daily for 3 days (Table 24-1). Single-dose antimicrobial therapy for bacteriuria has also been used with success.[11] The recurrence rate for all of these regimens is about 30 percent. Failure of single-dose regimens may be an indication of upper tract infection and the need for more protracted therapy, such as nitrofurantoin 100 mg at bedtime for 21 days.[12] For women with persistent or frequent recurrences of bacteriuria, suppressive therapy for the remainder of pregnancy may be indicated. The most commonly employed regimen is nitrofurantoin, 100 mg at bedtime.

Table 24-1

ANTIMICROBIAL REGIMENS FOR TREATMENT OF PREGNANT WOMEN WITH ASYMPTOMATIC BACTERIURIA OR CYSTITIS

Single dose
  Amoxicillin, 3 g*
  Ampicillin, 2 g*
  Cephalosporin, 2 g
  Nitrofurantoin, 200 mg
  Sulfonamide, 2 g
  Trimethoprim/sulfamethoxazole, 320/1600 mg

Three-day course
  Amoxicillin, 500 mg three times daily*
  Ampicillin, 250 mg four times daily*
  Cephalexin, 250 mg four times daily
  Nitrofurantoin, 50–100 mg four times daily
  Sulfonamide, 500 mg four times daily

Other
  Nitrofurantoin, 100 mg four times daily for 10 days

Treatment failures
  Nitrofurantoin, 100 mg four times daily for 21 days

Suppression for bacterial persistence or recurrence
  Nitrofurantoin, 100 mg at bedtime for remainder of
    pregnancy

*Increasing problems with community-acquired *E. coli* resistance to ampicillin and amoxicillin (15 to 20 percent) may make these regimens less desirable in the presence of this organism.

CYSTITIS

There is evidence that bladder infection during pregnancy develops without antecedent covert bacteriuria.[13] Typically, cystitis is characterized by dysuria, urgency, and frequency. There are few associated systemic findings. Usually there is pyuria as well as bacteriuria. Microscopic hematuria is common, and occasionally there is gross hematuria. While asymptomatic infection is associated with renal bacteriuria in half of the cases, more than 90 percent of the cases of cystitis are limited to the bladder.[13] Although cystitis is usually uncomplicated, the upper urinary tract may become involved by ascending infection. Certainly, 40 percent of pregnant women with acute pyelonephritis have preceding symptoms of lower tract infection.[14] Fakhoury and coworkers[15] described two pregnant women with severe hemorrhagic cystitis. They recommend continuous bladder irrigation; one woman required blood transfusions.

TREATMENT

Women with bacterial cystitis respond readily to any of several regimens (Table 24-1). Harris and Gilstrap[13] reported a 97 percent cure rate with a 10-day ampicillin regimen. Sulfonamides, nitrofurantoin, or a cephalosporin are also effective when given for 10 days. Recently, as with covert bacteriuria, there has been a trend to use a 3-day course of therapy. Single-dose therapy as described for asymptomatic bacteriuria has been shown effective for both nonpregnant and pregnant women, but concomitant pyelonephritis must be confidently excluded.

Frequency, urgency, dysuria, and pyuria accompanied by a "sterile" urine culture may be the consequence of urethritis caused by *Chlamydia trachomatis,* a common pathogen of the genitourinary tract. Mucopurulent cervicitis usually coexists. Erythromycin therapy usually is effective. Recently, single dose azithromycin (1 g) has been shown to be effective in eradicating *C. trachomatis* infections during pregnancy.

ACUTE PYELONEPHRITIS

Acute renal infection is the most common serious medical complication of pregnancy, occurring in 1 to 2 percent of pregnant women. Nearly 100,000 pregnant women are hospitalized in the United States each year for this complication. The population incidence varies and depends on the prevalence of covert bacteriuria and whether it is treated. For example, at Parkland Hospital, nearly 90 percent of women attend prenatal clinics where bacteriuria screening is performed and treatment given for the 8 percent who are infected. Before we began routine screening, nearly 3 percent of pregnancies were complicated by pyelonephritis; but with screening and attempts to eradicate bacteriuria, acute renal infection now complicates only about 1 percent of pregnancies. This is similar to the incidence cited earlier and reported by Gratacos and associates[4] after they instituted a screening program.

Pyelonephritis is more common after midpregnancy; it is unilateral and right-sided in more than half of cases, and bilateral in one fourth. In most women, renal parenchymal infection is caused by bacteria that ascend from the lower tract. Between 75 and 90 percent of renal infections are caused by bacteria that have P-fimbriae adhesins.[16]

CLINICAL FINDINGS

The onset of pyelonephritis is usually rather abrupt. Symptoms include fever, shaking chills, and aching pain in one or both lumbar regions. There is usually anorexia, nausea, and vomiting. The course of the disease may vary remarkably, with fever to as high as 42°C (107.6°F) and hypothermia to as low as 34°C (93.2°F). Tenderness can usually be elicited by percussion in one or both costovertebral angles. Although the diagnosis is usually apparent, pyelonephritis may be mistaken for labor, chorioamnionitis, appendicitis, placental abruption, or infarcted myoma, and—in the puerperium—for uterine infection and pelvic cellulitis.

The urinary sediment frequently contains many leukocytes, frequently in clumps, and numerous bacteria. In a survey of 190 women admitted to Parkland Hospital for pyelonephritis, *E coli* was isolated from the urine in 77 percent, *Klebsiella pneumoniae* in 11 percent, and *Enterobacter* or *Proteus* each in 4 percent.[17] Culture results from 120 women with antepartum pyelonephritis treated at Los Angeles County—University of Southern California Medical Center were similar to Parkland's experience.[18] About 15 percent of women with acute pyelonephritis also have bacteremia.

Almost all clinical findings in these women are ultimately caused by endotoxemia, and so are the serious complications of acute pyelonephritis (Table 24-2). A frequent and sometimes dramatic finding is thermoregulatory instability characterized by high spiking fever followed by hypothermia. Commonly, temperatures fluctuate from as low as 34°C (93.2°F) to as high as 42°C (107.6°F) (Fig. 24-2). Twickler and associates[19] have shown a significantly decreased systemic vascular resistance and increased cardiac output in these women with acute infection. These are mediated by *cytokines* elaborated by macrophages in response to endotoxin. They include interleukin-1, previously termed *endogenous pyrogen*, and tumor necrosis factor.[20]

MANAGEMENT

One scheme for management of the pregnant woman with acute pyelonephritis is shown in Table 24-3. MacMillan and Grimes[21] have questioned the clinical utility and cost-effectiveness of pretreatment urine and blood cultures. Because 15 percent of these women have bacteremia, they should be watched carefully to detect symptoms of endotoxin shock or its sequelae during the first day of therapy. Urinary output, blood pressure, and temperature are monitored closely. Intravenous hydration to ensure adequate urinary output is essential. High fever should be treated with a cooling blanket if necessary.

These serious urinary infections usually respond quickly to intravenous hydration and antimicrobial therapy. The choice of drug is empiric, and ampicillin, a cephalosporin, or an extended-spectrum penicillin is satisfactory. Ampicillin-resistant *E. coli* have become common, and Duff[22] reported a 27 percent clinical failure rate in 131 women given ampicillin. In a recent audit of urine cultures from 130 women admitted to Parkland Hospital for antepartum pyelonephritis, only half of *E. coli* strains were sensitive to ampicillin but 90 percent were sensitive to cefazolin.[23] Thus, many prefer to give gentamicin or another aminoglycoside

Table 24-2

MULTIPLE ORGAN SYSTEM DYSFUNCTION ASSOCIATED WITH ACUTE PYELONEPHRITIS DURING PREGNANCY

Thermoregulatory instability
   High spiking fevers
   Hypothermia

Transient renal dysfunction
   Elevated serum creatinine
   Decreased creatinine clearance

Hematologic dysfunction
   Hemolysis
   Anemia
   Thrombocytopenia

Pulmonary dysfunction
   Adult respiratory distress syndrome

if ampicillin is chosen. Serial determinations of serum creatinine are important if nephrotoxic drugs are administered. For all of these reasons, some prefer a cephalosporin or extended-spectrum penicillin, since these have been shown effective in 95 percent of such women.[24,25]

Clinical symptoms for the most part resolve during the first 2 days of therapy; but even though symptoms promptly abate, therapy is recommended for a total of 7 to 10 days. Cultures of urine usually become sterile within the first 24 h. Because changes in the urinary tract induced by pregnancy persist, relapse or reinfection are common and can be demonstrated in 30 to 40 percent following completion of treatment for pyelonephritis.[26,27] One method that may be used to detect recurrence is monthly urine cultures. If measures are not taken to ensure urine sterility, then nitrofurantoin, 100 mg at bedtime, may be given for the remainder of the pregnancy. Van Dorsten and coworkers[27] reported that this regimen reduces recurrence of bacteriuria to 8 percent.

OUTPATIENT MANAGEMENT

Angel and associates[28] described a randomized clinical trial in which they compared oral versus intravenous antimicrobial therapy for 90 women with antepartum pyelonephritis. Their purpose was to simulate outpatient therapy. They excluded women with underlying medical complications, those who could not tolerate oral medications, those with possible sepsis, and—at least retrospectively—those 15 percent

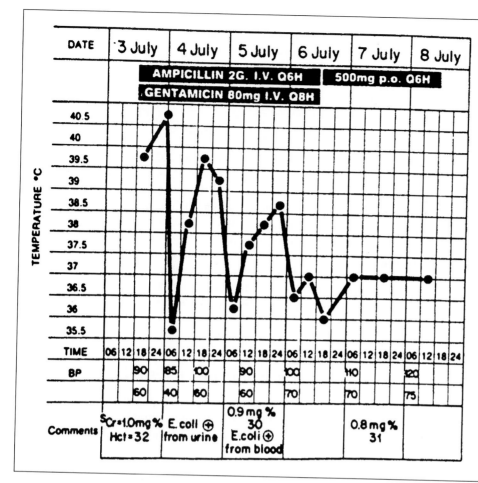

Figure 24-2

Vital signs graphic chart from a 25-year-old primigravida with acute pyelonephritis at 28 weeks' gestation. (From Lucas and Cunningham,[38] with permission.)

Table 24-3

MANAGEMENT OF THE PREGNANT WOMAN WITH ACUTE PYELONEPHRITIS

1. Hospitalization (see text)
2. Urine and blood cultures
3. Complete blood count, serum creatinine, and electrolytes
4. Monitor vital signs frequently, including urinary output (place indwelling bladder catheter if necessary)
5. Intravenous crystalloid to establish urinary output to at least 30 mL/h
6. Intravenous antimicrobial therapy
7. Chest x-ray if there is dyspnea or tachypnea
8. Repeat hematology and chemistry studies in 48 h
9. Change to oral antimicrobials when afebrile
10. Discharge after afebrile 24 h; consider antimicrobial therapy for 7 to 10 days
11. Urine culture 1 to 2 weeks after antimicrobial therapy completed

Source: Modified from Lucas and Cunningham,[12] with permission.

with bacteremia. These women generally did well; one in each group developed a serious complication: one had permeability pulmonary edema and the other developed hemolytic anemia. Sanchez-Ramos and coworkers[25] found that a single 1-g daily dose of intravenous ceftriaxone was effective therapy for hospitalized women. They suggested that such a regimen used with a 23-h stay may be ideal. Millar and colleagues[18] randomized 120 women less than 24 weeks' pregnant to inpatient versus outpatient treatment. The latter were observed for 4 to 24 h to verify that they could tolerate oral hydration. All of these women did well. In another study, Cook and collaborators[29] observed a 25 percent failure rate of inpatient oral therapy. Careful home health care and close follow-up are mandatory if these women are discharged before they are afebrile.

MANAGEMENT OF NONRESPONDERS

If clinical improvement is not obvious by 48 to 72 h or if complications ensue, then the patient should be evaluated for bacterial resistance or urinary tract obstruction. Pyelocalyceal dilatation, urinary calculi, and possibly intrarenal or perinephric abscesses may be visualized. Ultrasonography, "limited" computed tomography, or magnetic resonance imaging may be helpful for diagnosis (Fig. 24-3).

Thus, for the woman who remains substantively febrile after 72 h of appropriate therapy, a search for obstruction is launched. Sonography is the preferred method of diagnosis, and if findings are diagnostic of renal calculi, they are unlikely to be falsely positive. Conversely, the sensitivity of ultrasound to detect calculi is limited, and Hendricks and colleagues[30] identified only two-thirds of stones in pregnant women. If there is any doubt after the initial examination, plain abdominal radiography is indicated, because nearly 90 percent of renal stones are radiopaque. Possible benefits far outweigh the minimal fetal risk from radiation. If the results are negative, we recommend intravenous pyelography modified by the number of radiographs taken after contrast injection. The "one-shot pyelogram," in which a single radiograph is obtained 30 min after contrast injection, usually allows adequate imaging of the collecting system to detect stones or structural anomalies. Occasionally, a second or even a third radiograph may be indicated. Unilateral nonvisualization may be due to end-stage obstruction that may be visualized only with retrograde pyelography, which can often localize the source of obstruction.

Passage of a double-J ureteral stent will relieve the obstruction in most cases.[31] An example of this technique is shown in Fig. 24-4. If it is unsuccessful, then percutaneous nephrostomy is done. If this fails, surgical removal of renal stones is required for resolution of infection. If pyonephrosis is the source of continuing sepsis, removal of the infected kidney may be lifesaving.

COMPLICATIONS

RENAL DYSFUNCTION

In a prospective study of 220 women with antepartum pyelonephritis, Whalley and associates[32] found that nearly one-fourth had seriously diminished glomerular filtration rates. Fortunately, as shown in Fig. 24-5, renal dysfunction is transient and is usually reversible within several days, although it sometimes persists for weeks. There is good evidence that this is mediated by endotoxin lipopolysaccharide.[33] Management includes close observation with serial creatinine determination, treatment with intravenous fluids, and administration of antimicrobials without substantial nephrotoxicity (or with appropriate dosage reduction of those that are nephrotoxic).

HEMATOLOGIC DYSFUNCTION

Hematologic aberrations are common but seldom of clinical importance. For example, thrombocytopenia and minimally elevated fibrin split products in serum are frequently

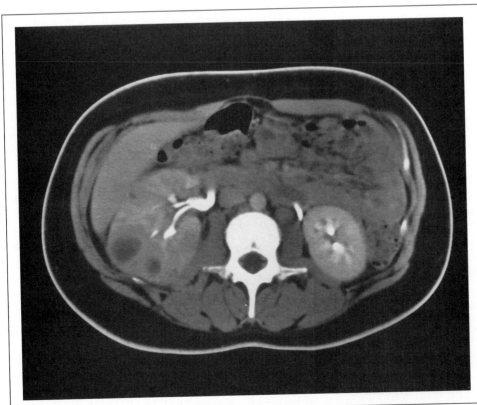

Figure 24-3

Magnetic resonance image taken in a woman 4 days postpartum. She had severe intrapartum pyelonephritis and her temperature still was spiking to 39°C (102.2°F) daily. The right kidney (*left side of photograph*) shows decreased enhancement and multiple areas of low density compatible with regional parenchymal involvement. With continued antimicrobial therapy, she was afebrile in 2 more days. (From Lucas and Cunningham,[38] with permission.)

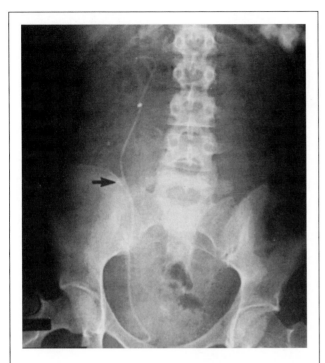

Figure 24-4

Abdominal x-ray in a woman 24 weeks' pregnant after passage of double-J stent to relieve obstruction caused by a right ureteral calculus *(arrow)*. The fetus is also visualized. (From Hendricks et al.,[30] with permission.)

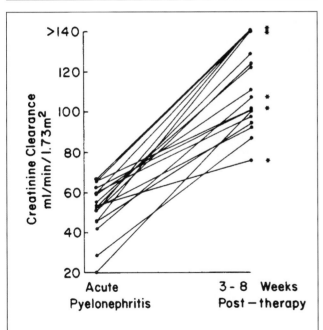

Figure 24-5

Glomerular filtration as determined by endogenous creatinine clearance in 18 pregnant women with acute pyelonephritis. These women had moderate to severe renal dysfunction, which approached normal by 3 to 8 weeks after start of therapy. (From Whalley et al.,[32] with permission.)

identified. In the rare case, endotoxin activates intravascular coagulation, and treatment of consumptive coagulopathy is directed mainly toward eliminating the infection. Unless operative intervention is planned, reversal of the coagulopathy follows such treatment and replacement of blood components is rarely necessary. Anemia is common with antepartum pyelonephritis and about one-third of women admitted will have a hematocrit of less than 30 percent.[8,34] There is now convincing evidence that endotoxin causes hemolysis.[34] Erythrocyte transfusions are seldom indicated in otherwise uncomplicated infection; however, we have found them necessary in nearly half of women with concomitant pulmonary injury (described below). More commonly, worrisome anemia develops after pyelonephritis, and it is not unusual for the hematocrit to reach 25 percent. Unless there is underlying chronic renal disease, restoration of the hemoglobin mass is usually prompt if there are adequate iron stores.

PULMONARY INJURY

Approximately 1 in 50 women with severe antepartum pyelonephritis develops evidence for pulmonary injury and respiratory insufficiency.[25,35] Importantly, Towers and associates[36] reported the incidence to be 1 in 12 if tocolysis was given to suppress concomitant uterine contractions. Endotoxin alters alveolar-capillary membrane permeability, with subsequent pulmonary edema. Fortunately, in most women, clinical manifestations are transient and respond promptly to increased inspired oxygen concentration. However, the adult respiratory distress syndrome is life-threatening; therefore attention should be given to the respiratory rate and other evidence of respiratory compromise or failure. Most women with pulmonary injury due to pyelonephritis have clinical manifestations within 48 h of admission, and tachypnea must be promptly investigated by chest radiograph and arterial blood gas analysis (Figs. 24-6*A* and *B*). Prompt recognition and appropriate respiratory therapy, which occasionally includes intubation and mechanical ventilation, prevents severe hypoxemia, which can cause fetal death or preterm labor.

As shown in Table 24-4, women with pulmonary capillary injury commonly have associated hematologic aberrations and renal dysfunction. These complications are more common in women with proven bacteremia, and it appears that infections caused by *K. pneumoniae* are usually more severe.[35,36] It is unclear whether prompt treatment with antimicrobials directed against this organism will prevent these complications. It is not possible to enumerate risk factors that prospectively identify a woman at risk for these complications. As shown in Table 24-4, patients tend to be more seriously ill; however, most factors that indicate severity of illness are recognized only in retrospect. In a similar study, Towers and colleagues[36] compared 11 women with antepartum pyelonephritis and pulmonary injury with 119 women with uncomplicated renal infection. Other signifi-

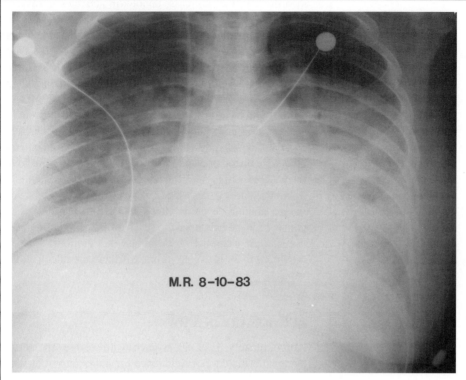

A

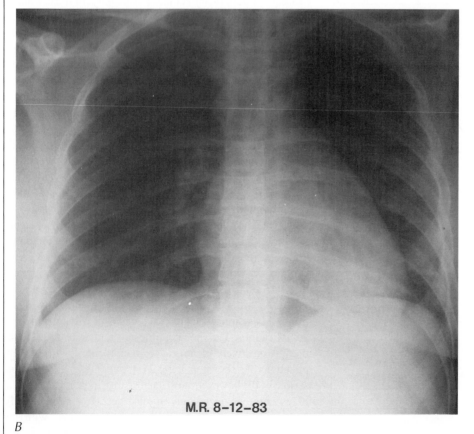

B

Figure 24-6

A. This 18-year-old multipara at 20 weeks' gestation had a normal radiograph at the time of admission (August 8). Respiratory distress 20 h later was accompanied by a left-sided pulmonary infiltrate which became bilateral by August 10. She had normal cardiovascular function as determined by pulmonary artery catheterization. *B*. By August 12, this patient's chest x-ray was normal.

Table 24-4

SELECTED FACTORS FOR PREGNANT WOMEN WITH PYELONEPHRITIS AND PULMONARY INJURY COMPARED WITH SIMILARLY INFECTED WOMEN WITHOUT RESPIRATORY DISTRESS

Factor	Respiratory Distress	No Distress	p Value
Symptoms, days (mean)	2.6	2.5	NS
Maximal temperature, °C (mean)	39.7	39.1	.002
Renal dysfunction, percent	57	20	.018
Hematocrit, percent (mean)	30.1	32.3	.012
Platelet count, μL Lowest (mean)	153,000	242,000	.02
Less than 100,000, percent	40	0	.003
Bacteremia, percent	43	22	.16
Klebsiella or *Proteus*, percent	40	13	.05
Days febrile (mean)	3.2	1.9	.004
Preterm delivery, percent	21	4	.10

Source: Modified from Cunningham et al.,[35] with permission.

cant predictive factors were fluid overload and use of to-colytic agents. Lung injury was more likely if tachycardia of more than 110 beats per minute coexisted with fever exceeding 39.4°C (103°F) in a woman at more than 20 weeks' gestation.

REFERENCES

1. Svanborg-Eden C, Hagberg L, Leffler H, Lonberg H: Recent progress in the understanding of the role of bacterial adhesion in the pathogenesis of urinary tract infection. *Infection* 10:327, 1982.
2. Hart AH, Pham T, Nowicki S, et al: Gestational pyelonephritis-associated *Escherichia coli* isolates represent a nonrandom, closely relation population. *Am J Obstet Gynecol* 174:983, 1996.
3. Whalley PJ: Bacteriuria of pregnancy. *Am J Obstet Gynecol* 97:723, 1967.
4. Gratacos E, Torres PJ, Vila J, et al: Screening and treatment of asymptomatic bacteriuria in pregnancy to prevent pyelonephritis. *J Infect Dis* 169:1390, 1994.
5. Rouse DJ, Andrews WW, Goldenberg RL, Owen J: Screening and treatment of asymptomatic bacteriuria of pregnancy to prevent pyelonephritis: A cost-effectiveness and cost-benefit analysis. *Obstet Gynecol* 86:119, 1995.
6. Romero R, Oyarzun E, Mazor M, et al: Meta-analysis of the relationship between asymptomatic bacteriuria and preterm delivery/low birth weight. *Obstet Gynecol* 73:576, 1989.
7. Schieve LA, Handler A, Hershaw R, et al: Urinary tract infection during pregnancy: Its association with maternal morbidity and perinatal outcome. *Am J Public Health* 84:405, 1994.
8. Gilstrap LC III, Leveno KJ, Cunningham FG, et al: Renal infection and pregnancy outcome. *Am J Obstet Gynecol* 141:708, 1981.
9. Kincaid-Smith P, Bullen M: Bacteriuria in pregnancy. *Lancet* 1:395, 1965.
10. Whalley PJ, Martin FG, Peters PC: Significance of asymptomatic bacteriuria detected during pregnancy. *JAMA* 198:879, 1965.
11. Andriole VT, Patterson TF: Epidemiology, natural history, and management of urinary tract infections in pregnancy. *Med Clin North Am* 75:359, 1991.
12. Lucas ML, Cunningham FG: Urinary tract infections complicating pregnancy, in *Williams Obstetrics*, 19th ed. Norwalk, CT: Appleton & Lange, Feb/March 1994, suppl 5.
13. Harris RE, Gilstrap LC III: Cystitis during pregnancy: A distinct clinical entity. *Obstet Gynecol* 57:578, 1981.
14. Gilstrap LC III, Cunningham FG, Whalley PJ: Acute pyelonephritis in pregnancy: An anterospective study. *Obstet Gynecol* 57:409, 1981.
15. Fakhoury GF, Daikoku NH, Parikh AR: Management of severe hemorrhagic cystitis in pregnancy: A report of two cases. *J Reprod Med* 39:485, 1994.
16. Stenqvist K, Sandberg T, Lidin-Janson G, et al: Virulence factors of *Escherichia coli* in urinary isolates from pregnant women. *J Infect Dis* 156:870, 1987.
17. Cunningham FG: Urinary tract infections complicating pregnancy. *Clin Obstet Gynecol* 1:891, 1988.
18. Millar LK, Wing DA, Paul RH, Grimes DA: Outpatient treatment of pyelonephritis in pregnancy: A randomized controlled trial. *Obstet Gynecol* 86:560, 1995.
19. Twickler DM, Lucas MJ, Bowe L, et al: Ultrasonographic evaluation of central and end-organ hemodynamics in antepartum pyelonephritis. *Am J Obstet Gynecol* 170:814, 1994.
20. Parrillo JE: Pathogenetic mechanisms of septic shock. *N Engl J Med* 328:1741, 1993.
21. MacMillan MC, Grimes DA: The limited usefulness of urine and blood cultures in treating pyelonephritis in pregnancy. *Obstet Gynecol* 78:745, 1991.
22. Duff P: Pyelonephritis in pregnancy. *Clin Obstet Gynecol* 27:17, 1984.
23. Horsager R, Cox S: Acute pyelonephritis: Outcomes and cost effectiveness of ampicillin and gentamicin therapy. *Am J Obstet Gynecol* 170:333, 1994.

24. Dunlow S, Duff P: Prevalence of antibiotic-resistant uropathogens in obstetric patients with acute pyelonephritis. *Obstet Gynecol* 76:241, 1990.

25. Sanchez-Ramos L, McAlpine KJ, Adair CD, et al: Pyelonephritis in pregnancy: Once-a-day ceftriaxone versus multiple doses of cefazolin. *Am J Obstet Gynecol* 172:129, 1995.

26. Cunningham FG, Morris GB, Mickal A: Acute pyelonephritis of pregnancy: A clinical review. *Obstet Gynecol* 42:112, 1973.

27. Van Dorsten JP, Lenke RR, Schifrin BS: Pyelonephritis in pregnancy: The role of in-hospital management and nitrofurantoin suppression. *J Reprod Med* 32:897, 1987.

28. Angel JL, O'Brien WF, Finan MA, et al: Acute pyelonephritis in pregnancy: A prospective study of oral versus intravenous antibiotic therapy. *Obstet Gynecol* 76:28, 1990.

29. Cook V, Herzog M, Hughes S, et al: Pyelonephritis in pregnancy: Oral versus IV antibiotics. *Am J Obstet Gynecol* 174:405, 1996.

30. Hendricks SK, Ross SO, Krieger JN: An algorithm for diagnosis and therapy of management and complications of urolithiasis during pregnancy. *Surg Gynecol Obstet* 172:49, 1991.

31. Rodriguez PN, Klein AS: Management of urolithiasis during pregnancy. *Surg Gynecol Obstet* 155:103, 1988.

32. Whalley PJ, Cunningham FG, Martin FG: Transient renal dysfunction associated with acute pyelonephritis of pregnancy. *Obstet Gynecol* 46:174, 1975.

33. Abraham E, Glauser MP, Butler T, et al: p55 tumor necrosis factor receptor fusion protein in the treatment of patients with severe sepsis and septic shock. A randomized controlled multicenter trial. *JAMA* 277:1531, 1997.

34. Cox SM, Shelburne P, Mason R, et al: Mechanisms of hemolysis and anemia associated with acute antepartum pyelonephritis. *Am J Obstet Gynecol* 164:587, 1991.

35. Cunningham FG, Lucas MJ, Hankins GDV: Pulmonary injury complicating antepartum pyelonephritis. *Am J Obstet Gynecol* 156:797, 1987.

36. Towers CV, Kaminskas CM, Garite TJ, et al: Pulmonary injury associated with antepartum pyelonephritis: Can patients at risk be identified? *Am J Obstet Gynecol* 164:974, 1991.

37. Roberts JA: Pathophysiology of pyelonephritis. *Infect Surg* Nov:633, 1986.

38. Lucas ML, Cunningham FG: Urinary infection in pregnancy. *Clin Obstet Gynecol* 36:855, 1993.

Chapter 25

NEUROLOGIC DISORDERS IN PREGNANCY

Bradley V. Vaughn

Imran Ali

Pregnancy increases the risk of neurologic complications, and each stage of pregnancy places the patient at risk for a variety of neurologic disorders. Although many common disorders are benign, neurologic complications account for one-third of maternal deaths. In addition, greater numbers of patients with preexisting neurologic disorders are becoming pregnant and present new challenges for the clinician. Many of these disorders can present with relatively acute symptoms. Knowledge about neurologic disorders during this vulnerable period will hopefully improve the probability for a good maternal and fetal outcome. This chapter reviews a spectrum of neurologic complications related to pregnancy and pregnancy in patients with neurologic disorders.

NEUROLOGIC LOCALIZATION

Localization of the neurologic deficits is paramount to determine the underlying etiology of neurologically related complaints. Table 25-1 and Fig. 25-1 outline basic patterns of neurologic deficits in central and peripheral lesions, allowing initial localization of the neurologic deficit. In general, the motor system exam is the most reliable and objective portion of the neurologic exam. The motor system can

be divided into two regions: the upper motor neuron (central nervous system) and the lower motor neuron (anterior horn cell, root, and peripheral nerve). Lesions of the upper motor neuron are characterized by hyperreflexia, extensor plantar response, and increased tone. Disorders of the lower motor neuron demonstrate loss of the deep tendon reflex, flexor plantar response, decreased muscle tone, and muscle wasting. Early in either upper or lower acute motor neuron lesions, patients may be flaccid.

COMA AND STUPOR

The presentation of stupor or coma in the pregnant patient raises concerns of possibly devastating etiologies. The workup should begin with a detailed history, physical exam, and laboratory evaluation. A complete neurologic examination will often give clues as to the diffuse or focal nature of neurologic injury.[1] Possible etiologies are listed in Table 25-2. Management of these patients includes rapid determination of possibly catastrophic reversible causes including hypoxemia, hypoglycemia, or drug intoxication, as listed in Table 25-3. Patients require supportive care until their conditions can be reversed. Once an etiology is determined, spe-

313

Table 25-1
LOCALIZATION OF NEUROLOGIC DEFICITS

Site	Findings
Cerebral hemisphere	Contralateral hemiparesis, central facial palsy, hemianopsia and sensory findings, contralateral hyperreflexia, extensor plantar–associated loss of cortical function (aphasia, agraphia, acalculi)
Brainstem lesion	Contralateral body hemiparesis and sensory findings, contralateral hyperreflexia, and extensor plantar response ipsilateral cranial nerve findings, ataxia, hyperventilation, pinpoint pupils
Spinal cord	Paraplegia or quadriplegia, hyperreflexia below lesion, sensory level, bilateral extensor plantar responses, bladder and rectal dysfunction
Neuropathy	Weakness, loss of reflex and muscle wasting (late finding) in distribution of the nerve, polyneuropathies associated with stocking-glove distribution of functional loss, usually flexor plantar or no response
Myopathy	Preservation of reflexes, flexor plantar response, no sensory deficits

cific therapy can be undertaken. Many of these disorders are further discussed below.

ARTERIAL STROKE IN PREGNANCY

The incidence of stroke is increased tenfold during pregnancy.[2] Most strokes occur in the latter half of pregnancy and in the postpartum period.[2] Patients with arterial infarcts usually present with sudden-onset focal neurologic deficits such as hemiparesis, aphasia, visual field defects, ataxia, diplopia, dysarthria, and dysphagia. The vascular territory affected determines the constellation of symptoms and signs corresponding to the area of infarcted brain. Therefore, patients with acute onset of focal neurologic deficits should be evaluated for possible ischemic injury. Establishing the presence of a stroke requires a complete neurologic examination

and consistent radiologic findings. Computed tomography (CT) provides rapid assessment, but the disadvantages are radiation exposure as well as relatively poor resolution. Frequently, CT scans are unremarkable acutely in an ischemic event. Magnetic resonance imaging (MRI) provides higher resolution and MR angiography is capable of noninvasive imaging of the cerebral vasculature. The effects of a magnetic field on the developing fetus are unknown, but at present MRI appears to be safe (see Appendix A2).

Rapid assessment in ischemic stroke is imperative to decrease the risk of irreversible damage. Early obstetric and neurologic consultation is necessary to confirm the diagnosis, define the etiology, and develop a management strategy.[2,3]

The diagnostic approach for stroke in pregnancy is similar to that of stroke in the young.[1] The etiologies of strokes can be divided into four major categories: embolic, thrombotic, vasculopathic, and miscellaneous (Table 25-4).

EMBOLIC STROKE

The onset of an embolic stroke usually occurs within seconds to minutes, and maximal deficit appears early in the course. Emboli may originate in the heart or large vessels and may be related to an arrhythmia, such as atrial fibrillation; an acquired cardiomyopathy, such as peripartum cardiomyopathy; or valvular heart disease. In recent years, numerous series have shown that a patent foramen ovale is a major risk factor in the young stroke patient and should be suspected when there is no other apparent cause. Valsalva maneuvers such as those occurring with delivery increase the risk that emboli will pass through a patent foramen ovale. Investigation of embolic infarcts requires a transthoracic and/or transesophageal echocardiogram. During echocardiography, Valsalva maneuvers and the introduction of small bubbles (bubble echocardiogram) may improve the chances of demonstrating the patent foramen. Holter monitoring as well as cardiac telemetry are useful in assessing for arrhythmias. Other causes of embolic stroke include amniotic fluid embolus and infective endocarditis.

THROMBOTIC STROKE

Patients with thrombotic strokes classically present with progression of neurologic deficits over minutes to hours, and they frequently wake up with the deficit. Some patients have a history of systemic vascular thrombosis or a family history of thrombotic disorders. Absence of such a history does not exclude the possibility of a hypercoagulable state. The most common of such states is the antiphospholipid antibody syndrome, which is also associated with spontaneous abortions as well as recurrent systemic thrombosis. Deficiencies of proteins C and S are also seen in this subgroup but are more frequently associated with venous thrombosis. Some researchers are concerned that protein C and S levels may decrease after delivery. Diagnosis requires a strong clinical sus-

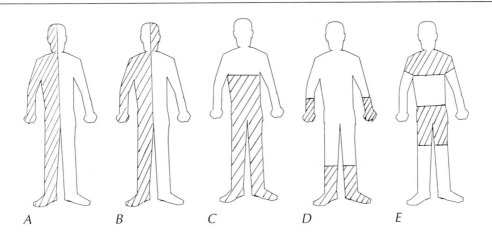

Figure 25-1

These five figures represent the classical distribution of neurologic deficits occurring with lesions of the nervous system. *A.* Lesion of the cerebral hemisphere with body and face findings contralateral to the lesion. *B.* Brainstem lesion with body contralateral and face ipsilateral to the lesion. *C.* Spinal cord lesion with motor and sensory level. *D.* Polyneuropathy with a stocking-glove distribution of sensory and motor deficits. *E.* Myopathy showing a proximal muscle weakness (but no sensory deficits).

Table 25-2

DIFFERENTIAL DIAGNOSIS OF COMA AND PERTINENT FINDINGS

Etiology	Neurologic Examination	Pertinent Findings
Anoxia	Nonfocal	May have posturing, seizures, and myoclonus
Carbon monoxide intoxication	Nonfocal	Carboxyhemoglobinemia
Hypoglycemia	Nonfocal	May have seizures, posturing, and sign of excessive sympathetic output, low serum glucose
Diabetic coma	Nonfocal	Fruity breath, Kussmal respiration, hyperglycemia, ketoacidosis, glycosuria, and ketonuria
Septic shock	Nonfocal	Hyperthermia, hypothermia, tachypnea, hypotension
Uremia	Nonfocal	Hypertension, uriniferous breath, asterixis, myoclonus, elevated BUN creatinine
Hepatic coma	Nonfocal	Jaundice, ascites, elevated bilirubin and NH_3, low serum protein, hypocoagulable state, asterixis
Addison disease	Nonfocal	Low serum cortisol; hyperkalemia and hyponatremia
Hypercapnia	Nonfocal; can cause papilledema	Elevated CO_2 and respiratory acidosis on blood gas; may have myoclonus or asterixis
Drug intoxication	Nonfocal	Variable depending on the agent
Meningitis	Nonfocal	Meningismus, fever, headache, inflammatory pattern on CSF examination
Status epilepticus	Nonfocal or focal	Electroencephalographic evidence of seizures, ongoing tonic-clonic activity or focal rhythmic twitching
Subarachnoid hemorrhage	Nonfocal or focal	Severe headache, meningismus, subhyaloid hemorrhage; CSF shows elevated red cells or xanthacromia; CT scan shows hemorrhage

(Continued)

Table 25-2 *(Continued)*

DIFFERENTIAL DIAGNOSIS OF COMA AND PERTINENT FINDINGS

Etiology	Neurologic Examination	Pertinent Findings
Eclampsia	Focal or nonfocal	Headache, seizures, hypertension, proteinuria
Hypertensive encephalopathy	Focal or nonfocal	Headache, flame hemorrhages in retina, convulsions, hypertension
Intracranial mass (tumor, abscess)	Focal deficit depending upon location of mass	Progressive headache, progressive neurologic deficits, papilledema or nausea and vomiting; MRI/CT scan demonstrates mass
Intraparenchymal hemorrhage	Focal depending upon location of hemorrhage	Sudden-onset symptoms, seizures, hypertension, headache; CT scan demonstrates hemorrhages
Subdural hemorrhage	Focal depending upon location of hemorrhage	Slow progression of symptoms, mild headache, history of trauma or anticoagulation; MRI/CT scan demonstrates subdural hemorrhage
Trauma	Focal or nonfocal	Battle signs or other evidence of trauma
Stroke, thrombotic	Focal findings depending upon distribution	Abrupt onset with progression of symptoms, more likely to occur in sleep; may not be seen early on CT scan
Stroke, embolic	Focal findings depending upon vasculature distribution Amniotic fluid embolus may be nonfocal	Sudden onset, maximal deficit soon after onset, may improve with time, possible risk of seizures; consider possible amniotic embolus, possible cardiac valvular or septal defect, arrhythmia; may not be seen early on CT scan
Central pontine myelinolysis	Focal or nonfocal	Intranuclear ophthalmoplegia related to rapid correction of hyponatremia
Encephalitis	Focal or nonfocal depending on area of cerebral injury	Seizures, confusion, and fever prior to coma; CSF shows an inflammatory pattern; MRI may show abnormality

picion. Testing must be done prior to starting anticoagulation to avoid lowering levels of protein C and S.

VASCULOPATHIC STROKE

Patients with vasculopathy may have premature atherosclerosis, vasculitides related to connective tissue disorders, vasculopathies associated with lupus erythematosus, thrombotic thrombocytopenic purpura, and/or Takayasu or fibromuscular dysplasia. The patient presentation in this group varies, but symptoms may wax and wane or present as multiple episodes. Any patient with multiple events without a clear cause needs a complete evaluation for vasculopathy. Evaluation in these situations is based on clinical assessment and identification of risk factors (for example, neck trauma and carotid dissection). Patients should have serologic evaluation for connective tissue disorders, syphilis, cholesterol lipid panel, carotid Dopplers, and MR angiography. Cerebral angiography is the gold standard for diagnosis of vas-

cular abnormalities, but this should be performed only if the risk is justified.

MISCELLANEOUS

Recreational drug use (e.g., cocaine, heroin, and amphetamines) may be associated with ischemic infarcts or hemorrhage. In addition, complicated migraine, eclampsia, alcohol abuse, or human immunodeficiency virus (HIV) infection may also be associated with occlusive cerebrovascular disease.

Management of ischemic strokes is rapidly changing with the advent of thrombolytic therapy and new neuroprotective agents currently in testing. Thrombolytic therapy is relatively contraindicated in pregnant patients, and most of the protocols for testing neuroprotective agents in stroke exclude pregnant women. Early recognition and intervention clearly improve the outlook of the patient with stroke. Vigorous hydration, oxygenation, and cardiac monitoring are the first resuscitative measures. Patients with fever must be evaluated

Table 25-3

MANAGEMENT OF COMA

Resuscitation
  Assess and maintain adequate airway, breathing, and circulation
  Immobilize neck until cervical spine injury has been excluded
  Pulse oximetry and oxygenation
  Monitor cardiac rhythm and obtain electrocardiogram
  Obtain core temperature

Initial treatment
  Begin crystalloid infusion
  Thiamine 100 mg IV
  Glucose test strip, administer 50% dextrose if hypoglycemic
  Use naloxone 0.4 mg IV if narcotics overdose is suspected

Evaluation
  Physical examination, pelvic and rectal examination
  Neurologic examination (assess for focality)
  Assess fetal heart tones and obtain obstetrics consultation

Diagnostics and treatment
  Complete blood count, type and screen, chemistries, toxicology panel, coagulation studies
  CT scan of head
  Treat seizures and infection
  Treat increased intracranial pressure
  Correct hypo- or hyperthermia
  Neurologic or neurosurgical consultation

Table 25-4

CATEGORIES OF ARTERIAL STROKES

Etiology	Classical Presentation
Embolic	Sudden onset (seconds to minutes), maximal deficit at onset, more likely to occur with patient active, higher risk of seizure
Thrombotic	More gradual onset (minutes to hours), more likely to occur with the patient asleep
Vasculopathy	Varied presentation, may wax and wane or include multiple events

for an infective source. Prompt and aggressive treatment of the fever and the presumptive source is required to avoid stroke extension. The benefits of heparin in acute stroke are controversial, but among all the anticoagulants, heparin is associated with the least risk during pregnancy. Low-molecular-weight heparin also does not appear to cross the placenta but has not been adequately studied as a therapy for stroke.[4] Anticoagulation is well accepted as preventing stroke in patients with atrial fibrillation and reduces the risk of repeat thrombosis in hypercoagulable states. Yet anticoagulation for these disorders in pregnant women has not been studied. Low-dose aspirin (81 mg) is possibly safe during the third trimester. All therapeutic options should be fully discussed with the patient and the consulting services prior to initiation of treatment.[2,3]

CEREBRAL VENOUS THROMBOSIS

Venous infarcts are more likely to occur during the third trimester of pregnancy or the postpartum period.[2,5] Patients usually present with headaches, papilledema, visual disturbances, and focal neurologic signs. Some patients present with partial seizures or even epilepsia partialis continua. The diagnosis requires a high index of suspicion and a complete neurologic evaluation. Although thrombosis most commonly involves the sagittal sinus, any venous structure may become thrombosed. Associated risk factors include dehydration, infection, and—rarely—a hypercoagulable state such as antithrombin III, protein C, or protein S deficiency. In most cases no obvious cause can be ascertained. As part of the evaluation, a MRI of the brain should be performed (Fig. 25-2). This study can be enhanced by MR venography. The scan may show an infarct with possible hemorrhage or swelling of the cerebrum. Frequently the medial parietal or occipital lobes are involved bilaterally. Cerebral angiography can confirm an occlusion of a large vessel and remains the most sensitive radiologic test.

Management requires intensive care admission, hydration, and monitoring of intracranial pressure. Heparin is an option to prevent extension of a clot but must be weighed against a significant risk of bleeding.[2,5]

INTRACRANIAL HEMORRHAGE IN PREGNANCY

The most common intracranial hemorrhagic complication of pregnancy is subarachnoid hemorrhage due to a ruptured cerebral aneurysm.[6] Subarachnoid hemorrhage is the third most common cause of nonobstetric maternal death. In pregnant patients with an unruptured cerebral aneurysm, the

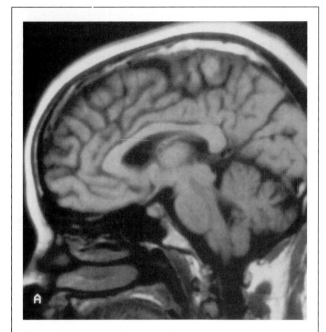

Figure 25-2

This T1 sagittal view of the MRI demonstrates thrombosis of the sagittal sinus as seen by the bright signal noted in the sinus above the parietal region.

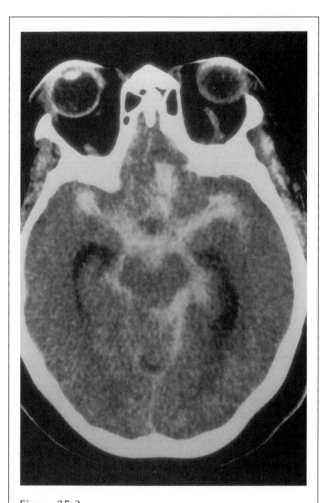

Figure 25-3

A CT scan taken from a patient with an acute subarachnoid hemorrhage. Note the higher density in the suprasellar area and region outlining the midbrain.

periods of greatest risk are the third trimester and the immediate postpartum period. Patients usually present with the worst headache of their lives, stiff neck, nausea, vomiting, third-nerve palsy, obtundation, seizures, and coma. Patients may also present with a sudden loss of consciousness that was preceded by a severe headache. On examination, findings of subhyaloid hemorrhages and nuchal rigidity may be noted. Prognosis is related to neurologic status at time of initial evaluation. Computed tomography will show acute subarachnoid blood better than MRI, especially in the first 24 h (Fig. 25-3). The CT scan may be unremarkable in 5 to 10 percent of patients and the cerebrospinal fluid (CSF) shows an increased count of red blood cells (RBCs) or possible xanthochromia. Angiography is the gold standard to identify the aneurysm.

The presentation of intracranial hemorrhage from an arteriovenous malformation is similar to that of an aneurysm, but focal neurologic symptoms and signs are more common due to parenchymal involvement. Hemorrhage occurs most often between 16 and 24 weeks of gestation or in the peripartum period and the risk of hemorrhage is 20 to 50 percent. Although rare in western societies, choriocarcinoma has a propensity to bleed and should be considered in the evaluation of subarachnoid and intraparenchymal hemorrhage.

Management requires early recognition, stabilization of the patient, and emergent neurosurgical consultation. Both neurosurgical and obstetric input are essential for good outcome. Patients frequently have increased intracranial pressure and may require ventriculostomy. Surgical clipping of

the aneurysm can be performed at any time in the pregnancy and is the only definitive treatment. If needed late in pregnancy, it may be combined with elective cesarean section. Accepted therapies such as calcium channel blockers (nimodipine) for prevention of vasospasm may be associated with significant risks in pregnancy and are best avoided. Vaginal delivery may increase the risk of hemorrhage in patients with known aneurysms or arteriovenous malformations; therefore elective cesarean section is recommended.

ECLAMPSIA: NEUROLOGIC CONSEQUENCES

Eclampsia is a poorly understood disorder characterized by hypertension, edema, proteinuria, and convulsions or encephalopathy, most likely related to systemic vasoconstric-

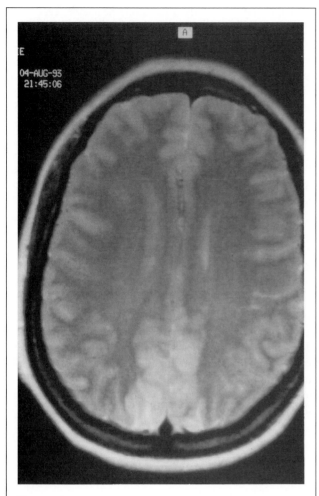

Figure 25-4

This axial MRI taken from a patient with eclampsia demonstrates the diffuse swelling in the gray matter, indicated by the brighter T2 signal, particularly in the occipital and parietal regions.

lieve that magnesium acts through neuromuscular blockade rather than as a true antiepileptogenic agent.[9] Phenytoin is an alternative for emergency management of seizures, and most patients do not require long-term anticonvulsants.[7,8] Other issues related to eclampsia are discussed in Chap. 7.

HEADACHE

Headache is a common ailment, especially in young women of childbearing age.[10] Several structures in the head can cause pain (Table 25-5). Migraine is the most common neurologic disorder in this age group. A complete assessment is required to exclude potentially fatal or devastating illnesses and to differentiate the various subtypes of headaches.[10–13] The presence of certain warning signs (Table 25-6) indicates that more extensive evaluation is required. A list of possible causes of headache is given in Table 25-7. New-onset headaches in pregnancy require careful evaluation. Pathologic etiologies such as mass lesions, cerebrovascular disease, meningeal processes, and eclampsia must be considered. Evaluation in these patients may include brain MRI, complete blood count with differential, erythrocyte sedimentation rate, lupus anticoagulant, anticardiolipin antibody, prothrombin time, and partial thromboplastin time.[11–13] Patients with meningeal signs or suspected hemorrhage should have emergent head CT scans and lumbar puncture if not contraindicated. In the third trimester, concern for cerebral venous thrombosis would warrant MRI with venography.[2]

In classic migraine, patients usually present with acute, unilateral, throbbing headache preceded by flashing lights or focal neurologic symptoms (migraine with aura). Common migraine is the same headache without the preceding aura. Any uncertainty about the diagnosis should lead to early neurologic consultation. Most patients have a prior history of similar headaches. Absence of such history is a cause for concern, as potentially serious disorders may mimic migraine.[10] Treatment of migraine headache requires consul-

tion. This disorder usually occurs during the second or third trimester but can also occur days after an uneventful pregnancy and delivery.[7,8] The presence of neurologic symptoms and signs (i.e., seizure) differentiate preeclampsia from eclampsia. This disorder is considered an obstetric emergency. Immediate stabilization and expeditious delivery of the fetus are the only definitive treatment. The neurologic changes include cerebral edema, most often in the parietooccipital region, associated with petechial hemorrhages (Fig. 25-4). Patients are clinically encephalopathic and frequently have convulsions. Either MRI or CT scan may show diffuse or focal edema, especially in the parietooccipital region. The scan may be completely normal in some cases.

Convulsions with eclampsia may cause fetal hypoxia and circulatory compromise. It is necessary to prevent seizure recurrence. There is considerable controversy over anticonvulsant therapy. Magnesium sulfate is the most frequently used anticonvulsant in eclampsia, but most neurologists be-

Table 25-5

STRUCTURES THAT CAN CAUSE HEADACHE

Skin
Muscle
Blood vessels
Periosteum
Peripheral nerves
Meninges
Sinuses

Table 25-6

WARNING SIGNS IN PATIENTS WITH HEADACHES

New onset in pregnancy
Focal neurologic deficit
Meningismus
Fever
Altered consciousness
Papilledema or signs of increased intracranial pressure
Headache different from previous headaches
Retinal hemorrhages

tation with an obstetrician and a neurologist, preferably one experienced in dealing with pregnancy. Most of the drugs effective in nonpregnant patients may have deleterious effects on the fetus, so caution must be exercised in prescribing medications.[13] Some physicians recommend short-term treatment with narcotics.

Patients presenting with bandlike or constricting bilateral headaches most likely have tension-type headache.[10] These patients usually do not appear ill and frequently have muscular tenderness over the scalp or neck. Historically, the headache is present daily, is of long duration, and is frequently associated with psychological stress. This variety of headache must be managed conservatively, sometimes using biofeedback or physical therapy.

Intracranial hemorrhage is a serious cause of headache. Patients may present with severe headache, stiff neck, loss of consciousness leading to coma, focal neurologic signs, or a convulsion. Rarely, patients may report hearing a "pop" just prior to the headache. They usually appear very sick,

Table 25-7

DIFFERENTIAL DIAGNOSIS OF HEADACHE

Migraine
Tension-type headache
Subarachnoid hemorrhage
Intraparenchymal hemorrhage
Cerebral venous thrombosis
CNS tumor
Pseudotumor cerebri
Sinus headache
Meningitis/encephalitis
Eclampsia

but some may have only a moderate headache, especially those with sentinel hemorrhages. Rapid diagnosis and intervention is essential to avoid devastating consequences.[6] Computed tomography is a reasonable first step in diagnosis and may show high density within the subarachnoid space (Fig. 25-3). Emergent neurosurgical consultation is necessary for appropriate intervention. Treatment is discussed in further detail above, under "Intracranial Hemorrhage in Pregnancy."

Pseudotumor cerebri is also called *benign intracranial hypertension* and primarily affects obese women and those with recent and significant weight gain. Patients usually have visual symptoms, such as transient loss of vision, in association with a diffuse, unremitting headache. Treatment in pregnancy is limited to cautious use of acetazolamide, the drug of choice in this disorder.[7] Other options include serial lumbar puncture as well as a short course of glucocorticoids.[7,13] In case of threat of optic nerve damage or blindness, neuroopthalmologic consultation should be obtained for emergent optic sheath fenestration.

Acute sinus headache may cause fever, postural headaches, and a purulent mucoid discharge. Occasionally, patients may note foul-smelling nasal drainage. Patients with tumor rarely present with isolated headaches but frequently appear ill or have progressive or subtle neurologic deficits. These findings indicate the need for brain imaging.

HEAD TRAUMA

Head trauma accounts for 20 percent of nonobstetric maternal deaths.[14,15] Closed or open head injury may result in intracranial hemorrhage and central nervous system (CNS) edema. These complications present the most acute neurologic danger for the patient. The patient's examination is a reasonable guide to the probability of good outcome. The Glasgow Coma Scale is a widely used screening tool for assessing brain function and has been correlated to outcome (Table 25-8). The scale ranges from the normal score of 15 to a minimum of 3. Individuals who have scores of 8 or less are considered to have suffered severe head injury. As outlined in Table 25-9, the management of these patients should be directed toward the assessment and therapy of the most dangerous complications first.

In the pregnant patient with head trauma, the effects on the fetus should be considered in evaluation and treatment.[14,15] Fetal demise and poor outcome are associated with the severity of maternal trauma.[14] Additionally, maternal systemic complications increase the risk of fetal complications. In every patient, the gestational age should be estimated and the mother should be checked for possible premature onset of labor. Patients who have evidence of increased intracranial pressure should be considered for intracranial pressure monitoring and CSF drainage. Hyperventilation and glucocorticoids do not appear beneficial. Mannitol, however, can

Table 25-8

GLASGOW COMA SCALE

Response	Score
Verbal	
None	1
Incomprehensible sounds	2
Inappropriate sounds	3
Confused	4
Oriented	5
Eye opening	
None	1
To pain	2
To speech	3
Spontaneously	4
Motor	
None	1
Abnormal extension	2
Abnormal flexion	3
Withdraws	4
Localizes	5

Table 25-9

MANAGEMENT OF PREGNANT PATIENTS WITH HEAD TRAUMA

Resuscitation
  Assess and maintain adequate airway, breathing, and circulation
  Immobilize neck until cervical spine injury has been excluded
  Pulse oximetry and oxygenation
  Monitor cardiac rhythm and obtain electrocardiogram
  Assess for other traumatic injuries
  Obtain core temperature

Initial treatment
  Begin crystalloid infusion
  Transfusion if needed

Evaluation
  Physical examination, pelvic, and rectal examination
  Neurologic examination including Glasgow Coma Scale
  Assess fetal heart tones and obtain obstetrics consultation
  Emergent neurosurgical consultation

Diagnostics and treatment
  Complete blood count, type and crossmatch, chemistries, toxicology panel, coagulation studies
  CT scan of head
  Treat seizures and infection
  Control intracranial pressure (mannitol should be used with caution)

cause fetal dehydration, contraction of blood volume, and bradycardia; its use during pregnancy should be restricted. In the event of maternal death or brain death, emergency cesarean section is indicated. This should be performed as early as possible to minimize fetal complications. Fetal demise or major morbidity has been associated with deliveries occurring 20 min after the cessation of maternal vital signs. Deliveries occurring in less than 5 min have been associated with excellent outcome[16] (see Chap. 29).

LOW BACK PAIN

Low back pain is a common symptom during pregnancy. For the majority of women, the discomfort does not represent a harbinger of significant pathology. Prospective studies have shown that 50 to 90 percent of women develop back pain during their pregnancy.[17–21] Approximately 9 percent of these women have back pain so severe that they have to discontinue work. Most back pain is worse in the evening and at night.[20] Risk factors include lack of antenatal exercise, advancing age and parity, poor posture, or improper lifting.

Several changes occur during pregnancy that make back pain more prevalent, including changes in posture and weight distribution.[17,19,21] Enlargement of the uterus and re-

laxation of the abdominal muscles produces a backward displacement of the spine and increases the work of the paraspinal muscles. Additionally, the effect of increased relaxin causes greater flexibility in ligaments and increases mobility of sacroiliac joints.

The diagnostic approach to low back pain in pregnant

Table 25-10

STRUCTURES THAT CAN CAUSE BACK PAIN

Skin
Muscle
Periosteum
Dura
Peripheral nerve or root
Abdominal or pelvic organs

women should be similar to that in other patients. Structures that can cause back pain are listed in Table 25-10. The history should include information regarding location and quality of pain, factors which aggravate and improve the discomfort, the diurnal pattern of the pain, and associated symptoms. Careful attention should be given to neurologic symptoms, especially weakness or bowel/bladder incontinence (Table 25-11). Women who awaken with acute back pain may have uterine compression of the inferior vena cava, causing blood to be shunted through the vertebral venous plexus. The physical exam should include examination of the back and specifically the area of pain. Supporting muscles and joints (especially the sacroiliac joints) should be examined for tenderness. Maneuvers such as pressing inward, moving the pelvic brim, or the Patrick test may aid in detecting sacroiliac joint pain.[23] Evaluation of the abdomen and pelvis should be performed considering the possibility of pancreatic disease, renal stones, or pathology involving the reproductive tracts. The patient should have a neurologic exam focused on the motor and sensory distributions of the lower extremities. The straight leg raising test may elicit pain; this is commonly associated with disk disease, hamstring muscle pain, and sacroiliac disease. The presence of fever with back pain should raise concern over possible infectious etiologies such as epidural abscess (a neurosurgical emergency) or diskitis, especially in diabetic or immuno-compromised patients.

Muscular pain is common, especially in the evening, when muscles have been fatigued, or after a day of improper lifting or posture. This discomfort is usually paraspinal in nature and is made worse by deep palpation of these muscles as well as by activation of these muscles. Bony joint pain may be demonstrated by movement of the sacroiliac joint or by putting pressure on the posterior facet joint by retroflexion of the back.[22]

The incidence of lumbar disk disease is unknown.[17,19–21] The biomechanical changes related to the pregnancy suggest that the incidence of disk disease should be high, but review of surgically proved cases suggests that it may be low. Lumbar disk disease may cause acute or persistent pain that may or may not radiate down the leg. Radiating pain does not confirm the diagnosis of disk disease, since these symptoms can be seen in peripheral nerve injury or muscular and sacroiliac joint disease. Neurologic deficits referable to a nerve root—such as dermatomal sensory loss, motor paralysis, absent reflex, or bowel or bladder incontinence—are significant findings. Motor paralysis or bowel/bladder incontinence are neurologic emergencies and warrant immediate evaluation for possible surgical intervention. Magnetic resonance imaging of the spinal canal and neural foramen is the most appropriate means of demonstrating the disk protrusion.

Treatment of the pregnant woman with back pain should be directed toward the underlying pathology. Recognition of an underlying emergency is paramount. Motor paralysis or bowel/bladder incontinence are neurologic emergencies and require immediate evaluation. Surgical therapy for disk disease is reserved for those with motor paralysis or bowel/bladder incontinence. Patients with partial paralysis referable to a root must be followed closely, and the risks and benefits of surgery should be weighed carefully. Injection of corticosteroids into the epidural space has been proposed as a safe and effective therapy for decreasing pain in disk disease.[19] For most women with back pain, common conservative therapies provide benefit, including short-term bed rest (3 days), daily low back exercises, the practice of good posture, and avoidance of situations that may exacerbate the pain. Patients with nighttime back pain should be advised to sleep in the lateral decubitus position to relieve compression of the vena cava. If conservative measures are unsuccessful, patients may try a longer period of strict bed rest (7 to 10 days), transcutaneous electrical nerve stimulation (TENS), and physical therapy, including lumbar support while sitting, frequent changes of position, application of heat or cold, and stretching exercises.[23]

Preventive measures should be encouraged in all pregnant women, especially those with a history of low back pain.[24,25] Begun prior to pregnancy, exercise, good posture, and observation of the basic biomechanical principles of the back are the mainstays of prevention. Exercise—including pelvic tilts, leg lifts, modified partial situps, walking, and swimming—are all aimed at strengthening the muscles and reducing the lordosis. Avoiding high heels, ensuring correct posture with minimal lordosis while walking or sitting, and proper lifting by flexing at the knees should decrease the risk of low back strain.

Table 25-11

DANGER SIGNS IN PATIENTS WITH BACK PAIN

Motor paralysis
Bowel or bladder incontinence
Abdominal or pelvic pain
Fever

FIRST SEIZURE

Approximately 10 percent of the population will have a seizure at some time during life. Yet epilepsy—defined as the recurrence of unprovoked seizures—occurs in only 1 percent of the population.[26] Seizures are the hallmark of a dis-

Table 25-12

PRECIPITANTS OF SEIZURES

Hypoglycemia
Electrolyte disturbance
Medication overdose
Hyperthermia
Trauma
Tumor
Stroke
Intracranial hemorrhage

turbance of the gray matter of the brain. Table 25-12 outlines several common precipitants; underlying focal cerebral insults such as stroke, hemorrhage, tumor, infection, or abscess are among them. Table 25-13 lists the steps for evaluation of a first seizure.

Patients with neurologic deficits on examination, abnormalities on brain imaging, and a family history of unprovoked seizures are at greater risk for recurrence of seizures and are more likely to eventually require anticonvulsants. Neurologic consultation should be obtained prior to initiating anticonvulsants. Pregnant patients need to be counseled on the risks related to epilepsy, recurrent generalized seizures, and teratogenic effects of anticonvulsants. In general, women with epilepsy have a greater risk of having children with malformations; and anticonvulsants appear to increase this risk, especially in the first trimester.[26,27] If an anticonvulsant is required, consensus guidelines suggest using the first-choice drug for the type of epilepsy in monother-

Table 25-13

EVALUATION OF FIRST SEIZURE

1. History and physican exam
2. Complete blood count and differential, glucose, electrolytes, calcium, magnesium, phosphorus, blood urea nitrogen, creatinine, prothrombin time, partial thromboplastin time
3. Electrocardiography and monitoring
4. MRI/CT scan; consider lumbar puncture
5. Neurologic consultation
6. Obstetric consultation
7. Electroencephalogram

apy at the lowest effective dose.[27] All pregnant patients taking anticonvulsants require daily folate supplementation to decrease the risk of fetal malformation.[27] For most patients, especially those who recover quickly from the first seizure and have no other neurologic findings, anticonvulsant therapy can be avoided. All seizure patients should be warned to avoid heights, the use of dangerous equipment, driving, and swimming.

THE PREGNANT PATIENT WITH EPILEPSY

Pregnancy has a variety of effects on epilepsy.[26–28] Usually the first and third trimesters are the most likely to be associated with increased seizures. The dramatic alterations in hormones, fluid balance, metabolism, sleep deprivation, and fatigue can increase the recurrence of seizures. Changes in drug absorption, fluid distribution, protein binding, blood volume, and renal and hepatic clearance contribute to the changes in blood levels, altering the availability of anticonvulsants to the brain. Due to these changes, total serum anticonvulsant levels decline during pregnancy and may remain decreased for 8 to 12 weeks after delivery. The levels of phenytoin, carbamazepine, and phenobarbital not bound to protein (free levels) decrease during pregnancy, whereas the levels of free valproate increase. For some medications, such as phenytoin, monitoring total and free (unbound portion) anticonvulsant levels can aid clinical management. All pregnant patients with epilepsy should be followed closely by a neurologist and an obstetrician.[27,28] Patients with epilepsy face an increased risk of miscarriage, fetal malformation, and premature delivery. Anticonvulsant medication appears to increase the risk of fetal malformation. When possible, patients with epilepsy should be treated by monotherapy at the lowest effective dosage and given folate supplementation. The vast majority of patients have uneventful pregnancies and over 90 percent deliver healthy children.

Delivery is a vulnerable time for patients with epilepsy.[27] Medication levels may fluctuate or drop near the time of delivery. This may be due to missed medication or poor absorption. Some patients may have seizures during or soon after delivery. Most of these seizures are usually short in duration, and supplemental anticonvulsant may be required. Vitamin K should be given prior to delivery to counteract depletion of vitamin K, which can occur with several anticonvulsants.

STATUS EPILEPTICUS

Definitions of status epilepticus vary. The classical definition of status epilepticus is *seizure activity lasting for more than 30 min.* Yet, patients with more than 10 min of seizure activity or two seizures without regaining consciousness should be treated as having status epilepticus.[29] This medical emergency requires immediate attention in order to avoid complications to the mother and fetus. Table 25-14 outlines a typical algorithm for management of status epilepticus. Intravenous loading doses of anticonvulsants should be calculated on the patient's current weight.[30]

Patients with status epilepticus generally have a history of seizures and are taking medication. If status epilepticus develops as the first seizure, a catastrophic event such as intracranial hemorrhage, tumor, or encephalitis is likely. Status epilepticus increases the risk of miscarriage and fetal demise. Greater seizure intensity and longer duration appear to affect the fetus adversely.

TUMORS

The management of intracranial tumors during pregnancy is difficult (Table 25-15). Mass lesions of the CNS may present with a variety of neurologic deficits, systemic complaints, and seizures. Termination of the pregnancy may be indicated in patients with progressive visual loss, signs of uncontrollable rising intracranial pressure, or frequent intractable generalized seizures.[31,32] Delivery complications include decreased cerebral perfusion or herniation because of the significant increases in intracranial pressure. Therefore, for intracranial tumors with potential mass effect, cesarean section is recommended.

Meningiomas are the most common tumors arising from the dura mater. These extra-axial tumors produce focal neurologic deficits or seizures by compressing or irritating the underlying tissue. Changes in hormonal levels and fluid volume may cause the meningioma to enlarge. Magnetic resonance imaging of the brain or enhanced CT will identify the mass. Surgical treatment can often be delayed until after delivery.[32]

Gliomas arise from the glial cells of the brain parenchyma and account for approximately 30 percent of intracranial tumors found during pregnancy. Gliomas may present during pregnancy with fatigue, nausea, vomiting, headache, seizures, or subtle focal neurologic deficits. These lesions are best seen on MR imaging of the brain. Biopsy of the lesion should be considered to differentiate the tumor from other infectious or granulomatous lesions. Dexamethasone can be used to reduce the vasogenic edema as well as some of the symptoms. The patient will have to be referred to a neurosurgeon and neurooncologist for further therapy.[32] Surgical excision of high-grade tumors should be considered early and chemotherapy should be avoided, if possible, until after the pregnancy. Anticonvulsants may be required following the onset of seizures.

Choriocarinoma is an aggressive trophoblastic tumor associated with cerebral metastasis.[31] Metastases may present with symptoms of stroke, intracranial hemorrhage, or seizures. Choriocarcinoma can also cause a wide range of radicular and peripheral nerve abnormalities by invading the lumbosacral plexus, vertebral bodies, neural foramen, or spinal canal.

Pituitary tumors usually produce amenorrhea and infertility and thus are uncommon in pregnant women.[33] Patients may present with headache and bitemporal visual loss. Magnetic resonance imaging of the brain will detect even small adenomas. Formal serial visual field tests should be performed to track the effect on the optic nerves. Declining visual acuity or progressive deterioration of visual fields is an indication for therapy. Patients with abrupt blindness need urgent intervention. Therapeutic options include transphenoidal surgery and radiation. Bromocrip-

Table 25-14
MANAGEMENT OF STATUS EPILEPTICS

	Time Frame
Resuscitation	0–5 min
Airway, breathing, circulation	
Oxygenate	
Initial examination	0–5 min
Brief history (especially anticonvulsant therapy)	
Brief physical exam (confirm seizure activity)	
Start IV (preferably two IV lines)	
Dextrose strip	
Complete blood count, blood chemistries, calcium, magnesium, anticonvulsant levels, toxicology panel	
Initial therapy	0–5 min
Lorazepam IV 0.05–0.1 mg/kg (may need to repeat in 20 min)	
Thiamine, glucose, or naloxone as indicated	
Phosphenytoin or phenytoin IV if not contraindicated. (15–20 mg/kg over 20 min with electrocardiography and blood pressure monitoring)	10–20 min
Further assessment	10–20 min
Assess fetal heart tone	
Neurology consultation	
Obstetric consultation	
Further therapy	30 min
Intubate patient (earlier may be necessary)	
Phenobarbital 20 mg/kg IV	

Table 25-15

BRAIN TUMORS

Tumor Type	Symptoms	Diagnostic Evaluation	Indications for Therapy	Therapy
Meningioma	Focal neurologic deficits, seizures	MRI or enhanced CT scan showing diffuse enhancing extraaxial lesion	Usually slow-growing, and therapy can be delayed until after delivery	Surgical excision, radiation for inoperable tumors
Gliomas	Fatigue, nausea, vomiting, headaches, seizures, and focal neurologic deficits	MRI, biopsy	Mass effect (vasogenic edema), seizures, high-grade tumors	Dexamethasone, anticonvulsants, surgical excision
Choriocarcinoma	Sudden-onset focal neurologic deficits, seizures, headache, intracranial hemorrhage, back pain, lower extremity weakness, bladder incontinence	MRI, pelvic ultrasound, serum and CSF chorionic gonadotropin levels with ratio of less than 60 to 1	Recognition of tumor	Surgical evacuation of tumor, whole-brain radiation, chemotherapy
Pituitary adenomas	Headaches, bitemporal visual field loss	MRI, CT scan of the sella, visual fields	Acute or progressive vision loss	Surgical excision, radiation for inoperable tumors

tine, a dopamine agonist, may be used to inhibit the growth of prolactin-secreting tumors and will also suppress lactation. Breast-feeding, however, may increase the size of prolactinomas.[34]

MOVEMENT DISORDERS

Movement disorders rarely occur during pregnancy.[35,36] Table 25-16 lists several movement disorders that may be seen in pregnancy. Neurologic consultation is usually not necessary in restless legs syndrome, the most common movement disorder associated with pregnancy.[35,36]

MULTIPLE SCLEROSIS AND OTHER DEMYELINATING DISORDERS

Multiple sclerosis is a relapsing-remitting demyelinating disorder of the CNS with usual onset between the ages of 20 and 35 years. It affects women twice as often as men.

Common symptoms include focal weakness, ataxia, paresthesias or dysesthesias, visual loss, incontinence, and incoordination. The disease has a variable and unpredictable clinical course.[32,37–39] Most multiple sclerosis attacks develop as progressive events occurring over a few days. Approximately 20 to 40 percent of patients relapse in the postpartum period, but pregnancy is not absolutely contraindicated.[32,37,38] The disease is not associated with a higher risk for the fetus or for the mother during labor or delivery. Epidural and other forms of anesthesia do not appear to pose a greater risk for these patients.

Acute exacerbations can occur at any time. Established treatment for acute exacerbation is intravenous methylprednisolone for 3 to 5 days followed by 7 to 10 days of oral prednisone taper. Such short courses of glucocorticoids are not likely to have a significant impact on pregnancy, but fetal complications such as adrenal insufficiency and virilization have been described. The effect of more aggressive immunosuppressive therapy is not known, and such therapy should be considered to be relatively contraindicated during pregnancy.

Metabolic stressors, fever, and infections (especially urinary tract infections) increase the likelihood of symptom recurrence. Breast-feeding is not contraindicated unless patients are taking immunosuppressive drugs, which are secreted into the breast milk.[32,39]

Table 25-16

MOVEMENT DISORDERS

Syndrome	Symptoms	Causes	Evaluation	Treatment
Restless legs	Crawling achy sensation improved with movement, associated with uncontrolled leg movement during rest and periodic limb movements during sleep	Folate deficiency, iron deficiency, uremia, peripheral vascular disease, arthritis, spinal cord lesions; stress, caffeine, and tricyclic medications can exacerbate symptoms	Serum iron, folate, blood urea nitrogen, creatinine levels; detailed neurologic exam to rule out central lesion	Withdraw from caffeine and tricyclic medications; stress reduction; biofeedback; folate, iron, vitamin E, gabapentin, dopaminergic agents, benzodiazepines
Chorea	Uncontrollable writhing or dancelike movements that may disappear during sleep; chorea gravidarium is reported to clear following delivery	Chorea gravidarium, sydenham chorea (rheumatic heart disease), systemic lupus erythematosus, medication induced (neuropsychiatric medications, especially antidopaminergic agents) hyperthyroidism, Wilson disease, vascular disease, meningovascular syphilis, Huntington disease, neuroacanthocytosis or adult onset Tay-Sachs disease	Detailed neurologic examination and consultation, slit-lamp exam of eyes, MRI, serum thyroid function tests, antinuclear antibodies, anticardiolipin antibody, lupus anticoagulant, serum copper and ceruloplasmin, fluorescent treponemal antibody, red cell morphology for acanthocytes	Benign chorea of pregnancy (chorea gravidarium) usually clears following delivery; cases involving violent movements may cause dehydration, malnutrition, or injury and should be seen by a neurologist for consideration of haloperidol or clonazepam
Dystonia	Posturing caused by increased tone in one or more extremities or neck; focal dystonias may cause spastic dysphonia, blepharospasm, or torticollis	Dopamine-blocking agents, idiopathic torsion dystonia	Detailed neurologic examination and consultation	Levodopa/carbidopa, diphenhydramine, consideration for injection of botulinum toxin A or administration of anticholinergic agents
Essential tremor	Oscillating movement of usually 5–10 Hz, accentuated with movement	Familial forms, idiopathic	Detailed neurologic examination	Withdraw tremor-producing medication: xanthines, sympathomimetics; is rarely disabling; in severe cases, may consider propranolol, primidone, or clonazepam

Table 25-16 (*Continued*)

MOVEMENT DISORDERS

Syndrome	Symptoms	Causes	Evaluation	Treatment
Parkinson's tremor	Resting oscillating movement of 3–5 Hz; improves with movement; patients also note difficulty initiating movements; hypokinesia, masklike face, smaller handwriting	Dopamine-blocking agents, vascular disease, idiopathic	Detailed neurologic examination and consultation; MRI for new-onset symptoms	Neurologic consultation

SPINAL CORD INJURY

Chronic spinal cord injury is associated with numerous issues that require a team approach, including the neurologic specialties, obstetrics, and rehabilitative medicine. Spinal cord–injured patients may go into labor and not have any associated pain, especially if the lesion is above T10; therefore it is recommended that these patients be routinely examined after 28 weeks for cervical effacement.[40,41] Spinal cord injury in itself is not an indication for cesarean section. Important issues include respiratory support for cervical lesions, recognition of autonomic instability (autonomic hyperreflexia or autonomic stress syndrome), prevention and early treatment of urinary tract infections, and prevention of unsupervised delivery. Severe autonomic instability can occur if the lesion is above T5–T6 (i.e., above the level of the splanchnic autonomic nerves); it is characterized by uncontrolled hypertension, throbbing headaches, sweating, and flushed skin. Cardiac arrhythmias can occur during labor or as a result of infection.[40,41] Intracranial hemorrhage can result. The use of regional anesthesia is necessary to control blood pressure. Beta blockers may also be helpful.

NEUROPATHY

Most neuropathies are compressive in nature. Table 25-17 lists common compressive neuropathies associated with pregnancy or delivery.[42,43] In general, a new-onset neuropathy requires a detailed neurologic examination to fully localize the lesion and rule out the possibility of a central lesion. Underlying causes of the polyneuropathies such as hypothyroidism or diabetes mellitus should also be excluded. Electromyography and nerve conduction studies may not demonstrate abnormalities until after 3 weeks of symptoms, but they are helpful in diagnosis and aid in predicting recovery.

Guillain-Barré syndrome (acute inflammatory polyradiculoneuropathy) is an inflammatory demyelinating neuropathy that can occur following an infection or surgery. The incidence is approximately 1.5 per 100,000 individuals and the disease course is unchanged by pregnancy.[44] It presents with stocking-glove or patchy numbness and weakness and loss of deep tendon reflexes. Patients can decompensate within hours to ventilatory dependence. The differential diagnosis includes toxic neuropathies, porphyria, vitamin deficiencies (B_{12}, folate), or hypothyroidism. Patients should be monitored closely in the hospital and preferably in the intensive care unit. Early plasma exchange aids in the recovery of neurologic function.[45] Intravenous immunoglobulins may be an alternative to plasma exchange.[46] Pregnant women with Guillain-Barré syndrome may require earlier ventilatory support due to loss of functional reserve capacity.[43] Patients more than 24 weeks pregnant should be positioned in the left lateral decubitus position to avoid compression of the inferior vena cava.

Parsonage Turner syndrome (neuralgic amyotrophy) is characterized by dramatic shoulder and upper extremity pain. The sensory symptoms are followed by weakness, usually involving the shoulder girdle muscles. Patients may require narcotic agents for severe pain. Sensory symptoms generally improve over several weeks, but motor recovery may take months.[47] Patients should be evaluated for possible radiculopathy and other compressive neuropathies.

Lumbosacral plexopathies are most commonly associated with direct compression, although invasive tumor such as choriocarcinoma should be considered. A complete obstetric examination including pelvic ultrasound may aid in the identification of invasive tumor.

Table 25-17

COMPRESSIVE NEUROPATHIES IN PREGNANCY

Nerve	Symptoms	Treatment
Facial (Bell palsy)	Facial weakness Possible hyperacousis Loss of taste Dull ache near the ear	Protect the eye from drying and damage
Median (carpal tunnel syndrome)	Thumb, index, and long finger numbness Wrist and shoulder pain especially at night	Wrist splinting Local injection of corticosteroids

Lateral femoral cutaneous
  (meralgia paresthetica)
	Hyperesthesia, numbness, and pain over
	  the lateral aspect of the thigh
		Local injection of corticosteroids

Femoral	Weakness of knee extension Anterior thigh parasthesia	Physical therapy for aid with gait
Obturator	Weakness of adduction of the thigh Pain of the medial thigh and groin	Physical therapy Nerve block for severe pain

Lumbosacral plexus or sciatic
  (tibial or peroneal portions)
	Weakness of foot dorsi- or plantarflexion
	Low back or shooting pain in posterior
	  leg
		Physical therapy
		Foot orthosis
		(If onset is during delivery, cesarean section may
		  be considered)

Peroneal (at the fibular head)	Foot drop of weakness of dorsiflexion of
	  the foot
	Numbness of anterior lateral lower leg
	  and dorsum of the foot
		Physical therapy
		Foot orthosis

Pudendal	Urinary incontinence Possible pelvic pain	

Women with preexisting peripheral neuropathies, especially diabetes, can present with several autonomic symptoms, such as orthostatic hypotension or gastroparesis.[48] Pregnancy does not appear to change the course of the diabetic neuropathy; control of glucose is the primary therapy.

MYASTHENIA GRAVIS

Myasthenia gravis is characterized by fatigable strength, causing fluctuating symptoms especially of the extraocular, facial, bulbar, and limb muscles. This autoimmune disorder is produced by a polyclonal antibody directed toward the nicotinic acetylcholine receptor and attenuating neuromuscular transmission. Acetylcholinesterase inhibitors such as pyridostigmine increase synaptic acetylcholine concentrations and thus diminish the symptoms related to fewer functional acetylcholine receptors. This disorder affects approximately 1 in 10,000 individuals.[49,50] The disease is more likely to affect women in the third decade, whereas men are more likely to be affected after the fifth decade.[49,50] The diagnosis of myasthenia gravis should be suggested by the history and physical exam. Intravenous edrophonium (10 mg) will often improve the objective clinical findings for a few minutes. Occasionally patients will need single-fiber electromyography studies to demonstrate the neuromuscular junction abnormality.[51] Approximately 80 percent of patients will have antibodies to the acetylcholine receptor, which can be detected on serologic exam.[52]

Pregnant women with myasthenia gravis are at risk for myasthenic or cholinergic crisis during pregnancy and postpartum (Table 25-18).[53] All patients with myasthenia gravis should be closely followed by a neurologist throughout their pregnancies. Approximately one-third of patients are unchanged during pregnancy, one-third improve, and one-third become worse.[52] Mortality rates for myasthenic mothers have been estimated at between 2 and 10 percent.[51] Myasthenic crises or exacerbations are characterized by progressive weakness and fatigability, which may become less responsive to the anticholinesterase therapy. Cholinergic crisis is characterized also by progressive weakness and increased salivation as well as by gastrointestinal hypermobility (vomiting, diarrhea, and abdominal cramping). Severe exacerbations or cholinergic crises can lead to respiratory failure. Myasthenic exacerbations require acute therapy to reduce antibody production. Emergent therapies include plasma exchange or intravenous immunoglobulins.[54,55] Patients also need to be educated about the possible side effects of therapies for myasthenia gravis, such as glucocorticoids, azathioprine, cyclosporine, plasma exchange, intravenous immunoglobulin, and thymectomy.[50,56] Cholinergic crisis results from overmedication with anticholinesterase inhibitors. Patients will require supportive care and a reduction of medication. Table 25-19 lists medications that can interfere with neuromuscular transmission.[57]

Delivery also carries risk for the myasthenic patient. The uterus is composed of smooth muscle, which does not utilize nicotinic receptors. However, the use of striated muscle in the second stage of labor may cause fatigue. Addition of an acetylcholinesterase inhibitor such as pyridostigmine may be helpful. Care should be taken to avoid the possibility of cholinergic crisis from an excess of acetylcholinesterase inhibitor which also produces weakness. During delivery, these medications should be given either intravenously or intramuscularly. Forceps delivery or cesarean section should

Table 25-19

MEDICATIONS THAT INTERFERE WITH NEUROMUSCULAR TRANSMISSION

Aminoglycosides	Magnesium sulfate
Tetracycline	Calcium channel blockers
Narcotics	Beta blockers
Lidocaine and	Quinidine
other local anesthetics	Quinine
Lithium	Neuromuscular blocking agents
Phenothiazines	

be considered early if the myasthenic patient starts to fatigue, but she should be given the opportunity to deliver vaginally if otherwise appropriate.[54] Anesthesia during the delivery should be used under close supervision. Medications such as benzodiazepines and narcotics may reduce the respiratory compensatory mechanism. Regional anesthesia is a safe method, and epidural anesthesia has been used successfully.[54] General anesthesia may be useful in patients undergoing cesarean section. Especially those patients with respiratory or bulbar symptoms need additional time to regain their respiratory competence and ventilatory independence following neuromuscular blockade.

Neonatal myasthenia gravis has been reported in approximately 10 percent of infants born to myasthenic mothers.[53,54] Passive transmission of the antibodies through the placenta accounts for development of the clinical syndrome. Infants usually present with symptoms within 24 h, but some may not show symptoms for 72 h. These infants may demonstrate generalized weakness, poor suck, meager cry, or respiratory distress. They require supportive care, and their condition should improve over the ensuing 3 to 4 weeks. Neonatal myasthenia gravis does not predict the subsequent development of myasthenia as an adult.[60]

Breast-feeding should be discussed with the patient. Antibodies and acetylcholinesterase inhibitors may be passed in the breast milk and thus affect the infant, but several mothers at our center have successfully breast-fed.[53,61] Mothers who are in an exacerbation, have high antibody titers, or who take high doses of medications may wish to avoid breast-feeding.

Table 25-18

MYASTHENIA IN PREGNANCY

During pregnancy	Myasthenic crisis
	Cholinergic crisis
	Medication-induced exacerbation
During delivery	Fatigability
	Increased weakness secondary to anesthetics
	Medication-induced weakness
Breast-feeding	Transfer of medication into milk
	Transfer of antibodies in milk (both of these are of unknown significance)
Postpartum	Neonatal myasthenia
	Hemorrhage
	Myasthenic crisis
	Cholinergic crisis
	Medication-induced exacerbation

MYOPATHY

Preexisting myopathies may have a significant effect on the pregnancy and may result in a variety of clinical problems.[43,56,62,63] Pertinent findings on neurologic exam are proximal muscle weakness, intact deep tendon reflexes, and no sensory deficits. The most treatable myopathies in adults are inflammatory in nature. Inflammatory myopathies such as polymyositis and dermatomyositis attack striated and cardiac muscle. These disorders are associated with a variety of autoimmune, malignant, and connective tissue disorders. New-onset disease can occur at any time but is more common in the first trimester. It is usually active throughout the pregnancy and remission may occur following delivery.[43,56] Preexisting disease is usually unaffected by the pregnancy but may flare especially in the third trimester. Little is known about pregnancy outcome, but in one report on 10 pregnancies in 7 women with polymyositis, there was a 60 percent rate of spontaneous abortion or fetal demise.[64] The benefit of treatment should be weighed against the risk. Patients with mild disease may not require therapy, whereas those with more aggressive disease should be considered for corticosteroid therapy or plasma exchange.[43,56] Patients should be closely comanaged by a neurologist and obstetrician during pregnancy.

MUSCLE CRAMPS

Muscle cramps are relatively common during pregnancy. They usually occur the night following exercise, fatigue, or dehydration. Rarely, cramps indicate an underlying problem such as hypothyroidism, uremia, electrolyte imbalance, amyotrophic lateral sclerosis, polio radiculopathy, or myopathy. Cramps are best treated with stretching of the affected muscle.[43,56]

CONNECTIVE TISSUE DISORDERS IN PREGNANCY

Systemic lupus erythematosus is a disorder predominantly affecting women of childbearing age. Neurologic complications occur in 50 percent of all patients with lupus, including seizures (18 to 70 percent), occlusive infarcts (32 to 43 percent), intracerebral hemorrhage (10 to 40 percent), encephalopathy (4 to 20 percent), myelopathy (2 to 8 percent), headaches (5 to 16 percent), and cranial and peripheral nerve palsies (5 to 10 percent).[65–67] The pathogenesis of this spectrum of disorders is poorly understood.

Lupus is associated with anticardiolipin antibodies and lupus anticoagulant.[65] These antibodies occur in about 50 percent of patients with lupus and predispose to recurrent venous or arterial thrombosis within and outside the CNS.[66,67] These antibodies are also associated with fetal heart block, stillbirth, and recurrent spontaneous abortions related to pla-

cental infarction. Frequently, these antibodies occur independently without lupus but with the same clinical profile. Recent data indicate that these patients require aggressive anticoagulation to prevent recurrent thromboses.

Data on the incidence of relapses during pregnancy are conflicting. The presence of antiphospholipid antibodies, a previous history of second-trimester abortion, and impaired renal function are poor prognostic indicators.[65] There is solid evidence now that patients with antiphospholipid antibodies require long-term anticoagulation.[66,67] Obstetric, neurologic, and rheumatologic consultation is essential for managing these very complicated patients. Other therapeutic options for CNS as well as peripheral disease include glucocorticoids, intravenous immunoglobulins, plasma exchange, azathioprine, and cyclophosphamide.

ACKNOWLEDGMENTS

The authors extend their thanks to Dr. Mauricio Castillo, who supplied the MRI and CT scan images for this chapter.

REFERENCES

1. Feldman E (ed): *Current Diagnosis in Neurology.* St. Louis: Mosby, 1994.
2. Donaldson JO, Lee NS: Arterial and venous stroke associated with pregnancy. *Neurol Clin* 12:3:583, 1994.
3. Wilterdink JL, Easton JD: *Cerebral Ischemia in Neurological Complications of Pregnancy.* New York: Raven Press, 1994, pp 1–23.
4. Carroll VS: Use of heparinoids to treat acute ischemic stroke. *Crit Care Nurs Clin North Am* 5:525, 1993.
5. Terhaar MF, Kaut K: Perinatal superior sagittal sinus venous thrombosis. *J Perinat Neonat Nurs* 7:35, 1993.
6. Dias MS, Selchar LN: Intracranial hemorrhage from aneurysms and arteriovenous malformations during pregnancy and the peurperium. *Neurosurgery* 27:855, 1990.
7. Fox MW, Harms RW, Davis D: Selected neurologic complications of pregnancy. *Mayo Clin Proc* 65:1595, 1990.
8. Kaplan PW, Repke JT: Eclampsia. *Neurol Clin* 12:3;565, 1994.
9. Donaldson JO: The case against magnesium sulfate for eclamptic convulsions. *Int J Obstet Anesth* 1:159, 1992.
10. Hainline B: Headache. *Neurol Clin* 12:443, 1994.
11. Goldstein PJ, Stern BJ (eds): *Neurologic Complications of Pregnancy,* 2d ed. Mount Kisco, NY: Futura, 1992.
12. Welch KMA: Migraine and epilepsy, in Devinsky O, Feldman E, Hainline B (eds): *Neurological Complications of Pregnancy.* New York: Raven Press, 1994, pp 77–82.
13. Reik L: Headaches in pregnancy. *Semin Neurol* 8:187, 1988.

14. Jordan BD: Maternal head trauma during pregnancy. *Adv Neurol* 64:131, 1994.

15. Kuhlmann RS, Cruikshank DP: Maternal trauma during pregnancy. *Clin Obstet Gynecol* 37:274, 1994.

16. Buschsbaum HJ, Cruikshank DP: Postmortem cesarean section, in Buschbaum HJ (ed): *Trauma in Pregnancy.* Philadelphia: Saunders, 1979, pp 236–249.

17. Berg G, Hammar M, Moller-Nielsen J, et al: Low back pain during pregnancy. *Obstet Gynecol* 71:71, 1988.

18. Nwuga VCB: Pregnancy and back pain among upper class Nigerian women. *Aust J Physiother* 28:8, 1982.

19. Hainline B: Low back pain in pregnancy. *Neurol Clin* 12:65, 1994.

20. Fast A, Weiss L, Parik S, Hertz G: Night backache in pregnancy: Hypothetical pathophysiological mechanisms. *Am J Phys Med Rehab* 68:227, 1989.

21. Spankus JD: The cause and treatment of low back pain during pregnancy. *Wis Med J* 64:303, 1965.

22. Caluneri M, Bird HA, Wright V: Changes in joint laxity occurring during pregnancy. *Ann Rheum Dis* 41:126, 1982.

23. Wade J: Obstetrical and gynaecological back and pelvic pains especially those contracted during pregnancy. *Acta Obstet Gynecol Scand* 41(suppl 2):11, 1962.

24. Mantle MJ, Holmes J, Currey HLF: Backache in pregnancy: II. Prophylactic influence of back care classes. *Rheumatol Rehabil* 202:27, 1981.

25. Fitzhugh ML, Newton M: Posture in pregnancy. *Am J Obstet Gynecol* 85:1091, 1963.

26. Yerby M, Devinsky O: Epilepsy and pregnancy, in Devinsky O, Feldman E, Hainline B (eds): *Neurological Complications of Pregnancy.* New York: Raven Press, 1994, pp 45–63.

27. Delgado-Escueta AV, Janz D: Consensus guidelines: Preconception counseling, management and care of the pregnant woman with epilepsy. *Neurology* 42(suppl 5):149, 1992.

28. Hiilesmaa VK: Pregnancy and birth in women with epilepsy. *Neurology* 42(suppl 5):8, 1992.

29. Treiman DM: Current treatment strategies in selected situations in epilepsy. *Epilepsia* 34(suppl 5):S17, 1993.

30. Jagoda A, Riggio S: Emergency department approach to managing seizures in pregnancy. *Ann Emerg Med* 20:80, 1991.

31. DeAngelis LM: Central nervous system neoplasms in pregnancy, in Devinsky O, Feldman E, Hainline B (eds): *Neurological Complications of Pregnancy.* New York: Raven Press, 1994, pp 139–152.

32. Weinreb HJ: Demyelinating and neoplastic diseases in pregnancy. *Neurol Clin* 12:509, 1994.

33. Finfer SR: Management of labour and delivery in patients with intracranial neoplasms. *Br J Anaesth* 67:784, 1991.

34. Prager D, Braunstein GD: Pituitary disorders in pregnancy, in Peterson LJ, Peterson CM (eds): *Endocrine disorders in pregnancy. Endocr Metab Clin North Am* 24:1, 1995.

35. Rogers JD, Fahn S: Movement disorders and pregnancy, in Devinsky O, Feldman E, Hainline B (eds): *Neurological Complications of Pregnancy.* New York: Raven Press, 1994, pp 163–178.

36. Golbe LI: Pregnancy and movement. *Neurol Clin* 12:497, 1994.

37. Birk K, Ford C, Smeltzer S, et al: The clinical course of multiple sclerosis during pregnancy and puerperium. *Arch Neurol* 47:738, 1990.

38. Poser S, Poser W: Multiple sclerosis and gestation. *Neurology* 33:1422, 1983.

39. Frith JA, McLeod JG: Pregnancy and multiple sclerosis. *J Neurol Neurosurg Psychiatry* 51:495, 1988.

40. Verduyn WH: Spinal cord injured women, pregnancy and delivery. *Paraplegia* 24:231, 1986.

41. Greenspoon JS, Paul RH: Paraplegia and quadriplegia: Special considerations during pregnancy and labor and delivery. *Am J Obstet Gynecol* 155:738, 1986.

42. Beric A: Peripheral nerve disorders in pregnancy, in Devinsky O, Feldman E, Hainline B (eds): *Neurological Complications of Pregnancy.* New York: Raven Press, 1994, pp 179–192.

43. Rosenbaum RB, Donaldson JO: Peripheral nerve and neuromuscular disorders. *Neurol Clin* 12:461, 1994.

44. Rodin A, Ferner R, Russell R: Guillain-Barré syndrome in pregnancy and the puerperium. *J Obstet Gynaecol* 9:39, 1988.

45. The Guillain-Barré Syndrome Study Group: Plasmaexchange and acute Guillain-Barré syndrome. *Neurology* 35:1096, 1985.

46. Kleyweg RP, van der Meche Meulstee J: Treatment of Guillain-Barré syndrome with high-dose gamma globulin. *Neurology* 38:1639, 1988.

47. Turner JWA, Parsonage MJ: Neuralgic amyotrophy (paralytis brachial neuritis) with special reference to prognosis. *Lancet* 2:209, 1957.

48. Steel JM: Autonomic neuropathy in pregnancy. *Diabetes Care* 12:170, 1989.

49. Kurtzke JF: Epidemiology of myasthenia gravis. *Adv Neurol* 19:545, 1978.

50. Sanders D, Howard J: Disorders of neuromuscular transmission, in Daroff and Bradley (eds): *Neurological Diseases.* Boston: Butterworth Heinemann, 1996, pp 1983–2002.

51. Sanders DB, Howard JF, Johns TR: Single fiber electromyography in myasthenia gravis. *Neurology* 29:68, 1979.

52. Lindstrom J, Shelton D, Fujii Y: Myasthenia gravis. *Adv Immunol* 42:233, 1988.

53. Plauche WC: Myasthenia gravis in mothers and their newborns. *Clin Obstet Gynaecol* 34:82, 1991.

54. Mitchell PJ, Bebbington M: Myasthenia gravis in pregnancy. *Obstet Gynecol* 80:178, 1992.

55. Esaon G, Landgraf F: Experience with intravenous immunoglobulin in myasthenia gravis: A review. *J Neurol Neurosurg Psychiatry* 57(suppl):55, 1994.

56. Gilchrist JM: Muscle disease in the pregnant woman, in Devinsky O, Feldman E, Hainline B (eds): *Neurological Complications of Pregnancy.* New York: Raven Press, 1994, pp 197–201.

57. Howard J: Adverse drug effects in neuromuscular transmission. *Semin Neurol* 10:89, 1990.

58. Baraka A: Anesthesia and myasthenia gravis. *Can J Anaesth* 39:476, 1992.

59. Breener T, Shahin R, Steiner I, Abramsky O: Presence of antiacetylcholine receptor antibody in human milk: Possible correlation with neonatal myasthenia gravis. *Autoimmunity* 12:315, 1992.

60. Ahlsten G, Lefvert AK, Osterman PO, et al: Follow-up study of muscle function in children of mothers with myasthenia gravis during pregnancy. *J Child Neurol* 7:264, 1992.

61. Varner M: Autoimmune disorders and pregnancy. *Semin Perinatol* 15:238, 1991.

62. Ville Y, Barbet JP, Pomidou A, et al: Limb girdle dystrophy and pregnancy: A case report. *J Gynecol Obstet Biol Reprod* 20:973, 1991.

63. Jaffe R, Mock M, Abramowitz J, Ben-Aderet N: Myotonic dystrophy and pregnancy: A review. *Obstet Gynecol Surv* 41:272, 1986.

64. Gutierrez G, Dagnino R, Mintz G: Polymyositis/dermatomyositis and pregnancy. *Arthritis Rheum* 27:291, 1984.

65. Out HJ, Bruinse HW, Christiaens GC, et al. A prospective, controlled multicenter study on the obstetric risks of pregnant women with antiphospholipid antibody. *Am J Obstet Gynecol* 167:26, 1992.

66. Futrell N, Millikan C: Neurological disorders of pregnancy: Connective tissue disorders. *Neurol Clin* 12:520, 1994.

67. Wong KL, Chan FY, Lee CP: Outcome of pregnancy in patients with systemic lupus erythematosus. *Arch Intern Med* 151:269, 1991.

Chapter 26

DERMATOLOGIC PROBLEMS ASSOCIATED WITH PREGNANCY

Lisa L. May

The cutaneous changes associated with pregnancy can be divided into three major groups: physiologic changes of pregnancy, dermatoses specific to pregnancy, and tumors of pregnancy. Each of these topics is discussed in this chapter. Other common skin eruptions such as allergic contact dermatitis and scabies also occur during pregnancy. Treatment of these disorders may vary from standard treatments, as certain medications should be avoided during pregnancy. This topic is also discussed briefly.

PHYSIOLOGIC CHANGES

Physiologic changes are those that occur so frequently in pregnant patients as to be considered almost normal. They are mentioned only briefly, because they are usually only of esthetic concern, they tend to resolve postpartum, and they rarely require treatment during pregnancy. A list of physiologic changes associated with pregnancy is given in Table 26-1. The three main types of physiologic changes are pigmentary changes, vascular changes, and hair changes.

Hyperpigmentation is one of the most common findings in pregnancy and is most pronounced on the areola, external

genitalia, and linea nigra (Fig. 26-1). Melasma, the "mask of pregnancy," is a specific type of hypermelanosis that occurs as blotchy, irregular pigmentation on the face. Melasma tends to be more pronounced in darker-pigmented skin. It usually regresses by 1 year after delivery. As sunlight may play an etiologic role, sunscreens should be used during pregnancy.[1] Oral contraceptives can exacerbate melasma.[2] Thus patients with pregnancy-associated melasma should be informed of this potential risk, because melasma due to oral contraceptives tends to be more persistent and less responsive to therapy.[3] Persistent melasma (i.e., after pregnancy) can be treated with any one or several of the following therapies: retin-A, hydrocortisone, hydroquinones, azelaic acid, chemical peels, or laser therapy.

Varicosities of the saphenous, vulval, and hemorrhoidal veins are also quite common. Patients should be counseled on ways to minimize these, including leg elevation, exercise, use of compression stockings, and avoidance of prolonged standing or sitting. Pregnancy gingivitis—consisting of erythema, edema, and easy bleeding of the gums—can be seen in 80 percent of pregnancies. This is thought to result from increased venous pressure due to compression by the gravid uterus.

Thickening of scalp hair during pregnancy is rarely a cause for complaint. Postpartum hair loss, however, can be

Table 26-1

PHYSIOLOGIC SKIN CHANGES ASSOCIATED WITH PREGNANCY

Localized hyperpigmentation (areola, genitalia, linea nigra)

Melasma

Striae gravidarum

Vascular
  Spider angiomas
  Palmar erythema
  Varicosities
  Gingivitis

Hair
  Thickening of scalp hair
  Hirsutism
  Postpartum telogen effluvium

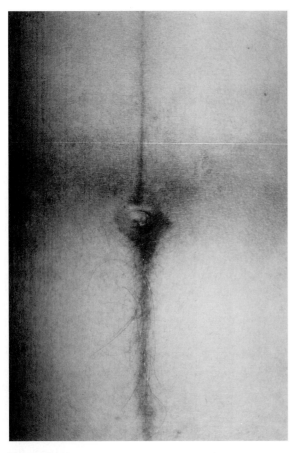

Figure 26-1

Linea nigra. The linea alba becomes darkened during pregnancy and gradually resolves postpartum.

alarming. This postpartum alopecia results from a telogen effluvium, which occurs between 1 and 5 months after delivery. Patients should be reassured that this hair loss is actually a precursor of new hair growth.

HERPES GESTATIONIS

Also known as pemphigoid gestationis, herpes gestationis (HG) is a rare vesiculobullous dermatosis of pregnancy sharing many features with bullous pemphigoid. The incidence is estimated to be between 1 per 1700 and 1 per 5000.[4] It usually develops during the first pregnancy but can begin during any pregnancy. When HG occurs after the first pregnancy, it appears to coincide with a change in sexual partners.[5] Herpes gestationis tends to recur in subsequent pregnancies with an earlier onset and more severe course. Flares with oral contraceptive use and menses also occur.

CLINICAL

This disorder typically begins in the second or third trimester. Initially, intensely pruritic urticarial papules and plaques develop. Tense vesicles and bullae form within these plaques or on normal skin (Fig. 26-2). The lesions may be annular or polycyclic or may even resemble erythema multiforme, with targetoid lesions. The majority of cases begin in the periumbilical region, with the abdomen, thighs, palms, and soles most commonly affected. Mucous membranes and the face are generally spared. These lesions will heal without scarring; however, postinflammatory hyperpigmentation is common.

LABORATORY AND PATHOLOGY

A majority of patients will have a leukocytosis with eosinophilia. Histology shows a subepidermal cleft with an inflammatory infiltrate consisting predominately of eosinophils. Direct immunofluorescence testing demonstrates linear C3 with or without IgG along the basement membrane zone.[6]

PATHOGENESIS

Herpes gestationis is an autoimmune vesiculobullous disease in which antibodies capable of fixing complement are directed against an 180-kDa basement membrane protein known as the *bullous pemphigoid antigen-2*.[7] The inciting event that leads to antibody formation remains unclear but appears to be hormonally influenced.[8]

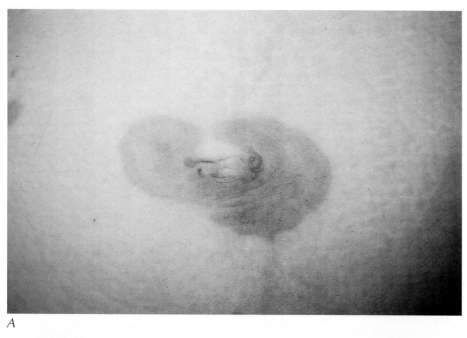

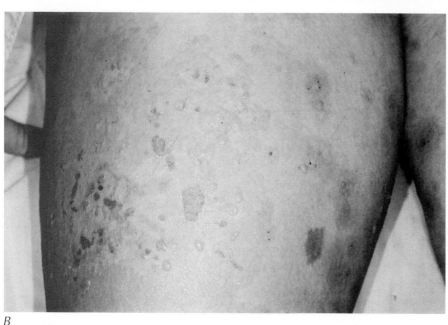

Figure 26-2

Herpes gestationis. *A*. Lesions often begin as urticarial plaques in the periumbilical area. *B*. Bullae and erosions on the thighs.

DIFFERENTIAL DIAGNOSIS

Herpes gestationis is the only pregnancy-associated dermatosis with bullae formation. Other blistering disorders, however, have been reported to begin during pregnancy. These include pemphigus vulgaris, pemphigus foliaceous, bullous drug eruption, and erythema multiforme. Bullous impetigo can certainly occur in pregnancy as well. Bacterial culture can be helpful; however, HG lesions can also become secondarily infected. Thus culture should not be the sole means of differentiating these two entities. Early lesions of HG must also be distinguished from pruritic ur-

ticarial papules and plaques of pregnancy. Pruritic urticarial papules and plaques of pregnancy tend to predominate in striae and to spare the periumbilical area. They may have vesicles, but bullae do not develop. Herpes gestationis may be differentiated from all of the above-mentioned disorders by skin biopsy for histology and direct immunofluorescence.

COURSE AND PROGNOSIS

After HG develops, the disease persists throughout the remainder of the pregnancy. Although flaring around the time of delivery is common, clearing of lesions is usually complete by 3 months after delivery. Patients may have long-lasting postinflammatory hyperpigmentation. Exacerbations may occur with menses, oral contraceptive use, and repeat pregnancies. Maternal prognosis is excellent in pemphigoid gestationis.

Less than 5 percent of newborns will develop vesiculobullous lesions, which, if present, are transient. The question of fetal morbidity and mortality has been debated. Although one report by Lawley showed an increase in fetal mortality,[9] no other studies have confirmed this. Other studies have shown an increase in prematurity and infants that are small for gestational age.[10–12] These patients need to be followed closely with antepartum fetal testing. It is not known whether treatment alters prognosis.

TREATMENT

Mild cases of HG can be treated with antihistamines and topical corticosteroids. Moderate to high doses of prednisone between 40 to 60 mg/day may be required in more severe disease. Complete tapering should not be attempted until after delivery. The patient may also require increased doses of prednisone in the immediate postpartum period to control for flaring of the disease after delivery.[3]

PRURITIC URTICARIAL PAPULES AND PLAQUES OF PREGNANCY

Synonyms include *polymorphic eruption of pregnancy, toxemic rash of pregnancy,* and *papular dermatitis of pregnancy.* This skin condition is a benign pruritic skin eruption of variable morphology developing late in pregnancy. Pruritic urticarial papules and plaques of pregnancy (PUPPP) constitutes the most common dermatosis specific for pregnancy, with an incidence estimated at 1 in 160.[13] This is a disease primarily of the first pregnancy, and 80 percent of patients with PUPPP are primigravidas.

CLINICAL

Pruritic urticarial papules and plaques of pregnancy tends to appear in the late third trimester but can begin anytime from the second trimester to 1 week postpartum. Intensely pruritic, blanchable, erythematous papules and urticarial plaques develop acutely. About 40 percent of patients develop papulovesicles, 20 percent have targetoid lesions, and 18 percent develop annular or polycyclic plaques.[13] The eruption is often confined to the striae initially. It commonly extends to the thighs, buttocks, upper arms, and lower thorax (Fig. 26-3). Despite the intense pruritus, excoriations are infrequent. No systemic manifestations have been reported.

LABORATORY AND PATHOLOGY

No laboratory abnormalities have been reported. Histology shows a nonspecific pattern with a superficial perivascular lymphohistiocytic infiltrate associated with papillary edema, spongiosis, and parakeratosis. Immunofluorescence is negative.

PATHOPHYSIOLOGY

No evidence supports an autoimmune or hormonal etiology. One theory is that the eruption is the result of an inflammatory response to damaged connective tissue in striae.[13] This theory is based on the observation that PUPPP is more likely to occur in patients with excessive maternal and fetal weight gain and in twin pregnancies.

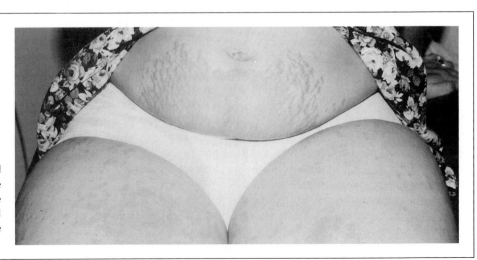

Figure 26-3

Pruritic urticarial papules and plaques of pregnancy. Note the predominance of lesions within the striae, sparing the periumbilical area in this primigravida. The thighs are also involved.

DIFFERENTIAL DIAGNOSIS

Herpes gestationis may initially be urticarial and thus be confused with PUPPP. Clinical differences between these two diseases were discussed previously. Another blistering disease, dermatitis herpetiformis, presents as pruritic vesicles and can be excluded by skin biopsy for histology and immunofluorescence. The targetoid lesions of PUPPP may also resemble erythema multiforme. Unlike erythema multiforme, PUPPP tends to spare the palms, soles, and oral mucosa. Skin biopsy can help differentiate between PUPPP, erythema multiforme, HG, and dermatitis herpetiformis. Scabies can also present as itchy papules and vesicles and thus must also be ruled out.

TREATMENT

Topical corticosteroids and oral antihistamines are usually sufficient to control symptoms. Occasionally, however, oral prednisone may be required.

COURSE AND PROGNOSIS

The eruption improves in 2 to 3 weeks after onset and usually clears quickly in the postpartum period. No maternal or fetal complications have been reported.

IMPETIGO HERPETIFORMIS

Also known as pustular psoriasis of pregnancy, impetigo herpetiformis (IH) is a rare form of pustular psoriasis with an acute onset without an antecedent history of psoriasis. It may be associated with severe maternal and fetal complications. Impetigo herpetiformis is a misnomer in that it is not related to either a bacterial or a herpesvirus infection.

CLINICAL

The onset of IH is usually in the third trimester, but it has been reported to begin as early as the first month.[14] The cutaneous eruption develops acutely and can be accompanied by fever, malaise, nausea, diarrhea, lymphadenopathy, and even tetany secondary to hypocalcemia. Impetigo herpetiformis begins as slightly pruritic erythema that rapidly enlarges and develops rings of pustules at the margins (Fig. 26-4). The pustules break down in the center to leave painful erosions. The eruption initially appears on the thighs, groin, and other intertriginous surfaces and then spreads to other parts of the body. Face, hands, and feet are rarely involved.

LABORATORY AND PATHOLOGY

Leukocytosis is a common finding. Hypocalcemia, hyperphosphatemia, and hypoparathyroidism have been reported and should be checked in patients suspected of having IH.

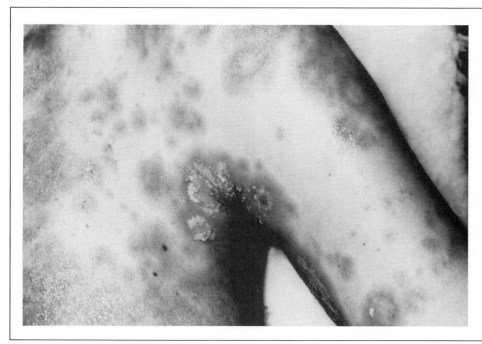

Figure 26-4

Impetigo herpetiformis. Erythematous plaques with pustules at the periphery.

Bacterial cultures of pustules are initially negative but are susceptible to secondary infection. Biopsies demonstrate a histologic picture identical to pustular psoriasis, with spongiform pustules filled with polymorphonuclear leukocytes in the upper layers of the epidermis. Immunofluorescence studies are negative.[3]

DIFFERENTIAL DIAGNOSIS

Herpes gestationis, dermatitis herpetiformis, impetigo, and subcorneal pustular dermatosis have a clinical resemblance to IH and must be excluded. A skin biopsy can help separate these entities, and is necessary to confirm the diagnosis.

PATHOPHYSIOLOGY

The etiology of IH is unknown.

COURSE AND PROGNOSIS

Impetigo herpetiformis tends to worsen as the pregnancy progresses. Resolution occurs rapidly after delivery or termination of pregnancy.

Prior to corticosteroids and antibiotics, maternal and fetal or neonatal deaths were frequent. Maternal mortality is now rare; however, fetal mortality may be increased despite control of the disease in the mother.[15] The etiology of the increased fetal mortality is not clear, although placental insufficiency has been suggested.[15]

TREATMENT

Treatment consists of fluid and electrolyte replacement, corticosteroids, antibiotics if secondary infection occurs, and fetal monitoring. Prednisone at high doses (60 to 80 mg/day) may be necessary. In severe cases with minimal response to the interventions mentioned above and evidence of maternal compromise or fetal distress, termination of the pregnancy may be indicated.[16]

PRURIGO OF PREGNANCY

Prurigo of pregnancy is another pruritic eruption that typically begins on the extremities in early pregnancy. Early-onset prurigo of pregnancy, prurigo gestationis, papular dermatosis of pregnancy, and pruritic folliculitis of pregnancy

are grouped under this diagnosis. Prurigo of pregnancy has been estimated to involve about 1 in every 300 pregnancies.[17] Its onset is usually during the second or third trimester, in contrast to PUPPP, which tends to occur in the last several weeks of pregnancy.

CLINICAL

Prurigo of pregnancy usually occurs on the extensor surfaces of the extremities as discrete excoriated or crusted papules (Fig. 26-5). Follicular involvement is variable. Pustules may be seen but vesicles are not.

LABORATORY AND PATHOLOGY

No laboratory abnormalities have been reported. Histology shows a nonspecific pattern with dermal edema, a lymphohistiocytic infiltrate with capillary damage but not vasculitis, spongiosis, parakeratosis, or crust formation.

PATHOPHYSIOLOGY

The etiology is unknown.

DIFFERENTIAL DIAGNOSIS

An earlier onset with a predilection for the extremities and lack of involvement of the striae favor the diagnosis of prurigo of pregnancy over PUPPP. Unlike PUPPP, the lesions of prurigo of pregnancy are often excoriated. If primary lesions are not present, these excoriations should be separated from cholestasis of pregnancy. Furthermore, cutaneous disorders not specific to pregnancy also enter into the diagnosis. In particular, scabies, contact dermatitis, and drug eruptions should be excluded.

COURSE AND PROGNOSIS

The eruption may continue for up to 3 months postpartum and may recur during subsequent pregnancies.[1] Prurigo of pregnancy is not associated with an increase in maternal or fetal morbidity or mortality.

TREATMENT

Treatment is symptomatic and consists of emollients, non-fluorinated topical corticosteroids, and oral antihistamines.

Figure 26-5

Prurigo of pregnancy. Note the excoriated discrete papules.

CHOLESTASIS OF PREGNANCY

Although not a disorder specific to the skin, cholestasis of pregnancy must be discussed in reviewing cutaneous disorders of pregnancy, because this entity should not be overlooked. Cholestasis of pregnancy is characterized by onset of pruritus during pregnancy with or without jaundice in the absence of primary cutaneous lesions. A mild anicteric form of cholestasis of pregnancy is often referred to as *pruritus gravidarum.* Cholestasis of pregnancy affects approximately 1 in 150 to 1 in 1300 pregnancies.[18,19] It is uncommon in Asians and African Americans but very common in Scandinavians and Chileans. About 15 percent of patients report a positive family history.[20]

CLINICAL

Pruritus begins in the second or third trimester and persists until delivery. Generalized excoriations may be the only overt sign of disease. The number of patients developing jaundice varies greatly from as high as 67 percent to less than 10 percent.[20]

LABORATORY AND HISTOLOGY

Serum bile acids are considered the most sensitive diagnostic test, with three times elevated levels in all women suspected of having cholestasis of pregnancy.[21] Of the routine liver function tests, alkaline phosphatase and aspartate aminotransferase

(AST) were the most sensitive, with mildly increased levels (less than four times normal) in approximately one-third of patients tested.[20] Bilirubin is elevated, but usually not above 5 mg/dL. Most is the direct, conjugated form. Hepatic ultrasonography is normal. A skin biopsy is not useful because no primary cutaneous lesions are present.

DIFFERENTIAL DIAGNOSIS

These patients do not have primary cutaneous lesions; thus if lesions other than excoriations are present, one must search for an alternative diagnosis. Other causes of jaundice and elevated liver function tests, especially viral or drug-induced hepatitis or gall bladder disease, should be excluded.

PATHOPHYSIOLOGY

Cholestasis of pregnancy is thought to result from estrogen and progesterone interference with hepatic excretion of bile acids. A genetic predisposition appears to exist.[1]

COURSE AND PROGNOSIS

The symptoms of cholestasis of pregnancy resolve rapidly after delivery; however, abnormal liver function tests may take 4 weeks to return to normal.[21] The condition may recur with subsequent pregnancies and oral contraceptive use.

Complications in the mother are low in cases of minimal

liver dysfunction, as evidenced by normal or minimal elevations of liver function tests and no sign of jaundice. Some studies have found a significantly higher incidence of preterm labor, fetal distress, low birth weight, and stillbirth.[22]

TREATMENT

In mild cases, emollients and antihistamines may be helpful. Cholestyramine (12 g/day in 3 to 4 divided doses) may be helpful in some patients. Because it is not absorbed, it is not harmful to the fetus; however cholestyramine prevents adsorption of fat-soluble vitamins (especially vitamin K), so a prothrombin time (PT) should be monitored. If the PT is prolonged, parenteral vitamin K should be administered. Because of the potential risk of fetal problems, these patients should be monitored closely during the third trimester.

SKIN TUMORS ASSOCIATED WITH PREGNANCY

GRANULOMA GRAVIDARUM

Granuloma gravidarum is a pyogenic granuloma occurring most commonly in the oral cavity. It typically presents as a friable red papule or nodule on the gingival surface next to a tooth or between two teeth (Fig. 26-6). Gingivitis is often present. The treatment for these lesions is surgical excision. Without treatment, the lesion usually regresses postpartum.

NEVI AND MALIGNANT MELANOMA

Nevi have been reported to undergo enlargement or color change by patient history in approximately one-third of pregnancies. When skin biopsies were performed on these lesions, there was no statistically significant level of atypia as compared with non-pregnant controls.[23] This finding implies that atypical change during pregnancy is uncommon.[24] Although subjective data suggest change in nevi during pregnancy, no objective prospective studies have been performed to date to document this change. Nevertheless, changing pigmented lesions with any atypical features should be biopsied to rule out the possibility of malignant melanoma.

The influence of previous, current, and subsequent pregnancies on the prognosis of malignant melanoma has also been debated. Numerous case reports have described development or rapid progression of melanoma during pregnancy. However, controlled studies have demonstrated increased tumor thickness at the time of diagnosis and a shorter disease-free interval but no difference in 5-year survival.[24] One study even showed a slightly better prognosis in those diagnosed during pregnancy.[25] The mechanism for the increased thickness of melanoma seen in pregnancy is unknown. Several theories have been proposed, including delay in diagnosis during pregnancy, an increase in hormones or growth factors, or a decrease in immune surveillance during pregnancy. Although few controlled studies have been performed, pregnancy prior to or after the development of melanoma does not seem to worsen the prognosis. Because the likelihood of recurrence is greatest during the first 2 years after the diagnosis of melanoma is made, it has been recommended that pregnancy be avoided during this time.[24]

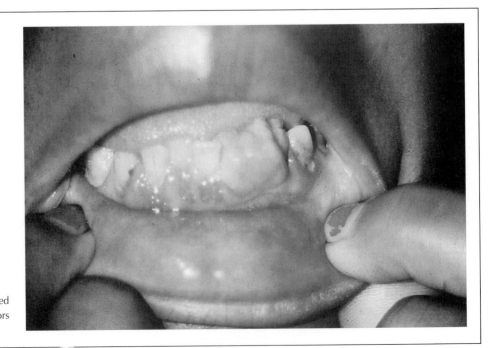

Figure 26-6

Granuloma gravidarum. Bright red papule located between incisors with background gingivitis.

TREATMENT DURING PREGNANCY

As in the case of any treatment during pregnancy, caution must be used in selecting a medication because of potential teratogenic or perinatal risks. A firm diagnosis must be established and the potential risks of a given therapy weighed carefully against potential benefits. This is especially important in dermatology, where diseases may be short-lived, have minimal morbidity, be cosmetic in nature, or can have treatment delayed until after delivery.

TOPICAL THERAPY

Some of the topical preparations that should be avoided in pregnancy include retinoids, salicylic acid, tar compounds, silver sulfadiazine (to large surface areas), podophyllin, and lindane. Two case reports in the literature suggest topical retinoids (Retin-A, Renova, Differin) can cause the same congenital malformations as those seen with Accutane.[26] Topical erythromycin and benzoyl peroxide can probably be used safely during pregnancy.

Topical corticosteroid use during pregnancy has not been associated with unfavorable outcomes. Low-potency nonfluorinated topical corticosteroids are thus considered safe and effective. Concern does exist, however, over the application of fluorinated topical corticosteroids to large surface areas. This caution is based on the effects of systemically administered glucocorticoids. The fluorinated glucocorticoids more readily cross the placenta and may be associated with a reduction in fetal growth.[27] Oral glucocorticoids like prednisone may be preferred in instances where large surface areas of skin are involved in the disease process (e.g., extensive allergic contact dermatitis).

ORAL THERAPY

Commonly used oral medications that should be avoided include tetracycline and related compounds as well as sulfonamides (near term). Oral retinoids (Accutane) have devastating teratogenic effects and are contraindicated during pregnancy. Oral antihistamines are probably safe to use during pregnancy.[27]

References

1. Demis DJ: *Clinical Dermatology.* New York: Harper & Row, 1997, Section 29-1, pp 1–18.
2. Resnick S: Melasma induced by oral contraceptive drugs. *JAMA* 199:95, 1967.
3. Winton GB, Lewis CW: Dermatoses of pregnancy. *J Am Acad Dermatol* 6:977, 1992.
4. Roger D, Vaillant L, Fignon A, et al: Specific pruritic diseases of pregnancy. *Arch Dermatol* 130:734, 1994.
5. Holmes RC, Black MM, Jeurecka W, et al: Clues to the aetiology and pathogenesis of herpes gestationis. *Br J Dermatol* 109:131, 1983.
6. Bushkell LL, Jordon RE, Goltz RW: Herpes gestationis. *Arch Dermatol* 110:65, 1974.
7. Morrison LH, Labib RS, et al: Herpes gestationis autoantibody recognize a 180kD human epidermal antigen. *J Clin Invest* 81:2023, 1988.
8. Lynch FW, Albrecht RJ: Hormonal factors in herpes gestationis. *Arch Dermatol* 93:446, 1966.
9. Lawley TJ, Stingl G, Katz SI: Fetal and maternal risk factors in herpes gestationis. *Arch Dermatol* 114:552, 1978.
10. Holmes RC, Black MM, Dann J, et al: A comparative study of toxic erythema of pregnancy and herpes gestationis. *Br J Dermatol* 106:499, 1982.
11. Shornick JK, Bangert JL, Freeman RG, et al: Herpes gestationis: Clinical and histologic features of twenty-eight cases. *J Am Acad Dermatol* 8:214, 1983.
12. Holmes RC, Black MM: The fetal prognosis in pemphigoid (herpes) gestationis. *Br J Dermatol* 110:67, 1984.
13. Holmes RC: Polymorphic eruption of pregnancy. *Semin Dermatol* 8:18, 1989.
14. Gligora M, Kolacio Z: Hormonal treatment of impetigo herpetiformis. *Br J Dermatol* 107:253, 1982.
15. Beveridge GW, Harkness RA, Livingston JRB: Impetigo herpetiformis in two successive pregnancies. *Br J Dermatol* 78:106, 1966.
16. Wolf Y, Groutz A, Walmar I, et al: Impetigo herpetiformis during pregnancy: Case report and review of the literature. *Acta Obstet Gynecol Scand* 74:229, 1995.
17. Black MM: Prurigo of pregnancy, papular dermatitis of pregnancy and pruritic folliculitis of pregnancy. *Semin Dermatol* 8:23, 1989.
18. Johnston WG, Baskett TF: Obstetric cholestasis. *Am J Obstet Gynecol* 133:299, 1979.
19. Wilson BR, Havercamp AD: Cholestatic jaundice of pregnancy: New perspectives. *Am J Obstet Gynecol* 54:650, 1979.
20. Berg B, Helm G, Petersohn L, Tryding N: Cholestasis of pregnancy. *Acta Obset Gynecol Scand* 65:107, 1986.
21. Shaw W, Frohlich J, Bernd AKW, Willms M: A prospective study of 18 patients with cholestasis of pregnancy. *Am J Obstet Gynecol* 142:621, 1982.
22. Johnson MB, Baskett TF: Obstetric cholestasis: A 14-year review. *Am J Obstet Gynecol* 133:299, 1979.
23. Foucar E, Bentley TJ, Laube DW, Rosai J: A histopathologic evaluation of nevocellular nevi in pregnancy. *Arch Dermatol* 121:350, 1985.
24. Driscoll MS, Grin-Jorgensen GM, Grant-Kels JM: Does pregnancy influence the prognosis of malignant melanoma? *J Am Acad Dermatol* 29:619, 1993.
25. Travers RL, Sober AJ, et al: Increased thickness of pregnancy-associated melanoma. *Br J Dermatol* 132:876, 1995.
26. Lipson AH, Collins F, Wester WS: Multiple congenital defects associated with maternal use of topical tretinoin. *Lancet* 314:1382, 1993.
27. Robert E, Scialli AR: Topical medications during pregnancy. *Reprod Toxicol* 8:197, 1994.

Chapter 27

MENTAL DISORDERS IN PREGNANCY AND THE POSTPARTUM PERIOD

Diana L. Dell
Diana O. Perkins
Linda M. Nicholas

The medical literature has often characterized a woman's pregnancy year as an emotionally quiet time, emphasizing its potential joys. As a result, psychiatric complications associated with pregnancy and the postpartum period are among the most underdiagnosed pregnancy-associated complications in modern obstetrics. Most often, a woman who develops symptoms of a mental illness during pregnancy or the postpartum period will first present to her primary-care physician. Life-threatening symptoms, including suicidality, mania, and psychotic symptoms often present in the emergency department setting. Recognition and treatment of psychiatric illness are essential for the proper care of pregnant and postpartum women.

MOOD DISORDERS

DESCRIPTION

The word *depression* can describe a wide range of conditions in pregnant as well as nonpregnant women. Depressed mood may reflect a normal reaction to loss or bereavement.

It may occur in response to adverse life events over which one has no control. It may also reflect a major depressive disorder, which is a serious but treatable condition. Therefore, the differential diagnosis of depressed mood is essential to the appropriate management and protection of the patient.

MAJOR DEPRESSIVE DISORDER

An episode of major depression may occur in the context of either major depressive disorder or bipolar disorder. It may develop in response to stressful life events or in the absence of a precipitating event. Symptoms reflect disturbance of biological functions, cognitive functions, and psychological well-being (Table 27-1). During an episode of major depression, behaviors governed by circadian rhythms—such as sleep, appetite, and energy level—are frequently disturbed. Depressed patients may have difficulty falling asleep; they may also experience early morning awakening or an increased need for sleep. Patients may report increased fatigue regardless of time spent sleeping. Changes related to eating include loss of appetite and weight; in severe cases, patients

Table 27-1

CRITERIA FOR MAJOR DEPRESSIVE EPISODE

A. Five (or more) of the following symptoms have been present during the same 2-week period, nearly every day, and represent a change from previous functioning; *at least one of the symptoms is either* (1) *depressed mood or* (2) *loss of interest or pleasure;*

   1. **Depressed mood most of the day, by subjective report (e.g., feels sad or empty) or observation made by others (e.g., appears tearful).** *Note:* **In children and adolescents, can be irritable mood.**

   2. **Markedly diminished interest or pleasure in all, or almost all, activities most of the day, by subjective report or observation** and 3 or 4 of the following, experienced nearly every day.

   3. Significant weight loss when not dieting or weight gain (e.g., a change of more than 5% of body weight in a month) or decrease or increase in appetite.

   4. Insomnia or hypersomnia.

   5. Psychomotor agitation or retardation (observable by others, not merely subjective feelings of restlessness or being slowed down).

   6. Fatigue or loss of energy.

   7. Feelings of worthlessness or excessive or inappropriate guilt (which may be delusional) (not merely self-reproach or guilt about being sick).

   8. Diminished ability to think or concentrate, or indecisiveness (either by subjective account or as observed by others).

   9. Recurrent thoughts of death (not just fear of dying), recurrent suicidal ideation without a specific plan, or a suicide attempt or a specific plan for committing suicide.

B. The symptoms do not meet criteria for a mixed episode.

C. The symptoms cause clinically significant distress or impairment in social, occupational, or other important areas of functioning.

D. The symptoms are not due to the direct physiologic effects of substance abuse, medication, or a general medical condition.

E. The symptoms are not better accounted for by bereavement, the symptoms persist for longer than 2 months, or are characterized by marked functional impairment, morbid preoccupation with worthlessness, suicidal ideation, psychotic symptoms, or psychomotor retardation.

Note: Do not include symptoms that are clearly due to a general medical condition or mood-incongruent delusions or hallucinations.
Source: American Psychiatric Association,[1] with permission.

---

may stop eating and drinking altogether. A subset of depressed patients may report symptoms of increased appetite and excessive weight gain. While not considered diagnostic of a major depression, gastrointestinal pain, bloating, belching, and constipation are also common symptoms in patients with major depression.

Cognitive changes generally affect attention and concentration. Patients complain of difficulty in organizing tasks, inability to complete assigned duties, and lack of mental energy. Thought content often reflects a sustained low mood, with pessimistic ideation about oneself, the world, and the future. A patient may show cognitive and motor slowing as well.

An impaired sense of psychological well-being may be reflected in pervasive worry or guilt about present or past events. A pervasive sense of worthlessness may reach delusional intensity. Active concerns about one's physical health are common, which may reflect a misunderstanding of the biological changes that occur with major depression. Patients with major depressive disorder always complain of a dysphoric mood (e.g., feeling "low," "down," "blue"), decreased interest in their usual activities, or inability to experience pleasure. This decline in interest often includes decreased interest in sexual activity. Importantly, thoughts about death or suicide occur frequently in major depressive disorder.

Severe major depressive disorder may also be associated with psychotic symptoms such as hallucinations or paranoid ideation. Psychotic symptoms may be the presenting feature of a major depressive illness or may be symptomatic of other medical conditions, as discussed below. These symptoms usually represent a medical emergency, often requiring immediate hospitalization.

BIPOLAR DISORDER

Bipolar disorder is evidenced by episodes of mania as well as symptoms of major depression. Mania is characterized by an expansive, elevated, elated, euphoric, or irritable mood. Cognitively, the patient experiences racing thoughts, flight of ideas, inflated self-esteem, grandiosity, distractibility, and sometimes delusions or hallucinations. His or her behavior may be marked by increased activity, excessive spending, pressured speech, intrusiveness, indiscretion, sexual promiscuity, and/or poor judgment. The patient often has decreased physical complaints, a decreased need for sleep, and increased energy. Hypomania is a milder form of these symptoms that, although less associated with impaired function, can also be quite disruptive. Treatment options for mania are discussed under treatment of psychotic disorders.

ADJUSTMENT DISORDERS

In modern psychiatry, disorders are defined by the scope, severity, and longevity of symptoms. At times a patient who is overwhelmed by a stressful life event may develop some of the characteristic symptoms of a major depression (e.g., depressed mood, trouble falling asleep) without meeting the full criteria. Here, a diagnosis of adjustment disorder with depressed mood may be more appropriate.[1] The diagnostic criteria for adjustment disorder are included in Table 27-2. Major depressive disorder is distinguished from adjustment disorder by (1) the number and severity of symptoms and (2) the fact that adjustment disorder is always a reaction to stressful life events, whereas major depressive disorder often occurs without a precipitating life event.

BEREAVEMENT

In response to loss or bereavement, patients may experience symptoms similar to those of a major depressive episode. Symptoms such as loss of appetite and insomnia may become severe, interfering with function. Normal grief reactions usually improve with time. When symptoms persist longer than 2 months, a major depression may have developed, and antidepressant treatment must be considered. Cultural values often serve to interpret "normality" for the duration and intensity of these symptoms.

NORMAL ADJUSTMENT TO PREGNANCY

The physical adjustment to the hormonal and physical changes associated with pregnancy may include fluctuations of mood, including sadness, unexplained tearfulness, or irritability (a condition sometimes referred to as "raging hormones" by patients or their partners). In addition, the pregnant patient may experience strong feelings about her pregnancy, including ambivalence about the changes pregnancy has made in her life. She may experience grief over the anticipated loss of her usual lifestyle and independence. These experiences are not pathologic but may be experienced as disruptive. Counseling explaining the normal change in mood is often helpful to reassure the pregnant woman.

EPIDEMIOLOGY OF MOOD DISORDERS IN PREGNANCY

Major depression is the most common psychiatric disorder among reproductive-age women. Its lifetime prevalence in the United States is between 9 and 20 percent.[2] Persons between the ages of 25 and 44 are at greatest risk, and rates for women are twice as high as those for men. It is estimated

---

Table 27-2

DIAGNOSTIC CRITERIA FOR ADJUSTMENT DISORDERS

A. The development of emotional or behavioral symptoms in response to an identifiable stressor(s) occurring within 3 months of the onset of the stressor(s).

B. These symptoms or behaviors are clinically significant as evidenced by either of the following:
1. Marked distress that is in excess of what would be expected from exposure to the stressor
2. Significant impairment in social or occupational (academic) functioning

C. The stress-related disturbance does not meet the criteria for another specific axis I disorder and is not merely an exacerbation of a preexisting axis I or axis II disorder.

D. The symptoms do not represent bereavement.

E. Once the stressor (or its consequences) has terminated, the symptoms do not persist for more than an additional 6 months.

Specify:
Acute: If the disturbance lasts less than 6 months
Chronic: If the disturbance lasts for 6 months or longer

Source: American Psychiatric Association,[1] with permission.

that 6.4 million U.S. women may have some form of depressive illness during any 6-month period.[3] The underdiagnosis of depression in women is a significant public health problem.

The incidence of depressive illness does not appear to increase during pregnancy, but it is no longer believed that the pregnant state provides protection against depressive illness. Since pregnancy does not confer protective benefits, the incidence of depression during pregnancy mirrors that in the general female population. Circumstances that may correlate with increased risk for depressive illness during pregnancy include a previous history of depressive illness, a positive family history, comorbid psychiatric diagnosis, development of a "high risk" pregnancy, detection of a fetal anomaly, prior pregnancy loss, inadequate social support, inadequate finances, a changing relationship with spouse and/or mother, and multiple changes in life events.[4] The period of greatest risk for major depression is during the first 9 weeks after delivery.[5] Risk of adjustment disorders may also be increased during pregnancy. Childbearing is a stressful life event for most women. Even when pregnancy is viewed as a positive, desired event, major life adjustments will be required throughout the pregnancy and postpartum period. Early identification and intervention in a woman experiencing an adjustment disorder may prevent the development of major depressive disorder.

ASSESSMENT OF DEPRESSIVE SYMPTOMS IN PREGNANCY

Complicating the diagnosis of major depression during pregnancy is the fact that many symptoms of major depression—such as trouble sleeping, fatigue, irritability, change in appetite, excessive nausea and vomiting, and poor concentration—are also common to the physical burden of pregnancy. The presence of any of these symptoms should prompt the clinician to inquire about other depressive symptoms. In particular, when a woman fails to meet the expected weight gain during pregnancy, major depressive disorder should be considered in the differential diagnosis. Routine screening for major depression in patients complaining of these symptoms is quick and simple. Table 27-3 gives examples of brief screening questions useful in assessing the hallmark symptoms of depressed mood and/or anhedonia. A positive response to any of these questions warrants a more careful evaluation. When a major depression occurs during pregnancy, the two most serious concerns that must be assessed are adequate nutrition and suicide risk.[4]

Often, a woman may be unwilling to discuss depressive symptoms with her physician spontaneously. A pregnant woman who begins to feel sadness or despair is often reluctant to mention these symptoms. She may not recognize the presence of a treatable disorder or may be hesitant to reveal what may be perceived as "unacceptable" feelings.

Medical conditions associated with depressive symptoms include thyroid disease, anemia, Vitamin B_{12} deficiency, folate deficiency, autoimmune disease, and substance abuse disorders. Physical examination and appropriate laboratory studies will rule out most of these causes of depressive symptoms (Table 27-4). As discussed below, evaluation for substance abuse should be part of routine management during prenatal care.

Women with a past history of major depressive disorder or mania are at high risk for recurrence of symptoms during the postpartum period. Practitioners should routinely ask about previous depression/mania in the initial prenatal evaluation. If this history is elicited, educational counseling during pregnancy should include early identification of symptoms. In addition, all routine obstetric visits should include screening for these warning signs, because the woman may not recognize the recurrence of depression.

Table 27-3

SCREENING QUESTIONS FOR MAJOR DEPRESSIVE DISORDER AND SUICIDALITY

For depressed mood:
Have you been feeling depressed or down most of the day, nearly every day?
If yes: Has that lasted for as long as 2 weeks?

For anhedonia:
Have you been a lot less interested in most things?
Are things a lot less enjoyable than they used to be? (Are things as much fun as they used to be?)
If yes: Has that lasted for as long as 2 weeks?

For suicidality:
Have things been so bad that you have been thinking you would be better off dead? Have you thought of actually killing yourself?
If yes: Have you thought of how you might kill yourself?

Source: First et al.,[45] with permission.

Table 27-4

LABORATORY EVALUATION OF DEPRESSIVE SYMPTOMS

Thyroid-stimulating hormone
Complete blood count
Level of vitamin B_{12}
Level of folate
Venereal Disease Research Laboratory testing (VDRL)
Toxicology screen
Serum chemistry (including liver and renal function)
Human immunodeficiency virus

DEPRESSIVE ILLNESS IN THE POSTPARTUM PERIOD

POSTPARTUM BLUES

It is not unusual for a woman to "get the blues" after delivery. The postpartum period may be characterized by mild subjective depression, affective lability, irritability, anxiety, and fatigue, often beginning on the third or fourth postpartum day. These symptoms usually remit within 1 to 2 days and may recur over the first few postpartum weeks. Brief supportive interventions to assess the patient's ability to cope with the demands of parenting and the adequacy of her support system usually suffice. Some women may need assistance with child care. A sleep-promoting agent, such as zolpidem, may help the new mother adjust to the disturbances in the sleep cycle that infant care often imposes.[6]

POSTPARTUM DEPRESSION

In contrast to postpartum blues, major depressive disorder with onset during the puerperium is a much more serious illness, with major implications for both mother and infant. The exact prevalence of postpartum depression is difficult to define since recent studies have found similar rates of depression in childbearing women and nonchildbearing controls.[7] It appears that in women with biological vulnerability to major depression, however, the postpartum period is a particularly high-risk period for emergence of symptoms. The onset of depressive symptoms in childbearing women is strongly clustered within the first 5 weeks postpartum.[5] Women with a history of a major depression or alcohol dependence prior to pregnancy are at particularly high risk of developing postpartum depression. In one study, 24 percent of women with a past major depression developed a postpartum major depression, compared with only 3 percent of women with no prior history.[5]

GRIEF RESPONSES TO PREGNANCY LOSS

Parents may begin forming attachments to the anticipated child very early in the pregnancy; however, fetal loss is common. Approximately 20 percent of recognized pregnancies are spontaneously lost in the first trimester and early second trimester. Additionally, there are 1.5 million induced abortions per year in the United States.[8] Grieving may be difficult after a miscarriage or stillbirth, since societal norms often do not validate the experience in a way that facilitates healing of the loss. Parents may grieve over the spontaneous loss of a 6-week fetus or a stillborn infant as intensely as they would grieve over any other major loss in their lives. For many young parents, it may be the first significant loss they experience.

Grieving following miscarriage or stillbirth is similar to the grieving process that follows the loss of a child. The normal process of bereavement may take up to 2 years to resolve. Abnormalities of bereavement may involve delayed onset of grief, symptoms that are more intense than usually encountered, prolonged symptoms, or "getting stuck" in one of the stages. The process of bereavement is more difficult when death is unexpected,[9] as typically occurs with miscarriage. It is also more difficult when the pregnancy was surrounded by marked ambivalence or when there are unresolved issues related to the events surrounding the pregnancy loss. Women who have experienced pregnancy loss have higher rates of depression, anxiety, and somatization during the first 6 months, compared to women who have given birth to live infants.[10] Support groups have been widely utilized and appear to be among the most helpful modalities for patients and their partners during this stressful life event.

When first told of the fetal death or major fetal anomaly, many parents experience shock and emotional numbing. They may express an unrealistic sense that "this is not really happening" and respond with denial and disbelief. If the obstetric condition is not an emergency, it can be very important at this stage to allow parents time to make an initial accommodation to their loss. They should be encouraged to make as many choices about the proposed obstetric intervention as feasible. This restores some sense of control in a situation where the parents may feel out of control. Clinical interventions may help them to go through the grief process. In particular, parents should be supported if they wish to see the products of conception after evacuation of the uterus. They should be encouraged to see and hold the stillborn infant after delivery; this is the only time they will ever have with their child. Seeing and holding it facilitates appropriate grieving by letting the parents claim the infant and establishing the reality of the loss. Photographs of the infant should be held on file in the event that the parents should want them after time has passed.[11]

As the experience becomes more "real," and the parents look for a reason for the loss, a searching stage emerges. This may take many forms: blaming themselves, blaming the caretakers or hospital, blaming God. The parents may experience vivid dreams about the baby or the birth process. Hallucinations or illusions of hearing an infant crying are not uncommon and are not considered pathologic. Parents may openly or unconsciously blame each other, which inhibits the grieving process and their ability to comfort each another. They may experience hostility toward other pregnant women and jealousy toward their live-born infants. They need to be assured that this is a normal experience and that it will lessen with the passage of time.[11]

With increasing acceptance of the loss comes disorientation. It often occurs some time after the death of the fetus/neonate. Social isolation by virtue of sadness and despair are common. Support groups of other patients and partners who have experienced perinatal loss are especially helpful at this stage. Major depression may develop, and patients may benefit from appropriate interventions. In particular, if disruption of occupational or academic functioning is severe or ongoing, psychotherapy and/or the use of antidepressants may be indicated. As time passes, an ongoing reorganization takes place: the parents begin to integrate the loss and return to their normal activities.[11]

PSYCHIATRIC COMPLICATIONS OF UNPLANNED PREGNANCY AND ABORTION

Unplanned pregnancies are common, with more than 6 million women becoming pregnant each year—roughly 11 percent of all reproductive-age women. Over half of all pregnancies are unintended or mistimed and about half of them will be electively aborted. Detection of an unwanted or mistimed pregnancy may precipitate an emotional crisis for the mother. Especially for the adolescent who becomes pregnant, issues relating to the discussion of sexuality with her parents, deciding whether to abort or carry the fetus, and the limited availability of reproductive services may result in debilitating ambivalence, disturbances of sleep or appetite, and suicide.[12]

Unplanned pregnancies are often more stressful than planned ones and pose a greater risk of an adverse outcome. For example, an unwanted pregnancy may lead to economic hardships. Often, the mother may delay receiving prenatal care and may not be compliant with medical recommendations. In particular, the fetus may be more likely to be exposed to harmful substances like tobacco and alcohol. The child produced by an unwanted pregnancy, as distinguished from a mistimed one, is at greater risk of being born at a low birth weight, of dying within its first year of life, of being abused, and of not receiving sufficient resources for healthy development.[12]

Before abortion was legalized, there was an accumulation of case reports of psychological impairment secondary to the abortion events (e.g., extreme pain, fear of dying, rape by the abortion provider).[13] Since abortion was legalized in 1972, most studies show that such negative emotional effects are usually transient.[14] Patients are at higher risk for depressive symptoms (usually as part of an adjustment disorder) following induced abortion if they (1) were pressured or coerced into abortion, (2) had marked ambivalence about their decision, (3) have limited social support, and (4) have had prior psychiatric illness.[12] Postpartum depression can occur following both spontaneous and induced abortion, at rates that are comparable to those noted during the postpartum period following live birth.

TREATMENT OF MAJOR DEPRESSION DURING PREGNANCY AND LACTATION

Issues with regard to treatment of the pregnant woman with major depression are centered around a complicated risk/benefit analysis. The clinician must consider the potential risk of the therapeutic modality to the fetus versus the risks to both the mother and fetus when the psychiatric disorder goes untreated.[4]

The most significant risks of untreated major depressive disorder include suicide, nutritional impairment secondary to disturbed appetite, and neglect of self-care, including poor compliance with prenatal and postpartum medical care. During the postpartum period, a woman with a major depression is at increased risk for neglect of her infant. In addition, major depression during pregnancy may have negative behavioral effects on the newborn, especially in causing neonatal irritability.[15] These are potentially serious and life-threatening sequelae that necessitate careful evaluation and appropriate intervention.

Treatment is usually done in an outpatient setting, although hospitalization must be considered when serious suicidal ideation is present or when the patient is incapacitated. Evaluation for suicidality begins with asking the patient about suicidal ideation, since patients are often reluctant to volunteer that information. Emergency psychiatric evaluation is mandated when suicidal ideation is present or suspected. Family members may be helpful in assessing suicidal potential.

Major depressive disorder responds to pharmacologic treatment and, when symptoms are mild to moderate, to cognitive behavioral therapy. The risks and benefits of both interventions should be discussed with the patient. Psychotherapy poses no risks to the fetus; often, a pregnant woman will choose a trial of cognitive therapy prior to pharmacologic treatment. Referral to an experienced therapist (psychiatrist, psychologist, or social worker) is appropriate when the primary-care clinician is not trained to do cognitively based psychotherapy. Patients will usually respond within 6 to 8 weeks of therapy. Other nonpharmacologic treatments that may be appropriate include light therapy (if the patient consistently becomes depressed in the winter) and sleep deprivation. Failure to respond to psychotherapy increases the likelihood that antidepressant medications may be required. In particular, if symptoms of major depression become debilitating and interfere with the physical health of the mother, the risk benefit of antidepressant treatment may favor medication treatment.

Numerous antidepressant medications are available (Table 27-5). The *selective serotonin reuptake inhibitors* (SSRIs)

Table 27-5

REPORTED TERATOGENICITY OF ANTIDEPRESSANT MEDICATION

Name	Trade Name	Class[c]	Fetal Risk	Neonatal Risk	Lactation Risk
Second-Generation Antidepressants: Selective Serotonin Reuptake Inhibitors (SSRIs)					
Fluoxetine[a]	Prozac	B	None reported	Preliminary data: no adverse effects	Excreted into breast milk
Fluvoxamine	Luvox	C	None reported	No data available	Excreted into breast milk
Paroxetine	Paxil	B	None reported	No data available	Excreted into breast milk
Sertraline	Zoloft	B	None reported	No data available	Excreted into breast milk
Second-Generation Antidepressants: Other					
Buproprion	Wellbutrin	B	None reported	No data available	Excreted into breast milk
Nefazadone	Serzone	C	None reported	No data available	Excretion into breast milk not known
Trazodone	Desyrel	C	None reported	No data available	Excreted into breast milk
Venlafaxine	Effexor	C	None reported	No data available	Excretion into breast milk not known
Tricyclic Antidepressants					
Nortriptyline[a]	Aventyl, Pamelor	D[b]	Reports of anomalies; causality unclear	No withdrawal ? Urinary retention	Excreted into breast milk
Desipramine[a]	Norpramin	C[b]	None reported	Withdrawal seizures reported	Excreted into breast milk
Amitriptyline	Elavil, Endep	D[b]	Reports of limb defects; causality unclear	No withdrawal	Excreted into breast milk
Amoxapine	Asendin	C	Inconclusive	No data available	Excreted into breast milk
Clomipramine	Anafranil	C	None reported	Withdrawal seizures reported	Excreted into breast milk
Doxepin	Sinequan	C[b]	Inconclusive	No withdrawal	Excreted into breast milk; infant respiratory depression reported
Imipramine	Tofranil	D[b]	Reports of anomalies; causality unclear	Withdrawal seizures reported	Excreted into breast milk
Maprotiline	Ludiomil	B	Inconclusive	No data available	Excreted into breast milk
Protriptyline	Vivactil	C[b]	No data available	No data available	No data available
Trimipramine	Surmontil	C	No data available	No data available	No data available
Monoamine Oxidase Inhibitors (MAOIs)					
Phenelzine	Nardil	C	Limited data; malformations noted	No data available	No data available
Tranylcypromine	Parmate	C	Limited data; malformations noted	No data available	No data available

[a]Consider for use as first-line agents.
[b]Drug not assigned to class by manufacturer; class assigned per Briggs et al (1994).[38]
[c]Refer to Chap. 16 for definitions of categories.
Source: Briggs et al.,[38] with permission.

are commonly used because of their minimal side effects and safety in overdose. Due to their relatively recent availability, there are only preliminary data regarding their safety during pregnancy: *fluoxetine* was introduced in 1988, *sertraline* in 1992, and *paroxetine* in 1993. More information is available on fluoxetine than on the other, newer SSRIs. Available studies and a postmarketing surveillance registry maintained by the manufacturer of fluoxetine show no evidence of increased risk of congenital anomalies. Very limited follow-up data are available. One follow-up study of children with in utero exposure to fluoxetine did not find any associated behavioral or cognitive effects of fluoxetine.[16] *Tricyclic* and *heterocyclic antidepressants* are older classes of antidepressants; therefore more information is available about the risks they may pose during pregnancy. There is no definitive evidence for teratogenicity associated with their use. Unfortunately, the side effects (dry mouth, blurred vision, tachycardia, constipation, mental slowing, sedation) are disturbing to many patients and compliance may be poor. *Nortriptyline* and *desipramine* are advantageous because they allow monitoring of serum levels, are associated with a lower risk of orthostatic hypotension, and have fewer anticholinergic side effects. Transient urinary retention and bowel obstruction have been observed in neonates exposed to high levels of these agents. The major disadvantage to their use is the high potential lethality secondary to overdose.[17] There are fewer data about the potential teratogenicity of the *monoamine oxidase inhibitors*. The side-effects profile includes orthostatic hypotension and potentially lethal hypertensive crisis secondary to noncompliance with strict dietary restraints. These potential adverse effects for the pregnant mother make the monoamine oxidase inhibitors a pharmacologic treatment of last resort in pregnancy.

Importantly, antidepressant medication needs to be adequately dosed. Underdosing of medication is unlikely to significantly reduce risk to the fetus and will not accomplish the goal of treatment of the major depression. Since patients who have experienced a major depression during pregnancy are at high risk of symptom exacerbation in the postpartum period, antidepressant medication should be continued for at least 6 months following delivery.

Electroconvulsive therapy (ECT) can be safely used during pregnancy and lactation. It may be administered in both inpatient and outpatient settings and offers the advantage of not exposing the fetus to long-term medications. It may be the treatment of choice for psychotic depression, especially in the first trimester.[18]

TREATMENT OF ADJUSTMENT DISORDERS AND BEREAVEMENT

Support groups have been widely utilized and appear to be among the most helpful modalities in helping patients and their partners to cope with bereavement. Individual supportive psychotherapy is also of benefit for many patients who are over-

whelmed by stressful life events or bereavement. Pharmacologic agents may play a limited role, helping patients cope with overwhelming anxiety. Judicious short-term use of benzodiazapines may be of value. In addition, agents such as zolpidem may be useful in treating transient insomnia.

ANXIETY DISORDERS

Anxiety is an unpleasant emotional state accompanied by subjective fear and objectively measurable physical effects (e.g., tachycardia, tachypnea, sweating). Feeling anxious is a normal reaction to stressful circumstances, including pregnancy, and often may actually be adaptive. Anxiety is pathologic when it causes marked distress or interferes with an individual's relationships or ability to function. Anxiety disorders are very common, with a lifetime prevalence of 24.9 percent and a 12-month prevalence of 17.2 percent.[19] Anxiety may also be a prominent feature in adjustment disorder, major depression, and other mental disorders.

PANIC ATTACKS

A person having a panic attack experiences a discrete period of intense fear or discomfort accompanied by four of the following symptoms: (1) palpitations, pounding heart, or accelerated heart rate; (2) sweating; (3) trembling or shaking; (4) sensations of shortness of breath or smothering; (5) feeling of choking; (6) chest pain or discomfort; (7) nausea or abdominal distress; (8) feeling dizzy, unsteady, light-headed, or faint; (9) derealization (feelings of unreality) or depersonalization (being detached from oneself); (10) fear of losing control or going crazy; (11) fear of dying; (12) paresthesias (numbness or tingling sensations); or (13) chills or hot flushes. Panic attacks develop abruptly and reach a peak within 10 min. They are common and may occur as isolated experiences in normal young adults or in connection with a variety of anxiety disorders. They are often easily treated, sometimes just with reassurance that the symptoms do not represent a serious physical illness. However, ongoing, untreated panic attacks can be severely debilitating.

PANIC DISORDER

Panic disorder is a common psychiatric disorder characterized by recurrent, unexpected panic attacks. The National Comorbidity Survey[19] reported lifetime and 12-month prevalences of 3.5 and 2.3 percent, respectively, for panic disorder. Panic disorder may occur with or without agoraphobia. *Agoraphobia* is defined as *anxiety about being in places or situations from which escape might be difficult (or embarrassing) or in which help may not be available in the event of a panic attack or panic-like symptoms.* Such situations are either avoided or endured with marked distress and anxiety about having an attack or experiencing symptoms.

The onset of symptoms occurs in young adulthood and affects women disproportionately. Patients with panic symptoms often initially present to emergency departments or primary-care clinics with physical complaints such as chest pain, shortness of breath, increased heart rate, numbness, and/or dizziness; they often fear that they are having a heart attack or stroke. Individuals with new onset of panic symptoms must be carefully evaluated to rule out medical conditions that mimic panic attacks. Pain, hypoxia, angina, myocardial infarction, substance abuse or withdrawal, hyperthyroidism, or pheochromocytoma can cause anxiety and panic symptoms.

OBSESSIVE COMPULSIVE DISORDER

Obsessive compulsive disorder (OCD) is characterized by recurrent obsessions or compulsions severe enough to be time-consuming, to cause marked distress, or to significantly interfere with an individual's functioning. Obsessive thoughts are usually disturbing. An example of an obsession is a recurrent thought of hurting a loved one, without anger or desire to harm that person. An example of a compulsion would be the impulse to wash one's hands over and over again or check locks numerous times.

ANXIETY DISORDERS IN PREGNANCY AND THE POSTPARTUM PERIOD

The effect of pregnancy on the course of panic disorder may be highly variable. A recent study examined the clinical course of 67 pregnancies occurring in 46 women with preexisting panic disorder.[20] In 43 percent of the pregnancies, women experienced improvement in their panic symptoms; in 33 percent, there was worsening; and in 23 percent there was no change. However, 63 percent of the pregnancies were associated with worsening of panic symptoms during the postpartum period, suggesting that women with panic disorder may be at risk for postpartum exacerbation. Other studies[21] have suggested that while women with mild symptoms may experience improvement, those with more severe illness may represent a subgroup at risk for persistence or worsening of symptoms.

Obsessive compulsive disorder is probably rare in pregnancy. Some reports, however, have suggested an association between pregnancy and the onset of OCD symptoms.[22,23]

TREATMENT OF ANXIETY DISORDERS

Panic disorder is effectively treated by pharmacologic agents, particularly antidepressant medication and/or benzodiazepines. Cognitive-behavioral techniques have also been shown to be effective. Since cognitive-behavioral therapy may have a medication-sparing effect, this modality may be especially useful prior to and during pregnancy.

For women who are taking benzodiazepines and are contemplating pregnancy, a plan for tapering benzodiazepines prior to conception should be discussed, since use of these medications during the first trimester has been associated with fetal anomalies (Table 27-6). In particular, studies have shown approximately a 12-fold increase in the risk for cleft palate, giving an absolute risk of about 7 per 1000 births (compared with a baseline risk of 6 per 10,000 births).[16] For patients already pregnant and using benzodiazepines, recommendations must be individualized. Benzodiazepines can produce withdrawal symptoms in the infant, so gradual tapering and discontinuation of these medications prior to delivery is recommended. Since the prospect of labor and delivery is anxiety-producing in its own right, this may not be possible with some patients. If a previously unmedicated patient requires pharmacotherapy, a tricyclic antidepressant or fluoxetine are reasonable choices for initial therapy. The severity of anxiety symptoms, presence of suicidality or comorbid mood disorder, concurrent medical conditions and medications, presenting stage of gestation, and other factors must be carefully considered. A retrospective study[21] has suggested that antipanic medication in the third trimester may have a protective effect in the puerperium. It has also been suggested that lactation may prevent postpartum exacerbation of anxiety disorders.[24]

Like panic disorder, OCD may benefit from cognitive-behavioral strategies, and these may be used as an alternative to medications during pregnancy. Obsessive compulsive disorder is specifically responsive to drugs that inhibit serotonin reuptake. When medication is necessary, fluoxetine is an effective and reasonable treatment. Clomipramine is an effective OCD therapy in nonpregnant women, but use during pregnancy is limited by its propensity to worsen orthostatic hypotension. Furthermore, its use during labor and delivery is contraindicated, secondary to reports of seizures in neonates born to mothers who have used clomipramine during late pregnancy.[25]

EATING DISORDERS IN PREGNANCY

Anorexia nervosa is a serious and sometimes fatal disorder occurring in approximately 1 percent of reproductive-age women. Women with anorexia nervosa suffer from self-imposed starvation in pursuit of thinness and a fear of fatness. *Bulimia nervosa* occurs in 1.7 percent of reproductive-age women and is characterized by episodic binge eating followed by efforts designed to reduce calorie absorption, including self-induced vomiting, use of laxatives or diuretics, or excessive exercise. Milder versions of eating disorders occur in another 3 to 5 percent of reproductive-age

Table 27-6

BENZODIAZEPINES AND OTHER ANXIOLYTICS

Name	Trade Name	Class[d]	Fetal Risk	Neonatal Risk	Lactation Risk
Chlordiazepoxide[a]	Librium	D[b]	Conflicting teratogenic data	Withdrawal observed, occurs early and late	Presumed excretion into human breast milk
Diazepam[a]	Valium	D[b]	Teratogenic effects reported	Floppy infant and withdrawal reported	Excreted into breast milk; infant sedation noted
Lorazepam[a]	Ativan	D	No teratogenic reports for this drug, but other drugs in class	Floppy infant and withdrawal reported	Excreted into breast milk
Alprazolam	Xanax	D	Reports of anomalies; causality unlikely	Withdrawal reported	Presumed excretion into human breast milk
Buspirone	BuSpar	B	No teratogenic effect reported	No data available	Excreted into breast milk in rats, no human data available
Clorazepate	Tranxene	D[b]	Reports of anomalies; causality unclear	Withdrawal observed	Presumed excretion into human breast milk
Flurazepam	Dalmane	X	Teratogenic effects for class of drug cited	Withdrawal predicted	Presumed excretion into human breast milk
Midazolam	Versed	D	No reports of use before third trimester	Hypotonic infant at delivery and 24 h	No data available
Temazepam	Restoril	X	Teratogenic effects for class of drug cited; ?IUFD[c] in combination with diphenhydramine	Floppy infant and withdrawal reported	Excreted into breast milk; infant sedation noted
Triazolam	Halcion	X	Teratogenic effects for class of drug cited	Withdrawal predicted	Excreted into breast milk

[a]Consider for use as first-line agents.
[b]Drug not assigned to class by manufacturer.
[c]IUFD = in utero fetal demise.
[d]Refer to Chap. 16 for class definitions.
Source: Briggs et al.,[38] with permission.

women.[26] Despite the relatively high prevalence and associated morbidity of these disorders, there have been few studies of their effects on the outcome of pregnancy.

Women with eating disorders are at increased risk for obstetric complications, including pregnancy-induced hypertension, forceps delivery, and cesarean section.[27,28] The offspring of these mothers are at risk for intrauterine growth retardation, congenital malformations, failure to thrive, and low Apgar scores.[29,30] For these reasons, women with eating disorders should be advised to avoid pregnancy until their symptoms are in remission or under control and their weight is normalized.

Women with eating disorders are often reluctant to volunteer information about their condition, and those with bulimia nervosa often appear to be of normal weight. As a result, practitioners may attribute episodes of weight loss, vomiting, electrolyte imbalance, or generalized gastrointestinal disturbances to the pregnancy itself. Women with

eating disorders who become pregnant will need close follow-up to ensure adequate nutrition and weight gain. Behavioral and possibly pharmacologic management may be helpful. Fluoxetine has recently been given an indication for the treatment of bulimia by the Food and Drug Administration. In extreme circumstances, hospitalization and feeding via nasogastric tube may become necessary.

PSYCHOSIS DURING PREGNANCY AND THE POSTPARTUM PERIOD

Psychotic symptoms include hallucinations, delusions, and severe disorganization of thought and behavior. Psychosis occurring during pregnancy and the postpartum period is most often a symptom of major depression, mania (bipolar disorder), or schizophrenia/schizoaffective disorder. Psychosis is a psychiatric emergency because the patient's poor judgment and behaviors may place both her and her fetus or newborn at risk.

PSYCHOSIS AND MANIA DURING PREGNANCY

Patients who have a chronic psychotic disorder or a past history of a psychotic illness continue to be at risk for psychosis during pregnancy. Patients with schizophrenia or bipolar disorder who become pregnant will often need close psychiatric and prenatal monitoring. Chronic symptoms, such as disorganization and paranoia, may interfere with the patient's ability to comply with prenatal care and to keep her medical appointments. In particular, pregnant patients with schizophrenia who develop complications of pregnancy may need more intense outpatient support in order to achieve adequate care. Psychiatric outreach services, including case management and home health nursing services, may be essential components of prenatal care.

Patients with bipolar disorder will be at risk of symptom exacerbation during pregnancy, especially if prophylactic medication (e.g., lithium carbonate, valproic acid, carbamazepine) is withheld. Manic symptoms—such as excessive energy, decreased need for sleep, sexual promiscuity, and engagement in other potentially dangerous behaviors— threaten the health and safety of both mother and fetus. Close monitoring by family and mental health professionals may be needed to reduce risk of dangerous behaviors. Psychiatric hospitalization may be needed.

PSYCHOSIS IN THE POSTPARTUM PERIOD

As in the case of patients at risk for major depression, the postpartum period likely represents a biologically vulnerable period for patients at risk for psychosis. Women may thus present with their first episode of psychosis in the postpartum period. A population-based study in Denmark found the risk of first-episode psychosis in the month following delivery to be 1 in every 2000 deliveries (25 cases) and in the year following delivery to be 1 in every 1000 deliveries (50 cases). About two-thirds of the cases met diagnostic criteria for major depression with psychotic features, with the other third split between mania and early schizophrenia.

Patients who develop first-onset psychosis in the postpartum period are at high risk for recurrent symptoms and dysfunction. While 40 percent of the women in the Danish registry had no further episodes in the 7- to 14-year follow-up period, 60 percent experienced at least one reoccurrence of a psychotic illness. Most women with recurrent illness developed nonpuerperal mania or depressive disorders; 4 percent had psychosis only in connection with subsequent deliveries. Postpartum psychotic illness led to chronic dis-

abling illness for one-third of the affected women. Close psychiatric follow-up is thus indicated for all women who experience a postpartum psychosis.

Psychosis in the pregnant and postpartum woman is a psychiatric emergency. Psychosis may result in disorganization and poor judgment, with the woman at risk for engaging in behaviors that are dangerous to her and her baby. For example, of the patients reviewed in the Danish registry, 10 percent had thoughts about killing their babies and a baby was put at risk in one instance.[31]

New-onset psychotic illness requires medical evaluation. Potential causes are similar to those of major depressive disorder; laboratory screening tests are listed in Table 27-4. In particular, substance abuse [phencyclidine hydrochloride (PCP), hallucinogens, cocaine] and many prescribed medications may result in transient psychosis.

TREATMENT OF PSYCHOSIS

ANTIPSYCHOTICS

Psychosis usually requires pharmacologic treatment; 12 medications are currently available in the United States for the treatment of psychosis (Table 27-7). The major benefit of treatment is minimizing the risk of symptom exacerbation. As discussed above, worsening of psychosis may result in poor prenatal care and dangerous psychotic behaviors that place both mother and child at risk. Thus, withholding pharmacologic treatment in psychotic pregnant or postpartum patients may pose significant risk to their health. In fact, psychotic illness has been suggested to be a risk factor for poor fetal outcome.[16] For most women, the potential benefits of antipsychotic treatment will outweigh the potential risks.

The risks that antipsychotic medications may pose to the fetus have not been systematically studied, but a meta-analysis of small studies is available.[16] Studies of pregnant women treated for hyperemesis with low-potency antipsychotics, particularly haloperidol, suggest no increased risk for birth defects in the fetus. Phenothiazines may pose a slightly increased risk of poor outcome. Newborns exposed to antipsychotics have been reported to have transient extrapyramidal symptoms, including increased muscle tone, tremor, motor restlessness, abnormal movements, and poor feeding.[32] Functional bowel obstruction has also been reported.[33] Despite the potential risk of these effects in newborns, cessation of antipsychotic medication is usually not indicated prior to delivery. Here, the risks of psychotic decompensation usually outweigh the potential for transient residual medication side effects in the newborn.

Patients with chronic psychotic illness should be maintained on their usual antipsychotic medication to minimize risk of relapse. Haloperidol should be considered first-line treatment in pregnant patients without a past pharmacologic treatment history because of more extensive experience with this drug, low risk of teratogenicity, and low risk of hy-

Table 27-7

ANTIPSYCHOTICS

Name	Trade Name	Class[d]	Fetal Risk	Neonatal Risk	Lactation Risk
Second-Generation Antipsychotics					
Risperidone[a]	Risperdal	C	Unknown	No data available	No human data available; animal studies worrisome
Olanzapine[a]	Zyprexa	C	Unknown	No data available	No human data available; animal studies worrisome
Clozapine	Clozaril	B	No teratogenic effects reported	No data available	Excreted into breast milk
First-Generation Antipsychotics					
Haloperidol[a]	Haldol	C	Reports of anomalies; causality unclear	No adverse events reported	Excreted into breast milk
Fluphenazine[a]	Prolixin	C[b]	Limited data; inconclusive	EPS[c]	No data available
Chlorpromazine	Thorazine	C[b]	Conflicting teratogenic data; probably safe in low doses	Prolonged jaundice, EPS, hyper- and hyporeflexia reported	Excreted into breast milk
Loxapine	Loxitane	C[b]	No data available	No data available	Excreted into breast milk in dogs, no human data
Molindone	Moban	C[b]	No data available	No data available	No data available
Perphenazine	Trilafon	C[b]	Conflicting teratogenic data; probably safe	No data available	Excreted into breast milk
Thioridazine	Mellaril	C[b]	Conflicting teratogenic data; probably safe	? EPS	No data available
Thiothixene	Navane	C[b]	No teratogenic effects reported	No data available	No data available
Trifluoperazine	Stelazine	C[b]	Conflicting teratogenic data; probably safe	? EPS	No data available

[a]Consider for use as first-line agents.
[b]Drug not assigned to class by manufacturer.
[c]EPS = extrapyramidal symptoms.
[d]Refer to Chap. 16 for class definitions.
Source: Briggs et al.,[38] with permission.

potension and other cardiovascular side effects in the pregnant woman.

Patients who develop psychosis in the postpartum period should be treated as any psychosis would be. The usual treatment of acute psychotic agitation includes haloperidol (dose of 2 to 5 mg orally or intramuscularly) and a benzodiazepine (e.g., lorazapam 1 to 2 mg every 2 to 4 h until sedation occurs, up to 10 mg/day). Choice of antipsychotic agent is usually based on prior response to treatment and tolerability of side effects. The newer, atypical antipsychotic agents (risperidone, olanzapine) may be preferable to the older agents because of their effectiveness and more favorable side-effect profiles.

MOOD STABILIZERS

Patients with schizophrenia, schizoaffective disorder, or mania may require a mood stabilizer, such as lithium, valproic acid, or carbamazepine (see Table 27-8). Lithium treatment during the first trimester increases the risk of Ebstein anomaly by 10- to 20-fold as compared with the risk in the general population. The absolute risk of Ebstein anomaly is very small, however, in the lithium-exposed fetus (1 in 1000 for the lithium-exposed fetus as compared with 1 in 20,000 in the unexposed fetus). Newborns exposed to lithium are at risk for "floppy infant" syndrome (cyanosis, hypertonicity).[34] A follow-up study of 60 lithium-exposed fetuses could

Table 27-8

MOOD STABILIZERS

Name	Trade Name	Class[b]	Fetal Risk	Neonatal Risk	Lactation Risk
Carbamazepine	Tegretol	C	Reports of anomalies; causality unclear	No data available	Excreted into breast milk
Lithium carbonate	Eskalith, Lithane, Lithobid	D[a]	Weak association with cardiac and neural tube anomalies	Transient lithium toxicity often noted	Excreted into breast milk (milk levels 40–50% of maternal serum levels)
Valproic acid	Depakote	D	Characteristic pattern of abnormalities reported	Hyperbilirubinemia, hyperglycemia	Excreted into breast milk

[a]Drug not assigned to class by manufacturer or multiple products listed.
[b]Refer to Chap. 16 for class definitions.
Source: Briggs et al.,[38] with permission.

not demonstrate long-term behavioral sequelae.[35] Treatment with valproic acid and carbamazepine has been associated with 15-fold increased risk of spina bifida (for exposed fetuses, the risk is estimated at 5 to 10 in 1000 births) and minor malformations (e.g., rotated ears).[16] One follow-up study failed to show long-term behavioral sequelae in carbamazepine-exposed fetuses.[36]

The risk/benefit analysis for women requiring mood stabilizers should include the severity of psychiatric illness, including past history of relapse risk if mood stabilizers have been discontinued. Women with severe, rapidly cycling mood swings may require mood-stabilizing medication throughout pregnancy. If the woman decides against this, lithium or other mood stabilizers should be slowly tapered, because this, compared with abrupt discontinuation, minimizes the risk of relapse. In addition, the dosage of lithium should be decreased by about one-third immediately prior to delivery to decease the risk of increases in the lithium level and subsequent lithium toxicity, which can occur secondary to changes in maternal blood volume after delivery.

SUBSTANCE ABUSE DISORDERS

Substance dependence or abuse occurs when a patient's pattern of use becomes maladaptive, causing impairment or distress. A patient must have at least three of the following seven symptoms to meet *substance dependence* criteria: (1) tolerance, (2) withdrawal, (3) taking more than intended, (4) a persistent desire or failure to control substance use, (5) spending a great deal of time getting the substance or recovering from its effects, (6) giving up other important ac-

tivities because of substance use, and (7) continued use despite knowing that the substance use was causing persistent health problems. A patient must have at least one of following symptoms to meet *substance abuse* criteria: (1) substance use causes the patient to fail to meet obligations, (2) recurrent use when dangerous (e.g., driving when intoxicated), (3) recurrent substance-related legal problems, or (4) continued use despite social or interpersonal problems related to substance intoxication.

ALCOHOL

Alcohol use during pregnancy has been identified as the leading preventable cause of birth defects.[37] Alcohol crosses the placental barrier freely at all stages of gestation. Fetal effects will be reflective of the gestational timing of alcohol exposure, genetically based differences in alcohol metabolism, the amount of alcohol consumed, and perhaps by the interaction of alcohol with other substances. Mild fetal alcohol syndrome has been induced by the consumption of as little as two drinks per day in early pregnancy. The complete syndrome is more likely when alcohol consumption exceeds four drinks per day. The complete fetal alcohol syndrome comprises a set of birth defects including craniofacial dysmorphology, prenatal and antenatal growth deficiencies, and central nervous system dysfunction. Other abnormalities include cardiac lesions, renal and genital defects, and hemangiomas, which have been reported in about 50 percent of infants. At 10-year follow up, it appeared that intellectual impairment was directly related to the degree of craniofacial abnormality. Behavioral problems are also commonly seen as long-term effects of fetal alcohol syndrome.[38] Alcohol passes freely into breast milk, and recent data indicate an untoward effect on psychomotor development

Table 27-9

"CAGE" SCREEN FOR
ALCOHOLISM

Have you ever:

C   thought you should CUT back on your drinking?

A   felt ANNOYED by people criticizing your drinking?

G   felt GUILTY or bad about your drinking?

E   had a morning EYE-OPENER to relieve hangover or
     nerves?

Note: A score of 2 or 3 indicates a high index of suspicion of alcohol dependence. A score of 4 is pathognomonic for dependence.
Source: From Ewing,[46] with permission.

in the neonate. Predicted short-term effects such as infant sedation are generally not noted at maternal blood alcohol levels less than 300 mg/dL.

Assessment of alcohol use or dependence should ideally be done in the preconceptional period, because fetal alcohol effects are most likely to occur early in pregnancy. Preconceptional evaluation allows for education of the patient about the teratogenic effects of alcohol and initiation of alcohol rehabilitation. The commonly used "CAGE" questions, shown in Table 27-9, have good reliability as a screening tool for alcohol dependence. When alcohol use or dependence is suspected, practitioners may elect to screen directly for the presence of alcohol in the blood or urine. Elevations in mean corpuscular volume and/or gammaglutamyl transferase are often seen in maternal alcohol abuse and may be "markers" predictive for fetal alcohol effects.[39]

Positive CAGE or laboratory screening should be followed by careful diagnostic assessment. Alcohol education and warnings about fetal anomalies may not be sufficient to promote abstinence in women who are chemically dependent. These patients will sometimes need detoxification prior to entering a rehabilitation program. Referral for treatment can be problematic, because many treatment centers will not accept pregnant women. Unemployment, lack of insurance, and lack of available care for other children may also be barriers to treatment.[40] Self-help groups like Alcoholics Anonymous and Women for Sobriety may have ongoing local programs, designed specifically for pregnancy, that can benefit these patients and their families.

NICOTINE

The effects of maternal smoking on birth weight and gestational length have been clearly documented over the last 10 years.[41] More recent attention has been directed toward defining the role that chronic exposure to nicotine may have on the developing fetal brain. Nicotine freely crosses the placenta, and there is good evidence that the human fetus may actually be exposed to higher nicotine concentrations than the smoking mother. Animal studies indicate fetal tolerance to nicotine and an increase in brain nicotinic receptors.[42] Animal data also indicate a positive association between chronic intrauterine exposure to nicotine and hyperactivity in the offspring. In humans, maternal smoking has also been associated with behavioral and cognitive impairment. A recent study suggests maternal smoking may also be a risk factor for attention deficit hyperactivity disorder (ADHD), which affects 6 to 9 percent of school-age children. This association remained statistically significant even after adjusting for socioeconomic status, parental IQ, and parental ADHD status. The study also confirmed that the children of mothers who smoked during pregnancy had lower IQ scores.[42]

MARIJUANA

The use of marijuana by pregnant women is common, with reports stating that from 3 to 16 percent of all pregnancies are exposed to the drug. The effect of marijuana exposure on the fetus remains unclear, primarily because of the frequency of multiple substance abuse. Possible marijuana-induced complications of pregnancy are controversial, with inconsistent findings in different studies. One significant confounding variable is concurrent use of marijuana and nicotine-containing products; both can independently produce the changes in birth weight and gestational length previously attributed to marijuana alone. Animal data from the 1960s and 1970s were inconclusive with regard to teratogenicity. In humans, most researchers have concluded either that marijuana does not produce structural defects or that the available data are insufficient to reach any conclusion.[38] Early concerns about chromosomal breaks associated with marijuana use have not been confirmed.

Of great concern, however, is the 1989 report noting a tenfold increase in rates of acute nonlymphoblastic leukemia among children exposed to marijuana in utero. The exposed children had an earlier mean age of onset (37.7 months versus 96.1 months; $p = .0007$) and a disproportionate share of monocytic or myelomonocytic morphology (70 percent versus 31 percent; $p = .02$). The reasons for these findings are unclear, but the possible presence of herbicides or pesticides on the marijuana cannot be excluded.[38]

Tetrahydrocannabinol (THC), the active ingredient in marijuana, is excreted into breast milk, and metaboiites are measurable in infant serum. Although no reports of adverse events secondary to exposure through breast milk have been reported, the American Academy of Pediatrics still considers breast-feeding contraindicated with ongoing marijuana use.[38]

COCAINE

Cocaine produces intense euphoria, disinhibition, an increased sense of competence as well as improved self-esteem. When used chronically, it produces less euphoria, but abstinence is associated with intense craving. Cocaine is often used in binges, which are followed by a post-intoxication "crash." The crash is characterized by an intensely dysphoric mood with marked anxiety. During this phase, many cocaine users will utilize alcohol, opiates, benzodiazepines, or other sedatives to relieve the dysphoria. This is followed by a period of withdrawal, usually marked by low-grade depression, disturbed sleep, and intense cocaine craving. From a psychiatric perspective, cocaine use may precipitate mania, delirium, delusional or hallucinatory states, and organic mood and personality disorders. It can also cause exacerbation of preexisting psychiatric disorders in susceptible individuals.[43]

Cocaine abuse is increasingly prevalent among pregnant women. Women who seek prenatal care late in gestation, show poor weight gain during pregnancy, have a history of chaotic lifestyles or family turmoil, complain of financial hardship inconsistent with their level of income, or reside in drug-infested high-crime neighborhoods should undergo voluntary drug testing for cocaine and other substances.[43] Cocaine is a sympathomimetic that produces hypertension and vasoconstriction directly via its cardiovascular activity. It crosses the placenta freely and can be found in numerous fetal tissues. It causes increased uterine vascular resistance, which decreases placental perfusion and may lead to fetal hypoxia. Both the hypoxia and direct effects of the cocaine have been observed to cause fetal tachycardia and hypertension.[38] Cocaine use in pregnancy has also been associated with spontaneous abortion, preterm labor, premature delivery, abruptio placentae, premature rupture of membranes, and maternal death. It has consistently been shown to be associated with intrauterine growth retardation and low birth weight. Fetal distress during labor is not uncommon in cocaine users and the increased incidence of meconium-stained amniotic fluid has been well documented. Distinct fetal anomalies associated with cocaine use are difficult to assess, primarily because of the high incidence of multiple substance abuse in this group. The possibility of higher than expected rates of urinary tract abnormalities has been investigated, with mixed results. Numerous instances of anomalies in the brain and gastrointestinal tract that appear to be secondary to vascular accidents have been reported. Ocular and facial abnormalities have also been reported.[38]

During the neonatal period, these infants tend to be irritable and tremulous, and they may experience muscular rigidity. Vomiting and diarrhea are also common. Symptoms begin on day 1 or 2 after birth, and are at maximum intensity by days 2 and 3. Increased rates of sudden infant death syndrome (SIDS) have been noted in cocaine-exposed infants during the first 6 months of life, but those data are not entirely clear.[38]

Breast-feeding is contraindicated among cocaine users. Signs of infant cocaine toxicity secondary to ingestion of breast milk after maternal cocaine use include irritability, vomiting, diarrhea, tremulousness, increased startle reflex, hyperreflexia with clonus, and marked lability of mood. Cocaine metabolites can be found in fetal urine for a protracted period following exposure via breast milk.[38]

OPIATES

In the United States, heroin exposure during pregnancy is confined to illegal use, although heroin is commercially available in other countries. Heroin crosses the placenta rapidly, but no well-defined syndrome of abnormalities has been associated with it. Acute maternal withdrawal will be associated with simultaneous fetal withdrawal, and intrauterine fetal demise can occur.

Methadone maintenance therapy is commonly used during pregnancy, and no increase in congenital anomalies has been noted among those taking methadone. The primary problems occur in the neonatal period, with withdrawal symptoms occurring in 60 to 90 percent of infants. Infants of opiate-addicted mothers are often small for gestational age. For reasons that are not yet clear, the infants of methadone-maintained mothers tend to have a higher birth weight than those of heroin-addicted mothers. This may reflect improved prenatal care in the methadone group.

Heroin crosses into breast milk in sufficient quantities to cause infant addiction. The American Academy of Pediatrics considers heroin abuse a contraindication to breast-feeding. Methadone concentrations in breast milk are sufficiently high to prevent withdrawal in breast-fed infants. But the American Academy of Pediatrics considers methadone to be compatible with breast-feeding provided that maternal doses do not exceed 20 mg/day. At least one infant death has been attributed to methadone obtained through breast milk.[38]

TREATMENT OF SUBSTANCE ABUSE IN PREGNANCY

In the course of prenatal care, women should be clearly informed about the hazards of alcohol, nicotine, and illicit drug use during pregnancy. The clinician should consider the threats that both the substance abuse and the lifestyle associated with it pose to the pregnant patient and her fetus. In particular, domestic violence, nutritional deficits, and poor weight gain are common in patients who use illegal substances or who are alcohol-dependent. Prenatal care is often absent or inadequate, and patients may be a risk for sexually transmitted diseases, with the attendant threats of primary transplacental infections like human immunodeficiency virus as well as secondary abnormalities like those seen in congenital syphilis.[43,44]

At the outset, patients should be encouraged to participate in regular prenatal care, since this single factor is positively related to higher birth weight and improved pregnancy outcome. Outpatient drug and alcohol rehabilitation programs designed specifically for pregnant women will often combine prenatal care and a battery of services including parenting classes, group therapy, counseling, and psychiatric management. In many areas, treatment centers designed specifically for pregnant patients have proved effective. Unfortunately, those resources are often inadequate to meet the high demand for their services. Unlike other areas of addiction medicine where being on a "wait list" for available facilities may not affect outcome, pregnant patients have more immediate needs and rehabilitation for them should not be delayed.

Hospitalization may be indicated when detoxification from alcohol is needed. Heroin detoxification should be delayed until after delivery, but methadone maintenance should be offered to these patients as soon as the diagnosis of opiate dependence has been made. Hospitalization may also be mandated for those patients with medical, obstetric, or psychiatric complications. During any initial period of hospitalization, close observation for evidence of withdrawal symptoms from other substances is essential.

Supportive therapies for these patients encourage breaking ties with the drug culture and with circumstances likely to cause recurrent use. Groups like Narcotics Anonymous, Alcoholics Anonymous, and Cocaine Anonymous provide a supportive environment as well as mutually supportive relationships with drug-free rehabilitating peers. They also employ cognitive-behavioral techniques designed to help the woman develop awareness that the drug abuse is a problem in her life and to help her overcome the recurring compulsion to use drugs or alcohol. The pregnant patient must also develop and maintain the awareness that she is responsible for the health and well-being of her infant.[43,44]

Involuntary drug testing and publicity surrounding cases of criminal prosecution for "prenatal child abuse" or for "delivery of controlled substances to a minor" (via the umbilical cord) has caused chemically dependent women to mistrust the health care system. Unfortunately, it also appears to have led to an increasing number of births to women who have had no prenatal care. Pregnant women may also fear losing custody of their existing children if they are known to use alcohol or drugs.[40]

Testing of neonatal blood and urine may be indicated if fetal alcohol syndrome is suspected at birth or signs of drug withdrawal appear in the neonatal period. This testing should not be undertaken lightly, because the removal of newborn infants from their mothers solely on the basis of positive drug test results has occurred in some jurisdictions.[40]

References

1. American Psychiatric Association: *Diagnostic and Statistical Manual of Mental Disorders,* 4th ed. (DSM-IV). Washington, DC: American Psychiatric Association, 1994.
2. Rinaldi RC: Screening for mood disorders. *J Fam Pract* 34:103, 1992.
3. Reiger DA, Hirschfeld RMA, Goodwin FK: The NIMH depression awareness, recognition, and treatment (D/ART) program: Structure, aims, and scientific basis. *Am J Psychiatry* 145:1351, 1988.
4. Miller LJ: Psychiatric disorders during pregnancy, in Stewart DE, Stotland NL (eds): *Psychological Aspects of Women's Health Care: The Interface between Psychiatry and Obstetrics and Gynecology.* Washington, DC: American Psychiatric Press, 1993, pp 55–70.
5. O'Hara MW: *Postpartum Depression: Causes and Consequences.* New York: Springer-Verlag, 1995.
6. Wilkie G, Shapiro CM: Sleep deprivation and the postnatal blues. *J Psychosom Res* 36:309, 1992.
7. Cox JL, Murray D, Chapman G: A controlled study of the onset, duration, and prevalence of postnatal depression. *Br J Psychiatry* 163:27, 1993.
8. American College of Obstetricians and Gynecologists. Early pregnancy loss. *ACOG Tech Bull* No. 212, Sept 1995.
9. Katona C, Robertson M: *Psychiatry at a Glance.* Oxford, England: Blackwell, 1995.
10. Janssen HJEM, Cuisinier MCJ, Hoogduin KAL, de Graauw KPHM: Controlled prospective study on the mental health of women following pregnancy loss. *Am J Psychiatry* 153:226, 1996.
11. American College of Obstetricians and Gynecologists: Grief related to perinatal death. *ACOG Tech Bull* No. 86, April 1985.
12. Brown SS, Eisenberg L (eds): *The Best Intentions: Unintended Pregnancy and the Well-Being of Children and Families.* Washington, DC: National Academy Press, 1995.
13. Miller LJ: Clinical strategies for the use of psychotropic drugs during pregnancy. *Psychiatr Med* 9:275, 1991.
14. Stotland NL: Induced abortion, in Stewart DE, Stotland NL (eds): *Psychological Aspects of Women's Health Care: The Interface between Psychiatry and Obstetrics and Gynecology.* Washington, DC: American Psychiatric Press, 1993, pp 207–225.
15. Zuckerman B, Bauchner H, Parker S, Cabral H: Maternal depressive symptoms during pregnancy and newborn irritability. *J Dev Behav Pediatr* 11:190, 1990.
16. Altschuler LL, Cohen LS, Szuba MP, et al: Pharmacologic management of psychiatric illness during pregnancy: Dilemmas and guidelines. *Am J Psychiatry* 153:592, 1996.

17. Rothschild AJ: Advances in the management of depression: Implications for the obstetrician/gynecologist. *Am J Obstet Gynecol* 173:659, 1995.

18. Ferrill MJ, Kehoe WA, Jacisin JJ: ECT during pregnancy: Physiologic and pharmacologic considerations. *Convuls Ther* 8:186, 1992.

19. Kessler RC, McGonagle KA, Zhao S, et al: Lifetime and 12-month prevalence of DSM-III-R psychiatric disorders in the United States. *Arch Gen Psychiatry* 51:8, 1994.

20. Northcott CJ, Stein MB: Panic disorder during pregnancy. *J Clin Psychiatry* 55:539, 1994.

21. Cohen LS, Sichel DA, Dimmock JA, Rosenbaum JF: Impact of pregnancy on panic disorder: A case series. *J Clin Psychiatry* 55:284, 1994.

22. Buttolph ML, Holland DA: Obsessive-compulsive disorders in pregnancy and childbirth, in Jenike MA, Baer L, Minichiello WE (eds): *Obsessive-Compulsive Disorders: Theory and Management*, 2d ed. Chicago: Year Book, 1990, pp 89–97.

23. Neziroglu F, Anemone R, Yaryura-Tobias JA: Onset of obsessive-compulsive disorder in pregnancy. *Am J Psychiatry* 149:947, 1992.

24. Klein DF: Commentary: Pregnancy and panic disorder. *J Clin Psychiatry* 55:293, 1994.

25. Cowe L, Lloyd DJ, Dawling S: Neonatal convulsions caused by withdrawal from maternal clomipramine. *Br J Med* 284:1837, 1982.

26. Stewart DE, Raskin J, Garfinkel PE, et al: Anorexia nervosa, bulimia and pregnancy. *Am J Obstet Gynecol* 157:1194, 1987.

27. Lemberg R, Phillips J: The impact of pregnancy on anorexia nervosa and bulimia. *Int J Eating Dis* 8:285, 1989.

28. Stewart DE, Robinson E, Goldbloom DS, Wright C: Infertility and eating disorders. *Am J Obstet Gynecol* 163:1196, 1990.

29. Treasure JL, Russell GF: Intrauterine growth and neonatal weight gain in babies of women with anorexia nervosa. *Br Med J Clin Res* 296:1038, 1988.

30. Hediger ML, Scholl TO, Belsky DH, et al: Patterns of weight gain in adolescent pregnancy: Effects on birth weight and preterm delivery. *Obstet Gynecol* 74:6, 1989.

31. Videbech P, Gouliaev G: First admission with puerperal psychosis: 7–14 years of follow-up. *Acta Psychiatr Scand* 91:167, 1995.

32. Auerbach JG, Hans SL, Marcus J, Maeir S: Maternal psychotropic medication and neonatal behavior. *Neurotoxicol Teratol* 14:399, 1992.

33. Falterman LG, Richardson DJ: Small left colon syndrome associated with maternal ingestion of psychotropic drugs. *J Pediatr* 97:300, 1980.

34. Woody JN, London WL, Wilbanks GD: Lithium toxicity in a newborn. *Pediatrics* 47:94, 1971.

35. Schou M: What happened to the lithium babies? A follow-up study of children born without malformation. *Acta Psychiatr Scand* 54:193, 1976.

36. Scolnick D, Nulman I, Rover J, et al: Neurodevelopment of children exposed in utero to phenytoin and carbamazepine monotherapy. *JAMA* 271:767, 1994.

37. Centers for Disease Control and Prevention: Fetal alcohol syndrome—United States, 1979–1992. *MMWR* 42:339, 1993.

38. Briggs GG, Freeman RK, Yaffe SJ: *Drugs in Pregnancy and Lactation: A Reference Guide to Fetal and Neonatal Risk*, 4th ed. Baltimore: Williams & Wilkins, 1994.

39. Ylikorkala O, Stenman U, Halmesmaki E: Gammaglutamyl transferase and mean cell volume reveal maternal alcohol abuse and fetal alcohol effects. *Am J Obstet Gynecol* 157:344, 1987.

40. Blume S, Russell M: Alcohol and substance abuse in the practice of obstetrics and gynecology, in Stewart DE, Stotland NL (eds): *Psychological Aspects of Women's Health Care: The Interface between Psychiatry and Obstetrics and Gynecology*. Washington, DC: American Psychiatric Press, 1993, pp 391-409.

41. American College of Obstetricians and Gynecologists: Smoking and reproductive health. *ACOG Tech Bull* No. 180, May 1993.

42. Milberger SSD, Biederman J, Faraone SV, et al: Is maternal smoking during pregnancy a risk factor for attention deficit hyperactivity disorder in children? *Am J Psychiatry* 153:1138, 1996.

43. James ME, Coles CD: Cocaine abuse during pregnancy: Psychiatric considerations. *Gen Hosp Psychiatry* 13:399, 1991.

44. American College of Obstetricians and Gynecologists: Domestic violence. *ACOG Tech Bull* No. 209, Aug 1995.

45. First MB, Spitzer RL, Gibbon M, Williams JBW: *Structured Clinical Interview for DSM-IV Axis I Disorders*. Research version, patient edition (SCID-I/P). New York: Biometrics Research, New York State Psychiatric Institute, 1996.

46. Ewing JA: Detecting alcoholism: The CAGE questionnaire. *JAMA* 14:1905, 1984.

Chapter 28

CARDIOVASCULAR DISORDERS IN PREGNANCY

Beth S. Rosenberg

Pregnancy is associated with a myriad of physiologic alterations. Over the course of the 38 to 40 week gestational period, there are marked changes that may have significant effects on hemodynamic function. Cardiovascular decompensation may result when previously asymptomatic pathology becomes challenged by these changes or when a cardiovascular disorder presents for the first (or only) time during pregnancy. Cardiovascular disorders in pregnancy often present a significant challenge to the clinician because many of the usual diagnostic and therapeutic modalities pose a threat to the health of the developing fetus.

The most common cardiovascular disorders likely to become manifest during pregnancy are hypertension, valvular and congenital heart disease, dysrhythmias, cardiomyopathies, arterial dissection, and ischemic heart disease. The signs and symptoms, diagnosis, treatment, and follow-up for each of these disorders are addressed in this chapter.

In prior sections, the anatomy and physiology of normal pregnancy were discussed in detail. It is the plasma volume expansion, increased heart rate and cardiac output, reduced systemic vascular resistance, and progesterone hormonal predominance that are most often responsible for cardiovascular compromise from preexisting cardiac disease. However, disease that prevents any of these hemodynamic and/or hormonal adaptations from occurring may also compromise maternal and fetal health.

HYPERTENSION

PATHOPHYSIOLOGY

Normally, pregnancy is associated with minimal to slight decrease in the systolic blood pressure, while the diastolic blood pressure typically decreases by approximately 10 mmHg during the second trimester and returns to prepregnancy values during the third trimester. Hypertension (defined as a blood pressure of $\geq 140/90$ or an increase of $\geq 30/15$ mmHg over the prepregnant blood pressure) that occurs in a gravid woman may be relatively benign, requiring no intervention beyond close follow-up, or may be life-threatening to both the mother and baby. Hypertension is the most frequently diagnosed cardiovascular disorder in pregnancy, occurring in 10 to 15 percent.[1] As in the nonpregnant state, essential hypertension and secondary hypertension may be present. The underlying cause of essential hypertension remains unknown, whereas secondary hypertension is due to some treatable underlying pathologic process such as renal artery stenosis, hyperthyroidism, pheochromocytoma, or aldosteronism. The other hypertensive syndromes associated specifically with pregnancy are transient hypertension and preeclampsia. Transient hypertension develops during pregnancy or in the first 24 h postpartum.

Preeclampsia typically occurs after the 20th week of gestation and is classically associated with proteinuria and edema. The pathophysiology of hypertension classified as preeclampsia is quite different from those disorders discussed thus far. See Chapter 7 for further discussion.

The pathologic process underlying preeclampsia involves a defect in placentation, which ultimately results in abnormal cardiovascular adaptations. In contrast to the normal adaptations in pregnancy, the preeclamptic woman will demonstrate a decrease in plasma volume and cardiac output with an increase in systemic vascular resistance. This failure of appropriate cardiovascular adaptation results in inadequate perfusion of vital organs—such as the placenta, liver, brain, and kidneys—and may therefore threaten not only the pregnancy and fetal development but also the life and health of the mother.

DIAGNOSIS AND DIFFERENTIAL DIAGNOSIS

In general, earlier diagnosis of hypertension will improve the likelihood of appropriate management. Classification of the type of hypertension (i.e., chronic, transient, preeclampsia) as well as assessment of end-organ damage will be important for determining what treatment, if any, is necessary. The diagnosis of hypertension should not be based on a single blood pressure measurement. Rather, a minimum of two measurements separated in time by at least 4 h is necessary. A clear diagnosis of chronic hypertension can be made only in women who have known hypertension prior to pregnancy. Transient hypertension, which may be diagnosed at any point in the pregnancy, should be viewed as a retrospective diagnosis for two reasons: (1) in women diagnosed with hypertension after the 20th week, preeclampsia should not be ruled out until after delivery, and (2) in women diagnosed with hypertension during the first half of the pregnancy, preexisting or chronic hypertension and both essential and secondary hypertension must be included in the differential diagnosis. Illicit drug use (particularly cocaine or amphetamines) should be considered in the differential diagnosis of hypertension in general and during pregnancy as well.

LABORATORY TESTS

Once the diagnosis of hypertension has been made, based upon repeat resting measurements, several laboratory tests should be ordered to determine if there is evidence of end-organ damage, because such a finding would mandate medical treatment of the elevated blood pressure.

Renal function is evaluated with a urinalysis, electrolytes, blood urea nitrogen (BUN), and creatinine. Abnormalities in any of these tests will require further evaluation and referral to a high-risk obstetric center. Liver function tests,

platelet count, and a peripheral blood smear to rule out hepatic dysfunction, thrombocytopenia, and microangiopathic changes, respectively, are necessary to determine if the HELLP* syndrome (discussed in greater detail in Chap. 3) is present. A 12-lead electrocardiogram (ECG) will help rule out cardiac dysfunction. If this ECG is abnormal or there are signs or symptoms of cardiovascular compromise, a two-dimensional (2D) echocardiogram should be obtained. As with other evidence of end-organ damage, abnormalities in cardiac function require specialized follow-up in a high-risk obstetric center and evaluation by a cardiologist. Fundoscopic examination will be necessary to rule out hypertensive retinopathy or other evidence of ophthalmic end-organ damage. Finally, in the case of markedly elevated blood pressure (where pheochromocytoma or illicit drug use might be in the differential diagnosis) a 24-h urine catecholamine measurement and serum/urine toxicology screens should be done.

TREATMENT, DISCHARGE INSTRUCTIONS, AND FOLLOW-UP INTERVAL

Treatment of hypertension in the pregnant woman will depend on the type, severity, and presence or absence of end-organ damage. Women with chronic hypertension (diagnosed prior to or in the first 20 weeks of pregnancy) should ideally begin their treatment prior to pregnancy with adjustment in their antihypertensive regimen to exclude angiotensin-converting enzyme (ACE) inhibitors and diuretics (if possible). In women who are diagnosed with hypertension of mild or moderate severity (ranging from 140 to 160/90 to 100 mmHg) but without evidence of end-organ damage, no medical treatment is necessary. However, when there is evidence of end-organ damage, antihypertensive therapy is necessary. Preeclampsia should always remain in the differential diagnosis when a women is diagnosed with hypertension during or after the 20th week and will require diligent follow-up, as outlined in Chap. 7.

In general, methyldopa (Aldomet) is the drug of choice in the management of hypertension during pregnancy because it has been the most extensively studied antihypertensive agent in this setting. If methyldopa is contraindicated, poorly tolerated, or ineffective, labetalol or nifedipine (sustained release) are acceptable alternatives. The goal of medical therapy in this setting is to maintain the diastolic blood pressure in the 80 to 90 mmHg range. Further information on the use of these drugs during pregnancy may be found in Chap. 7.

During pregnancy, a blood pressure ≥160/110 mmHg after the 20th week of gestation defines severe preeclampsia and frequently requires urgent intervention. Such severe hyper-

---

*HELLP = hemolysis, elevated liver enzymes, and low platelet count.

tension increases the maternal risk of stroke and cardiovascular morbidity and compromises placental blood flow. In this setting, parenteral antihypertensive drug therapy in a unit where blood pressure may be closely monitored is the treatment of choice. If fetal viability and lung maturity are confirmed, delivery is suggested once the blood pressure is brought under control. The goal in treatment of severe hypertension is to maintain the mean arterial pressure in the range of 105 to 125 mmHg (or diastolic pressure of 90 to 105 mmHg). The agents of choice include hydralazine (2.5 mg IV, then 5 to 10 mg every 20 min to a maximum of 40 mg) or labetalol (initially 20 mg IV, then 40 to 80 mg IV every 10 min until the goal is reached or until a cumulative amount of 300 mg has been given). Diazoxide (parenteral) and nifedipine (sublingual) are now not used because of their potential to cause a precipitous reduction in blood pressure. Nitroprusside (parenteral) is considered a third-line agent because of its potential for cyanide toxicity in the neonate, but it may be used for a short (less than 1 h) period if the hypertensive emergency is considered life-threatening to both mother and fetus. The dose is 0.25 μg/kg per min infusion, and may be increased by 0.25 μg/kg per min every 5 min.

Hypertension in pregnancy requires close follow-up, whether it is medically treated or not. The potential for end-organ damage and/or preeclampsia to develop is always present. Compliance with medical treatment, clinical follow-up, and bed rest (if recommended) is imperative. Clinical follow-up should be arranged for every 3 to 4 weeks through the 24th week, then biweekly through the 34th week, then weekly until delivery. At the follow-up visits, seated blood pressure, fundoscopic examination, cardiac and pulmonary auscultation, uterine measurement, and urinalysis should always be performed. Additionally, at every third visit, a fetal ultrasound, liver function tests (LFT), electrolytes, blood urea nitrogen (BUN), creatinine, and platelet count should be obtained to maximize the possibility of an uncomplicated pregnancy, delivery, and postpartum period.

INDICATIONS FOR SPECIALTY CONSULTATION AND HOSPITALIZATION

Referral to an obstetrics center/specialist is recommended if a woman is diagnosed with preeclampsia or to a high-risk obstetrics center if there is evidence of end-organ damage secondary to hypertension. Additionally, women that are treated for a hypertensive emergency should be followed by a high-risk obstetrics specialist.

The primary indications for hospitalization for hypertension during pregnancy are (1) severe hypertension (>162/100) requiring parenteral therapy; (2) acute onset of end-organ damage, such as acute renal failure, acute liver failure, pulmonary edema, or stroke; or (3) inability or unwillingness of the patient to comply with treatment, which could endanger the life of the mother and/or fetus. Indications for hospital-

ization of the woman with preeclampsia or eclampsia are discussed in Chap. 7.

VALVULAR DISEASE AND CONGENITAL HEART DISEASE

PATHOPHYSIOLOGY

In their review of cardiac surgery experience during pregnancy, published in 1994, Chambers and Clark[2] reported that approximately 1 to 4 percent of pregnancies in the United States are complicated by some type of cardiac disease; rheumatic heart disease (RHD) is the most common. They state that because of a significant reduction in the incidence of childhood rheumatic fever and improvements in both medical and surgical management of congenital heart disease (CHD) resulting in improved survival, the ratio of RHD to CHD had decreased from 16:1 in 1954 to 3:1 in 1967. This ratio is probably closer to 1:1 at the present time in the United States. Although valvular heart disease and CHD are rarely encountered in the pregnant woman, their effects with respect to both fetal and maternal morbidity and mortality can be devastating. Although many women will present after having previously been diagnosed and treated, at least some will be diagnosed for the first time when they seek medical attention for the pregnancy. Thus, when a pregnant woman develops symptoms of excessive shortness of breath, dyspnea on exertion, palpitations, or even chest discomfort, valvular heart disease and previously undiagnosed congenital heart disease must be in the differential diagnosis.

Valvular heart disease may be caused by rheumatic fever, congenital abnormalities, or bacterial endocarditis. Acute or subacute bacterial endocarditis is actually very rare during pregnancy; therefore this disorder is not discussed in detail. Antibiotic prophylaxis is addressed later in this section.

Valvular disease caused by rheumatic fever presents most often as mitral stenosis (90 percent).[3] Mitral insufficiency—usually in combination with mitral stenosis (6.6 percent), aortic insufficiency (2.5 percent), and aortic stenosis (1 percent)—are the other major causes of valvular heart disease during pregnancy. Tricuspid and pulmonic valve disease secondary to rheumatic fever is usually found in combination with one of the previously listed abnormalities; these are not discussed as individual entities here. Mitral stenosis should be high on the list of possible diagnoses for any pregnant woman who develops acute dyspnea, orthopnea, or paroxysmal nocturnal dyspnea (PND). Complications can include left atrial enlargement with the resultant development of atrial fibrillation as well as atrial thrombus and subsequent thromboembolic events (including cerebrovascular, renovascular, and coronary vascular emboli). Left atrial enlargement develops as the gradient across a narrowed valve orifice increases. The normal transvalvular gradient in pregnancy should not exceed 5 mmHg. However, in the stenosed mitral valve, both the tachycardia and the plasma volume will result in a significant increase in the left atrial pressure, causing left atrial enlargement and an elevated mitral valvular gradient. These hemodynamic changes occur relatively early in pregnancy and can create symptoms even with mild mitral stenosis. Pulmonary edema is occasionally the first sign of mitral stenosis during pregnancy. This complication will occur as the transvalvular gradient exceeds the normal maximal value in pregnancy of 12 to 13 mmHg. It can also occur if atrial fibrillation develops or with sudden increases in volume, as occurs in the immediate postpartum period with the autotransfusion that ensues. Aortic insufficiency and mitral insufficiency are usually well tolerated during pregnancy when they are isolated lesions. However, they are usually found in combination with mitral stenosis, which is then the disorder that will require management. Aortic stenosis may actually be improved with pregnancy (because of the increased plasma volume, resulting in improved cardiac output) if the degree of stenosis is mild. However, in the case of significant (or severe) aortic stenosis, maternal mortality may be as high as 15 percent. This high mortality rate is due to the fact that in severe aortic stenosis (where the transvalvular gradient approaches and/or exceeds 70 mmHg), the cardiac output is highly dependent on the circulating blood volume. Therefore, a sudden volume loss or loss of capacitance, as in the case of unexpected hemorrhage or epidural anesthesia without prehydration, can be fatal. There is also an increased incidence of ventricular arrhythmias if left ventricular hypertrophy develops secondary to aortic stenosis.

Pregnancy in the woman with a prosthetic valve in place can result in a variety of complications, most of which are secondary to the anticoagulation necessary to prevent thrombosis of the valve. All of these women should already be followed by a cardiologist and a high-risk obstetrician (prior to conception) who, together with the patient, can develop the safest option(s) for management during pregnancy. The reader is referred to the review by Sullivan[4] for a discussion of this topic in depth.

Congenital heart disease, usually surgically corrected, is now seen almost as frequently as rheumatic heart disease in pregnant women. The pathophysiology of CHD is as varied as the different entities themselves. Space limitations do not permit an exhaustive discussion here, but, there are several key points worth mentioning. Although some women with a history of CHD will tolerate the course of pregnancy without much difficulty, there are others (often with pulmonary hypertension) in whom the maternal mortality rate approaches 50 percent.[5] There is also an increased risk (ranging from 2.5 to 50 percent) of CHD in the fetus. The most commonly encountered CHD in women of childbearing age are atrial septal defect (ASD), which may be corrected or uncorrected; ventricular septal defect (VSD), which is usually surgically corrected by this age; patent ductus arteriosus (PDA), which is usually corrected; pulmonic stenosis;

bicuspid aortic valve; coarctation of the aorta; Marfan syndrome; and tetrology of Fallot (TOF). Tetralogy of Fallot is usually repaired surgically, but frequently with persistent abnormalities such as pulmonic insufficiency, right ventricular outflow tract obstruction, and conduction system disease. Although most women of childbearing age with a history of CHD will tolerate pregnancy without significant untoward events, there are specific instances when a woman should be advised against conception or against proceeding with a pregnancy in progress. These instances include pulmonary hypertension (primary or secondary to Eisenmenger syndrome), where maternal mortality may exceed 50 percent; unrepaired coarctation of the aorta (where the risk of aortic dissection/rupture is high); and Marfan syndrome with aortic dilatation ($\geq$40 mm) at baseline. A key point regarding these particular disorders is that if a pregnant woman presents with chest pain, the differential diagnosis—especially if CHD is at all possible—must include not only cardiac ischemia and pulmonary embolism but also pulmonary hypertension and aortic dissection. The final key point is that if a woman is not already being followed by a high-risk obstetrics team and a cardiologist and she has a known history or is suspected of having either valvular or congenital heart disease, she should be referred for that type of follow-up as soon as it can be arranged.

DIAGNOSIS AND LABORATORY TESTS

The diagnosis of any of the disorders discussed above begins with a complete history and physical examination. The history should include any family history of CHD (in a parent or sibling) as well as a complete medical history and review of systems. The physical examination must include auscultation of the lungs, where rales might suggest heart failure; palpation and auscultation of the heart, where a right ventricular heave might suggest pulmonary hypertension or an abnormal murmur might suggest the presence of previously undiagnosed valvular disease or CHD; and careful examination of the pulses, where a "water hammer" pulse at the carotids might suggest severe aortic insufficiency, or diminished peripheral pulses might suggest mitral stenosis. The importance of a thorough history and physical examination for the diagnosis of these disorders or complications secondary to these disorders during pregnancy cannot be overemphasized.

There are no specific laboratory tests that will be of value in arriving at a diagnosis of valvular or congenital heart disease in the pregnant woman. However, periodic arterial blood gas analyses will be necessary for ongoing evaluation and management of the patient with cyanotic CHD (i.e., tetralogy of Fallot).

Rarely, cases of infectious endocarditis develop or present during pregnancy. In this circumstance, a history of fever, malaise, and myalgias accompanied by a new or enhanced murmur on physical examination or symptoms of heart failure should suggest infectious endocarditis. The diagnosis is confirmed by two or more positive blood cultures or noncardiac stigmata of bacterial endocarditis, such as retinal emboli (manifest as Roth spots), Janeway lesions, or Osler nodes (embolic lesions found on the hands and/or feet), and splinter hemorrhages (found in nail beds, suggesting emboli). These signs of infectious endocarditis occur as a result of embolization of small fragments of vegetations that may develop on left heart valves (e.g., aortic or mitral valve) and are virtually pathognomonic for this disease process. Other less specific laboratory tests that might suggest this diagnosis include an elevated white blood cell count (WBC) and an elevated erythrocyte sedimentation rate (ESR).

The transthoracic 2D echocardiogram is valuable in the assessment of cardiac structure and function. This imaging method evaluates valvular structure and function and identifies septal defects and shunts as well as many congenital disorders. It poses no risk to the mother or fetus. The addition of Doppler ultrasound can provide essential information regarding transvalvular gradients (as in the case of mitral or aortic stenosis) as well as pulmonary artery pressure. A fetal echocardiogram is also obtained at the 18th to 20th week in women with congenital heart disease, to rule out fetal CHD. Cardiac catheterization, on the other hand, should be used with caution, because it may cause risk to the developing fetus due to radiation exposure (see Appendix A-2). The radiation exposure can be minimized (but not entirely eliminated) by the use of a lead shield/apron. Obviously, cardiac catheterization should be limited to those women in whom 2D echocardiography fails to provide enough diagnostic information and for those in whom surgery is likely. Magnetic resonance imaging (MRI) can be helpful in diagnosing CHD and defining associated anatomy, but it has not been extensively studied in early pregnancy.

TREATMENT

Few general rules can be made regarding treatment of pregnant women with valvular heart disease or CHD. One rule that generally applies to such women (with the single exception of those with surgically repaired ASDs) is that they will require peripartum endocarditis antibiotic prophylaxis. Women with a history of mitral valve prolapse and mitral regurgitation should also receive antibiotic prophylaxis (Table 28-1).[6] Beyond this general recommendation, treatment will depend on the specific disorder, its severity, and the functional abilities of the individual woman. Functional ability (when described according to New York Heart Association class) appears to correlate well with prognosis, both with respect to maternal mortality and the success of the pregnancy. Women with New York Heart Association class I or II have a <1 percent mortality rate associated with pregnancy and tend to progress through the pregnancy without significant problems, regardless of the specific valvular lesion or congenital disorder (Table 28-2). Women with class

---

Table 28-1

AMERICAN HEART ASSOCIATION RECOMMENDATIONS FOR PREVENTION OF BACTERIAL ENDOCARDITIS

Infection present at the time of vaginal delivery should prompt antibiotic prophylaxis if any of the following lesions is present:

Prosthetic heart valves of any type[a]
Prior bacterial endocarditis[a]
Most structural cardiac abnormalities[b]
Rheumatic valvular disease (corrected or uncorrected)
Hypertrophic cardiomyopathy
Mitral valve prolapse with valvular regurgitation

The recommended antibiotic regimen for genitourinary procedures is ampicillin 2 g plus gentamicin 1.5 mg/kg (not to exceed 80 mg) 30 min before the procedure and up to 8 h. If the patient is allergic, substitute vancomycin 1 g for ampicillin (no repeat dose necessary).

---

[a]Although antibiotic prophylaxis is *not* recommended for uncomplicated vaginal delivery, some physicians recommend prophylaxis for low-risk procedures in individuals with prosthetic heart valves or prior endocarditis.
[b]Common exceptions: Isolated secundum atrial septal defect, mitral valve prolapse without regurgitation, prior rheumatic fever without valvular defect, or physiologic heart murmur.
Source: Adapted from Dajani AS, et al,[6] with permission.

Table 28-2

NEW YORK HEART ASSOCIATION CLINICAL CLASSIFICATION

Class	Limitations
I	None. No angina or symptoms of cardiac insufficiency even with vigorous activity.
II	Physical activity. Comfortable at rest, but develops symptoms with ordinary activity. Symptoms may include chest pain, dyspnea, excessive fatigue, or palpitations.
III	Marked limitation of physical activity. Comfortable at rest, but develops symptoms with less than ordinary activity.
IV	Symptomatic at rest and unable to perform any physical activity without discomfort.

III or IV symptoms may require frequent hospitalizations and hemodynamic monitoring during their pregnancies and have mortality rates in the 5 to 15 percent range.

DISCHARGE INSTRUCTIONS AND FOLLOW-UP INTERVAL

Most women who present during pregnancy with signs or symptoms of decompensation secondary to valvular heart disease or CHD will require hospitalization, possibly until the time of delivery. Some of those women may require invasive hemodynamic monitoring (with a pulmonary artery catheter) or a corrective procedure (i.e., valvuloplasty or cardiac surgery). Clearly, pregnancy in these women is a management challenge to be undertaken only by a team that should include at least a cardiologist, a high-risk obstetrician, and an anesthesiologist.

INDICATIONS FOR SPECIALTY CONSULTATION AND HOSPITALIZATION

The indications for specialty consultation have already been discussed. However, the indications for hospitalization are worth enumerating. They include signs/symptoms of pulmonary edema; fever with a new or worsening murmur, which might suggest endocarditis; hemoptysis, which could suggest the development of pulmonary hypertension; chest pain or worsening dyspnea for which there is no obvious explanation; and cyanosis, which might reflect worsening of a previously stable right-to-left shunt or reversal of a previous left-to-right shunt.

DYSRHYTHMIAS

PATHOPHYSIOLOGY

The pregnant woman who presents with complaints of palpitations and syncope or near syncope should be evaluated for the presence of a sustained dysrhythmia. Life-threatening rhythm disturbances are unusual in the pregnant female in the absence of cardiomyopathy, ischemia, valvular heart disease, CHD, or other structural abnormalities. However, there are dysrhythmias that may result in hypotension, thus threatening placental/fetal blood flow. The most common rhythm disturbances diagnosed during pregnancy include atrial premature beats, ectopic atrial tachycardia, paroxysmal supraventricular tachycardia (PSVT), ventricular premature beats, and ventricular tachycardia.[7] Any of these dysrhythmias may occur in a structurally normal heart at any time during the pregnancy; PSVT is actually seen more frequently in pregnancy and may be a first-time presentation.

It may also be seen in previously diagnosed patients who may develop more frequent, more sustained, or faster episodes. The etiology of these rhythm disturbances in the pregnant woman with a structurally normal heart is not entirely clear. It has been suggested that changes in volume status might increase myocardial irritability. The increase in the resting heart rate may shorten myocardial refractoriness, thus decreasing the threshold for premature beats and tachyarrhythmias. Increased emotional and physical stress may also predispose the woman to these dysrhythmias.

The more uncommon rhythm disturbances seen during pregnancy include atrial flutter, atrial fibrillation, Wolfe-Parkinson-White syndrome, and symptomatic bradycardia. These abnormalities occur almost exclusively in structurally abnormal hearts. The one exception is the sinus bradycardia or sinus arrest that may occur in the supine hypotensive syndrome of pregnancy. An excellent recent review of this entity and treatment is offered by Kinsella and Lohmann.[8]

DIAGNOSIS AND DIFFERENTIAL DIAGNOSIS

In the pregnant woman who complains of excessive shortness of breath, palpitations, syncope, or near syncope, the presence of some type of rhythm disturbance should be considered. If the woman complains of these symptoms but is not acutely symptomatic, a reasonable diagnostic workup would include a 12-lead ECG and 24- or 48-h Holter monitoring (depending on the frequency of her symptoms). The first step in treating a dysrhythmia is to identify it. In the case of atrial premature beats, ectopic atrial tachycardia, and ventricular premature beats, no further diagnostic workup is necessary. Any other rhythm disturbance will require at least a 2D echocardiogram to rule out structural abnormalities.

In the woman who is acutely symptomatic upon presentation, a 12-lead ECG with a rhythm strip may be all that is necessary to make a definitive diagnosis. The next diagnostic step in this setting will be to determine if the woman is hemodynamically stable or unstable. This differentiation will influence the early treatment of the rhythm disturbance.

LABORATORY TESTS

Most or not all of the diagnostic workup of the patient with a rhythm disturbance has been described in the preceding section. However, the treatment of some of these dysrhythmias may be guided by a few laboratory tests. First, it is important to realize that along with the changes in volume status that occur with pregnancy comes the potential for electrolyte imbalances. The most important (and perhaps only necessary) laboratory test is serum electrolytes, including sodium, potassium, chloride, magnesium, phosphorus, and calcium. Significant abnormalities in any of these laboratory values can predispose an individual to rhythm disturbances.

TREATMENT

The treatment of a rhythm disturbance that presents during pregnancy is dependent on the nature of the dysrhythmia and whether or not the woman is hemodynamically stable. In the case of a hemodynamically unstable patient or one with sustained tachyarrhythmias that are refractory to medical treatment, electrical DC cardioversion will be necessary. The risk of inducing a dysrhythmia in the fetus is minimal because very little of the electrical energy will actually reach the fetus and its fibrillatory threshold is relatively high. Nonetheless, fetal heart rate monitoring during treatment of maternal dysrhythmias is highly recommended.[7]

Medical therapy may be utilized to terminate a dysrhythmia and/or maintain sinus rhythm. The choice of agent is somewhat limited by the potential harm that the drug may do to the developing fetus. In general, the safest agents that have been used extensively in pregnancy include digoxin, beta blockers, and quinidine. Adenosine, which is found endogenously and is used to terminate sustained PSVT, is also relatively safe, although its potential to cause complete heart block and/or other bradyarrhythmias in the mother and fetus mandates fetal heart rate monitoring if this agent is used. The other tachyarrhythmia that may require urgent medical therapy is ventricular tachycardia in the patient who is alert and relatively stable hemodynamically. In this setting intravenous lidocaine would be the drug of choice. Bradyarrhythmias are rarely encountered antepartum or during labor and delivery. In the pregnant woman, these dysrhythmias are usually the result of a congenital or acquired heart block and should be treated with either temporary or permanent transvenous pacing, which is considered safe in pregnancy. Dosing of these drugs is similar to that in the nonpregnant patient.

DISCHARGE INSTRUCTIONS AND FOLLOW-UP INTERVAL

Any woman who requires treatment of a dysrhythmia (medical or otherwise) during pregnancy should be referred to a cardiologist and a high-risk obstetrician and followed by them. The follow-up with the cardiologist, at least, should be arranged for no later than 1 week after discharge. The patient should be instructed to take any prescribed medication strictly as directed and should immediately contact the responsible cardiologist for recurrence of symptoms or side effects from the medicine.

INDICATIONS FOR HOSPITALIZATION

Hospitalization should be considered for the patient who presents with a sustained dysrhythmia that requires any type of intervention (medical or electrical) for reversal or suppression. This will be necessary for three reasons: (1) to ensure that the rhythm disturbance does not recur; (2) to assess for the occurrence of any untoward side effects in the mother; and (3) to monitor fetal heart rate to ensure that there are no untoward effects in the fetus. The patient should be admitted to a telemetry bed, where both the fetal and maternal heart rhythms can be continuously monitored for a minimum of 24 h. Hospitalization for more than 48 h is rarely necessary unless the abnormal rhythm recurs or there are untoward side effects from the medication prescribed.

CARDIOMYOPATHIES

PATHOPHYSIOLOGY

Congestive heart failure and pulmonary edema may occur in association with a variety of circumstances in the pregnant woman, including any of the general disorders discussed thus far. Additionally, underlying cardiomyopathy must be included in the differential diagnosis for any pregnant woman who presents with new-onset heart failure. Fortunately, cardiomyopathy in the young woman of childbearing age is rare. There are many different types of cardiomyopathy, including hypertensive, alcoholic, ischemic, viral, drug-induced, hypertrophic, and idiopathic, but very few of these will be encountered in the young woman of childbearing age. Peripartum cardiomyopathy (PPCM) is probably less common than the types listed above, but it should be considered when a young woman with a history of pregnancy presents with signs and/or symptoms of heart failure. The specific etiology of PPCM remains an enigma. However, several risk factors have been identified. Lampert and Lang[9] have suggested that PPCM is more likely to occur in women with a history of multiple pregnancies, women of African American descent, women bearing twins, and women with a history of preeclampsia, cocaine abuse, enterovirus infection, selenium deficiency, or postpartum hypertension.

DIAGNOSIS AND DIFFERENTIAL DIAGNOSIS

Four criteria are suggested for the diagnosis of PPCM. These include (1) development of heart failure during the last month of pregnancy or within 5 months of delivery; (2) no other identifiable cause for heart failure; (3) no evidence of heart disease prior to the last month of pregnancy; and (4) evidence of left ventricular systolic dysfunction by 2D echocardiogram.[9] These criteria are worth bearing in mind, since women with other types of cardiomyopathy or CHD will typically manifest symptoms of heart failure during the second trimester of the pregnancy, when the hemodynamic challenges are greatest. The most common time of development of symptoms of PPCM is in the postpartum period (about 75 percent of diagnosed PPCM), when there are substantial changes in hemodynamic and fluid status. The differential diagnosis of the woman who presents with symptoms of heart failure in the last month of pregnancy or during the first 5 months of the postpartum period should include PPCM as well as the other causes listed earlier. Additionally, sepsis, drug toxicity, and metabolic disorders should be considered and ruled out.

LABORATORY TESTS

The laboratory tests that will be useful in this setting are those that will help to narrow the differential diagnosis. Appropriate laboratory tests would include a CBC and blood cultures, to rule out sepsis; basic electrolytes and an arterial blood gas, to rule out a metabolic disorder or pulmonary process; cardiac enzymes, to rule out acute myocardial infarction; and toxicity screens for illicit and therapeutic drugs.

The 2D echocardiogram is critical for establishing the diagnosis and for evaluating the effects of treatment on the failing heart. Right heart catheterization (via pulmonary artery catheter) is useful for both diagnosis and monitoring during labor and delivery if the woman presents antepartum. Left heart catheterization, on the other hand, is frequently postponed until after delivery, because it involves radiation, which could pose risks to the fetus. It is also useful to obtain a radionuclide ventriculogram, but as in the case of left heart catheterization, this is frequently postponed until after delivery. Endomyocardial biopsy is not recommended because it is not likely to alter the course of treatment significantly.

TREATMENT

Treatment of PPCM is not markedly different from that for other dilated, congestive cardiomyopathies. Medical therapy will include sodium restriction, diuretics, digoxin, and afterload-reducing agents. In the cardiomyopathy that presents during pregnancy, the afterload agent of choice will be hydralazine; but after delivery, ACE inhibitors should be used because of their proven benefits in heart failure. If the echocardiogram demonstrates a left ventricular thrombus, intravenous or subcutaneous heparin should be instituted (antepartum) and converted to warfarin sodium (postpartum). There continues to be a debate regarding the use of immunosuppressive agents in the setting of idiopathic cardiomyopathy and PPCM, but there is currently no conclusive evidence that this is beneficial, so this type of therapy is not recommended at this time. Until fairly recently, bed rest was recommended as adjunctive therapy for the treatment of PPCM. However, the risk of developing deep venous thrombosis with resultant pulmonary embolism outweighs any possible benefit of this treatment. Therefore, bed rest is not recommended as part of the treatment plan for PPCM.

DISCHARGE INSTRUCTIONS, FOLLOW-UP INTERVAL, INDICATIONS FOR SPECIALTY CONSULTATION AND HOSPITALIZATION

The woman diagnosed with PPCM will require very close follow-up by a cardiologist, since the mortality rate associated with this disease is in the range of 25 to 50 percent and approximately 50 percent of those deaths occur within 3 months of the initial onset of symptoms.[9] If PPCM is diagnosed prior to delivery, hospitalization until delivery is a reasonable approach, given the complexity of the symptoms and treatment of the disease. While the patient is hospitalized, consultation with both a cardiologist and a high-risk obstetrician should be undertaken to optimize the health of both mother and fetus. Upon discharge, follow-up with the cardiologist should be arranged. Women with newly diagnosed PPCM must be carefully instructed in how and when to take their medications, what type of diet to consume (i.e., sodium and fluid restrictions), and to weigh themselves at the same time every day (to pick up signs of excess fluid retention as early as possible). It is important to realize that the best chance for optimal recovery of cardiac function is with aggressive medical therapy in the first 3 to 6 months after the diagnosis of PPCM.

ISCHEMIC HEART DISEASE

PATHOPHYSIOLOGY

Myocardial infarction (MI) in the pregnant woman is another very rare cardiovascular disorder, but it is associated with a relatively high mortality rate (as high as 40 percent during the second trimester) in both the mother and the fetus.[10] It is likely that as women postpone the age of childbearing to the late 30s and early 40s, MI in the pregnant woman may be seen more frequently. The factors relative to pregnancy that might increase the risk of MI include the hemodynamic changes that occur during pregnancy, the stress of labor and delivery, and the hemodynamic changes seen in the immediate postpartum period. In the pregnant woman, the most common cause of MI is coronary atherosclerosis, followed by coronary artery spasm. Other etiologies include thromboembolism, coronary artery dissection, arteritis, and cocaine use. In general, the same risk factors that predispose others to MI will predispose the pregnant woman to MI. These include smoking, hypertension, preeclampsia, hyperlipidemia, diabetes mellitus, and a family history of premature coronary artery disease.

DIAGNOSIS AND DIFFERENTIAL DIAGNOSIS

The classic symptom of MI is chest pain accompanied by diaphoresis and possibly nausea and vomiting. However, in the pregnant woman, chest pain may occur in a variety of circumstances. The differential diagnosis of chest pain must include acute MI, pulmonary embolism, aortic dissection, and gastroesophageal reflux. The best way to diagnose an MI is unchanged by pregnancy, i.e., a 12-lead ECG and cardiac enzymes.

LABORATORY TESTS

The most useful laboratory tests in the woman suspected of having an acute MI are the creatine kinase (CK) and CK isoenzymes, which will be elevated by 6 to 8 h after the onset of an acute MI. However, it should be noted that these enzymes may be elevated following labor and delivery because of a cross reaction in the assays with enzymes from the uterus (in the case of a cesarean section) and/or the placenta. Lactic dehydrogenase (LD) and the LD isoenzymes (particularly LD_1 and LD_2 isoenzymes), which rise later than the CK (peaking at 18 to 24 h) may be helpful in some situations. More recently, troponin-T has been used to confirm acute MI; this enzyme may, however, be elevated in the setting of unstable angina without infarction and may not be widely available. Additional laboratory tests that may be helpful in the management of the patient with an acute MI are serum chemistries, which will help detect electrolyte abnormalities that may predispose toward lethal ventricular tachyarrhythmias; CBC, to rule out anemia; and a fasting lipid profile, to assess for hyperlipidemia. Cardiac catheterization should be reserved for use until after delivery unless the pregnant woman is hemodynamically unstable, has recurrent ischemia, or shows evidence of extensive myocardium at risk.

TREATMENT

The pregnant woman who presents with an acute MI should be admitted to a cardiac care unit and is generally treated as she would be if she was not pregnant, with the following exceptions. Thrombolytic agents (streptokinase, tPA) are contraindicated in pregnancy. Beta blockers, nitrates, morphine, and heparin should be used as in the nonpregnant woman, but care must be taken to monitor blood pressure carefully, since hypotension will threaten placental perfusion. The use of aspirin is not without risk to the fetus. Soderlin et al.[10] present some of the pros and cons of aspirin use in this setting, concluding that low-dose aspirin can probably be used safely after the 13th week of pregnancy, when the threat of teratogenesis is no longer present.

DISCHARGE INSTRUCTIONS AND FOLLOW-UP INTERVAL

When the pregnant woman who has had an MI is discharged from the hospital, instructions must be given regarding the proper use of prescribed medications; low-fat, low-sodium, low-cholesterol (American Heart Association) diet; physical activity; and signs/symptoms to be aware of. Risk-factor modification including smoking cessation, blood pressure control, stress management, and lipid elevation management is crucial, since recurrent MI during pregnancy carries a mortality rate as high as 75 percent. This individual will probably require weekly follow-up to ensure optimal compliance with the recommendations listed above. Cardiac rehabilitation is a valuable adjunct to the usual follow-up, although the physical activity goals will have to be modified in the pregnant woman until after delivery.

INDICATIONS FOR SPECIALTY CONSULTATION AND HOSPITALIZATION

Hospitalization is necessary in the case of any pregnant woman suspected of having an acute MI because of the relatively high maternal and fetal mortality rates. However, whether an MI is ruled in or ruled out, the index of suspicion for myocardial ischemia (i.e., unstable angina) may be high. In that case consultation from a cardiologist must be obtained prior to discharge.

ARTERIAL DISSECTION

PATHOPHYSIOLOGY

Changes in arterial integrity that occur during pregnancy are the result of hormonal alterations. These hormonal effects on arterial structure are described in depth by Nolte et al.[11] and include changes in the composition of the ground substance, fragmentation of reticulum fibers, and loss of the normal corrugation of the internal elastic lamina. Similar findings have also been reported in women taking oral contraceptives. It has been hypothesized that the hemodynamic stress associated with pregnancy combined with the structural changes in the vessels of pregnant women can predispose some of them to the rare occurrence of arterial dissection or aneurysm with subsequent rupture. The most common sites of aneurysm and/or dissection are the thoracic aorta, iliac artery, splenic artery, and cerebral artery. Coronary, renal, and ovarian artery dissections and/or ruptures have also been reported. This type of vascular disorder is seen more in grand multiparas than in other instances. Most ruptures or dissections that occur in association with pregnancy occur during the third trimester or the early postpartum period.

DIAGNOSIS, DIFFERENTIAL DIAGNOSIS, AND LABORATORY TESTS

Although arterial dissection and rupture during pregnancy are exceedingly rare, maternal and fetal survival are even rarer. Therefore early diagnosis is essential for any chance of survival. The key step in making this diagnosis is to consider it a possibility. The differential diagnosis would include myocardial infarction, mesenteric ischemia, cholecystitis, pancreatitis, and peptic ulcer disease as well as arterial dissection and arterial rupture. The patient who presents with an arterial dissection will often be hypertensive initially, whereas the individual with an arterial rupture will generally be profoundly hypotensive. A complete examination of the patient's pulses as well as blood pressures in both arms is important to further evaluate the patient. A widened mediastinum found upon chest x-ray might suggest an aortic dissection. If the patient can be stabilized, magnetic resonance imaging of the chest and abdomen will confirm the diagnosis of dissection and determine its extent. In the case of profound hypotension, a low hematocrit will support the diagnosis of arterial rupture. Other recommended laboratory tests include those that were suggested in the previous section (under "Myocardial Ischemia"), since MI is in the differential. If extensive aortic dissection is suspected, evaluation of renal function (BUN and creatinine) will be important to rule out renal artery involvement. A coagulation panel should be obtained as well as blood type and cross-match for at least four units of packed RBCs.

TREATMENT

Once the diagnosis of arterial rupture is made, the only treatment with the potential to preserve the life of the mother and possibly her fetus is emergent surgical repair. It is therefore prudent to involve the vascular surgeon in the case as soon as arterial rupture is considered. Arterial dissection, on the other hand, may be treated medically with elective surgical repair at a later date, or it may also require emergent surgical intervention. Medical therapy for confirmed arterial dissection consists primarily of lowering the blood pressure. Intravenous nitroprusside should be utilized emergently, and once optimal control of blood pressure has been attained, another agent may be started

(such as labetalol or esmolol) while the patient is weaned off nitroprusside. Obviously, the pregnant woman with an arterial dissection will require close observation in an intensive care unit and consultation with vascular surgery, anesthesiology, cardiology, and high-risk obstetrics. Continuous fetal monitoring should be initiated in the viable gestation (i.e., 24 to 26 weeks).

DISCHARGE INSTRUCTIONS AND FOLLOW-UP INTERVAL

Once the diagnosis of arterial rupture or arterial dissection has been made, it is unlikely that the patient will be discharged prior to delivery. Therefore, this discussion is limited to those women who survive and are postpartum. In this setting, the woman will require discharge instructions similar to those recommended for the woman discharged following an acute MI. Modification of those risk factors that can be modified (i.e., smoking, hypertension, hyperlipidemia) should be addressed upon discharge. Follow-up should be arranged with both the cardiologist and the vascular surgeon within 1 month of discharge.

References

1. Gallery EDM: Hypertension in pregnancy—Practical management recommendations. *Drugs* 49:555, 1995.
2. Chambers EC, Clark SL: Cardiac surgery during pregnancy. *Clin Obstet Gynecol* 37:316, 1994.
3. Brady K, Duff P: Rheumatic heart disease in pregnancy. *Clin Obstet Gynecol* 32:21, 1989.
4. Sullivan HJ: Valvular heart surgery during pregnancy. *Surg Clin North Am* 75:59, 1995.
5. Perloff JK: Congenital heart disease and pregnancy. *Clin Cardiol* 17:579, 1994.
6. Dajani AJ, Bisno AL, Chung KJ: Prevention of bacterial endocarditis. *JAMA* 264:2919, 1990.
7. Page RL: Treatment of arrhythmias during pregnancy. *Am Heart J* 130:871, 1995.
8. Kinsella SM, Lohmann G: Supine hypotensive syndrome. *Obstet Gynecol* 83:774, 1994.
9. Lampert MB, Lang RM: Peripartum cardiomyopathy. *Am Heart J* 130:860, 1995.
10. Soderlin MK, Purhonen S, Haring P, et al: Myocardial infarction in a parturient. *Anaesthesia* 49:870, 1994.
11. Nolte JE, Rutherford RB, Nawaz S, et al: Arterial dissections associated with pregnancy. *J Vasc Surg* 21:515, 1995.

Chapter 29

CARDIOPULMONARY RESUSCITATION DURING PREGNANCY AND PERIMORTEM CESAREAN SECTION

Vern L. Katz

GENERAL PRINCIPLES OF MANAGEMENT

One of the most difficult aspects of the cardiopulmonary resuscitation (CPR) of a pregnant woman is concern for the viability and the health of the fetus. There are two guiding principles for performing CPR on a pregnant woman. First, the successful resuscitation of the mother should precede all else as the primary guiding principle of these efforts,[1-4] and all of the medications, resuscitation, and electrocardioversion protocols should follow exactly as in the nonpregnant woman. While the first guiding principle is *saving the mother's life,* the second is *concern for the life of the fetus.* The great majority of cardiac arrests in pregnant women will be from nonresuscitatable causes such as massive trauma, fatal pulmonary emboli, or intracranial hemorrhage. (It is rare for a pregnant woman to have a myocardial infarction.) Thus, because most cardiac arrests are nonresuscitatable, the physician performing CPR must be alert and ready to deliver the fetus emergently during the CPR.[5-9] For example,

if a mother arrives in the emergency department with an obvious nonresuscitatable cause, such as severe head and chest trauma, emergency cesarean delivery should be undertaken immediately in the emergency department. However, if it is questionable whether the mother can be resuscitated, then cardiopulmonary resuscitation should be performed prior to delivery. One may rely on the 4-minute rule for emergency cesarean delivery.[5] This rule states that if the peripheral pulses are not felt by 4 min after CPR is begun, a cesarean delivery should be performed. A rapid cesarean procedure should allow delivery of the neonate within 1 min. Thus, 5 min after the maternal arrest, resuscitation of the neonate may begin. The 4-minute rule is based on the concept that neurologic damage to the fetus begins to occur after it is deprived of oxygen for 4 min. Thus, consideration of fetal health and viability necessitates rapid delivery. Although the fetus may often survive periods of hypoxia for several minutes, efforts to deliver the fetus should be made at this point. This type of delivery has been termed a *perimortem cesarean delivery.*[5] During a perimortem cesarean, resuscitative efforts should be continued on the mother.[5-12] If the

371

mother can be resuscitated with resumption of cardiac output, then there is no need for cesarean delivery. Performing a perimortem cesarean section as part of CPR of the mother may improve resuscitative results for the mother by improving cardiac output.

PHYSIOLOGIC ADAPTATIONS OF PREGNANCY THAT MAY AFFECT CARDIOPULMONARY RESUSCITATION

The pregnant woman adapts to the demands of the uteroplacental-fetal unit by rapidly expanding cardiac output and blood volume and by decreasing systemic vascular resistance. These maternal physiologic adaptations have less of an impact on CPR than one might expect.[5–12] The primary physical change that does affect CPR is postural. Beyond 24 weeks of gestation, the uterus begins to compress the vena cava and, as pregnancy progresses, compresses the aorta as well (Fig. 29-1). Late in the third trimester, with the mother in the supine position, cardiac return may be decreased by up to 70 percent resulting in a decrease of cardiac output by 25 to 30 percent.[5–12] The postural effect of aortocaval compression necessitates repositioning of the mother during any medical evaluation in the last half of pregnancy, whether she is in the emergency department for a minor trauma, being transported to the radiology department, or most importantly, being resuscitated.[1–14] The effect of aortocaval compression on CPR is profound. The implication of this postural effect is that the mother must either be tilted or the uterus displaced off the vena cava in order to perform adequate cardiopulmonary resuscitation[1–14] (Fig. 29-1B).

In determining the duration of gestation of the mother (as described previously), one may use the rule of finger breadths (Fig. 29-2). For example, the uterine fundus may be palpated at the umbilicus at 20 weeks of gestation. The uterus grows about 1 cm per week after this point. After measuring the distance between the top of the uterine fundus and the umbilicus, the clinician may add 2 weeks (to the initial 20 weeks) for every finger breadth above the umbilicus. (For instance, if the top of the fundus is four finger breadths above the umbilicus, the estimated gestational age is 28 weeks.) This is helpful both in establishing whether there will be aortocaval compression and in determining viability. The vena cava and aorta bifurcate into the iliac vessels at the level of the umbilicus; until the uterine mass is appreciably higher than this level (about 4 cm), there is almost no aortocaval compression. Viability occurs generally at 24 to 26 weeks of gestation. Thus, if the fundus is below the umbilicus or only one or two finger breadths above the umbilicus, the pregnancy may be considered not viable.

The second aspect of maternal physiologic change of pregnancy that affects cardiac resuscitation is respiratory adaptation.[5,9,14] During pregnancy, progesterone and the expanding uterus lead to significant effects on the respiratory drive and the respiratory system. These have been discussed in detail in Chap. 2. The mild respiratory alkalosis and increased respirations will not affect CPR. However, the de-

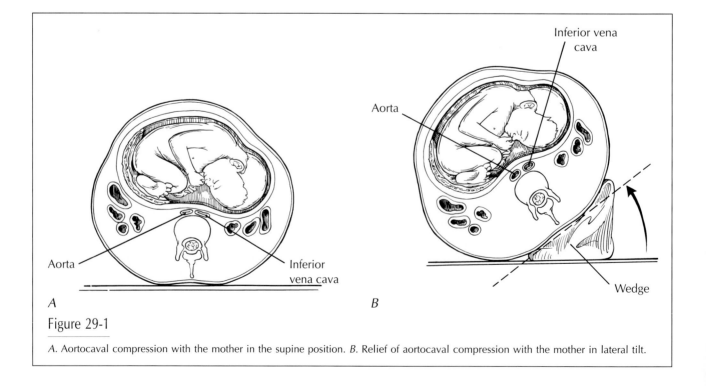

Figure 29-1

A. Aortocaval compression with the mother in the supine position. B. Relief of aortocaval compression with the mother in lateral tilt.

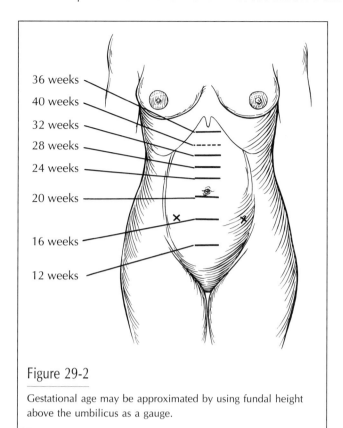

Figure 29-2

Gestational age may be approximated by using fundal height above the umbilicus as a gauge.

crease in functional residual volume and functional reserve that occurs during pregnancy does affect cardiopulmonary resuscitation. The obtunded mother, particularly the mother who has developed a respiratory arrest, will become anoxic more quickly than the nonpregnant patient, since the pregnant woman has less functional reserve. Thus, resumption of respirations with adequate oxygenation takes on a greater urgency. Prompt ventilation with 100% oxygen is both safe and necessary in the mother with respiratory compromise.

Progesterone decreases smooth muscle activity, resulting in prolonged gastric emptying time during pregnancy. The enlarging uterus in late pregnancy also distorts the gastrointestinal tract. Thus, early endotracheal intubation to protect the airway from aspiration is an integral part of cardiopulmonary resuscitation, despite the natural hesitancy to intubate a semiconscious pregnant woman.[5-13]

The expanded cardiac volume that leads to the most profound physiologic changes in pregnancy does not greatly affect CPR. However, the mother will divert blood flow to vital organs, brain, heart, and adrenals at the expense of the pregnant uterus. This can result in a normal blood pressure but with low uteroplacental perfusion, a situation made worse with the mother in the supine position, when cardiac output will be diminished and preferentially directed to areas above the diaphragm.

In summary, for the clinician, anatomic and physiologic changes of pregnancy must be considered during maternal CPR. When the pregnant patient needs resuscitation, ges-

tational age must be considered. However, when records are unavailable, the gestational age may be estimated by using the finger-breadth rule. After 24 weeks, the supine position should be avoided. Early intubation with appropriate ventilation with 100% oxygen is also critically important in resuscitating the pregnant woman.

MANAGEMENT OF CARDIOPULMONARY ARREST IN PREGNANCY—HISTORICAL OVERVIEW

Until about 10 years ago, cardiopulmonary resuscitation of the pregnant woman was carried out in the traditional fashion. After the mother was considered unresuscitatable and CPR discontinued, a check for fetal viability was performed. If a fetal heart rate was auscultated, a postmortem cesarean section was performed. With this approach, most infants died within a few days from profound neurologic damage. In the mid-1980s, it was recognized that chest massage was uniquely unsatisfactory in restoring adequate cardiac output to the pregnant victim of cardiac arrest and her fetus. Several examples in the literature described women with what was considered electromechanical dissociation.[5] After emergency cesarean delivery, cardiac output improved. Algorithms were then developed to perform cesarean delivery as part of the cardiopulmonary resuscitation.[6-13] Throughout the past decade, cesarean delivery has become accepted as part of the normal resuscitation of the pregnant woman if her peripheral pulses could not be obtained.

INITIAL EVALUATION AND MANAGEMENT

The essence of care of the obtunded and severely traumatized pregnant patient is similar in most respects to that of the nonpregnant patient. However, preparation for any potential problems concerning the fetus is an important aspect of care. If there is adequate notification from the transporting personnel, it is preferable to have an obstetrician or pediatrician present when the pregnant woman arrives at the emergency department. If the traumatized patient—whether obtunded or already undergoing CPR—arrives with sufficient notification, immediate consultation with pediatric and obstetric staff should be obtained if available.

Policies should be developed in all emergency departments to address the issue of CPR during pregnancy. Cardiopulmonary resuscitation should be performed in the emergency department without movement into an operating suite. However, certain aspects of the resuscitation may necessitate surgical procedures. Part of the CPR may be a perimortem cesarean section. Thus, if possible, a pregnant woman should be assessed in the trauma room, with the facilities to perform the surgical procedures immediately available. The materials for perimortem cesarean section are readily found in the trauma suite (including scalpel, clamps, Mayo scissors, large bandage scissors, suture, and needle holders; see Table 29-1). Materials for resuscitation of the baby must also be available, including a radiant warmer, neonatal laryngoscope with functioning batteries and lights, neonatal intubation tubes, cord clamp, scissors, bulb syringe, neonatal Ambu Bag with tubing, oxygen source, and suction source (see Chap. 12 for resuscitation of the neonate). Materials for resuscitation of the baby delivered in an emergent situation are also in the standard resuscitation pack. Notification of pediatrics will aid in the resuscitation, since there will be two patients requiring attention after an emergent delivery.

The first step in the management of the pregnant woman who may be developing a cardiac arrest is similar to that in the nonpregnant patient. If the patient is responsive, she should be placed in the left lateral decubitus position, protecting the cervical spine if necessary. If she is on a spine board, she should be tilted, either by placing a rolled towel under one edge of the backboard or by assigning someone to displace the uterus manually. If she is unresponsive, the ABCs must be attended to (airway, breathing, and circulation). As this is being done, the code team, anesthesia, obstetrics, and pediatric staff should be called in. The positioning of the pregnant patient's head to facilitate breathing is similar to that in the nonpregnant patient; intubation should be performed early in the resuscitation in order to protect the airway from regurgitation secondary to delayed gastric emptying of pregnancy. If the pregnant woman is not breathing, she should be given two slow breaths with 100% oxygen while checking for pulses. In the absence of a palpable pulse, CPR should be initiated immediately. If a pulse is present, intravenous fluid should be started as well as oxygen and endotracheal intubation. During initial management, we cannot emphasize strongly enough the importance of keeping the patient in a lateral tilt position. The most appropriate intravenous fluids to use are lactated Ringer's solution or normal saline, because rapid infusion of dextrose may result in fetal acidemia.

BASIC CARDIAC RESUSCITATION TECHNIQUES

Prior to 24 weeks of gestation, the approach to basic CPR is essentially the same for pregnant and nonpregnant patients. After 24 weeks of gestation, CPR is modified by the need to perform an emergency cesarean during resuscitation and the avoidance of supine positioning. The techniques described in the American Heart Association textbook for basic life support should be followed, with the same algorithms for ratio of chest compression to respiration.[14] Because of the changes of pregnancy, the stomach contents should be assumed to be full; therefore the airway should be secured with an endotracheal tube as soon as possible.

The determination of cardiac arrest is the same as in a nonpregnant patient and is determined by palpation of the pulse.[14] The carotid pulse may be palpated in a similar fashion as in the nonpregnant patient. Chest compressions should be initiated and performed in a similar manner in pregnancy and nonpregnancy, with compression along the lower half of the sternum. The person performing the CPR should push directly down over the sternum. Importantly, the victim's head should be below the level of compressions and not elevated. The fingers of the resuscitator may be extended or interlaced, but fingers should not be used in compression. The resuscitator's elbows should be locked and the shoulders should be over the outstretched hands. The sternum should be depressed 1½ to 2 in., as in the nonpregnant patient. Compressions should be performed at approximately 80 to 100/min. It is rare that there would be only one person performing compressions in the emergency department; however, a 15-to-2 ratio of compressions to breathing is appropriate in one-person resuscitation. Almost always, there are several people performing CPR and the 5-to-1 compression-to-ventilation ratio should then be observed.

For women who are known to be beyond 24 weeks of gestation or in situations where the uterus is palpable above the umbilicus, the mother should be placed in a lateral tilt or the uterus should be displaced.

There are essentially two techniques for displacement of the pregnant uterus. Unfortunately, both involve positioning of the mother such that chest compression becomes less effective.[5–14] The first technique for displacement involves placing a wedge under the abdomen, preferably under the right side. The woman is thus tilted toward the left. This will most often involve some tilting of the chest, making chest

---

Table 29-1

EQUIPMENT FOR A PERIMORTEM CESAREAN DELIVERY

Scalpel
Bandage scissors
Mayo scissors
Toothed forceps
Richardson retractors
Needle drivers
Suture

compressions more difficult. The second technique involves having an assistant lift the uterus off the vena cava. This is very difficult to do for more than a few seconds and most often takes a large person who will often be lifting the whole body up. Alternatively, the pregnant uterus can be displaced laterally—manually pushing the uterus off the great vessels.

An extremely important aspect of positioning is the determination of pulses. If pulses cannot be palpated along the femoral arteries at the inguinal ligament, one must assume that effective cardiac output is not being maintained. Pulses that are occurring in the neck but not in the femoral arteries may reflect inadequate blood flow to the uterus. If a cesarean section is performed as part of or during resuscitation, basic CPR should be continued throughout the procedure and for an extended period of time afterwards. It has been well documented that, after an emergency cesarean section, some patients gain enough venous return because of displacement of the pregnant uterus away from the vena cava that cardiac output may increase to the point where successful resuscitation becomes possible. The point of continuing CPR until after a cesarean section cannot be stressed enough.

Another aspect of basic CPR that bears mentioning includes the fact that, late in pregnancy, the diaphragm will be displaced upward, as will the liver and spleen. Thus, it becomes even more important that appropriate CPR be performed and that the hands not slide low on the sternum, because this may lead to liver trauma. This further complicates the issue of positioning of the patient.

The American Heart Association has stated that during chest compression, cardiac output is at best 25 to 33 percent of normal.[14] With aortocaval compression from the pregnant uterus, there may be as much as a two-thirds drop in cardiac output. Thus, with CPR and the mother in a supine position in the latter half of pregnancy, there may be as little as a 10 percent cardiac output.[5–14] Radiologic studies have shown that immediately after cesarean birth, aortocaval compression is ended. If peripheral pulses cannot be felt despite normal rhythm or despite chest compressions, then the resuscitation demands cesarean delivery.

Cesarean delivery of a fetus after maternal death is a well-documented operation and postmortem cesarean delivery is a part of mythology and popular folklore throughout the world. The current medical literature includes numerous instances of well-documented, successful postmortem deliveries with successful, intact survival of babies up to 30 min after cardiac arrest.[5–14] The great majority of infant survival occurs with delivery within 5 to 10 min of cardiac arrest. This underlies the rationale for a prompt cesarean delivery to save a neurologically intact baby. The rationale for prompt cesarean delivery is not only to allow ex utero resuscitation of the baby but to relieve aortocaval compression. Marx documented the need for prompt resuscitation in five cases of cardiac arrest that occurred secondary to anesthetic complications at the time of elective procedures during pregnancy.[5]

Three women had CPR initiated with immediate cesarean section. The mothers and infants did well. Two mothers had CPR but cesarean delivery was delayed; these women suffered neurologic sequelae. Other authors have also documented the successful use of perimortem delivery in returning maternal cardiac output.

Consideration for the fetus is a guiding principle of CPR in pregnancy. If cardiac output as determined by peripheral pulsations cannot be returned within 4 min, the emergency physician should initiate a cesarean delivery. If an obstetrician is present, he or she may perform it. If not, the emergency physician should perform it while ancillary staff continues CPR.

ADVANCED CARDIAC LIFE SUPPORT

The limitations and performance of advanced cardiac life support are the same for pregnant women and nonpregnant individuals. Algorithms such as those developed by the American Heart Association should be followed as if the patient were not pregnant.[15]

Advanced cardiac life support is dependent on continuity between basic and advanced support. As chest compressions and ventilation are being performed, evaluation of the cardiac rhythm is begun. The need for use of the defibrillator is part of the initial evaluation.[15] Defibrillation is necessary if the mother is supine and has a sinus rhythm but is pulseless. Prior to defibrillation, she should be put into lateral tilt. If she has an arrhythmia requiring rapid cardioversion—specifically ventricular fibrillation, ventricular tachycardia, or ventricular asystole—defibrillation should be initiated as quickly as possible. Pregnancy is not a contraindication to electrical cardioversion. Defibrillation is performed in the same way for the pregnant as for the nonpregnant patient.[1–4,6–15] There are multiple reports in the literature documenting the safety of defibrillation during pregnancy. The guiding principle of maternal resuscitation is that the fetus is most likely to do well if the maternal resuscitation efforts are successful. The positioning of the conductor pads is the same in pregnancy as in nonpregnancy. The success of resuscitation depends on the establishment of appropriate cardiac rhythm as soon as possible. Thus, the emergency physician should not hesitate to use the defibrillator as appropriate. Many times the trauma patient will be brought in having been defibrillated by the emergency medical technicians (EMTs). The technique of three defibrillations, as in the algorithms used by the American Heart Association's algorithm for cardiac life support, is similar in pregnancy and nonpregnancy. The pulse should be assessed. If the mother's pulses cannot be palpated, CPR should be initiated and/or continued while the defibrillator is connected. Up to three shocks may be given, beginning at 200, 300, and 360 J. If the patient remains pulseless, resuscitation should be continued for 1 min, the cardiac rhythm reassessed, and three-shock defibrillation repeated if necessary. If ventricular fibrillation or ventricular tachycardia is noted, epinephrine should be given (1 mg IV push) and then defibrillation repeated. Basic cardiac chest compression should be continued, with a recheck for ventricular fibrillation or ventricular tachycardia after 1 min. This should be repeated as necessary.

During the first 4 min of CPR, 16-gauge or larger intravenous lines should be placed and normal saline or lactated Ringer's solution infused rapidly. The medications used for bradycardia, asystole, and tachycardia are all appropriate for use in the emergency situation in pregnancy.[14,15] Many agents can be administered through the endotracheal tube as well as the intravenous line. Lidocaine, beta blockers, atropine, beta-adrenergic agents, calcium channel blockers, alpha and beta agonists, epinephrine, norepinephrine, dopamine, dobutamine, calcium, digitalis, narcotics, nitroglycerine, and nitroprusside are all acceptable agents during pregnancy (Table 29-2). These agents may be used as appropriate. While medications are being given, it is important to check whether basic chest compressions are producing femoral pulses. If there is adequate electrical activity but pulses are absent, the emergency physician should move toward performing a cesarean delivery. Pulseless electrical activity (PEA) or electromechanical disassociation has several etiologies, from hypovolemia to pneumothorax to pulmonary embolism. Many of these may be causing the arrest in the pregnant woman. Additionally, pregnancy itself may be a cause of PEA.[15]

It is possible that, prior to the mother's cardiac arrest or cardiac damage, there was enough cerebral or cardiac damage to prevent the recovery of adequate myocardial function. In such cases, the emergency physician should proceed

with a cesarean delivery in order to save the fetus. It is not necessary to check for fetal viability, because this wastes time. If the patient is brought in pulseless with CPR already begun, the degree of fetal compromise is difficult to assess rapidly. It is very difficult, in the middle of a resuscitation, to assess for fetal heart rate. If the fetal heart rate is very slow, for example, it may be missed by auscultation. To stop the cardiac resuscitation of the mother in order to document fetal viability is inappropriate. Thus, in the pulseless cardiac arrest patient, cesarean delivery should be initiated whether fetal viability is established or not. There are numerous documentations in the literature of the resuscitation of fetuses (with intact recovery) with maternal arrests up to 25 to 30 min after the arrest.[5-13] Thus, even if the mother is brought in to the emergency department with ongoing CPR, cesarean delivery should be performed. The cesarean delivery may start immediately if cardiac resuscitation has been initiated prior to arrival in the emergency department. If there are adequate pulsations in the mother with CPR, attempts to establish independent, maternal cardiac activity should be continued and it is not necessary to perform a cesarean delivery.

Occasionally, the emergency physician will encounter a patient who is not in a full cardiopulmonary arrest but close to a respiratory arrest. Endotracheal intubation with initiation of ventilation should be considered in a pregnant patient who is approaching respiratory failure.[9-11] The initiation of mechanical respirations in a pregnant woman with pulmonary extremis will be helpful to both mother and fetus.

PERFORMING A PERIMORTEM CESAREAN DELIVERY: TIMING OF THE PROCEDURE

A perimortem cesarean section should be initiated within 4 min of maternal cardiac arrest.[5-9] If a woman is brought in to the emergency department and CPR has been ongoing in the field, a cesarean delivery may be performed immediately.

As discussed above, there is a double rationale for performing the perimortem section as part of resuscitation: First, the pregnant woman is essentially two patients, the fetus and the mother. Although fetuses can survive as long as 30 min after maternal cardiac arrest, the greatest likelihood of fetal survival as well as intact survival requires neonatal resuscitation rapidly (4 to 5 min) after maternal cardiac arrest. This is because the fetus has compensatory mechanisms to prevent injury and brain damage.[5-13] Many of the situations leading to maternal cardiac arrest have already produced maternal respiratory depression and thus the fetus is already relatively hypoxic. The second reason for performing a cesarean section is that one of the greatest hindrances to effective CPR is the inability to obtain adequate cardiac output. As described above, attempts may be made to displace the uterus off the vena cava; however, these are usually only partially

Table 29-2

MEDICATIONS AND DOSAGES COMMONLY USED FOR RESUSCITATION

Medication	Dosage
Atropine	0.5–1.0 mg IV
Epinephrine	1.0–5.0 mg IV
Norepinephrine	2–12 μg/min IV
Dopamine	1–5 μg/kg/min IV
Dobutamine	2–20 μg/kg/min IV
Isoproterenol	2–10 μg/min IV
Nitroprusside	0.1 μg/kg/min IV
Nitroglycerine	0.3–0.4 mg sublingual
Furosemide	20–40 mg IV
Adenosine	6-mg bolus IV
Lidocaine	1.0–1.5 mg/kg IV
Procainamide	20–30 mg/min IV

Source: Adapted from Ref. 15.

successful. Any alteration of a victim's supine position during chest compression leads to decreased effectiveness. Thus, if the cause of the cardiac arrest is *reversible*—as from cerebrovascular accidents, pulmonary emboli, drug overdoses, or other forms of shock—the greatest likelihood of performing adequate resuscitation will be with the uterus emptied by cesarean section. If the cause of the cardiac arrest is *irreversible*—as in the case of a massive myocardial infarction or, more commonly, chest or head trauma—the sooner the baby is delivered, the better the chance the baby has. It will obviously not hurt the mother with irreversible cardiac arrest to perform a cesarean delivery.

TECHNIQUE OF PERIMORTEM CESAREAN DELIVERY

Once the decision to perform the cesarean delivery is made, the mother should not be moved to an operating suite. There is no need to scrub the abdomen. The important aspect of the emergency delivery is speed. There is no need to administer anesthesia. The cesarean delivery will be relatively bloodless, since there is no cardiac output. Any emergency physician may perform the cesarean delivery. If a surgeon or obstetrician is present, he or she is most able to perform it. As stated above, chest compressions and ventilation should be continued throughout the procedure and after the delivery.

The abdominal incision should be made from approximately 4 to 5 cm below the xyphoid to 2 to 3 cm above the pubis (Fig. 29-3*A*). The incision should be stopped at the pubic hairline. The incision is made through the midline and taken down through the subcutaneous tissue and fascia. The rectus muscles are separated bluntly in the midline and the peritoneum is entered with a midline incision, usually below the umbilicus. The incision is then continued superiorly and inferiorly (Fig. 29-3*B*). Care should be taken not to injure the bladder at the inferiormost aspect of the peritoneal incision (Fig. 29-3*B*). Once the peritoneal cavity is entered along the midline, the uterus will be readily visible. A vertical incision from the top of the uterine fundus to immediately above the opaque insertion of the bladder is simplest (Fig. 29-3*C*). The fetus should then be delivered from the abdomen, quickly dried, and resuscitated in the fashion of an emergency delivery (Fig. 29-3*D*). A key point is that the success of the cesarean delivery demands a rapid incision and rapid delivery. Rapid delivery is best obtained with large abdominal and uterine incisions.

After delivery of the infant, the placenta should be delivered from the uterus. The uterus should be cleaned of membranes with a sponge or towel (Fig. 29-3*E*). While CPR is continued, the uterus can be closed either by a surgical assistant or by the primary physician. The uterus should be closed in one or two layers with a large suture in a running locking stitch. The stitch may be either #0 or #1 semiperma-

nent ligature, such as Vicryl or Dexon, on a large needle. It will usually take two layers to close the uterus. The most important aspect of this procedure is rapid closure. If the mother can be resuscitated and pulses return, she must be stabilized and transferred as quickly as possible. If she is not resuscitatable, as from massive chest or head trauma, multilayered closure may not be necessary. Normally, after the uterus is closed, the fascia and peritoneum may be closed rapidly with a bulk closure and running stitch. This closure should be with a permanent or semipermanent suture. A #0 or #1 Maxon or Proline is appropriate. The subcutaneous tissue does not need to be closed. The skin can be closed either with clips or with a running 2-0 stitch that may be revised later. Again, the rapidity of the procedure and the continuation of the code is important for the mother's survival.

If necessary—prior to closure of the fascia—the liver, intestines, and other organs may be rapidly inspected to ensure that they have not been affected by trauma. If resuscitation of the mother appears to be successful, broad-spectrum antibiotics should be given. A third-generation penicillin with beta-lactamase inhibitors may be used. A third-generation cephalosporin may also be used. After the mother is resuscitated, she should be transferred to the intensive care unit and managed in the same way as any other victim of cardiac arrest or trauma.

The decision to perform a perimortem cesarean delivery is very difficult for the nonobstetrician. It is highly traumatic for the emergency physician as well as the emergency staff. We strongly recommend that a postresuscitation conference be held after any resuscitation of a pregnant trauma victim. Whether or not a perimortem cesarean section is performed, such a conference held within a week to 10 days is helpful. All health providers involved, including EMTs, should be invited. This conference may function both as a quality assurance as well as an educational conference. A facilitator, chaplain, or other support staff may also be invited. The double tragedy of losing a mother and a fetus or the tragedy of losing one of them may be very difficult for the emergency staff. During the conference, a discussion of the principles of therapy and resuscitation for the emergency staff as well as discussion of the protocols involved in the case functions to both teach and relieve the emotional stress involved.

LEGAL AND ETHICAL CONSIDERATIONS FOR PERIMORTEM DELIVERY

At the time of the writing of this chapter, there had never been litigation regarding the performance of a perimortem section. Legal questions *have* arisen when a perimortem cesarean delivery was not performed. However, to our knowledge, no litigation has arisen regarding those issues. It is inappropriate to try to obtain consent for perimortem delivery, since the life of the patient depends on prompt action. In truth, the health

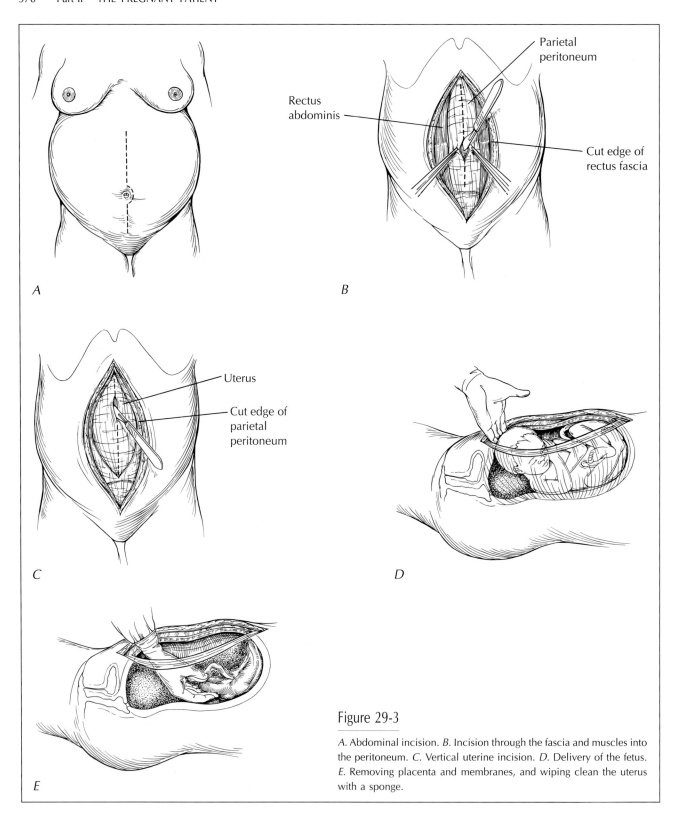

Parietal
peritoneum

Rectus
abdominis

Cut edge of
rectus fascia

A

B

Uterus

Cut edge of
parietal
peritoneum

C

D

E

Figure 29-3

A. Abdominal incision. *B.* Incision through the fascia and muscles into
the peritoneum. *C.* Vertical uterine incision. *D.* Delivery of the fetus.
E. Removing placenta and membranes, and wiping clean the uterus
with a sponge.

of both the mother and fetus may be positively influenced by
the perimortem section. The emergency physician would not
stop or break away from resuscitation in order to obtain consent for open cardiac massage; similarly, it would be inappropriate to do this to perform a perimortem cesarean delivery. Since the performance of the cesarean section is part of
the resuscitation and this has been documented throughout the
literature, it is well within the standard of care to perform such
an operation. Indeed, the timely performance (i.e., within 4
to 5 min of arrest) constitutes optimal care.

At least two ethical principles are involved advocating the performance of the perimortem cesarean delivery. The first is the principle of beneficence. This principle involves always acting for the good of the patient. Since the pregnant mother represents two patients, the performance of a cesarean delivery in order to save the baby and potentially aid in resuscitating the mother by eliminating aortocaval compression works for the benefit of both the mother and fetus. The ethical principle of doing no harm or absence of malfeasance is also upheld in performing this operation. No major blood vessels and no nerves are encountered during the cesarean delivery, given the nature of the operation. Thus, the long-term health of the mother is in no way potentially compromised by performing this operation. Cesarean delivery does not represent a life-threatening operation, and in the setting of cardiac arrest may represent a helpful aspect of resuscitation.

SUMMARY

The underlying principle of cardiac resuscitation of the pregnant woman is the concern for both mother and fetus. Prior to viability, the life of the fetus is totally dependent on the successful resuscitation of the mother. After viability, the two patients must be considered independently. The primary aspects of resuscitation will not harm the fetus as long as cardiac output is maintained; if a perimortem cesarean is indicated as part of resuscitation, this obviously is beneficial for the fetus/neonate.

References

1. Special resuscitation situations. *JAMA* 268:2242, 1992.
2. Dildy GA, Clark SL: Cardiac arrest during pregnancy. *Obstet Gynecol Clin North Am* 22:303, 1995.
3. Satin AJ, Hankins GDV: Cardiopulmonary resuscitation in pregnancy, in Clark SL, Cotton DB, Hankins GDV, Phelan JP (eds): *Critical Care Obstetrics,* 2d ed. Boston: Blackwell, 1987, pp 579–596.
4. Roth A, Elkayam U: Acute myocardial infarction associated with pregnancy. *Ann Intern Med* 125:751, 1996.
5. Katz VL, Dotters DJ, Droegemueller W: Perimortem cesarean delivery. *Obstet Gynecol* 68:571, 1986.
6. Esposito TJ: Trauma during pregnancy. *Emerg Med Clin North Am* 12:167, 1994.
7. Lanoix R, Akkapeddi V, Goldfeder B: Perimortem cesarean section: Case reports and recommendations. *Acad Emerg Med* 2:1063, 1995.
8. Neufeld JDG: Trauma in pregnancy, what if . . . ? *Emerg Med Clin North Am* 11:207, 1993.
9. Pearlman MD, Cunningham FG: Trauma in pregnancy, in Cunningham FG, MacDonald PC, Gant NF, et al (eds): *Williams Obstetrics,* 19th ed. Oct/Nov 1996, suppl PM-1179-21.
10. Garry D, Leikin E, Fleisher AG, Tejani N: Acute myocardial infarction in pregnancy with subsequent medical and surgical management. *Obstet Gynecol* 87:802, 1996.
11. Sherman HF, Scott LM, Rosemurgy AS: Changes affecting the initial evaluation and care of the pregnant trauma victim. *J Emerg Med* 8:575, 1990.
12. Selden BS, Burke TJ: Complete maternal and fetal recovery after prolonged cardiac arrest. *Ann Emerg Med* 17:346, 1988.
13. Lopez-Zeno JA, Carlo WA, O'Grady JP, Fanaroff AA: Infant survival following delayed postmortem cesarean delivery. *Obstet Gynecol* 76:991, 1990.
14. Chandra NC, et al: *Textbook of Basic Life Support for Healthcare Providers.* New York: American Heart Association, 1994.
15. Cummins RO (ed.): *Textbook of Advanced Cardiac Life Support.* New York: American Heart Association, 1997.

PART III

EMERGENCY GYNECOLOGIC DISORDERS IN THE PEDIATRIC PATIENT AND ADOLESCENT

Chapter 30

METHODS OF GYNECOLOGIC EXAMINATION IN THE YOUNG PATIENT

David Rosen

The techniques used to perform gynecologic examinations of young patients in the emergency department are not substantially different from those used in the examination of older patients. Adequate preparation of the patient (and family), appropriate equipment and lighting, an unhurried approach, and sensitivity to the needs of the patient are important in either setting. Still, the clinician examining younger patients faces additional challenges not typically encountered in the care of adult women. Younger patients will likely be unaccustomed to examination of their genitalia and therefore may well be more uncomfortable or fearful than older patients. Providers, too, may be uncomfortable with the gynecologic examination of younger patients. Issues for providers include general discomfort in caring for younger patients, reluctance to broach difficult topics such as sexuality or potential abuse, lack of experience with the prepubertal or adolescent examination, and uncertainty in distinguishing between normal, variant, and abnormal findings.

In fact, the confident and prepared examiner should have little difficulty examining most younger patients. Preparation of the patient and her family are critical, and patience in this area will be well rewarded. Proper equipment—including appropriately sized vaginal specula, ample lighting, and a private, quiet, conducive environment—are essential.

The clinician should be confident of his or her basic examination skills and familiar with developmental gynecologic anatomy. Finally, the clinician should anticipate and preempt difficult examinations. Care should be taken not to inadvertently traumatize younger patients in order to complete an examination. When patients do not appear able to cooperate, early consideration should be given to the use of conscious sedation or examination under anesthesia. Evaluation of alleged or suspected sexual abuse of children is best managed by a specialized team with expertise and experience in seeing these patients.

THE DECISION TO EXAMINE A YOUNGER PATIENT

It is important for the clinician to recognize that examination of the genitalia is likely to be uncomfortable for younger patients, psychologically if not physically. Many preadolescent and adolescent girls will have infrequently (or never) had their genitalia examined by their primary care provider.

Understandably, then, discomfort arises not only from a fear of the unknown but also from a stranger's sudden focus on the patient's "private parts." The latter will be especially true if the examination is being performed in the setting of alleged or suspected sexual abuse. Older children and young adolescents may be extraordinarily modest and reluctant to expose themselves for the examination. For adolescents, the complaint that brought them to the emergency department may involve disclosing behaviors that are private, potentially embarrassing to the patient, and possibly unknown to the parents. Here, assurances of confidentiality are required before the patient will reveal the actual facts of the situation. Table 30-1 lists common indications for examination of the genitalia in this age group.

Although there may be reluctance on the part of patients, families, and clinicians, and despite the potential difficulties in accomplishing the evaluation, gynecologic examinations should not be avoided or deferred when they are clinically indicated. Anecdotes abound in which significant pathology was missed and definitive diagnosis delayed because of a clinician's unwillingness to examine the genitalia. Similarly, in a recent study, 76 percent of girls seeking evaluation for blunt urogenital trauma had injuries worse than originally suspected once an adequate examination was performed.[1] If the emergency department examiner feels unprepared to perform the examination properly, or if subsequent evaluation by a specialist is expected, early consultation is appropriate so that a single satisfactory examination might be done in place of serial examinations by multiple providers.

Table 30-1

COMMON INDICATIONS FOR EXAMINATION OF THE GENITALIA IN THE ACUTE CARE SETTING

Vaginal discharge in the prepubescent girl
Vaginal bleeding in the prepubescent girl
Other vulvovaginal complaints

Hypermenorrhea and/or dysfunctional uterine bleeding

Suspected sexually transmitted infection
Suspected complications of pregnancy
Suspected ovarian cyst and/or torsion
Pelvic pain

Genitourinary trauma

Suspected child sexual abuse

Rape

PREPARING FOR THE EXAMINATION

APPROPRIATE SETTING AND EQUIPMENT

Ideally, the younger patient should be evaluated in a private setting, free from distractions and interruptions. Patients should be reassured that there will be no sudden intrusions, and all efforts should be made to ensure that this is the case. Private rooms, rather than curtained examination areas, should be used if at all possible. Adequate space should be available for the patient, the examiner, a parent or other supportive person, and a chaperone/assistant.

An adequate examination table with adjustable stirrups is required. For patient comfort, it is considerate to pad the stirrups. Seating should be available for the parent and should be suitable in the event that the examination will be conducted with a small child in the parent's lap. Ample lighting is needed, preferably from a light source that remains cool. A fiberoptic light source is ideal, and it should be mobile to accommodate examinations that are not performed on the examination table.

A wide range of vaginal specula should be readily available (Fig. 30-1). A Pederson speculum is optimal for most adolescent examinations, while some adolescents will be more easily examined using the narrower Huffman speculum. For prepubertal children, the small Pederson speculum can sometimes be used, but more often visualization of the vagina will require the use of a smaller instrument such as a nasal speculum, a veterinary otoscope, or even a regular pediatric otoscope (without the ear speculum in place).

Supplies should be available to test for common infections such as *Neisseria gonorrhoeae*, *Chlamydia trachomatis*, and herpes simplex virus. In many facilities, these tests will usually be done using a DNA genetic probe, immunofluorescence, or other nonculture techniques. Nevertheless, culture media should be available, since nonculture methods are not sufficiently reliable for use in the investigation of sexual abuse. Small calcium alginate swabs on flexible shafts should be available to aid in obtaining cultures from small children. Remember, calcium alginate swabs are toxic to *C. trachomatis* if cultures are being used as opposed to antigen detection or DNA probes (see Appendix A3).

A variety of strategies have been described to facilitate the sampling of vaginal secretions from children too young to tolerate a speculum examination or even a vaginal swab. One technique employs a "catheter within a catheter" to instill and reaspirate sterile nonbacteriostatic saline from the vagina (see "Examination of the Young Child").

PREPARATION OF THE FAMILY

The decision to perform a gynecologic examination on a younger patient should be based on specific clinical hy-

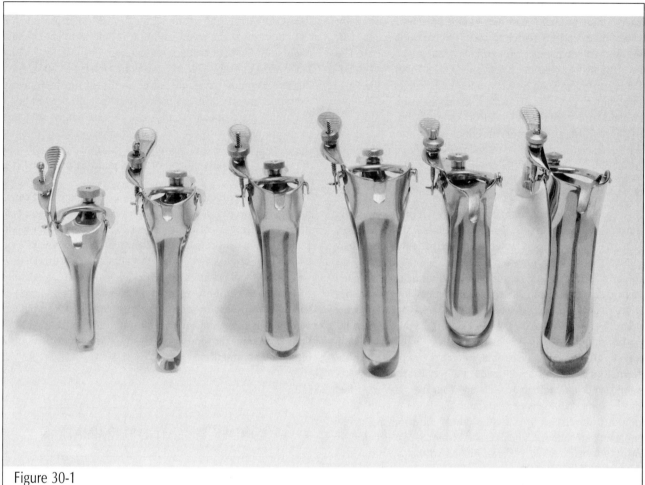

Figure 30-1

Photo showing a variety of speculum widths and lengths.

potheses that must be conclusively evaluated. Understandably, many families are anxious when the examination is suggested and will need to be reassured prior to the examination. Most families respond well to an understandable explanation of the clinical suspicions being explored as well as a careful description of exactly what will be done and why. Families must be helped to understand that the proposed examination is the most appropriate way to answer the clinical question. Parents are concerned that the child's examination will be identical to the complete pelvic examination with which they are most familiar, so it is important to describe the limited nature of the examination that will be done. Families are concerned that the procedure will hurt, so it is crucial to emphasize that it is unlikely to be painful. It is helpful to point out that instruments and equipment especially designed for children will be used. Finally, because some families are worried about hymenal integrity, it can be advantageous to address this issue explicitly. Important reassurance can be given by a statement such as: "We will only do those parts of the examination that are appropriate

for your daughter's body; we will certainly not 'break' or 'tear' any tissue."

PREPARATION OF THE PATIENT

Adequate preparation of the patient is the single most important step in ensuring a successful gynecologic examination. A carefully conducted history offers an opportunity for the examiner to establish rapport with the patient. Talking directly to the child or adolescent is important. Clinicians who only infrequently care for pediatric patients are surprised at how well even very young children can describe their symptoms, answer questions, assent to procedures, and in general participate fully in their own care. Willingness to involve the child in the earlier parts of the visit are well rewarded later, when the child can choose to cooperate or not.

With adolescent patients, confidentiality should be discussed early in the visit and the visit should be structured so that there is some opportunity for history to be obtained from the patient alone. Often, vital information is elicited once confidentiality is assured, and the presenting complaint takes on an entirely different focus. Some adolescents will present with no parents or guardians in attendance at all. The rules related to confidentiality and consent with minor patients vary from state to state and are governed by the "mature minor" doctrine. However, every state in the United States permits clinicians to deliver reproductive health care to minors without parental consent or notification as long as the adolescents are capable of understanding and making informed decisions about their own care.[2]

When families are present, clinicians frequently worry that parents will be reluctant or unwilling to permit private discussions with their daughter. In practice, this is usually not problematic. Parents are usually quite willing to allow the clinician to speak privately with the patient; in fact, parents are usually delighted to have the clinician address the topics of sexuality and reproductive health they presume are to be discussed behind closed doors. Parents do want the opportunity to provide information they feel is relevant, they want assurances that they will be informed of any serious or life-threatening diagnoses, they want to be involved in any significant decision making, and they expect to be informed of the plans being made. Parents nearly always respond well to a statement such as "Your daughter may feel more comfortable answering some questions in private, so now I'd like to ask you to step out of the room for a few moments so that she and I can talk alone. We'll certainly bring you back when we are finished so that you can hear what we think is going on and our plans to take care of it."

The examination itself should be preceded by a complete and clear description of exactly what will be done, using simple and unambiguous language. Medical jargon should be avoided; stirrups are "foot-holders," cultures are "tests," and lesions are "sores." For very young children, it is helpful to know what words they use to denote their genitalia and to use these same words. The clinician should be alert for nonverbal cues suggesting confusion, apprehension, or discomfort and should offer additional support or explanation when necessary. For both children and adolescents, it is often helpful to demonstrate the equipment that will be used, if only to prove that there are no hidden needles.

Because of the psychosexual connotations of the genitalia and prevailing societal expectations of modesty, there is a perceived loss of control and sense of vulnerability inherent in exposure of the perineum for a gynecologic examination. To the extent possible, clinicians should endeavor to restore patients' sense of control in order to increase their comfort during the examination. Patients, for example, should be encouraged to make as many choices as possible about the conduct of their examination. Even very young patients can help to determine how they will be positioned for their examination, who will be present in the room, or even the color of their gown. Similarly, it is important for patients to retain final authority over what will or will not be done to their bodies. Patients can be told to say *"stop"* if, during the ex-

amination, something hurts, they feel uncomfortable, or they want to interrupt the examination for any other reason.

In describing the examination, it is helpful to specifically endorse feelings of embarrassment, nervousness, and reluctance. One can say: "Nearly everyone is nervous about having this examination done, but when it's all finished, nearly everyone says it wasn't as bad as they thought it would be." One must state unequivocally that "It won't hurt" and that the examination will stop if it does. If appropriate, it is sometimes effective for the examiner to say that he or she will "just look." Of course, none of this should be promised if it is not true.

With older patients, when a more comprehensive examination is expected, it is not enough to outline *what* you will do but also important to describe how, why, and with what. For patients who have never had a previous gynecologic exam, it is appreciated when the clinician can offer some sense of how the examination will *feel* as well as an account of what will be done. While a thorough explanation sometimes requires a considerable investment of time, that investment is more than repaid by a more relaxed and cooperative patient and consequently by a smoother and more efficient examination.

CONDUCTING THE EXAMINATION

With proper preparation and a modicum of skill, clinicians should have little trouble in examining most children and adolescents successfully and productively. Patients are more relaxed and comfortable when the clinician is confident and unhurried. The examiner should be decisive but not forceful. Evaluation of the uncooperative patient is discussed below.

POSITIONING THE PATIENT

A relevant general physical examination should be performed prior to examination of the genitalia. This information can be useful not only in making an accurate diagnosis but also in further establishing rapport and trust. The physical examination moves the clinician closer to the patient and allows the clinician to demonstrate sensitivity and gentleness prior to the gynecologic portion of the examination.

Examination of the genitalia can be successfully accomplished with patients positioned in a variety of ways. With older children and adolescents, the dorsal lithotomy position, with the feet in adjustable stirrups, is preferred. This position is usually at least somewhat familiar to patients and can be managed by most without much difficulty or distress. For younger patients, there are other options to consider. Children are offered the choice of being examined on the table or in their parent's (usually their mother's) lap. If the examining table is chosen, children are given the choice of putting their feet into the stirrups or in the frog-leg position. Examinations done with the child arranged in the mother's lap are rarely limiting and offer some advantages. The mother may be seated in a chair (Fig. 30-2A) or, better, may lie on the examining table with or without her feet in stirrups (Figs. 30-2B and C). The child lies in the mother's lap, reclining against her chest. The child's legs are abducted and draped across the mother's thighs, or they are arranged in

the frog-leg position. With hands resting gently on the child's legs, the mother can help to keep the legs abducted during the examination. Frequently, children are more easily able to lie still when positioned with their parent.

Examining the child in the knee-chest position is sometimes very helpful. This position usually allows very satisfactory visualization of the vagina and is most useful to exclude vaginal foreign bodies, to investigate complaints of vaginal discharge, or to assess the posterior hymenal margin

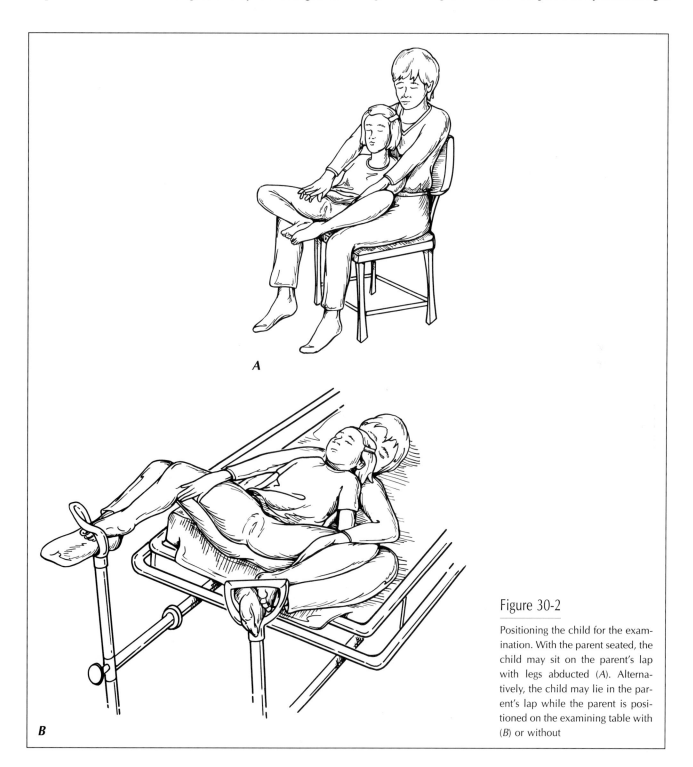

A

B

Figure 30-2

Positioning the child for the examination. With the parent seated, the child may sit on the parent's lap with legs abducted (A). Alternatively, the child may lie in the parent's lap while the parent is positioned on the examining table with (B) or without

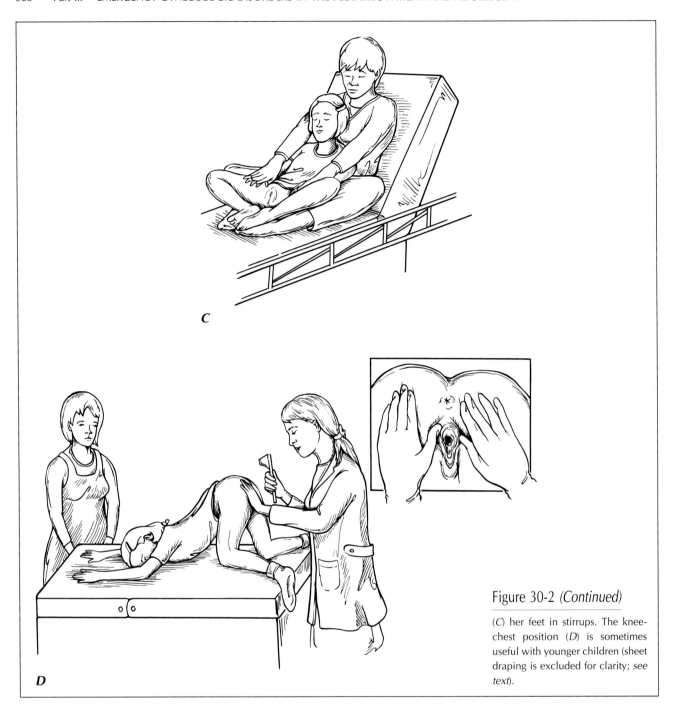

C

Figure 30-2 *(Continued)*

(*C*) her feet in stirrups. The knee-chest position (*D*) is sometimes useful with younger children (sheet draping is excluded for clarity; *see text*).

D

when sexual abuse is suspected. The knee-chest examination is more suitable for younger children than for older children or adolescents; the latter are usually reluctant to position themselves in this way. Children are draped with a sheet and are asked to lie prone on the examining table. While remaining draped, they are asked to raise the buttocks while simultaneously stretching the arms out toward the front and pulling the chest down toward the table (Fig. 30-2*D*). This position is not unlike that of a cat trying to stretch; children who have cats are quickly in place, while others may require

more help in arranging themselves. The parent is positioned at the child's head. Once in the knee-chest position, the child should be encouraged to relax and to let her back sag down toward the table. The examiner retracts the buttocks laterally and upward. As the muscles relax, the introitus likewise relaxes and, with adequate illumination, the vaginal canal (and sometimes the cervix) can be visualized. Relaxation also permits optimal visualization of the margin of the hymenal orifice and findings not seen using supine examination techniques are sometimes discovered.

EXAMINATION OF THE YOUNG CHILD

The young child is usually examined in the mother's lap or with the mother present. A security object, favorite toy, or stuffed animal can help make the child more comfortable during her examination. The specific presenting complaint will direct the focus and extent of the examination. In general, the vulva should be examined for signs of trauma or other abnormalities. The skin should be evaluated for lesions suggestive of infection (e.g., *Candida* or human papilloma virus), infestation (e.g., scabies), or primary dermatologic conditions (e.g., eczema). The presence and configuration of pubic hair should be recorded.

The vaginal introitus is exposed by gently separating the buttocks or thighs. The clitoris, urethral meatus, fossa navicularis, posterior fourchette, and hymen should be inspected in turn for any abnormalities. Clitoromegaly (width of the clitoral glans >5 mm) should be identified. The hymenal configuration should be noted (Fig. 30-3) and unexpected anomalies of the hymenal orifice carefully described. The

technique of labial traction may afford a more useful view of the hymen: the examiner gently grasps the labia majora with the thumb and forefinger of each hand and pulls outward and slightly laterally (Fig. 30-4). When done correctly, this is painless for the patient. The presence or absence of estrogen effect should be noted. The unestrogenized hymen is thin, red, and delicate, while the estrogenized hymen is dull pink, thickened, and redundant or folded. Estrogen effects may be noted well before breast budding occurs. Measurements of the hymenal orifice are controversial; at best, they are dynamic and dependent on positioning, patient relaxation, and the method of the examination. A popular rule of thumb suggests that the largest dimension of the normal hymenal orifice should be no greater than 1 mm for every year of age: thus, a normal 7-year-old girl might have a hymenal orifice of 7 mm. This guideline is generally helpful, but it should not be applied strictly; normal hymenal dimensions in a variety of examining circumstances have been published.[3] If the hymenal orifice cannot be visualized or is obscured by folds of hymenal tissue, the examiner may use a cotton or calcium alginate swab to gently probe until it is

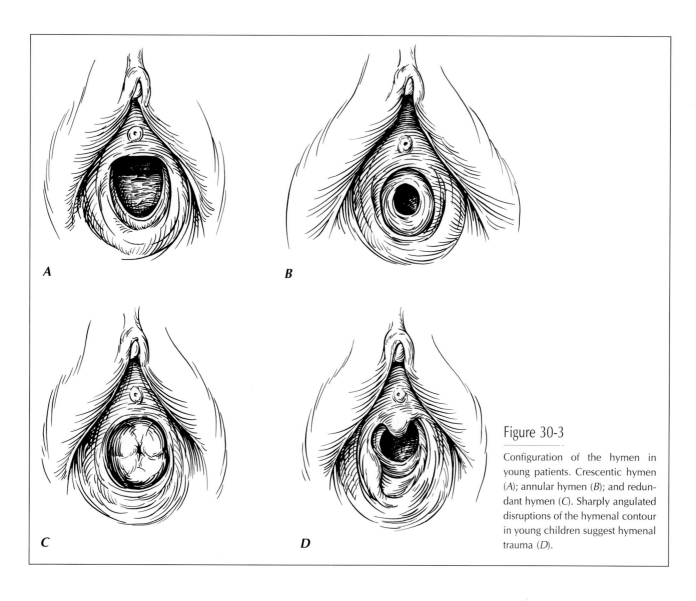

Figure 30-3

Configuration of the hymen in young patients. Crescentic hymen (*A*); annular hymen (*B*); and redundant hymen (*C*). Sharply angulated disruptions of the hymenal contour in young children suggest hymenal trauma (*D*).

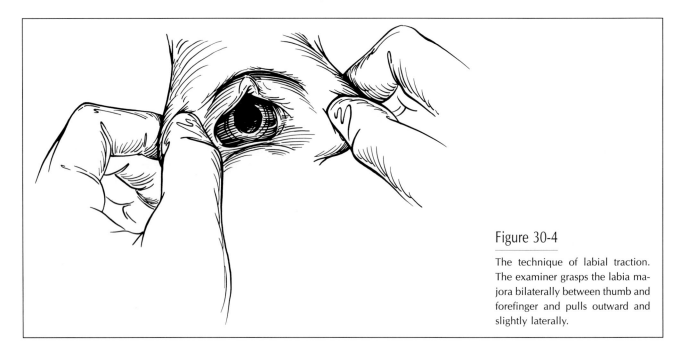

Figure 30-4

The technique of labial traction. The examiner grasps the labia majora bilaterally between thumb and forefinger and pulls outward and slightly laterally.

visualized. Saturating the swab with 2% viscous lidocaine may be helpful; the patient should be told she will feel this maneuver but that it should not hurt.

Though they may be required in some circumstances, speculum examinations of the vagina are not routinely done in prepubertal children. Likewise, digital bimanual examinations are generally not indicated. When the vagina must be visualized, examination with sedation or under anesthesia should be strongly considered, and consultation is warranted to ensure that the most experienced examiner makes the best diagnostic use of the examination. When the possibility of a pelvic mass is suspected, a rectoabdominal examination can provide nearly the same information as the vaginal bimanual examination in prepubertal patients. Not surprisingly, children have no enthusiasm for rectal examinations. Nevertheless, these can usually be managed without anesthesia or sedation in cooperative older children.

For patients whose chief complaint is vaginal discharge, various techniques have been described to collect vaginal secretions for analysis. When discharge is copious, small swabs for specimen collection can frequently be introduced through the hymenal orifice without undue difficulty or patient discomfort. In other settings, however, use of swabs can be uncomfortable or even painful when applied to the atrophic vaginal mucosa of younger children. Pokorny[4] has described a technique that can be helpful in these situations. A catheter within a catheter is constructed using the hub and tubing of a butterfly intravenous catheter and the distal 4 in. of a #12 red rubber urinary catheter. Using sterile technique, the needle end of the intravenous catheter is removed and slipped into the length of bladder catheter. A tuberculin syringe filled with 1.0 mL of sterile nonbacteriostatic saline is

attached to the hub of the assembly. The procedure is carried out in the supine frog-leg position after explaining to the child, in language that she can understand, that her vagina will be "washed with water." The vaginal introitus is exposed, and the catheter is introduced 2 to 3 cm into the vagina. Saline is injected and aspirated several times to ensure adequate mixing with vaginal secretions. The entire apparatus is then quickly removed.

EXAMINATION OF THE ADOLESCENT

As discussed above, gynecologic examination of the adolescent should be undertaken only after a comprehensive confidential history has been obtained from the adolescent alone. Important components of the interview include age of menarche, menstrual history, (frequency, duration, and volume of flow), sexual history and current sexual activity, history of previous sexually transmitted diseases, and previous gynecologic care (of which parents may be unaware). The examiner should be sensitive to patient concerns related to privacy, body image, and sexuality. Modesty should be respected. Some patients will ask for a female examiner, and these requests should be accommodated insofar as possible. General preparation of the patient for her examination has already been discussed. For adolescents being examined for the first time, it is generally worthwhile to describe the examination in considerable detail. Emphasizing that this examination is done routinely on adolescents and that it is an examination that the patient will have done routinely throughout her life can sometimes help to normalize the experience.

Conduct of the actual examination is largely similar to the

examination done in adult women. It is typical to have a chaperone present for the examination; the adolescent may or may not want her mother, sister, or friend present as well. The examination can be used as an opportunity to educate. Normal anatomy, sexual maturation, menstrual physiology, and similar topics may all be addressed as part of the visit. However, the nature of the presenting complaint, pain or discomfort, or patient receptiveness may all mitigate against the possibility of providing much in the way of education during the acute visit. It is often sufficient for the clinician to use the word "normal" frequently in describing the examination as it proceeds.

The examination is conducted in the dorsal lithotomy position with the feet in stirrups. Tanner stage (Figure 30-5) is recorded and careful inspection for anatomic variations or congenital anomalies is done, particularly in the girl being examined for the first time. The external genitalia are examined for evidence of trauma, infection, or other unusual findings. Clitoromegaly, inguinal lymphadenopathy, or hernias should be identified.

The hymen in adolescent girls is likely to be folded and redundant. Its orifice may not be fully visible, or it may appear smaller than it actually is. As in younger patients, a moistened swab can be helpful in delineating the size and contour of the hymenal orifice. In adolescent patients being examined for the first time, it is frequently helpful to perform a digital vaginal examination prior to a speculum examination. One finger is used rather than two. A lubricated examining finger is less uncomfortable than a speculum and affords the examiner an opportunity to locate the cervix prior to insertion of the speculum. However, the use of lubricant precludes obtaining a satisfactory Pap smear or cultures.

For most adolescents, the straight blades of a Pederson speculum offer the best compromise between patient comfort and adequate visualization of the vagina. Some patients will tolerate the wider Graves speculum; the narrower Huffman speculum is appropriate for younger adolescents and when the hymenal orifice is smaller. The smallest pediatric specula are seldom adequate in adolescent patients, as their short length does not permit visualization of the cervix. Specula should be warmed and may be lubricated with water. Physiologic leukorrhea is a common finding in premenarchal adolescents and should not be confused with pathologic processes. Cervical ectropion, in which columnar cervical epithelium is everted onto the visible portion of the cervix, is also fairly common and should not be mistaken for cervical pathology (see Chapter 35, color plate 1). In young women who are sexually active, wet prep and cultures for *Chlamydia* and *N. gonorrhoeae* are usually appropriate. Pap smears may also be obtained in appropriate clinical settings or to avoid the need for a subsequent examination.

Bimanual examination is usually done with a single examining finger. The presence of cervical motion tenderness should be ascertained. The uterus and adenexae should be palpated for enlargement, discrete masses, or tenderness. Pa-

tients being examined for the first time may have difficulty distinguishing between the discomfort of the examination itself and the tenderness being sought. The examiner might say: "You will feel me press very hard on your belly. I need you to tell me whether I am pressing on something sore or whether you just feel me pressing deeply." For the most part, rectovaginal examinations are not required in adolescent patients.

SPECIAL SITUATIONS

THE UNCOOPERATIVE PATIENT OR FAMILY

When the reason for a gynecologic examination is clearly presented and the family and patient have been adequately prepared, truly uncooperative patients should be rare. In the setting of the uncooperative patient or family, the clinician should first attempt to ascertain precisely the reason for the reticence. Often, a particular concern will be at issue—one that can be resolved through additional reassurance, education, or a modification in the exam protocol. One can ask the patient (or family): "What is it about the examination that has you most worried? Maybe we can find some way to get around that for you."

Sexual abuse should also be specifically considered when concerns about the examination are unexplained or seem exaggerated. Sexual abuse may be directly or indirectly responsible for the presenting complaint, or it may have occurred far in the past and be unrelated to the current visit. Still, even remote sexual abuse can be associated with unresolved issues and may make such patients very apprehensive about the proposed examination. Patients are not always willing to disclose previous abuse to an unfamiliar provider in the emergency department; clinicians should not discount the possibility of abuse even when it is explicitly denied by patients.

If the patient's anxieties or concerns about the examination cannot be ascertained or assuaged, the help of family should be enlisted. Often, it is useful to leave the room of an uncooperative patient and allow the family some time alone. A clearer picture of the situation may emerge once the parent has had an opportunity to talk privately with the child or adolescent. For very young children, persuasion with stickers or other treats can be remarkably effective. Preadolescents and younger adolescents are often intensely modest and will be more cooperative once they are reassured that their modesty will be preserved.

Needless to say, no child or adolescent should be examined forcibly. The rights of patients to control their own bodies must be respected. Moreover, it is unlikely that an examination will be productive in the child who is resistant, tensing the muscles (including those of the perineum), and who is unwilling to relax. In such patients, an examination using sedation should be considered.

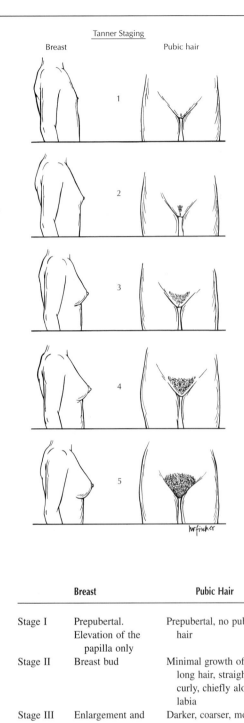

	Breast	Pubic Hair
Stage I	Prepubertal. Elevation of the papilla only	Prepubertal, no pubic hair
Stage II	Breast bud	Minimal growth of long hair, straight or curly, chiefly along the labia
Stage III	Enlargement and elevation of the breast and areola	Darker, coarser, more curly hair over the pubis
Stage IV	Areola and papilla form a secondary mound on the breast	Considerable hair growth of adult type but not hair on the medial thighs
Stage V	Adult breast	Adult configuration pubic hair with growth onto the medial thighs

Figure 30-5

Tanner staging.

EVALUATION OF ALLEGED OR SUSPECTED SEXUAL ABUSE

The evaluation of the sexually abused child is discussed in detail in Chapter 32. Most abused children can readily be examined using the same principles and techniques already described. Some children will be especially fearful of being examined; others, especially very young children, will be surprisingly compliant. When it is determined that the alleged or suspected abuse occurred at some time in the past, the examination may best be deferred to an established clinic or team specifically organized to evaluate these patients. Conversely, patients seen acutely (within 72 hours) after alleged or suspected abuse should be examined immediately and may require a formal forensic examination (using a "rape kit"). These examinations can be traumatic for patients, upsetting for families, and emotionally charged for examiners as well. Ordinarily, the forensic examination is done soon after the assault and therefore at an especially vulnerable time for the patient. Sedation for the examination may be considered especially in the immediate aftermath of the assault, for young children, or for patients who are obviously distressed.

Forensic examinations are time-consuming and require careful documentation and meticulous attention to procedures. For evidence to be admissible in court, the chain of custody must be strictly guarded. The complete examination includes a full-body survey with photographs, fingernail scrapings, pubic hair combing, plucked hair, and the collection of duplicate swabs of all specimens. All bacteriologic studies should be true cultures and not genetic probes, immunofluorescent assays, or other non-culture methods. Subsequent screening for syphilis, human immunodeficiency virus, and hepatitis B is based on the history of the alleged abuse. Morning-after contraception may be offered in appropriate clinical settings (see Chap. 48).

SEDATION

Examination using conscious sedation or general anesthesia should be considered when these modalities would alleviate significant discomfort and/or pain, when they would help to minimize negative psychological responses to the examination or treatment, or in other settings in which examinations could not otherwise be performed.[5] Typically, sedation is most frequently indicated in the evaluation of very young children, in the evaluation of developmentally delayed children (who may not understand the nature of the examination), or when potentially noxious procedures may be required. Only conscious sedation is discussed in detail; however, general anesthesia is a reasonable alternative when conscious sedation is not available or in situations where extensive instrumentation is anticipated.

Safety concerns have prompted recent guidelines for conscious sedation from the American Academy of Pediatrics.[5]

When used in children, all sedative agents are dosed by weight and care must be taken to avoid overdosage (Table 30-2). Resuscitation equipment and personnel trained in pediatric resuscitation should be immediately available. While sedated, a patient's vital signs and oxygen saturation should be continuously monitored, to prevent airway and respiratory compromise. Continuous ECG monitoring is indicated for patients with a history of cardiac disease.

Choice of specific sedative agents will be determined by the nature of the examination to be conducted and its expected duration. Patient age can sometimes influence the choice of sedative but more often affects the route of administration. Because each agent will have its own unique properties, potential adverse effects, and idiosyncrasies, it is best when consultation and assistance are available from clinicians experienced in the use of these potent drugs. Specialists in pediatric emergency medicine usually have the most expertise and experience with the use of these agents in the emergency department.

Fentanyl citrate is a narcotic that is now used in outpatient settings. Its onset of action is short, its duration of action is brief, and it has potent analgesic and sedative effects, making it ideal for short, painful procedures. Its short half-life and potency make it possible to precisely titrate the drug to the desired clinical effect. Fentanyl is usually used parenterally, but it is now available in lollipop form.[6] Respiratory depression can occur with fentanyl, is dose-dependent, and is more likely when other respiratory depressants are used concurrently. It is rapidly reversed by naloxone. Other adverse effects of fentanyl include facial pruritus, nausea and vomiting, and—rarely—anaphylaxis and profound muscular rigidity that can make ventilation difficult. Fentanyl does not cause hypotension or cardiovascular depression.

Midazolam is a short-acting benzodiazepine with sedative, anxiolytic, amnestic, and relaxant properties, but it has no analgesic effect. It has a rapid onset and a brief duration of action. Midazolam is suitable for brief, mildly noxious procedures. It can be given by nearly any route, including parenterally, intramuscularly, per rectum, and intranasally. Onset of action is dependent on the route of administration, usually 5 to 15 min. Respiratory depression is the most common adverse effect and is dose-dependent. Respiratory depression can be temporarily reversed by flumazenil, though this antagonist is not formally approved for use in children.

Ketamine is a dissociative agent with sedative, analgesic, and amnestic effects. It is useful for a wide range of diagnostic and therapeutic procedures but is short-acting. Ketamine may given by multiple routes but is usually used intravenously or intramuscularly. Onset is usually immediate when given intravenously, 5 to 10 min when given intramuscularly, and longer when administered by mouth. The dissociative state produced by ketamine may cause a trance-like effect whereby children appear to be wide awake and staring. The duration of action is 15 to 20 min. Side effects from ketamine include involuntary eye movements and motor activity as well as breath-holding during induction. Because ketamine is a secretagogue, it is recommended that atropine be administered concurrently (in the same syringe). Emergence dysphoria and nightmares occur commonly in

Table 30-2

USEFUL DRUGS FOR THE CONSCIOUS SEDATION OF PATIENTS IN THE EMERGENCY DEPARTMENT

Agent	Dose	Supplement	Onset	Duration
Fentanyl				
IV	1–3 μg/kg (over 3–5 min)	0.5 μg/kg	3–5 min	30–40 min
PO		n/a	Variable	Variable
Midazolam				
IV	0.15 mg/kg	0.02 mg/kg	3–10 min	30–45 min
IM	0.15 mg/kg	0.1 mg/kg	5–15 min	30–45 min
PO	0.5 mg/kg	n/a	10–30 min	Variable
Intranasal	0.2–0.3 mg/kg	n/a	5–10 min	30–45 min
PR	0.2–0.3 mg/kg	n/a	5–10 min	30–45 min
Ketamine				
IV	1–2 mg/kg		seconds	15 min
IM	2–4 mg/kg		5–10 min	20 min
PO			Variable	Variable

n/a = not appropriate.

adults but less commonly (if at all) in children. These can be prevented by the administration of benzodiazepines. Concurrent medication with midazolam is recommended, especially in older children and adolescents. Laryngospasm has been reported rarely. Ketamine does not cause respiratory or hemodynamic compromise.

Several other sedating agents can be useful in the emergency department. Short-acting barbiturates such as *methohexital* provide deep sedation but usually require intravenous or intramuscular administration. As with other barbiturates, respiratory and cardiac depression can occur and are dose-dependent. Use of these agents is limited by their brief duration and action and by the potential for adverse effects. When available, *nitrous oxide* can be easily administered, provides reliable analgesia, and has few adverse effects. However, nitrous oxide is not available for regular use in many emergency departments. Some older sedation protocols can no longer be recommended for routine use in children. Both chloral hydrate and "cocktails" of meperidine/promethazine/chlorpromazine ("DPT") were extensively used in the past to sedate children in the emergency department. These agents are seldom used today because of difficulties related to unreliable onset, prolonged sedation, and adverse effects.

References

1. Lynch JM, Gardner MJ, Albanese CT: Blunt urogenital trauma in prepubescent female patients: More than meets the eye. *Pediatr Emerg Care* 11:372, 1995.
2. Levenberg PB, Elster AB: *Guidelines for Adolescent Preventive Services: Implementation and Resource Manual.* Chicago: American Medical Association, 1995, pp 112–118.
3. McCann J, Voris J, Simon M, Wells R: Comparison of genital examination techniques in prepubertal girls. *Pediatrics* 85:182, 1990.
4. Pokorny SF, Stormer J: Atraumatic removal of secretions from the prepubertal vagina. *Am J Obstet Gynecol* 156:581, 1987.
5. American Academy of Pediatrics Committee on Drugs: Guidelines for monitoring and management of pediatric patients during and after sedation for diagnostic and therapeutic procedures. *Pediatrics* 89:1110, 1992.
6. Schutzman SA, Burg J, Leibelt E, et al: Oral transmucosal fentanyl citrate for premedication of children undergoing laceration repair. *Ann Emerg Med* 24:1059, 1994.

Chapter 31

VAGINAL BLEEDING AND DISCHARGE IN THE PEDIATRIC AND ADOLESCENT AGE GROUPS

Elisabeth H. Quint

VULVOVAGINITIS AND VAGINAL BLEEDING IN THE PREMENARCHAL GIRL

The genital tract of the prepubertal child is quite different from that of a woman of reproductive age. At birth, the vaginal mucosa is thick and estrogenized, because of intrauterine exposure to maternal estrogen. After several days, the estrogen level drops and the vaginal mucosa changes into a smooth, atrophic, thin, and delicate tissue. The pH is between 6.5 and 7.5, and there should be no visible vaginal discharge or bleeding in a healthy prepubertal female. However, there are two points in the developmental timetable when noticeable discharge may be present. The first is in the neonatal period when white mucoid discharge may be present because of circulating maternal estrogens. As the estrogen levels fall, the discharge disappears, but there may be a small uterine estrogen withdrawal bleed. This should all disappear by 6 weeks of age. The typical prepubertal appearance of vulvovaginal atrophy without discharge or bleeding remains throughout childhood, until ovarian stimulation occurs. At this time a noticeable whitish or yellow discharge may appear, which is nonodorous and not irritating. Reassurance for the patient and the parents is in order in these circumstances.

PATHOPHYSIOLOGY

Prepubertal girls are at relative risk for vulvovaginitis because of the proximity of vagina and anus, the lack of protective hair and labial fat pads, and the lack of estrogenization. Other potential contributing factors to vulvovaginitis in this age group are obesity, tight-fitting jeans or leotards, harsh soaps and bubble baths as well as poor hygiene. The normal flora of the prepubertal child has been studied and includes lactobacilli, alpha-hemolytic streptococci, and diptheroids. Other common isolates include *Escherichia coli, Klebsiella,* and other streptococci.[1,2] Etiologies for

Table 31-1

ETIOLOGIES OF VAGINAL DISCHARGE IN THE PREPUBERTAL CHILD

Nonspecific vulvovaginitis
Specific vulvovaginitis
   Candida albicans
   Respiratory pathogens
      Group A β-streptococcus
      Streptococcus pneumoniae
      Neisseria meningitides
      Branhamella catarrhalis
      Staphylococcus aureus
      Haemophilus influenzae
   Enteric
      Shigella
      Yersinia
      Escherichia coli
   Sexually transmitted diseases
      Neisseria gonorrhoeae
      Chlamydia trachomatis
      Herpes simplex
      Trichomonas
      Condyloma acuminatum
Pinworms
Foreign body
Polyps, tumors
Vulvar skin disease (lichen sclerosus, contact dermatitis, psoriasis)
Systemic illness
Trauma
Prolapsed urethra
Congenital anomalies (ectopic ureter, double vagina with fistula)

Table 31-2

ETIOLOGIES FOR VAGINAL BLEEDING IN THE PREPUBERTAL CHILD (REFERRAL POPULATION)

		Incidence
Associated with precocious puberty		21%
True	Idiopathic	
	Cerebral disorders	
	Tuberous sclerosis	
	Congenital adrenal hyperplasia	
	Primary hypothyroidism	
Pseudo	Ovarian tumors	
	Adrenal tumors	
	McCune-Albright syndrome	
	Gonadotropic producing tumors	
	Iatrogenic	
Not associated with precocious puberty		
Neonatal hormonal withdrawal		
Vaginitis (e.g., shigella, *Streptococcus pyogenes*)		6%
Vulvar lesions (e.g., lichen sclerosus, condyloma)		10%
Trauma		8%
Accidental		
Sexual abuse		
Foreign body		
Tumors		21%
Urethral polyps/prolapse		10%
Precocious menarche		
Unknown		25%

Source: Hill NCW, Oppenheimer LW, Morton KE: The aetiology of vaginal bleeding in children. A 20-year review. *Br J Obstet Gynaecol* 96:467, 1989.

vaginal discharge are described in Table 31-1. Inflammation combined with a lack of estrogen can cause labial agglutination, where the labia minora become adherent either in part or completely.

Vaginal bleeding in a prepubertal child is always abnormal after 3 or 4 weeks of age. The etiologies are listed in Table 31-2. Most bleeding in premenarchal girls occurs not because of major trauma but because of vulvovaginitis (especially due to Shigella or group A beta streptococci), scratching, or the introduction of a vaginal foreign body.

HISTORY AND PHYSICAL EXAMINATION

The diagnosis of vaginal bleeding and discharge in the premenarchal child relies heavily on a detailed history. If the main complaint is discharge, the characteristics of the discharge are important: color (bloody, green, yellow), consis-

tency (watery, flocculent), duration (more than 1 month is usually a nonspecific discharge), associated pruritus (vulvar or anal), odor (fecal, fishy), and staining of underwear. Has there been previous treatment and has it been effective? Is there a recent history of infection or use of antibiotics? Are there indications for suspicion of sexual abuse, including behavioral changes, abdominal pain, headaches, enuresis? Obtain information on perineal hygiene, including wiping from front to back, use of harsh soaps and bubble baths, and urinating with the knees together, which increases urinary reflux in the vagina.

If the presenting complaint is vaginal bleeding, the history should focus on the circumstances of bleeding, times of recurrence, and associated symptoms like pain (see Fig. 31-1). Acceleration of weight and height or other signs of puberty suggest precocious puberty. Relevant history includes trauma, sexual abuse, history of foreign body, blood dyscrasias, and other medical problems.

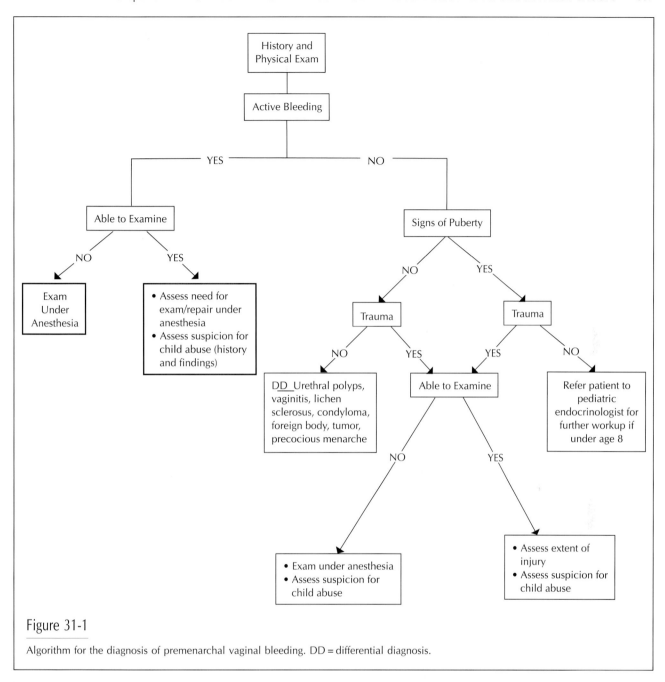

Figure 31-1

Algorithm for the diagnosis of premenarchal vaginal bleeding. DD = differential diagnosis.

The physical examination for vaginal discharge and bleeding must include special attention to Tanner staging of breasts, pubic and axillary hair, and the external genitalia. (see Fig. 30–5). Look for the presence of pubic hair, clitoral size, signs of estrogenization (lush pink vulva and vaginal tissue as opposed to thin, red skin), discharge, bleeding, and any signs of trauma. Note the degree of perineal hygiene and perianal excoriation (suggestive of pinworm). Describe the type of hymen and look for signs of sexual abuse (described in Chaps. 30 and 32). An attempt to see inside the vagina can be made by using the knee-chest position and an otoscope. With deep inspiration in the knee-chest position, the cervix or foreign bodies can sometimes be identified.

A rectoabdominal exam can be performed in the frog-leg position by inserting a well-lubricated index or little finger into the rectum and placing the other hand on the abdomen. In the premenarchal girl, only a small button cervix should be felt (ratio of uterus to cervix = 1:2). As the rectal finger is removed, the vagina is milked for evidence of blood or discharge.

DIFFERENTIAL DIAGNOSIS

The most common etiology of vaginal discharge is non-specific vaginitis. In the case of a specific vaginitis, respiratory, enteric, and sexually transmitted pathogens are the major etiologic agents. *Shigella* and *Yersinia* can produce bloody vaginal discharge, sometimes associated with diarrhea. *Candida* in prepubertal girls is uncommon unless it is associated with risk factors such as antibiotic use or diabetes mellitus. If there is suspicion that *Neisseria gonorrhoeae* or *Chlamydia trachomatis* may be causing the discharge, a culture-proved diagnosis is crucial to pursue prosecution and positive results must be reported to local authorities.[3–6] These infections may be acquired by colonization at birth from a mother with an active infection, but they rarely persist beyond 12 to 24 months.[6,7] Genital herpes caused by herpes simplex types 1 and 2 has been reported in children. The clinical presentation is similar to that described in adults, with painful vesicles and ulceration developing after an incubation period of 2 to 20 days. A primary infection can cause inguinal adenopathy, fever, malaise, headache, and significant discomfort with urination. Although the virus has been described as surviving in water and on plastic surfaces,[8] the majority of cases are thought to be sexually transmitted.[9,10] When a child presents with genital herpes, other sites, like the oropharynx and the hands, must be carefully inspected. When both oral and genital lesions are present, the chance of autotransmission increases. The differential diagnosis of ulcerative lesions includes varicella, herpes zoster, dermatitis, trauma, and *Candida*. Trichomoniasis, causing a frothy yellow-green discharge, is fairly uncommon in the unestrogenized premenarchal child.[11] Approximately 5 percent of infants of mothers with vaginal trichomoniasis will become infected perinatally.[12] Beyond the first few weeks of life, it is highly suspicious for sexual abuse; therefore a complete investigation must be undertaken.[13] Bacterial vaginosis (BV) generally presents as a thin grayish discharge with a fishy odor. It is caused by a mixed collection of organisms, including *Gardnerella vaginalis*, *Bacteroides* species, and *Mobilincus*. It is unclear how often BV is associated with sexual abuse. Bacterial vaginosis has been described in asymptomatic girls,[2] as well as in 25 percent of abused children compared to 4 percent in a case-control study.[14]

The diagnosis of labial agglutination or labial adhesions was reported in 1.4 percent of infants,[15] usually occurring between the ages of 2 months and 2 years. If the agglutination is partial, it is commonly posterior; if complete, a tiny opening just below the clitoris is usually present (Fig. 31-2). The condition is usually asymptomatic but may present with dysuria, urinary retention, or urinary tract infections. It can be confused with vaginal agenesis, but the presence of a midline raphe makes the diagnosis clear. Other differential diagnoses include lichen sclerosus and childhood cicatricial pemphigoid.

Condyloma acuminatum (genital warts) is caused by the human papilloma virus, usually types 6 and 11 in this age group.[16] It can be transmitted perinatally (up to the age of 2 or 3 years) as well as by sexual abuse.[17] The literature is unclear about the exact age limit, but more than 50 percent of children with genital or anal warts have histories of sexual abuse.[18–20] Therefore, every child presenting with genital warts, regardless of age, deserves a sexual abuse evaluation. The diagnosis is usually made by careful clinical inspection. The application of 3 to 5% acetic acid reveals the characteristic white appearance of the lesions; after it is applied, more

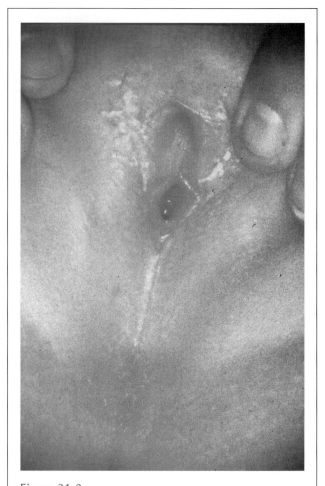

Figure 31-2

Labial agglutination in a 9-year-old girl. (Photograph courtesy of S.F. Smith, M.D. and the North American Society for Pediatric and Adolescent Gynegology, with permission.)

condylomata may become apparent. The differential diagnosis includes *condyloma latum* due to syphilis, perineal tumors, prolapsed urethra, and molluscum contagiosum.

Trauma is usually evident from history and examination. Examination of a child with active bleeding from the vulva can be performed by wiping 2% lidocaine jelly on the cut and then irrigating with warm water from a syringe. If the complete extent of the wound cannot be assessed or the injury does not fit the description of the accident, an exam under sedation or anesthesia is imperative (see Chap. 30). A straddle injury usually causes ecchymoses in the vulva and periclitoral folds. A hymenal tear is very uncommon without a penetrating injury (caused by a nail or a broomstick); in the absence of such a history, sexual abuse should be suspected.

Precocious puberty is defined as sexual development before the age of 8. The causes are numerous (see Table 30-2) and referral to an endocrinologist is appropriate.

Lichen sclerosus is a skin disease of unknown etiology. It can present with itching, dysuria, irritation, and occasionally bleeding. On examination, the skin is atrophic and parchmentlike, with flat ivory-colored papules that can coalesce into plaques and with occasionally ulcers, inflammation, and hemorrhages (Fig. 31-3). There may be an hourglass configuration involving the anus.[21] Secondary infection can occur, especially if itching has been present (Fig. 31-4). The differential diagnosis includes vaginitis, pinworm, sexual abuse, and vitiligo.

A urethral prolapse usually presents with bleeding and complaints of dysuria as well as pain after coughing, straining, or trauma. Occasionally it can lead to urinary retention. The urethral mucosa protrudes through the meatus and presents as a red-blue friable annular (doughnut-shaped) mass (Fig. 31-5).[22]

Foreign bodies present with vaginal discharge or bleeding, occasionally associated with a foul odor. Sometimes the diagnosis can be made in the outpatient setting; often an examination under anesthesia is necessary to confirm the foreign body and for its removal.

Tumors are uncommon in this age group. The most common neoplasm is sarcoma botryoides or embryonal rhabdomyosarcoma.[23] This is a rare tumor in very young girls, involving the vagina, uterus, bladder, or urethra. The symptoms include vaginal discharge, bleeding, abdominal pain, mass, or passage of grapelike tissue. Ninety percent of these tumors occur before age 5. Sarcoma botryoides grows very rapidly and has a poor prognosis unless it is diagnosed early and aggressively treated with a combination of surgery, chemotherapy, and radiation.[24]

Blood dyscrasias are an uncommon source of vaginal bleeding but should be considered if there are other signs of bleeding, such as epistaxis, petechiae, or hematomas.

Precocious menarche is an uncommon diagnosis, defined as cyclical vaginal bleeding without signs of pubertal development, and is considered to be a response to transient production of estrogen by the ovary.[25] It is a self-limiting disease that can last several months. Since it is a diagnosis of exclusion, it is important to rule out all other causes of vaginal bleeding first. The evaluation of a premenarchal girl with vaginal bleeding is described in the algorithm (Fig. 31-1).

LABORATORY TESTS

If vaginal discharge is persistent or purulent, a Gram stain, wet preparation, and cultures should be done. The specimen can be obtained by inserting a soft plastic eyedropper, a small urethral catheter, or a cotton swab moistened with nonbacteriostatic saline gently through the hymenal opening to aspirate vaginal secretions. If no discharge is present, 1 or 2 drops of saline can be introduced into the vagina and then aspirated.[26] The secretions are mixed with 1 or 2 drops of saline and then a drop is placed on a glass slide under the microscope to be examined for leukocytes, motile trichomonads, or clue cells of BV. A second drop of secretions is mixed with a drop of 10% potassium hydroxide (KOH) on another slide. The release of an amine odor is helpful in the diagnosis of BV, and the KOH slide is examined for the hyphae or budding of *Candida*. A culture for *N. gonorrhoeae* is done on the modified Thayer-Martin medium at the time of examination.[3] A *Chlamydia* culture can be performed for persistent vaginal discharge if there is suspicion of sexual abuse. Since enzyme immunoassays

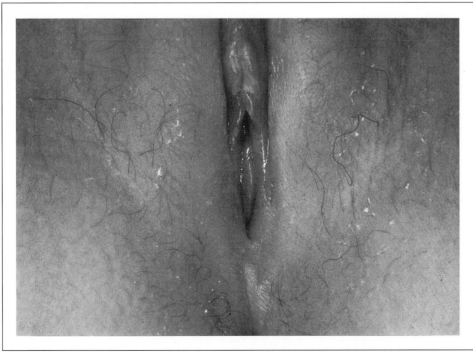

Figure 31-3

Lichen sclerosus in an 8-year-old girl, with distribution around the labia and parchment-like skin.

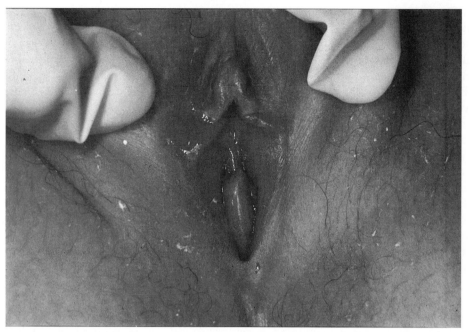

Figure 31-4

Same patient as in Fig. 31-3. With traction, the ulcers became apparent.

and direct fluorescence slides may yield false-positive results, the culture is the preferred test for medicolegal purposes.[4-6] Cultures for other organisms are done by sending the cotton applicator in an aerobic transport tube for aerobic cultures (see Appendix A-3).

If anal itching is the presenting symptom, screening for pinworms should be done. Material is obtained in the morning by pressing the sticky side of a piece of cellophane tape against the perianal area. The tape is then placed against a slide and the slide examined for the characteristic eggs. If there is suspicion of genital herpes, a culture must be obtained, preferably after unroofing one of the vesicles. However, this can be false-positive in a cross reaction with varicella. False-negative results may also be seen if specimens are obtained from lesions with decreased shedding (e.g., crusted or recurrent lesions, see Fig. A3-1).

If the amount of vaginal bleeding has been significant or the patient appears unusually pale, blood for a hematocrit and hemoglobin should be sent.

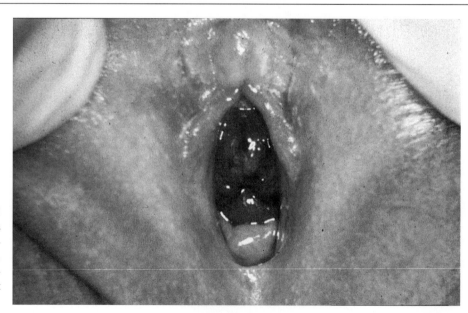

Figure 31-5

Urethral prolapse in a prepubertal girl. A friable, red, annular mass is present around the urethra. (Photograph courtesy of M.A. Finkel, D.O. and the North American Society for Pediatric and Adolescent Gynecology, with permission.)

TREATMENT

For nonspecific vaginitis it is important to stress hygiene measures to the parents. These include good perineal hygiene (including wiping from front to back), unscented soap products, cotton underpants, no tight-fitting clothes, and urinating with the legs spread apart. For treatment of persistent nonspecific vulvovaginitis, a broad-spectrum antibiotic (amoxicillin or cephalexin) is used for 14 days. If this is unsuccessful, an estrogen cream applied daily may help. If the discharge is still persistent, an exam under anesthesia may be performed to rule out a foreign body. In very persistent and select cases, referral to a specialist in pediatrics or gynecology is appropriate. For a specific vaginitis caused by *Shigella* or *Yersinia*, trimethoprim/sulfamethoxazole, one tablet (8 mg/40 mg)/kg per day orally for 7 days, is prescribed. *Candida* can be treated with topical nystatin, miconazole, or clotrimazole cream. Oral fluconazole has been used to treat fungal infections in children with human immunodeficiency virus (HIV) infection,[27] but it is currently not recommended for the pediatric age group with vaginal candidiasis. *Neisseria gonorrhoeae* is usually treated with 125 mg ceftriaxone intramuscularly. If the child is over 8 years old, doxycycline 100 mg orally twice a day for 7 days is added. In younger children, *C. trachomatis* is treated with erythromycin, 50 mg/kg per day for 10 days. Treatment of genital herpes in children should be individualized. For symptomatic primary genital herpes in adults, acyclovir can shorten the duration of symptoms, particularly if given soon after onset. Because acyclovir is unlabeled for use in children less than 2 years old, some clinicians choose to treat symptomatically with sitzbaths and local care. Bacterial superinfection may require antibiotics with activity against both *Streptococcus* and *Staphylococcus*. Trichomoniasis is treated with metronidazole 15 mg/kg per day in divided doses for 7 days. This same dose can also be used for the treatment of bacterial vaginosis.

The treatment of labial adhesions consists of estrogen cream applied daily with gentle outward traction by the parent or other caregiver (Fig. 31-6). Forceful separation should be avoided. The cream makes the tissues thicker and the separation is usually complete in 7 to 14 days. After that, continued use of emollients for several months is recommended to prevent recurrence. If this is unsuccessful and there are urinary symptoms, separation under anesthesia is recommended. Genital condylomata are usually treated under general anesthesia with carbon dioxide laser. Occasionally, in a mature, cooperative girl with only a few lesions, treatment in the outpatient setting with trichloroacetic acid may be tried. The failure rate ranges from 29 to 50 percent.[28,29] Podophyllin should be avoided in the pediatric age group.

The treatment of lichen sclerosus consists of instituting perineal hygiene measures (see above) and the use of mild to moderately potent topical glucocorticoids. If the condition is severe, occasionally highly potent glucocorticoids, like clobetasol propionate 0.05%, are used for short periods of time (2 to 3 weeks). Longer use can lead to atrophy and skin breakdown. Antibiotics can be used for secondary in-

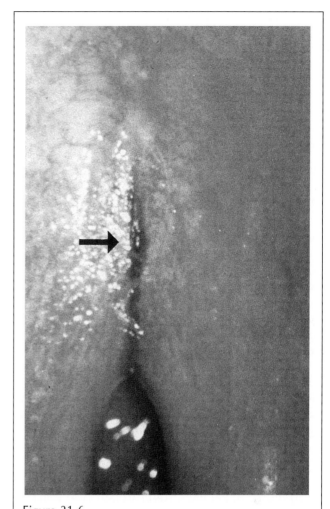

Figure 31-6

Labial agglutination. With traction, the white line becomes clearly visible. Estrogen cream can be applied while traction is held on the labia. (Photograph courtesy of Pediatric and Adolescent Gynecology, Little, Brown Company, Inc. with permission.)

fection due to excoriations from scratching. Some studies have shown a spontaneous improvement with adolescence.[21] Urethral prolapse is usually treated by nonsurgical means like sitzbaths, 2 weeks of daily topical estrogen, and oral antibiotics for secondary infection. If there are large areas of necrosis, surgical resection is usually needed.

If a foreign body is evident on physical examination, an attempt can be made to retrieve it in the emergency department. Toilet paper can be removed with a moistened cotton-tipped applicator or with irrigation. To irrigate, place a small catheter in the vagina and rinse it out thoroughly with normal saline. Depending on the age and cooperation of the child, this may need to be done under sedation or anesthesia. (see Chap. 30).

FOLLOW-UP

For most patients with vaginitis, follow-up is indicated only if the condition persists or returns, in which case the patient can be instructed to see her pediatrician. The patient with suspected sexually transmitted disease or trauma due to sexual abuse will need to be reported to the local authorities—child protective services (CPS)—and follow-up of all cultures will be necessary. The patient's pediatrician or the local CPS will need to be involved for long-term follow-up.

Referral to a pediatrician for follow-up of chronic conditions like lichen sclerosus, labial agglutination, and urethral prolapse should be arranged.

INDICATIONS FOR HOSPITALIZATION

Most patients with the diagnosis of vaginal discharge or vaginal bleeding will be diagnosed and treated as outpatients with follow-up as needed. In certain circumstances, however, the physician may not be able to make the diagnosis without an examination under anesthesia. If the patient is bleeding profusely and the wound or source of bleeding cannot be adequately assessed, the pediatric surgeon, gynecologist, or urologist needs to be consulted for an exam under anesthesia and possible repair. On occasion, a patient may come in with severe vulvar discomfort (e.g., severe lichen sclerosus) and it will be impossible to perform an examination and make a diagnosis. Depending on the patient's age, conscious sedation or an examination under anesthesia can be performed to make a diagnosis, perform biopsies, or treat the condition.

VAGINAL BLEEDING AND VULVOVAGINITIS IN THE ADOLESCENT

Menstrual disorders and vulvovaginitis are among the most common complaints of adolescents. In contrast to the nonspecific etiology of vaginitis in the prepubertal child, vaginitis and vaginal discharge in the adolescent usually have a specific etiology, most commonly related to sexual contact.

Menstrual irregularities are most commonly due to dysfunctional uterine bleeding—defined as excessive, prolonged, or unpatterned bleeding from the endometrium without an organic cause. The normal menstrual cycle usually consists of a mean interval of 28 days ($\pm$6 days) with a mean duration of 4 days ($\pm$2 to 3 days). Normal blood loss is around 30 mL per cycle with an upper limit of 80 mL. Table 31-3 gives the differential diagnosis of abnormal uterine bleeding.

PATHOPHYSIOLOGY

Some 6 to 12 months before menarche, the physiologic vaginal secretions increase and cause a leukorrhea due to normal desquamation of epithelial cells secondary to estrogen effect. After puberty, the vaginal flora resembles that of an adult. Vaginal secretions consist of the products of vaginal

---

Table 31-3

DIFFERENTIAL DIAGNOSIS OF DYSFUNCTIONAL UTERINE BLEEDING

Pregnancy complications
  Abortion
  Ectopic pregnancy
  Trophoblastic disease
Benign and malignant neoplasms of the genital tract
  Cervical polyp
  Vaginal adenosis
  Vaginal carcinoma
  Cervical carcinoma
  Granulosa–theca cell tumors
  Endometriosis
  Leiomyoma
Genital tract infection
  Vaginitis
  Cervicitis
  Vaginal foreign body
  Intrauterine contraceptive device
  Salpingo-oophoritis
Endocrinopathies
  Polycystic ovarian disease
  Hyperprolactinemia
  Hypothyroidism
  Hyperthyroidism
Administration of drugs or hormones
Trauma
Coagulation disorders
  Idiopathic thrombocytopenic purpura
  Von Willebrand disease
  Thallasemia
Chronic systemic illness
  Liver cirrhosis
  Renal failure

---

transudation, endocervical mucous secretions, endometrial and tubal fluids, exfoliated cells, and fluids from several glands. The vaginal flora is dependent upon pH and glycogen-glucose availability for bacteria. Under normal circumstances, the fermentation of glycogen to organic acids leads to a pH of 3.8 to 4.5. This environment favors mainly lactobacilli.[30] Changes in pH or glycogen status affect the lactobacilli, thereby permitting other organisms to grow. Common causes for such changes include antibiotics, douches, alkaline secretions during menses, oral contraceptives, poorly controlled diabetes mellitus, and multiple sexual partners. Estrogen production during adolescence can also lead to a prominent ectropion, and these exposed columnar cervical cells are more susceptible to infection with N. gonor-

rhoeae or *C. trachomatis*. Therefore, it becomes clear that teenagers are at risk for vaginitis as well as sexually transmitted diseases.

Approximately 10 to 15 percent of all gynecologic patients have dysfunctional uterine bleeding (DUB), but it is more commonly seen in adolescents. The etiology of adolescent DUB involves slow maturation of the hypothalamic-pituitary-ovarian axis. This is especially true for the first 18 months after menarche in the adolescent female, as the cycles are usually anovulatory.[31] Although menarche occurs, on the average, at 12.8 years of age in the United States, up to 5 more years may be needed for regular ovulatory cycles to occur.[32]

Normal ovulation involves a regular cyclical production of estradiol, initiating ovarian follicular growth and endometrial proliferation, and, following ovulation, the production of a significant increase in progesterone, which stabilizes the endometrium. Without ovulation and subsequent progesterone production, a state of unopposed estrogen occurs. This causes dilation of the spiral arterial supply in the endometrium, with resultant endometrial growth and associated abnormal height without proper structural support, the result of which is a spontaneous superficial breakage with random asynchronous bleeding. Eventually, increased estrogen has a negative effect on the hypothalamic-pituitary ovarian axis, causing a decrease in follicle stimulating hormone (FSH) and luteinizing hormone (LH) as well as estrogen. This results in a vasoconstriction and collapse of the thickened hyperplastic endometrial lining, with heavy and often prolonged bleeding. In anovulatory cycles, the estrogen levels can be either high or low. With chronic high levels, there is intermittent heavy bleeding, and chronically low levels may result in prolonged light bleeding.

DIAGNOSIS

The presenting symptoms of vulvovaginitis in adolescents usually include vaginal discharge with color ranging from yellow or white to greenish-brown. The vulva can be very erythematous and irritated, causing pruritus, dysuria, or superficial dyspareunia. Pelvic pain, abnormal bleeding, or associated symptoms like fevers may indicate an ascending upper genital tract infection. The history should focus on the characteristics of the discharge; color, odor, pruritus, and duration. Additional information should be obtained regarding menstrual cycles, especially age at menarche, regularity, cycle length and duration, and heaviness of flow. Obtain information on the use of douches, tampons, and medications. The past medical history must include specific information regarding possible endocrinologic abnormalities. The subject of sexual activity must be approached in a friendly, nonthreatening matter and confidentiality assured early on in the visit. It is preferable that the young women be questioned about sexual activity, number of sexual partners, sexual practices, and dyspareunia without the parents present. Open-

ended questions such as "Do you have a boyfriend?" can be used to establish communication early on. The physical examination may be the patient's first pelvic examination. Taking time to explain the procedure is essential. The initial examination includes inspection of the genitalia and noting of Tanner staging. (see Table 30–5). Any signs of inflammation, scratch effects, trauma, or discharge are noted. After this, the labia are gently separated and the hymen and vestibule examined. Whether or not a speculum is used for the sampling of the discharge depends on the size of the hymeneal opening, the use of tampons, and previous sexual activity. If an adolescent is not sexually active, a moistened cotton swab can be used to obtain cultures and a specimen for wet mount. If she has used tampons in the past, it is usually possible to use a Hufman speculum (narrow but long, as opposed to a pediatric speculum, which is narrow and short) to visualize the cervix and obtain cultures. With the speculum in place it is also possible to assess the cervix and the presence and volume of active bleeding. Cultures for *Chlamydia* and gonorrhea need to be taken from every sexually active teenager and, if possible, a Pap smear should be obtained if not performed within the last year. A rectoabdominal or vaginoabdominal bimanual exam is done to detect uterine or adnexal tenderness as well as to rule out any masses.

The most common causes of vaginal discharge in a teenager are candidiasis, bacterial vaginosis, and the sexually transmitted diseases trichomoniasis, gonorrhea, and chlamydial infections. *Candida albicans* is found in 85 to 90 percent of all candidal infections,[33] but noncandidal specimens are becoming more prevalent. Vulvovaginal candidiasis usually presents with severe pruritus in association with a white or yellow floccular discharge. Examination reveals erythema of the vulva, sometimes associated with satellite lesions on the thigh. Bacterial vaginosis accounts for one-third of all vaginitis and commonly presents with a thin grayish discharge with a foul, fishy odor. An acute inflammatory reaction and pruritus are rare. Bacterial vaginosis is not considered a sexually transmitted disease, since its prevalence in sexually active and virginal women is similar.[34] *Trichomonas vaginalis* accounts for 15 to 20 percent of all vulvovaginitis[35] and is considered a sexually transmitted disease. The patient usually presents with a copious, frothy, yellow-green discharge and can have accompanying dysuria and pruritus. On examination, the patient may have punctuate hemorrhages on the vagina and cervix. The other sexually transmitted diseases, gonorrhea and chlamydial infection, are discussed in Chap. 42.

The most common type of abnormal bleeding in teenagers is anovulatory bleeding, due to the immaturity of the hypothalamic-pituitary-ovarian axis. If a girl appears to be bleeding extremely heavily starting at the very first period and necessitating blood transfusions, coagulopathy must be considered in the differential diagnosis. Blood loss in the normal menstrual cycle is self-limited due to the action of platelets and fibrin. Individuals with thrombocytopenia or coagulation deficiency may thus have problems with excessive menstrual bleeding. A 9-year review examined all hospital admissions for acute menorrhagia and determined that 19 percent were the result of primary coagulation disorders, including idiopathic thrombocytopenic purpura and Von Willebrand disease.[36] Of the adolescents presenting with severe menorrhagia or hemoglobin less than 10, some 25 percent were found to have a coagulation disorder; of those presenting with menorrhagia at the first menses, 50 percent were found to have a coagulation disorder.[36]

The possibility of pregnancy should be considered in any adolescent with abnormal bleeding, and a pregnancy test is mandatory even if the patient denies sexual intercourse. Any trauma, infection, or neoplasm can cause abnormal uterine bleeding. Vaginitis, vaginal trauma, a foreign body, or a vaginal neoplasm may cause bleeding that may be assumed by the patient to be uterine in origin. The patient with a foreign body in the vagina generally presents with a bloody, malodorous discharge. Cervical polyps, cervical carcinoma, and cervical inflammation can cause bleeding. Finally, uterine pathology may lead to abnormal bleeding, including endometritis, polyps, and, rarely in this age group, fibroids. Among the endocrinologic disorders that can cause abnormal bleeding, thyroid disease is the most common. In general, hypothyroidism presents with hypermenorrhea and hyperthyroidism presents with hypomenorrhea. Hyperprolactinemia caused by a prolactinoma or certain medications can lead to anovulation and abnormal uterine bleeding. Other diseases to be ruled out are congenital adrenal hyperplasia, Cushing syndrome, hepatic dysfunction, and adrenal insufficiency. Abnormal uterine bleeding in adolescents can be caused by eating disorders, stress, exercise, and weight loss. Common medications (e.g., seizure medications) that increase the cytochrome P450 mechanisms in the liver increase the metabolism of glucocorticoid hormones and can result in dysfunctional uterine bleeding.

LABORATORY TESTS

For the adolescent presenting with vaginal discharge, a cervical Gram stain, cultures for gonorrhea and chlamydial infection, and a wet preparation should be performed. A specimen from the vaginal secretions is obtained with a speculum and is mixed with 1 or 2 drops of saline. The pH balance of the vagina is tested. A pH of >4.5 is more consistent with *Trichomonas* or BV, while a pH <4.5 is consistent with a candidal infection. A drop is placed on a glass slide under the microscope to be examined for the moving trichomonads or clue cells consistent with bacterial vaginosis. Clue cells are stippled vaginal epithelial cells, the borders of which appear obscured by bacteria. Mobiluncus bacterial rods with their characteristic corkscrew movement may be present in the case of a bacterial vaginosis infection. Another drop of secretions is mixed with a drop of 10% KOH on a slide. The release of amine odor (fishy smell, called

whiff test) is used to help in the diagnosis of bacterial vaginosis and the slide is examined for the hyphae and buds of candida. A culture for *N. gonorrhoeae* is done on the modified Thayer-Martin media at the time of examination. A chlamydial culture is done for persistent vaginal discharge and by suspicion of sexual abuse.

For abnormal vaginal bleeding, the initial laboratory studies should include a CBC with platelets. A coagulation profile is recommended if the patient is having acute hemorrhage or has a hemoglobin of less than 10. This should include PT, PTT, and bleeding time. A pregnancy test should also be obtained. If there is any evidence of endocrinologic abnormality, a TSH prolactin, and androgen as well as pituitary imaging studies may be considered. Screening for sexually transmitted diseases should be performed. A pelvic ultrasound can be obtained if there is a high level of suspicion for an anatomic abnormality or if it is impossible to perform a pelvic exam.

TREATMENT

The treatment of choice for candidiasis is intravaginal antimycotic preparations for 3 to 7 days. Usually the imidazoles (miconazole, buconazole, or clotrimzoale) or triazoles (terconazole) are used.[37] In adolescents, the shorter course is associated with better compliance. A newer oral treatment is now available (fluconazole 150 mg given once).[38]

For BV, the treatment can be oral (metronidazole 500 mg twice a day for 7 days) or intravaginal (metronidazole gel twice a day for 5 days). A single 2-g oral dose increases compliance but has lower cure rates.[35] Clindamycin cream 2% for 7 days is an alternative treatment regimen.[39] *Trichomonas* is treated by the oral rather than intravaginal route to eradicate reservoirs in the urethra and periurethral tissues. The 7-day regimen of 250 mg three times a day has a 95 percent cure rate; the one-time 2-g dose has a cure rate of 88 percent. Sexual partners should be treated simultaneously.[40]

Gonorrhea and chlamydial infections are usually treated at the same time and the guidelines of the Centers for Disease Control and Prevention are recommended for this (see Chap. 42).

The goals of therapy for menorrhagia once other pathology has been ruled out is to stop the bleeding, restore synchrony to the endometrium, and replenish iron stores. Most often this can be achieved with estrogen and/or progesterone therapy. The algorithm (Fig. 31-7) outlines the management of dysfunctional uterine bleeding in a systematic fashion.

Irregular vaginal bleeding may be controlled with oral contraceptives; usually a 35-μg ethinyl estradiol preparation is adequate. If anovulatory bleeding is the cause of bleeding, it is also possible to substitute only the missing progestin. Progestins (such as medroxyprogesterone 10 mg) are prescribed for 10 days to induce stromal stability, which is then followed by a withdrawal flow. Disadvantages of this treatment, however, are that the patient is not protected from

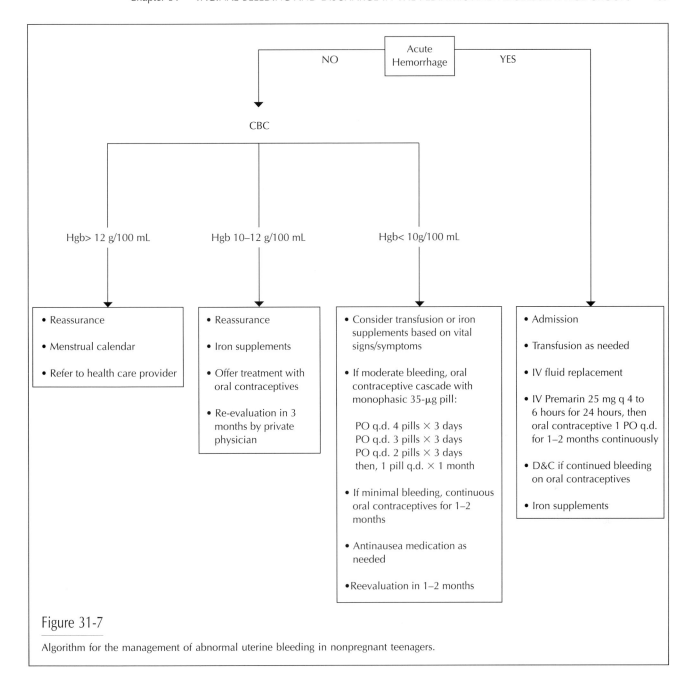

Figure 31-7

Algorithm for the management of abnormal uterine bleeding in nonpregnant teenagers.

pregnancy if she is sexually active and irregular bleeding can occur if the patient ovulates. If atrophic uterine lining is suspected because of prolonged bleeding, sometimes confirmed by an endometrial stripe on ultrasound of only several millimeters, the patient will require estrogen treatment before progestins are given. The estrogen can be given in the form of oral contraceptives or conjugated estrogen (such as Premarin) 2.5 mg for 7 days. For acute, severe menorrhagia, a 50-μg oral contraceptive can be used. The patient may take one pill, four times a day for 1 to 5 days and then be tapered down to one pill per day. Alternatively, intravenous Premarin, 25 mg every 4 to 6 h for 24 h, may be used if the bleeding is acute, the patient is hemodynamically unstable, and admission to the hospital is being considered.[41]

Alternative treatments include prostaglandin inhibitors, which alter the balance between thromboxane and prostacyclin. They may be used as an addition to hormonal therapy or alone if bleeding is not excessive. All patients with anemia should also be treated with iron supplements. A dilatation and curettage is generally not considered unless medical therapy is not successful.

FOLLOW-UP

If the symptoms of the vaginitis resolve with appropriate treatment and are not due to a sexually transmitted disease, no further follow-up is indicated. For the adolescent with gonorrhea and chlamydial infection, it is important to do a follow-up culture for a test of cure after treatment, and this must be arranged for. This visit can also be used to continue education and review birth control options.

The teenager with abnormal bleeding must establish a relationship with a health care provider for long-term follow-up. This can be a gynecologist, pediatrician, or adolescent specialist. The majority of patients with abnormal uterine bleeding will convert to normal menstrual cycles spontaneously within 1 to 2 years. However, the prognosis of patients with acute anemia as well as continued irregular bleeding after several years of treatment is more guarded. A 25-year prospective evaluation of adolescents with dysfunctional uterine bleeding showed that 60 percent continued bleeding for 2 years after initial onset. Persistent problems were noted in 50 percent of patients after 4 years and then 30 percent after 10 years.[42]

INDICATIONS FOR HOSPITALIZATION

An ascending infection due to gonorrhea and/or *Chlamydia*, causing pelvic inflammatory disease, is indication for hospitalization (see Chap. 44).

The adolescent patient who bleeds to the point of needing blood transfusions and intravenous estrogen will have to be admitted by the gynecology or pediatric service for close monitoring and workup.

References

1. Paradik JE, Campa JM, Friedman HM, Grishmuth G: Vulvovaginitis in premenarchal girls: Clinical features and diagnostic evaluation. *Pediatrics* 70:193, 1982.
2. Hammerschlag MR, Albert S, Rosner I, et al: Microbiology of vagina in children: Normal and potentially pathogenic organisms. *Pediatrics* 68:57, 1978.
3. Whittington WL, Rice RJ, Biddle JW, et al: Incorrect identification of *Neisseria gonorrhoeae* from infants and children. *Pediatr Infect Dis* 7:3, 1988.
4. Alexander ER: Misidentification of sexually transmitted organisms in children: Medicolegal implications. *Pediatr Infect Dis* 7:1, 1988.
5. Ingram DL, White ST, Occhiuti AC, et al: Childhood vaginal infections: Association of *Chlamydia trachomatis* with sexual contact. *Pediatr Infect Dis* 5:226, 1986.
6. Fuster CD, Neinstein LS: Vaginal *Chlamydia trachomatis* prevalence in sexually abused prepubertal girls. *Pediatrics* 79:235, 1987.
7. Bell TA, Stamm WE, Kuo CC, et al: Delayed appearance of *Chlamydia trachomatis* infection acquired at birth. *Pediatr Infect Dis J* 6:928, 1987.
8. Nerurkar LS, West F, May M, et al: Survival of herpes simplex virus in water specimens collected from hot tubs in spa facilities and on plastic surfaces. *JAMA* 250:3081, 1983.
9. Gushurst CA: The problem of genital herpes in prepubertal children. *Am J Dis Child* 139:542, 1985.
10. Hibbard RA: Herpetic vulvovaginitis and child abuse. *Am J Dis Child* 139:542, 1985.
11. Jones JG, Yamauchi T, Lambert B: *Trichomonas vaginalis* infestation in sexually abused girls. *Am J Dis Child* 139:846, 1985.
12. Al-Salihi FL, Curran JP, Wang J: Neonatal *Trichomonas vaginalis:* Report of three cases and review of the literature. *Pediatrics* 53:196, 1974.
13. Ross JD, Scott GR, Busuttil A: *Trichomonas vaginalis* infection in prepubertal girls. *Med Sci Law* 33:82, 1993.
14. Hammerschlag MR, Cummings M, Doraiswamy B, et al: Nonspecific vaginitis following sexual abuse in children. *Pediatrics* 75:1028, 1985.
15. Christensen EH, Oster J: Adhesions of the labia minora (synechia vulvae) in childhood. A review and report of fourteen cases. *Acta Paediatr Scand* 60:709, 1971.
16. Goerzen JL, Robertson DI, Inoue M, Trevenen CL: Detection of HPV DNA in genital condylomata acuminata in female prepubertal children. *Adolesc Pediatr Gynecol* 2:224, 1989.
17. Gutman LT, Herman-Giddens ME, Phelps WC: Transmission of human genital papillomavirus disease: Comparison of data from adults and children. *Pediatrics* 91:31, 1993.
18. Obalek S, Jablonska S, Favre M, et al: Condylomata acuminata in children: Frequent association with human papillomaviruses responsible for cutaneous warts. *J Am Acad Dermatol* 23:205, 1990.
19. Hanson RM, Glasson M, McCrossin I, et al: Anogenital warts in childhood. *Child Abuse Neglect* 13:225, 1989.
20. Foster LD: Human papillomavirus infections in children. *Pediatr Ann* 23:354, 1994.
21. Berth-Jones J, Graham-Brown RAC, Burns DA: Lichen sclerosus et atrophicus—A review of 15 cases in young girls. *Clin Exp Dermatol* 16:14, 1991.
22. Capraro VJ, Bayonet-Rivera NP, Magosas I: Vulvar tumor in children due to prolapse of urethral mucosa. *Am J Obstet Gynecol* 108:572, 1970.
23. Maurer HM: The Intergroup Rhabdomyosarcoma Study: Update, November 1978. *NCI Monogr* 56:61, 1981.
24. Flamant F, Gerbaulet A, Nihoul-Fekete C, et al: Long-term sequelae of conservative treatment by surgery, brachytherapy, and chemotherapy for vulvar and vaginal rhabdomyosarcoma in children. *J Clin Oncol* 8:1847, 1990.
25. Blanco-Garcia M, Evain-Brion D, Roger M, et al: Isolated menses in prepubertal girls. *Pediatrics* 76:43, 1985.
26. Paradise JE, Compos JM, Friedman HM, Frishmuth G: Vulvovaginitis in premenarchal girls: Clinical features and diagnostic evaluation. *Pediatrics* 70:193, 1982.
27. Nahata MC, Brady MT: Pharmacokinetics of fluconazole after oral administration in children with human immunodeficiency virus infection. *Eur J Clin Pharmacol* 48:291, 1995.

28. Hanson RM, Glasson M, McCrossin I, et al: Anogenital warts in childhood. *Child Abuse Neglect* 13:225, 1989.

29. Gale C, Muram D: The surgical treatment of condyloma acuminata in children. *Adolesc Pediatr Gynecol* 3:189, 1990.

30. Fredrich EG: Vaginitis. *Am J Obstet Gynecol* 152:247, 1985.

31. Venturoli S, Porcu E, Fabbri R, et al: Menstrual irregularities in adolescents: Hormonal patterns and ovarian morphology. *Horm Res* 24:269, 1986.

32. McDonough PG, Gant P: Dysfunctional bleeding in the adolescent, in Barwin BN, Belisle S (eds): *Adolescent Gynecology and Sexuality.* New York: Masson, 1982.

33. Sobel JD: Vaginal infections in adult women. *Med Clin North Am* 74:1573, 1990.

34. Bump RC, Bueshing WJ: Bacterial vaginosis in virginal and sexually active adolescent females: Evidence against exclusive sexual transmission. *Am J Obstet Gynecol* 1988.

35. Sobel JD. Vaginal infections in adult women. *Med Clin North Am* 74:1573, 1990.

36. Claessens EA, Cowell CA: Acute adolescent menorrhagia. *Am J Obstet Gynecol* 139:277, 1981.

37. Horowitz BJ: Mycotic vulvovaginitis. A broad overview. *Am J Obstet Gynecol* 165:1188, 1991.

38. Perry CM, Whittington R, McTavish D: Fluconazole: An update of its antimicrobial activity, pharmacokinetic properties and therapeutic use in vaginal candidiasis. *Drugs* 49:9984, 1995.

39. Hillier S, Krohn MA, Watts H, et al: Microbiologic efficacy of intravaginal clindamycin cream for the treatment of bacterial vaginosis. *Obstet Gynecol* 76:407, 1990.

40. Lossick JG, Kent HL: Trichomoniasis: Trends in diagnosis and management. *Am J Obstet Gynecol* 165:1217, 1991.

41. DeVore GR, Owens O, Kase N: Use of intravenous Premarin for the treatment of dysfunctional uterine bleeding—Double blind, randomized control study. *Obstet Gynecol* 59:285, 1982.

42. Southam AL, Richart RM: The prognosis for adolescents with menstrual abnormalities. *Am J Obstet Gynecol* 94:637, 1966.

Chapter 32

SEXUAL ABUSE AND ASSAULT IN THE PEDIATRIC PATIENT

Susan F. Pokorny

The emergency department physician plays a vital role in the evaluation and management of survivors of childhood sexual abuse and assault. This role is strengthened if the physician remembers two important principles: (1) treatment for both the psychosocial and physical aspects of the sexual assault or abuse begins with the first encounter and (2) the physician cannot and should not attempt to become "the judge and jury" for the case. The physician's role is that of a healer; he or she is also the one responsible for examining the "scene of the crime." The first principle, that of healing, is occasionally forgotten in the context of forensic and psychosocial pressures; however, the physician must never forget that the patient's needs far outweigh the needs of the legal system. The second principle, that of avoiding judgments, goes counter to the physician's habit of making decisions and therefore deserves special emphasis. To be effective, the physician must become a team member in a very complex psychosocial and legal system that attempts to aid the survivors of childhood sexual assault and abuse.

In initiating an evaluation, it is important for the physician to avoid drawing conclusions prematurely, as, for example, by assuming that abuse has occurred merely because an examination for childhood sexual abuse has been requested by the police or another responsible agency. In such a case, the physician is much more likely to find physical evidence compatible with childhood sexual abuse. On the other hand, physicians have sometimes ig-

nored physical findings or behavioral changes suggestive of childhood sexual abuse simply because the child or caretaker has failed to give an explicit history of such abuse.

Other provider biases relate to whether the physician views his or her role as that of the victim's primary care-taker or as that of a specialist and expert witness for the forensic legal system. These diverse provider roles have a major impact on whether a genital examination is performed and in what degree of detail. Once the physician has agreed to consider evaluating a child for childhood sexual abuse, however, he or she must accept the responsibility of coordinating all findings and reports with other agencies and professionals in the community responsible for the protection of children and the prosecution of criminals.

This interaction with other social agencies presents the physician with several awkward dilemmas. For example, traditional doctor/patient confidentiality is violated. The physician may also have insufficient knowledge of forensic techniques and studies and of the young female's anal and genital anatomy at various stages of development. Furthermore, a history of a sexual assault or abuse is not taken in the same way as the traditional medical history. A much more occult concern, but nevertheless a real one, is the provider's awareness of the limited reimbursement potential for involvement in forensic examinations as well as the possibility of future disruptions of his or her practice by the demands of the legal system.

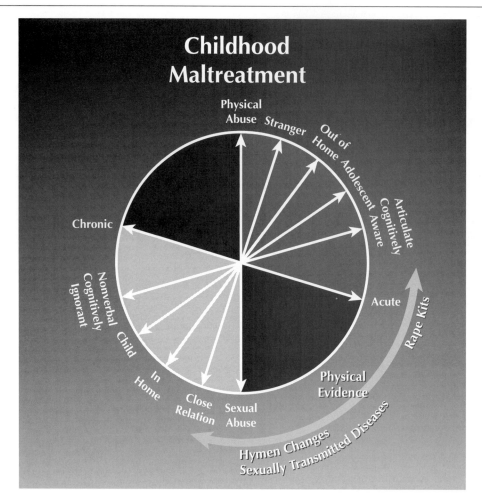

Figure 32-1

The spectrum of childhood maltreatment.

SPECTRUM OF CHILDHOOD SEXUAL ABUSE

Childhood sexual abuse is one of the whole spectrum of entities classed under *childhood maltreatment* (Fig. 32-1). It is very important for the clinician to understand these wide environmental spectrums in which childhood mistreatment occurs. Where on the spectrum of situations a patient is at the time the clinician first addresses the issue will affect the manner in which the evaluation is performed as regards its detail and the timing of its various aspects. These spectrums of childhood maltreatment range from clear cases of physical abuse to sexual abuse. The perpetrator can range from a total stranger to a very close caretaker—from a frightening individual to one seen by the child as loving and caring. The maltreatment might occur inside or outside the home. Childhood maltreatment covers the spectrum from the new-born period to adolescence; because of this age range, the patient may be able to offer an explicit history of the maltreatment or she may be too young to put it into words. Also the manner in which the abuse is perceived varies with the child's cognitive development. Finally, childhood maltreatment can be on an acute basis, or it can be chronic.

A 12-year-old who has entered puberty and is attacked and raped by a stranger is going to be much more willing to report the incident and to comply with a forensic evaluation if she is able to understand that the evaluation will vindicate her. Because this is an acute episode and she has experienced estrogen stimulation of her lower genital tract, a physical evidentiary evaluation including completion of a rape kit should be performed as quickly as possible. Because of her young age, however, a speculum does not necessarily have to be used to obtain vaginal specimens; use of a Q-tip or vaginal lavage with a soft catheter can and should be substituted in many cases.

Another 12-year-old of the same physical and cognitive development who may have been in a clandestine sexually abusive situation for years with an elderly, respected member of the household will not be quite as ready to verbalize her experience because she is aware of its inappropriateness. She might, therefore, not be as willing to comply with a physical examination. The clinician would then have to decide whether or not to perform the exam under anesthesia to complete the rape kit. The latter might be the correct choice if there is a strong possibility of finding debris (i.e., sperm, semen, the assailant's pubic hair, etc.) on the patient's body, which would support the caretaker's suspicion or allegations that abuse has occurred.

Yet another 12-year-old of the same cognitive development might be the one to make the "outcry" that an elderly, respected relative was abusing her. Unfortunately, in many of these situations, the abuse has occurred weeks or months earlier and a forensic rape kit would serve no purpose, since no incriminating debris would remain on the patient's body.

If another 12-year-old with the same physical development had cognitive delays (mental retardation) and abuse was strongly suspected by a caretaker, an attempt to complete a forensic rape kit should be made, since the time of the event is uncertain; but again, the examiner would have to weigh whether or not to proceed to an examination under anesthesia *if* the child were noncompliant.

Another 12-year-old may have no cognitive delays but may not have entered puberty. The same guidelines for timing the abuse or assault dictate whether or not to proceed with a rape kit. However, because the child is prepubertal, the typical pelvic examination would be waived and the examiner should document the details of the external genital anatomy, particularly the hymenal anatomy (Fig. 32-2). That

is not to say that a vaginal specimen should not be obtained, but because of the patient's prepubertal status, the clinician should use a soft rubber catheter to get a vaginal wash and forgo use of a speculum to get a cervical specimen.[1]

It should be noted that only a very small percentage of reported cases of childhood sexual abuse result in medical evidentiary examinations. In one community in 1993, where the majority of physical examinations were provided by a single agency, only 600 of 6000 reported cases of childhood sexual abuse led to physical examinations.[2] This study indicates to some degree the reluctance of the medical community to become involved in these complex evaluations. It should be noted, however, that if the medical community were more often involved, more cases would be "substantiated" by being reported from or involved with the medical community than if they were handled entirely outside the medical community. When the medical community was involved, 40 percent of evaluations were "indicated" and 60 percent were "unfounded"; when other resources without the help of the medical community were involved with the evaluation and management of these cases, only 29 percent were "indicated" and 71 percent were "unfounded."[2]

The vast majority of claims of childhood sexual abuse are temporally remote from the time of the abuse. This is based on a variety of cognitive issues: the child might not initially realize that the abuse was inappropriate, or the child might have been threatened by the assailant and out of fear did not initially report the assault. In these cases, physical changes of the external genital area (Figs. 32-2 and 32-3) and documentation of sexually transmitted diseases become the important areas of investigation for the physician, not the completion of a rape kit. It is only when the episode of abuse has occurred within the preceding 3 to 5 days that a foren-

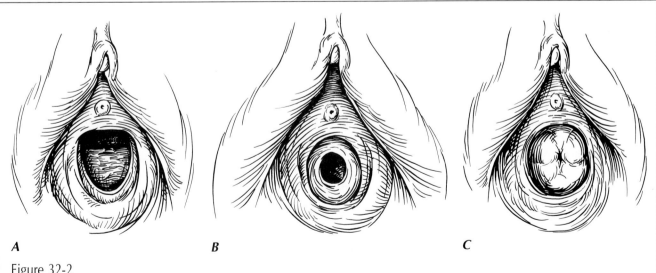

Figure 32-2

Variations of intact hymen configuration in childhood. (From Pokorny SF: Configuration of the prepubertal hymen. *Am J Obstet Gynecol* 157:950, 1987, with permission.)

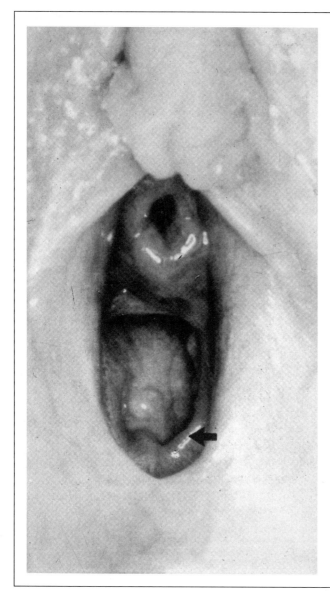

Figure 32-3

Remnants of the hymen in a 7-year-old girl years after multiple episodes of penile-vaginal penetration. (From Pokorny SF: Pediatric Vulvovaginitis, in Kaufman RH, Faro S (eds): *Benign Diseases of the Vagina and Vulva*. St. Louis: Mosby, 1994, p 49, with permission.)

sic rape kit should be completed; within this time frame, there might be evidence remaining on the child's body that would substantiate her story or the history given by a caretaker. Rape kits would be very unlikely to yield any meaningful evidence if the abuse had occurred weeks before the child was brought in for an examination.

The legal definition of whether a new forensic study can be used in court is based on the "relevancy test." This legal doctrine states that novel scientific data are similar to other expert testimony, allowing the data to be admitted into a court of law, but it also allows the data to be attacked by cross examination and reputation. Another legal proceeding that has had an impact on DNA fingerprinting is the Frye test, which states ". . . the thing from which the deduction is made must be sufficiently established to have gained general acceptance in the particular field to which it belongs." Certainly DNA fingerprinting has become a standardized

part of forensic studies as evidenced by certain high-profile, media-covered forensic cases in the last few years. Nevertheless, the contribution that DNA fingerprinting can make in substantiating a patient's allegations of sexual abuse or assault will be disregarded if the material obtained for DNA analysis is not handled in a proper manner.

THE EXAMINATION AND COLLECTION OF FORENSIC MATERIAL

The most important aspect of evaluating and managing a child in the emergency department is the treatment of any acute physical or genital injuries. In-depth interviews are not encouraged in the anxiety-laden atmosphere of an emergency department when an acute genital injury is involved. Questions, if necessary, should be carefully phrased in an open-ended manner and care must be taken not to place words or ideas into the mind of a young survivor. Leading questions can hurt future prosecution efforts. The examiner should query the child with statements such as "tell me what happened" followed by "tell me more" or "and then what happened" and then write the history of what the child thought had occurred verbatim in the chart. There was a time when many emergency department examiners used "anatomically correct dolls" in an effort to get the child to reveal, with less anxiety, details about the sexual assault. These dolls however, were not truly anatomically correct and because of their unusual configurations caught the attention of many young children, tending to evoke misleading statements. It is probably best not to use them unless the clinician has had special training.

When the abuse has occurred weeks or months earlier, many communities have designated evaluation and treatment centers for survivors of sexual assault and abuse. These centers offer a less anxiety-producing environment for the child than an emergency department. In these situations, the examiner's role is to document any anatomic evidence that could be compatible with sexual assault or abuse as well as the presence or absence of any sexually transmitted diseases related to the child's genital symptoms. There are many good photographic resources that can aid in the documentation of these nonacute injuries.[3]

Depending on the degree of certainty for the potential of finding debris on the child's body, as stated in the earlier examples, the physician should consider an examination under anesthesia or a "standby" anesthesia procedure, such as the use of ketamine for the collection of the forensic rape kit material, especially if it appears the examination and collection of materials would be traumatic to the child (see Chap. 30).

The environment in which the rape kit is collected and processed—including a system for maintaining a "chain of evidence"—is very important. Material for rape kits must be handled in such a manner as to assure the court of law that nobody could have tampered with the evidence, either at the time the evidence was collected or as the evidence was transported to the forensic laboratory; this is called the *chain of evidence.* Once a rape kit is open and until it is properly sealed, the provider must have the ability to swear in a court of law that the material was not out of his or her sight or in any other circumstance in which it might have been altered. This, for example, precludes the provider from initiating the rape kit, leaving the room to care for another patient, or leaving the room to go to a microscope to look for motile sperm in a specimen and then returning to the room to complete obtaining materials for the rape kit. This makes it necessary, if specimens are to be examined for motile sperm, to have the microscope within the room in which the forensic rape kit is being prepared. The physician or provider preparing the rape kit must be strict about not allowing other individuals to enter or leave the room during the process of completing the rape kit; should individuals come in and out of the room during the processing of the forensic rape kit, that fact can be presented to a jury and will raise doubt about the reliability of the evidence obtained.

Rape kits are standardized and protocol-driven and vary from community to community. In essence, they consist of a series of swabs and containers that must be adequately labeled with the provider's signature and the survivor's mark and placed in a sealed kit that is then closed with "evidentiary tape." Actually obtaining specimens for rape kits is relatively simple, and written instructions for the multiple steps whereby rape kits are prepared are part of the package. Whenever possible, it is advisable to obtain two specimens of each sample; both the plaintiff and defendant frequently ask to have their own specific forensic laboratories examine the samples. Most of the rape kit is designed to document foreign material on the survivor's body that will substantiate his or her story. It is therefore important to have the survivor undress on a white piece of paper so that any sand, mud, debris, hair, etc., that may be loose on his or her body can be collected and noted, and placed in the rape kit.

Hair is not a positive identifier, but is a comparative identifier of the patient and the assailant. Therefore any loose hair found in the pubic region is placed in a separate bag. Then, if she has reached pubarche, pubic hair from the survivor are placed in the rape kit. Hair can identify individuals by their race, sex, blood type, and hair color. Clothing is best examined while it is on the patient and any tears in the clothing can be matched with body trauma; if at all possible, these findings should be photographed. If there is strong evidence that there is material on the clothing that would substantiate the patient's history, the clothing should be marked and placed in paper bags and sent to the forensic lab. Should clothing be saved for further forensic studies, it should be placed in a paper bag as opposed to a plastic bag since semen will mildew in a moisture-sealed container. Emergency departments must be prepared to provide clothing to be worn home by rape survivors.

Some emergency departments have Wood's lamps, which are used to identify semen on both the body and the clothes. Semen produces a fluorescent color when under a Wood's lamp. The examiner should be aware that certain fungal infections or mildew in clothing will also fluoresce.

Sperm should be looked for in the patient's vagina, in the endocervical mucus, in the rectum, and along the gingival line of the mouth. If there is strong suspicion that the episode was recent, doing a wet-mount preparation from these areas in search of motile sperm would be very important in timing the assault. Routinely, these specimens are taken, air-dried, and ultimately studied in the forensic laboratory for both whole sperm and sperm particles. Depending on the age and maturity of the patient, speculum exams may not be possible; they may also be impossible because of the patient's fright and anxiety. Nevertheless, a wet-mount specimen can be obtained from the vagina with a cotton swab or a vaginal aspirator. Sperm remain motile for 8 to 12 h if they are not in a "hostile environment." For example, if the survivor is on birth control pills, sperm do not remain motile as long. Specimens of endocervical mucus can reveal motile sperm and/or sperm particles for up to several days.

All specimens should be air-dried. Specimens are examined for seminal fluid as well as sperm. If any seminal fluid is on other parts of the patient's body than the vagina or rectum, it can be removed by gently wiping the skin with a moistened 2- by 2-in. gauze pad. This is then allowed to dry, placed in a separate package, and identified, including the body locations from which it came. Seminal fluid is examined for acid phosphatase plus choline, which prove conclusively that the material is seminal fluid. The material is also examined for prostatic antigens; this is a very important means of confirming the assault if the assailant is aspermic or has had a vasectomy.

All specimens—hair, fingernail scrapings, saliva, vaginal fluids, and blood—are examined for blood-group antigens. There are a certain number of females in the general population who do not secrete blood-group antigens into their vaginal pool or other body secretions such as saliva; they are the so-called nonsecretors. It is more expeditious to examine vaginal specimens for blood-group antigens than to subject them to forensic DNA typing. Therefore, if blood-group antigens are found in the vaginal pool and the patient is found to be a nonsecretor, there is no doubt that the blood-group antigens in the vaginal pool came from the assailant. One way to determine whether the patient is a nonsecretor is to obtain a specimen of her saliva by requesting that she chew on a 2- by 2-in. gauze pad, allowing it to air-dry, and placing it in a separate paper container. Some 80 to 85 percent of survivors secrete their blood-group antigens into their saliva and therefore also into their vaginal secretions.

Besides obtaining all of the above-mentioned materials for forensic studies, the physician must attend to the survivor's other needs. Should the survivor, for example, not have urinated since the moment of the assault, having the survivor urinate into a sterile bedpan for collection of that urine specimen can be extremely helpful; if properly handled and spun down, that specimen might contain sperm.

Urinalysis is also occasionally used to determine whether the patient was under the influence of drugs; this information can be valuable in terms of explaining why she was not able to give a detailed account of the assault. Blood work can be obtained to determine if the patient was under the influence of drugs or alcohol and to determine, at the time of examination, the patient's serology and status regarding both infection with human immunodeficiency virus (HIV) and pregnancy. Genital cultures for sexually transmitted diseases are not routinely obtained in the adult survivor, but should there be any suspicion of their presence, they should be obtained from the survivor of childhood assault. All extra tests must be obtained on an individualized and informed basis.

MANAGEMENT OF INJURIES

In the emergency department setting, evaluating acute genital injuries is also an important consideration because many genital injuries described as "accidents" are actually due to sexual assault. Details on the performance of the genital examination are provided in Chap. 30. On the other hand, genuinely accidental genital injuries may be mistakenly attributed to sexual assault simply because of overconcern on the part of the child's caretaker. Emergency department providers must therefore be able to determine whether the presenting genital injuries are compatible with the history as stated.

In a series of 32 acute genital injuries that involved an identifiable wound or acute bleeding, the vast majority of wounds due to sexual assault were *midline* vestibular injuries that *transected the hymen* (Fig. 32-4). In this series there were only three such injuries that were *not* attributed to sexual assault; these were three minor injuries involving a "direct hit," occurring as the child fell directly onto the sharp object that transected the hymen. The other genital injuries in this series did not involve the hymenal orifice and were primarily located away from the vestibular floor.[4]

Chronic sexual abuse will lead to a retraction of the hymenal tissues into nubbins or remnants of this tissue (Fig. 32-3). An explanation should be sought if a child undergoing a genital examination for any reason is noted to have these findings, as they are very strong evidence of stretch trauma occurring at the vaginal orifice.

The emergency department physician should understand the effects of estrogen on the tissues of the lower genital tract throughout childhood and early adolescence.[5] The presence of estrogen allows genital tissues to stretch. For example, estrogen has a tremendous impact on the vaginal tissues during pregnancy, allowing passage of a term-size infant with minimal vaginal trauma. By the same token, prepubertal children lack estrogen stimulation; therefore their genital tissues are much more likely to be torn, traumatized, and altered by any type of stretch trauma—a speculum, an adult finger, or an erect penis.

It is important to understand this impact of estrogen, because the older child—for example a very young and virginal teenager—who has sufficient estrogen can be sexually assaulted with little physical evidence of trauma to the lower genital tract. This is particularly true if such a child is not seen in the immediate postassault period and even more so in the overweight young teenager who has even higher levels of unopposed estrogen than a thin peripubertal girl.

In addition to estrogen effect, the amount of laceration seen after childhood sexual assaults is determined by the acuteness of the assault; if the abuse has been occurring over a long period of time, with gradual dilatation of the vaginal orifice by the assailant, there is less likelihood of laceration.

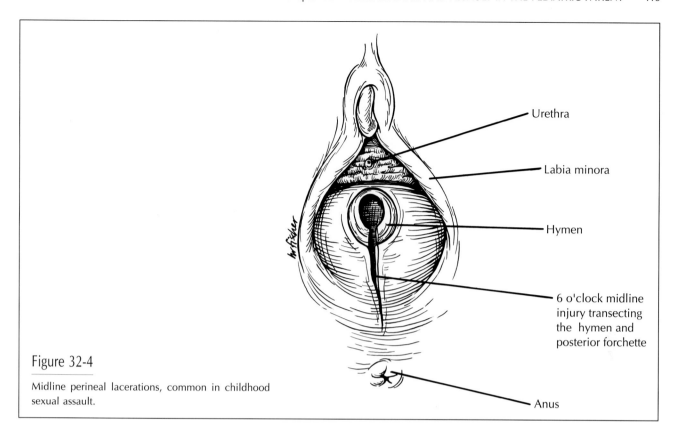

Urethra

Labia minora

Hymen

6 o'clock midline
injury transecting
the hymen and
posterior forchette

Anus

Figure 32-4

Midline perineal lacerations, common in childhood
sexual assault.

References

1. Pokorny S, Stormer J: Atraumatic removal of secretions from the prepubertal vagina. *Am J Obstet Gynecol* 156: 581, 1987.
2. Kerns DL, Terman DL, Larson CS: The role of physicians in reporting and evaluating childhood sexual abuse cases, in Behrman RE (ed): *The Future of Children: Sexual Abuse of Children.* Los Altos, CA: The David and Lucille Packard Foundation, 1994, pp 122, 126.
3. Pokorny SF, Heger A, Emans SJ, et al (eds): *Evaluation of the Sexually Abused Child: A Medical Textbook and Photographic Atlas.* New York: Oxford University Press, 1992.
4. Pokorny SF, Pokorny WJ, Kramer W: Acute genital injuries in prepubertal females. *Am J Obstet Gynecol* 166:1461, 1992.
5. Yordan EE, Yordan RA: The hymen and Tanner staging of the breast. *Adolesc Pediatr Gynecol* 5:76, 1992.

Chapter 33

COMMON GENITOURINARY PROBLEMS IN THE PEDIATRIC AND ADOLESCENT FEMALE

Monica Sifuentes

Genitourinary conditions in children and adolescents often create a diagnostic dilemma for several reasons. First, for most conditions, symptoms vary according to the age of the patient. Second, congenital lesions may initially manifest themselves in this age group—for example, a first-time urinary tract infection (UTI) due to vesicoureteral reflux or obstruction of the ureteropelvic junction. Furthermore, because of the similarity of symptoms, many of these problems can be confused with each other. Is the right-lower-quadrant pain in the premenarchal female consistent with appendicitis, ovarian torsion, or UTI? Even more complex is the case of the adolescent female who may be sexually active. Is her diffuse lower abdominal pain a simple cystitis or pelvic inflammatory disease (PID)? Delaying the correct diagnosis often results in increased morbidity and, rarely, mortality for the young patient. Therefore, evaluations must be thorough, complete, and timely.

URINARY TRACT INFECTION

Urinary tract infection is a common condition seen in children and adolescents. It is the most common serious bacterial illness among febrile infants and young children who present without an obvious source of infection.[1,2] Because the majority of symptomatic UTIs will occur during the first decade of life,[3] it is essential that those who evaluate infants, children, and adolescents recognize the signs and symptoms of UTI and be aware of the long-term consequences associated with recurrent, unrecognized, or inappropriately treated UTIs. The ongoing challenge for the clinician remains to differentiate between lower urinary tract disease (cystitis) and involvement of the upper urinary tract (pyelonephritis). Timely diagnosis and the proper management of both of these conditions will prevent morbidity and decrease the need for more expensive medical care in the future, such as dialysis or renal transplantation.[4]

EPIDEMIOLOGY

It is difficult to establish the true rate of UTI in infants and children, since as many as 40 percent of infections are asymptomatic.[5] Multiple studies have demonstrated, however, that the prevalence of symptomatic UTIs in pediatric patients varies with age and gender.[5–7] During the neonatal period, there is a male predominance seen primarily in uncircumcised boys. When both genders are taken into account, UTIs occur in approximately 0.1 to 2 percent of infants to age 3 months.

Urinary tract infections become more common in females later in infancy and childhood, with approximately 1 percent of school-aged girls developing symptomatic infections each year.[6] Overall, a prevalence of 1.5 to 2 percent in 1- to 5-year-olds has been reported.[8] Male:female ratios for school-age children are approximately 1:4 and 1:25 for symptomatic and asymptomatic infections, respectively.[5]

The incidence of UTI increases during adolescence, when females become sexually active.[6] In the United States, 7 percent of 15-year-old females report ever having had sexual intercourse; this figure rises to 27 percent by age 17 and 55 percent by age 19.[9] And 10 to 20 percent of females have at least one episode of cystitis during adolescence or young adulthood.[10]

Among febrile infants and young children, the prevalence of UTI has been reported to be between 4 and 7.5 percent. In a recent prospective study of 945 febrile infants less than 1 year of age (temperature >38.3°C (>100.9°F), 5.3 percent were diagnosed with UTI.[1] It is interesting to note that 17 percent of white female infants with a temperature >39°C (>102.2°F) had a UTI, significantly more than any other group of infants by sex, race, and temperature.[1] In this same study, 30 percent of infants who had initially received diagnoses other than UTI were ultimately found to have a positive urine culture. Studies such as this have led to the universal recommendation that UTI should always be considered in the differential diagnosis of fever during the first year of life.

RISK FACTORS

Anatomic abnormalities of the urinary tract are an important risk factor in the development of UTIs in children and adolescents. They include vesicoureteral reflux (VUR) and obstructive lesions such as obstruction of the ureterovesical or ureteropelvic junction. Posterior urethral valves also lead to obstruction but rarely occur in females.

Nonstructural risk factors for the development of UTI in females include constipation, stool incontinence, poor hygiene, use of chemical irritants such as bubble baths, pinworms, dysfunctional voiding (infrequent or incomplete voiding), sexual abuse, sexual intercourse, and the use of diaphragms. Indwelling urethral catheterization and the presence of a neurogenic bladder are also risk factors.[4,6,11] In some instances, existing perineal flora directly colonize the urethra; in others, trauma to the urethra leads to bladder colonization and the subsequent development of a urinary infection.

A familial risk factor for UTI is the presence of VUR in a parent or sibling. Up to 45 percent of siblings of children with persistent VUR will have reflux themselves, compared with less than 1 percent of the general population.[12]

Last, a positive history of UTI is an additional risk factor, since UTI recurs in approximately 30 percent of children after an acute infection. This is especially important if the child has had three or more previous UTIs, as the risk then increases to 75 percent.[5] Chronic conditions such as obstructive and reflux nephropathy can result from recurrent infections.

PATHOPHYSIOLOGY

A combination of both bacterial and individual host factors ultimately contributes to the development of UTIs in children and adolescents. In neonates, infections are usually bloodborne and bacteria are hematogenously spread to the kidneys. In older female children and adolescents, the usual route is by ascension of bacteria via the short urethra directly into the bladder; these bacteria are augmented by the abundance of vaginal and rectal microorganisms in the periurethral area. Any condition that leads to urinary stasis may predispose to the development of cystitis in certain hosts. Vesicoureteral reflux, obstructive uropathies, renal stones, and abnormal bladder emptying are examples of such conditions.[4,8]

Although viral organisms such as adenovirus have been known to cause hemorrhagic cystitis, bacterial enteric pathogens cause most urinary infections. By far the most common bacterial organism is *Escherichia coli,* which is responsible for 80 to 90 percent of acute UTIs in children and adolescents. Specific cell wall properties of pathogenic *E. coli* prevent it from being cleared from the bladder during voiding. The *E. coli* organisms adhere to the uroepithelium of the bladder via receptor-specific pili or fimbriae emanating from the bacterial cell wall. Because adherent bacteria cause a decrease in ureteral motility, *E. coli* with P-fimbriae are able to ascend to the kidney and cause infection.[13] This process leads to pyelonephritis in most young children. In contrast, the *E. coli* found in UTIs of patients with VUR and scarring do not have P-fimbriae.[7] Other cell-surface structures and properties of *E. coli* have also been identified as important in the pathogenesis of UTI, including hemolysin production, O and K antigenic serotypes, and colicin.[5,7]

In pyelonephritis, as bacteria reach the kidney, complement is activated and stimulates chemotaxis. Granulocytes are then activated, leading to phagocytosis of bacteria. The aggregation of granulocytes causes microabscesses and occlusion of capillaries, which results in ischemia and anaerobic metabolism. Superoxide and toxic oxygen radicals are then produced as the ischemic renal tissue is reperfused. These substances damage tissue, which may result in cell death, the formation of scars, and the permanent loss of functional renal tissue.[13]

Other gram-negative organisms that can cause UTIs in healthy children and adolescents are *Klebsiella, Proteus,* and *Enterobacter* species. Gram-positive cocci include enterococci and *Staphylococcus epidermidis,* which are seen primarily in adolescents.[7] In addition, *Staphylococcus saprophyticus,* a coagulase-negative staphylococcus, has also been recognized as a common cause of UTI in sexually active adolescents and young women.[6,10] In certain cases, different organisms must be considered, given the particular circumstance. For instance, infections by *Staphylococcus aureus* and *S. epidermidis* are associated with indwelling catheters or shunts.[4,8] Chronic infections or infections in patients receiving antimicrobial suppression are frequently caused by *Proteus, Pseudomonas,* or *Candida* species or enterococci.[5] Among children with recurrent UTIs, organisms other than *E. coli* are encountered with increased frequency.[14]

DIFFERENTIAL DIAGNOSIS

Multiple conditions may mimic UTI in females, but the differential diagnosis can be tailored depending upon the age of the patient. Symptomatic urinary tract infections are associated with a number of complaints such as low-grade fever and abdominal pain as well as nausea and vomiting. Other gastrointestinal complaints may include persistent diarrhea. The classic urinary symptoms—dysuria, increased hesitancy, frequency, or urgency—and the sudden onset of enuresis are seen only in older children and adolescents. Particularly in young children and infants, the presentation is much more subtle. Nonspecific symptoms include poor feeding, irritability, recurrent vomiting, and poor weight gain. Any of these symptoms can indicate lower as well as upper tract disease. In older children, however, upper tract disease is usually accompanied by more serious constitutional symptoms like high fever, chills, costovertebral or lower abdominal tenderness, and dehydration (Table 33-1).

Emergent conditions leading to an acute abdomen, such as appendicitis or ovarian torsion, can usually be sorted out in the older child and adolescent by taking a careful history. Important historical points include when the pain began; its current quality, duration, and location; its association with other symptoms (i.e., anorexia, nausea and vomiting); and whether the pain is migratory. Pain that began in the epigastrium and has migrated to the right lower quadrant asso-

Table 33-1

COMMON SIGNS AND SYMPTOMS OF URINARY TRACT INFECTION

Neonates	Infants/Children	School-Age Children/ Adolescents
Poor feeding	Fever	Abdominal pain
Lethargy	Vomiting	Enuresis
Irritability	Diarrhea	Fever and/or chills
Jaundice	Abdominal pain	Dysuria
Vomiting	Failure to thrive	Urgency
Persistent diarrhea	Foul or strong-smelling urine	Frequency
Fever or hypothermia		Hematuria
Poor weight gain		Flank pain

Source: Adapted from Todd[6] and Batisky.[4]

ciated with anorexia and nausea is much more suggestive of appendicitis. A previous history of intermittent pain is more consistent with an ovarian process; a history of UTI in the past increases the likelihood of a recurrent UTI. In addition, in a pubescent female, ectopic pregnancy must be considered. Congenital bowel disorders such as intussusceptions and volvulus are also in the differential diagnosis.

Less emergent conditions like pinworm infestations may involve the vagina in addition to the anus and can cause severe itching. This may lead to local excoriation from scratching and dysuria as the urine touches the raw perineal surface during voiding. A careful examination of the perineum will rule out this entity.

DIAGNOSTIC WORKUP

HISTORY AND PHYSICAL EXAMINATION

The evaluation of a child or adolescent suspected of having a UTI begins with a history that focuses on current symptoms, the presence of predisposing conditions (VUR, obstructive lesions), and a past history of UTI. A voiding history is also important to obtain since poor habits such as infrequent or incomplete voiding or poor hygiene can predispose to UTI. Dysfunctional voiding may be manifest by urinary dribbling, daytime enuresis, or a weak urine stream at the time of micturition.[6] With regard to the adolescent, a menstrual as well as sexual history should be obtained.

In all patients overall growth should be noted, since renal insufficiency can lead to poor growth; the blood pressure should also be checked for hypertension. The physical examination should include an assessment of the patient's hydration status and general clinical appearance. Any evidence of costovertebral tenderness, lower abdominal or suprapubic pain, abdominal masses (congenital anomaly of the kidney), and edema should be noted. The external genitalia should be examined for any obvious anomalies, vaginal discharge, erythema, or inflammation. In addition, labial adhesions or local irritation should be documented as they may be etiologic (e.g., labial adhesions resulting in poor urinary outflow) or may provide clues as to etiology (e.g., periurethral excoriations associated with pinworms).

LABORATORY DATA

Controversy exists regarding whether an acute infection can be readily diagnosed or excluded by urine dipstick or microscopic analysis alone.

URINE DIPSTICK

It is well established that a positive dipstick for nitrites, leukocyte esterase, or blood may be indicative of UTI. The leukocyte esterase test detects esterase released from leukocytes, an indirect test for the presence of white blood cells.[15] The nitrite test is more specific and is positive when nitrate is converted to nitrite in the bladder by certain bacteria. Since most gram-negative organisms are capable of reducing nitrates to nitrites, the dipstick will be positive in most UTIs. Most gram-positive organisms, however, are not capable of reducing nitrates and nitrites will not be detected.[15]

A recent study performed in an emergency department (ED) examined the correlation between a negative urine dipstick for leukocyte esterase and nitrite and the presence of bacteria and white blood cells (WBCs) microscopically. Three hundred urinalyses from ED patients were studied prospectively, and all patient charts documenting a negative dipstick for leukocyte esterase or nitrites and a positive clinical microscopy urinalysis were reviewed. At the lower range of sensitivity stated by the manufacturer (10 WBCs per high-power field), the authors found 56 percent of the dipstick WBC esterase results to be falsely negative. In addition, 64 percent of patients with moderate bacteriuria on microscopy had a falsely negative dipstick for nitrites. Fifty-eight percent of patients who had falsely negative leukocyte esterase results and 62 percent with falsely negative nitrite dipsticks ultimately had positive urine cultures from the ED. It was concluded that the sensitivity of the dipstick is low as compared with urine culture.[16]

In children below the age of 2, the false negative rate is too high to use the urine dipstick as a primary screen for deciding when to get a culture or when to make a diagnosis of UTI without a culture.[1,17] The differences between adult women and young children and the usefulness of the dipstick may be related to the degree of pyuria in the two age groups, the enzyme content of immature leukocytes, or

both.[2] In addition, bacteria must be present in the bladder for sufficient time to reduce nitrates to nitrites, which yield a positive test result. Thus, the urine dipstick for nitrites is particularly useful in first-morning or concentrated urine specimens where the bacteria have had sufficient time (4 to 6 h) to metabolize the nitrate to nitrite. The low sensitivity of dipstick nitrite testing in young children may be the result of random urine sampling usually obtained by catheter rather than the first-morning voids frequently recommended for adult women.[2]

Microscopic urinalysis is important for the detection of significant numbers of WBCs, red blood cells, casts, and bacteria. The presence of pyuria or hematuria is more indirect evidence of UTI and is neither sensitive nor specific.[6] More than 100 bacteria per high-powered field corresponds to $>10^5$ colony-forming units per milliliter on culture. This demonstration of bacteria microscopically is the most reliable and fastest means of establishing the diagnosis of UTI before the urine culture is available.[5]

In the febrile child under age 1, neither pertinent clinical signs or symptoms nor leukocytes and bacteria on microscopic exam of the urine are accurate predictors of positive urine culture results.[1,2] It is therefore recommended that in all febrile infants who are suspected of having a UTI, urine culture be performed in addition to both a urine dipstick and microscopic analysis.

URINE CULTURE

In neonates and infants, the most accurate method of obtaining a urine specimen is by percutaneous suprapubic bladder aspiration or urethral catheterization.[5,14] The urine should then immediately be sent to the laboratory for culture and sensitivity. Bagged specimens are not recommended in infants and young children, since culture results are often contaminated, making them unreliable and uninterpretable.[5,7] More importantly, a diagnosis of UTI made from these specimens generally leads to a costly, unnecessary workup of the urinary tract. In the young, non-toilet-trained female, urethral catheterization is often necessary to make an accurate diagnosis. In toilet-trained school-age and adolescent females, carefully collected midstream urine specimens are acceptable.

Normally, urine should be sterile, so one simple definition of UTI is the growth of bacterial colonies from the urine. The number of bacteria believed to be significant, however, will vary with the method used to collect the urine.[4] In addition, the concentration of bacteria in the urine may be influenced by how long the urine has been in the bladder, the rate of production of urine, and how the specimen is stored after it has been collected.[13]

As in adults, a positive urine culture is the gold standard for making a diagnosis of UTI in female children and adolescents. Any growth from a suprapubic tap aspiration is evidence of an infection; $\geq 10^4$ colonies from an "in-and-out" catheterization should be considered positive; and $\geq 10^5$

colonies from a midstream "clean-catch" urine collection is diagnostic of UTI. The presence of multiple organisms or skin flora usually indicates contamination of the urine specimen except in adolescent females, where *S. saprophyticus* and *epidermidis* can cause symptomatic UTI. In addition, some patients with structural urologic abnormalities may, in fact, have polymicrobial infections. Urine sensitivities are important to assure appropriate antibiotic coverage and should be obtained on all urine specimens.

BLOOD TESTS

Routine blood tests such as a serum blood urea nitrogen (BUN) and creatinine are not necessary in an uncomplicated first episode of UTI. If the patient is being hospitalized, however, or if there is a previous history of urinary infections, these studies may be obtained to evaluate renal function. In addition, a complete blood count (CBC) and blood culture should be obtained if the infant or child is febrile ($\geq$39.5°C, $\geq$103.1°F) or requires hospitalization. The incidence of urosepsis is lower in older, non-toxic-appearing children and adolescents, so the additional blood work is often not necessary or cost-effective.

PROCEDURES

SUPRAPUBIC BLADDER ASPIRATION

A suprapubic bladder aspiration may be performed in children less than 2 years of age in the following manner: place the infant or child in the supine position and prep the skin above the symphysis pubis with surgical soap. Using a 1.5-in. 23-gauge needle attached to a 5-mL syringe, insert the needle in the midline approximately 2 to 4 cm (1 to 2 fingerbreaths) above the symphysis pubis. While applying gentle negative pressure, advance the needle at about a 20° angle cephalad an appropriate distance through the bladder wall until urine is obtained. Remove at least 3 mL of urine to be sent for dipstick, microscopic analysis, and culture. The risk of intestinal perforation as well as other complications is minimal with this procedure. Contraindications include a bleeding diathesis or an empty bladder. Although local anesthesia may be used, it sometimes initiates voiding. Gentle pressure with a finger over the urethral meatus may prevent reflex voiding.[6]

BLADDER CATHETERIZATION

Bladder catheterization in the infant or younger child should be attempted atraumatically on the parent's lap or on the examination table. The labia majora, labia minora, and periurethral area should be cleansed with surgical soap and wiped with sterile gauze. A sterile 5-Fr feeding tube is then carefully inserted into the urethra until urine flow is appreciated. The first drops of urine should be discarded, since urethral microorganisms may have been forced into the blad-

der. A later aliquot of at least 3 mL of urine is then collected in a sterile container and promptly sent to the laboratory for microscopic analysis, culture, and sensitivity. It is imperative to indicate on the laboratory slip that it is a catheterized specimen. This procedure is not usually associated with an increased risk of nosocomial infection.

RADIOGRAPHIC STUDIES

Emergent radiographic studies are not necessary either to make a diagnosis of UTI or to treat it adequately. Plain films of the abdomen are superfluous and expose the patient to unnecessary radiation. Other studies such as ultrasounds, cystoureterograms, and nuclear renal cortical scans are useful during the subsequent radiographic workup of the infant or child with UTI but are rarely helpful acutely. Functional and structural abnormalities of the urinary tract are often diagnosed at that time.[4,8]

Of note is that renal cortical imaging is gaining acceptance by some authors for initially detecting renal parenchymal involvement (pyelonephritis).[3] This may be particularly helpful in young preverbal patients or when it is clinically difficult to distinguish between cystitis and pyelonephritis. The importance of making this distinction early in the course of the illness is that pyelonephritis and recurrent UTI in young children have been associated with a risk of subsequent renal damage. The technique of renal cortical scintigraphy involves the intravenous injection of a radiopharmaceutical such as dimercaptosuccinic acid (DMSA) labeled with the radionuclide technetium 99m. The study provides an image of both kidneys and an estimate of the proportion contributed by each kidney to total renal function. The image also reflects any vascular changes that affect the uptake of DMSA by the proximal renal tubules.[18] Focal or diffuse areas of decreased cortical uptake of tracer without any loss of volume indicate the presence of pyelonephritis. Areas of decreased uptake in association with volume loss represent old scars.[3]

TREATMENT

ACUTE INFECTIONS

The outpatient management of uncomplicated UTI is straightforward. Generally, a single broad-spectrum oral agent that will adequately cover what is likely to be the causative organism is recommended. If the infection is recurrent, the antibiotic coverage should take into account sensitivity studies on the organism that caused the infection(s) in the past. Antibiotic duration for young and school-age children is 10 days. Since it is often difficult to localize the infection in this age group and there have been very few studies of prepubertal girls with acute cystitis, single-dose or short-course therapy is currently not recommended.

A study by Madrigal et al. of 132 children with uncomplicated first-time UTIs was conducted to compare bacteriologic cure rates for a single-dose regimen and a multiple-dose regimen.[19] Although the authors reported no difference in cure rates, a statistically significant recurrence rate of 20.5 percent was noted in children who received the single-dose regimen compared to those who were given longer treatment.

Single-dose oral therapy may be used in the adolescent female with an uncomplicated UTI; it consists of either amoxicillin 3.0 g or trimethoprim/sulfamethoxazole (TMP/SMX) 320 mg/1600 mg (two double-strength tablets). A 3-day oral regimen with TMP/SMX or nitrofurantoin has also been suggested. The advantages of single-dose treatment include increased compliance with medication and follow-up, decreased cost and side effects, as well as a more rapid resolution of symptoms. In a study in female adolescents of single-dose versus conventional 10-day therapy, cure rates were approximately equal with sensitive organisms. However, 20 percent of patients developed candidal vaginitis in association with the longer treatment.[20] Side effects such as vaginitis will almost certainly contribute to poor compliance in the adolescent population.

The preferred drug for conventional oral administration is TMP/SMX because of its excellent absorption and tissue penetration. In addition, most urinary pathogens causing uncomplicated UTIs are highly susceptible to TMP/SMX.[5] Other oral antibiotics that can be used are sulfisoxazole, amoxicillin, nitrofurantoin, cephalexin, and cefixime (Table 33-2).[5,6,14] In some communities, amoxicillin is no longer used because of strains of *E. coli* that are resistant.

Initial treatment with one dose of intramuscular ceftriaxone or gentamicin has also been proposed by some authors to ensure an immediate cessation of bacterial proliferation in renal tissue. This is followed by the initiation of an oral agent within the next 12 to 18 h.[14]

Symptomatic treatments are important for patient comfort and compliance. Phenazopyridine hydrochloride (Pyridium) may be used for 2 days in older children and adolescents as a urinary analgesic. The dose is 12 mg/kg over 24 h divided T.I.D. for children 6 to 12 years of age and 200 mg T.I.D. for adolescent women. Patients should be warned about the change in urine color that accompanies pyridium use. It should not be used for longer than 48 h because of the risk of methemoglobinemia, hemolytic anemia, and other toxic reactions.[14] Although there are conflicting reports on the mechanism by which cranberry juice produces a bacteriostatic effect, drinking large amounts of it has been shown to be beneficial in the reduction of bacteriuria. Proposed explanations include acidification of the urine and the inhibition of bacterial adherence to mucosal surfaces.[21] Antipyretics (acetaminophen or ibuprofen) can be used to control fever, which may persist for the first 24 to 48 h after beginning antimicrobial therapy. Finally, sitzbaths in warm water for 20 to 30 min three to four times a day may offer relief of dysuria.[14]

RECURRENT INFECTIONS

Treatment for recurrent infections or in children at risk for recurrent infections should include a consideration of the organisms responsible for previous infections as well as the antibiotics to which the child has recently been exposed.

ANTIBIOTIC PROPHYLAXIS

Nitrofurantoin or TMP/SMX in suppressive doses (1 to 2 mg/kg per day) is recommended in the interim between the completion of acute therapy and the performance of the VCUG following UTI. Antimicrobial prophylaxis reduces the risk of reinfection and avoids the problem of the interpretation of reflux in the presence of cystitis.[5,14,22] In children with VUR, suppressive doses of antibiotics are continued for 1 year following the acute infection since this is the time when the likelihood of recurrence is highest.[7,14]

The risk of repeat infection may occur in 25 to 50 percent of children during the first year following the initial UTI. Therefore, repeat urine cultures should be obtained initially at 1- to 2-month intervals and then at 3- to 4-month intervals for at least 1 year or until reflux resolves.[7]

RADIOGRAPHIC FOLLOW-UP

Should all UTIs be evaluated radiographically? Guidelines for pursuing radiographic studies in patients with UTI have been developed and include: (1) the first febrile UTI in girls younger than 3 to 5 years; (2) older girls of any age with recurrent UTIs; and (3) the child with suspected pyelonephritis.[4,5,22,23] Girls older than 10 should have at least a second UTI before any studies are initiated. In most cases, sexually active adolescents do not warrant a radiologic

Table 33-2

OUTPATIENT TREATMENT OF URINARY TRACT INFECTION

Antibiotic	Dose/Interval
Trimethoprim/ sulfamethoxazole (Bactrim)	8–10 mg/kg TMP PO b.i.d. for 10 days
Amoxicillin	20–40 mg/kg PO t.i.d. for 10 days
Cefixime (Supras)	8 mg/kg PO q.d. for 10 days
Cephalexin (Keflex)	20–50 mg/kg PO q.i.d. for 10 days
Nitrofurantoin (Macrodantin)	5–7 mg/kg PO q.i.d. for 10 days
Sulfisoxazole	120–150 mg/kg PO q4–6h for 10

workup. An exception is if the adolescent has two to three episodes of cystitis in a 12- to 18-month period.[14]

The reason for imaging the renal tract after an infection is to look for a cause and detect renal damage early so that appropriate long-term management can be instituted.[18] The investigation is undertaken to ascertain whether the kidneys are normal, involved, or at risk of scarring; whether VUR is present and to what degree; and to identify outflow obstruction requiring surgical treatment, such as posterior urethral valves.[4,24]

Ultrasound is useful for imaging the upper urinary tract and may determine gross structural defects, obstructive lesions, positional abnormalities of the kidneys (ectopic kidneys), and renal size and shape. Advantages of ultrasound are that it is noninvasive and imparts no radiation. However, ultrasonography alone is not adequate for the investigation of UTI, since it does not detect either VUR, renal scars, or inflammation.

A voiding cystoureterogram or contrast VCUG provides the most comprehensive assessment of the lower urinary tract but does not provide any information about kidney structure and function. A voiding cystoureterogram allows for grading of the severity of reflux, identifies bladder diverticula, measures bladder capacity and residual urine, and visualizes the urethra. The value of identifying reflux is to guide medical management so that the risk of renal scarring from persistent reflux and recurrent infection is minimized.[18] This procedure requires that the child be catheterized while contrast material is infused into the bladder. Both the rapidity and severity of VUR are assessed fluoroscopically. The degree of reflux is reported as grades I through V. Advantages of this particular procedure are that it offers a detailed anatomic definition of the collecting system, bladder, and urethra as well as an accurate assessment of the degree of reflux. The major disadvantage is the high dose of radiation exposure to the gonads.[4]

Radionuclide cystography (nuclear cystogram) is available as an alternative to a contrast VCUG and may be used to determine the presence of reflux. This method of imaging is more appropriate for the evaluation of young females, since the radiation dose to the gonads is 1 percent that of standard fluoroscopy used during contrast VCUG. The disadvantage is that a nuclear cystogram cannot define urethral or bladder wall anomalies. Fortunately, urethral abnormalities are relatively rare in girls.[3,25] Intravenous pyelography (IVP; excretory urogram) is usually not indicated unless one is concerned about ureteral duplication, a ureterocele, or some other ureteral anomaly.

INDICATIONS FOR ADMISSION AND SPECIALTY CONSULTATION

In considering the possibility of inpatient treatment, several factors must be taken into account: (1) the patient's clinical appearance; (2) the age of the patient (the risk of permanent renal damage as a consequence of infection is inversely related to the child's age); and (3) compliance and the reliability of follow-up.[13] Parenteral antibiotics may be required in infants less than 2 to 3 months of age; suspected pyelonephritis at any age (complicated UTI); patients who are moderately or severely dehydrated, appear toxic, or are in shock; in patients with a history of recurrent infection or known renal disease; and in those with an infection involving an organism that is resistant to oral antibiotics. Hospitalization should also be considered when there is no improvement on oral therapy or symptoms are worsening.

Hospitalized patients should initially be treated with two antibiotics that provide broad-spectrum coverage for both gram-negative and gram-positive organisms, such as ampicillin and gentamicin. A third-generation cephalosporin, cefotaxime or ceftriaxone, may also be used. Ceftriaxone should not be used in neonates or jaundiced patients because of the displacement of bilirubin from albumin and biliary sludge pseudolithiasis.[14]

Most children and adolescents can be evaluated, treated, and followed without nephrologic or urologic consultation. Specialty consultation should be considered for patients with evidence of urinary tract obstruction, renal scarring, significant voiding problems, or anatomic abnormalities. In addition, children at any age with a solitary, small, or atrophic kidney or who have hypertension should be referred to the specialist for consultation.[14] Both pediatric nephrology and urology consultations are also necessary in patients with known high-grade reflux (grades III through V), since its management remains controversial. A recently completed study from the International Vesicoureteral Reflux Study Group revealed there was no difference in the rate of renal scarring between prophylactic medical treatment and surgery in these children.[7,8]

DISCHARGE INSTRUCTIONS AND FOLLOW-UP INTERVAL

In the infant and younger child, a follow-up culture should be obtained within 48 to 72 h after initiation of antibiotic treatment. This is especially important for the patient with recurrent infection or for those who are not improving symptomatically (persistent fever, vomiting, abdominal pain). Modification of antibiotic therapy may be necessary at this time, depending on the bacterial sensitivity tests.

If the younger child is doing well and repeat urinalysis and culture do not suggest persistent infection, oral antibiotics are continued to complete a 10-day course. School-age children and adolescents do not necessarily need a follow-up culture if it is a first-time uncomplicated UTI and they are improving clinically.

Both upper and lower UTIs in young females mandate complete evaluation for urinary anomalies and reflux at follow-up.[7,14,22] Therefore, after finishing the 10-day antibiotic regimen for the acute infection, the child should be placed on a suppressive dose of antibiotics until structural or obstructive anomalies are ruled out by voiding cystouretero-gram (VCUG).

OVARIAN TORSION

Torsion of the uterine adnexa is a well-described surgical emergency that can involve the fallopian tube and ovary either separately or together. Although reported as occurring rarely in prepubescent girls, torsion should be a serious consideration in the differential diagnosis of acute abdominal pain and genitourinary problems in female children and adolescents. Its clinical diagnosis is often uncertain, however, leading to multiple unnecessary tests and delays in surgical intervention.[26] Early recognition of this condition, including an accurate preoperative diagnosis, is imperative to ensure the salvage of a compromised ovary in this vulnerable population.[27]

EPIDEMIOLOGY

Torsion of a normal ovary occasionally occurs in women of childbearing age, but some authors suggest that the highest incidence is in children before menarche.[28] Approximately 15 percent of adnexal torsion occurs during infancy or childhood,[29] with the majority of cases seen in the 7- to 10-year-old group, and many of these cases do not involve either a tumor or cyst.[29] Torsion of a normal ovary or tube is not a rare occurrence. In one study at U.S.C. Women's Hospital, nearly 20 percent of cases involved normal adnexa.[26] In diseased ovaries, rates of torsion do not seem to vary with the type of tumor present. Rates of ovarian torsion are reported as 9.5 per 100 women with neoplasms of epithelial origin, 13.6 for germ-cell neoplasms, and 10.5 for stromal neoplasms.[30]

A predominance of right-sided adnexal involvement is reported in the literature.[27] It is unclear whether there is an anatomic reason for this or whether suspicion of appendicitis leads to the more frequent diagnosis of right-sided lesions. One possible anatomic explanation for the predilection to the right ovary is the availability of more space on the right as compared to the left, which is occupied by the sigmoid colon.[31] Regardless, given the lower index of suspicion, many left-sided adnexal torsions are probably missed.[27]

RISK FACTORS

The most common antecedent of adnexal torsion is a benign ovarian neoplasm. In a series of 861 women with a postoperative diagnosis of ovarian neoplasm, benign cystic teratoma was the most common diagnosis, especially in young women, accounting for 44 percent of all neoplasms.[32] Also

called *dermoid tumor,* benign cystic teratoma represents 38.6 percent of benign ovarian neoplasms in children and adolescents, with approximately 50 percent diagnosed incidentally during laparotomy or on x-ray of the pelvis.[33]

The histologic type of ovarian tumor does not appear to affect the rate of adnexal torsion, and torsion rarely involves cancer.[30] What does appear to predispose to torsion is the size and mobility of the tumor. Benign ovarian neoplasms carry a 12.9-fold increased risk of being involved in adnexal torsion as compared with malignant ovarian neoplasms. In addition, neoplasms of low malignant potential carry an 8.7-fold increased risk of torsion, although this may not be statistically significant.[30] The reasons for this discrepancy are unclear. One hypothesis is that malignant neoplasms are just less common in young women and children.[32] Others relate the low probability of torsion by malignant neoplasms to their ability to adhere to local structures by inflammation, adhesions, or local invasion.[30]

In many series, however, torsion does not involve a neoplasm, and in children and adolescents, a majority of cases occur in normal adnexa. Of note is that physiologic ovarian cysts (e.g., hemorrhagic corpus luteum) may also be associated with torsion.[26,27,31,33]

PATHOPHYSIOLOGY

Torsion of the fallopian tube or ovary and paraovarian cysts or some combination of all three may occur.[31] Excessive mobility of the child's normal adnexa purportedly predisposes the ovary to torsion. It has also been suggested that follicular cysts, a normal feature of prepubescent ovaries, may produce ovarian enlargement.[28] Other proposed mechanisms of torsion include anatomic abnormalities of the fallopian tube or ovary, such as an elongated mesosalpinx or increased weight of the fallopian tube secondary to venous blood congestion, edema, or an ectopic pregnancy. In conditions like pregnancy and menstruation, there is increased venous congestion. It has also been suggested that in the presence of a small infantile uterus with a relatively large ovary, changes in intraabdominal pressure or sudden movements can start a twist of the adnexa. Other etiologies for ovarian torsion that are more common in older women include pregnancy (displacement of the adnexa by the growing uterus and increased vascularity); gynecologic surgery (abdominal and laparoscopic tubal ligation); and induction of ovulation (iatrogenic ovarian hyperstimulation).[27,31,35]

In the initial stages of torsion, only venous and lymphatic drainage is impaired. The ovary increases in volume after a few days and appears on ultrasound as a solid mass because of vascular engorgement and stromal edema.[33] Later, venous and then arterial thrombosis develops along with subsequent infarction of the adnexa.[38] If torsion is intermittent, the ovarian engorgement may regress rapidly.[33] In 1891, Kuestner observed that twisting of the adnexal pedicle generally occurred as follows: the pedicle on the patient's left side will be rotated to the right in a clockwise direction; the pedicle on the right side will rotate to the left in a counterclockwise direction. The majority of reported cases of ovarian torsion have confirmed this.[35]

DIFFERENTIAL DIAGNOSIS

The differential diagnosis in a female with acute lower-quadrant pain is extensive. More importantly, many of the conditions require immediate surgical intervention. Because it may be difficult to distinguish between them, especially in the adolescent female, each serious diagnosis must be carefully considered and excluded on the basis of a focused history and thorough physical examination.

In right adnexal torsion, the most common erroneous diagnosis is acute appendicitis. Adnexal torsion, unlike appendicitis, is characterized by the acute onset of pain localized immediately to the right or left lower quadrant without preliminary migration from the epigastric region. In torsion, the pain may also be localized to the iliac fossa and radiate to the pubis, thigh, or lower back. Nausea and vomiting are usually associated with the pain and begin when the pain starts, unlike appendicitis, where nausea and vomiting typically follow the onset of pain.[31] In addition, more than half the patients with ovarian torsion complain of previous episodes of pain.[27,31] Nonspecific symptoms such as anorexia, constipation, tenesmus, and dysuria may accompany either condition and usually do not help in differentiating between the two.

Pelvic inflammatory disease or salpingitis generally presents with acute lower abdominal or pelvic pain and can be confused with ovarian torsion in the sexually active adolescent. If salpingitis is suspected in a premenarchal or virginal female, an inquiry regarding sexual abuse must be made. One symptom that favors the diagnosis of PID over adnexal torsion is the presence of abnormal vaginal bleeding or discharge. On physical examination, it may be more difficult to distinguish these two entities, since lower abdominal pain, adnexal tenderness, and an adnexal mass occur in a majority of both cases. Cervical motion tenderness is more prominent in PID. Ultrasound may be helpful if a solid unilateral adnexal mass is seen (favors torsion) or a multiloculated thick wall cyst is seen (favors tuboovarian abscess).

Early intrauterine pregnancy, hemorrhagic corpus luteum, and tubal pregnancies may each be confused with adnexal torsion.[31] Pregnancy must be ruled out if there is a history of amenorrhea, any menstrual irregularity, and sexual activity and is readily done by using a sensitive serum assay for beta human chorionic gonadotropin (β-hCG). Ultrasound can be used to detect the presence of a gestational sac or fetal pole as early as the third or fourth postovulatory week.[31] Consideration of ectopic pregnancy may delay the diagnosis of torsion. An abnormal pregnancy is suspected when serially measured levels of β-hCG fail to increase at least 1.7-fold in 48 h.[31,37]

Ovarian cysts and tumors are usually asymptomatic and are not painful unless the ovarian capsule is markedly stretched. Large (>7 cm), complex, or solid ovarian masses usually require surgical exploration.[31] Ultrasound may be useful to evaluate a tender adnexal mass, identifying a small, simple physiologic cyst to be followed clinically. Hemorrhage into an ovarian cyst may be seen as a solid adnexal mass associated with fluid in the cul-de-sac. Since this is a nonspecific finding, other conditions must be considered, such as ovarian neoplasm, ectopic pregnancy, and ovarian torsion if there is an atypical history associated with lower abdominal pain.[31]

When the lower abdominal pain is predominantly left-sided and there is also infection, ureteral calculi or gastrointestinal colonic disease should be considered.[31,35] If less localized, lower abdominal pain may be due to ovulation (mittelschmerz) in pubertal girls, suggested by onset in midcycle. Finally, cystitis can present with diffuse lower abdominal pain in all age groups.

DIAGNOSTIC WORKUP

HISTORY AND PHYSICAL EXAMINATION

Since the signs and symptoms of ovarian torsion can be nonspecific, the clinician must maintain a high index of suspicion in all women with lower abdominal pain. Almost all patients will experience some type of abdominal, pelvic, or flank pain, which is often sudden in onset, unilateral, and severe. The pain may also be crampy, colicky, or intermittent. Nausea and vomiting may be coincident with or may follow the onset of pain and are fairly common.[27] A palpable adnexal mass occurs in at least 50 percent of patients with torsion[28]; there may also be moderate leukocytosis associated with low-grade ($<38°C$, $<100.4°F$) fever. Anywhere from 10 to 50 percent of patients have had intermittent torsion over a period of time, as suggested by a history of repeated attacks of pain interspersed with asymptomatic intervals.[26,27,31]

Chronic torsion may have a more gradual onset of symptoms. In cases of incomplete torsion, symptoms may be intermittent as the adnexa spontaneously twist and untwist.[31]

During the pelvic examination, the uterus is often displaced to the affected side, and a palpable mass is typically present on rectal or bimanual exam. Other abdominal findings may include rebound tenderness, rigidity, decreased bowel sounds, and distention. If the patient is seen late in the course of torsion, peritonitis with accompanying rigidity may prevent the mass from being fully appreciated. Fever ($>38°C$, $>100.4°F$) is unusual unless there is abscess formation or necrosis.[31]

LABORATORY DATA

Ancillary tests do not seem to play a prominent role in the diagnosis of adnexal torsion, although a few tests may be performed to rule out other conditions. A negative serum or urine pregnancy test should be documented in the pubescent female, a CBC may reveal leukocytosis (which is nonspecific), and a urine dipstick and microscopic analysis should be performed to rule out the possibility of UTI. If there is strong suspicion of ovarian torsion, waiting for urine culture results is not advisable, as the timely diagnosis of ovarian torsion is important in preserving ovarian viability. A decreased hematocrit is uncommon, even though adnexal torsion is often associated with intraabdominal serosanguinous fluid. Culdocentesis is usually negative and, given other noninvasive radiographic modalities to detect fluid in the cul-de-sac, is not necessary in the pediatric patient.

RADIOGRAPHIC STUDIES

An abdominal x-ray may identify the characteristics of an abdominal mass: displacement of bowel and/or ureters or the presence of structured radioopacities (e.g., teeth in a benign cystic teratoma). An abdominal x-ray should not be used to confirm the presence of a mass that is already clinically evident, since this will only delay surgery and expose the patient to unnecessary radiation.

Ultrasonography confirms the presence of an adnexal mass and can characterize its consistency. Findings may include a solid, complex, or cystic mass[31,33] or, in some instances, small cystic structures around the periphery of the ovary.[27] Follicular enlargement in the cortical zone has been noted and is attributed to transudation of fluid into the follicle of the congested ovary.[38,39] The twisted ovary may range in size from just above normal (3 to 4 cm) to massively enlarged (>10 cm).[38] Additionally, with a history consistent with torsion, if the sonographer is able to demonstrate a separate, normal-appearing ovary on the side of the pain the likelihood of fallopian tube or parovarian cyst torsion should be considered.[26] Advantages of ultrasound in the evaluation of pelvic masses include convenience, accuracy, lack of ionizing radiation, noninvasiveness, and cost-effectiveness.[31]

Transvaginal color Doppler sonography may be useful, but its role in the early diagnosis of adnexal torsion has not been completely established. Some authors propose that if normal blood flow is seen on the color Doppler study, ovarian torsion can be ruled out.[31] However, others believe that it is the absence of flow that is more definitive for adnexal torsion, indicating complete venous as well as arterial occlusion. Early in torsion, venous and lymphatic stasis typically occurs. Later, venous and then arterial thrombosis develops along with the subsequent infarction of the adnexum. Given this sequence of events, it becomes apparent that persistent arterial flow may be seen via Doppler during the early or less complete stages of torsion.[38]

Recent studies have looked at the role of MRI in the evaluation of pelvic masses in adolescents.[34] Advantages include more favorable acceptance by patients and families, since the procedure is noninvasive and there is no exposure to ionizing radiation. In addition, MRI can be performed regardless of the patient's habitus, and a full bladder is not required. Furthermore, MRI does not require hospitalization or anesthesia and is less costly than laparoscopy. The disadvantages are apparent when MRI is compared with ultrasonography, as MRI is much more costly, its availability is limited, it is less comfortable for the patient and more time-consuming, and it does not offer the multiple variation of planes and inclinations offered by the experienced sonographer.[34] In general, computed tomography (CT) and MRI are usually not required for diagnosing ovarian torsion in the acute setting, but some radiographic findings are diagnostic for subacute presentations.[40]

TREATMENT

When the condition is recognized, the treatment for ovarian torsion is emergency laparotomy or laparoscopy and, since most patients are prepubertal or of reproductive age, preservation of tubes and ovaries is the main objective.[26] The routine use of diagnostic laparoscopy allows for the direct visualization of the pelvic structures[31] and for cultures of the intraperitoneal exudate to be obtained if the diagnosis of PID is entertained. It is also an effective means of reducing the number of unnecessary laparotomies when a diagnosis of torsion is uncertain.[26] Very experienced laparoscopists can fully manage adnexal torsion through the laparoscope.

The management of the twisted adnexum is somewhat controversial, especially if there has been a delay in diagnosis. Although in the past most women were treated by salpingo-oophorectomy because of concern that untwisting of the adnexum might precipitate thromboembolic events such as a pulmonary embolus,[41] a more conservative approach has now been reported. Since most of the affected women are young, thromboembolic phenomenon rarely occur, and most torsions do not involve a malignant neoplasm.[26] At least an initial attempt to untwist the adnexum has been proposed to allow for preservation of the ovary and/or tube and is meeting with increased acceptance in all but necrotic adnexal torsions.[41] Hemorrhagic infarction of the ovary and fallopian tube or an obvious gangrenous adnexum requires surgical removal without untwisting the pedicle.[31,35]

If torsion occurs in a normal ovary and oviduct in a young patient, the physician should be aware of the possibility of its recurrence and consider fixation of the other mesosalpinx. Plication may anchor a mobile oviduct and prevent further torsion and infarction. The disadvantage of plication is that, in some cases, it may lead to tubal compromise and theoretically to future problems with fertility.[35] In a patient with a benign neoplasm associated with ovarian torsion, cystectomy followed by ovarian plication is preferred if the ovary is viable.

INDICATIONS FOR ADMISSION AND SPECIALTY CONSULTATION

The presence of a palpable abdominal mass should not delay surgical consultation and operation in the patient with symptoms consistent with adnexal torsion. The challenge remains to distinguish ovarian torsion from other more common causes of acute abdominal pain in children and adolescents. Direct visualization remains the only means of definitive diagnosis; therefore a gynecologist or surgeon should be notified early in the course of the workup.

PELVIC INFLAMMATORY DISEASE

Pelvic inflammatory disease (PID) involves infection of the uterus, fallopian tubes, and adjacent pelvic structures that is not associated with surgery or pregnancy (see Chap. 44). Also known as salpingitis, it is reported that one out of every seven to eight sexually active adolescent females is affected.[42,43] Risk factors for PID in this age group include young age (<19 years old), multiple sexual partners, intrauterine device (three- to fivefold increased risk), previous episode of salpingitis, and douching.[43–47] The medical consequences of PID are significant: it is a direct cause of infertility, is associated with ectopic pregnancy, and contributes to long-term sequelae such as chronic abdominal pain, dyspareunia, and adhesions. Infection occurs by the contiguous spread of microorganisms from the lower genital tract via the endometrial cavity to the upper genital tract (fallopian tubes), resulting in inflammation, scarring, and crypt formation in the fallopian tubes.[44] The etiology of acute salpingitis is polymicrobial: responsible organisms include *Neisseria gonorrhoeae, Chlamydia trachomatis,* and mixed anaerobic-aerobic bacteria.

The diagnosis of PID is difficult, since not all adolescents will present with the classic findings of lower abdominal pain, adnexal tenderness, the presence of a mass, fever, and an elevated sedimentation rate. The most common presenting symptom is diffuse, bilateral lower abdominal pain, although in some cases the pain may be unilateral. Unilateral right-sided pain can be confused with acute appendicitis. Therefore, maintaining a high index of suspicion and inquiring about sexual activity, number of partners, and a previous history of STDs will aid the clinician in making an accurate diagnosis. Other complaints might include an abnormal vaginal discharge or bleeding, nausea, vomiting, dysuria, dyspareunia, and fever or chills. The timing of the last menstrual cycle is also important historical information, since both chlamydial and gonococcal disease tend to occur during the first half of the menstrual cycle.[45] Suggested criteria for the diagnosis of acute salpingitis are listed in Table 33-3. Based on these criteria, the clinician should decide on

---

Table 33-3

CLINICAL CRITERIA: DIAGNOSIS OF ACUTE PELVIC INFLAMMATORY DISEASE

The following three minimum clinical criteria should be present:
1. Lower abdominal tenderness
2. Adnexal tenderness
3. Cervical motion tenderness

Additional criteria may be used to increase the specificity of the diagnosis. They include:

Routine criteria:
1. Oral temperature >38.3°C (100.9°F)
2. Abnormal cervical or vaginal discharge
3. Elevated erythrocyte sedimentation rate
4. Elevated C-reactive protein
5. Laboratory documentation of cervical infection with *N. gonorrhoeae* or *C. trachomatis*

Elaborate criteria:
1. Histopathologic evidence of endometritis on endometrial biopsy
2. Tuboovarian abscess on sonography or other radiologic tests
3. Laparoscopic abnormalities consistent with PID

Source: Centers for Disease Control and Prevention,[49] with permission.

---

the likelihood of PID and consider other conditions in the differential, such as isolated lower genital tract infection (e.g., cervicitis or vaginitis), ectopic pregnancy, torsion or rupture of an adnexal mass, acute appendicitis, and endometriosis.[48]

Appropriate laboratory tests include a CBC with differential, erythrocyte sedimentation rate (ESR), urinalysis, pregnancy test, and testing for gonococcal and chlamydial infection. A Gram stain of the endocervix for gram-negative intracellular diplococci may also be helpful, though a positive Gram stain is found in only about one-half to two-thirds of women with cervical gonorrhea.

An abdominal and pelvic ultrasound is necessary if the diagnosis is unclear, a pelvic mass is palpated, or ectopic pregnancy is a possibility.[46] A gynecology consult is appropriate in the adolescent, particularly in those young women whose diagnosis is uncertain, whose illness is severe, or whose symptoms are prolonged. If there is any doubt about the diagnosis, the current recommendation is to treat for presumptive PID.

Admission to the hospital is recommended for all adolescents with PID, since compliance is often an issue and long-term sequelae of untreated or incompletely treated disease are serious.[46] Other reasons for inpatient management are the need to reassess the patient's condition to make certain that surgical conditions such as appendicitis or ectopic pregnancy are not present (see Table 44-5 for a complete list).[43] Current treatment guidelines for inpatient treatment from the Centers for Disease Control and Prevention (CDC) are cefoxitin 2 g IV q6h (or cefotetan 2 g q12h) and doxycycline 100 mg PO or IV q12h. An alternative regimen is clindamycin 900 mg IV q8h and gentamicin 2 mg/kg IV or IM loading dose followed by a maintenance dose of 1.5 mg/kg IV or IM q8h.[49] Parenteral antibiotics should be continued for at least 48 h after the patient improves clinically, although some authors advocate a full 7 to 10 days of inpatient therapy to ensure eradication of all organisms.[43] If the decision is made to complete treatment on an outpatient basis, the patient should be discharged home on oral doxycycline 100 mg b.i.d. or clindamycin 450 mg PO q.i.d. to complete a 14-day course.[48,49]

OVARIAN CYSTS

Functional ovarian cysts are common during adolescence and include follicular as well as corpus luteum cysts. Although simple cysts are usually small (less than 5 cm) and asymptomatic, larger cysts can occur and may be complicated by torsion, rupture, or bleeding.[51] The pubertal adolescent may present with acute lower abdominal pain on the side of the involved ovary,[52] or the pain may be described as gradual and steady.[51] Knowledge of the relationship of the onset of pain to the patient's own normal menstrual cycle is helpful in the diagnosis and management of the adolescent with abdominal pain.

In the normal menstrual cycle, follicle-stimulating hormone (FSH) recruits a cohort of approximately twenty ovarian follicles to begin maturation and produce estrogen. The rise in estrogen leads to a surge in both FSH and luteinizing hormone (LH), which triggers ovulation, leading one dominant follicle to release an ovum while the others regress. Following ovulation, a corpus luteum is formed, which secretes both estrogen and progesterone. The life span of the corpus is constant at about 12 to 14 days; if fertilization does not occur, it will involute, causing a decrease in the levels of estrogen and progesterone. With the decrease in progesterone, the endometrium is shed and menstruation occurs.[53,54]

FOLLICULAR CYSTS

Follicular cysts are the most common types of persistent physiologic ovarian cysts. They result from either failure of the dominant follicle to ovulate or from failure of other fol-

licles to undergo normal atresia.[55] Their average diameter is small (approximately 1 to 2 cm),[52] but they may become large (6 to 8 cm).[55] Usually follicular cysts are asymptomatic and are found incidentally on routine pelvic examination or by ultrasound if this is performed for some other reason. In addition, menstrual irregularities may occur in some patients from estrogen production by the cysts or failure of the corpus luteum to develop.[52,55] If symptoms do occur, pain is usually transient, self-limited, and associated with ovulation. Large cysts may rupture (leading to a transient peritonitis that resolves in 24 h)[56] or undergo torsion (leading to acute lower abdominal pain).

The treatment of an isolated episode of pain from a symptomatic follicular cyst is observation. Both parents and the patient should be told that all young women of reproductive age have ovarian cysts and their presence does not indicate pathology. Since most functional cysts will resolve spontaneously over 4 to 8 weeks, the adolescent should be reexamined during a subsequent menstrual cycle by her primary physician. If the pain is recurrent, oral contraceptives are recommended to suppress follicular activity.[52]

A gynecology consult should be obtained for the adolescent with acute lower abdominal pain and a tender adnexal mass or evidence of peritonitis on physical examination. Other conditions in the differential include appendicitis, ovarian torsion, PID, a hemorrhagic cyst, and ectopic pregnancy. An ultrasound can be extremely helpful in identifying the cyst. Laparoscopy should be performed if the diagnosis is uncertain and after a urine pregnancy test is done.

CORPUS LUTEUM CYSTS

Corpus luteum cysts are less common than follicular cysts but may be seen more frequently on an acute basis because they are larger than follicular cysts and their propensity for rupture can cause intraperitoneal hemorrhage.[52,55,56] They result from abnormal, persistently functioning corpora lutea and are considered cysts when their diameter is greater than 3 cm.[56] Corpus luteum cysts are usually large (5 to 10 cm in diameter) and often associated with hemorrhage into the cyst.[55] Like follicular cysts, most corpus luteum cysts are asymptomatic, occasionally manifesting themselves as brief bouts of unilateral, sharp lower abdominal pain prior to menses.[51] Symptomatic cysts, however, may delay menses or produce heavy vaginal bleeding from prolonged progesterone production. The management of small luteal cysts is essentially the same as that for small follicular cysts. Surgical intervention is usually not necessary, since bleeding is usually minimal and of short duration.[52]

Large cysts may cause acute lower abdominal pain from rupture complicated by ovarian hemorrhage and often require surgical intervention.[52,55,56] Peritoneal signs may also be present, depending on whether the hemorrhage is intraovarian or extraovarian.[51] A gynecologic consultation should be obtained early in these patients, especially if significant bleeding is suspected or if the diagnosis is inconsistent with the clinical picture. A urine or serum test for β-hCG should be performed to exclude ectopic pregnancy. Conservative surgical therapy has been advocated that involves cystectomy and/or cauterization of the bleeding vessels. Oophorectomy is not required to obtain hemostasis.[56]

URETHRAL PROLAPSE

Urethral prolapse is a symmetric eversion of the distal urethral mucosa through the meatus (Fig. 33-1). It is seen primarily in prepubertal African American females but has also been reported in postmenopausal women. Multiple predisposing factors have been suggested and remain controversial, including trauma (straddle injuries, sexual abuse, catheterization, blows to the abdomen, and auto accidents) and medical conditions accompanied by increases in intraabdominal pressure (constipation, diarrhea, prolonged spasmodic coughing).[57–62] Poorly developed smooth muscle supports of the urethra have been cited as the cause for prolapse in girls with increased abdominal pressure.[62] In addition, urethral prolapse has been associated with UTI. Some have postulated that the etiology of prolapse is related to estrogen deficiency or a hypoestrogen state, given the ages of

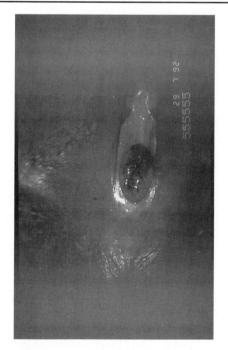

Figure 33-1

Urethral prolapse. Photograph courtesy of Dr. Carol Berkowitz, Harbor–UCLA Medical Center.

the females seen with this condition and its response to topical estrogen cream.[63,64]

DIFFERENTIAL DIAGNOSIS

Although the definitive diagnosis of urethral prolapse is made on the basis of the physical examination, other less common conditions in the differential diagnosis include urethral polyps, papilloma, carbuncle, prolapsed ureterocele, condyloma, sarcoma botryoides (rhabdomyosarcoma), and periurethral abscess.[62,65] A complete, circular, "doughnut-shaped" mass in the anterior introitus with a central opening, however, is pathognomonic for urethral prolapse.

DIAGNOSTIC WORKUP

HISTORY AND PHYSICAL EXAMINATION

The young child with urethral prolapse is often asymptomatic, with the diagnosis made on routine physical examination of the genitalia by the pediatrician. In the emergency setting, a child may complain of hematuria or vaginal bleeding or spotting on the underwear. Symptoms consistent with UTI (dysuria, urinary frequency, or urinary retention) can also be seen if the urethra becomes very inflamed.[63] Pain in the genital area is not common, however.

Upon examination of the genitalia, a cherry-red, circular, symmetric mass is seen superior to the hymenal opening (Fig. 33-1). A central umbilicated area represents the urethral opening. To verify this, a small urinary catheter may be carefully introduced into this central opening. Occasionally, if the prolapse is large enough (2 to 3 cm), the vaginal introitus may be difficult to visualize.[62] The prolapse may also appear to be fungating and neoplastic, depending on the degree of inflammation, edema, and necrosis of urethral mucosa.[64]

LABORATORY DATA

A urinalysis is indicated to rule out UTI if the diagnosis is unclear. Red blood cells may be present, but the culture will be negative. No other laboratory or radiographic studies are indicated, since urethral prolapse is a clinical diagnosis.

TREATMENT AND DISCHARGE INSTRUCTIONS

The treatment of urethral prolapse depends on the degree of prolapse. For minimal prolapse (only a small amount of protuberant tissue that appears viable), an emollient (e.g., petroleum jelly, povidone-iodine, or neomycin ointment) to the area and warm sitzbaths are all that is usually indicated. The parents should be reassured that resolution will probably occur within 1 to 2 weeks. Topical estrogen cream can also be applied twice daily for 1 to 2 weeks following sitzbaths. Some authors have reported the successful use of oral antibiotics in conjunction with the other treatment modalities.[57] Manual reduction is not recommended, since it is painful and may be difficult to accomplish.[57,63] Urethral prolapse can recur weeks to months after conservative medical management,[62] but recurrence rates are as high as 67 percent. Larger prolapses (2 to 3 cm in diameter) or those associated with necrosis require urgent urologic consultation (see below).

FOLLOW-UP INTERVAL

Young girls with urethral prolapse should be seen by their primary-care provider in 1 to 2 weeks or sooner if the patient becomes symptomatic, is not improving, or there is worsening in her clinical course. Some families may choose to see their physicians sooner and should be encouraged to do so if there is any concern about the diagnosis or treatment plan.

INDICATIONS FOR ADMISSION AND SPECIALTY CONSULTATION

A urologist should be consulted for patients with large fungating or necrotic masses, with recurrences, and where the diagnosis is uncertain or the patient is not improving. Numerous surgical procedures have been reported, with most including excision of necrotic tissue and repair of the remaining viable tissue. Patients requiring urologic consultation will have the procedure done under general anesthesia, but most young healthy girls will not require overnight hospitalization. Recurrence is rare following surgical treatment.[62]

Social service consultation should be requested if there is any suggestion or disclosure of sexual abuse.

References

1. Hoberman A, Chao HP, Keller DM, et al: Prevalence of urinary tract infections in febrile infants. *J Pediatr* 123:17, 1993.
2. Hoberman A, Wald ER, Reynolds EA, et al: Pyuria and bactiuria in urine specimens obtained by catheter from young children with fever. *J Pediatr* 124:513, 1994.
3. Andrich MP, Majd M: Diagnostic imaging in the evaluation of the first urinary tract infection in infants and young children. *Pediatrics* 90:436, 1992.
4. Batisky D: Pediatric urinary tract infections. *Pediatr Ann* 25:266, 1996.
5. McCracken GH: Diagnosis and management of acute urinary tract infections in infants and children. *Pediatr Infect Dis J* 6:107, 1987.
6. Todd JK: Management of urinary tract infections: Children are different. *Pediatr Rev* 16:190, 1995.
7. Anand SK: Urinary tract infections, in Berkowitz CD (ed): *Pediatrics: A Primary Care Approach.* Philadelphia: Saunders, 1996, pp 275–278.
8. Lerner GR: Urinary tract infections in children. *Pediatr Ann* 23:463, 1994.
9. Shafer MA, Sweet RL: Pelvic inflammatory disease in adolescent females. *Adolesc Med* 1:545, 1990.
10. Neinstein LS: Genitourinary tract infections, in Neinstein LS (ed): *Adolescent Health Care.* Baltimore: Williams & Wilkins, 1991, pp 365–375.
11. Hooton TM, Scholes D, Hughes JP, et al: A prospective study of risk factors for symptomatic urinary tract infection in young women. *N Engl J Med* 335:468, 1996.
12. Van den Abbeele AD, Treves ST, Lebowitz RL, et al: Vesicoureteral reflux in asymptomatic siblings of patients with known reflux: Radionuclide cystography. *Pediatrics* 79:147, 1987.
13. Shapiro ED: Infections of the urinary tract. *Pediatr Infect Dis J* 11:165, 1992.
14. Hellerstein S: Urinary tract infections. *Pediatr Clin North Am* 42:1433, 1995.
15. Lohr JA: Use of routine urinalysis in making a presumptive diagnosis of urinary tract infection in children. *Pediatr Infect Dis J* 10:646, 1991.
16. Propp DA, Weber D, Ciesla ML: Reliability of a urine dipstick in emergency department patients. *Ann Emerg Med* 18:560, 1989.
17. Shaw KN, Hexter D, McGowan KL, et al: Clinical evaluation of a rapid screening test for urinary infections in children. *J Pediatr* 118:733, 1991.
18. Smellie JM, Rigden SPA: Pitfalls in the investigation of children with urinary tract infection. *Arch Dis Child* 72:251, 1995.
19. Madrigal G, Odio CM, Mohs E, et al: Single dose antibiotic therapy is not as effective as conventional regimens for management of acute urinary tract infections in children. *Pediatr Infect Dis J* 7:316, 1988.
20. Fine JS, Jacobson MS: Single-dose versus conventional therapy of urinary tract infections in female adolescents. *Pediatrics* 75:916, 1985.
21. Avorn J, Monane M, Gurwitz JH, et al: Reduction of bacteriuria and pyuria after ingestion of cranberry juice. *JAMA* 271:751, 1994.
22. Hellerstein S: Evolving concepts in the evaluation of the child with a urinary tract infection. *J Pediatr* 124:589, 1994.
23. Altemeier WA: A backward look at urinary tract infections. *Pediatr Ann* 24:255, 1996..
24. Smellie JM, Rigden SPA, Prescod NP: Urinary tract infection: A comparison of four methods of investigation. *Arch Dis Child* 72:247, 1995.
25. Conway JJ, Cohn RA: Evolving role of nuclear medicine for the diagnosis and management of urinary tract infection. *J Pediatr* 124:87, 1994.

26. Hibbard LT: Adnexal torsion. *Am J Obstet Gynecol* 152:456, 1985.

27. Spigland N, Ducharme JC, Yazbeck S: Adnexal torsion in children. *J Pediatr Surg* 24:974, 1989.

28. Bowen A: Ovarian torsion diagnosed by ultrasonography. *South Med J* 78:1376, 1985.

29. Adelman S, Benson CD, Hertzler JH: Surgical lesions of the ovary in infant and childhood. *Surg Gynecol Obstet* 141:219, 1975.

30. Sommerville M, Grimes DA, Koonings PP, et al: Ovarian neoplasms and the risk of adnexal torsion. *Am J Obstet Gynecol* 164:577, 1991.

31. Merritt DF: Torsion of the uterine adnexa: A review. *Adolesc Pediatr Gynecol* 4:3, 1991.

32. Koonings PP, Campbell K, Grimes DA, Mishell DR Jr: Relative frequency of primary neoplasms: A 10-year review. *Obstet Gynecol* 74:921, 1989.

33. Fedele L, Dorta M: Diagnostic imaging, in JS Sanfilippo (ed): *Pediatric and Adolescent Gynecology*. Philadelphia: Saunders, 1994, pp 441–466.

34. Fedele L, Dorta M, Brioschi D, et al: Magnetic resonance evaluation of gynecologic masses in adolescents. *Adolesc Pediatr Gynecol* 3:83, 1990.

35. Wakamatsu M, Wolf P, Benirschke K: Bilateral torsion of the normal ovary and oviduct in a young girl. *J Fam Pract* 28:101, 1989.

36. Sanfilippo JS: Chronic pelvic pain: Medical and surgical approach, in JS Sanfilippo (ed): *Pediatric and Adolescent Gynecology*. Philadelphia: Saunders, 1994, pp 635–653.

37. Ammerman S, Shafer MA, Snyder D: Ectopic pregnancy in adolescents: A clinical review for pediatricians. *J Pediatr* 117:677, 1990.

38. Gordon JD, Hopkins KL: Adnexal torsion: Color Doppler diagnosis and laparoscopic treatment. *Fertil Steril* 61:383, 1994.

39. Rosado W, Trambert M, Gosink B, et al: Adnexal torsion: Diagnosis by using Doppler sonography. *Am J Radiol* 159:1251, 1992.

40. Kimura I, Togashi K, Kawakami S, et al: Ovarian torsion: CT and MRI imaging appearances. *Radiology* 190:337, 1994.

41. Zweizig J: Conservative management of adnexal torsion. *Am J Obstet Gynecol* 168:1791, 1993.

42. Grisanti KA: Gastrointestinal disorders: Abdominal pain, in Barkin RM (ed): *Pediatric Emergency Medicine*. St Louis: Mosby–Year Book, 1992, pp 728–737.

43. Rosenfeld WD: Sexually transmitted diseases in adolescents: Update 1991. *Pediatr Ann* 20:303, 1991.

44. Gittes EB, Irwin CE: Sexually transmitted diseases in adolescents. *Pediatr Rev* 14:180, 1993.

45. McCormack WM: Pelvic inflammatory disease. *N Engl J Med* 330:115, 1994.

46. Shafer MA, Sweet RL: Pelvic inflammatory disease in adolescent females. *Adolesc Med* 1:545, 1990.

47. Shafer MA: Sexually transmitted diseases in adolescents: Prevention, diagnosis, and treatment in pediatric practice. *Adolesc Health Update* 6:1, 1994.

48. Woodhead JC, et al: Evaluation and management of abdominal and pelvic pain, in Strasburger VC (ed): *Basic Adolescent Gynecology: An Office Guide*. Baltimore: Urban & Schwarzenberg, 1990, pp 173–229.

49. Centers for Disease Control and Prevention: 1993 Sexually transmitted diseases—Treatment guidelines. *MMWR* 42:RR-14, 1993.

50. Drugs for sexually transmitted diseases. *Med Lett* 37:117, 1995.

51. Ludwig S, Selbst SM, Lavelle J: Adolescent emergency conditions, in McAnarney ER, et al (eds): *Textbook of Emergency Medicine*. Philadelphia: Saunders, 1992, pp 932–954.

52. Woodhead JC, et al: Evaluation and management of abdominal and pelvic pain, in Strasburger VC (ed): *Basic Adolescent Gynecology: An Office Guide*. Baltimore: Urban & Schwarzenberg, 1990, pp 173–229.

53. Coupey SM, Ahlstrom P: Common menstrual disorders. *Pediatr Clin North Am* 36:551, 1989.

54. Wenning JB: Genital tract cysts and tumors, in McAnarney ER, et al (eds): *Textbook of Emergency Medicine*. Philadelphia: Saunders, 1992, pp 672–674.

55. Neinstein LS: Polycystic ovary syndrome and ovarian cysts and tumors, in Neinstein LS (ed): *Adolescent Health Care: A Practical Guide*. Baltimore: Williams & Wilkins, 1984, pp 679–686.

56. Horowitz IR, Sainz de la Cuesta R: Benign and malignant tumors of the ovary, in Carpenter SEK, Rock JA (eds): *Pediatric and Adolescent Gynecology*. New York: Raven Press, 1992, pp 397–416.

57. Richardson DA, Hajj S, Herbst AL: Medical treatment of urethral prolapse in children. *Obstet Gynecol* 59:69, 1982.

58. Anveden-Hertzberg L, Gauderer MW, Elder JS: Urethral prolapse in children: An often misdiagnosed cause of urogenital bleeding in girls. *Pediatr Emerg Care* 11:212, 1995.

59. Fernandes ET, Dekermacher S, Sabadin MA, et al: Urethral prolapse in children. *Urology* 41:240, 1993.

60. Jerkins GR, Verheek K, Noe HN: Treatment of girls with urethral prolapse. *J Urol* 132:732, 1984.

61. Mercer LJ, Mueller CM, Hajj SN: Medical management of urethral prolapse in the premenarchal female. *Adolesc Pediatr Gynecol* 1:181, 1988.

62. Sirnick A, Melzer-Lange M: Gynecologic and obstetric disorders, in Barkin RM (ed): *Pediatric Emergency Medicine*. St Louis: Mosby–Year Book, 1992, pp 796–827.

63. Baldwin DD, Landa HM: Common problems in pediatric gynecology. *Urol Clin North Am* 22:161, 1995.

64. Pokorny SF: Prepubertal vulvovaginopathies. *Obstet Gynecol Clin North Am* 19:39, 1992.

65. Lowe FC, Hill GS, Jeffs RD, et al: Urethral prolapse in children: Insights into etiology and management. *J Urol* 135:100, 1986.

PART IV

EMERGENCY GYNECOLOGIC DISORDERS IN THE REPRODUCTIVE AGE

Chapter 34

CLINICAL ANATOMY

John O. L. DeLancey

SUBCUTANEOUS TISSUES OF THE VULVA

The structures of the vulva lie on the pubic bones and extend caudally under their arch (Fig. 34-1). They consist of the mons, labia, clitoris, and vestibule and associated erectile structures and their muscles. The mons comprises hair-bearing skin over a cushion of adipose tissue, which lies on the pubic bones. Extending posteriorly from the mons, the labia majora are composed of similar hair-bearing skin and adipose tissue, which contains the termination of the round ligaments of the uterus and the obliterated processus vaginalis (canal of Nuck). The round ligament may give rise to leiomyomas in this region; the obliterated processus vaginalis can be a dilated embryonic remnant in the adult.

Between the two labia majora, the labia minora, vestibule, and glans clitoris can be seen. The labia minora are hairless skin folds, each of which splits anteriorly to run over and under the glans of the clitoris. The more anterior folds unite to form the hood-shaped prepuce of the clitoris, while the posterior folds insert into the underside of the glans as the frenulum. Preclitoral abscess often arises from an infection beginning under the hood of the clitoris and presents as a fluctuant mass over the glans. The most anatomic point to drain it is in the cleft between the hood and the glans. Incising the hood in the midline carries the risk of permanently exposing the sensitive glans; therefore opening along the normal cleavage plane is to be preferred.

In the posterior lateral aspect of the vestibule, the duct of the major vestibular gland can be seen 3 to 4 mm outside the hymenal ring (Fig. 34-1). Abscess arising in the duct of Bartholin's gland is common and presents frequently in the emergency department. The duct abscess points toward the normal duct orifice posteriorly and laterally in the vestibule, lying at the 5 or 7 o'clock position. More lateral drainage

will involve a deeper and bloodier dissection, and posterior draining, if too deep, can injure the rectum.

The minor vestibular gland openings are found along a line extending anteriorly from the site of Bartholin's duct, parallel to the hymenal ring and extending toward the urethral orifice. The urethra protrudes slightly through the vestibular skin anterior to the vagina and posterior to the clitoris. Its orifice is flanked on either side by two small labia. Skene's ducts open into the inner aspect of these labia and can be cystically dilated in some women; such a duct will present as a fluid-filled mass lateral to the external urethral meatus, usually deviating the external urinary orifice to the side opposite the cyst. These cysts usually do not require drainage unless they are large or symptomatic. These glands can be involved in gonococcal infections and therapy with antibiotics is curative.

Within the skin of the vulva are specialized glands that can become enlarged and thereby require surgical removal. The holocrine sebaceous glands in the labia majora are associated with hair shafts; in the labia minora they are freestanding. They lie close to the surface, and this explains their easy recognition with minimal enlargement. In addition, lateral to the introitus and anus, there are high densities of apocrine sweat glands in addition to the normal eccrine sweat glands. The former structures undergo cyclic change with the menstrual cycle, having increased secretory activity in the premenstrual period. They can become chronically infected as hidradenitis suppurativa or neoplastically enlarged as hidradenomas. The eccrine sweat glands present in the vulvar skin rarely present abnormalities but can form palpable masses as syringomas.

The hymenal ring lies at the junction of the introitus and vagina. There is tremendous variation in its development and configuration (Fig. 32-2). It is not uncommon for young girls to be brought to emergency departments with a question of possible sexual assault. This is a serious matter and requires

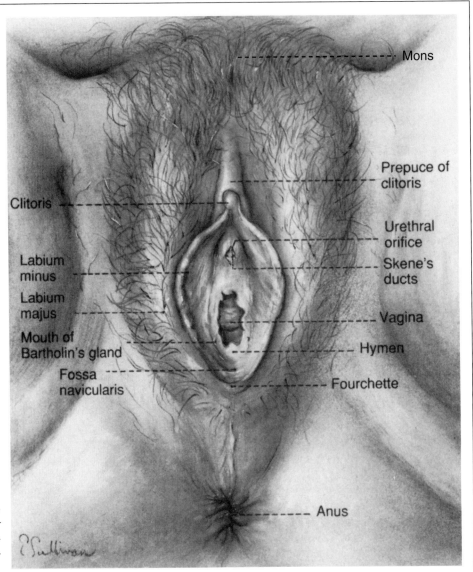

Figure 34-1

External genitalia. [From Rock JA, Thompson JD (eds): *TeLinde's Operative Gynecology,* 8th ed. Philadelphia: Lippincott-Raven, 1997, with permission.]

discretion. In the absence of recent injury, it may be difficult for those unused to examining young girls to know definitively if the vagina has been penetrated. Advice from a gynecologist or pediatric sexual abuse specialist should be sought when available.

Deeper within the vulvar tissues lies the clitoris, whose midline shaft and paired crura lie on the pubic symphisis and extend along the caudal margins of the inferior pubic rami. The paired vestibular bulbs lie beneath the vestibular skin on either side of the introitus and are made up of erectile tissue. The ischiocavernosus muscles cover the crura of the clitoris, while the bulbocavernosus muscles lie on the vestibular bulbs (Fig. 34-2). There are a few muscle fibers that originate in common with the ischiocavernosus muscles from the ischial tuberosity and run medially to the perineal body. These are called the *superficial transverse perineal muscles.* The paired vestibular bulbs lie immediately under the vestibular skin and are composed of erectile tissue. They

are covered by the bulbocavernosus muscles, which originate in the perineal body and lie over their lateral surfaces. These muscles, along with the ischiocavernosus muscles, insert into the body of the clitoris and act to pull it downward. In a woman with suspected neurologic damage to the caudal nerves, watching to see if the clitoris is pulled downward during contraction and assessment of its motion following stroking of the perineal skin (the bulbocavernosus reflex) can help test the integrity of the sacral roots.

Traumatic injury to the vulva is common. Straddle injuries occur when a fall brings the vulva into contact with a bike bar or fence rail, tearing the skin over the pubic rami, lacerating the deeper structures, or causing a hematoma to form. Blood collections in the superficial space tend to track anteriorly onto the abdominal wall and are limited by the peripheral attachments of Colles' fascia.[1] This subcutaneous fascia has lateral attachment to the ischiopubic rami and dorsal attachment to the posterior edge of the perineal membrane (or urogenital di-

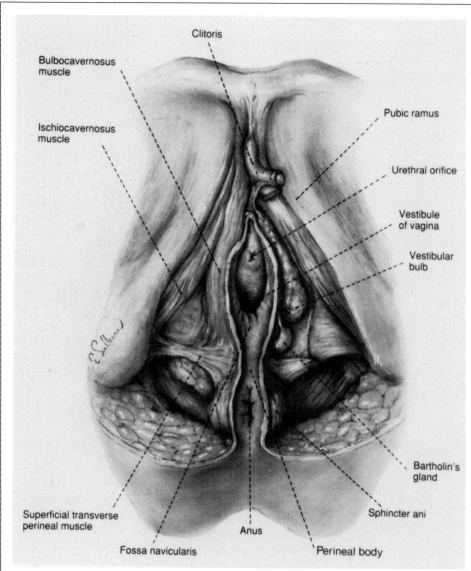

Clitoris

Bulbocavernosus
muscle

Ischiocavernosus
muscle

Pubic ramus

Urethral orifice

Vestibule
of vagina

Vestibular
bulb

Bartholin's
gland

Sphincter ani

Superficial transverse
perineal muscle

Anus

Fossa navicularis

Perineal body

Figure 34-2

Deep structures within the vulva.
[From Rock JA, Thompson JD (eds):
TeLinde's Operative Gynecology,
8th ed. Philadelphia: Lippincott-
Raven, 1997, with permission.]

aphragm), so that blood in the deep subcutaneous space cannot track beyond these attachments. The open ventral margin, however, allows blood to track into the subcutaneous tissues of the abdominal wall. Trauma to the erectile tissue of the vestibular bulb or clitoris can result in massive bleeding from these erectile bodies and requires immediate direct compression followed by urgent surgical repair.

PUDENDAL NERVE AND VESSELS

The pudendal nerve is the sensory and motor nerve of the perineum.[2] Its course and distribution in the perineum parallel the pudendal artery and veins, which connect with the internal iliac vessels (Fig. 34-3). The nerve arises from the sacral plexus (S2-S4) and the vessels originate from the anterior division of the internal iliac artery.

There are three branches of the pudendal nerve and vessels: the clitoral, perineal, and inferior hemorrhoidal branches. They supply the clitoris, the subcutaneous tissues of the vulva, and the bulbocavernosus, ischiocavernosus, and transverse perineal muscles. The pudendal nerve and vessels also supply the skin of the inner portions of the labia majora, the labia minora, and the vestibule. The inferior hemorrhoidal branch goes to the external anal sphincter and perianal skin. Pudendal nerve block performed by perforating the sacrospinous ligament at the tip of the ischial spine proves useful not only to decrease pain during vaginal birth but also for local anesthesia during emergency procedures involving the perineal skin (Fig. 34-4).

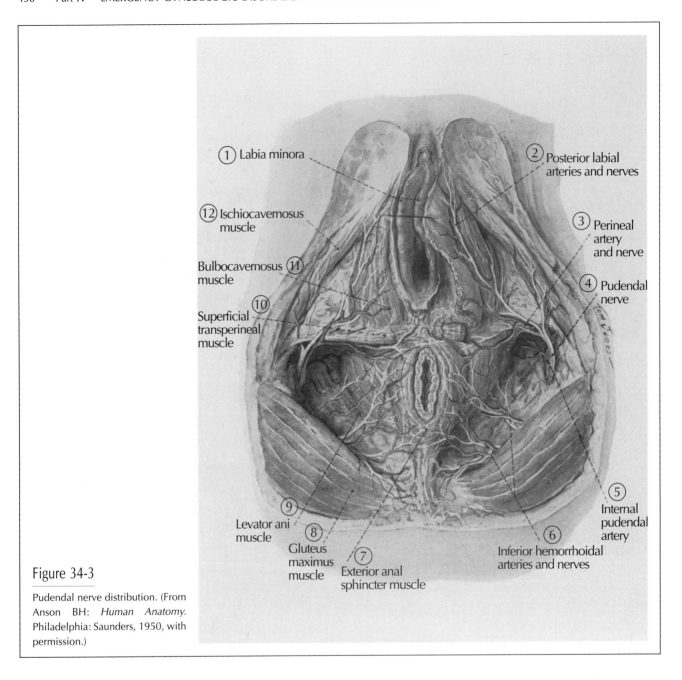

Figure 34-3

Pudendal nerve distribution. (From Anson BH: *Human Anatomy.* Philadelphia: Saunders, 1950, with permission.)

① Labia minora
② Posterior labial arteries and nerves
③ Perineal artery and nerve
④ Pudendal nerve
⑤ Internal pudendal artery
⑥ Inferior hemorrhoidal arteries and nerves
⑦ Exterior anal sphincter muscle
⑧ Gluteus maximus muscle
⑨ Levator ani muscle
⑩ Superficial transperineal muscle
⑪ Bulbocavernosus muscle
⑫ Ischiocavernosus muscle

PERINEAL BODY AND ANAL SPHINCTERS

Within the area bounded by the lower posterior vaginal wall, the perineal skin, and the anus is a mass of connective tissue called the *perineal body*.[3] The term *central tendon of the perineum* has also been applied to this structure and is quite descriptive, suggesting its role as a central point into which a number of muscles insert.

The perineal body is attached to the inferior pubic rami and ischial tuberosities through the perineal membrane and superficial transverse perineal muscles. Anterolaterally, the perineal body receives the insertion of the bulbocavernosus muscles. The upper portions of the perineal body, on its lateral margins, are connected with some of the fibers of the pelvic diaphragm. Posteriorly, the perineal body is attached to the coccyx by the external anal sphincter, which is embedded in the perineal body anteriorly and is attached at its other end to the coccyx. All of these connections anchor the perineal body and its surrounding structures to the bony pelvis and help keep it in place.

The external anal sphincter lies in the posterior triangle of the perineum (Fig. 34-5). It has a teardrop shape with a point tethered on the coccyx dorsally and the loop extending between the rectum and vagina. The circular external

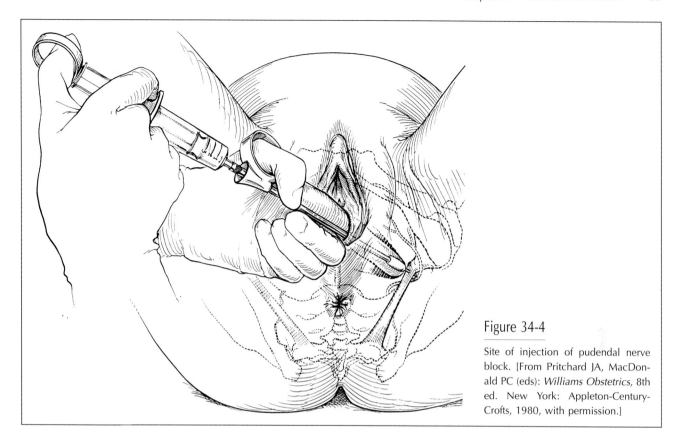

Figure 34-4

Site of injection of pudendal nerve block. [From Pritchard JA, MacDonald PC (eds): *Williams Obstetrics,* 8th ed. New York: Appleton-Century-Crofts, 1980, with permission.]

orifice of the anal canal is attributed to a subcutaneous component that does encircle the anal canal, but the majority of the external sphincter is a loop that pulls dorsally on the anal canal.

The internal anal sphincter is a thickening in the circular muscle of the anal wall. It lies just inside the external anal sphincter and is separated from it by a visible intersphincteric groove. It can be identified just beneath the anal submucosa in repair of a chronic fourth-degree laceration of the perineum. The longitudinal layer of the bowel, along with some fibers of the levator ani, separate the external and internal sphincters.

Lacerations of the perineal body occur frequently at the time of vaginal delivery, during some sexual assaults, or after perineal trauma. An anatomic reconstruction is needed to restore structural continuity and function to this important region. The depth of a laceration should be explored to look for a separated anal sphincter muscle, which is normally between the vaginal canal and anal canal, just below the perianal skin. If complete transection of the perineal body has occurred, so that the anal canal is opened, the internal anal sphincter, which lies between the external sphincter and anal canal, must also have been separated and must be repaired. As the repair is accomplished, care should be taken to close the connective tissue under the mucosa so as to reunite the supportive tissues in the midline and to restore the support provided by the perineal body.

PELVIC MUSCLES

The obturator internus arises from the inner surface of the obturator foramen and membrane and leaves the pelvis through the lesser sciatic foramen to insert into the medial surface of the greater trochanter (Fig. 34-6). The piriformis takes its origin from the anterior aspect of the sacrum and passes through the greater sciatic foramen to insert into the upper border of the greater trochanter. A muscle strain in either of these muscles can lead to discomfort in the pelvic area and may present to the emergency department as low abdominal, hip, or pelvic pain. Palpating the tender muscle anterolaterally just cephalad to the inferior pubic ramus in the case of the obturator internus and posterior and superior to the ischial spine and sacrospinous ligament in the case of the piriformis muscle assists in making this diagnosis. Both of these pelvic wall muscles are lateral rotators and abductors of the thigh, and maneuvers that stretch them may reproduce the pain and confirm the nature of the problem. This muscle pain can pose a diagnostic dilemma when focus is placed on searching for a visceral cause of pelvic pain. Simply entertaining this diagnosis, however, allows the clinician to make the diagnosis easily through reproducing the patient's complaint by palpating the tender muscle.

The opening between the bones and muscles of the pelvic

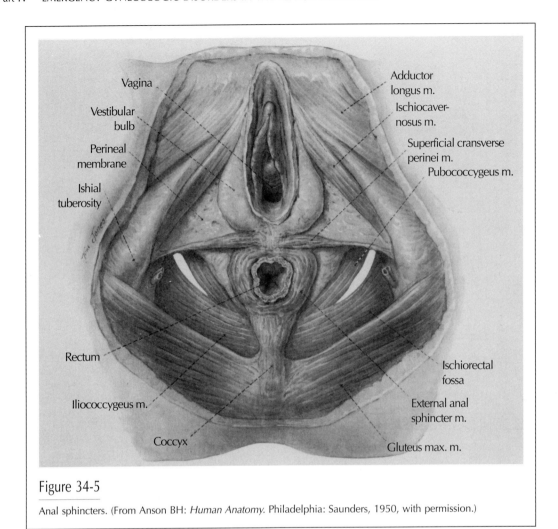

Figure 34-5

Anal sphincters. (From Anson BH: *Human Anatomy.* Philadelphia: Saunders, 1950, with permission.)

wall is spanned by the muscles of the pelvic diaphragm: the pubococcygeus, the iliococcygeus, the puborectalis, and the coccygeus muscles.[4] The most medial of these muscles is the puborectalis/pubococcygeus complex (Figs. 34-4 and 34-5). The pubococcygeus portion of these muscles has an insertion into the anococcygel raphe and the superior surface of the coccyx, while the puborectalis represents those inferior fibers that pass behind and also insert into the rectum. Some women develop pain in these muscles from recent vigorous use of Kegel's exercises in much the same way that someone beginning a program of running may have sore legs. This can lead a woman to seek care for dyspareunia.[5]

PELVIC ORGANS

VAGINA

The vagina is a pliable hollow viscus whose shape is determined by the structures surrounding it and by its attachments to the pelvic wall (Figs. 34-7 and 34-8). These attachments are to the lateral margins of the vagina, so that its lumen is a transverse slit, with the anterior and posterior walls in contact with one another. The lower portion of the vagina is constricted as it passes through the urogenital hiatus in the levator ani. The upper vagina is more capacious. The cervix lies within the anterior vaginal wall, making the vagina shorter anteriorly than posteriorly by approximately 3 cm, with the former being 7 to 9 cm in length. There is, however, great variability in this dimension. The bladder and urethra lie in contact with the anterior vaginal wall, making them accessible to palpation during pelvic examination, while the rectum lies posteriorly and can also be felt through the vaginal wall.

Deep lacerations of the vaginal canal can involve the structures adjacent to the vaginal canal. In the upper vagina anteriorly, both the bladder and the ureters lie immediately adjacent to the vagina and may be injured along with the vagina (Fig. 34-8). In instances where there is a deep laceration in the upper vagina, care should be taken to inspect this area to make sure that no injury to the bladder or ureters has occurred. Instillation of a dilute methylene blue solution

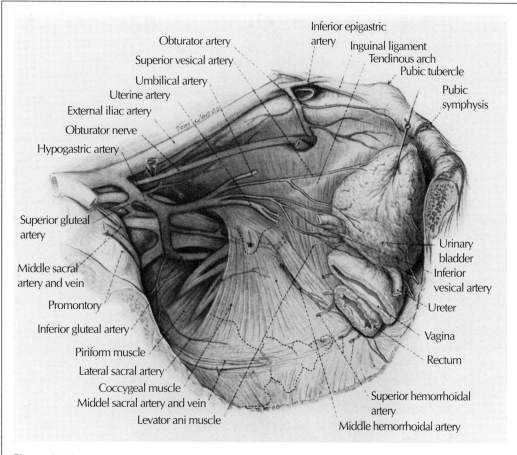

Figure 34-6

Structures of the pelvic wall, including obturator internis piriformis. (From Anson BH: *Human Anatomy*. Philadelphia: Saunders, 1950, with permission.)

into the bladder allows recognition of bladder injury when this contrast material is seen in the vagina. Ureteral injury is somewhat more difficult to detect. Visualization of clear fluid coming from the wound in the absence of a bladder laceration implies a ureteral injury, but intravenous pyelography or cystoscopy with retrograde contrast injection would be needed to confirm this. Nearer the introitus, the urethra causes a bulge in the anterior vaginal wall. Masses present in this area may represent a urethral diverticulum that can be infected, can carry a stone, or may simply be an asymptomatic finding.

The posterior vaginal wall has different anatomic relationships in its upper and lower portions. The upper vagina lies adjacent to the cul de sac of Douglas for the 4 cm below the vaginal cervical junction (Fig. 34-7). This anatomic relationship allows a needle to be placed transvaginally into the cul de sac (culdocentesis). In women with an upper vaginal laceration, consideration must be given to intestinal injury. Although not universally present, it is a possible accompaniment of this type of trauma and should be considered. The lower portion of the vagina lies immediately ad-

jacent to the rectum. Rectal damage can be assessed simply with a rectal examination, and this should be performed whenever a laceration involves the posterior vaginal wall.

The vagina becomes narrowed and smooth in postmenopausal women not on estrogen and who are not sexually active. This is not a reason for particular concern but may explain problems that arise when they wish to resume sexual intercourse.

UTERUS: CORPUS AND CERVIX

The uterus is a fibromuscular organ whose shape, weight, and dimensions vary considerably depending on both estrogenic stimulation and previous parturition (Fig. 34-9). It has two portions, an upper muscular corpus and lower fibrous cervix. In the reproductive-age woman, the corpus is considerably larger than the cervix; but before menarche and after the menopause, the corpus and cervix are relatively similar in size. Within the corpus, there is a triangularly shaped endometrial cavity surrounded by a thick muscular

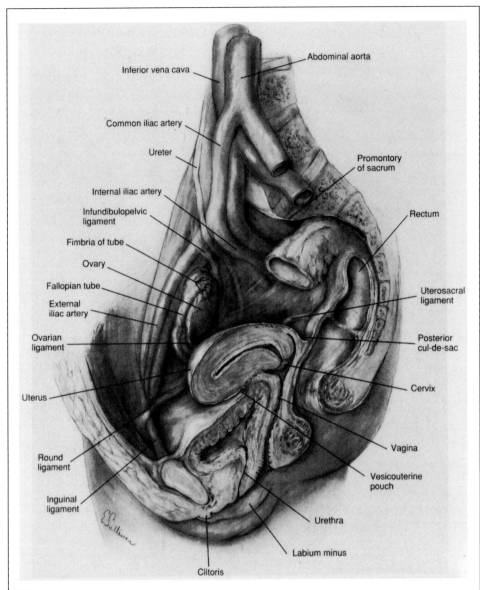

Figure 34-7

Sagittal section of the pelvis showing adjacent relationships. [From Rock JA, Thompson JD (eds): *TeLinde's Operative Gynecology,* 8th ed. Philadelphia: Lippincott-Raven, 1997, with permission.]

wall. That portion of the corpus which extends above the top of the endometrial cavity (i.e., above the insertions of the fallopian tubes) is called the *uterine fundus.*

The uterus is lined by a unique mucosa, the *endometrium.* It has both a columnar epithelium, which forms glands, and a specialized stroma. The superficial portion of this layer undergoes cyclic change with the menstrual cycle. Spasm of hormonally sensitive spiral arterioles lying within the endometrium causes shedding of this layer at the end of each cycle, but a deeper basal layer of the endometrium remains to regenerate a new lining. Separate arteries supply the basal endometrium, explaining its preservation at the time of menses.

The cervix is divided into two portions: the portio vaginalis, which is that part protruding into the vagina, and the portio supravaginalis, which lies above the vagina and below the corpus. The upper border of the cervical canal is marked by the internal os, where the narrow cervical canal widens out into the endometrial cavity. The cervix contains numerous gland clefts. When the orifice of one of these clefts become occluded, cystic dilatation occurs, resulting in the common nabothian cyst. These cysts can be small and numerous or single and large. Collections of large numbers of these cysts can substantially enlarge the cervix and give it a hard, firm consistency. Confirmation that this was caused by cystic dilatation can be made by aspirating one of the cysts

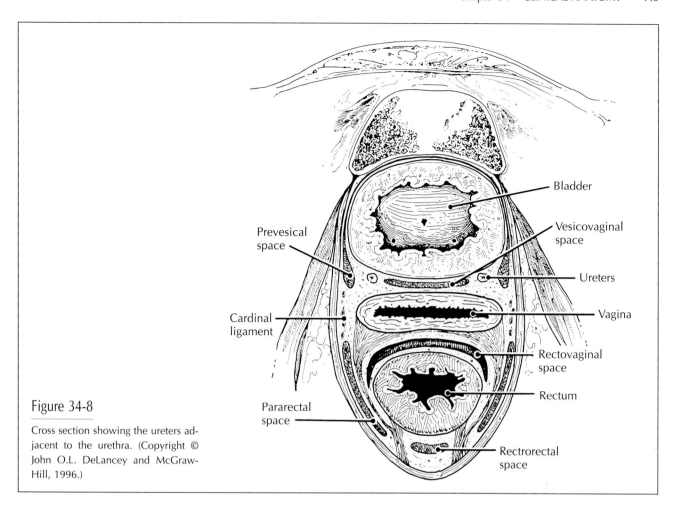

Figure 34-8

Cross section showing the ureters adjacent to the urethra. (Copyright © John O.L. DeLancey and McGraw-Hill, 1996.)

with an 18-gauge needle. Return of thick mucus confirms that the enlargement is caused by nabothian cysts. These cysts are rarely if ever the cause of any discomfort and are an incidental finding.

The cervix changes its appearance substantially during pregnancy. It becomes cyanotic and swollen. The bright-red glandular tissue of the endocervical canal pushes downward and outward so that it becomes visible at the external orifice of the cervix. This is a normal physiologic ectropion associated with pregnancy. It is often also seen with oral contraceptive use. Unlike cervical cancer, which usually produces a firm and scirrhous distortion of the cervix, this is smooth and soft. If there is concern about cervical cancer, biopsy of the lesion is indicated.

ADNEXAL STRUCTURES AND BROAD LIGAMENT

The fallopian tubes are paired tubular structures 7 to 12 cm in length. Each has four recognizable portions. At the uterus, the tube passes through the cornu as an interstitial portion. Upon emerging from the corpus, a narrow isthmic portion begins with a narrow lumen and thick muscular wall. Proceeding toward the abdominal end, next is the ampulla, which has an expanding lumen and more convoluted mucosa. The fimbriated end of the tube has a great number of frondlike projections to provide a wide surface for ovum pickup. The distal end of the fallopian tube is attached to the ovary by the fimbria ovarica, which is a smooth muscle band responsible for bringing the fimbria and ovary close to one another at the time of ovulation. The outer layer of the tube's muscularis is composed of longitudinal fibers; the inner layer has a circular orientation. Ectopic pregnancy occurs most frequently in the fallopian tube. Because of the varying distensibility of the tube, depending on its varying diameter, there are great variations in the time when tubal pregnancy presents.

The lateral pole of the ovary is attached to the pelvic wall by the infundibulopelvic ligament and the ovarian artery and vein contained therein. Medially it is connected to the uterus through the uteroovarian ligament. During reproductive life, it measures approximately 2.5 to 5 cm long, 1.5 to 3 cm in thickness, and 0.7 to 1 cm in width, varying with its state of activity or suppression, as with oral contraceptive medications. Functional cysts of the ovary are common and present either as incidental findings on pelvic examination or may cause pain resulting in a visit to the emergency department. Adnexal enlargement requires knowledgeable

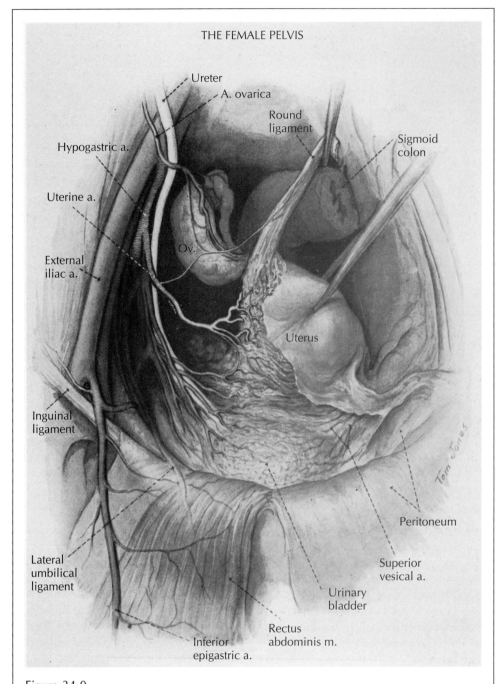

THE FEMALE PELVIS

Figure 34-9

Uterus, adjacent structures, and their blood supply. (From Anson BH: *Human Anatomy*. Philadelphia: Saunders, 1950, with permission.)

consultation because of the competing need (1) to avoid intervening unnecessarily in a woman who has a normal but unusually large hemorrhagic corpus luteum while (2) not neglecting a bleeding corpus luteum, ovarian torsion, or malignancy.

The round ligaments are extensions of the uterine musculature and represent the homologue of the gubernaculum testis. They begin as broad bands arising on each lateral aspect of the anterior corpus. Pain from muscular spasm in these structures presents as abdominal pain during pregnancy, is usually associated with movement, and is usually not associated with other abdominal symptoms.

BLOOD SUPPLY AND LYMPHATICS OF THE GENITAL TRACT

The blood supply to the genital organs comes from the ovarian arteries and the uterine and vaginal branches of the internal iliac.[6] A continuous arterial arcade connects these vessels on the lateral border of the adnexa, uterus, and vagina. The blood supply of the upper adnexal structures comes from the ovarian arteries, which arise from the anterior surface of the aorta just below the level of the renal arteries. The accompanying plexus of veins drains into the vena cava on the right and the renal vein on the left.

The uterine artery originates from the internal iliac artery. It usually arises independently from this source but may have a common origin with either the internal pudendal or vagi-

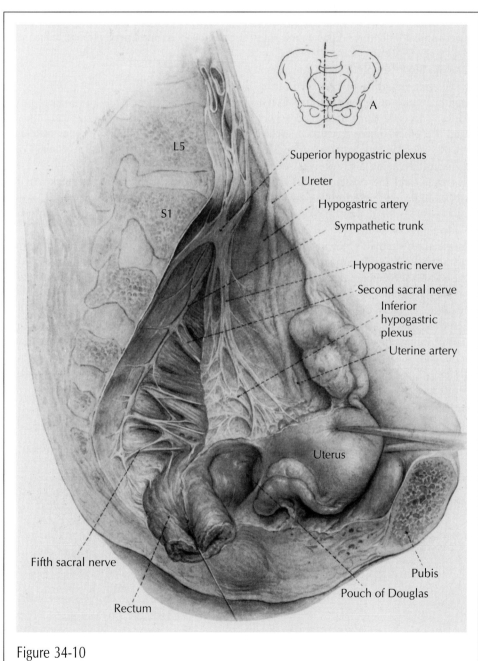

Figure 34-10

Innervation of the uterus. (From Anson BH: *Human Anatomy.* Philadelphia: Saunders, 1950, with permission.)

nal artery. It joins the uterus at approximately the junction of the corpus and cervix, but this position varies considerably both with the individual and also with the amount of upward or downward traction on the uterus. Accompanying each uterine artery are several large uterine veins that drain the corpus and cervix.

Upon arriving at the lateral border of the uterus (after passing over the ureter and giving off a small branch to this structure), the uterine artery flows into the side of the marginal artery that runs along the side of the uterus. Through this connection it sends blood both upward toward the corpus and downward to the cervix. As the marginal artery continues along the lateral aspect of the cervix, it eventually crosses over the cervicovaginal junction and lies on the side of the vagina.

The vagina receives its blood supply from a downward extension of the uterine artery along the lateral sulci of the vagina and from a vaginal branch of the internal iliac artery. These form an anastomotic arcade along the lateral aspect of the vagina at 3 and 9 o'clock. There are also branches from these vessels that merge along the anterior and posterior vaginal walls. The distal vagina also receives supply from the pudendal vessels, and the posterior wall has a contribution from the middle and inferior hemorrhoidal vessels.

Laceration of the lateral portion of the uterus, cervix, and upper vagina causes the most dramatic bleeding. Also, in women presenting to an emergency department after hysterectomy with profuse vaginal bleeding, the source of the bleeding is usually along the lateral margin of the vagina at the vaginal cuff. Therefore, in lacerations within this area, the lateral aspect should be searched first for the site of the bleeding vessel. During termination of pregnancy, a lateral laceration of the uterus can cause profound bleeding. This may well be retroperitoneal and not disclosed through the cervix or uterus. Therefore, a woman with a relatively small amount of bleeding who has systemic evidence of more profound blood loss should be evaluated to determine whether blood has accumulated in the retroperitoneal space beside the uterus.

The uterus receives its nerve supply from the uterovaginal plexus (Frankenhauser's ganglion), which lies in the connective tissue of the cardinal ligament, and through nerves accompanying the ovarian blood vessels (Fig. 34-10).[7] The uterovaginal plexus connects to the central nervous system through the hypogastric nerves and hypogastric plexus. Injection of local anesthetic agents through the lateral vaginal fornix blocks conduction of pain through this region and greatly reduces the discomfort of cervical dilation. It does not, however, blunt perception of pain from the uterine corpus.

References

1. Tobin CE, Benjamin JA: Anatomic and clinical-re-evaluation of Camper's, Scarpa's and Colles' fasciae. *Surg Gynecol Obstet* 88:545, 1949.
2. Klink EW: Perineal nerve block: An anatomic and clinical study in the female. *Obstet Gynecol* 1:137, 1953.
3. Oh C, Kark E: Anatomy of the perineal body. *Dis Colon Rectum* 16:444, 1973.
4. Dickinson RL: Studies of the levator ani muscle. *Am J Dis Women* 22:897, 1889.
5. DeLancey JOL, Sampselle CM, Punch MR: Kegel dyspareunia: Levator ani myalgia caused by overexertion. *Obstet Gynecol* 82:658, 1993.
6. Roberts WH, Krishingner GL: Comparative study of human internal iliac artery based on Adachi classification. *Anat Rec* 158:191, 1967.
7. Krantz KE: Innervation of the human uterus. *Ann NY Acad Sci* 75:770, 1959.

Chapter 35

THE ABNORMAL SPECULUM EXAMINATION

Lauren B. Zoschnick

The vaginal speculum exam is an important component of the diagnosis and treatment of pelvic complaints in women. The focus of this chapter is first to define the anatomy and its variations as it relates to age, pregnancy and anatomic distortions. In addition, benign cervical conditions, tumors, pseudotumors and cysts, intraepithelial neoplasia and invasive carcinomas of the cervix are described.

Visualization of the cervix is of paramount importance in defining gynecologic disease. The patient's trust and compliance are foremost in obtaining an optimal view. Adequate lighting can be obtained with an overhead lamp, a lighted speculum, or a head lamp. Choosing the proper size speculum while keeping the woman's comfort in mind is helpful. Often, particularly in reproductive-age multiparous women, the view of the cervix can be obstructed by the protruding or patulous lateral vaginal walls. This can be remedied by placement of a lateral side-wall retractor or fashioning a similar device by placing a condom over a bivalve speculum and perforating the tip for visualization. Finally, insertion of the speculum is much more successful if one is aware that the axis of the vagina is almost horizontal in the standing position and that one should attempt to place the speculum blades in this axis along the posterior vaginal wall. This will serve two purposes: first, to aid in finding the cervix readily, and, second, to avoid causing discomfort to the patient. If there is difficulty in visualizing the cervix, a helpful clue is recognizing that the anterior vaginal wall has significantly more rugal folds than the posterior wall.

NORMAL ANATOMY

The cervix is the lower, cylinder-shaped portion of the uterus. It is predominantly fibrous and pale pink in color. The vagina is attached to the middle portion of the cervix, dividing it into an upper, supravaginal segment and a lower, visible segment called the *portio vaginalis.*

The endocervical canal is fusiform in shape, its widest portion being in this mid-segment. Cervical length and the width of the portio vaginalis vary; on average, the length is 2.5 to 3.0 cm and the width 3 to 4 cm. The dimensions are hormonally dependent, as is seen in menopausal and prepubertal women with a narrowing of the external os.[1]

The portio vaginalis is covered distally by squamous epithelium, which is typically pale pink in color. More proximally, at the opening to the endocervical canal or external os, is the columnar epithelium. This is a single layer of columnar and cuboidal cells arranged in many folds and crypts. It appears reddish in color secondary to the reflection of light off the underlying capillaries; grossly, under low magnification, it looks like a cluster of grapes.[2]

The junction between the distal squamous epithelium and the proximal columnar epithelium is called the *transformation zone.* This is most often visible in reproductive-age women and is more pronounced in pregnancy and with exogenous estrogen use (e.g., oral contraceptives) and diethylstilbestrol (DES) exposure *in utero* (see Color Plate 1).*

The accentuation of the transformation zone in the above circumstances can be associated with contact bleeding and is often referred to as *cervical ectropion.* Its appears as a velvety-red circular patch centered on the portio vaginalis. It should also be remembered that this transformation zone is the region where dysplastic changes begin in the presence of the human papillomavirus (HPV).

The stroma of the cervix is composed of collagenous connective tissue in a mucopolysacchride substance. It is a more rigid structure than the uterus, as it contains only about 15 percent muscle and a small amount of elastin; it is composed mostly of fibrous tissue.[1]

VARIATIONS

The appearance of the cervix can vary greatly. In pregnancy, the cervix can appear bluish (see Color Plate 2); prolapse or herniation of the uterus and cervix can often be accompanied by benign pressure ulcerations, cystoceles, and rectoceles or enteroceles.

On speculum examination in the emergency department, foreign bodies are often found in the vagina. In addition to tampons, diaphragms, and ruptured condoms, intrauterine device (IUD) strings can be visualized protruding from the external os. The two types of IUDs currently prescribed in the United States are the Paragard and the Progestacert. The former utilizes a white monofilament thread while the other has a blue-black thread (see Color Plate 3).[3]

BENIGN DISEASES OF THE CERVIX

Cervicitis can be divided into noninfectious and infectious etiologies. Noninfectious cervicitis can be chemical or mechanical in origin. It may be caused by, for example, diaphragms, douches, foreign bodies, pessaries, IUDs, and tampons.

Inflammation of the cervix or cervicitis, both noninfectious and infectious, is often misinterpreted on gross inspection, cytology, and histology. Because of this, the older terms—such as *acute, chronic,* and *follicular cervicitis*—are being employed less commonly. An alternative approach, particularly for infectious cervicitis, is to consider the site of the infection. Infectious cervicitis results from a variety of organisms, including bacteria *(Chlamydia trachomatis, Neisseria gonorrhoeae, Mycobacterium tuberculosis),* fungi *(Candida albicans, Candida glabrata),* viruses (herpes simplex virus, HPV), and protozoa *(Trichomonas vaginalis).*[4]

Endocervical infections—usually due to *N. gonorrhoeae* or *Chlamydia trachomatis*—are also called *mucopurulent cervicitis* (Color Plate 4). Two simple objective criteria are used to make the diagnosis. First is visualization of a yellow-green endocervical exudate and, second, the presence of 10 or more neutrophils per $\times 100$ microscopic field.[5] In addition, the cervix often appears erythematous, edematous, and friable, resulting in easy bleeding upon contact with a cotton swab. Of clinical importance is the fact that 50 to 60 percent of women with mucopurulent cervicitis are found to have *C. trachomatis* on culture of the endocervical canal.[1]

BENIGN TUMORS

Endocervical polyps are the most common benign neoplastic growths of the cervix. They are most commonly found in multiparous women in their 40s and 50s. The majority are smooth reddish-purple and bleed easily when touched. Their size varies from a few millimeters to several centimeters in diameter and can be solitary or multiple (see Color Plate 5). Polyps can arise from the portio vaginalis; these are called *cervical polyps.*

Usual symptoms of endometrial or cervical polyps include intermenstrual bleeding, particularly after coitus, though many women are asymptomatic. Polyps are thought to occur as a response to inflammation. Both focal hyperplasia and localized proliferation of cervical cells occur as a response to inflammation. Malignant degeneration is rare.[4]

Cervical leiomyomas are smooth, firm, usually solitary masses. Although 3 to 8 percent of all myomas are cervical, the majority of cervical myomas actually arise from the isthmic portion of the uterus and cannot be visualized on speculum exam. Most are small and asymptomatic. Larger myomas can produce symptoms of dysuria, urinary urgency or frequency, urethral obstruction, and dyspareunia. On occasion, a pedunculated myoma may protrude through the external os. These lesions are often associated with ulceration and infection.[1]

TUMOR-LIKE LESIONS

Microglandular hyperplasia can resemble cervical polyps and range from 1 cm to 2 cm in size (see Color Plate 6). Likewise, they can be associated with postcoital spotting or bleeding. Most occur in women with a history of oral contraceptive use or pregnancy or in postpartum patients.[4]

Endometriosis appears as one or more bluish or reddish nodules (see Color Plate 7). These nodules are a few millimeters in diameter and can be seen on the portio vaginalis or in the endocervical canal.[6] Occasionally, these lesions may be large or cystic; they can produce abnormal vaginal bleeding.

*All Color Plates cited in this chapter appear between pages 460–461.

DIETHYLSTILBESTROL

A number of nonneoplastic abnormalities of the cervix and vagina are found in women exposed to diethylstilbestrol (DES) in utero. It is estimated that 3 million U.S. women were given DES to prevent pregnancy complications of abortion and prematurity from the 1940s through the 1960s. In 1971, after the discovery that a number of these DES-exposed women had clear-cell adenocarcinoma of the vagina, the use of estrogens including DES during pregnancy was discontinued in the United States.[7] Though clear-cell adenocarcinoma of the cervix is an unusual malignancy, even in DES-exposed women (less than 1 in 1000), a number of nonneoplastic conditions of the cervix and vagina are frequently found in DES-exposed women. These include vaginal adenosis and extensive cervical ectropion, structural changes such as cervical hoods (cockscombs), collars (rims), pseudopolyps, and vaginal ridges (see Color Plate 8). Adenosis of the cervix and vagina affects 30 to 40 percent of DES-exposed women.[8] The appearance of adenosis is similar to that of the grapelike clustering of columnar epithelium lining the endocervical canal. This appearance on the cervix is again referred to as *ectropion.* The red, granular spots or patches in the vagina are more common on the anterior wall and generally conform to the upper third of the vagina.

CYSTS

Nabothian cysts are a common finding on the cervix of reproductive-age women. They are subepithelial cysts of endocervical mucus and form in the transformation zone when mucus-excreting endocervical crypts become blocked, forming cysts that are white or yellow in color and semiopaque and translucent in appearance. Nabothian cysts vary from 0.3 to 3 cm in diameter (see Color Plate 9). These mucus-containing cysts are a result of the process of metaplasia when endocervical cells are transformed into squamous epithelium as a result of the acid environment. Nabothian cysts are usually asymptomatic.

In contrast, epithelial inclusion cysts are more commonly found in the vagina and occasionally on the portio vaginalis. They are the most common cystic structures of the vagina and are found in the posterior or lateral walls of the lower third of the vagina. They vary in size from 1 to 3 cm and are frequently found at the site of a previous episiotomy or, following hysterectomy at the vaginal apex.

Inclusion cysts are lines by stratified squamous epithelium and contain a thick yellow substance formed by degenerating squamous cells.[9] That is, a small tag of cervical or vaginal epithelium becomes buried beneath the surrounding epithelium. The vast majority of these cysts are also asymptomatic.

Finally, there is a group of cysts found in the vagina that are embryonic in origin. These soft, thin-walled cysts are often referred to as *Gartner's ducts* and can be mesonephric, paramesonephric, or of urogenital sinus origin. These embryonic cysts are 1 to 5 cm in diameter and are most commonly single. They are most often found in the upper half of the vagina and are present in approximately 0.5 percent of women. Occasionally, a large cyst can cause symptoms, including vaginal pain and urinary complaints.

PRECANCEROUS LESIONS

Intraepithelial neoplasia is a term widely used to describe precancerous or dysplastic abnormalities of the cervix, vagina, and vulva. This terminology has recently been expanded in the development of the Bethesda classification of cervical abnormalities.[10] The spectrum of intraepithelial neoplasia includes low- and high-grade squamous intraepithelial neoplasia. See Table 35-1.

These lesions are linked to HPV infection, causing these cellular preinvasive changes as well as the potential for progression to invasive squamous cell carcinoma.[11] Lesions associated with HPV are generally not seen on speculum examination without the application of acetic acid or Lugol's solution. This is typically done at the time of colposcopy. On occasion, a white plaque, or "leukoplakia," is present on the portio vaginalis.

Table 35-1

SPECTRUM OF INTRAEPITHELIAL NEOPLASIA

Condyloma
CIN[a] I (mild dysplasia)—Low grade squamous intraepithelial lesion
CIN II (moderate dysplasia)
CIN III (severe dysplasia)   } High-grade intraepithelial lesion
Carcinoma in situ
Invasive squamous cell carcinoma

[a]Cervical intraepithelial neoplasia

CARCINOMA OF THE CERVIX

Squamous carcinomas make up 85 to 90 percent of cervical cancers, while 10 to 15 percent are adenocarcinomas. Occasionally, both cancers can be found in the same individual. Women with squamous carcinomas of the cervix typically present with abnormal vaginal bleeding or a brown discharge, frequently citing a prolonged interval since their last Pap smear. The average age of development of invasive cervical cancer is 1 to 10 years after the onset of dysplasia, emphasizing the preinvasive and progressive nature of dysplastic cervical lesions. The appearance of invasive squamous carcinoma can include friability and contact bleeding, cervical enlargement, tortuous capillaries, and ulceration[12] (see Color Plate 10).

ADENOCARCINOMA IN SITU

Adenocarcinomas of the cervix occur in women of all ages. They do not appear to have a viral etiology, nor are they associated with sexual transmission. They, like the squamous carcinomas, have a variety of histologic types. A rare but important variety is clear-cell adenocarcinoma, which can be associated with DES exposure, much like vaginal clear-cell carcinoma; but these lesions may also develop in the absence of DES.

Unfortunately, adenocarcinoma of the cervix is not associated with any symptoms or grossly visible signs, like squamous carcinomas; a recent study suggests poorer survival in all stages as compared with squamous-cell carcinoma.

CONCLUSION

Visualization of the cervix and vagina will often contribute to the diagnosis of women's pelvic complaints. Adequate visualization is accomplished with proper lighting, appropriate instrumentation, knowledge of the anatomy, and a co-operative patient. Knowledge of a variety of benign conditions as well as cervical neoplasms will assist in the diagnosis of both vague and specific symptoms. This will be of further help to emergency physicians and other providers in directing these women to appropriate follow-up when necessary.

References

1. Herbst AL, Mishell DR, Stenchever MA, Droegemuller WM: *Comprehensive Gynecology*, 2d ed. St Louis: Mosby, 1992.
2. Jordan JA, Singer A: *The Cervix*. Philadelphia: Saunders, 1976.
3. *Physicians' Desk Reference*, 51st ed. Montvale, NJ: Medical Economics Company, 1997.
4. Kurnan RJ: *Blaustein's Pathology of the Female Genital Tract*, 3d ed. New York: Springer-Verlag, 1988.
5. Brunham RL, Paavonen J, Stevens CE, et al: Mucopurulent cervicitis—The ignored counterpart in women of urethritis. *N Engl J Med* 311:1, 1984.
6. Bardner HL: Cervical and vaginal endometriosis. *Clin Obstet Gynecol* 9:358, 1960.
7. Herbst AL, Ulfelden H, Poskanzer DC: Adenocarcinoma of the vagina: Association of maternal stibestrol therapy with tumor appearance in young women. *N Engl J Med* 284:878, 1971.
8. Robby SJ, Kauffman RH, Pratt J, et al: Pathological findings in young women enrolled in national cooperative diethylstilbestrol adenosis project (DESAP). *Obstet Gynecol* 53:309, 1979.
9. Fluhman CF: *The Cervix Uteri and Its Diseases*. Philadelphia: Saunders, 1961.
10. Tabbara S, Saleh ADM, Andersen WA, Barber SR, Taylor PT, Crum CP: The Bethesda classification for squamous intraepithelial lesions: Histologic, cytologic and viral correlates. *Obstet Gynecol* 79:338–346, 1992.
11. Schiffman MH: Recent progress in defining the epidemiology of human papillomavirus infection and cervical neoplasia. *J Natl Cancer Inst* 84:394–398, 1992.
12. Piver SM: Diagnosis and management of invasive cervical carcinomas. *ACOG Tech Bull* December 1989; no. 138.

Chapter 36

DISEASES OF THE BREAST

David Allen August
Vernon K. Sondak

It has been estimated that at some time in their lives, as many as 30 percent of women in the United States see a physician with a chief complaint relating to their breasts. Almost all women have either palpable breast irregularities or breast tenderness at some time during their reproductive years. Pregnancy and lactation are periods during which breast symptoms, physical examination signs, and clinical problems are particularly common. Despite the frequency of breast findings and symptoms, urgent problems are unusual and emergencies truly rare.

Public awareness of the frequency and potential consequences of a diagnosis of breast cancer, however, assures that almost all new breast problems are perceived as emergencies by the patient. The goals of initial evaluation of women presenting in primary- or urgent-care settings with signs and symptoms of breast disease are as follows:

- Identify and treat the rare, true emergency conditions of the breast.
- Identify and treat the uncommon urgent conditions of the breast.
- Efficiently initiate appropriate evaluation (and occasionally treatment) of routine breast problems that present to an emergency department or urgent-care setting.
- Identify potential breast cancers, initiate preliminary evaluation, and arrange referral to a specialist.
- Avoid unnecessary evaluation and referral when appropriate.
- Provide appropriate reassurance to the patient when a cancer diagnosis is unlikely.
- Arrange appropriate follow-up to assure proper evaluation and treatment.

The major pitfall in the diagnosis of breast diseases is failure to recognize the potential presence of a malignancy and to arrange for appropriate evaluation and follow-up.

This chapter discusses common breast problems that may be encountered by emergency department and primary care clinicians (physicians, nurses, and physicians' assistants) who work with women. Emphasis is placed upon recognition of typical histories and signs and symptoms, and upon initiation of simple diagnostic and therapeutic interventions that will either definitively treat problems or facilitate subsequent workup and treatment by a specialist.

BREAST DEVELOPMENT, ANATOMY, AND PHYSIOLOGY

BREAST DEVELOPMENT

Breast development begins in utero with the appearance of the milk line during the fifth week of gestation. Initially, this ridge of tissue runs from the base of the upper limb to the base of the lower limb; subsequently, over several weeks, all but the thoracic portion regresses. For as long as 1 month after birth, in utero exposure to maternal hormones may stimulate the neonatal breast to produce colostrum ("witch's milk"). From this point, aside from minor development of the ductal system, the breast is quiescent until puberty.

Failure of proper regression of the milk line leads to the most common congenital breast anomaly, accessory breast

451

tissue. This tissue, most often just an accessory nipple (polythelia), may be found anywhere along the milk line, from axilla to groin. Actual accessory breast tissue separate from the main breast mound (polymastia) is most commonly found in the axilla. Abnormal regression of the milk line

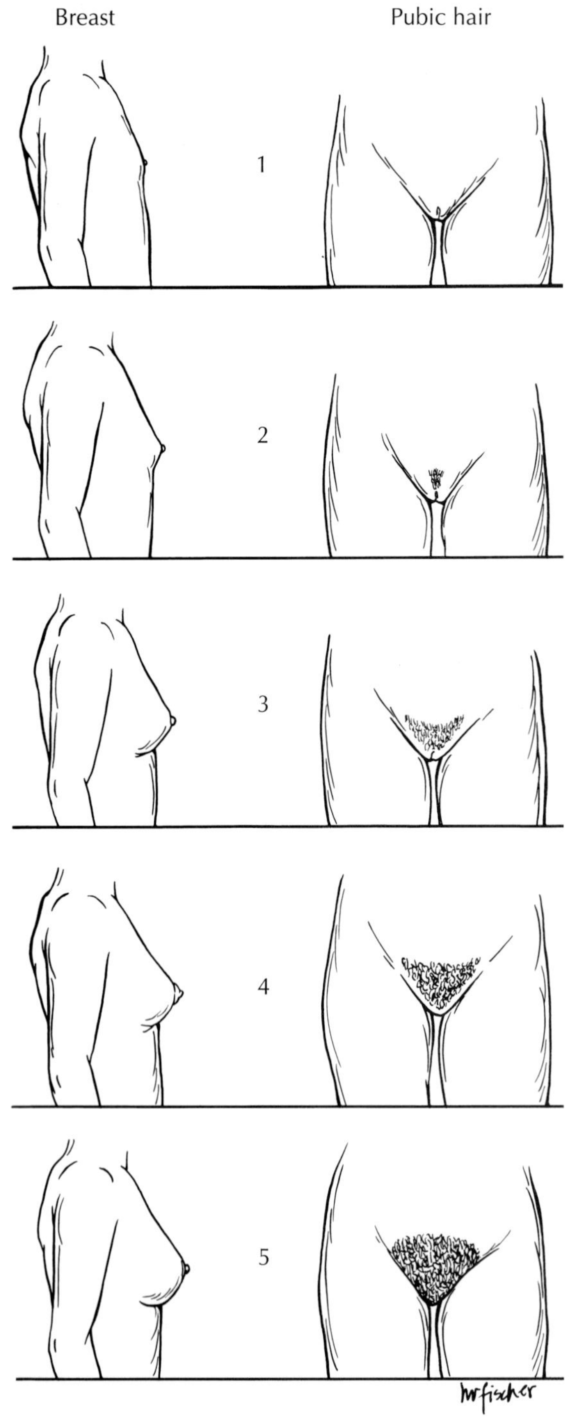

Figure 36-1

The stages of breast development as described by Tanner.[1] (From August DA, Sondak VK,[2] with permission.)

may lead to breast hypoplasia or (rarely) complete absence of the breast (amastia).

At puberty, the female breast bud undergoes a series of changes that culminate in the adult appearance. Injury to the breast bud prior to puberty and completion of full breast development can lead to asymmetric hypoplasia or even total absence of an adult breast mound. As described by Tanner (Fig. 36-1), adult breast development begins at about age 10 with elevation of the nipple (Tanner stage 1).[1] Subsequently, the breast mound begins to appear (stage 2), the breast enlarges and areolar size and pigmentation increase (stage 3), the areolar mound projects outward (stage 4), and finally the areolar mound regresses to form the final adult contour (around age 15, stage 5). The high levels of unopposed estrogen present soon after menarche initiate these events. Progesterone secretion as ovulatory cycles begin 1 to 2 years later allows full breast maturation to occur.

ADULT ANATOMY

The breast sits on the anterior chest wall, extending from the sternocostal junction medially to the midaxillary line laterally and from the second to the sixth ribs in the midclavicular line. The axillary tail of Spence, an extension of breast tissue into the axilla, gives the breast a teardrop shape. The nipple-areolar complex is variably centered on the breast mound. The areola is a relatively flat area of pigmented skin that is usually well demarcated from the surrounding breast skin. Montgomery's tubercles, evident as numerous small protuberances on the areola, are the openings of sebaceous glands that lubricate the nipple during breast-feeding.

The entire breast is richly supplied with sensory nerves, particularly the nipple. The arterial supply to the breast arises from branches off the internal mammary, lateral thoracic, thoracodorsal, and subscapular arteries. The venous anatomy is noteworthy for a plexus of veins that begins in the subareolar region and drains into the intercostal, internal mammary, and axillary veins. The lymphatic drainage of the breast is primarily to the axilla, with a small portion going to internal mammary lymph nodes. Lymph flow is not anatomically restricted; lymph draining to the axilla and to the internal mammary chain can originate in any quadrant of the breast.

BREAST PHYSIOLOGY

Cyclic changes in pituitary trophic factors and circulating hormones associated with the menstrual cycle influence female breast morphology and physiology (Fig. 36-2).[2] Breast engorgement and tenderness are at a minimum 5 to 7 days after menstruation. At this point in the cycle, breast palpation is most sensitive for detecting masses and most comfortable for the patient. Ductal, secretory, and vascular events and associated interlobular edema cause the breast swelling,

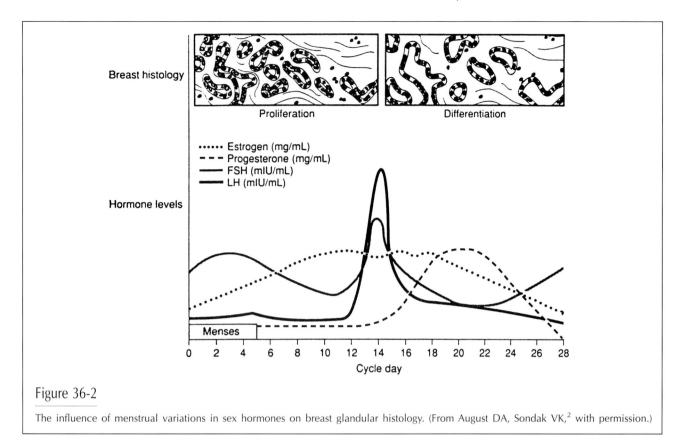

Figure 36-2

The influence of menstrual variations in sex hormones on breast glandular histology. (From August DA, Sondak VK,[2] with permission.)

engorgement, and tenderness associated with the premenstrual phase. At the onset of menstruation, the rapid decline in circulating sex hormone levels leads to breast involution. Because the degree of proliferation and involution varies from cycle to cycle and between different areas of the breast, all cycling women have some breast nodularity.

During pregnancy, marked glandular growth occurs under the influence of estrogen, progesterone, placental lactogen, prolactin, and chorionic gonadotropin. These changes, which begin early in the first trimester, prepare the breasts for milk production at parturition. By parturition, the combined effects of vascular engorgement, epithelial proliferation, and colostrum accumulation may triple the size of the breast. The abrupt change in hormonal milieu that occurs with delivery leads to the production and secretion of colostrum, followed after 4 to 5 days by milk rich in lipid, protein, carbohydrate, and immunoglobulin. The nursing infant's tactile stimulation of the nipple-areolar complex maintains milk production. Throughout lactation, the breasts remain engorged and nodular, making examination and assessment difficult. The presence of nutrient-rich milk during lactation facilitates bacterial overgrowth, should obstruction to flow from any of the major ducts occur. Obstructive mastopathy most often occurs secondary to areolar inflammation and accounts for the susceptibility to suppurative mastitis during nursing. Postlactational involution of the breast occurs during the 3 months after cessation of nursing. The breast gradually approaches its nulliparous state,

but this process is not complete because some glandular hypertrophy persists indefinitely.

In contrast to the events that occur when lactation ceases, the mammary involution occurring with menopause involves actual loss of glandular tissue. Ultimately, the postmenopausal breast consists largely of fat, connective tissue, and mammary ducts, with only sparse lobular elements.

HISTORY AND PHYSICAL EXAMINATION

The superficial location of the breast on the chest wall facilitates the breast examination but can also contribute to anxiety and frustration for the patient. A thorough breast examination should be reassuring to the patient and, if the findings warrant, permit formulation of diagnostic and treatment strategies that the patient understands and supports.

PATIENT HISTORY

Most patients seek medical attention because of breast-related tenderness or a lump. The patient should be questioned about the presence of a lump and related symptoms and about symptoms in the normal breast parenchyma. The presence and character of a nipple discharge should be elicited.

The relation of symptoms to the menstrual cycle or hormone therapy is important. Complaints that vary with menses suggest a benign cause. Cancers are often asymptomatic. Changes that the patient notes on breast self-examination may be significant and should be correlated with the menstrual cycle.

In the emergent/urgent-care setting, the primary objectives of breast evaluation are recognition of acute (trauma, suppurative infections) and subacute (locally advanced breast cancer) situations and identification of potentially malignant lesions. The former should be obvious by history and examination. Assessment of the patient's breast cancer risk will help assess the possibility of a malignancy. However, it must also be remembered that most women who develop breast cancer have no obvious risk factors beyond the two strongest, female gender and age. More than 50 percent of breast cancers occur in women 65 years of age or older. In contrast, adenocarcinoma of the breast is virtually never seen before age 20, and women under age 30 make up fewer than 1 percent of all breast cancer patients.[3] After gender and age, family history and the presence of "precursor lesions" found on a prior breast biopsy are the most significant predictors of cancer risk. If the family history discloses that a relative has had breast cancer, the relationship to the patient, the age at diagnosis of the relative, and whether the cancer was bilateral should be noted. The nature of previous breast problems and histologic findings from prior breast surgeries should be queried. Menstrual and reproductive histories, radiation exposure, and current or prior hormone use may also be relevant (estrogen use, in particular, may alter the texture of the breast on examination).

PHYSICAL EXAMINATION

Physical examination of the breasts is easiest during the week after menses, when breast tenderness and engorgement are at a minimum. The supraclavicular spaces and the anterior and posterior cervical lymph node chains should be palpated routinely as part of the breast exam. Next, with the patient fully disrobed from the waist up, the breasts are observed and compared (Fig. 36-3). Minor size differences are common and of no significance. Note should be made of skin changes, dimpling, or nipple abnormalities. Subtle abnormalities in the lower quadrants may be accentuated by having the patient raise her arms above her head and by pectoral muscle contraction. The axillae, including lymph nodes and the mammary tissue in the axillary tail, are best examined in the sitting position. Note should be made of the number, size, consistency, and mobility of any palpable lymph nodes.

Palpation is best performed with the patient supine. Placement of the patient's ipsilateral hand behind her head pulls the lateral quadrants and tail of the breast onto the chest wall, facilitating compression on the thoracic cage. Palpation must proceed in an orderly fashion to ensure that the

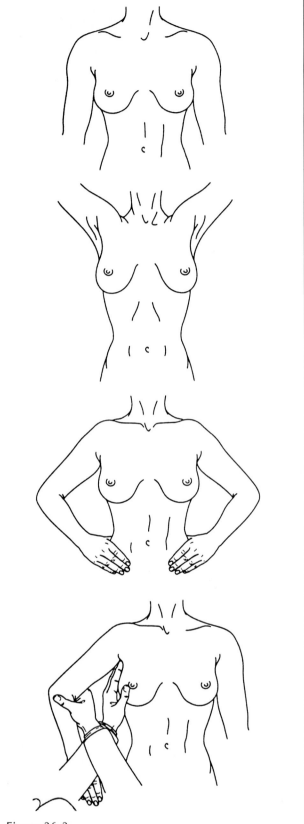

Figure 36-3

Positioning for examination of the breasts. (From August DA, Sondak VK,[2] with permission.)

whole breast is covered. Asymmetry in glandular consistency between breasts should be noted. Discrete or dominant nodules and thickenings should be described by their location (clock-face position and distance from nipple), consistency, borders, and size. Palpation is completed by gently squeezing the nipple-areolar complex to detect subareolar masses and latent nipple discharge. The character of a discharge is significant; milky, serous, or green-brown discharges are almost always benign in origin (fibrocystic changes). Although bloody discharge most often results from a benign intraductal papilloma, it may mark an underlying cancer and should be evaluated further.

BREAST IMAGING

Breast imaging techniques are most often used for breast cancer screening and to look for synchronous, clinically occult disease when a patient presents with a palpable breast abnormality. Because these uses are rarely pressing, the role of breast imaging in an acute/urgent-care setting is limited. However, appropriate use of mammography and breast ultrasound occasionally provides diagnostic clues that can facilitate the planning of a cost-effective evaluation; in some instances, they may even provide diagnostic certainty. Additionally, knowledge of current recommendations and controversies concerning the use of screening mammography can help clinicians to educate patients and promote patient participation in health maintenance. It must be remembered that breast imaging methods are complements to, not substitutes for, a thorough history and physical examination. Reliance on the results of mammography and breast ultrasound outside of the context provided by a history and physical examination can result in missed diagnosis of malignant lesions, with potentially disastrous consequences.

The low level of radiation exposure associated with mammograms performed using dedicated equipment in certified centers (about 1 mGy to the glandular tissue per study) assures that mammography is safe. It is most helpful in women over age 40, when the incidence of breast cancer begins to rise sharply and the sensitivity of the test increases as the dense parenchymal tissue of young women is progressively replaced by fatty tissue. Although sensitive, mammography is not specific. Only about 25 percent of nonpalpable lesions detected mammographically are found to be malignant at biopsy. Conversely, as many as 15 percent of palpable breast cancers may be undetectable mammographically. In the evaluation of a woman presenting with a palpable mass or other clinical abnormality, mammography may help establish a diagnosis (Fig. 36-4). Mammography should be performed before biopsy in all women over the age of 30 years to detect synchronous, nonpalpable ipsilateral or contralateral disease. Otherwise, mammography is rarely indicated before

age 35 except when a diagnosis of breast cancer has already been established.

Routine screening mammography decreases breast cancer-related mortality in asymptomatic women over the age of 50.[4] Prospective, randomized trials have yet to definitively assess the ability of mammography to reduce breast cancer mortality in women aged 40 to 50. Currently, the American Cancer Society recommends that mammographic screening begin at age 40 (Table 36-1).[5] The Board of Scientific Counselors of the National Cancer Institute has taken a more individualized approach, suggesting that women under age 50 discuss the indications for screening mammography with their primary health care provider.[6]

Ultrasonography uses high-resolution, 1- to 10-MHz acoustic waves to image the breast. The most important feature of ultrasound is its ability to distinguish between cystic and solid masses. It is not an effective screening test for breast cancer. Clinically, breast ultrasound is most helpful in premenopausal women to confirm the diagnosis of a cyst or in women under age 30 to support a clinical impression of fibroadenoma (see below). It may also be helpful to identify and facilitate treatment of breast abscesses.

Breast ductography (injection of radioopaque contrast material into a breast duct to help determine the cause of a nipple discharge) is rarely indicated. Thermography has largely been discredited. Breast MRI and positron emission tomography (PET) may have important clinical uses in the future; these modalities are currently under intensive investigation.[7]

Table 36-1	
AMERICAN CANCER SOCIETY RECOMMENDATIONS FOR BREAST CANCER SCREENING	
Age, years	**Recommendation**
20–39	BSE[a] monthly
	Clinical exam every 3 years[b]
40–49	BSE monthly
	Clinical exam annually
	Mammography every 1–2 years
50 and older	BSE monthly
	Clinical exam annually
	Mammography annually

[a]Breast self-examination.
[b]Physical examination by a trained clinician.
Source: Dodd,[5] with permission.

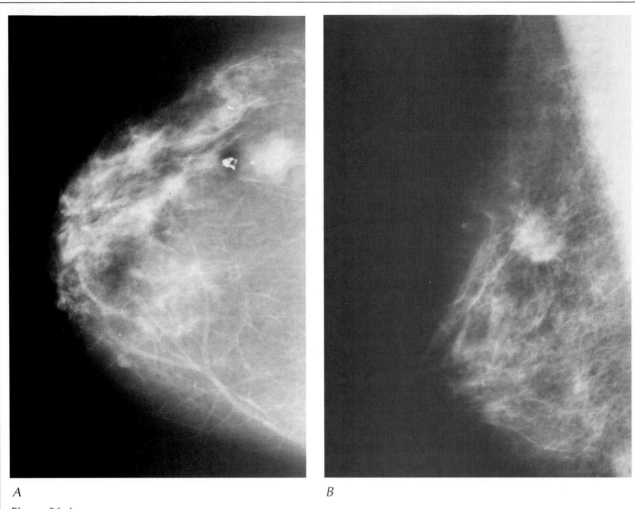

A

B

Figure 36-4

Mammograms showing (*A*) a typical fibroadenoma with "popcorn" calcifications and (*B*) a typical cancer with increased density and irregular, spiculated borders. (Courtesy of Dr. Irv Litt, Radiology Group of New Brunswick, NJ.)

DIAGNOSTIC PROCEDURES

FINE-NEEDLE ASPIRATION BIOPSY

INDICATIONS.   Fine-needle aspiration biopsy (FNAB) permits rapid, minimally invasive diagnosis of many palpable breast masses. The incidence of false-positive diagnosis of cancer is generally less than 0.5 percent; the sensitivity (percentage of actual cancers detected) is approximately 80 percent.[8] False-negative findings are caused by inadequate sampling (missing the lesion), improper processing of the specimen, or inability of the cytologist to make a definite diagnosis. Fine-needle aspiration biopsy should be used to aid in the diagnosis of palpable breast masses. It permits immediate, cost-effective differentiation of breast cysts (characterized by aspiration of nonbloody fluid with complete resolution of the mass) from potentially malignant lesions

(containing bloody fluid or no fluid at all). When the latter are encountered, FNAB permits sampling of cellular material for cytologic analysis. A diagnostic FNAB reveals cells showing a specific benign entity or cells that are unequivocally malignant. Findings such as normal or benign epithelial or fat cells or of acellular, atypical, or suspicious material are nondiagnostic and mandate further evaluation (generally surgical biopsy). The FNAB technique may also be used to confirm the presence of pus when a breast abscess is suspected.

EQUIPMENT.   Alcohol wipes, sterile gauze, 1% plain lidocaine, a 21-gauge needle on a 10-mL syringe, microscope slides and holders, a phlebotomy test tube containing heparin, cytologic spray fixative, and an adhesive strip bandage.

PROCEDURE.   Fine-needle aspiration biopsy is carried out with a 21-gauge needle on a 10-mL syringe (Fig. 36-5).[9] After the skin is anesthetized with lidocaine, the aspirating needle is positioned in the lesion and short bursts of suction are applied to the syringe. A number of passes are made through the mass, and the needle is removed from the breast after suction is released. The sample is extruded onto a glass slide and stabilized with aerosolized fixative. Three to five milliliters of unpreserved saline are then drawn up through the needle into the syringe and evacuated into the heparinized phlebotomy tube to permit analysis of a cytologic cell block.

COMPLICATIONS.   Ecchymosis.

AFTERCARE.   None.

CORE-NEEDLE BIOPSY

INDICATIONS.   Core-needle biopsy (CNB) permits rapid, minimally invasive histologic diagnosis of many palpable breast masses. The incidence of false-positive diagnosis of cancer is near zero; the sensitivity is approximately 80 percent.[10] As with FNAB, any CNB that is not definitively diagnostic of either a cancer or a specific benign entity necessitates further workup. Core-needle biopsy should be used for biopsy of larger breast masses (approximately 2 cm or greater) that are probably cancerous. Because it obtains a histologic sample, CNB is more definitive than FNAB and permits determination of the tumor's hormone receptor status. It is, however, slightly more invasive and causes more immediate discomfort.

EQUIPMENT.   Betadine, sterile gauze, 1% plain lidocaine, a 1-mm by 1-cm Tru-cut needle, no. 11 blade, formalin-containing specimen cup, adhesive wound-closure strips (Steri-Strips), and an adhesive strip bandage.

PROCEDURE.   After prepping and anesthetizing the skin using sterile technique, a 1- to 2-mm incision is made in the skin with the no. 11 blade. The site of the incision should be chosen so that the trajectory of the Tru-cut needle is tangential to the chest wall, avoiding possible injury to underlying structures. Generally, two or three specimens are obtained. Because it is difficult to anesthetize a solid mass fully, the patient should be informed that each needle pass may cause a sharp, stabbing pain lasting several seconds. The skin incision is closed using a wound-closure strip.

COMPLICATIONS.   Ecchymosis, hematoma.

AFTERCARE.   Keep dry for 24 h.

PUNCH BIOPSY OF THE SKIN

INDICATIONS.   A punch biopsy (PB) is used to establish a histologic diagnosis of a lesion in the skin overlying the breast. Most often, it is used to confirm a clinical diagnosis of either inflammatory breast cancer (revealed by the presence of breast cancer cells in dermal lymphatics) or of skin invasion by an underlying cancer.

EQUIPMENT.   Betadine, sterile gauze, 1% plain lidocaine, 3-, 4-, or 6-mm disposable biopsy punch, small scissors and forceps, formalin-containing specimen cup, adhesive wound-closure strips (Steri-Strips), and an adhesive strip bandage.

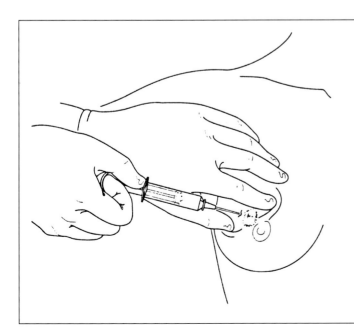

Figure 36-5

The technique of fine-needle aspiration of a breast mass. (From August DA, Sondak VK,[2] with permission.)

PROCEDURE.   After the skin is prepped and anesthetized using sterile technique, the biopsy punch is positioned on the lesion and rotated between the thumb and forefinger while moderate pressure is applied. This is done until the cutting edge of the punch incises the full thickness of the skin. The scissors and forceps are then used to detach the base of the specimen from the underlying subcutaneous tissue. The skin defect is closed using a wound-closure strip or a single 3-0 nylon suture.

COMPLICATIONS.   Ecchymosis, hematoma, bleeding.

AFTERCARE.   Keep dry for 24 h.

OTHER TISSUE-SAMPLING TECHNIQUES

Other techniques used to biopsy suspicious breast lesions include x-ray guided stereotactic biopsy, surgical biopsy of palpable masses (incisional or excisional), and wire-localization surgical biopsy of nonpalpable breast masses. Although these techniques are not used in urgent-care settings, knowledge of them can help to plan the evaluation of a woman presenting with a mass requiring tissue diagnosis or to manage resulting complications. X-ray guided stereotactic biopsy is used to obtain either a cytologic or core-needle tissue sample of a nonpalpable mass detected mammographically. Special mammography equipment is used to guide the biopsy needle into the suspicious lesion.[7] Both incisional and excisional breast biopsy are formal operative procedures. Incisional biopsy involves removal of a portion of a mass and is reserved for lesions too large (generally greater than 3 cm) to be easily excised for diagnostic purposes. Excisional biopsy removes an entire lesion, which permits optimal diagnostic evaluation.[2] Virtually all of these procedures may be performed under local anesthesia in an outpatient setting. Wire-localization biopsy is performed for nonpalpable lesions detected mammographically. A wire is placed into the breast under mammographic guidance immediately preoperatively so that the wire tip is adjacent to the lesion. This guides the surgeon to the proper area to biopsy.[11]

TRUE BREAST EMERGENCIES

TRAUMA

Isolated blunt trauma to the breast is uncommon but can occur during motor vehicle accidents or from other types of direct force applied to the chest wall.[12,13] Most commonly, blunt trauma to the breast is seen in association with multiple thoracic injuries, including rib fractures, and is often ac-companied by extensive ecchymoses. The widespread use of shoulder restraints has likely resulted in some increase in the incidence of these types of breast injuries. There are rare reports of subcutaneous breast rupture[12,13] or rupture of silicone implants in women who have undergone prior augmentation mammoplasty.[14] In the absence of a history of a motor vehicle accident, the presence of a significant isolated breast injury is very unusual and should raise the possibility of abuse. Occasionally, breast cancer may mimic breast trauma; a high index of suspicion is necessary in the absence of a clear history of recent, significant blunt-force injury. Traumatic breast injuries, whether isolated or associated with multiple trauma, rarely require specific therapy. The long-term sequelae of breast trauma, however—including hematoma, fat necrosis, Mondor's disease, and posttraumatic mammographic abnormalities—may require medical attention.

Most of the signs and symptoms of breast trauma resolve within 4 to 6 weeks of injury. Persistent abnormalities beyond that time or the presence of a mass after minimal trauma without accompanying ecchymosis must be viewed with suspicion. Persistent posttraumatic lesions may represent fat necrosis, but they may also represent breast cancer. A significant percentage of women with breast cancer may remember a coincidental but etiologically unrelated event of breast trauma. Persistent sequelae of breast trauma may include the presence of a nonpalpable mass, architectural distortion of the breast tissue, or microcalcifications detected on routine mammography. Unless serial mammograms confirm the etiology of the radiographic findings as dating to the trauma, a biopsy procedure is usually required to exclude the possibility of interval development of a malignancy.

BREAST HEMATOMA

Hematomas occur most commonly following breast biopsy or other surgical procedures.[15] They usually present as painful, tender masses with overlying ecchymoses and generally resolve over a period of several weeks. Fortunately, progressive hematomas sufficiently large to require intervention are very rare. Severe hematomas are more commonly encountered in patients with coagulation disorders or who are taking anticoagulant medications. Rarely, breast hematomas can be seen in the absence of a history of trauma or coagulopathy due to hemorrhage into a breast cyst. Late rupture or infection of a breast hematoma may occur as the hematoma liquefies. Rupture may occur as late as several months after surgery in patients undergoing postoperative breast irradiation.

Whenever possible, prevention of hematoma formation—through the achievement of meticulous hemostasis during breast surgery and correction of coagulation abnormalities prior to invasive procedures on the breast—is better than treatment. For the patient who presents in an acute-care setting with a breast hematoma after minor trauma or a recent invasive procedure, an initial determination must be made whether the hematoma is expanding or tensely distended and at a risk of rupture. Expanding hematomas, especially those occurring within 48 h after surgery, often signify the presence of ongoing bleeding. In such patients, consideration should be given to reoperation for evacuation of the hematoma and ligation of bleeding vessels. Tense, painful hematomas—particularly those occurring more than 48 h after the initiating trauma—are not likely to be associated with a discrete bleeding vessel. Moreover, the clot tends to diffuse through the breast parenchyma and is not readily amenable to surgical evacuation. For these reasons, hematomas presenting later in their course are generally best managed conservatively, with analgesics and a support bra along with correction of any coagulation defects that may be present. Aspiration is generally not effective until the hematoma begins to liquefy. Infected hematomas can sometimes be managed by the combination of percutaneous drainage (usually with a drainage catheter placed into the center of the cavity under ultrasound guidance) and systemic antibiotics, but open drainage and packing are generally indicated.

BREAST INFECTIONS

Inflammatory and infectious processes involving the breast are relatively uncommon but represent a frequent cause of acute care visits. Whenever infectious mastitis or a breast abscess is suspected clinically, the possibility of an inflammatory carcinoma must also be entertained. Any inflammatory process that does not respond completely and promptly to antibiotics or drainage should be subjected to biopsy to rule out cancer. It also is sound practice to biopsy the abscess wall whenever open surgical drainage is performed. If there is doubt about whether an inflammatory process is indicative of a breast cancer, prompt referral to a specialist is indicated.

Lactation and periductal mastitis (see below) are risk factors for development of breast infections. Infection complicates breast-feeding in 1 to 10 percent of women, but these lactational infections account for fewer than 10 percent of all breast infections.[16] *Staphylococcus aureus* is by far the most common pathogen. Nursing women are most vulnerable to infection during the first month of breast-feeding, when the skin of the nipples is most easily damaged, and much later, when the child has teeth that may traumatize the nipples.

Acute infections of the breast generally present with erythema, edema, tenderness, malaise, and fever. Differentiation between mastitis (soft tissue infection of the breast, usually associated with cellulitis of the overlying skin) and breast abscess (a purulent breast infection that may present with the signs and symptoms of mastitis or may demonstrate only focal reaction to the underlying purulent collection and is usually accompanied by palpable fluctuance) is usually straightforward, but may at times be difficult. The distinction is important, because mastitis is best treated with antibiotics alone, whereas an abscess requires surgical drainage (with or without antibiotic coverage, depending upon the extent of the local and systemic reaction). If the presence of an abscess is suspected, this can be confirmed by either aspiration of the fluctuant area (a 16-gauge needle may be necessary to aspirate what is often thick, creamy material), or with the use of breast ultrasound.

Many breast infections begin as cellulitis without abscess formation. If they are recognized at this stage, antibiotic treatment with a first-generation cephalosporin (such as cephalexin 500 po q.i.d. for 7 days) or an antistaphylococcal penicillin (e.g., dicloxacillin 250 mg q.i.d. for 7 days) is frequently successful. Small, periareolar abscesses may often simply be incised and drained if there is no associated generalized erythema or tenderness. In either case, the infection should respond rapidly to therapy, with at least partial resolution within 48 h. Clinical follow-up in person or by telephone within 48 to 72 h is appropriate.

Occasionally, either abscess or simple mastitis may present with obvious signs of regional or systemic toxicity. Immediate surgical consultation for consideration of admission is indicated in the presence of a fever greater than 38.5°C (101.3°F), a white blood cell count greater than 15,000/mm^3, generalized erythema or edema of the breast, and in immunocompromised hosts (patients with diabetes, those receiving chemotherapy or glucocorticoids, and patients with a prior history of breast irradiation). Parenteral antibiotics useful in this setting include cefazolin 1 g IV q8h or nafcillin 2g IV q4h. It is here that rare but serious complications of breast infections such as necrotizing soft tissue involvement or bacteremia may develop.

When an abscess is suspected, percutaneous aspiration is often the most efficient method to confirm the diagnosis, and it permits bacterial culture and sensitivity testing. Although some have tried nonoperative management of breast abscesses, open surgical drainage is the most prudent and effective treatment. Generally, because of the significant inflammation and the sensitivity of the breast, adequate open drainage and biopsy requires either general anesthesia or significant systemic sedation. Hence, immediate referral to a surgeon is often preferable to attempting drainage in the outpatient, acute-care setting using only local anesthesia. In the United States, many women who develop infections while lactating cease breast-feeding, but there is no absolute requirement to do so. Nursing is often difficult for several days on the affected side; the breast should be mechanically emptied and the infant fed from the other breast until nursing can recommence.

Nonlactational infections other than those associated with periductal mastitis are unusual and should raise the specter of inflammatory cancer. Spontaneous, chronic breast infections can occur secondary to unusual pathogens, such as actinomycosis, tuberculosis, and syphilis. Acute, noninfectious mastitis can be seen secondary to a variety of inflammatory processes, such as systemic lupus erythematosus, or it can complicate fibrocystic changes. In the latter cases, the source of the inflammation is presumed to be a ruptured breast cyst.

PERIOPERATIVE COMPLICATIONS

The most frequent complications that may present following breast surgery include hemorrhage, hematoma, infection, drain problems, and seroma formation.[2] Immediate postoperative hemorrhage is best evaluated and treated by the operating surgeon. Exsanguinating hemorrhage is rare. Expanding hematomas may occur but can usually be controlled with direct pressure until emergency care by a specialist can be arranged. Stable hematomas are best managed with analgesics and a well-fitted bra. Wound infections may be handled on an ambulatory basis with an oral first-generation cephalosporin if there is no abscess to be drained, systemic signs of toxicity are limited [temperature less than 39°C (102.2°F) and white blood cell count less than 15,000 mm^3], and the patient is not immunocompromised. Daily follow-up is necessary to assess response to treatment. Worsening signs of cellulitis or systemic response to infection, development of purulence, or failure to improve after 48 h suggest a need for referral to a specialist for evaluation and possible inpatient treatment. Postsurgical abscesses are treated in much the same way as spontaneous abscesses, as discussed above.

Most surgeons use closed-system suction drains following major breast surgery to prevent seroma formation in the axillary space and beneath chest wall skin flaps. Infections occurring in relation to drains generally require drain removal and antibiotic therapy; any fluid collections that develop in this setting subsequent to drain removal usually require drainage either by repeated aspiration or incision. Drains may become clogged with either clotted blood or tissue debris. This can lead to leakage of serous fluid around the drain, repeatedly soaking the overlying dressing. Many of these blockages resolve spontaneously over 12 to 24 h and require no specific intervention other than reassurance. For drain blockages that persist, "milking" of the drain tubing often clears the blockage and restores normal closed drainage. If this maneuver fails, drain removal is generally necessary, with subsequent percutaneous aspiration of a seroma if one forms.

Following planned removal of drains, seromas may form. If they are small and asymptomatic, no treatment is required. For larger (greater than approximately 50 mL) or symptomatic seromas, sterile percutaneous aspiration using a large syringe connected to a three-way stopcock (to allow emptying of the syringe if the seroma volume is too large) and a 20-gauge needle is appropriate. Repeated aspiration is often required.

URGENT CONDITIONS FREQUENTLY SEEN IN ACUTE-CARE SETTINGS

Urgent conditions of the breast include entities that do not truly require urgent or emergent evaluation or treatment but that commonly present de novo to urgent-care clinicians and are often perceived by patients as emergent. Knowledge of these conditions can facilitate prompt and efficient evaluation and in some circumstances allow definitive diagnosis and treatment of problems that cause patients discomfort and anxiety.

FAT NECROSIS

Trauma to fat within the breast can incite an inflammatory response leading to fat necrosis.[15] In only about half of cases, however, is a traumatic event recalled. Fat necrosis can easily be confused with carcinoma, as it may present with a palpable mass and even skin dimpling and retraction. While no specific treatment is required for fat necrosis, the presence of cancer must be excluded. Referral to a specialist is indicated for persistent or new masses, even in the face of recent or remote trauma.

MONDOR'S DISEASE

Thrombophlebitis of one of the superficial veins of the breast, known as *Mondor's disease,* results in a palpable, cordlike mass in the breast. Most cases have no identifiable cause, but strenuous exercise, vein ligation, or coagulation during a breast biopsy can be causative. Patients with Mondor's disease may complain of burning breast pain. Physical examination reveals a characteristic cordlike mass in the superficial subcutaneous tissue of the breast, most commonly in the lower breast. Skin retraction and dimpling may be present. Because of the skin changes and the palpable mass, Mondor's disease can be mistaken for cancer. Mammography can be helpful in establishing the diagnosis. Mondor's disease is benign and self-limited, so no specific treatment is required. A nonsteroidal anti-inflammatory drug often provides symptomatic relief.

MASTODYNIA

One of the most common urgent presentations of women with benign breast disease is mastodynia, also called *mastalgia.*[2] The discomfort may be either constant or cyclical, waxing or waning with the menstrual cycle. Cyclical breast pain is generally related to hormonally induced changes in the breast tissue (fibrocystic changes) and is rarely associated with breast cancer, but a specific cause for the pain should

COLOR PLATES*

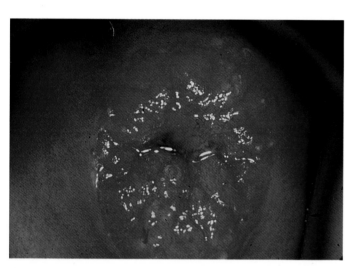

Plate 1 (Chap. 35, page 448)   Cervical ectropion. The cervical transformation zone in a woman on oral contraceptives. Note the prominent eversion of endocervical cells covering more than one half of the portio vaginalis. *(Photograph courtesy of John R. G. Gosling slide collection)*

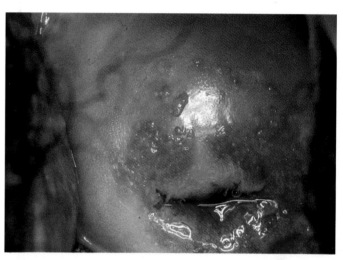

Plate 2 (Chap. 35, page 448)   Positive Chadwick sign. Note the bluish hue of the pregnant cervix. *(Photograph courtesy of John R. G. Gosling slide collection)*

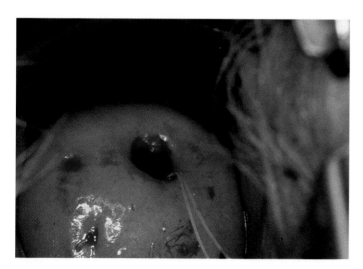

Plate 3 (Chap. 35, page 448)   Paragard IUD string protruding from the cervix.

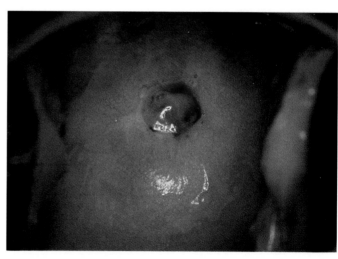

Plate 4 (Chap. 35, page 448)   Mucopurulent cervicitis. *(Photograph courtesy of Mark D. Pearlman, M.D.)*

*All Color Plates are cited in Chapter 35, on pages 448, 449, and 450.

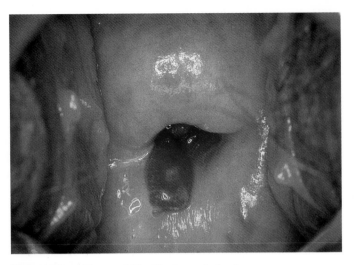

Plate 5 (Chap. 35, page 448)   Single cervical polyp.

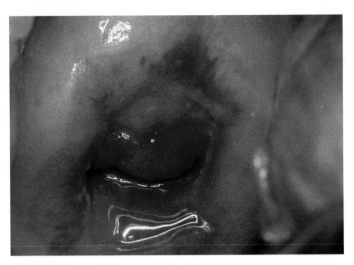

Plate 6 (Chap. 35, page 448)   Microglandular hyperplasia. Similar in appearance to a cervical polyp, this lesion is protruding into the os from the upper lip of the cervix.

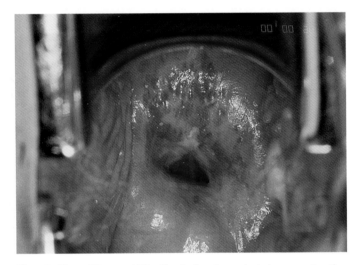

Plate 7 (Chap. 35, page 448)   Cervical endometriosis in a menstruating woman. Note the red papules on the portio vaginalis which contain blood and endometrial tissue.

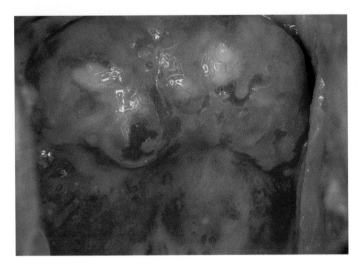

Plate 8 (Chap. 35, page 449)   DES exposure. The upper portion of this cervix demonstrates a collar-like appearance. Note the acetowhite changes after the application of 5% acetic acid. Also note the two Nabothian cysts on the right upper segment of the portio vaginalis.

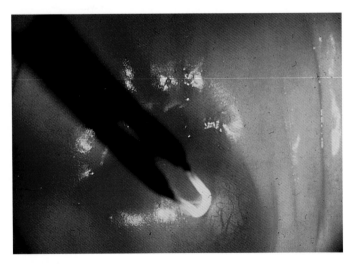

Plate 9 (Chap. 35, page 449)   Nabothian cyst. The forcep is pointed to the raised, round cyst which is yellow-white in color. Note the distinct capillaries branching over the surface of the cyst. *(Photograph courtesy of John R. G. Gosling slide collection)*

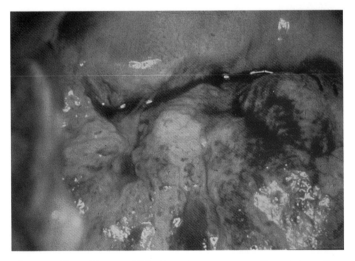

Plate 10 (Chap. 35, page 450)   Invasive squamous cell carcinoma. Note the abnormal vasculature and hemorrhage on the posterior cervical lip. *(Photograph courtesy of John R. G. Gosling slide collection)*

be sought in all cases. The timing of the pain relative to the menstrual cycle is important. Cyclical mastodynia is usually most severe in the days leading up to the menstrual period and decreases or resolves completely following menstruation. The pain may be referred to the axilla, underarm, or scapula. Constant pain not related to the menstrual cycle may be due to an infection or cyst. Once physical examination and mammography, when appropriate, have ruled out a mass lesion, most patients with cyclical mastodynia require no treatment beyond reassurance. Mastodynia that begins cyclically but progresses to become constant and severe, however, often requires specific treatment by a specialist.

The initial physical examination should verify that the pain is in fact originating in the breast. Costochondritis of the upper ribs (Tietze's syndrome) may be perceived by the patient as breast pain. Reproduction of the pain by palpating the affected ribs allows the diagnosis of costochondritis to be made. This is a self-limited condition; nonsteroidal anti-inflammatory drugs are indicated if the pain is severe. In rare instances, pain of cervical nerve root or even cardiac origin can be referred to the breast.

In most women with mastodynia, examination reveals tender, nodular breasts, suggesting a diagnosis of fibrocystic changes. The examiner must determine whether a discrete mass, distinct from the surrounding breast tissue, is present. A tender mass can arise from a benign process (e.g., a cyst or confluent area of fibrocystic changes). Although less likely, a cancer in association with fibrocystic changes may also present as a tender mass. The evaluation of a discrete breast mass is described elsewhere in this chapter.

After appropriate steps have been taken to rule out malignancy, a key aspect of the treatment of mastodynia is reassuring the patient that she does not have breast cancer. Patients should be counseled about fibrocystic breast changes and reassured that the symptoms are neither due to cancer nor indicative of an increased risk for developing cancer. For most patients, occasional use of nonsteroidal anti-inflammatory drugs is the only therapy required. Prescription analgesics, particularly narcotics, should not be used. Symptoms severe enough to prompt consideration of using such drugs mandate a more complete evaluation and use of specific therapy. This should generally be provided by a specialist who is able to follow the patient long-term.

The relationship between methylxanthines (particularly caffeine) and breast pain/nodularity is controversial. Some women unequivocally experience subjective symptomatic improvement and report a decrease in breast nodularity upon reducing or eliminating caffeine intake. Therefore, it is reasonable to advise patients with cyclical mastodynia—particularly those with very nodular breasts—to eliminate intake of caffeine-containing beverages (coffee, tea, colas) and foods (primarily chocolate) as much as possible for a period of several months. At the end of that time, the patient is best able to judge whether there has been sufficient subjective improvement to justify further caffeine abstention. In addition, these patients should be urged to stop smoking, be-

cause nicotine is purported to worsen mastodynia. A variety of medications have been advocated for the treatment of mastodynia (Table 36-2). Given the subjective nature of the complaints and the high likelihood of relief just with reassurance, it is difficult to determine the precise contribution of most of these drugs. Vitamin E or other vitamin supplements have not been shown to be beneficial in randomized trials, although anecdotal cases of benefit abound.

Hormonal agents have been used extensively to treat mastodynia. Given the side effects and need for long-term treatment for severe mastodynia, such therapy should be provided by a specialist in breast diseases.

PALPABLE BREAST MASS

Despite the importance of mammography in the screening and diagnosis of breast cancer, the majority of breast cancers (65 to 80 percent) still present as a palpable mass[17] (Table 36-3). Initial evaluation of a breast lump should always include performance of a thorough history and physical examination.[2,18] Because of the high incidence of cancer in postmenopausal women, evaluation of masses in this group is straightforward. Any discrete mass or thickening in

---

Table 36-2

PHARMACOLOGIC TREATMENT OF MASTODYNIA

Agent	Mode of Action	Comment
Caffeine avoidance	Unknown	Efficacy anecdotal
Vitamin E	Unknown	Efficacy anecdotal
Birth control pills	Regulates menstrual cycle	Trial and error to find proper dose May exacerbate pain
Danazol	Weak androgen	Very effective Virilizing effects and liver toxicity dose-limiting Should be prescribed by a specialist
Tamoxifen	Antiestrogen	Efficacy anecdotal Complications potentially significant Should be prescribed by a specialist
Evening primose oil	Unknown	Available over the counter Efficacy moderate

Table 36-3

EVALUATION OF A PALPABLE BREAST MASS

Age	Study	Result	Action
Less than 30 years	Ultrasound or FNAB	Cyst	Reasses for recurrence in 4–8 weeks
		Solid and well circumscribed or cytology diagnostic of fibroadenoma	Referral to specialist to follow likely fibroadenoma
		Cystic and solid, irregular borders, or does not totally resolve with FNAB aspiration	Referral for surgical biopsy
30 years to meno-pause	Bilateral mammo-grams FNAB[a]	Cyst	Reassess for recurrence in 4–8 weeks
		Solid	Referral for surgical biopsy unless cytology diagnostic of fibroadenoma
Postmenopausal	Bilateral mammo-grams		Definitive tissue diagnosis

[a]Fine needle aspiration biopsy.

a postmenopausal woman that is not well documented in prior exams must be assumed to be cancer until proved otherwise. After bilateral mammograms are obtained, definitive tissue diagnosis is indicated by means of FNAB, CNB, or surgical biopsy. In the setting of an urgent visit, the evaluation may be facilitated by obtaining bilateral mammograms (if not performed in the previous 4 months) and appropriate use of either FNAB or CNB. Referral to a specialist (a general surgeon or surgical oncologist) is indicated.

If a woman under age 30 has a well-circumscribed breast mass, fibrocystic changes or a fibroadenoma should be suspected. Breast ultrasound may confirm the presence of a simple cyst; FNAB may also confirm a simple cyst or demonstrate cells diagnostic of a fibroadenoma. In this age group, simple cysts that do not recur after aspiration do not require special follow-up. Patients with solid masses, even those with cytologically proved fibroadenomas, should be referred to a specialist for further evaluation and follow-up. Even under age 30, some 1 to 4 percent of women undergoing breast biopsy are found to have cancer. Diagnostic vigilance, even in younger women, is crucial.[19]

The presence of cycling glandular tissue in premenopausal women makes evaluation of breast masses in these patients more problematic. Bilateral mammography for these women over age 30 is important. Surgical biopsy is indicated unless imaging techniques and either FNAB or CNB definitively reveal either a simple cyst or a fibroadenoma. A cyst that yields nonbloody fluid and completely disappears with aspiration may be assumed to be benign. The fluid is generally serous, green, or brown and need not be analyzed cytologically unless it appears to contain blood. If, at 6-week follow-up, the cyst has not recurred, no further evaluation is necessary. After mammograms and (if appro-

priate) an FNAB or CNB, referral to a specialist for all non-cystic lesions is indicated.

ABNORMAL MAMMOGRAM

Patients may present after undergoing screening mammography that reveals "an abnormality." Findings on mammography may range from clearly benign (not requiring any further evaluation) to almost diagnostic of cancer. When patients seek urgent-care evaluation for mammographic abnormalities, a thorough history and physical examination should be performed. Next, the original mammograms must be reviewed by a qualified radiologist. Often, additional mammographic views (magnification or cone-down views to better characterize microcalcifications and parenchymal densities) or a breast ultrasound may be obtained. These may result in sufficient characterization of an abnormality such that either no further workup or 4- to 6-month radiologic follow-up is all that is necessary. Furthermore, these additional views will assist a specialist if added radiographic workup suggests a possible malignancy, indicating that a referral is needed.

FIBROCYSTIC CHANGES

The nodularity and/or tenderness experienced by all women during their reproductive years, as a result of cyclic glandular responses to the hormonal variations of the menstrual cycle, are referred to as *fibrocystic breast changes*. Many women present for evaluation if these symptoms become more pronounced or lead to anxiety over the possibility of breast cancer. Even if the history and physical examination in patients presenting with these complaints are normal, bilateral screening mammography should be performed if they are over age 40. If the evaluation does not reveal anything suggestive of a malignancy, reassurance that fibrocystic symptoms are common and not related to breast cancer or risk of development of breast cancer is all that is required. Decrease of caffeine intake and occasional use of a nonsteroidal anti-inflammatory drug may provide some symptomatic relief of breast tenderness. Women with recurring symptoms, especially severe symptoms, who have abnormal examinations or who remain anxious should be referred to a specialist for further evaluation and support.

NIPPLE DISCHARGE

Discharges from the nipple are quite common. When the discharge is neither milky nor bloody, it may be assumed to be physiologic ("fibrocystic") in origin and no further workup is required. Postpartum, milk may continue to be secreted for as long as 2 years after breast-feeding has stopped, particularly with breast stimulation. Such stimulated milky discharges are of little consequences, and patients can safely be reassured. On rare occasions, a bilateral, spontaneous milky nipple discharge can be indicative of hyperprolactinemia resulting from either medications or a pituitary adenoma. Evaluation by a specialist is indicated. Unilateral nipple discharges that contain blood are usually caused by a benign intraductal papilloma. However, because a bloody discharge may occasionally be indicative of an underlying breast cancer, a sample of the discharge should be obtained on a microscope slide for cytologic evaluation. Referral to a specialist is indicated for a bloody nipple discharge.

NIPPLE IRRITATION

Nipple irritation may be caused by repeated vigorous rubbing, by overexposure to the sun (sunburn), or by chronic abrasion, as might be seen in a braless runner wearing a sweat-soaked shirt. The nipples are easily protected from chronic abrasion by application of a small dab of petroleum jelly or use of protective pads inserted into the cups of a support bra. Nipple irritation, however, may also be indicative of Paget's disease, which is heralded by the appearance of a weeping, eczematoid lesion of the nipple. There may be accompanying edema and inflammation. Nipple biopsy reveals malignant cells within the milk ducts. This lesion is almost always associated with an underlying carcinoma. Because these changes may transiently respond to topical treatments, there is often significant delay in diagnosis.[20] For weeping lesions, a smear obtained for cytologic analysis may prove diagnostic. When Paget's disease is suspected, referral to a specialist is indicated. Bilateral mammography may facilitate subsequent workup.

AXILLARY LYMPHADENOPATHY

Benign, palpable axillary lymphadenopathy is a common finding on physical examination. In women with unilateral axillary adenopathy—particularly if the nodes are multiple, hard, and/or greater than 1.5 cm in diameter—the possibility of breast cancer metastatic to axillary nodes must be considered. This is true even if careful physical examination does not reveal a palpable breast abnormality. Bilateral mammograms are indicated. If the level of suspicion is high, FNAB of an axillary lymph node may expedite subsequent evaluation. Regardless, unless the palpable nodes are benign in the opinion of the examiner, referral to a specialist should be made.

PERIDUCTAL MASTITIS (MAMMARY DUCT ECTASIA)

Periductal mastitis, also called *plasma cell mastitis* or *mammary duct ectasia,* is an uncommon benign disorder characterized by dilated (ectatic) mammary ducts with inspissated secretions and marked periductal inflammation. It generally presents as noncyclical mastodynia associated with nipple retraction or discharge. In severe cases, subareolar abscesses form and can burrow through the skin at the areolar border to form mammary duct fistulas. Younger women tend to present with inflammatory and infectious processes, such as recurrent subareolar abscesses, while perimenopausal and postmenopausal women are more likely to present with nipple discharge and retraction or sterile subareolar masses.

For older women who present with the typical thick, white, creamy nipple discharge, reassurance may be the only treatment needed. For other modes of presentation (bloody discharge, nipple retraction, mammary duct fistula, or recurrent abscesses), referral to a specialist for differentiation from a malignant entity and definitive treatment should be suggested.

INFLAMMATORY BREAST CANCER

Of all of the potential presentations of a breast malignancy, *inflammatory breast cancer* is the one most likely to mimic an acute condition.[2] This term is applied to a subset of patients with locally advanced (stage III) breast cancer wherein permeation of dermal lymphatics by tumor leads to edema and erythema of the breast, which can easily be mistaken for infectious mastitis. Specifically, patients present with a clinical syndrome that includes breast warmth, tenderness, edema, and erythema. The combination of swelling and redness results in an orange-peel appearance of the overlying skin *(peau d'orange).* In those cases where there is no underlying mass and palpable axillary lymph nodes are not present, the risk of misclassifying the problem as an infectious process is greatest. The histologic hallmark of inflammatory breast cancer is dermal lymphatic invasion demonstrable on skin biopsy, although the clinical syndrome may be present in the absence of this biopsy finding. The signs of inflammatory breast cancer must not be mistaken for indicators of a benign infectious or inflammatory process; prompt mammography and biopsy of the skin and any palpable or radiographic breast lesions are required. Similarly, any diagnosis of an infectious breast condition must be promptly reconsidered if there is not an initial good response to antibiotics or if there is persistence despite apparently good treatment.

Other forms of locally advanced breast cancer present in the urgent-care setting. Stage III breast cancers are characterized by (1) the presence of a large (>5 cm) primary tumor with clinically involved axillary lymph nodes; (2) inflammatory cancers as already described; and (3) the presence of certain other "grave signs"—namely, breast edema, skin ulceration (as opposed to dimpling), fixation of the tumor to the chest wall (not just the pectoralis muscles), palpable axillary nodes larger than 2.5 cm in diameter or fixed to one another, satellite tumor nodules in the ipsilateral breast, or the presence of arm edema. Treatment of patients with locally advanced breast cancer generally involves initial systemic chemotherapy followed by surgery and/or radiation therapy. Immediate recognition of locally advanced breast cancer and prompt referral to a specialist is mandatory. Bilateral mammography and FNAB or CNB upon initial presentation can facilitate subsequent efficient evaluation by the specialist.

STRONG FAMILY HISTORY

In the course of a routine history and physical examination or during evaluation of an otherwise apparently benign breast abnormality, it may be discovered that a patient has a striking family history of breast cancer. Such histories are characterized by the presence of multiple first-degree relatives, grandmothers, aunts, and/or first cousins with premenopausal breast cancer. Additional indicators of significant familial risk include bilateral breast cancer and presence of ovarian cancer as well. Women with these factors in their family history should be referred to a specialist (surgeon, medical oncologist, or geneticist) well versed in the issues of familial breast cancer for further evaluation, counseling, surveillance, and risk management.[21,22]

BREAST DISEASES OF EXTRAMAMMARY ORIGIN

A variety of problems may arise in the nonglandular portions of the breast. Diseases of the skin overlying the breast should be treated as dermatologic problems, not breast disorders. A variety of neoplasms of mesenchymal origin may arise in the breast. Fibromatosis (desmoid tumors), fat necro-

sis, foreign-body reactions, sarcoidosis, lymphoma, and various infections (including those of mycobacterial origin) have also been described. Mondor's disease was mentioned previously. Because the breast is responsive to hormonal influences, endocrine abnormalities may produce mammary sequelae. Most common is galactorrhea resulting from abnormal elaboration of prolactin secondary to a pituitary adenoma, a thyroid disorder, or medications. Measurement of a serum prolactin level is appropriate in women with onset of new, bilateral galactorrhea who have not lactated within the prior year.

REFERRAL TO SPECIALISTS

Because breast problems are so common and because of the clinical and demographic overlaps in the spectra of benign and malignant breast disease, evaluation of breast disorders can be challenging. Attention to a few principles of referral (Table 36-4) can help to assure efficient, high-quality patient care and to avoid a failure to diagnose a breast cancer.

A referral should be considered when diagnostic uncertainty remains after completion of the history, physical examination, and simple laboratory and radiographic studies; cancer cannot be ruled out with a high degree of certainty; a problem is chronic or recurring; follow-up beyond a single, simple additional visit is likely to be required; subsequent multidisciplinary care involving more than one medical specialty is likely to be required; the patient is overly anxious or suspicious, or is behaving inappropriately; and when you as the examining clinician are uncertain or unsettled.

Specialists in breast disease must often accept diagnostic

Table 36-4

REFERRAL TO SPECIALISTS

- Refer when there is diagnostic uncertainty after initial studies are obtained, when cancer cannot be definitively ruled out, when a problem is chronic or recurring, when follow-up is likely to be extended, when multidisciplinary care will likely be needed, and when you or the patient are uncertain or uncomfortable.
- Obtain basic studies.
- Defer complex or expensive studies to the specialist.
- Speak directly with the specialist about the referral.
- Assist the patient to gather all pertinent written records, original mammograms and reports, and pathology slides and reports.

uncertainty ("I'm 99 percent but not 100 percent sure that . . ."). They must explain that uncertainty in a manner that adequately informs the patient but does not inappropriately frighten her. This often requires a degree of knowledge and confidence that is only gained from experience. Furthermore, it requires adequate time to spend with the patient (and possibly her family). It is unreasonable to expect that these conditions can routinely be met in an acute/urgent-care setting.

Referrals are most effective when the appropriate basic studies have been completed (history, physical exam, mammograms, ultrasound, possible FNAB or CNB) but before any further diagnostic or therapeutic studies are planned. Assisting patients to gather the necessary materials (progress notes, breast imaging reports and original films, cytology/pathology reports and slides) promotes goodwill, facilitates the task of the specialist, and makes it more likely that the patient will receive a complete evaluation in one visit with the specialist.

Most helpful is direct contact between the referring clinician and the specialist, in person or by telephone. This allows communication of the nuances of the referral, begins the process of formally passing responsibility for the patient on to the specialist, and facilitates subsequent communication between the specialist and the referring clinician.

RECORD KEEPING

Meticulous record keeping is important to facilitate continuity of care, assure appropriate follow-up, and minimize risk of medicolegal liability. All patient encounters must be documented. Mention should be made not only of pertinent findings in the history and physical examination but also of pertinent negatives. In addition to the chief complaint and history of present illness, breast cancer risk factors (age, menopausal status, reproductive history, family history, and history of prior breast problems) should be documented. The physical examination record should include evidence of a general physical exam as well as the important elements of a breast exam (axillary, supraclavicular, and cervical nodes; appearance of breasts upright and supine; appearance of nipple-areolar complexes; findings on palpation; and results of gentle squeezing of the nipples). Physical examination findings are best described in terms of location (position on clock face and distance from nipple, often best captured in a diagram), size, consistency (hard/soft, tender, fixed/mobile), and symmetry with the opposite breast.

Laboratory test and imaging results should be summarized in the encounter note. Verbal reports should be identified as such. Discussions with radiologists and other consultants and referrals to specialists should be documented.

Finally, discussions with the patient should be noted. Particular concerns and anxieties voiced by the patient should be recorded. Instructions to patients and follow-up appointments made or recommended should be documented. Attention to these issues protects both the patient and the clinician.

MEDICOLEGAL LIABILITY AND RISK MANAGEMENT

As summarized by Kern, delay in the diagnosis of breast cancer was the leading cause of claims and lawsuits against physicians for misdiagnosed conditions between 1985 and 1990.[23] Delayed diagnosis of breast cancer resulted in 542 claims during this period, resulting in a total payout of over $100 million. Obstetrician/gynecologists and primary care practitioners were among the most common defendants in these cases.

The typical profile of a patient who sustains a delayed diagnosis of breast cancer includes age less than 40; presentation with a self-discovered, painless mass; physical examination noting a mass felt to be benign because of the patient's age; negative mammogram (present in approximately 15 percent of all cases of breast cancer); working diagnosis of fibrocystic changes; referral to a specialist not recommended; and no attempt made to obtain tissue.[23]

For the primary care clinician, these facts emphasize that adherence to a few simple principles can avoid missed diagnoses of breast cancer. For any woman presenting with a breast problem, a diagnosis of cancer must be considered regardless of patient age. The physical exam and breast imaging studies are complementary; a normal mammogram in the presence of a palpable breast mass does not rule out the possibility of cancer. Tissue diagnosis is the only definitive means of ruling in or out the possibility of breast cancer. Finally, when either the clinician or the patient is in doubt, referral to a specialist is always the safest course of action.

References

1. Tanner JM: *Growth at Adolescence*. Oxford, England: Blackwell, 1962, p 35.
2. August DA, Sondak VK: Breast disease, in Greenfield LJ (ed): *Surgery: Scientific Principles and Practice*. Philadelphia: Lippincott, 1996, pp 1357–1415.
3. Henderson IC: Breast cancer, in Murphy GP, Lawrence W, Lenhard RE (eds): *American Cancer Society Textbook of Clinical Oncology*. Atlanta: American Cancer Society, 1995, pp 198–219.
4. Kerlikowske K, Grady D, Rubin SM, et al: Efficacy of screening mammography: A meta-analysis. *JAMA* 273:149, 1995.
5. Dodd GD: American Cancer Society guidelines on

screening for breast cancer. An overview. *CA* 42:177, 1992.

6. Kaluzny AD, Rimer B, Harris R: Commentary: The National Cancer Institute and guideline development. Lessons from the breast cancer screening controversy. *J Natl Cancer Inst* 86:901, 1994.

7. D'Orsi CJ, Adler DD, Ikeda DM, et al: Breast imaging. *Radiology* 190:936, 1994.

8. Layfield LJ, Glasgow BJ, Cramer H: Fine-needle aspiration in the management of breast masses. *Pathol Annu* 24(part 2):23, 1989.

9. Cady B: How to perform breast biopsies. *Surg Oncol Clin North Am* 4:47, 1995.

10. Foster RS Jr: Techniques for diagnosis of palpable breast masses, in Harris JR, Lippman ME, Morrow M, Hellman S (eds): *Breast Diseases.* Philadelphia: Lippincott-Raven, 1996, pp 133–138.

11. Campbell ID, Royle GT, Coddington R, et al: Technique and results of localization biopsy in a breast screening programme. *Br J Surg* 78:1113, 1991.

12. Eastwood D: Subcutaneous rupture of the breast: A seat belt injury. *Br J Surg* 59:491, 1972.

13. Dawes R, Smallwood J, Taylor I: Seat belt injury to the female breast. *Br J Surg* 73:106, 1986.

14. Bellon A, Cowley R, Hoopes J: Blunt chest trauma: Evaluation of the augmented breast. *J Trauma* 20:982, 1980.

15. Magnant CM: Fat necrosis, hematoma, and trauma, in Harris JR, Lippman ME, Morrow M, Hellman S (eds): *Breast Diseases.* Philadelphia: Lippincott-Raven, 1996, pp 61–65.

16. Tanabe KK: Duct ectasia, periductal mastitis, and infections, in Harris JR, Lippman ME, Morrow M, Hellman S (eds): *Breast Diseases.* Philadelphia: Lippincott-Raven, 1996, pp 49–54.

17. Rosato FE, Rosenberg AL: Examination techniques: Role of the physician and patient in evaluating breast diseases, in Bland KI, Copeland EM (eds): *The Breast: Comprehensive Management of Benign and Malignant Diseases.* Philadelphia: Saunders, 1991, pp 409–418.

18. Donegan WL: Evaluation of a palpable breast mass. *N Engl J Med* 327:937, 1992.

19. Ferguson CM, Powell RW: Breast masses in young women. *Arch Surg* 124:1338, 1989.

20. Duda RB: Paget disease, in Harris JR, Lippman ME, Morrow M, Hellman S (eds): *Breast Diseases.* Philadelphia: Lippincott-Raven, 1996, pp 870–876.

21. Biesecker BB, Boehnke M, Calzone K, et al: Genetic counseling for families with inherited susceptibility to breast and ovarian cancer. *JAMA* 269:1970, 1993.

22. King M-C, Rowell S, Love SM: Inherited breast and ovarian cancer: What are the risks? What are the choices? *JAMA* 269:1975, 1993.

23. Kern KA: Preventing the delayed diagnosis of breast cancer through medical litigation analysis. *Surg Oncol Clin North Am* 3:101, 1994.

Chapter 37

AMENORRHEA: A PRACTICAL APPROACH TO MANAGEMENT

Gregory M. Christman

Cheryl J. Paradis

Amenorrhea is defined as the absence of cyclic menstrual flow. This definition can further be divided with the clinical definitions of primary and secondary amenorrhea. *Primary amenorrhea* is the failure to achieve menses by age 14 in the absence of secondary sexual characteristics or the lack of menses by age 16 in the presence of secondary sexual characteristics. *Secondary amenorrhea* is characterized as the absence of menses for a duration equivalent to three cycle intervals or 6 months in a woman who had previously been menstruating.

Menstruation is a process that generally occurs at regular intervals as a result of the integration of hormonal signals between the hypothalamus, pituitary, and ovaries. The ovaries must be capable of responding to signals from the pituitary and the hypothalamus must be capable of responding to the feedback signals received from the ovary. It is essential to have a functioning outflow tract, including a patent vagina, endocervix, and uterus, as well as an endometrium capable of responding to steroid hormones from the ovary. If there is an abnormality at any step in this cascade that hinders the ability to produce or respond to the needed hormone signals, the result is amenorrhea.

Briefly, the menstrual cycle can be divided into three phases—the follicular phase, the ovulatory phase, and the luteal phase (see Fig. 38-1). The function of the follicular phase is to select and mature an oocyte for ovulation. This selection is initiated by follicle-stimulating hormone (FSH), which is secreted by the anterior pituitary. Decreasing estradiol and progesterone resulting from the demise of the corpus luteum at the time of menses removes the negative inhibition of estradiol and progesterone on the pulse generator of the gonadotrophin-releasing hormone (GnRH) in the hypothalamus. This mechanism allows the hypothalamus to secrete more pulses of GnRH, which, in turn, stimulates the anterior pituitary to release luteinizing hormone (LH) and FSH. The low levels of estradiol in the early follicular phase allow the preferential release of FSH over LH from the pituitary in response to each pulse of GnRH, and FSH acts on the granulosa cells in the follicles to stimulate the production of estradiol. Initially multiple follicles are stimulated by FSH and the level of estradiol rises. A dominant follicle is then selected, the exact mechanism of which is still unknown. Local changes in the dominant follicle under the stimulation of both FSH and estradiol induce the formation of luteinizing hormone receptors on the dominant follicle. Increasing levels of estradiol then exhibit a positive feedback on the hypothalamus to further enhance the secretion of GnRH. Rapidly increasing estradiol levels exert a positive feedback on the anterior pituitary to preferentially secrete LH in response to GnRH. Luteinizing hormone acts on the granulosa cells in the dominant follicle to start the production of progesterone, mature the oocyte to prepare for fertilization, and induce enzymes along with the rapid accumulation of follicular fluid to induce follicular rupture. The luteal phase of the menstrual cycle is characterized by the formation of a corpus luteum and the production of progesterone. Increasing progesterone levels then act as a negative feedback mechanism on the hypothalamus and the anterior pituitary to decrease the pulsatile production of GnRH and decrease the secreted levels of FSH. In the absence of pregnancy, the levels of estradiol and progesterone diminish when the functional life span of the corpus luteum is completed. When a critical threshold is reached, low estradiol and progesterone levels allow the anterior pituitary to release stores of FSH produced in the prior luteal phase as the increasing GnRH pulse frequency allows the cycle to commence once again.

The growth and secretion of the endometrium is regulated by the steroid hormones produced by the ovaries during the described cycle. During the follicular phase of the menstrual cycle, the endometrium is in the proliferative phase. Estradiol produced by the follicle in the proliferative phase stimulates the growth of the glands and the stroma of the endomestrium. During the luteal phase of the menstrual cycle, the endometrium is in the secretory phase. The secretion of progesterone, the dominant hormone during this phase of the cycle, acts to halt the growth of the glands and stroma of the endometrium, and under progesterone's influence the glands become tortuous and filled with secretions. If fertilization and implantation do not occur, the blood vessels of the endometrium, in response to the demise of the corpus luteum, undergo vasospasm, which subsequently causes necrosis and shedding of the uterine lining.

As a physician or caregiver evaluating patients in the emergency department or acute care clinic, you will undoubtedly encounter patients with complaints of amenorrhea, both primary and secondary. As the initial evaluating physician or caregiver, you will need to be aware of the differential diagnosis of primary or secondary amenorrhea and the various laboratory tests and studies used to help establish a diagnosis. Although the varied possibilities in the differential diagnosis of amenorrhea appears overwhelming and foreboding (Table 37-1), this chapter presents a practical and cost-effective approach to the initial diagnosis and treatment of patients presenting with amenorrhea. Patients with amenorrhea may eventually need a referral to a surgeon, psychiatrist, gynecologist, or medical or reproductive endocrinologist; however, an accurate and timely initial evaluation and workup will expedite appropriate initial care by the astute provider of emergency health care.

PRIMARY AMENORRHEA

In the patient presenting with primary amenorrhea, it is essential to obtain a thorough history and physical examination. Broad considerations include pregnancy, outflow tract disorders, gonadal failure, genetic and congenital disorders of sexual differentiation, central nervous system (CNS) disease, stress, systemic medical disease, or constitutional delay.

The history obtained should focus on developmental history, growth and sexual differentiation, diet, exercise, psychological stresses, family history—especially as it relates to genetic disorders and maturation, evidence of increased androgen production, galactorrhea, or evidence of other endocrine abnormalities.

The physical examination in these patients is crucial, since the key to determining the diagnosis generally lies in documenting the presence or absence of secondary sexual characteristics, the patient's estrogen status, and the presence or absence of a functioning reproductive tract. As shown in Table 37-2, patients presenting with primary amenorrhea can be divided into four groups based on the presence or absence of appropriate secondary sexual characteristics and the presence of a uterus. This classification system can often serve as the basis for determining which initial tests would be valuable in the emergency department setting to determine the diagnosis and the appropriate resources for referral in patients with primary amenorrhea.

As you will recall, a series of interactions between the hypothalamus, pituitary gland, ovaries, and adrenal glands initiate puberty. The textbook definition of delayed puberty is the absence of pubertal onset at an age of development that is 2.5 standard deviations from the mean. This includes the absence of thelarche or breast development by age 13 and menarche by age 16.[1] The pubertal transition from childhood to adulthood usually takes 3 to 5 years. It is initiated by reactivation of the hypothalamic-pituitary-ovarian (HPO) axis by an unclear mechanism and is marked by increased gonadal steroid and adrenal androgen production. The first sign of puberty is generally breast development, starting at 8 to 10 years of age, soon followed by adrenarche (the development of pubic and axillary hair), although adrenarche may be the first sign of puberty in approximately 20 percent of girls. Menarche or the onset of the first menstrual period occurs late in puberty (average age 12.8 years in the United States) and is usually the result of estrogen withdrawal without ovulation in initial bleeding episodes. The pubertal transition of pubic and axillary hair changes of adrenarche and breast development during thelarche can best be documented on examination using the classification system of Tanner (Table 37-3).

Normal physiologic causes of primary amenorrhea include pregnancy and constitutional delay. A serum or urine pregnancy test should be obtained in any sexually active pa-

Table 37-1

DIFFERENTIAL DIAGNOSIS OF AMENORRHEA

I. Anatomic defects (outflow tract)
  A. Labial agglutination/fusion
  B. Imperforate hymen
  C. Transverse vaginal septum
  D. Cervical agenesis—isolated
  E. Cervical stenosis—iatrogenic
  F. Vaginal agenesis—isolated
  G. Müllerian agenesis (Mayer-Rokitansky-Kuster-Hauser syndrome)
  H. Complete androgen resistance (testicular feminization)
  I. Endometrial hypoplasia or aplasia—congenital
  J. Asherman's syndrome (uterine synechiae)
II. Ovarian failure (hypergonadotropic hypogonadism)
  A. Gonadal agenesis
  B. Gonadal dysgenesis
    1. Abnormal karyotype
      a. Turner syndrome 45,X
      b. Mosaicism
    2. Normal karyotype
      a. Pure gonadal dysgenesis
        i. 46,XX
        ii. 46,XY (Swyer syndrome)
  C. Ovarian enzymatic deficiency
    1. 17(-Hydroxylase deficiency)
    2. 17, 20a-Lyase deficiency
  D. Premature ovarian failure
    1. Idiopathic—premature aging
    2. Injury
      a. Mumps oophoritis
      b. Radiation
      c. Chemotherapy
    3. Resistant ovary (Savage syndrome)
    4. Autoimmune disease
    5. Galactosemia
III. Chronic anovulation with estrogen present
  A. PCOS
  B. Adrenal disease
    1. Cushing's syndrome
    2. Adult-onset adrenal hyperplasia
  C. Ovarian tumors
    1. Granulosa–theca cell tumors
    2. Brenner tumors
    3. Cystic teratomas
    4. Mucinous/serous cystadenomas
    5. Krukenberg tumor

IV. Chronic anovulation with estrogen absent (hypogonadotropic hypogonadism)
  A. Hypothalamic
    1. Tumors
      a. Craniopharyngioma
      b. Germinoma
      c. Hamartoma
      d. Hand-Schüller-Christian disease
      e. Teratoma
      f. Endodermal sinus tumors
      g. Metastatic carcinoma
    2. Infection and other disorders
      a. Tuberculosis
      b. Syphilis
      c. Encephalitis/meningitis
      d. Sarcoidosis
      e. Kallmann's syndrome
      f. Idiopathic hypogonadotropic hypogonadism
      g. Chronic debilitating disease
    3. Functional
      a. Stress
      b. Weight loss/diet
      c. Malnutrition
      d. Psychological eating disorders (anorexia nervosa, bulimia)
      e. Severe exercise
  B. Pituitary
    1. Tumors
      a. Prolactinomas
      b. Other hormone-secreting pituitary tumors (ACTH, thyrotropin-stimulating hormone, growth hormone)
      c. Nonfunctional tumors (craniopharyngioma)
      d. Metastatic carcinoma
    2. Space-occupying lesions
      a. Empty sella
      b. Arterial aneurysm
    3. Necrosis
      a. Sheehan syndrome
      b. Panhypopituitarism
    4. Inflammatory/infiltrative
      a. Sarcoidosis
      b. Hemochromatosis

Table 37-2

EVALUATION OF PRIMARY AMENORRHEA

Group 1: Normal secondary sexual characteristics, absent uterus

Initial screening test: testosterone

Low testosterone levels; mullerian agenesis (Mayer-Rokitansky-Kuster-Hauser syndrome)

Male levels of testosterone: testicular feminization (androgen-insensitivity syndrome)

Confirmatory test: XY karyotype

Group 2: Absent secondary sexual characteristics, absent uterus

Screening test: karyotype

Testicular regression or gonadal enzyme deficiency

Group 3: Absent secondary sexual characteristics, uterus present

Screening test: follicle-stimulating hormone (FSH)

Low levels of FSH: (hypogonadotropic hypogonadism) Kallman syndrome, CNS lesions, anorexia nervosa, chronic disease

High levels of FSH: (gonadal dysgenesis) Turner syndrome, XX or XY gonadal dysgenesis, gonadal enzyme deficiency

Confirmatory test: karyotype

Group 4: Normal secondary sexual characteristics, uterus present

Evaluate as secondary amenorrhea (see Table 37-5)

Table 37-3

EVALUATION OF SECONDARY SEXUAL CHARACTERISTICS
(See Fig. 30-5, Chap. 30)

- Tanner stage 1: Preadolescent elevation of papillae, normal vellous hair resembles adult in type but covers smaller areas
- Tanner stage 2: Elevation of breast and papillae as small mounds with enlargement of areolar diameter. Sparse growth of long, slightly pigmented downing hair along labia.
- Tanner stage 3: Enlargement and elevation of breast and areola without separation of contours. Darker, coarser, and curlier hair growing sparsely over public area.
- Tanner stage 4: Areola and papillae project from breast to form a secondary mound. Pubic hair appears.
- Tanner stage 5: Mature projection of papillae only with recession of areola into general contour of breast. Adult pubic axillary hair distribution.

Source: Adapted from Tanner,[1] with permission.

---

tient complaining of amenorrhea, including primary amenorrhea, since it is physiologically possible in some cases to ovulate prior to the first menstrual period. Constitutional delay as a diagnosis for primary amenorrhea is one of exclusion, and a diagnosis and cause (if possible) of primary amenorrhea should be established in all patients without evidence of secondary sexual changes by age 13 or lack of menses by age 16 even in the presence of normal secondary sexual development.

DIAGNOSTIC APPROACH TO PATIENTS WITH PRIMARY AMENORRHEA

The four groups into which patients presenting with primary amenorrhea are divided include (1) normal secondary sexual characteristics, absent uterus; (2) absent secondary sexual characteristics, absent uterus; (3) absent secondary sexual characteristics, uterus present; and (4) normal secondary sexual characteristics, uterus present (Table 37-2). In patients characterized as belonging to group 1, the absence

of the uterus and the presence of secondary sexual characteristics generally limits the possibilities to either müllerian agenesis or testicular feminization. The easiest way of discriminating between these two possibilities is to document a high level of testosterone (in the adult male reference range) in patients with testicular feminization (also called *androgen insensitivity*). Although not absolutely required, a peripheral blood karyotype after the testosterone results are available would provide further documentation of the diagnosis, with an XY karyotype in androgen insensitivity and XO in müllerian agenesis. Group 2 patients are rare and generally represent a diagnosis of either testicular regression, which can be confirmed on a peripheral blood karyotype, or perhaps a rare gonadal enzyme deficiency best evaluated by a medical or reproductive endocrinologist. Group 3 patients lack secondary sexual characteristics and have a palpable uterus on exam. The most cost-effective initial test in this group is an FSH level. An FSH level ≥40 mIU/mL in any patient over 12 years of age generally indicates primary ovarian failure as a result of gonadal dysgenesis. This is the case because, although the hypothalamus and pituitary in patients with gonadal dysgenesis undergo activation in puberty at the same time as in normal adolescents, the lack of negative feedback from an abnormal streak gonad causes a rapid rise in FSH to menopausal levels. In patients with a low FSH (≤5 mIU/mL), causes of hypogonadotropic hypogonadism must be considered, such as Kallman syndrome, stress or anorexia nervosa, a CNS lesion, or the effects of chronic illness. Group 4 patients are indistinguishable on examination from patients presenting with secondary amenorrhea with the presence of both a palpable uterus and secondary sexual characteristics. Fortunately, the diagnostic approach to this group is identical to the approach that is discussed under "Secondary Amenorrhea," below (see Table 37-5).

CONGENITAL MÜLLERIAN ANOMALIES

Patients with müllerian abnormalities characterized by outflow obstruction or agenesis will have normal secondary sexual characteristics, however, they fail to undergo menarche. Upon laboratory evaluation, these patients will exhibit eugonadotropic eugondasim (i.e., normal pituitary and ovarian function). Outflow tract defects as a cause of primary amenorrhea include imperforate hymen, transvaginal septum, vaginal agenesis and the syndrome of müllerian agenesis (Mayer-Rokitansky-Kuster-Hauser Syndrome). Patients with outflow obstruction may present with cyclic abdominal or pelvic pain and/or a bulge in the vagina or a pelvic mass (Fig. 37-1). These patients should be reassured and referred to a gynecologist for surgical correction. The treatment of distal outflow obstruction is simple surgical excision of the imperforate hymen or transverse septum.

Müllerian agenesis (Mayer-Rokitansky-Kuster-Hauser syndrome) should be suspected in any patient who presents with normal secondary sexual characteristics and an undetected uterus on physical exam. The incidence of müllerian agenesis is 1 in 4000 to 10,000 female births. The findings on physical examination should be confirmed by ultrasound or MRI on a nonemergent basis to determine those cases with the presence of a uterus and vaginal agenesis who would be candidates for surgical reconstruction. There is a strong association of urinary (25 to 50 percent) and skeletal (10 to 15 percent) anomalies coinciding with müllerian agenesis, and these patients will need evaluation with an intravenous pyelogram (IVP). In these patients, a neovagina may ultimately be fashioned with graduated dilators[2] or surgically with the McIndo procedure.[3] Both of these procedures are done just prior to the desired onset of sexual activity, usually under the supervision of a reproductive endocrinologist.

ANDROGEN INSENSITIVITY SYNDROME

Androgen insensitivity syndrome is included in the category of anatomic anomalies, although it could also be included with gonadal dysfunction. These patients will often present with the complaint of primary amenorrhea. They will also complain of absent secondary sexual characteristics except for the presence of apparently normal breast development. Physical examination is significant for the absence of pubic hair, a blind vaginal pouch, absence of the uterus, and possible inguinal hernias that are actually undescended testicles. Laboratory tests indicate a high level of testosterone in the adult male reference range and an elevated LH. A 46XY

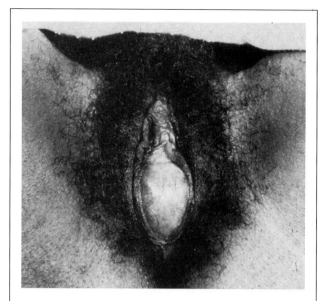

Figure 37-1

Imperforate hymen with associated hematocolpos. (From Baramkita *J Reprod Med* 29:376, 1984, with permission.)

karyotype is additional evidence supporting the diagnosis. The pathophysiology of this disorder involves end-organ insensitivity to androgens and includes either absence of the receptor, receptor defects, or postreceptor abnormalities. These patients should eventually be referred to a gynecologist. Bilateral gonadectomy is recommended after puberty and breast development because of an increased risk of malignant transformation of the gonad.[4] These patients will also need the institution of estrogen replacement following the gonadectomy.

GONADAL DYSGENESIS AND PRIMARY GONADAL FAILURE

Patients who have a gonadal abnormality as the etiology for their amenorrhea will present with elevated levels of FSH and the absence of secondary sexual characteristics. These patients have hypergonadotropic hypogonadism. Gonadal abnormalities may be congenital or acquired. Ovarian failure due to congenital abnormalities include gonadal agenesis/dysgenesis and genetic disorders in steroid production. Acquired etiologies of gonadal failure include radiation, chemotherapy, infections such as mumps oophoritis, or autoimmune processes. Although these acquired etiologies may cause primary amenorrhea, they are usually associated with secondary amenorrhea and therefore will be discussed further under "Secondary Amenorrhea," below.

Turner syndrome is the most common form of gonadal dysgenesis. These patients are usually diagnosed prior to puberty rather than presenting primarily with a complaint of amenorrhea secondary to the classic stigmata of Turner syndrome found upon clinical examination. However, if a patient presents with the complaint of primary amenorrhea and examination reveals short stature, webbing of the neck, shieldlike chest with widely spaced nipples, and absent secondary sexual characteristics, a karyotype should be obtained. The usually karyotype is 45X transmitted with a sporadic nonfamilial inheritance. Other karyotypes include mosaics of 45X/46XX, 45X/46XY, or 45X/47XXX. The necessity of obtaining a peripheral karyotype cannot be stressed enough. If there is a Y chromosome, the chances of gonadal germ-cell malignancy are great. Treatment of women with Turner syndrome under the care of a gynecologist should consist of continued evaluation for cardiac and renal anomalies, screening for hypertension, and the replacement of estrogen. In adolescence, estrogen replacement must be weighed against the possibility that the epiphyseal plates will close early, thus jeopardizing the patient's growth. For this reason consultation with a pediatric endocrinologist is advised for the appropriate use of estrogen replacement, oxandrolone, and growth hormone in teenagers with Turner syndrome so as to maximize height.[5]

HYPOGONADOTROPIC HYPOGONADISM

The largest group of patients with amenorrhea comprises those with chronic anovulation. These patients may have defects in the hypothalamus, pituitary gland, thyroid, or adrenal gland or disorders relating to glucocorticoid feedback mechanisms (Table 37-4). These patients will present to the emergency department with the complaint of amenorrhea and clinical symptoms associated with the etiology of their anovulation. On physical examination, they are noted to have absent secondary sexual characteristics. Laboratory tests demonstrate low levels of FSH; therefore these patients are considered to have hypogonadotropic hypogonadism.

Hypothalamic defects include several etiologies, such as tumors and infection, and functional derangements due to such things as stress, severe weight loss and malnutrition, excessive exercise, and eating disorders. Tumors and infections can cause secondary amenorrhea and are discussed under "Secondary Amenorrhea," below.

Functional disorders of the hypothalamus are common causes of primary amenorrhea. For example, anorexia nervosa, consisting of an obsession with diet and exercise and a distorted body image, is a very serious medical problem in adolescents and is often associated with amenorrhea. Other symptoms in anorexia include depression, fatigue, and constipation. Physical examination reveals an emaciated patient who is often hypotensive. Lanugo hair and dry skin may also be noted. The exact mechanism of amenorrhea in anorexia nervosa is not known with certainty; however, most investigators feel that these patients have diminished pulsatile secretion of GnRH as mediated by increased central opioid tone. Psychiatric referral and counseling may be lifesaving in these patients, and all those suspected of having this disorder should be referred to a caregiver experienced in dealing with it.

Table 37-4

REFERENCE GUIDE—ASSESSMENT AND TREATMENT OF HYPOGONADOTROPIC HYPOGONADISM

Etiology
 Hypothalamic causes
  Stress
  Severe exercise
  Weight loss (anorexia/bulimia)
  Hyperprolactinemia (see above)
  CNS lesion
  Radiation, infection, or trauma

 Pituitary causes
  Sheehan's syndrome
  Pituitary apoplexy (embolus or infarct)
  Other causes (vasculitis, sickle cell anemia, lymphoma)

Evaluation
 Physical examination
 History (ask about eating disorders)
 CNS imaging (if no supporting history is elicited)
 Evidence of a low estradiol and a normal or low FSH

Treatment
 Treat systemic or psychiatric disorders
 Hormonal replacement therapy
 Ovulation induction: clomiphene citrate, GnRH pumps,
  gonadotropins

Both exercise and stress are felt to play a role in amenorrhea and hypothalamic suppression. Competitive athletes and individuals who participate in strenuous exercise or highly demanding activities may present with the complaint of primary amenorrhea. As in the case of anorexia nervosa, the supposed pathophysiologic mechanism appears to be the central inhibition of GnRH release by endogenous opioids. These patients should be referred to a gynecologist who can treat their exercise-induced hypoestrogenemic state with exogenous estrogen to avoid the possibility of exercise-induced stress fractures and bone loss.

Patients with Kallmann syndrome also have primary amenorrhea and absent secondary sexual characteristics. These patients often present with an impaired sense of smell. They will have a low FSH and a normal karyotype. This syndrome is associated with absent or hypoplastic olfactory sulci on MRI scan and isolated GnRH deficiency as a result of abnormal migration of GnRH neurons to the hypothalamus.[6] Kallmann syndrome is inherited as an autosomal dominant trait and is frequently associated with color blindness and the anosmia already mentioned as well as, occasionally, midline facial defects such as cleft lip or palate. These patients should be referred to a gynecologist for cyclic estrogen and progesterone therapy or to a reproductive endocrinologist for pulsatile GnRH replacement or gonadotropin therapy if future fertility is desired.

Lesions of the pituitary gland and stalk may also cause amenorrhea secondary to tumors, space-occupying lesions, necrosis, or inflammatory/infiltrative processes, and are discussed under Secondary Amenorrhea.

SECONDARY AMENORRHEA

Secondary amenorrhea is much more common than primary amenorrhea. As in the case of patients presenting to the emergency department with a complaint of primary amenorrhea, the importance of a thorough history and physical examination cannot be overstated. The history should include a detailed account of the patient's gynecologic background including but not limited to the age of menarche, the prior pattern of menses (regular or irregular), previous occurrences of amenorrhea, the presence of hirsutism, and recent sexual activity. The patient should be questioned regarding the presence or absence of perimenopausal vasomotor symptoms, the age of menopause of family members, whether the loss of periods was abrupt or was preceded by a period of menstrual irregularity, weight loss or gain, stress, strenuous exercise, or neurologic symptoms. It is also important to record the presence of any medical illnesses or any recent change in the patient's health.

The physical examination should focus on the presence of neurologic deficits, abnormalities found upon pelvic examination, galactorrhea, and signs of hypoestrogenemia or hyperandrogenemia. As previously stated, for any patient presenting to the emergency room with the complaint of amenorrhea, the possibility of pregnancy must be ruled out. This is easily accomplished with a rapid urine or serum pregnancy test. The presence of amenorrhea and abdominal pain is a common presentation for ectopic pregnancy; however, most ectopic pregnancies become symptomatic within several weeks of the missed period and therefore do not meet the classic definition of secondary amenorrhea, as these patients would have a delay in menses greater than three times the duration of prior cycles. The possibility of a ruptured ectopic pregnancy with a negative serum pregnancy test has been reported but is extremely rare, and a negative pregnancy test should be considered as reasonable proof that an ectopic pregnancy does not exist.

DIAGNOSTIC APPROACH TO PATIENTS WITH SECONDARY AMENORRHEA

Like primary amenorrhea, secondary amenorrhea can be divided into four categories: (1) physiologic and endocrine abnormalities, (2) anatomic abnormalities, (3) gonadal abnormalities, and (4) chronic anovulation. In addition to having laboratory screening tests performed, a woman presenting with secondary amenorrhea will often be given a progestin challenge test. In the normal menstrual cycle, progesterone is the predominate hormone produced in the luteal phase. It halts the growth of the endometrium (through the interference of estrogen), causes increased secretion by the glands of the endometrium, and initiates menstrual bleeding upon its withdrawal. The function of the progestin challenge is twofold. First, it provides information about the patient's estrogen status and, second, it indicates whether the outflow tract is patent. This helps to further categorize the etiology of the secondary amenorrhea. A positive withdrawal bleed suggests anovulation as the etiology of the amenorrhea. It also confirms a functional outflow tract and a reactive estrogen-primed endometrium. A negative withdrawal bleed indicates a problem in the outflow tract or the fact that insufficient estradiol is reaching the endometrium. Estrogen and progesterone are often given to patients with negative progestin challenge tests to assure appropriate hormonal preparation of the endometrium. A positive withdrawal bleed then establishes the diagnosis that the amenorrhea is the result of deficient estrogen stimulation of the endometrium. A negative withdrawal bleed indicates an outflow tract obstruction.

In Table 37-5, the approach to the patient with secondary amenorrhea is reviewed. The initial tests include a rapid serum pregnancy test followed by a careful history and physical examination. If historical factors indicate that the patient would be at risk for Asherman's syndrome or iatrogenic cervical stenosis, she should be referred to a gynecologist for workup and treatment. The next appropriate screens would include an androgen profile (testosterone, DHEA-S, and 17-OH progesterone) if there is a prior history of irregular cycles or examination evidence of hirsutism. If not, the patient should be screened with an FSH and referred to a gynecologist or endocrinologist for further review. The FSH will be valuable to the consultant or to any individual completing the evaluation since a high FSH (>20 mIU/mL) will indicate the possibility of ovarian failure, whereas a low or normal FSH test (<10 mIU/mL) will be consistent with thyroid deficiency, hyperprolactinemia, or other etiologies of chronic anovulation. The follow-up tests for a normal FSH level include a PRL to exclude the possibility of a prolactinoma or hyperprolactinemia; a TSH test should also be obtained to rule out hypothyroidism. If both the TSH and PRL are elevated and the PRL is <150 ng/mL, hypothyroidism should be treated first for a period of 3 months before the PRL is rechecked unless there are visual or neurologic symptoms suggesting the rare situation of coexistent hyperprolactinemia and hypothyroidism. If no abnormalities are noted on the TSH and PRL tests, a progestin withdrawal should be performed using medroxyprogesterone 10 mg PO q.d. for 10 to 14 days. If the progestin challenge reveals a withdrawal bleeding response—even if the bleeding is scant or light—the patient should be screened with an androgen

Table 37-5

EVALUATION OF SECONDARY AMENORRHEA

1. Exclude pregnancy
2. Careful history and physical exam
   a. History consistent with iatrogenic cervical stenosis or Asherman's syndrome; obtain an hysterosalpingogram and/or transvaginal ultrasound.
   b. If there is hirsutism, enlarged ovaries, and/or prior irregular cycles: obtain serum for T, DHEA-S, 17-OH P.
   c. If there are signs or symptoms of estrogen deficiency, obtain serum FSH.
3. FSH screening test
   a. If elevated FSH (>40 mIU/mL) (hypergonadotropic hypogonadism): possibilities include gonadal dysgenesis and premature ovarian failure. Refer for further workup.
   b. If normal or low FSH: possibilities include chronic anovulation with estrogen present (PCOS—50% lack signs of hirsutism, thyroid deficiency, and estrogen-secreting ovarian lesions) or chronic anovulation with estrogen deficiency (CNS lesions, hypothalamic amenorrhea, or hyperprolactinemia).
4. Follow-up for a normal or low FSH test
   a. Obtain TSH and prolactin
      • If TSH is elevated, work up for hypothyroidism; If PRL is also elevated, repeat 1 month after thyroid replacement.
      • If PRL is elevated with a normal TSH, evaluate for hyperprolactinemia.
   b. Progestin withdrawal bleed [medroxyprogesterone acetate 10 mg PO for 10 days]
      • If positive: T, DHEA-S, 17-OH P.
      • If negative and evidence of a normal TSH, PRL: obtain *T, DHEA-S, 17-OH P, plus E2*. If E2 < 30 pg/mL, schedule CNS imaging studies. If E2 ≥ 30 pg/mL, provide estrogen plus progestin withdrawal [conjugated estrogens (Premarin) 2.5 mg PO for 25 days plus Provera 10 mg PO days 16–25]. If no withdrawal bleed is elicited, evaluate for CNS lesions and causes of hypogonadotropic, hypogonadism.

Key: T = testosterone; DHEAS = dihydroepiandrosteredione sulfate; 17-OHP = 17 hydroxyprogesterone; FSH = follicle-stimulating hormone; E2 = estradiol; PRL = prolactin; PCOS = polycystic ovarian syndrome.

profile to determine whether there is any elevation consistent with polycystic ovarian disease. A negative progestin withdrawal bleed should be followed by an androgen profile in addition to an estradiol level. If the estradiol level is in the menopausal range (<30 pg/mL), a CT scan should be performed to exclude the possibility of CNS lesions. If the estradiol is greater than 30 pg/mL, the patient should undergo a trial of estrogen priming using conjugated estrogens 1.25 to 2.5 mg PO q.d. for 25 days plus medroxyprogesterone administered 10 mg PO q.d. during the last 10 days of estrogen administration. If no bleeding occurs, the patient should be referred to a gynecologist for suspected Asherman's syndrome or outflow tract obstruction. The presence of a withdrawal bleed only after estrogen priming should alert the clinician to reconsider the possibility of CNS lesions or other causes of hypogonadotropic hypogonadism.

ASHERMAN'S SYNDROME

Asherman's syndrome, or intrauterine adhesions, may result from several causes (Table 37-6). The most common is physical trauma after a dilation and curettage, especially after a pregnancy in the postpartum period. The history will usually identify a postpartum or postabortal dilation and curettage procedure. Less commonly, a prior cesarean section, myomectomy, or metroplasty may be the reported cause. Infectious etiologies include tuberculosis and schistosomiasis in third-world countries, with pelvic inflammatory disease and intrauterine device–related endometritis being a more-common infectious etiology in the United States. Laboratory values are completely normal in these patients, indicating eugonadotropic eugonadism. Modalities used to diagnose Asherman's syndrome include hysterosalpingography, transvaginal ultrasound, and hysteroscopy. The treatment of Asherman's syndrome is hysteroscopy, with lysis of the intrauterine adhesions.

PREMATURE OVARIAN FAILURE

Premature ovarian failure is a common cause of secondary amenorrhea and may be related to congenital or environmental causes (Table 37-7). Patients will present with complaints of secondary amenorrhea and menopausal symptoms of hot flashes, mood swings, vaginal dryness, and insomnia. The laboratory evaluation will reveal an elevated FSH and decreased estradiol levels. The basic underlying pathophysiology is an acceleration of the normally occurring process of oocyte atresia. Chromosomal abnormalities are among the most common causes of premature ovarian failure.[7] As discussed earlier, chromosomal abnormalities generally present as primary amenorrhea; however, in patients who have mosaic karyotypes—45X/46XX or 47XXX—there may be spontaneous ovulation and subsequent menses. These patients will then present with secondary amenorrhea.

Table 37-6

REFERENCE GUIDE—ASSESSMENT AND TREATMENT OF ASHERMAN SYNDROME OR OUTFLOW TRACT OBSTRUCTION

Definition: Amenorrhea secondary to intrauterine adhesions

Causes
    D&C (usually postpartum)
    Infectious (tuberculosis, endometritis, schistosomiasis)

Evaluation and treatment
    Hysterosalpingogram
    Transvaginal ultrasound
    Diagnostic or operative hysteroscopy

Table 37-7

REFERENCE GUIDE—ASSESSMENT AND TREATMENT OF PREMATURE OVARIAN FAILURE

Definition: Low estrogen and high FSH (>40 mIU/mL) before 40 years of age

Causes
  1. Abnormal karyotype—45,X/47,XXY / mosaics XX/X, XX/XY
  2. Autoimmune—often associated with other autoimmune conditions or endocrine deficiencies
  3. Infectious—TB, mumps oophoritis
  4. Radiation therapy or chemotherapy

Evaluation
  1. History and physical
  2. Laboratory
      a. E2 in menopausal range (<20 pg/mL)
      b. FSH > 40 mIU/mL
      c. Karyotype for women < 35 years) of age
      d. Screen for associated endocrine deficiencies: hypothyroidism (TSH, T4, antithyroid antibodies), Addison's disease (A.M. cortisol, ACTH test), hypoparathyroidism (calcium, phosphorus), pernicious anemia (CBC), and diabetes (fasting blood sugar).

Treatment
  1. Hormonal replacement therapy (HRT) with cyclic progestins.
  2. Screening and clinical suspicion for associated autoimmune diseases and endocrine deficiencies.
  3. Avoid gonadotropin ovulation induction due to poor success rates. Remember HRT is not a means of contraception.

In a patient with premature ovarian failure, a karyotype must be checked to determine if an intraabdominal gonad is present containing the 46XY mosaic so as to eliminate the potential malignant transformation of the ovary with a germ-cell tumor.

Autoimmune disorders and endocrinopathies are frequently associated with premature ovarian failure. Approximately 13 to 66 percent of patients with premature ovarian failure will exhibit signs of other autoimmune diseases or endocrinopathies.[8] Hypothyroidism, Addison's disease, myasthenia gravis, pernicious anemia, and hypoparathyroidism are just a few of the autoimmune diseases that have been associated with premature ovarian failure. The mechanism of premature ovarian failure in these patient is felt to be secondary to the presence of antiovarian antibodies. In patients who do not have an autoimmune disorder but have premature ovarian failure, antiovarian bodies are not identified.[9]

Patients with premature ovarian failure may also present secondary to prior environmental or medical exposure to radiation or chemotherapy. Women with Hodgkin and non-Hodgkin lymphoma are often treated with pelvic radiation, resulting in increased rates of early ovarian failure. The rate of ovarian failure depends on the dose of radiation. Doses between 250 and 500 rads cause a 60 percent sterilization rate, with doses between 500 and 800 rads causing a 70 percent sterilization rate and doses greater than 800 rads causing a sterilization rate close to 100 percent.[10] Chemotherapy regimens have also been noted to cause ovarian failure, with the alkylating regimens being the most damaging and most extensively studied. The damage of alkylating chemotherapy occurs primarily at the granulosa cell layer of follicles. In patients conceiving after chemotherapy, there appears to be no proven increased risk of birth defects, suggesting that little overall long-term damage to oocytes occurs as a result of this toxicity. This toxicity is age-related, with higher ovarian failure rates noted in older patients receiving equivalent doses of alkylating chemotherapy.

A rarer etiology of premature ovarian failure is galactosemia, an inherited error of galactose metabolism due to congenital deficiency of galactosyl-1-phosphate uridyltransferase, with resultant increased circulating levels of galactose 1-phosphate and galactose. The mechanism of ovarian failure in this disease process is undetermined but, it is rapidly disappearing as an etiology of amenorrhea due to newborn screening programs and appropriate diet manipulation.

Premature ovarian failure is most often a disorder of unknown cause, and it remains a diagnosis of exclusion. Laboratory evaluation of patients with premature ovarian failure includes tests for the known multiple etiologies and screens for the commonly associated autoimmune diseases (including Hashimoto's thyroiditis, adrenal insufficiency, hypoparathyroidism and pernicious anemia, and diabetes) with the determination of TSH, T4, antithyroid antibodies, A. M. cortisol or ACTH stimulation test, calcium, phosphorus, complete blood count, and a fasting blood sugar.

Treatment of patients with premature ovarian failure is based on the underlying etiology. All of these patients, secondary to their premature ovarian failure and resultant hypoestrogenemia, require cyclic estrogen and progesterone treatment. If fertility is desired, ovulation-induction agents may be used, but the success rate is extremely poor. Spontaneous pregnancies have been reported on hormonal replacement therapy; therefore, if pregnancy is not desired, patients should be advised to use a backup form of contraception or be replaced with oral contraceptives.

CENTRAL NERVOUS SYSTEM LESIONS AND SHEEHAN'S SYNDROME

A common category of abnormalities causing secondary amenorrhea is chronic anovulation, which may be caused by disorders of the hypothalamus, pituitary or various hormone feedback mechanisms. These patients will present to the emergency department with the complaint of secondary amenorrhea and clinical symptoms associated with the etiology of their anovulation. Hypothalamic etiologies for chronic anovulation and amenorrhea include tumors, infections, and infiltrative etiologies, and functional derangement of the hypothalamus and pituitary. Tumors of the hypothalamus include germinomas, hamartomas, teratomas, endodermal sinus tumors, and metastatic carcinoma. Infectious etiologies can include tuberculosis and syphilis, and infiltrative diseases include sarcoidosis and hemochromatosis. These patients will often present first with the complaint of secondary amenorrhea but may possibly be discovered to exhibit the life-threatening condition of panhypotituitarism. They may commonly exhibit neurologic deficits, headache, or galactorrhea.

Laboratory evaluation of these patients exhibits hypogonadotrophic hypogonadism and elevated prolactin if there is associated compression of the pituitary stalk. It is important to remember that dopamine serves as an inhibitory factor for prolactin release; therefore, since it is the only inhibitory factor transiting the pituitary stalk, prolactin is commonly elevated in tumors affecting transport of trophic factors through the stalk where inhibition of stimulatory factors causes a lack of production and secretion of all other pituitary hormones. If these patients exhibit signs of panhypopituitarism, thyroid and adrenal functions need to be tested and hormone replacement therapy instituted if necessary. The mechanism behind the amenorrhea in these patients is suppression of GnRH either through mass effect, causing decreased secretion in the portal blood system, or destruction of the pituitary gland, causing decreased pro-

duction of LH and FSH. If GnRH cannot affect the pituitary, there will not be any release of FSH or LH and anovulation will result.

Craniopharyngioma is a benign tumor derived from Rathke's pouch, originating from the pituitary stalk. These tumors occur predominantly in the young, the majority of patients being less than 20 years of age. These patients exhibit varying degrees of pituitary dysfunction. The characteristic signs of this tumor are growth retardation, diabetes insipidus, and hypogonadism. Treatment is surgical removal with radiotherapy and hormone replacement therapy as necessary.

Hypopituitarism may also be due to necrosis of the pituitary gland. Sheehan's syndrome occurs secondary to necrosis, affecting the anterior lobe of the pituitary gland primarily. Pituitary infarctions may occur as a result of severe postpartum hemorrhage and hypovolemia. The necrosis may involve varying amounts of the anterior lobe of the pituitary; the posterior lobe is almost never affected. The GH, LH, and FSH secretory cells are almost always damaged because of their location in the pituitary. These patients will present to the emergency department with the complaint of secondary amenorrhea and failure to lactate after a delivery complicated by severe hemorrhage. The clinician will also see varying signs and/or symptoms of other trophic deficiencies depending on the extent of the necrosis. These patients will need to have cyclic replacement of estrogen and progesterone as well as other hormones in which they are deficient.

STRESS, ILLNESS, WEIGHT LOSS, AND SECONDARY AMENORRHEA

Functional disorders affecting the ability of the hypothalamus to release GnRH include stress, weight loss, severe dieting, psychological eating disorders, and strenuous exercise. Chronic medical illnesses may also be associated with functional derangement of the hypothalamus, causing secondary amenorrhea. Patients with hypothalamic dysfunction need cyclic estrogen and progesterone. These patients will present to the emergency department with the complaint of secondary amenorrhea, neurologic deficits, and complaints related to their underlying disorder.

HYPERPROLACTINEMIA

Hyperprolactinemia as a cause of chronic anovulation and amenorrhea may be due to various etiologies (Table 37-8). These etiologies include pituitary adenomas, nipple or chest wall stimulation (including postthoractomy scars), suckling, breast implants, and herpes zoster. Hypothyroidism, renal failure due to decreased renal clearance, medications, and ectopic production from lung and renal tumors are all recognized etiologies of hyperprolactinemia.

Patients with hyperprolactinemia will usually present to the emergency department with the complaint of amenorrhea and/or glactorrhea. If the etiology is a prolactinoma

Table 37-8

REFERENCE GUIDE—ASSESSMENT AND TREATMENT OF HYPERPROLACTINEMIA

Incidence: One-third of patients presenting with secondary amenorrhea will have hyperprolactinemia; however, only 50 percent of hyperprolactinemia/amenorrhea patients will have galactorrhea.

Causes
  1. Pituitary adenomas
  2. Nipple or chest wall stimulation
  3. Hypothyroidism
  4. Renal failure
  5. Ectopic production (lung and renal tumors, leiomyomata)
  6. Medications:
      a. Dopamine antagonists (metaclopramide, tricyclic antidepressants, antipsychotics, phenothiazines)
      b. Uptake inhibitors (imipramine, amphetamine)
      c. Catecholamine-depleting agents (methyldopa, reserpine)
      d. Estrogens (oral contraceptives, hormonal replacement therapy, pregnancy)
      e. Progestins (Depo-Provera)

with suprasellar pressure or extension, patients may present with visual field defects.

The laboratory evaluation consists of a TSH level and a PRL level. If both are elevated, hypothyroidism must be addressed and treated, with the PRL level repeated after several months of treatment prior to assuming that it is secondary to any pathology of the pituitary. A patient who is hypothyroid and has an elevated TSH has an elevated PRL secondary to stimulation by an elevated TRH level, which stimulates both TSH and PRL release.

The mechanism whereby an elevated PRL level causes amenorrhea centers around its interference with pulsatile GnRH secretion. This interference ultimately disrupts FSH and LH release, causing amenorrhea. Prolactin-secreting adenomas or prolactinomas are the most common of the adenomas discovered in the pituitary gland. They are divided into microadenomas, which are less than 1 cm in diameter, and macroadenomas, which are larger than 1 cm in diameter. The patient who has a macroadenoma should be screened carefully for visual field deficits and symptoms of lower extension into the sinuses, as indicated by the leakage of cerebrospinal fluid.

The treatment options available to patients with prolactin-secreting adenomas are expectant management, medical management (i.e., suppression of prolactin-using dopamine agonists), or surgical therapy, usually transphenoidal resection. Currently, transphenoidal surgery is usually reserved for prolactinomas that progress on medical suppression, macroadenomas with extension, or macroadenomas in patients who plan to attempt pregnancy. The decision to treat or observe is based largely on the symptoms that a patient is experiencing and the ability of that patient to tolerate those symptoms.

Bromocriptine is the dopamine agonist used in the medical treatment of symptomatic prolactinomas. It binds directly to dopamine receptors and thereby suppresses pituitary prolactin secretion. These drugs may have significant side effects including nausea, headaches, and orthostatic hypotension. Some patients also experience vomiting and abdominal cramping. Bromocriptine doses should be increased slowly so that tolerance can build enough to prevent these side effects; almost all patients can adjust to the side effects if they are given a slow start.

In a review of multiple clinical trials, it was determined that 80 percent of patients with amenorrhea/galactorrhea and hyperprolactinemia without demonstrable tumors had resumption of menses when treated with bromocriptine. Average treatment time to resumption of menses was only 5 to 7 weeks. Patients usually have resumption of menses before the suppression of galactorrhea with bromocriptine therapy is completely effective.[11]

Monitoring of patients of prolactinomas consists of taking an annual PRL level in patients with microadenomas and an MRI of the pituitary if the PRL level increases, if the patient is not on bromocriptine therapy, if bromocriptine fails to keep prolactin suppressed, or if new neurologic symptoms develop. Macroadenomas are generally followed with yearly MRI scans and prolactin levels.

Other hormone-secreting tumors of the pituitary that may cause amenorrhea and increased prolactin secretion include ACTH- and growth hormone–secreting tumors. If one suspects Cushing's disease or acromegly, a 24-h urine for free cortisol and a measurement of ACTH should be obtained to rule out Cushing's disease and a growth hormone and insulin-like growth factor I level should be obtained while the patient is fasting. Empty sella syndrome may also cause amenorrhea. These patients have a distortion of the pituitary gland caused by an invasion of the arachnoid from the sella turcica, producing a small hernia-filled space containing cerebrospinal fluid. These patients often have elevated PRL levels and a coexistent prolactinoma.

POLYCYSTIC OVARY SYNDROME

Polycystic ovary syndrome is a symptom complex consisting of amenorrhea/oligoamenorrhea, hirsutism, obesity, and enlarged polycystic ovaries (Table 37-9). This syndrome was first described by Stein and Leventhal in 1935.[12] Many etiologies of chronic anovulation and the appearance of polycystic ovaries on ultrasound exist and include adrenal disorders, hyperprolactinemia, ovarian tumors and the syndrome of polycystic ovary disease. The pathophysiology of this disease often centers around an alteration in the feedback mechanisms of the hypothalamic-pituitary-ovarian axis.[13] Luteinizing hormone is increased; therefore the production of androgens is also increased. This is reflected in elevated levels of free or total testosterone, androstenedione,

dihydroepiandrosterone, dihydroepiandrosterone sulfate, 17-hydroxyprogesterone, and estrone. Estrone is increased as a result of peripheral conversion of the increased androstenedione by aromatase in peripheral adipose tissue. Sex hormone–binding globulin levels are generally decreased secondary to the increased levels of testosterone and the negative impact testosterone has on the hepatic production of sex hormone–binding globulin. Therefore free estradiol is increased in women with polycystic ovary disease as a result of decreased binding. Both estrone and estradiol act by positive feedback to further increase LH release. They also act as negative feedback regulators on FSH release. This causes numerous follicles in the ovary to remain immature or to undergo atresia; their inability to progress to dominant follicles results in a failure of ovulation.

Laboratory values obtained to evaluate polycystic ovary syndrome include an elevated LH, normal or low FSH, decreased SHBG (sex hormone binding globulin) and an elevated testosterone level. If there is suspicion of congenital adrenal hyperplasia, an ACTH stimulation test should be performed with the measurement of 17-hydroxyprogesterone, which would be increased with a 21-hydroxylase deficiency. If Cushing's disease is suspected, a 24-h urine should be ob-

---

Table 37-9

REFERENCE GUIDE—ASSESSMENT AND TREATMENT OF POLYCYSTIC OVARY SYNDROME

Definition: chronic anovulation with normal circulating estrogen levels with or without elevated circulating androgens.

Etiologies
1. Congenital adrenal hyperplasia (CAH)
2. Cushing's syndrome
3. Insulin receptor defect/hyperinsulinemia (HAIR-AN syndrome)
4. Hyperprolactinemia
5. Ovarian tumors
6. Polycystic ovarian disease

Clinical signs:
1. obesity, 40%;
2. hirsutism, 50%;
3. abnormal uterine bleeding, 30%;
4. infertility 65%.

Laboratory findings: increased luteinizing hormone (LH), decreased sex hormone–binding globulin, elevated free E2 and testosterone.

Treatment principles
1. Treat systemic diseases and exclude the possibility of a virilizing neoplasm.
2. Use of oral contraceptives for treatment of hirsutism. Add aldactone for an unsatisfactory cosmetic response to OCPs. Use cyclic progestins for treatment of anovulation or dysfunctional uterine bleeding.
3. Induce ovulation if fertility is desired.

Key: HAIR-AN = hyperandrogenism, insulin resistance, acanthosis nigricans; OCPs = oral contraceptive pills.

tained to evaluate free cortisol excretion. An elevated level would confirm the diagnosis.

The treatment of patients with hyperandrogenic anovulation is based on the etiology of the chronic anovulation. Patients who are found to have polycystic ovary disease must be cycled with oral contraceptives or progestins to prevent endometrial hyperplasia secondary to chronic unopposed estrogen secretion. In cases of hirsutism, patients may be treated with aldactone or oral contraceptives for an improved cosmetic appearance. If fertility is desired, these patients will need ovulation induction agents, including clomiphene citrate, or exogenous gonadotropins. Patients with polycystic ovarian disease desiring pregnancy who fail to ovulate on clomiphene citrate should be referred to a reproductive endocrinologist secondary to the higher risk of ovarian hyperstimulation syndrome when exogenous gonadotropins are administered.[14]

References

1. Tanner JM: *Growth in Adolescence,* 2d ed. Boston: Blackwell, 1962.
2. Pinsky L: A community of human malformation syndromes involving the mullerian ducts, distal extremities, urinary tract and ears. *Teratology* 9:65, 1974.
3. Wabrek AJ, Millard PR, Wilson WB Jr, Pion RJ: Creation of a neovagina by the Frank nonoperative method. *Obstet Gynecol* 37:408, 1971.
4. Bates GW: *Adolescent Amenorrhea in Pediatric and Adolescent Gynecology.* New York: Raven Press, 1992, p 169.
5. Christman GM: Turner's syndrome—adulthood: Reproductive health care and options. *Adolesc Pediatr Gynecol* 2:181, 1989.
6. Schwanzel-Fukuda M, Pfaff DW: Origin of luteinizing hormone-releasing hormone neurons. *Nature* 338:161, 1989.
7. Jewelewicz RJ, Schwartz M: Premature ovarian failure. *Bull NY Acad Med* 62:219, 1986.
8. Alper MM, Garner PR, Seibel MM: Premature ovarian failure—Current concepts. *J Reprod Med* 31:699, 1986.
9. Tang VW, Faiman C: Premature ovarian failure: A search for a circulating factor against gonadotropin receptors. *Am J Obstet Gynecol* 146:816, 1983.
10. Asch P: The influence of radiation on fertility in men. *Br J Radiol* 53:271, 1980.
11. Cuellar FGG: Bromocriptine mesylate (Parlodel) in the management of amenorrhea/galactorrhea associated with hyperprolactinemia. *Obstet Gynecol* 55:278, 1980.
12. Stein IF, Leventhal ML: Amenorrhea associated with bilateral polycystic ovaries. *Am J Obstet Gynecol* 29:181, 1935.
13. Christman GM, Randolph JF Jr, Kelch RP, Marshall JC: Reduction of gonadotropin-releasing hormone pulse frequency is associated with subsequent selective follicle stimulating hormone secretion in women with polycystic ovarian disease. *J Clin Endocrinol Metab* 72:1278, 1991.
14. Christman GM, Hammond MG: Ovulation induction in the hyperandrogenic woman. *Infertil Reprod Med Clin North Am* 2:547, 1991.

Chapter 38

ABNORMAL UTERINE BLEEDING

Ellen C. Wells

Abnormal uterine bleeding (AUB) refers to any bleeding from the uterus that is excessive in duration, frequency, or amount. The goals of the physician treating AUB are to (1) control the immediate bleeding if necessary, (2) determine the cause, and (3) prevent similar episodes from occurring. The first goal may be accomplished while the evaluation to determine the etiology is still in progress. However, a diagnosis will be important to accomplish the third goal, which commonly involves reestablishing cyclic bleeding. Since the initial presentation for most women will be a complaint of vaginal bleeding, the first step will be to determine if the bleeding is originating in the endometrial lining of the uterus or is extrauterine in origin. The second step in managing AUB will be to determine if the bleeding is superimposed on an ovulatory cycle or is anovulatory in nature.

PATHOPHYSIOLOGY

THE NORMAL MENSTRUAL CYCLE

The normal menstrual cycle occurs at regular intervals ranging from 21 to 35 days and lasting from 3 to 7 days. The normal hormonal fluctuations of the idealized 28-day cycle are shown in Fig. 38-1. Cycle days are numbered beginning with the first day of bleeding, and the interval is recorded as the time between the first day of one bleeding episode until the first day of the next bleeding episode. The mean menstrual blood loss in normal women is approximately 35 mL, with 78 percent of the blood loss occurring in the first

2 days. Individuals with blood loss greater than 80 mL have significantly lower mean hemoglobin, hematocrit, and serum iron levels; therefore this is considered "excessive" (hypermenorrhea or menorrhagia). The number of pads or tampons a patient uses may be useful information, as it indicates the impact of the problem on the woman's life. However, it has been shown that there is no direct correlation between menstrual blood loss and the subjective assessment of blood loss by the number of pads or tampons used or the number of days of bleeding.

In the normal menstrual cycle, using a 28-day cycle, for example, the first 14 days represent the phase of follicular development within the ovary to produce an oocyte in anticipation of ovulation (Fig. 38-1). Estrogen production by granulosa cells lining the developing follicle is the stimulus for regeneration of the endometrium to cover denuded areas from the previous menstruation. With continued estrogen stimulation, the endometrium becomes *proliferative,* reaching a height of 3 to 5 mm. In response to estrogen production by the ovary, the pituitary gland produces a midcycle surge of luteinizing hormone (LH) and follicle-stimulating hormone (FSH), resulting in the release of a mature oocyte. The corpus luteum then forms within the collapsed capsule. It has a life span of approximately 14 days, producing a shift from the production of mostly estrogen to mostly progesterone. With progesterone stimulation, the endometrium maintains its preovulatory height, but it continues to mature within this *secretory phase,* preparing for implantation. If fertilization and implantation occur, an embryo will release human chorionic gonadogropin (hCG) into the circulation, which will prompt the corpus luteum to continue producing estrogen and progesterone to maintain the early pregnancy. Without the stimulus of the hCG, the corpus luteum will

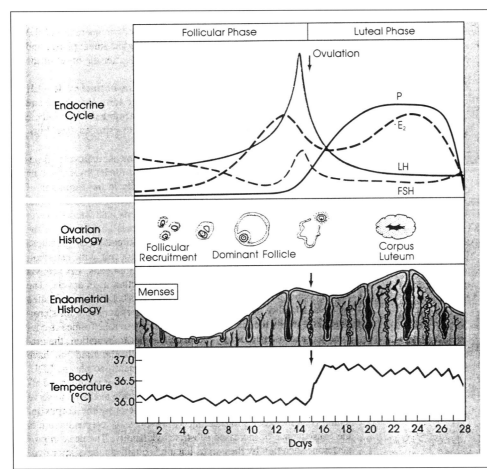

Figure 38-1

Graphic representation of the interrelationship between ovarian hormones (estradiol and progesterone) and pituitary hormones (follicle stimulating hormone and luteinizing hormone). [From Carr BR, Wilson JD: Disorders of the ovary and female reproductive tract, in Isselbacher KJ, Braunwald E, Wilson JD, et al (eds): *Harrison's Principles of Internal Medicine*, 13th ed. New York: McGraw-Hill,1994, p 2022.]

regress and estrogen and progesterone production will decline. The loss of estrogen and progesterone stimulation to the endometrium results in vasoconstrictive changes within the spiral arterials supplying the endometrium, with subsequent endometrial ischemia and sloughing. Release of prostaglandins and other biochemical mediators in response to this results in uterine contraction and the characteristic "cramping" of an ovulatory menstruation. Follicle stimulating hormone from the pituitary gland then rises in response to the low estrogen levels, stimulating the ovary to renewed follicular activity and beginning the next cycle.

CHARACTERISTICS OF ABNORMAL UTERINE BLEEDING

Abnormal uterine bleeding includes several different patterns that fall outside the regular cyclic, predictable menses characteristic of ovulatory cycles. Bleeding patterns that fall within the normal range but are perceived as longer, excessive, or "different" compared with a normal cycle for that individual patient may warrant further investigation. *Hypermenorrhea (menorrhagia)* is defined as cyclic menstrual bleeding that is excessive in duration or amount. It may be secondary to anatomic uterine abnormalities such as leiomyomas, polyps, or an abnormal endometrium, as may occur with unopposed estrogen stimulation associated with anovulation or from endometrial hyperplasia. *Oligomenorrhea* refers to bleeding or light spotting that occurs at intervals greater than 35 days. *Metrorrhagia* is bleeding that occurs at irregular frequent intervals. *Menometrorrhagia* is excessive and prolonged bleeding at frequent and irregular intervals. Other terms that may be helpful in characterizing abnormal bleeding include *intermenstrual bleeding* and *postcoital spotting* or *bleeding.* Intermenstrual bleeding implies that the bleeding is noted in addition to and between normal cyclic menses. This bleeding should be grouped as ovulatory (or midcycle), premenstrual, or postmenstrual if such a pattern exists. Postcoital spotting denotes the pattern of bleeding after intercourse and implies potential cervical pathology.

DIAGNOSIS

EXTRAUTERINE SOURCES OF BLEEDING

In evaluating women with complaints of vaginal bleeding, it is important to evaluate other extrauterine potential sources of bleeding. Cervical lesions such as carcinoma, polyps, or condylomata may be visualized. Eversion of the squamo-columnar junction (ectropion), as seen with the use of oral contraceptive pills or with pregnancy, may be a source of bleeding secondary to trauma. Cervical infection with *Chlamydia* creates a friable inflammatory eversion that bleeds readily when touched. The vagina may contain a carcinoma, sarcoma, or adenosis. Lacerations from trauma or coitus may occur at the introitus or deep within the vagina. Vaginal infections or retained foreign bodies such as pessaries or tampons may produce local irritation with bleeding. Lower urinary tract lesions such as urethral caruncles or infected urethral diverticula as well as lower GI sources such as hemorrhoids or anal fissures should be excluded.

OVULATORY ABNORMAL UTERINE BLEEDING

Abnormal ovulatory uterine bleeding is generally characterized as having a regular cyclic component preceded by such symptoms as breast tenderness, bloating, or dysmenorrhea, but an extra component of bleeding is superimposed. Cyclic hormonal factors can cause this, such as bleeding at midcycle during ovulation, when estrogen levels decrease slightly, or polymenorrhea due to follicular or luteal phase shortening. Premenstrual staining or delayed menses may be due to irregular endometrial shedding, as with an inadequate luteal phase or a persistent corpus luteum, respectively.

Organic pelvic disease such as endometriosis, pelvic inflammatory disease, or certain ovarian neoplasms can potentially disrupt the normal cycle. Several lesions or abnormalities within the uterus may present as abnormal uterine bleeding. Uterine leiomyomas, particularly those with a submucosal location, may be associated with necrotic overlying endometrium or produce contralateral pressure necrosis within the endometrial cavity. Their presence may also inhibit the normal vasoconstriction of spiral arterials at menses. Endometrial polyps, hyperplasia, or malignancy may produce hypermenorrhea or intermenstrual bleeding. Adenomyosis, or the invasion of benign endometrial glands and stroma into the myometrium, can cause hypermenorrhea and secondary dysmenorrhea. Chronic endometritis may present as intermenstrual spotting, with a tender uterus on exam and plasma cells on biopsy. Iatrogenic factors such as the presence of an intrauterine device may also contribute to abnormal bleeding. Fig. 38-2 summarizes various causes of AUB.

Pregnancy-related events should always be considered in reproductive-age women with abnormal bleeding. These women will often describe otherwise normal cyclic menses. Persistent bleeding after a recent pregnancy would suggest endometritis or retained products of conception. A sensitive serum or urine β-hCG determination will detect an early pregnancy. First-trimester bleeding with an intrauterine pregnancy may represent a threatened or missed abortion if the cervical os is closed versus an incomplete or inevitable abortion if the cervical os is open (*see* Chap. 4).

It is important to obtain a β-hCG determination on any reproductive age woman in which pregnancy is even a remote possibility in order to quickly and accurately diagnose pregnancy related bleeding, especially ectopic pregnancy. These women generally present with delayed menses, spotting, and unilateral pain. Ultrasound commonly reveals an adnexal mass with no intrauterine pregnancy. If ruptured, increased fluid will be seen in the cul de sac.

Blood dyscrasias including platelet abnormalities from thrombocytopenia purpura, leukemia, and von Willebrand's disease may present as abnormal or heavy bleeding, usually in adolescence. Claessens and Cowell[1] reported fifty-nine cases of acute menorrhagia in adolescence in which twenty percent were found to have underlying coagulation disorders. Women with such coagulation disorders may give histories of recurrent unexplained menorrhagia, bleeding with tooth extractions, easy bruising, epistaxis, or a family history of bleeding disorder. Iatrogenic factors such as anticoagulant therapy will produce similar symptoms.

ANOVULATORY ABNORMAL UTERINE BLEEDING

Anovulatory bleeding results from an endometrium which, in the absence of luteal phase progesterone, is in a chronically estrogen stimulated proliferative state. This thickened tissue bleeds irregularly and sheds incompletely as estradiol levels fluctuate during waves of follicular development. Anovulatory bleeding is typically irregular with long intervals between periods (e.g., 6 to 8 weeks), and frequently heavy. Protracted periods of anovulation increase the risk of endometrial hyperplasia and endometrial adenocarcinoma. Anovulatory cycles are frequently encountered in the perimenarchal adolescent due to delayed, asynchronous, or abnormal hypothalamic maturation, and in the perimenopausal woman with failing ovarian function. Periods of physical or psychological stresses including medical illnesses, malnutrition, and intense physical exercise regimens may directly affect the hypothalamus. Rapid weight gain or weight loss may have a similar effect. These can present as either AUB or amenorrhea. Hormonally mediated medical illnesses which disrupt the ovulatory cycle producing abnormal uterine bleeding or amenorrhea include hyperprolactinemia, hypothyroidism, hyperthyroidism, Cushing's disease, and adrenal hyperfunction including congenital adrenal hyperplasia and late onset adrenal hyperplasia.

Causes of Vaginal Bleeding

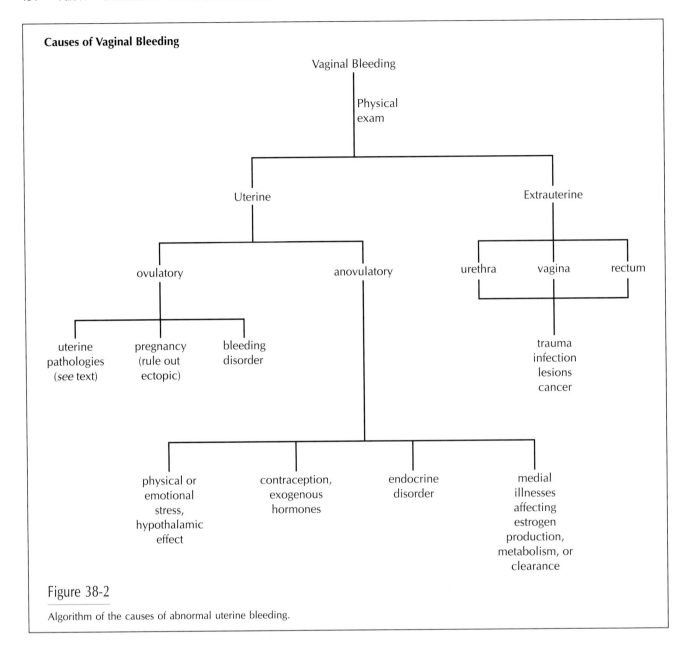

Figure 38-2

Algorithm of the causes of abnormal uterine bleeding.

Polycystic ovarian syndrome represents a spectrum of disease in which mild hyperandrogenism is present with an increased luteal hormone to follicular-stimulating hormone ratio. The classic triad for these patients is obesity, hirsutism, and oligomenorrhea. When menses does occur, it can be particularly heavy and prolonged. The initiating factors for this syndrome are not clearly understood and variants exist which do not directly match the classic description.

Exogenous hormone use, often specifically initiated to prevent ovulation as a means of contraception, can be a potential source of abnormal bleeding. Oral contraceptive pills typically contain both estrogen and progesterone for 21 days followed by 7 days of placebo in which withdrawal bleeding occurs. Levonorgestrel subdermal implants (Norplant),

depomedroxyprogesterone injections (DepoProvera), and progesterone-only birth control pills provide continuous progesterone stimulation superimposed on the woman's indogenous estrogen production. Because ovulation does not occur, irregular bleeding is related to the relationship between these two hormonal levels and their effect on sustaining the endometrium. The prolonged progesterone-dominant effect of these methods results in a thin endometrium which may present as amenorrhea or as atrophic bleeding. These abnormal bleeding situations will respond best by adding or increasing the estrogen component (*see* Chap. 48). Finally, liver disease such as cirrhosis or hepatitis as well as chronic renal failure may contribute to abnormal bleeding patterns due to changes in the metabolism and clearance of estrogen.

EVALUATION

HISTORY

In the reproductive-age woman, abnormal bleeding associated with pregnancy or contraception use are common, and this information should be gathered early in the history. The patient's age, number of previous pregnancies and outcomes, current sexual activity, and method of contraception should be elicited. Her last menstrual period and menstrual pattern in the past should be discussed. The frequency, quantity, duration, and pattern of her abnormal bleeding should be collected, as well as premenstrual or pregnancy symptoms. (Any relationship of pain or bleeding to bowel movements or urination should be recorded.) Characteristics of ovulatory versus anovulatory bleeding, as discussed above, will be helpful at this point in directing further questioning. A history of concurrent diseases—such as liver or renal disease, endocrinopathies, and bleeding disorders—should be addressed. Recent illnesses, psychological or emotional stress, and recent weight change should be elicited. Any pain including quantity, quality, location, and duration should be assessed.

It is extremely important to consider the possibility of pregnancy-related bleeding in any reproductive-age women who presents with lower abdominal pain and bleeding. An ectopic pregnancy is life-threatening, and the timing of diagnosis in some cases may be crucial. Testing for β-hCG is imperative, even in situations when the likelihood of pregnancy appears remote. Pregnancy in women with a previous history of tubal ligation, tubal surgery, previous ectopic pregnancy, previous pelvic inflammatory disease, endometriosis, or use of an intrauterine device (IUD) should be investigated thoroughly and followed closely until the diagnosis of ectopic pregnancy is either excluded or confirmed.

PHYSICAL EXAMINATION

Vital signs are imperative to evaluate hemodynamic status and should be obtained after the presenting complaint and before any further history is taken. Tachycardia, hypotension, or orthostatic changes would prompt the physician to quickly evaluate the cause of bleeding for immediate control. Components of the general physical examination may point to chronic diseases, thyroid abnormalities, obesity, hirsutism, or signs of Cushing syndrome. The abdominal examination should be directed to identify any areas of tenderness, the presence of bowel sounds, signs of peritoneal irritation, and any evidence of masses or ascites. Rebound or guarding should increase the suspicion for pelvic infection or hemoperitoneum. The pelvic examination should differentiate the source of bleeding, including urethral, vulvar, or rectal origins. The vagina should be inspected for lacerations, fissures, lesions, infection, or foreign body. The cervix should be evaluated for polyps, inflammation, ulcers, or lesions. Cancer as well as sexually transmitted diseases such as condyloma acuminata from human papillomavirus,

condyloma lata from syphilis, or mucopurulent or bloody cervical discharge from chlamydial infection or gonorrhea should be considered. Blood or tissue protruding through the os or an IUD string should be noted. Pedunculated intrauterine leiomyomas or polyps can sometimes be expelled through the cervix, with subsequent infection and bleeding. In pregnant patients, it is important to determine whether the cervical os is opened or closed. Bimanual examination will assist in determining uterine size and detecting uterine leiomyomas as well as the presence of any adnexal masses. Cervical motion tenderness is suggestive of pelvic inflammatory or adnexal disease. A slightly enlarged, boggy uterus with adnexal fullness and a bulging cul-de-sac from hemoperitoneum may be seen with ectopic pregnancy. Uterine tenderness can also be present in PID, septic abortion, endometriosis, and adenomyosis. Rectovaginal examination will assist in assessing the cul-de-sac, a retroverted uterus, or posterior masses and may allow palpation of uterosacral ligament nodularity, which is sometimes present in endometriosis.

TESTS AND STUDIES FOR DIAGNOSIS

Two laboratory tests that should be performed immediately in cases of acute and heavy bleeding include a β-hCG and a complete blood count. The β-hCG determinations performed on the urine will be accurate detecting levels as low as 25 mIU/mL. Serum β-hCG determinations will detect levels down to 5 mIU/mL. If pregnancy is detected, a quantitative β-hCG determination will be important, as this value can be followed serially to determine if it is rising appropriately. In a normal early pregnancy, the β-hCG value generally doubles in 48 hours, with a lower limit of normal demonstrating a rise of at least 66 percent over 48 hours. Values that do not rise appropriately or decline are indicative of ectopic pregnancy or a failed intrauterine pregnancy. The β-hCG values may also be correlated with ultrasound findings in patients in whom serial values are not available (see Chapters 3 and 4). A complete blood count will document the presence and severity of anemia, and the white blood cell count is a marker for infection. In interpreting this hemoglobin and hematocrit with acute blood loss, it should be remembered that equilibration may not have occurred and values may be falsely reassuring. Serum iron and ferritin studies may also be useful to assess iron stores in chronic AUB. Coagulation studies should be considered in severe bleeding present from adolescence and in patients who have a family history of bleeding disorders. Studies that can be useful in determining the etiology of AUB in women with anovulatory uterine bleeding include TSH and prolactin.

A biopsy should be obtained of abnormal lesions of the vulva, vagina, or cervix, being careful not to biopsy vascular lesions (e.g., varices or hemangiomas). Consultation with a gynecologist may be helpful prior to biopsy. A recent or current Pap smear is not an adequate screen if a cervical lesion is actually seen, and a biopsy should be performed. In women over age 35 with uterine bleeding, an endometrial biopsy should be considered, since in them the risk of hyperplasia and endometrial adenocarcinoma are increased (Table 38-1, Fig. 38-3). However, a biopsy should not be performed until the results of the pregnancy test are available and negative. In general, this procedure should be performed by the person (service) who will follow-up the pathology report.

Transvaginal sonography can be extremely valuable in the evaluation of women with AUB. Total uterine size can be measured and the presence of any intrauterine leiomyomas determined. Even small leiomyomas that encroach on the endometrial cavity (i.e., submucosal or intracavitary) may play significant roles in abnormal bleeding (Fig. 38-4). The thickness and characteristics of the endometrial tissue may be evaluated. Increased fluid within the cavity or polyps may be seen (Fig. 38-5). The amount of tissue present within the endometrial cavity may be helpful with therapeutic decisions, in that a very thin lining may respond best to estrogen therapy (Fig. 38-6), but a very thick lining may respond better with removal by dilatation and curettage (Fig. 38-7). Progesterone withdrawal can also be used to manage thick linings if neoplasm is ruled out (e.g., by endometrial biopsy).

Transvaginal sonography is particularly helpful in early pregnancy and possible ectopic pregnancy (see Chap. 3 for a detailed discussion of ectopic pregnancy). Transvaginal sonography may also detect ovarian cysts associated with cul-de-sac fluid, particularly a hemorrhagic corpus luteum, which may present as adnexal pain in early pregnancy. Culdocentesis is less commonly performed now that ultrasound is available to assess cul-de-sac fluid (Table 38-2, Fig. 38-8). The presence of nonclotting blood on culdocentesis is diagnostic of hemoperitoneum.

Hysteroscopy is a valuable tool in the diagnosis of patients with abnormal uterine bleeding (Fig. 38-9). Hysteroscopically directed biopsies of lesions or hysteroscopic resections can be performed. Gimpelson and Rappold[2] have demonstrated that dilatation and curettage alone may miss 10 to 25 percent of lesions within the uterine cavity.

TREATMENT OF ABNORMAL UTERINE BLEEDING

ACUTE MANAGEMENT

Immediate evaluation and management are necessary in episodes of acute hemorrhage. An accurate assessment of vital signs and orthostatic changes should be made. Stabilization in the acute phase may require intravenous hydration and venous access with a crossmatch and complete blood count being obtained. A Foley catheter for monitoring urine output will help ascertain the degree of volume depletion in instances of acute blood loss. Pregnancy, neoplasia, and blood dyscrasias should be assessed early within

---

Table 38-1

ENDOMETRIAL BIOPSY

Indications:
1. Evaluate abnormal uterine bleeding
2. Assess ovulation
3. Evaluate for luteal-phase defects
4. Diagnose chronic endometritis

Contraindications:
1. Pregnancy
2. IUD (relative)
3. Acute pelvic infection
4. Profuse bleeding
5. Unfamiliarity with procedure

Possible adverse effects:
   Infection, bleeding, uterine perforation with injury to bladder or bowel, vasovagal reflex

Equipment needed:
   Speculum
   Povidone/iodine solution
   Tenaculum
   Uterine sound
   Pipelle (uterine curette or sampler)
   Formalin

Procedure:
1. Perform a pelvic examination to assess uterine size and position. Obtain a sensitive pregnancy test.
2. Obtain informed consent. Place the patient in the dorsal lithotomy position. Insert the speculum and prep the cervix with povidone/iodine.
3. Place the tenaculum on the anterior cervical lip for traction.
4. Insert the Pipelle to the fundus, at which point you should meet resistance. Markings on the Pipelle are in 1-cm increments. The Pipelle will enter to 5 to 7 cm in a normal-size uterus. Resistance at less than 3 cm implies that you have not yet passed the internal cervical os (Fig. 38-7).
5. A uterine sound may be necessary to find the cavity. Excessive force will increase the risk of perforation or creation of a false passage.
6. Upon adequate placement, the inner stem of the Pipelle is withdrawn, creating negative pressure. The instrument is then moved from the fundus to the lower uterine segments in at least four separate areas to obtain an adequate sample.
7. The Pipelle is removed and the sample placed in formalin.

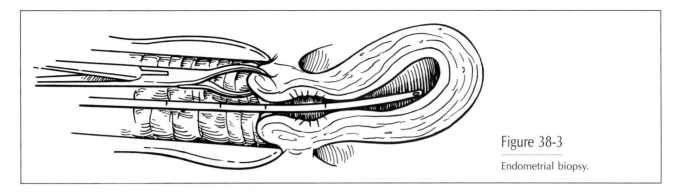

Figure 38-3

Endometrial biopsy.

this group. Occasionally, women with depleted iron stores from long-standing anovulation will present with acute hypovolemia from an anovulatory bleeding cycle.

Hypovolemia is an indication for dilatation and curettage with sharp or suction curette. Uterine packing in these cases is not recommended, as it may increase the risk of infection and hide continued bleeding. Dilatation and curettage is also recommended for acute bleeding in women over the age of 35, as this age group faces a greater risk of pathologic changes. It should be noted that in women with anovulatory uterine bleeding, the dilatation and curettage may slow the bleeding but does not change the underlying pathophysiology. Long-term management is necessary following control of the acute bleeding episode.

In women who experience an acute episode of bleeding but are hemodynamically stable, medical management may be initiated. The underlying question with management options is how quickly the bleeding must be stopped. The management approach within this group is to stabilize the en-

dometrium, slowing or stopping acute bleeding, and allowing a subsequent episode of controlled bleeding. In women with prolonged bleeding and a thin endometrium by ultrasound, treatment with estrogen will stimulate the growth of denuded, raw surfaces. Estrogen also has the advantage of temporarily stabilizing even the thickened, estrogen-stimulated endometrium. If women in this category are not significantly improved in 24 hours or develop hypovolemia, dilatation and curettage is recommended. Estrogen therapy may be given as oral conjugated estrogen 10 mg/day (2.5 mg q.i.d.) or 25 mg IV q4h. DeVore and colleagues[3] found that oral and intravenous routes of estrogen were equally effective in stopping bleeding. Bleeding generally stopped after the second dose by either route of medication. They attributed this time interval to the time needed to induce mitosis and growth within the endometrium. Oral therapy is therefore appropriate in women who are able to take oral medications. Medroxyprogesterone acetate 10 mg/day is added as soon as the bleeding subsides. Conjugated estro-

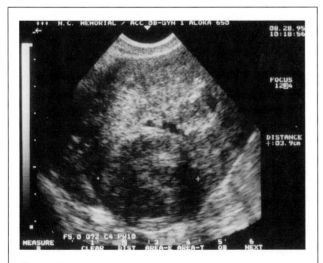

Figure 38-4

A leiomyoma measuring 3.9 cm is located immediately adjacent to the endometrial cavity, outlined by crosses.

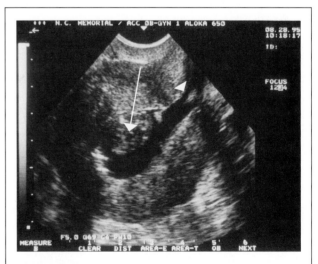

Figure 38-5

An endometrial cavity containing a polyp (*long arrow*). Visualization is enhanced by hydrosonography. Catheter tip for fluid injection is seen in the endocervical canal (*arrowhead*).

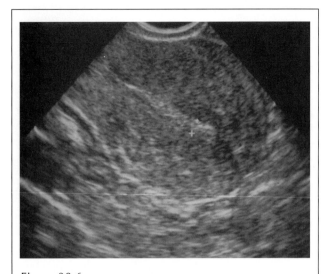

Figure 38-6

Thin endometrial stripe (measured between calipers, outlined by crosses).

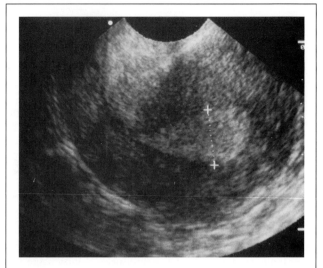

Figure 38-7

Thick endometrial stripe (measured between calipers, outlined by crosses).

Table 38-2

CULDOCENTESIS

Indications:
1. Hypovolemia with suspected hemoperitoneum
2. Cul-de-sac fluid visualized by ultrasound
3. Acute abdominal pain

Contraindications:
1. No fluid in cul-de-sac by ultrasound
2. Pelvic or cul-de-sac mass which would pose risk for perforation

Possible adverse effects:
   Infection, hemorrhage, perforated viscus

Equipment needed:
   Speculum
   Sterile cotton swabs
   Povidone/iodine solution
   Lidocaine, 1%
   Spinal needle, 18-gauge
   Two 10-mL syringes
   Tenaculum

Procedure:
1. Place the patient in the lithotomy position with the back of the table elevated.
2. Perform a bimanual pelvic examination to determine uterine position and assess for pelvic or cul-de-sac masses.
3. After obtaining informed consent, place the speculum and prep the upper vagina and cervix with povidone/iodine solution.
4. Inject the submucosa of the posterior cervix and vaginal fornix with 1% lidocaine.
5. Grasp the posterior cervix with the tenaculum and lift it anteriorly to expose the posterior fornix.
6. Fill a 10-mL syringe with 2 mL of saline and attache an 18-gauge needle.
7. With traction on the tenaculum, move the needle forward through the posterior fornix with a deliberate thrust.
8. Apply negative pressure and rotate the needle until fluid or blood is obtained.
9. A second pass may be made if the first is nondiagnostic (no fluid obtained).

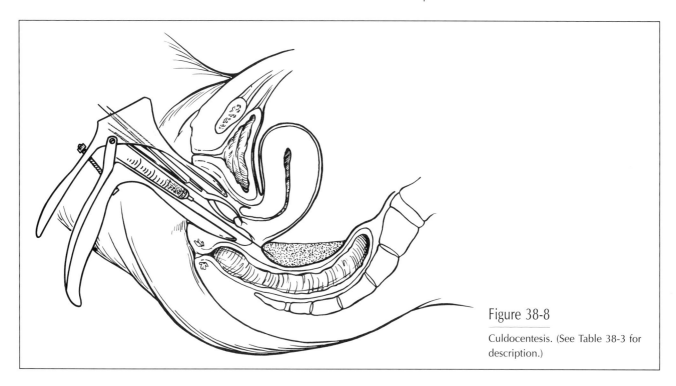

Figure 38-8

Culdocentesis. (See Table 38-3 for description.)

gen and progesterone are continued for 7 to 10 days. At that point both estrogen and progesterone are stopped, with a synchronized withdrawal bleed. If the endometrial lining has been thick, this bleed may be heavy but should not be prolonged.

Several regimens have been promoted to stop subacute bleeding using oral contraceptive pills. These regimens are

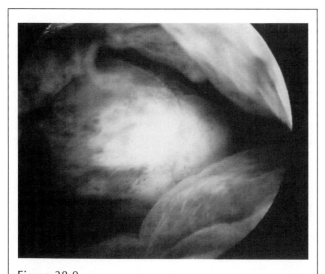

Figure 38-9

Hysteroscopy reveals an endometrial polyp with surrounding lush endometrium.

very useful for nonpregnant women without anatomic abnormalities as a cause for their bleeding. Theoretically the progesterone in these pills will decrease estrogen receptors and therefore may not stop the bleeding quite as rapidly as estrogen alone during the initial phase, followed by the addition of progesterone. Two common regimens are (1) four tablets a day for a week followed by withdrawal bleeding and (2) a slow taper using a single pack of birth control pills—4 tablets a day for 2 days, 3 tablets a day for 2 days, 2 tablets a day for 2 days, and then 1 tablet a day for the last 3 days. A fixed (monophasic) oral contraceptive pill should be used (e.g., ethinyl estradiol 35 μg and norethindrone 1 mg). These regimens may be difficult for some women due to the nausea produced by the high estrogen dose. It should be remembered that the withdrawal of estrogen or progesterone or a sudden drop in the level of either one of these hormones can produce repeated withdrawal bleeding.

In women with anovulatory bleeding and an adequate hematocrit (e.g., above 28 percent), particularly with persistent light bleeding or spotting, progesterone therapy alone may be employed. Medroxyprogesterone acetate 10 mg/day for 10 days simulates the luteal phase in the estrogen-primed endometrium. Its use stabilizes and matures the endometrium, as in the secretory phase. The discontinuation of progesterone provokes withdrawal bleeding. This withdrawal bleeding may be heavy secondary to the large amount of tissue present, but it should not be prolonged, as the endometrium is in synchrony. Withdrawal bleeding usually occurs at 3 to 10 days after discontinuation of progesterone.

The patient should be warned that she should expect bleeding with discontinuation of progesterone and that it may be heavy. This is sometimes referred to as a *medical curettage.*

In women on prolonged oral contraceptive use or continuous progesterone contraception, such as the progesterone-only pill, levonorgestrel subdermal implants (Norplant), or depomedroxyprogesterone (DepoProvera), the endometrial lining may be very thin, and the addition of estrogen will decrease symptoms of breakthrough bleeding. Breakthrough bleeding or spotting during the first three cycles at the initiation of oral contraceptive therapy may resolve with subsequent cycles. Therefore, any treatment during this time would be based on the severity of symptoms and their effect on the woman. A more extensive discussion of hormonal contraceptive–related bleeding may be found in Chap. 48.

LONG-TERM MANAGEMENT

Anovulation is frequently a chronic problem, and long-term therapy is essential. If contraception is needed, an oral contraceptive pill is an excellent choice. If pregnancy is desired, clomiphene citrate may be used to induce ovulation. Medroxyprogesterone acetate 10 mg/day for 10 days each month may be used to produce scheduled bleeding in women who are at no risk for pregnancy, are using a barrier method, or have a contraindication to estrogen use. Observation without pharmacological management is suitable for women with isolated or infrequent episodes of anovulation. A progesterone IUD is an option in women who are ovulatory and has been associated with a decreased menstrual blood loss. A histologic diagnosis of complex hyperplasia may require higher doses of progesterone for therapy and repeat biopsy for follow up. Complex hyperplasia is associated with a 2 percent risk of subsequent cancer. Hyperplasia with atypia is associated with an even higher risk of endometrial cancer. This risk also increases with age. Higher progesterone doses (e.g., megestrol acetate, or Megace, 40 mg/day) or hysterectomy are recommended. Referral to a gynecologist is recommended for this management.

Other hormone-based therapies that have been promoted for the management of anovulatory bleeding include the use of danazol 200 to 400 mg/day. This therapy is associated with weight gain and acne. Women may still ovulate on this medication. There is a decrease in menstrual blood loss, but expense and moderate side effects limit its use. Gonadotropin-releasing hormone agonists may play a role in the management for some women by suppressing gonadotrophin secretion from the pituitary gland and subsequently lowering serum estradiol levels. The resultant amenorrhea may improve anemia by allowing an adequate time interval for hemoglobin and hematocrit to return to normal. Major drawbacks are menopausal side effects, the drug's expense, and the fact that it should not be used longer than 6 months because of the risk of bone loss. Add-back therapy

with low-dose estrogen and progesterone decreases this effect but has not been evaluated in controlled, prospective trials.

Nonsteroidal anti-inflammatory drugs have been shown to be effective in decreasing menstrual blood loss. Alterations in prostaglandin synthesis and release appear to occur in women with both anovulatory and ovulatory abnormal bleeding. In women with normal menstruation, the ratio of prostaglandin F2 alpha (causing vasoconstriction) to prostaglandin E2 (causing vasodilatation) steadily increases from midcycle to menses. Nonsteroidal anti-inflammatory drugs administered during menses to women with menorrhagia and ovulatory AUB may alter these ratios and reduce mean menstrual blood loss by 20 to 50 percent[4]; reduced blood loss has also been demonstrated in the presence of anovulation, myomas, IUDs, and von Willebrand disease. Nonsteroidal anti-inflammatory drugs may play a role not only in vasoconstriction in the decidua basalis but also in platelet aggregation, as they affect thromboxane and prostacyclin pathways, hence their potential use in von Willebrand disease.

SURGICAL THERAPY

Hysteroscopic evaluation of the endometrium can be useful not only for diagnosis but also therapy. Removal of polyps, directed biopsies, or resection of intracavitary myomas may be performed. Endometrial ablation may also be performed with hysteroscopic guidance. This therapy is considered when no underlying pathology exists and medical therapy has been unsuccessful. It should not be performed in women who desire future childbearing. In this procedure, the basal layers of the endometrium are destroyed using laser or electrical energy or heat, preventing regeneration. This results in complete amenorrhea in about 50 percent of women and reduced bleeding in another 40 percent of women with menorrhagia. Results are improved if the endometrium is suppressed with GnRH agonists, danazol, or medroxyprogesterone for 4 to 6 weeks and worse if there are anatomic causes of bleeding (e.g., leiomyomata). A theoretical concern with this method is that an isolated area of residual endometrium could progress to carcinoma without recognition in an otherwise obliterated cavity. Longer follow-up will be needed with these patients to further assess this risk.

Hysterectomy is generally reserved for women with persistent abnormal bleeding who have not responded adequately to medical therapy or in the presence of malignancy. It may also be the treatment chosen by some women with endometrial hyperplasia with atypia or on weighing other considerations, such as age and desire for future childbearing. Hysterectomy or myomectomy are important options for women with AUB, enlarging uterine leiomyomas, or the presence of other symptoms related to leiomyoma.

References

1. Claessens EA, Cowell CA: Acute adolescent menorrhagia. *Am J Obstet Gynecol* 139:277, 1981.
2. Gimpelson RJ, Rappold HO: A comparative study between panoramic hysteroscopy with directed biopsies and dilatation and curettage. *Am J Obstet Gynecol* 158:489, 1988.
3. DeVore GR, Owens O, Kase N: Use of intravenous Premarin in the treatment of dysfunctional uterine bleeding: A double-blind randomized control study. *Obstet Gynecol* 59:285, 1982.
4. Vargyas JM, Campeau JD, Mishell DA: Treatment of menorrhagia with meclofenamate sodium. *Am J Obstet Gynecol* 157:944, 1987.
5. Townsend DE, Ricart RM, Paskowitz RA, Woolford RE: Rollerball coagulation of the endometrium. *Obstet Gynecol* 76:310, 1990.

Chapter 39

EMERGENCY DISORDERS INVOLVING THE VULVA

Raymond H. Kaufman

A basic tenet in the management of women with vulvar disease is that a correct diagnosis must be established before treatment is instituted. A careful history and physical examination is paramount in making this diagnosis. However, unless the diagnosis is clear-cut, in many instances vulvar biopsy is required before a diagnosis can be established. But in dealing with acute emergencies involving the vulva, a biopsy will shed little light in clarifying the management plan necessary to deal with this emergency. Nevertheless, certain laboratory tests can be of value in the emergency department setting. The simplest and one that will be used most often is a wet-mount preparation utilizing saline and potassium hydroxide mounts to exclude various vaginitidies as a cause of the vulvar symptoms. In addition, a scraping taken from a vulvar lesion that is then placed in potassium hydroxide solution can be of value in excluding fungal infection as the source of the vulvar symptoms. When the latter is performed, the scraping is easily taken using the edge of a scalpel blade. The material obtained is then placed on a glass slide, to which 15 to 20% potassium hydroxide is added. Gently heating the slide over a flame is of benefit in dissolving keratinized material. The specimen is then cover-slipped and examined under the microscope using both low and high power magnification.

PRURITUS

The most common cause of acute vulvar pruritus is related to either a vaginal candidiasis or trichomoniasis. This subject is discussed in Chap. 43. The nonneoplastic epithelial disorders—which include lichen simplex chronicus, lichen sclerosus, and other dermatoses such as eczema, psoriasis, and sebhorreic dermatitis—are a frequent cause of vulvar pruritus. Rarely, however, is this pruritus of such an acute degree that it requires emergency treatment. However, a patient will occasionally have such intense and persistent pruritus that she will seek emergency care for relief of this symptom. The nonneoplastic epithelial disorders are classified on the basis of gross and histopathologic changes, as follows: (1) squamous cell hyperplasia (formerly hyperplastic dystrophy), incorporating lichen simplex chronicus; (2) lichen sclerosus; (3) other dermatoses.

SQUAMOUS CELL HYPERPLASIA

Frequently, areas of squamous cell hyperplasia are localized, elevated, and well delineated, but more often, these changes

493

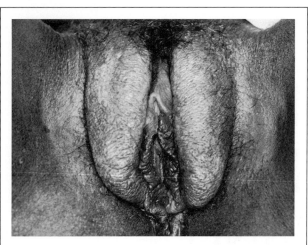

Figure 39-1

Squamous cell hyperplasia. This patient had experienced vulvar pruritus for many years. Thickening, lichenification, and whitening of the tissue is evident. The patient presented with acute exacerbation of the pruritus.

are quite diffuse, resulting in significant thickening, lichenification, and both red and white appearance of the vulvar tissues (Fig. 39-1). Fissures and excoriations are quite common secondary to chronic scratching. Scrapings for the presence of fungi should be taken from such lesions to exclude fungal infection as the underlying cause of the patient's symptoms. The differential diagnosis includes contact allergic and irritant dermatitis, lichen sclerosus, and fungal infections involving the vulvar tissue.

TREATMENT

If an eczematous type of vulvitis is present as the result of infected excoriations or irritants in previously used medications, wet dressings with an agent such as aluminum acetate (Burow's solution) applied to the vulva three or four times daily will be beneficial. Topical application of corticosteroids is also effective in alleviating pruritus. The high- or medium-potency glucocorticoids such as 0.025 or 0.01% fluocinolone acetonide or 0.01% triamcinolone acetonide are effective in relieving pruritus. The drug should be applied two or three times daily; however, it should not be used on a continuous basis for more than several weeks, since secondary changes may develop or these patients may have a "rebound" effect when the medication is discontinued. If a fungal infection is found involving the vulva, it should be treated separately with one of the antifungal agents such as clotrimazole 1% cream or ketoconazole 2% cream twice daily for a period of 1 to 2 weeks. Warm sitzbaths are also extremely effective in alleviating pruritus. It is generally advisable for the patient to take a warm sitzbath, adequately

dry the vulva, and then apply a topical agent for relief of pruritus.

LICHEN SCLEROSUS

The gross appearance of lichen sclerosus is often characteristic. In well-developed and classical lesions, the skin has a crinkled, "cigarette paper" or parchment-like appearance (Fig. 39-2). The changes commonly extend around the anus in a figure-eight configuration. Often, there is edema of the clitoral foreskin, which completely hides the clitoris. Phimosis of the clitoris may be seen late in the course of the disease. The labia minora often fuse with the labia majora and are not identifiable as such. Splitting of the skin in the midline is often observed. Fissures may also develop in the natural folds of the skin and in the posterior fourchette. Small ecchymotic areas and areas of telangiectasia may be noted within the skin and mucosa. The diagnosis of lichen sclerous is best confirmed on vulvar biopsy; however, the patient should be referred to her primary-care physician for this procedure.

TREATMENT

Clobetazol 0.05% is effective in alleviating the symptom of pruritus as well as causing regression of the lichen sclerosus. Of interest is the fact that relatively long term use of this potent steroid usually does not result in some of the secondary changes seen when glucocorticoids are used for a long period of time on the vulva. When utilized, clobetazol should be applied twice daily for 1 month, at bedtime for 2 months, and then twice weekly for 3 months. Follow-up examination should be carried out after 1 month of therapy. The patient should also be referred to her primary-care physician for vulvar biopsy to confirm the diagnosis.

CONTACT IRRITANT AND ALLERGIC DERMATITIS

Contact dermatitis is an inflammatory reaction of the skin to a primary irritant or an allergenic substance. It is often difficult to distinguish the two. Many individuals reporting that they are allergic to a substance have really had contact irritant reactions.

Most instances of contact dermatitis involving the vulva are truly primary irritant responses. Patients usually complain of marked irritation, itching, and burning. Significant edema, formation of vesicles, and even bullae are often seen (Fig. 39-3). Contact dermatitis should not be confused with a primary herpes infection. Often the reaction is so severe that the patient finds the symptoms to be intolerable and requires immediate attention. Vesiculation and ulceration are most often induced by primary irritants used in strong sub-

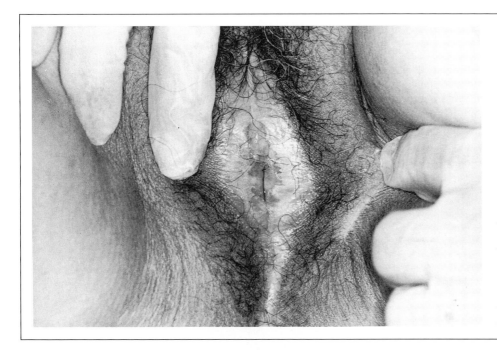

Figure 39-2

Lichen sclerosus with introital stricture. This patient had long-standing vulvar pruritus. She presented in the emergency department complaining of severe pain when coitus was attempted, which was a result of the marked introital stenosis.

stances over a prolonged period or by allergenic substances. The severity of the reaction is influenced by the sensitivity of the patient to the substance with which she has come into contact. Occasionally, urinary retention may develop in association with a severe reaction and occasionally painful regional lymph-adenitis may be experienced.

DIAGNOSIS

A careful history is often of help in establishing the diagnosis. Have the patient's vulvar tissues been in contact with any chemicals or medications? Have they been exposed, as occasionally happens, to poison oak or poison ivy? The oleoresins produced by poison ivy and poison oak result in classical allergic contact dermatitis. The allergen is usually transmitted to the vulvar tissues by contaminated hands and less often by direct contact. The period between contact with the allergen and the eruption varies from several hours to several days. The symptoms and findings are similar for this type of reaction and for contact irritant reactions.

Contact and allergic vulvitis must be differentiated from a variety of eruptions including squamous cell hyperplasia, acute candidiasis, trichomoniasis, tinea cruris, and herpes simplex virus infections.

TREATMENT

Mild reactions usually subside rapidly after the causative agent is withdrawn, so that aggressive therapy is not necessary. When the patient has a severe, painful reaction, immediate institution of therapy is usually indicated after a diagnosis of contact vulvovaginitis is established and an infectious cause for the problem is eliminated. Wet com-

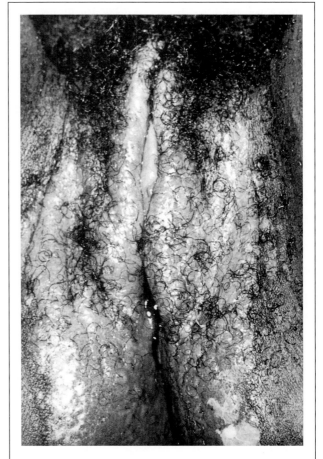

Figure 39-3

Severe contact vulvitis. This severe reaction developed 4 days after injudicious use of podophyllum. (From Kaufman R, Faro S: *Benign Diseases of the Vulva and Vagina.* St Louis: Mosby–Year Book, 1994, with permission.)

presses of aluminum acetate (Burow's solution 1:20) may provide rapid relief of symptoms. After 1 or 2 days of wet compresses, a previously weeping, tender lesion may become dry, clean, and less painful. Then, the topical application of a corticosteroid cream or lotion will often relieve the patient's symptoms and bring about rapid improvement in the lesions. Allergic reactions respond more rapidly to corticosteroids than to any other therapeutic agent. Systemic glucocorticoids are often necessary and are quite effective in the presence of a severe allergic reaction, such as seen with poison ivy or poison oak. They are best administered in diminishing doses over a 2- or 3-week period.

ACUTE PAIN

BARTHOLIN ABSCESS

Contrary to frequent teaching, most Bartholin abscesses result from a nongonococcal infection of Bartholin duct cysts. Culture taken from the abscess contents usually reveals a wide spectrum of organisms. *Escherichia coli* is the organism found most often. Bartholin abscesses often develop in preexisting duct cysts but can occur in the absence of a cyst. It is possible that obstruction of the Bartholin duct, possibly due to inspissated mucus, may lead to the development of bartholinitis and subsequent abscess. Bartholin abscesses generally develop in women of reproductive age. In older women, associated cellulitis, necrotizing fasciitis, or, rarely, tumor should be ruled out.

SYMPTOMS

Exquisite pain and tenderness are the primary symptoms seen in the presence of a Bartholin abscess. Some abscesses develop slowly, occasionally over a week or longer, and give rise only to mild symptoms as they slowly develop. Occasionally, this type of abscess may spontaneously regress, although usually it will continue to enlarge and spontaneously drain. Most commonly, the Bartholin abscess develops rapidly; within 2 or 3 days, marked edema, swelling, pain, and tenderness become evident (Fig. 39-4). These abscesses may undergo spontaneous rupture within 72 hours if they are not surgically drained.

Swelling and redness over the site of the affected gland is usually obvious. Associated severe lateral edema may also be present. The abscess is usually palpable as an exquisitely tender, fluctuant mass.

TREATMENT

Occasionally, the early treatment of bartholinitis with broad-spectrum antibiotics may prevent abscess formation. However, the typical infected Bartholin gland is usually not seen

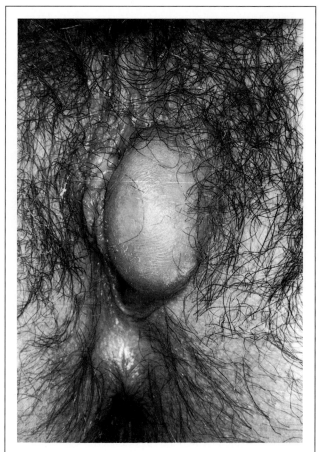

Figure 39-4

Bartholin abscess. Marked swelling and redness is noted on the patient's left vulva. This encompasses the region of the Bartholin gland and extends up the entire side of the labia. (From Kaufman R, Faro S: *Benign Diseases of the Vulva and Vagina.* St Louis: Mosby–Year Book, 1994, with permission.)

at this stage of development. Most often, patients will present with an exquisitely tender, hyperemic, fluctuant mass. Under these circumstances, incision and drainage are necessary and can easily be performed in an outpatient setting. Prior to making the incision, the point of planned entry into the abscess may be infiltrated with 1 to 2 mL of 1% lidocaine, although usually this is not required. Ethyl chloride spray can be used over the puncture site for local anesthesia. The incision into the abscess should be made along the medial aspect of the fluctuant mass. If one traces the labium minus into the swelling, it will be noted that the swelling is equally distributed lateral and medial to the plane of the labium minus. The incision should be made just lateral to the hymenal ring in the region where the Bartholin duct orifice is found. Care should be taken not to make the incision over the keratinized labial skin as a chronic, externally draining Bartholin gland may result. A stab incision is made into the abscess cavity and extended for several millimeters in each direction, allowing drainage of the purulent material. A sterile swab should rapidly be inserted into the cavity and material obtained for both aerobic and anaerobic cultures as well as gonococci. Once the purulent material has drained, a small, curved clamp should be inserted into the abscess cavity and any loculations still present broken up. Suture marsupialization of the abscess cavity at this time is not recommended. However, the insertion of a Word catheter (Fig. 39-5) into the cavity will often result in a functional marsupialization resulting in the development of a new orifice from the Bartholin gland. The Word catheter is the size of a #10 Foley catheter with a stem 1 in. long and a single barrel. A solid stopper is attached to one end and a 5-mL latex inflatable balloon is attached to the other. The catheter is inserted into the abscess cavity and the bulb is inflated with 2 to 4 mL of water. The end of the catheter is then tucked up into the lower vagina, where it can be left in place. Usually, the catheter should remain in place for a period of 4 to 6 weeks. The patient may engage in all activities, including intercourse, with the catheter in place.

POSTOPERATIVE CARE

The patient should be instructed to take warm sitzbaths for 15 to 20 min three or four times daily for the next 72 hours. She should be started on antibiotics and continue them until the edema and erythema have disappeared. Initiating therapy with ampicillin 500 mg q6h or ampicillin/sulbactam 500 mg q8h pending report of the culture and sensitivity is recommended.

NECROTIZING FASCIITIS

Necrotizing faciitis of the vulva is a severe soft tissue infection that has high morbidity and mortality if not recognized early. This infection is uncommon, can be difficult to recognize, and can progress insidiously or rapidly. Although most commonly affecting diabetics, necrotizing fasciitis must also be suspected in post menopausal women with abscesses involving the vulva or Bartholin glands.[1-3] Other risk factors include vascular insufficiency, immunocompromised states, surgical incisions, cutaneous trauma, and decubitus ulcers. Necrotizing fasciitis is a polymicrobial infection.

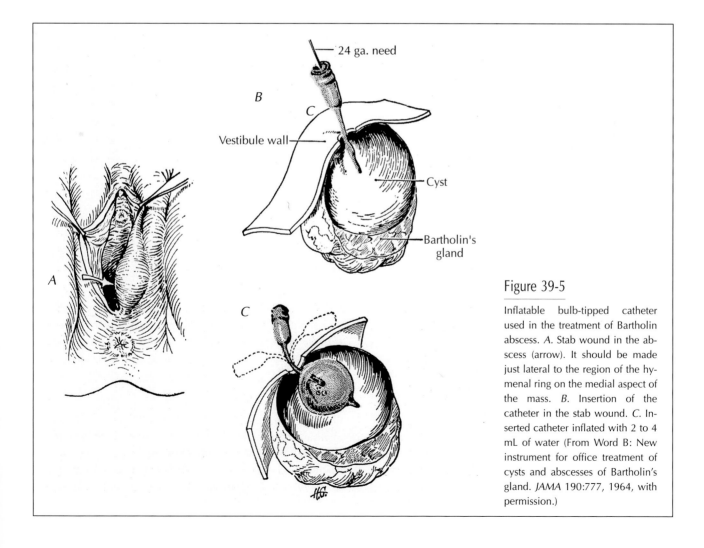

Figure 39-5

Inflatable bulb-tipped catheter used in the treatment of Bartholin abscess. *A.* Stab wound in the abscess (arrow). It should be made just lateral to the region of the hymenal ring on the medial aspect of the mass. *B.* Insertion of the catheter in the stab wound. *C.* Inserted catheter inflated with 2 to 4 mL of water (From Word B: New instrument for office treatment of cysts and abscesses of Bartholin's gland. *JAMA* 190:777, 1964, with permission.)

Aerobic organisms consume oxygen in the infected tissue, providing a more desirable environment for anaerobic organisms to proliferate.

Necrotizing fasciitis is an infection of the subcutaneous tissues that spreads along fascial planes. It is characterized by severe tenderness, edema, and necrosis of subcutaneous tissues. The overlying skin may not be initially involved, or it may be erythematous or violaceous. As infection progresses and nutrient vessels thrombose, bullae and cutaneous necrosis develop. Purulent exudate or pustules are usually not present, and crepitance is a late finding. Numbness may occur in the involved area secondary to infarction of cutaneous nerves. Fever, leukocytosis, and systemic toxicity are late signs.

Once the clinical diagnosis is suspected, antibiotics should be given and the gynecologist consulted for aggressive surgical debridement. Antibiotics alone are insufficient without debridement. A comprehensive antibiotic regimen should be given that provides coverage against mixed anaerobes, enterococci, and group A streptococci. It should include the use of expanded-spectrum penicillins and cephalosporins, clindamycin, or metronidazole, and an aminoglycoside.

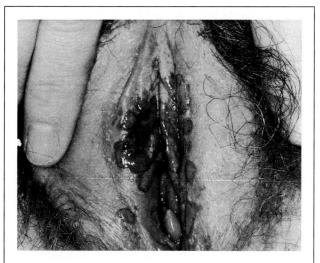

Figure 39-6

Primary herpes genitalis. One week after the development of herpes genitalis, multiple painful, shallow ulcers are seen. (From Kaufman RH, et al: Clinical features of herpes genitalis. *Cancer Res* 33:446, 1973, with permission.)

HERPES GENITALIS

Occasionally, an initial primary herpes infection will cause the patient such discomfort that she will require immediate evaluation and treatment. The type 2 herpes simplex virus (HSV-2) is usually transmitted by direct sexual contact, and the symptoms associated with an initial primary infection usually develop between 3 and 7 days after contact with the virus. Often, an initial infection may be mild or even completely asymptomatic, but occasionally patients develop severe, disabling symptoms. The patient may complain of severe vulvar pain and tenderness. She may also experience severe dysuria and urinary retention. Inguinal and pelvic pain related to lymphadenopathy is frequently observed with primary infection. Systemic symptoms of headache, generalized aching, and malaise with fever are also common.

The lesions seen in a primary herpes infection are frequently extensive and involve the labia majora, labia minora, perianal skin, vestibule of the vulva, and possibly the vaginal as well as the cervical mucosa. Profuse watery discharge can also be present with primary infection. Early in the course of the disease, multiple vesicles may be scattered over these areas, but they rapidly rupture and leave shallow, ulcerated areas (Fig. 39-6). Lesions may coalesce to form large bullae that subsequently lead to the development of large ulcers. Superficial ulcerations may be seen in the ectocervix and within the vagina. Occasionally, a fungating necrotic mass may be seen covering the ectocervix. The latter can easily be confused with invasive cervical carcinoma. Under these circumstances, the cervix may be exquisitely tender, may bleed easily, and, when it is manipulated, can provoke severe pelvic

pain. Inguinal lymphadenopathy is usually present. The primary lesions may persist for 2 to 6 weeks unless immediate therapy is instituted.

Occasionally, meningitis and encephalitis may be seen in association with a primary infection. The patient under these circumstances usually complains of severe headache, neck stiffness, and/or blurring of vision. If the sacral plexus is involved, acute urinary retention can result. However, the commonest reason for urinary retention is infection involving the urethra and bladder.

DIAGNOSIS

Usually, the diagnosis of a primary genital herpetic infection is obvious. However, other vesicular ulcerative lesions involving the vulva may be confused with it. Herpes zoster may also present with painful vesicles and ulcers; however, the diagnosis is apparent when it is observed that the lesions are unilateral in distribution and generally follow the course of nerve distribution to the vulva. Herpes genitalis may also be confused with multiple syphilitic chancres, chancroid, vaccinia, and possibly Behçet syndrome. In an outpatient facility, the diagnosis can often be established by performing a Tzanck smear. A scraping can be taken from one of the ulcers or from the base of an unroofed vesicle. The vesicular fluid alone should not be used to make this preparation. Viral inclusion bodies may be present in the nuclei of desquamated cells. However, the diagnosis is best confirmed by obtaining cultures directly from the ulcers or from vesicular fluid. Once the specimen is obtained, the cotton-tipped swab should be placed in Eagle's medium containing 2 to 10% fetal bovine serum and antibiotics. The specimen should rapidly be transmitted to the laboratory, where the virus can easily be isolated in tissue culture. If immediate transportation is not possible, the culture tube should be kept in a refrigerator at 4°C (39.2°F) until it can be transported to the laboratory. Cultures should not be frozen.

TREATMENT

Acyclovir has been available for a number of years in the management of patients with genital herpetic infections. This drug and other similar medications such as valacyclovir and famciclovir have proved to be effective in shortening the duration of clinical symptoms as well as the duration of viral shedding. The sooner treatment is instituted after the onset of symptoms, the more effective it will be. The usual oral dose of acyclovir recommended is 200 mg five times daily for 10 days for primary HSV infections (or valacyclovir 500 mg b.i.d. or famciclovir 125 mg b.i.d.). Therapy depends upon the duration of the patient's symptoms and viral shedding. Patients with severe primary genital herpes or disseminated infection, including meningitis, should be treated with intravenous acyclovir 5 to 10 mg/kg q8h. Therapy in such severely ill patients should be continued for 5 to 7 days. Recurrent HSV is treated with acyclovir 200 mg 5 times a day for 5 days (*see* Chap. 42).

FOLLOW-UP

Patients should be advised that there is at least a 50 to 60 percent chance that they will have recurrent episodes of genital herpesvirus infections. If recurrences occur frequently, they can be controlled by the use of suppressive therapy with acyclovir or valacyclovir. In addition, the patient should be counseled regarding the possible risks associated with vaginal delivery in the presence of an active herpesvirus infection.

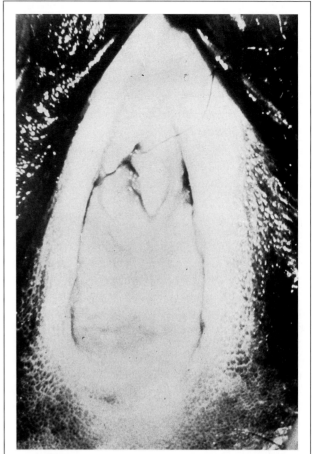

Figure 39-7

Imperforate hymen in a 14-year-old girl. She had been having increasingly severe lower abdominal pain for several months.

IMPERFORATE HYMEN

Often, an imperforate hymen is not recognized until after puberty, when retention of menstrual blood becomes troublesome. As the child menstruates each month, larger amounts of blood accumulate within the vagina, which slowly becomes distended to form a hematocolpos. Eventually, the cervix may become dilated with the accumulation of blood, giving rise to hematometria and hematosalpinx. The patient will often complain of increasingly severe cyclic lower abdominal pain; occasionally, a large, tender mass will be palpated arising from the pelvis. Associated bladder pressure, frequency, and urinary retention may develop. The diagnosis can be determined if an imperforate hymen is found (Fig. 39-7). A history of cyclic lower abdominal cramping pain not associated with menses in a young woman in the pubertal age range should make the examining physician suspicious of such a problem. Associated amenorrhea, urinary retention, lower abdominal pain, and a palpable pelvic mass should prompt the examiner to do a careful examination of the external genitalia as well as a rectal examination. Ultrasonography will be of considerable help in establishing the diagnosis of hematocolpos. Usually, examination will reveal an intact hymen to be bulging outward. Occasionally, if the hymen is firm and fibrotic, this will not be observed. However, rectal examination should help to confirm the diagnosis of a hematocolpos.

TREATMENT

A cruciate incision should be made at the introitus through the hymen. If significant bleeding is noted coming from the edges of the hymen, the edges can be oversewn with a fine, absorbable suture. Because the external and internal genitalia of these patients are susceptible to infection in the presence of old blood, strict aseptic conditions should be maintained and prophylactic antibiotics given prior to starting the operative procedure. Following drainage of the hematocolpos, a bimanual examination should be avoided because of the risk of infection. Instead, it should be done at a later time.

ACUTE VULVAR EDEMA

Acute vulvar edema is an uncommon occurrence, with multiple causes. In the postpartum patient, the sudden occurrence of unilateral vulvar edema associated with a significantly elevated white blood cell count may foreshadow the development of necrotizing fasciitis. Prompt diagnosis and radical surgical excision are necessary. Significant bilateral labial edema occurring during the third trimester of pregnancy or in the postpartum period is occasionally associated with a hypertensive disorder of pregnancy. Bed rest and appropriate management of toxemia is the recommended treatment.

Seasonal edema of the vulva may occur in some individuals with hay fever. It may also be seen in association with peritoneal dialysis, as well as the intraperitoneal installation of dextran 70 (Hyskon). The latter is still used by some gynecologic surgeons following pelvic surgery in the belief that it may be of some benefit in preventing postoperative adhesions. This edema will slowly resolve as the dextran is absorbed. Severe cutaneous edema is also occasionally seen in association with vulvovaginal candidiasis. This often is associated with physical findings suggesting an intravaginal candidal infection causing a white, cheesy discharge. Saline and potassium hydroxide (KOH) wet-mount preparations will be of help in establishing this diagnosis. Regardless of the cause of the acute vulvar edema, bed rest and perineal ice packs are useful therapeutic measures. Once the specific etiology is established, it will require treatment (i.e., for acute candidiasis, an oral antifungal agent or the intravaginal instillation of an antifungal agent, plus the topical application of an antifungal agent).

HEMORRHAGE

Acute hemorrhage arising from the vulva is most unusual. However, this may occasionally be seen in association with vulvar carcinoma. A tumor large enough to result in acute hemorrhage will usually be obvious on physical examination. A thorough pelvic examination, however, should still be performed to exclude the possibility of bleeding from the vagina, cervix, or uterine fundus. If obvious bleeding is seen coming from the carcinoma, the bleeding site should be identified and the bleeding controlled either by coagulation or a figure-eight suture. Unfortunately, if there is significant tu-

mor necrosis, it may be difficult to place a suture that will provide hemostasis.

On rare occasions, a large varicose vein may rupture, with subsequent hemorrhage. This is most likely to occur after acute trauma to the vulva. When this occurs, the bleeding vessels need to be identified and a suture ligature placed around the bleeding site.

TRAUMA

Because of its location, the vulva is seldom injured accidentally. The injuries most commonly seen are in the prepubertal female and usually result from straddling injuries. Rape is also a not uncommon cause of acute trauma to the vulvovaginal tissues (see Chap. 46).

Traumatic injuries in the adult are occasionally seen following an automobile or motorcycle accident and are usually associated with trauma elsewhere, such as pelvic fractures. Pelvic examination should be done in women with severe multisystem trauma, particularly if there has been a pelvic fracture, to identify potential vaginal, vulvar, or perineal injury. Occasionally, injuries occur following insertion of a foreign body into the vagina by the patient or a second party. Injuries to the vulva are usually manifest as hematomata and/or lacerations.

LACERATION

Laceration of the vulva and vagina is likely to occur after a violent fall on a slender object such as a stake or by impalement on the handlebars of a motorcycle or bicycle. Such injuries may extend through the vagina into adjacent organs such as the rectum, bladder, urethra, and cul-de-sac. When this occurs, hemorrhage may be severe. When multiple lacerations are seen primarily within the vagina, a foreign body should be looked for as the cause. Not uncommonly, remnants of metal, glass, or plastic objects may be found within the vagina as well as in the paravaginal tissues. Anterior, posterior, and lateral x-rays should be taken to locate any radioopaque object. In most instances, when hemorrhage is severe, control of the hemorrhage and repair of the defects should be performed in the operating room under appropriate anesthesia. If a vaginal laceration is bleeding profusely, the vagina can temporarily be packed with sterile plain gauze. The surgical treatment of these lacerations should be directed toward restoration of normal anatomy. The bleeding blood vessels should be ligated and the tissue edges carefully approximated. In the presence of severe traumatic injuries involving the vulva and vagina, careful evaluation of the rectum and bladder for injury should also be carried out. If the injury extends through the cul-de-sac, a laparotomy will be required, since injury to the small or large intestine may well have occurred and will require appropriate repair.

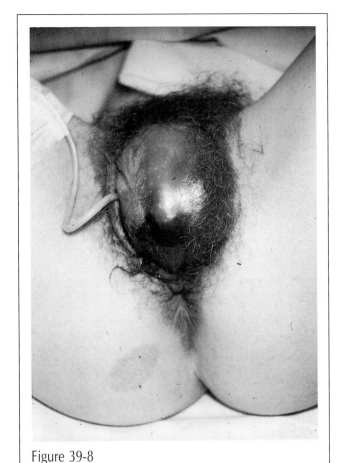

Figure 39-8

Vulvular hematoma.

Lacerations involving the vulva and vagina of the child require special consideration. Forcible examination of a child should never be attempted. In the presence of pain, significant bleeding, or evident laceration, the child should be examined in the operating room under anesthesia. Lacerations should be repaired by careful approximation of the tissue edges.

HEMATOMA

Hematomas of the vulva most commonly occur during childbirth and occasionally secondary to retracted blood vessels following an episiotomy. Not uncommonly, they may be clinically manifest after the patient has been discharged from the hospital following delivery. This is especially true because of the short postpartum stay allowed to most women today. The hematoma is manifest by swelling and tenderness, and if it is large, by significant pain. Usually such hematomas are small, although occasionally they may become extensive and extend from the vulva through the paravaginal tissues and into the broad ligament. The skin over a large hematoma is often black, shiny, and edematous (Fig. 39-8). When there is extensive extravasation into the tissue spaces, the blood loss may be significant enough to result in hemorrhagic shock. Nonpuerperal hematomas are almost invariably secondary to trauma, and these patients will usually present with such a history.

TREATMENT

Small hematomas with an intact surface can usually be managed by careful observation for evidence of continued enlargement. Bed rest with the application of an ice pack for 12 to 24 h is advisable. If the hematoma continues to enlarge, it will then be necessary to incise the mass, evacuate the blood clot, find the bleeding blood vessels, and ligate them. This is best performed in the operating room setting by a gynecologist. Occasionally, bleeding is diffuse and obvious vessels causing the hematoma cannot be identified. Under these circumstances, the cavity of the hematoma should be carefully packed. Appropriate antibiotic coverage should be given (e.g., cefotetan, ampicillin/sulbactam, or clindamycin and gentamicin), since infection will often develop. Large hematomas should be evacuated. As a general rule, hematomata larger than 5 to 10 cm in diameter should be evacuated, since the risk of complications in such patients is greater than when the hematomas are smaller. Conservative management of large vulvar hematomas often result in the need for subsequent operative interventions because of secondary infection; it may also require transfusions as opposed to when they are managed surgically.

References

1. Stephenson H, Dotters DJ, Katz V, et al. Necrotizing fasciitis of the vulva. *Am J Obstet Gynecol* 166:1324, 1992.
2. Addison WA, Livengood CH III, Hill GB, et al. Necrotizing fasciitis of vulvar origin in diabetic patients. *Obstet Gynecol* 63:473, 1984.
3. Roberts DB. Necrotizing fasciitis of the vulva. *Am J Obstet Gynecol* 157:568, 1987.

Chapter 40

ABDOMINAL AND PELVIC PAIN

Kathy Y. Jones
Veronica T. Mallett

One of the most difficult diagnostic dilemmas in clinical medicine is posed by the woman of reproductive age with complaints of abdominal or pelvic pain. The differential diagnosis encompasses not only diseases of the reproductive tract but also of the gastrointestinal and urinary tracts. Many of the presenting symptoms are similar and overlapping. The patient's first encounter with the primary clinician offers the best opportunity to make the correct diagnosis and avoids overlooking life-threatening conditions for those more benign. Often, patients are seen by multiple services until being admitted to "rule out" a series of conditions. Unfortunately, this type of shifting back and forth can lead to increased morbidity and mortality, as appropriate treatment may be delayed. For example, the woman in whom appendicitis is diagnosed in a timely fashion has minimal morbidity and almost no mortality, with preservation of reproductive function. In contrast, if recognition is delayed until perforation of the appendix, postoperative morbidity is increased and spread of infection can lead to tubal scarring and loss of fertility.

In general, common causes of lower abdominal pain in women have been grouped into three categories: pregnancy-related, gynecological, and nongynecological. The list of potential diagnoses is extensive and it can be difficult to determine into which of these categories a patient's condition falls. In an effort to facilitate a diagnostic approach, these conditions can be classified according to the onset of pain—acute versus chronic. Acute causes of lower abdominal pain can be further subdivided into two general categories, non-inflammatory and inflammatory, based on the presence or absence of fever. To allow the classification of the pain, it is useful to review the origin and nature of abdominal pain. Knowledge of the nature of pain will help to refine likely diagnostic possibilities.

The objective of this chapter is to outline a reasonable approach to the evaluation and management of common conditions known to cause lower abdominal pain in women of reproductive age and older women. This diagnostic approach focuses on presenting symptoms, history taking, clinical features, laboratory tests, and diagnostic procedures found essential to reach the correct diagnosis.

PATHOPHYSIOLOGY

PAIN DUE TO PERITONEAL IRRITATION

Inflammation of the peritoneum is a major source of abdominal pain. Localized peritonitis results from the extension of inflammation to the peritoneum from an adjacent organ such as inflamed uterus and tube, appendix, or gallbladder. Generalized peritoneal irritation can occur with a leaking abscess or contaminated contents of the colon, or it may be sterile, as with exposure to gastric or pancreatic juices. When generalized, peritonitis causes reflex spasms of the overlying muscles, resulting in rigidity and tenderness

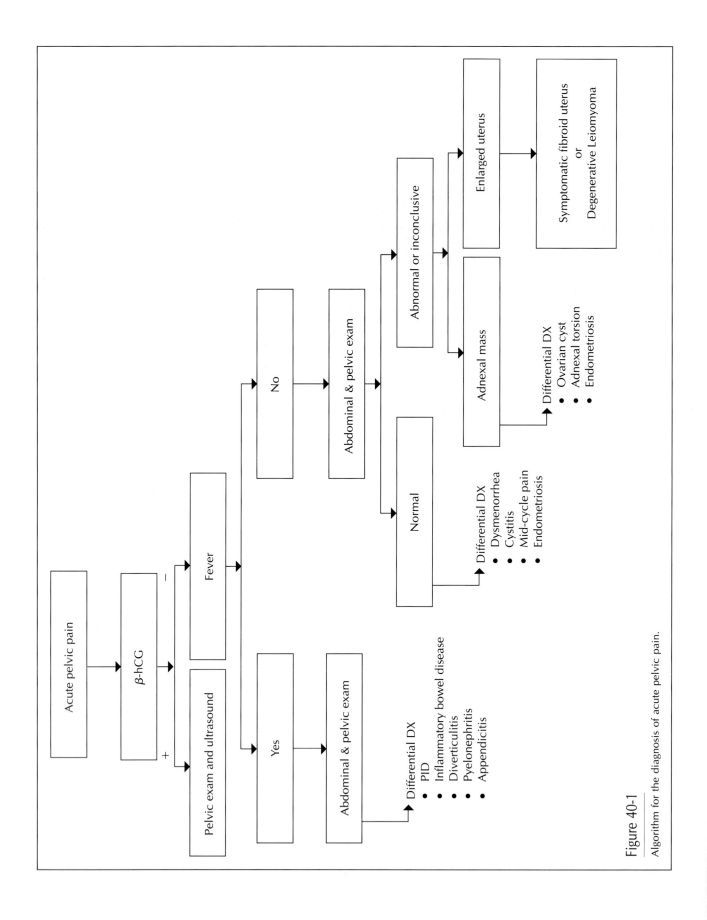

Figure 40-1

Algorithm for the diagnosis of acute pelvic pain.

of the abdominal wall; it manifests itself as rebound tenderness and guarding.

PAIN DUE TO ISCHEMIA

Any type of ischemia—be it somatic, visceral, or cardiac—causes pain. In the reproductive age female, noncardiac causes such as adnexal torsion, bowel strangulation due to adhesion or, rarely, volvulus predominate. In the older female, cardiac or vascular causes are important.

PAIN DUE TO TENSION

Tension in the muscles of the gut or ureter occurs as a result of distention or spasm. *Colic* refers to the wavelike pain associated with a forceful peristaltic reaction. Irritative substances of viral origin or attempts at forcing luminal contents through an obstruction lead to this characteristic pain. Disorders of the upper GI tract or female reproductive organs do not cause colic-like pain. Rapid stretching of the capsule of a solid organ—e.g., the ovary, liver, spleen or kidney—also produces pain. However, slow distention of the capsule of some solid organs (e. g., ovarian neoplasms) is frequently not associated with pain.

HISTORY

The approach to women presenting with abdominal pain follows the basic clinical model directing attention to history, focused physical examination, and laboratory data. The key to making the correct diagnosis begins with careful scrutiny of the patient's history. Important historical data are listed in Table 40-1. The age of the patient is the first diagnostic clue, as certain conditions have a higher prevalence in a particular age group. For example, pelvic inflammatory disease (PID), tuboovarian abscess (TOA), and appendicitis are more common among reproductive-age women. Whereas, diverticular disease is much more common in women in the seventh or eighth decade of life.

The next step entails obtaining an accurate account of the presenting symptoms. The onset, character, location, and duration of the pain are important in delineating which organ system is involved.

ONSET OF PAIN

Pain of sudden onset suggests an acute event. Major consideration are perforation of a hollow viscus, such as a bowel perforation; sudden vascular compromise such as torsion of an ovarian/adnexal mass; or rupture of an ovarian cyst.

Table 40-1

HISTORICAL DATA IN THE EVALUATION OF ACUTE PELVIC PAIN

Age

Characteristics of pain
   Onset/duration
   Palliative/aggravating factors

Associated symptoms
   Urinary symptoms
   Gastrointestinal symptoms
   Fever
   Abdominal bleeding
   Vaginal discharge

Menstrual history

Obstetrical history

Gynecological history
   Pelvic inflammatory disease
   Ectopic pregnancy
   Sexually transmitted diseases
   Fibroid tumors
   Ovarian cysts

Contraceptive history
   Intrauterine device
   Oral contraceptive
   Barrier methods

Surgical history

Social history
   Marital status
   Number of sexual partners
   Current sexual activity

Events such as obstruction of a hollow viscus or inflammation of visceral walls are more gradual in nature. These include appendicitis, salpingitis, and cholecystitis. Pain from these processes takes several hours to reach its peak. These patients will describe a progressive worsening as opposed to immediate, severe pain.

CHARACTER OF PAIN

Patients often describe abdominal and pelvic pain as sharp, dull, achy or throbbing. The character of the pain may provide some clue as to the underlying mechanism. For example, cramping is the major response of the uterus to noxious stimuli. Colic is characteristic of obstruction of a hollow viscus. Pleuritic pain originating in the abdomen is most often the result of an inflamed diaphragm or irritation of the diaphragm as it moves against an inflamed organ or peritoneum. This process can be seen in PID, or acute cholecystitis, or a bleeding, ruptured, ectopic pregnancy.

LOCATION AND RADIATION OF PAIN

Severe abdominal pain that becomes generalized, either gradually or rapidly, is often caused by leakage of irritating fluid into the peritoneal cavity. Irritation is often caused by pus, blood, bile, or gastric juice. Pain that is more localized may offer an indication of the organ involved.

1. Distention of the stomach or upper small intestine produces pain that is in the midline or to the right, just below the xiphoid and above the umbilicus.
2. Small intestinal pain may be periumbilical. Acute appendicitis classically presents with periumbilical pain that localizes to the right lower quadrant.
3. Colon pain is often referred to the midline between the symphysis and umbilicus. Pain along the large intestine may be localized to the site.
4. Pancreatic pain is midepigastric and spreads to the back.
5. Gallbladder distention produces midepigastric pain, eventually spreading to the right upper quadrant. Radiation can be at the right scapula or the shoulder.
6. Rectosigmoid distention produces suprapubic pain, as does bladder distention and cystitis.
7. Threatened inevitable and incomplete abortions are generally accompanied by midline or bilateral lower abdominal pain, usually of a crampy, intermittent nature.
8. Ectopic pregnancy is generally associated with unilateral, continuous, crampy pain that paradoxically may suddenly improve once rupture has occurred.
9. Pelvic inflammatory disease frequently presents with pain that is usually bilateral, dull, and aching in nature and often radiates to the lower back or upper thighs. With a unilateral TOA, the pain may be more severe on the side of involvement.
10. Degenerating myoma will frequently cause sharp, stabbing, or aching pain in the region of the myoma.
11. Corpus luteal and simple ovarian cysts, once ruptured, will produce generalized, aching pain increasing in severity over time, especially if continued bleeding occurs.
12. In the case of adnexal or ovarian torsion, the pain is characteristically colicky, throbbing, or gripping in nature but with an intermittent "waxing and waning" course and a predisposition for the right side.
13. Pain due to urinary calculi can present with colicky, severe flank pain or pain in the inguinal region depending on the location of the calculus.

ASSOCIATED SYMPTOMS

Once the clinician has assessed the presenting symptoms of pain, associated symptoms accompanying the pain syndrome may help to devise the working differential diagnosis. The most common symptoms include fever, anorexia, nausea and vomiting, diarrhea, vaginal discharge, and vaginal bleeding. Other symptoms consist of dysuria, frequency, and dyspareunia. Fever, coupled with symptoms of peritoneal irritation should suggest inflammatory disorders—e.g., PID, TOA, appendicitis, or leaking hollow viscus. Nausea, vomiting, and anorexia are nonspecific symptoms of peritoneal irritation that can be associated with inflammatory conditions as well as hemoperitoneum. Two-thirds of women with ovarian torsion have associated nausea and vomiting. Diarrhea, usually bloody, is a hallmark for diverticulitis, certain infectious diseases (e.g., *Shigella*), and inflammatory bowel disease. Keep in mind that acute episodes of terminal ileitis can mimic acute appendicitis. Complaints of vaginal discharge may be indicative of a sexually transmitted cervicitis associated with PID. Patients complaining of vaginal bleeding should alert the clinician to either pregnancy-related disorders, abnormalities of the menstrual cycle, or certain uterine or cervical abnormalities. Once pregnancy is ruled out, the physician should concentrate on potential etiologies such as dysmenorrhea, dysfunctional uterine bleeding (DUB), symptomatic fibroids, and endometriosis.

MENSTRUAL HISTORY

Menstrual history gives the clinician a sense of the cycle's regularity and duration as well as the average blood loss. It is important to ask the patient if her menstrual cycle has changed since menarche in reference to frequency, length of bleeding, dysmenorrhea or cramps, blood loss, and passage of clots. Patients experiencing primary dysmenorrhea will express a history of severe cramps or "painful periods" since the time of menarche. These patients also can present with accompanying symptoms of nausea and vomiting, headache, diarrhea, and lower backache. Severe dysmenorrhea can be a common symptom when endometriosis is present. Women with symptomatic uterine leiomyomas frequently have long but regular cycles associated with excessive blood loss and passage of clots. Patients with DUB and chronic anovulation typically give a long history of irregular menstrual cycles. If menses occurs only once every 3 to 4 months, it is not unusual for vaginal bleeding episodes to last for 14 to 30 days. Amenorrhea following a normal menstrual intervals strongly suggests the possibility of pregnancy, but "normal menses" does not necessarily rule out pregnancy.

GYNECOLOGIC HISTORY

A patient's obstetric and gynecologic history can be a source of critical diagnostic clues. Past surgical history helps to establish a risk of bowel obstruction or adhesive disease. Adhesive disease in the pelvis or abdomen can be a source of abdominal pain. A history of voluntary or spontaneous abortion and ectopic pregnancy is useful in establishing the likelihood of a pregnancy-related disorder. Patients with a history of an ectopic pregnancy have an increased risk for an ectopic gestation in subsequent pregnancies. It is also important to establish previously diagnosed gynecologic disorders such as ovarian cysts, endometriosis and uterine fibroids. A past history of sexually transmitted diseases (STDs), PID, and multiple sexual partners predisposes patients to the development of PID and TOA.

CONTRACEPTIVE HISTORY

The patient's method of contraception can also be of diagnostic value, especially in the reproductive-age female. The risk of acute PID may be reduced by approximately 50 percent in patients taking oral contraceptive pills or using barrier methods of contraception on a regular basis. Additionally, women using oral contraceptives are at less risk for complications of functional ovarian cysts secondary to cessation of ovulation. Although prior or present use of an intrauterine contraceptive device (IUD) is a well-established risk factor for acute PID, it does not increase the absolute risk for developing an ectopic pregnancy. However, pregnancy that occurs with an IUD in place has a tenfold increased risk of being extrauterine in location. Similarly, a pregnancy that occurs after tubal surgery has a higher chance of being an ectopic. Finally, absence or inconsistent use of contraception should raise the specter of pregnancy or STDs.

SOCIAL HISTORY

The detail of a patient's social history is not often completely explored. In order to accurately assess a patient's propensity for certain gynecological disorders, this area requires thorough investigation. Specific questions examining the number of sexual partners in the last year, type and frequency of sexual activity, as well as the most recent sexual encounter can be helpful in evaluating abdominal pain. Patients with acute PID frequently give a history of recent unprotected sexual intercourse. Patients in a monogamous relationship are less likely to develop acute PID.

PHYSICAL EXAMINATION

After history taking is complete, a careful history examination should be performed. This should include evaluation for the presence of fever; orthostatic changes in blood pressure and heart rate; abdominal and pelvic tenderness; signs of peritoneal irritation (rigidity, rebound tenderness); shoulder pain; vaginal and cervical discharge; cervical erythema; cervical motion tenderness (CMT); uterine size, shape, and consistency; adnexal masses and tenderness; cul-de-sac masses; rectal masses; and nodularity of the uterosacral ligaments. The evaluation for these abnormalities requires not only abdominal palpation but also a speculum examination, bimanual examination, and rectovaginal examination.

OBSERVATION OF THE PATIENT

Observation is an important first step in assessing the woman with abdominal or pelvic pain and is frequently a major clue to determining the severity of her condition. Is the patient restless, as seen commonly with colic, or does she lie immobile in a semi-Fowler's position, as is seen with pelvic inflammatory disease? Is there evidence to suggest impending shock or vascular collapse? Is she chatting or does she prefer to be undisturbed? Taking the time to make such observations can help to guide the extent and rapidity of the workup.

SIGNS OF VASCULAR COLLAPSE

In many disorders presenting as an "acute abdomen," there is a rapid translocation of blood or fluid from the vascular space to the peritoneal cavity or intestinal lumen. Rapid, weak pulse, hypotension, orthostatic changes in blood pressure, moist skin, and restlessness are signs of shock. Early recognition of these signs and vigorous fluid replacement will improve prognosis regardless of the etiology. If a hemoperitoneum is suspected or vigorous vaginal bleeding is occurring, rapid fluid replacement sometimes with blood products is critical. Examples of such disorders are the ruptured ectopic pregnancy, intestinal obstruction, and acute peritonitis.

EXAMINATION OF THE ABDOMEN

In performing an examination of the abdomen for the complaint of abdominal pain, one should make the following observations:

1. Are there signs of peritoneal irritation? This is determined by the presence of abdominal rigidity, rebound tenderness, or involuntary guarding.
2. Character of bowel sounds: Are they hyperactive? Do they come in rushes as in intestinal obstructions, or are they silent, as with peritonitis? They may be present early in the course of ischemia but disappear as the process evolves.
3. Is there a mass or free fluid in the abdomen? If this is suspected, radiography or ultrasonography are indicated.

PELVIC AND RECTAL EXAMINATION

A normal uterus should feel similar in size and consistency to an inverted pear. If the uterus feels larger or is irregular in shape, consider pregnancy or uterine leiomyoma. Prior to menopause, the ovaries are easily palpable in a thin female. After menopause, the adnexa and ovaries should not be palpable. Upon rectovaginal examination, the posterior surface of the uterus, uterosacral ligaments and cul-de-sac can be palpated.

The pelvic exam is sometimes difficult to complete or interpret secondary to adnexal tenderness, which occurs with any type of peritoneal irritation or stretching of the capsule of a visceral organ. The pelvic examination can be helpful to detect: (1) a discrete, palpable adnexal mass; (2) an enlarged uterus; (3) a cul-de-sac mass; or (4) a bulging cul-de-sac due to fluid accumulation. If a patient tells of a history of delayed menses and has an adnexal mass, the diagnosis is an ectopic pregnancy until proven otherwise. If an adnexal mass is detected in the absence of vaginal bleeding and pregnancy, ovarian cysts and adnexal torsion are likely diagnoses. If the diagnosis of pregnancy has been eliminated, an enlarged uterus and vaginal bleeding suggest the presence of uterine leiomyoma. Women with dysmenorrhea usually have normal pelvic findings except for mild uterine tenderness. A cul-de-sac mass or bulging should alert the physician to the possibility of intraperitoneal bleeding, presence of purulent exudate, or abscess as well as a space-occupying lesions such as an ovarian cyst, endometriomas, or fibroid tumors. These abnormal findings warrant further evaluation with diagnostic imaging such as ultrasonography and possibly culdocentesis.

Rectal examinations can be helpful if abdominal examination is unremarkable. A rectal exam may occasionally demonstrate a tender localized mass, as in appendicitis or diverticulitis. In addition, blood in the stool, occult or frank, suggests pathology in the gut.

Table 40-2

DIFFERENTIAL DIAGNOSIS OF ACUTE GYNECOLOGIC INTRAABDOMINAL DISEASE

	Clinical and Laboratory Findings					
Disease	CBC	Urinalysis	Pregnancy Test	Culdocentesis	Fever	Nausea and Vomiting
Ruptured ectopic pregnancy	Hematocrit low after treatment of hypovolemia	Red blood cells rare	Positive. β-hCG low for gestational age	High hematocrit. Defibrinated, nonclotting sample with no platelets. Crenated red blood cells	No	Unusual
Salpingitis	Rising white blood cell count	White blood cells occasionally present	Generally negative	Yellow, turbid fluid with many white blood cells and some bacteria	Progressively worsening; spiking	Gradual onset with ileus
Hemorrhagic ovarian cyst	Hematocrit may be low after treatment or hypovolemia	Normal	Usually negative	Hematocrit generally less than 10%	No	Rare
Torsion of adnexa	Normal	Normal	Generally negative	Minimal clear fluid if obtained early	No	Rare
Degenerating leiomyoma	Normal or elevated white blood cell count	Normal	Generally negative	Normal clear fluid	Possibly	Rare

Table 40-3

DIFFERENTIAL DIAGNOSIS OF ACUTE NONGYNECOLOGIC INTRAABDOMINAL DISEASE

Disease	Clinical and Laboratory Findings					
	CBC	Urinalysis	Pregnancy Test	Culdocentesis	Fever	Nausea and Vomiting
Appendicitis	Normal early; high white blood cell count later	Normal	If patient is pregnant, presentation of disease is typical	Yellow, turbid fluid with many white blood cells and no bacteria	Not early in course	Yes
Retrocecal appendicitis	Normal early; high white blood cell count later	Many white blood cells if abscess forms	Not helpful	May be normal	Yes in advanced disease	Variable
Regional enteritis (Crohn's disease)	High white blood cell count	Normal	Not helpful	Yellow, turbid fluid with many white blood cells	Yes, if severe	Yes, if severe. Recent history of diarrhea
Colonic diverticulitis	High white blood cell count	Normal	Not helpful	Yellow, turbid fluid with many white blood cells and no bacteria	Yes, if severe	Variable
Bowel obstruction	High if ischemic bowel damage is present	Normal	Not helpful	Increased amount of fluid with many white blood cells if bowel is ischemic	Only if bowel is ischemic	Yes

Source: Adapted from Pernoll: *Current Obstetrics and Gynecology: Diagnosis and Treatment.* 7th ed, 1991.

LABORATORY EVALUATION

The diagnostic workup of a woman in the reproductive age group with abdominal or pelvic pain usually requires basic laboratory tests, which should include a complete blood count (CBC), urinalysis, and serum or urine beta human chorionic gonadotropin (β-hCG). The results of the tests should be an integral part of the decision tree as the ultimate diagnosis is formulated. Referring to Tables 40-2 and 40-3, the CBC (noting an elevated WBC) is helpful in identifying inflammatory conditions such as PID, TOA, appendicitis, inflammatory bowel disease, or diverticulitis. A low hematocrit or falling serial hematocrit is suggestive of ongoing bleeding, which can occur with a ruptured ectopic pregnancy or actively bleeding ruptured ovarian cyst. Severe anemia can also be seen with long-standing menorrhagia from

fibroid tumors. The β-hCG is crucial to the diagnosis of pregnancy-related conditions. The urinalysis is helpful in suggesting the diagnosis of acute cystitis or renal calculi by the presence of WBCs or blood, respectively. Cultures for gonorrhea and chlamydia should be obtained from the cervix during the speculum examination.

IMAGING

ULTRASONOGRAPHY

Ultrasonography is a useful diagnostic tool in the evaluation of lower abdominal and pelvic pain. It can be used to evaluate the abdomen and pelvis when patients are unable to cooperate with bimanual pelvic examination. Additionally, it can characterize a pelvic mass, adnexal mass, or uterine size and assess the presence of fluid in the cul-de-sac. It is not as helpful in evaluating conditions of the gastrointestinal tract in the lower abdomen. Ultrasound can also verify an intrauterine gestation. A transvaginal sonogram should be used to evaluate the pelvis and cul-de-sac. If the ultrasonic features suggest the presence of fluid in the cul de sac without a mass, then culdocentesis can be attempted.

RADIOGRAPHIC EXAMINATION

Flat-plate and upright radiographs of the abdomen should be obtained in any woman whose acute abdominal pain is generalized or above the pelvic brim. Findings that may clarify the diagnosis include free air under the diaphragm, indicating a perforated viscus; absent psoas shadow, suggesting retroperitoneal bleeding; small bowel air fluid levels, suggesting small bowel obstruction, a paralytic or mechanical ileus; or large bowel gas and/or fluid levels suggesting volvulus or obstruction.

MANAGEMENT AND SPECIALTY REFERRAL

Certain clinical features, laboratory tests, and diagnostic procedures have been used to help determine the etiology of acute lower abdominal pain. These consists of fever, anorexia, nausea and vomiting, WBCs, serum hCG, hematocrit, urinalysis, culdocentesis, and abdominal/pelvic ultrasound. Tables 40-2 and 40-3 provide a synopsis of each of the above findings in relation to gynecologic and nongynecologic diseases. Fever is a key feature that can be used to identify an inflammatory process. If fever is present and is associated with an elevated WBC, consideration must be given to the potential diagnosis of PID, appendicitis, pyelonephritis or inflammatory bowel disease. Consultation with both the gynecologic and surgical services is appropriate, especially since PID and appendicitis are often difficult to differentiate from each other. Both of these conditions can, on pelvic examination, have cervical motion tenderness (CMT) and other signs of peritoneal irritation. Sometimes right-sided tenderness upon rectal examination can be a distinguishing feature in favor of appendicitis. Suspicion of inflammatory bowel disease and diverticulitis require other radiologic and diagnostic procedures such as barium enema, upper gastrointestinal series, and colonoscopy with biopsy for definitive diagnosis.

If the patient does not exhibit fever and an elevated WBC, the focus of the diagnostic approach should be aimed at noninflammatory conditions. The presence or absence of vaginal bleeding can be used to direct decision making. If pregnancy is confirmed by a positive hCG in the setting of lower abdominal pain with or without vaginal bleeding, then abortion, ectopic pregnancy, and hemorrhagic corpus luteum of pregnancy must be considered. Pelvic examination can be informative if the uterus is enlarged corresponding to gestational age estimated by the last menstrual period. Uterine size that does not correspond to the estimated gestational age in conjunction with an adnexal mass is highly suspicious for an ectopic pregnancy. Serum quantitative β-hCG is helpful to obtain the diagnosis when used in conjunction with ultrasound findings of the endometrial cavity.

Symptoms of vaginal bleeding with a negative pregnancy test and a normal pelvic examination can be found in patients with DUB, dysmenorrhea, and endometriosis. Dysfunctional uterine bleeding in the adolescent and young adult can present with massive hemorrhage and severe anemia. These patients should be stabilized with intravenous fluids or blood products as needed. Coagulopathies, particularly platelet dysfunction, can manifest as irregular heavy vaginal bleeding. Management of DUB is covered in Chapter 38.

The pain syndrome associated with dysmenorrhea responds well to nonsteroidal anti-inflammatory drugs (e.g., naproxen, ibuprofen, ketoprofen, etc). The patient should expect reduction in the severity of symptoms within 2 hours of taking the medication. The patient should be instructed to take the medication every 6 to 8 hours with meals and to continue the medication for at least 3 to 4 days. A follow-up appointment should be made with her primary-care physician or gynecologist in the next few days.

In women with vaginal bleeding and a negative pregnancy test, the findings of an abnormal or inconclusive pelvic examination requires careful consideration. The pelvic exam may reveal either an enlarged uterus, an adnexal mass, or both. In the absence of pregnancy, an enlarged uterus usually suggests the presence of leiomyomas. These tumors can be asymptomatic or can cause varying degree of pelvic pressure and pain as well as heavy vaginal bleeding with menses. With a small to moderate amount of bleeding and a stable hemoglobin, the patient can be managed in a similar fashion as with DUB. The use of NSAIDs may decrease bleeding and also provide relief for any associated dysmenorrhea. The patient can be discharged home with instructions to follow up in the office with her gynecologist. Acute hemorrhage can be temporized with dilatation and curettage of the uterus, requiring gynecologic consultation. Dilatation and curettage serves a twofold purpose. First, it gives the clinician a histologic diagnosis useful for future management. Second, the procedure allows the clinician to obtain information concerning the size and shape of the endometrial cavity as well as to remove the superficial lining of the endometrium. Postoperatively, the patient can be managed with oral contraceptives or progesterone alone. Once bleeding is minimized, the patient can be discharged on these medications with instruction for follow-up in her gynecologist's office. Ultrasonography should be performed when the pelvic exam is abnormal or difficult to characterize, to verify uterine size or the presence of fibroids, characterize the endometrial thickness (which may be suggestive of a polyp or neoplasia), and to evaluate the ovaries.

A pelvic exam that reveals an adnexal mass or fullness in the setting of severe dysmenorrhea suggests the possibility of endometriosis. When endometriosis involves the ovaries, collections of hemolyzed blood can become loculated in the ovarian capsule. These collections are called *endometriomas* and can be palpated as large, fixed adnexal masses. Ultrasound evaluation of the pelvis will show thick-walled cysts with septations and debris. However, an endometrioma, TOA, and hemorrhagic cyst can sometimes be difficult to distinguish solely on sonographic characteristics. Definitive diagnosis requires surgical intervention, most commonly laparoscopy. In the acute setting, endometriosis with severe dysmenorrhea can be treated with NSAIDs. Patients can be discharged home with strict instructions to return to the ED if pain is unresponsive to pain medications or becomes more intense. In the meantime, the patient should schedule a follow-up appointment within 3 to 4 days for counseling and further management.

When the patient does not have vaginal bleeding and pregnancy is excluded, the diagnostic directive is based on the pelvic exam. In the case of a normal pelvic examination and midcycle menstrual status, the diagnosis of mittelschmerz should be considered. There are no diagnostic studies useful for diagnosis, and the treatment is medical, with analgesics or NSAIDs. Patients should be instructed that the pain will dissipate spontaneously and to keep a calendar noting any relationship between the timing of the pain and phase of menstrual cycle. When the pelvic exam is abnormal, revealing an adnexal mass, ovarian cysts and ovarian torsion should be considered. In the reproductive-age woman, these cysts include ovarian endometriomas, corpus luteum cysts, benign cystic teratomas (dermoid cysts), dysfunctional follicular cysts, and serous or mucinous cystadenomas. Uncommonly, ovarian carcinoma can be present in this age group. Evaluation and diagnosis of ovarian cancer is discussed in Chap. 55. Each of these cysts exhibits distinguishing features upon ultrasound evaluation though none are pathognomonic. If a cyst is detected on examination and confirmed with ultrasonography, conservative management is appropriate when there is no evidence of torsion or active bleeding. These patients can be given NSAIDs and should be instructed to follow-up with their gynecologist in the office as soon as possible. If the cyst, with the exception of the dermoid cyst, has ruptured without evidence of ongoing bleeding, the patient can be discharged home with analgesics. Again, instruct the patient to follow-up with her primary-care practitioner or gynecologist. In case of the ruptured dermoid cyst, chemical peritonitis is common and the presenting signs and symptoms are sufficient to warrant emergent surgical intervention. The diagnosis of ovarian torsion is usually established clinically unless Doppler-flow ultrasonography is available. Some authors have utilized color Doppler to establish lack of arterial blood flow. If the diagnosis is considered, gynecologic consultation is necessary. Laparoscopic treatment with untwisting of the adnexa and conservation of the ovary is usually successful. Occasionally, the adnexal tissue is infarcted requiring removal of the involved structures.

When an enlarged, irregularly shaped uterus is found and there is point tenderness over a discrete mass suggestive of a leiomyoma or "fibroid," the diagnosis of degenerating fibroids should be entertained. This should be confirmed with a gynecologic consultation and ultrasound evaluation of the pelvis. Ultrasonographic features of a fibroid uterus include discrete hypoechoic areas within the walls of the uterus as well as other such areas signifying calcifications. The pain syndrome can again be treated with NSAIDs. The patient can be discharged home with instructions to follow up with her gynecologist.

Suggested Readings

1. Dunton C: Torsion of the ovary, in Benrubi G (ed): *Obstetric and Gynecologic Emergencies.* Philadelphia: Lippincott, 1994, pp 275–281.

2. Fales W, Overton D: Abdominal pain, in Tintinalli J, Ruiz E, Krome R (eds): *Emergency Medicine: A Comprehensive Study Guide,* 4th ed. New York: McGraw-Hill, 1996, pp 217–221.

3. Lewandowski G: Nongynecologic infectious and inflammatory diseases in the pelvis, in Copeland L (ed): *Textbook of Gynecology.* Philadelphia: Saunders, 1993, pp 586–591.

4. Mallett V: Gynecologic emergencies, in Tintinalli J, Ruiz E, Krome R (eds): *Emergency Medicine: A Comprehensive Study Guide,* 4th ed. New York: McGraw-Hill, 1996, pp 555–561.

5. Moss T, Cuschieri R: Management of women presenting to the accident and emergency department with lower abdominal pain (letter; comment). *Ann R Coll Surg Engl* 77:396, 1994.

6. Mueller BA, Daling JR, Moore DE, et al.: Appendectomy and the risk of tubal infertility. *N Engl J Med* 315:1506, 1986.

7. Powers R, Guertler A: Abdominal pain in the ED: Stability and change over 20 years. *Am J Emerg Med* 13:301, 1995.

8. Quan M: Diagnosis of acute pelvic pain. *J Fam Pract* 35:422, 1992.

9. Summers P, Pearson J: Medical and surgical considerations in gynecology, in *Current Obstetrics and Gynecology: Diagnosis and Treatment.* Norwalk, CT: Appleton & Large, 1991, pp 866–871.

Chapter 41

PELVIC MASSES

Ellen C. Wells

The discovery of a pelvic mass in a reproductive-age woman may be precipitated by symptoms of pain, pressure, fullness, or increasing abdominal girth. Associated symptoms such as urinary frequency or constipation provide clues to location but do not clearly delineate the tissue of origin, as they may be generated secondary to external pressure on these organ systems. Determining the exact organ from which the mass originates is the most direct way of formulating an appropriate differential diagnosis and proceeding with a timely conclusion and plan.

The presence of a pelvic mass identified on a routine exam or noted as an incidental finding during an evaluation for another complaint deserves appropriate but not necessarily emergent evaluation. Similarly, many complaints associated with pelvic masses are gradually progressive over a number of months and represent the effect of growth on surrounding pelvic functions. The timing of presentation is dependent on when enough symptoms are generated that the woman recognizes a change. An outpatient evaluation is again appropriate.

Masses that present with pain may necessitate admission, depending on the severity of pain, the presence of an acute abdomen, the potential need for immediate surgical attention, or for infections with abscess requiring intravenous antibiotics. Ectopic pregnancy must be considered and a pregnancy test should be performed in any reproductive-age woman with pain and a mass. An intrauterine pregnancy with pain also requires thorough evaluation and may necessitate hospitalization.

DIFFERENTIAL DIAGNOSES

UTERINE MASSES

Masses of uterine origin will be palpable contiguous with the cervix on bimanual exam and, depending on size, be detectable in the abdomen above the level of the pubic symphysis. Pregnancy should be considered in any reproductive-age woman with an enlarged uterus on exam. Particular attention should be directed to her last menstrual period and her contraceptive method. A 6-week gestation may be palpable as a mildly enlarged, boggy uterus. The diagnosis can be confirmed with a positive pregnancy test or an ultrasound showing an intrauterine gestational sac. A 12-week gestation will produce uterine enlargement that fills the pelvis and rises to the level of the pubic symphysis. At this gestation, fetal heart tones can frequently be heard with Doppler. A uterus that is enlarged to the level of the umbilicus would be consistent with a 20-week gestation. By this time fetal movements have frequently been perceived by the woman and fetal heart tones can be heard with a fetoscope. An unsuspected, but somewhat advanced pregnancy may be encountered in adolescence, in obese women, and in women with oligomenorrhea.

Uterine leiomyomas are a common cause of uterine enlargement. Leiomyomas, or myomas, are benign tumors of muscle cell origin and are the most frequent pelvic tumors in women. They occur in one of four white women and one of two black women and are commonly multiple. Locations within the uterus include subserosal, intramural, submucosal, and cervical. Myomas are also occasionally found within the pelvis without a direct attachment to the uterus. The etiology of uterine leiomyomas is incompletely understood. Each tumor results from proliferation of a single muscle cell. The cell of origin may be from a small embryonic rest or from the smooth muscle of blood vessels. The stimulus for growth is also unclear. The role of estrogen as a stimulus has been explored. Estrogen receptors are found in higher concentration in myomas than in the surrounding myometrium. Most myomas decrease in size during hypoestrogenic states such as menopause or during therapy with gonadotropin-releasing hormone (GnRH) agonists (e.g., leuprolide or naferilin). Myomas often enlarge during early pregnancy, with stabilization in size occurring in later pregnancy. Myomas may enlarge with the use of oral contraceptive pills. However, it is also noted that many women with small myomas show no growth under the influence of even high circulating estrogen levels.

Pelvic pain and abnormal uterine vaginal bleeding are the commonest symptoms associated with myomas. One of three women with myomas experiences pelvic pain. Secondary dysmenorrhea is the most frequent complaint. Symptoms of pelvic heaviness or dull aching are common. Myomas with rapid growth (e.g., during pregnancy) may present with severe pain and even localized peritoneal irritation from acute degeneration. This occurs secondary to central necrosis as the tumor outgrows its blood supply. An anterior myoma pressing on the bladder may produce symptoms of urinary frequency and urgency. Abnormal bleeding, usually presenting as hypermenorrhea is reported by 30 percent of women with myomas.

The incidence of leiomyosarcomas in women felt to have leiomyomas is low. Leibsohn[1] reported a series of 1429 hysterectomies with a preoperative diagnosis of leiomyomas in which leiomyosarcomas were found histologically in 0.49 percent. Rapid growth of leiomyomas at any age or growth of myomas after menopause should raise the suspicion of malignancy. Rapid growth in the reproductive-age woman should also alert the physician to the possibility of a pregnancy within a myomatous uterus.

A pelvic mass associated with pain in an adolescent around the time of menarche may be the first presentation of a congenital uterine anomaly. A transverse vaginal septum or an imperforate hymen may present with cyclic monthly pain without menstruation and may progress to a significant pelvic mass consisting of a hematocolpos and hematometra with marked pelvic and rectal pressure. Cyclic pain with menses and a pelvic mass in adolescence may represent a bicornuate uterus with one noncommunicating uterine horn (Fig. 41-1).

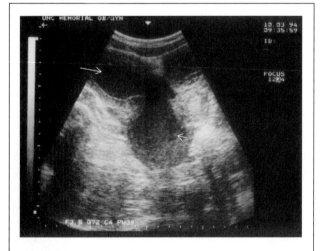

Figure 41-1

Noncommunicating uterine horn (*top left, long arrow*) with hematometra and (*lower midline, short arrow*) hematocolpos.

OVARIAN NEOPLASM

A palpable but otherwise asymptomatic adnexal mass should raise suspicion of an ovarian neoplasm. Benign cystic teratomas, or dermoid cysts, are among the most common ovarian neoplasms. Histologically, these slow-growing tumors are found to contain elements from all three germ cell layers. They occur in all age groups, and are common in teenagers and young adults. They are bilateral in 10 to 15 percent.

Benign teratomas frequently contain a thick sebaceous fluid as well as hair, muscle fibers, cartilage, bone, and teeth. Although they are frequently discovered incidentally, they may produce acute symptoms with rupture, which causes a severe chemical granulomatous peritonitis, or with torsion, which occurs secondary to their size and increased weight. Approximately 1 to 2 percent of dermoid cysts undergo malignant transformation, usually in women over age 40. The malignant component is generally a squamous carcinoma. Rarely, ovarian teratomas will contain functioning thyroid tissue (struma ovarii), causing hyperthyroidism. Other benign ovarian tumors encountered in reproductive-age women include serous cystadenomas, fibromas, and Brenner tumors. Malignant ovarian neoplasms may also occur in reproductive-age women, but most occur in menopausal women. In early stages, these adnexal masses may be mobile with no evidence of ascites, but at advanced stages they will commonly be fixed with accompanying ascites.

OVARIAN CYST

Ovarian cysts are a common cause of adnexal enlargement associated with pain. The term *functional cyst* is often used in this setting, and although dysfunction might be a better description, the term is simply used to convey the association of this cystic enlargement with the components of normal cyclic ovarian function. Normal ovarian follicles reach a size of about 2.0 to 2.5 cm prior to ovulation. Therefore, the term *follicular cyst* should be used to refer to cystic structures within the ovary that are greater than 2.5 to 3 cm in diameter. Follicular cysts may reach 8 to 10 cm in size and generally regress spontaneously in 1 to 3 months. The stretching of the ovarian capsule due to the size of the cyst is the general source of discomfort. Cysts may rupture during examination or with intercourse. Rupture is generally associated with an immediate sharp pain that which may resolve rapidly or gradually improve over several days. Peritoneal signs may be present due to irritation from cyst fluid or blood.

Corpus luteum cysts are less common than follicular cysts. A normal corpus luteum may be up to 3 cm in diameter. Therefore, corpus luteum cysts are described as structures greater than 3 cm in diameter originating from the corpus luteum. In the normal development of a corpus luteum, capillaries invade the granulosa cells and produce a spontaneous but limited bleeding that fills the central cavity. This blood is subsequently absorbed, forming a small cystic space. If hemorrhage is excessive, the cystic space enlarges, stretching the ovarian capsule and causing pain. An unruptured follicular or hemorrhagic cyst may continue to produce symptoms of pain throughout the remainder of the cycle. It will commonly regress after the cycle is complete and hemorrhagic contents will gradually be resorbed. If a hemorrhagic cyst ruptures, a sharp pain as well as peritoneal irritation from the blood will be noted. Bleeding after rupture is usually self-limited. Rarely, women with anemia, marked or persistent pain, hypovolemia, or marked cul-de-sac fluid will require admission for observation, serial hematocrits, or operative intervention.

TORSION

Torsion of the ovary or of the ovary and fallopian tube is a twist or turn of the ovarian attachments through the uteroovarian ligament to the uterus and through the infundibulopelvic ligament to the pelvic side wall, which compromises ovarian blood supply. A woman with adnexal torsion will present with acute, severe, unilateral lower abdominal and pelvic pain. She may relate the onset of pain to an abrupt change in position. A palpable adnexal mass is demonstrated in over 90 percent of patients. Progressive enlargement may occur as arterial blood flow continues, but venous flow is compromised. At the point of arterial compromise, infarction occurs. Associated symptoms include nausea and vomiting, with acute appendicitis or small bowel obstruction in the differential diagnosis. With infarction, an elevated white blood cell count and low-grade fever may be present.

Torsion may occur within a normal adnexa, though any process resulting in ovarian enlargement increases the risk of torsion. Approximately 50 to 60 percent of women with adnexal torsion will be found to have ovarian tumors, with dermoids being the most frequently encountered.[2] Ovarian enlargement from other ovarian cysts, ovulation induction, and paraovarian cysts is also seen in patients with ovarian torsion. Torsion of a malignant ovarian tumor is rare, as the ovarian mass is usually fixed in the pelvis.

ENDOMETRIOSIS

Endometriosis is a disease process in which endometrial glands and stroma develop outside the endometrial cavity. Implants of glands and stroma initially produce cyclic pain associated with menses, which may progress to pelvic adhesive disease resulting in pain throughout the cycle. Endometriosis within the ovarian capsule produces cystic structures called *endometriomas,* which may range from a few millimeters up to 5 to 10 cm in diameter. These are often called *chocolate cysts* due to the thick brown hemosiderin-laden fluid within the cyst. A pelvic exam may reveal tender, enlarged ovaries that are commonly adherent to surrounding structures.

TUBOOVARIAN ABSCESSES

Pelvic inflammatory disease refers to inflammation caused by an infection in the upper genital tracts. This includes endometriosis, salpingitis, oophoritis, myometritis, parametritis, and peritonitis. A tuboovarian complex (see Chap. 44) is defined as a collection of infected fluid within an anatomic space created by adherence of adjacent organs, including the fallopian tubes, ovaries, and sometimes the intestines. Acute pelvic inflammatory disease is usually a polymicrobial infection caused by organisms ascending from the vagina and cervix. Bacterial organisms include *Neisseria gonorrhoeae, Chlamydia trachomatis,* endogenous aerobic and anaerobic bacteria, and perhaps genital mycoplasmal species. Women with pelvic inflammatory disease will commonly have fever, an elevated erythrocyte sedimentation rate, cervical motion tenderness, and bilateral adnexal tenderness with or without masses.[3] Indications for hospitalization in patients with pelvic inflammatory disease include presence of a tuboovarian complex or abscess, pregnancy, uncertain diagnosis, gastrointestinal symptoms, and peritonitis in the upper quadrants. Positive human immunodeficiency virus (HIV) status, recent operative or diagnostic procedures, and inadequate response to outpatient therapy are also reasons for hospital admission.

Women with a history of pelvic inflammatory disease may have sequelae of pelvic adhesive disease presenting as chronic or recurrent pelvic pain with the involved adnexus palpable as a pelvic mass. Approximately 20 percent of women with acute pelvic infections subsequently develop chronic pelvic pain. Recurrent acute pelvic inflammatory disease is experienced by approximately 25 percent of women.

PELVIC MASSES OF RECTAL OR LOWER GASTROINTESTINAL ORIGIN

Pelvic masses presenting in patients with weight loss, anemia, or specific GI symptoms may have a lower GI or rectal origin. Diverticulitis may present with fever and pain localized to the left lower quadrant. A tender, sausage-like, fixed mass may be palpable in the left adnexus on exam. The pathologic change in diverticulitis is a focal area of inflammation in the wall of a diverticulum, usually at its apex, which develops in response to the irritating presence of inspissated fecal material. Appendicitis should be considered in women who present with right-lower-quadrant pain. Anorexia is common, and nausea and vomiting may occur. The pain of appendicitis is initially periumbilical in location but moves to the right lower quadrant. A low-grade fever is typical. The white blood cell count is usually mildly elevated. Examination will reveal tenderness in the right lower quadrant with peritoneal signs present. A mass or fullness may be palpable, depending on the degree of inflammation and adherence of the appendix to surrounding structures. Often no mass is palpable.

Colorectal cancer is a concern in patients, particularly those over 50 years of age, who present with a fixed pelvic mass, history of change in bowel habits, and/or blood in the stool. Carcinomas of the large bowel are predominantly adenocarcinomas and begin as intramucosal epithelial lesions usually arising in adenomatous polyps or glands. Further growth penetrates the muscularis mucosa, invading lymphatic and vascular channels to involve regional lymph nodes and adjacent structures. These cancers may have long periods of silent growth before producing bowel symptoms. Symptoms are typically nonspecific but may present as a change in bowel habit, melena, or rectal bleeding. Abdominal pain, bloating, constipation and diarrhea are more indicative of partial bowel obstruction present in a quite advanced colon carcinoma.

RETROPERITONEAL OR EXTRAPERITONEAL MASSES

Some types of lymphoma, particularly subtypes of diffuse non-Hodgkin's lymphoma, may come to medical attention because of an abdominal mass, splenomegaly, or a gastrointestinal mass with symptoms associated with space-occupying growth. These symptoms include chronic pain, abdominal fullness, early satiety, obstruction, or even gastrointestinal hemorrhage. A mass that is fixed and appears to arise from the pelvic side wall or retroperitoneal space also suggests the diagnosis of lymphoma. However, lymphomas are an unusual cause of pelvic mass.

EVALUATION

HISTORY

The initial history in any reproductive-age woman with abdominal or pelvic complaints should include her age, gravidity, parity, last menstrual period, status of sexual activity, and type of contraception. Symptoms that correlate with the size of the mass may include pressure, fullness, early satiety, or increasing abdominal girth. Conditions producing uterine enlargement may be associated with urinary frequency, urgency, and even stress urinary incontinence. Masses at the level of the cervix or the lower uterine segment or masses exerting pressure at the pelvic brim may present with ureteral obstruction or hydronephrosis and flank discomfort. Masses in the cul-de-sac from the uterus, adnexa, or lower gastrointestinal tract may present as rectal pressure, deep dyspareunia, or fullness and constipation. It is somewhat disturbing to realize that a number of etiolo-

gies for pelvic masses may progress to advanced stages with relatively few symptoms until size alone brings them to the attention of the patient or physician.

In women who present with pain the quality, quantity, location, and duration are all important. The activity associated with the onset of pain should be elicited. An adnexus may twist with a sudden change in position. A common presentation of pain for a woman with a ruptured ovarian cyst is during sexual intercourse. Some 75 percent of women with symptoms of pelvic inflammatory disease develop this disorder within a few days after menses. A ruptured cyst may present as an acute unilateral pain which subsides gradually over time. Torsion and appendicitis can present as acute, unremitting unilateral pain often associated with nausea and vomiting. Bowel obstruction may present in a manner very similar to torsion. A differentiating factor may be that the pain in the bowel obstruction is more colicky or crampy, with waves of pain followed by intervals of relief. Women with any of these sources of pain commonly maintain a fetal position during the interview. Associated gastrointestinal symptoms may include loss of appetite, nausea and/or vomiting, and diarrhea. Any recent fever or chills should be elicited. The presence of flank pain, dysuria, urgency, or frequency should be identified, as urinary tract infection is extremely common.

In addition to the last menstrual period, contraceptive method, and sexual activity, the normal menstrual pattern should be established. If the patient has had any similar pain before, it should be determined whether this was related sequentially to any particular time in her menstrual cycle. It should be noted whether she has a new sexual partner. Previous abdominal or pelvic surgeries, particularly histories of tubal ligation, previous ectopic pregnancy, tubal reconstructive surgery, or gastrointestinal surgery should be elicited. Past gynecologic or gastrointestinal disorders should be noted, such as history of infertility, previous pelvic inflammatory disease, diverticulosis, or polyps. Pertinent family history would include site-specific ovarian cancer, breast and ovarian cancer clusters (BrCa 1) or Lynch syndrome II with family members having colorectal cancer in association with ovarian and/or endometrial cancers.

PHYSICAL EXAMINATION

The physical examination begins with an initial assessment of vital signs. Blood pressure and pulse with orthostatic changes may demonstrate evidence of hypovolemia from acute hemorrhage. An elevated temperature may support a diagnosis of infection. An acute abdomen with fever should alert one to the possibility of a ruptured tuboovarian abscess or a ruptured appendix, which could progress rapidly to sepsis.

The abdomen should be inspected for evidence of distention. Ascites may be determined by shifting dullness or a fluid wave. The presence or absence of bowel sounds should be documented. The upper and lower abdomen should be assessed for masses. Mobility of any masses should also be assessed. Enlarged ovaries, particularly if mobile, may present in the upper abdomen on occasion. These might be missed if the physician relied solely on a pelvic exam. The degree and location of tenderness should be elicited as well as signs of rebound and voluntary or involuntary guarding. The inguinal area should be assessed for lymph nodes.

A pelvic exam is best performed when the bladder is empty, since a distended bladder may be misdiagnosed as a pelvic mass. Even when bladder fullness is recognized, its presence may distort or mask an underlying pelvic mass. A full bladder may lift the uterus and ovaries further away from the vaginal hand, limiting the bimanual examination. A speculum exam should be performed to evaluate the cervix for any evidence of irritation, ulceration, bleeding, or mass. A mucopurulent discharge from the cervix may be examined under the microscope to determine the presence of gram-negative intracellular diplococci (*N. gonorrhoeae*) or to evaluate the number of white blood cells per high-power field (possible *C. trachomatis*). Cultures should be obtained at this time for *N. gonorrhoeae* and *C. trachomatis* in any patient for whom pelvic inflammatory disease is in the differential diagnosis. Bimanual exam allows palpation of the cervix for size and shape as well as any evidence of parametrial extension of induration or fullness. The uterine size, shape, and mobility may also be determined. A "fixed pelvis" with a firm mass effect that extends from side wall to side wall with limited or no mobility suggests extensive pelvic adhesive disease, severe endometriosis, or cancer. A midline nodular mass may be consistent with uterine leiomyomas but could also contain an underlying ovarian enlargement. This differentiation often cannot be determined simply by bimanual examination. Similarly, a pedunculated myoma may be confused with an adnexal mass (Fig. 41-2). Direct and rebound tenderness should be assessed in both the right and left adnexa. The presence of cervical motion tenderness is suspicious for adnexal disease (e.g., acute salpingitis), as movement of the cervix causes stretching across this tissue. In women with marked tenderness, the bimanual examination may be limited and inadequate to determine the presence of a mass. Cul-de-sac fluid or a cul-de-sac mass can best be determined by rectovaginal examination. Similarly, the size and shape of a retroverted uterus can best be determined with a rectal finger. Dissection of an abscess may also occur into the rectovaginal septum. Careful perianal and rectal examination is also necessary to identify perianal or rectal abscesses. The stool should be tested for occult blood. Diverticular abscesses and colon cancer are more likely to be found in the left lower quadrant or cul-de-sac areas; 70 percent of colon cancers are within reach of the examining finger.

An enlarged but soft and boggy uterus may be palpable in early pregnancy. First-trimester pregnancy presenting with midline cramping and vaginal bleeding should be assessed for the possibility of spontaneous abortion. If the cervical os is closed and the bleeding is not profuse, the woman may be followed expectantly for threatened abortion. Follow-up studies including transvaginal sonography and serial quantitative human chorionic gonadotrophin (βCG) values will aid in determining the viability of the pregnancy. Early pregnancy with adnexal pain with or without a mass and associated with light bleeding should be evaluated for the potential of an ectopic pregnancy. These women may give a history of previous pelvic inflammatory disease, previous tubal reconstructive surgery, or previous tubal ligation. A corpus luteum cyst may also present similarly in early pregnancy. Early pregnancy complications are covered in detail in Chaps. 3 and 4.

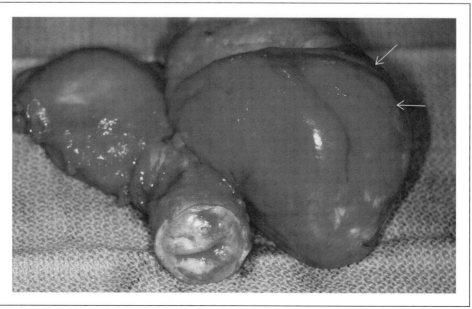

Figure 41-2

A large myoma, arising from the lower uterine segment, extended into the right adnexa.

In adolescence, a pelvic mass and pain should be evaluated for uterine anomalies. A noncommunicating uterine horn may present as cyclic pelvic pain and a pelvic mass. A transverse vaginal septum will be notable on exam as a bulging membrane within the vagina with no cervix visible. Similarly, an imperforate hymen will demonstrate a bulge at the introitus without a vaginal opening. The cervix or uterus can be palpated on rectal exam.

LABORATORY TESTS AND DIAGNOSTIC STUDIES

A hemoglobin, hematocrit, pregnancy test, and white blood cell count should be performed in the initial evaluation. Cultures for gonorrhea and chlamydial infection may be obtained at the time of speculum examination. For suspected ovarian neoplasms, the tumor-associated antigen CA-125, carcinoembryonic antigen (CEA), human chorionic gonadotrophin (hCG), and alpha-fetoprotein (AFP) are useful markers. The CA-125 may be mildly elevated in a number of disease processes that irritate the peritoneal cavity, most notably in endometriosis. It is generally markedly elevated in women with ovarian adenocarcinoma. The CEA is commonly elevated in colon cancer and may be elevated in some ovarian neoplasms. Both hCG and AFP may be elevated in younger patients with malignant teratomas or other germ-cell tumors.

Transvaginal sonography can be extremely helpful in the evaluation of a pelvic mass and is particularly useful in differentiating enlargement of the uterus from that of the ovaries. In the evaluation of female pelvic organs, sonography is usually better and less expensive than computed tomography (CT) or MRI studies. In cases of early pregnancy, a gestational sac may be seen as early as 5 weeks and a fetal pole with cardiac activity at 6 weeks. Ectopic pregnancies may also be visualized within the adnexa, sometimes as an echogenic ring surrounding a small fluid sac. A β-hCG value combined with ultrasound is also helpful in diagnosing an ectopic pregnancy. An intrauterine gestational sac is usually visualized by vaginal sonography when β-hCG values reach 1000. Therefore, the suspicion for ectopic pregnancy increases with β-hCG values at or above this level without visualizing an intrauterine gestation.

Uterine leiomyomas have a distinctive ultrasound pattern within or arising from the uterus (Fig. 41-3). Characteristics of adnexal masses are extremely helpful in differentiating masses of ovarian and fallopian tube origin. A simple cystic structure is consistent with a follicular or corpus luteum cyst (Fig. 41-4A). Recent hemorrhage into an ovarian cyst has a characteristic cobweb pattern (Fig. 41-4B). Benign cystic teratomas contain echogenic material that forms layers consistent with its mucinous secretions as well as areas of calcification from teeth and bone, which may also be seen with conventional radiography. Endometriomas often have a homogeneous ground-glass appearance (Fig. 41-4C). A cystic, tubular, or sausage-shaped structure may represent a

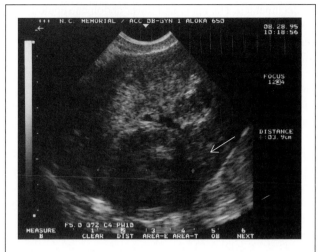

Figure 41-3

Transvaginal sonography reveals a circular pattern within the myometrium consistent with a myoma (*arrow*).

hydrosalpinx. Complex adnexal masses with cystic and solid components with obvious distortion of the normal architecture may be seen with a number of diagnoses, including pelvic adhesive disease, tuboovarian abscess, endometriosis, ectopic pregnancy, or ovarian cancer.

Identification of the organ system with which the mass is associated is important in determining not only the diagnosis but also which specialty services may be required for consultation. In cases where cervical, uterine, or ovarian cancer is suspected, a CT scan is helpful in demonstrating the presence or absence of lymph node involvement, ureteral obstruction, ascites, liver metastasis, or associated pelvic masses. In potential gastrointestinal sources, a CT scan may be beneficial, but may also require barium enema or flexible sigmoidoscopy or colonoscopy.

TREATMENT

In a woman who presents with acute, relentless abdominal pain and a mass, immediate gynecologic or surgical consultation is imperative. It is particularly important to rule out ectopic pregnancy, as a delay in this diagnosis may produce significant morbidity or mortality. Hospitalization is generally required in this setting due to the potential of immediate surgical management or, in cases of an uncertain diagnosis, close observation. Peritoneal lavage or culdocentesis may give a rapid diagnosis of hemoperitoneum. Diagnostic laparoscopy can be helpful in evaluating the presence of hemoperitoneum as well as inspecting the pelvis, the appendix, and the gallbladder.

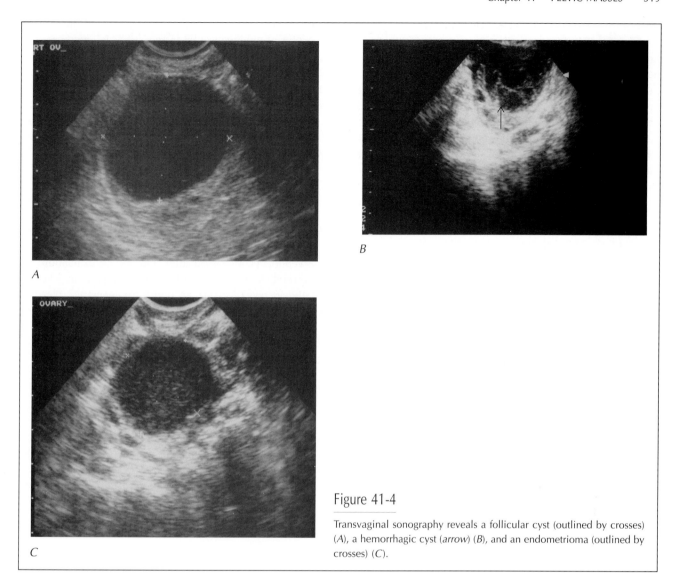

Figure 41-4

Transvaginal sonography reveals a follicular cyst (outlined by crosses) (*A*), a hemorrhagic cyst (*arrow*) (*B*), and an endometrioma (outlined by crosses) (*C*).

If a mass is detected but the patient is otherwise stable, follow-up with a gynecologist is recommended for continued evaluation on an outpatient basis. These women may later be surgical candidates once their evaluation is complete and these results as well as options of management have been thoroughly discussed with the patient and her family.

COMPLICATIONS OF PREGNANCY (see also Chaps. 3 and 4)

In women who present with a pelvic mass and are found to be pregnant, the management depends on any symptoms present. If there are no symptoms of vaginal bleeding or pain, the woman should be referred to an obstetrician to begin or continue her antepartum care. If she has any risk factors for ectopic pregnancy, she should be seen for her initial obstetric evaluation within the next week. Often, follow up is arranged in 48 hours to follow serial β-hCG levels. In women who present with a diagnosis of pregnancy and a mass associated with pain or bleeding, immediate consultation should be obtained to begin the assessment for pregnancy viability and rule out ectopic pregnancy. If an intact intrauterine pregnancy is identified by ultrasound and the cervical os is closed on examination, a threatened abortion is diagnosed and expected management recommended. Women are often placed on "pelvic rest," meaning temporary abstinence from sexual activity and no strenuous physical activity. There is no evidence, however, that these limitations change the natural course of the pregnancy.

In women with a gestational sac by ultrasound but with an open os or those with tissue protruding through an open os, a diagnosis of inevitable or incomplete abortion would be appropriate. These women may need dilatation and curettage to complete this process in a timely manner, particularly if their bleeding has been prolonged or profuse. A quantitative β-hCG will be an important value to obtain in any woman in whom the viability of pregnancy is uncertain. In a normal early pregnancy, the β-hCG value doubles in 48 hours, with the lower limit of normal demonstrating a rise of at least 60 percent over 48 hours. Values that do not rise appropriately or decline are indicative of a failed intrauterine pregnancy or potential ectopic pregnancy. The β-hCG values may also be correlated with ultrasound findings in patients in whom serial values are not available, as previously discussed. Women who are pregnant and present with adnexal pain and bleeding for whom an intrauterine pregnancy is not visualized should be followed with β-hCG values and gynecologic consultation. Diagnostic laparoscopy is particularly useful in suspected ectopic pregnancy. Marked fluid in the cul-de-sac on ultrasound or a positive peritoneal lavage or culdocentesis warrant immediate surgical intervention.

UTERINE LEIOMYOMAS

Treatment of uterine leiomyomas depends on both their size and the severity of the symptoms they produce. Small myomas in an intramural or subserosal location may produce minimal or no symptoms and may be followed expectantly for any evidence of growth. Myomas that create uterine enlargement consistent with or greater than a 12-week gestation, particularly those associated with symptoms or excessive bleeding, should be considered for removal. In addition, their size limits the ability of an examiner to adequately evaluate the ovaries on routine examination. Depending on their shape and location, they may also cause obstruction of the ureters at the level of the pelvic brim or cervix. Uterine leiomyomas may also produce severe dysmenorrhea as well as irregular bleeding and menorrhagia. Nonsteroidal anti-inflammatory drugs decrease prostaglandin release, reducing menstrual pain and decreasing menstrual blood loss. Medroxyprogesterone acetate or depo-medroxyprogesterone acetate may control symptoms by regulating menses or producing amenorrhea. Gonadotropin-releasing hormone agonist therapy decreases the size of uterine leiomyomas by as much as 60 percent.[4] Women also experience amenorrhea on this therapy, with a subsequent rise in their hematocrit. Limitations of GnRH agonist therapy include hot flashes and other menopausal symptoms. Its use is generally limited to 6 months, as use beyond this point is associated with bone loss. The reduction in size of uterine leiomyomas does not persist after discontinuation of therapy and virtually all leiomyomas return to their pretreatment size. Surgical options include myomectomy, which involves removing the individual leiomyomas without complete removal of the uterus, versus hysterectomy. The blood loss at the time of surgery is generally higher with myomectomy than with hysterectomy. Among women followed after myomectomy, approximately 25 to 30 percent subsequently undergo a second surgical procedure for recurrent myomas and symptoms. Women who have not completed childbearing may choose myomectomy over hysterectomy despite the increased intraoperative blood loss and potential recurrent symptoms. Women who are followed expectantly should have ultrasound evaluation of the ovaries on a regular basis if the ad-

nexa are not easily palpable on examination. Hysteroscopic resection of submucosal or intracavitary leiomyomas may be used for therapeutic relief in appropriate patients. Women who present with acute pain due to degenerating leiomyomas may be managed with nonsteroidal anti-inflammatory drugs or may require narcotic analgesics in the initial period. Common times for presentation of degenerating leiomyomas are during pregnancy and in the immediate postpartum period.

UTERINE ANOMALIES

In adolescents who present with congenital uterine or lower genital tract anomalies as a source of pelvic mass, surgical intervention is warranted after appropriate evaluation. An imperforate hymen or transverse vaginal septum may be surgically opened to create an outlet for menstrual bleeding (Fig. 41-5). A symptomatic noncommunicating uterine horn will require removal. These women face an increased risk of endometriosis due to the retrograde menstruation that has commonly occurred prior to their diagnosis.

ADNEXAL MASSES

Adnexal masses that, on evaluation, are felt to be consistent with benign ovarian neoplasms will be treated surgically with removal via ovarian cystectomy or unilateral oophorectomy. Frozen section is extremely useful in these instances, as a borderline tumor or carcinoma may then be appropriately staged and lymph node sampling obtained.

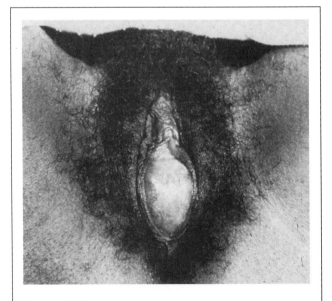

Figure 41-5

Imperforate hymen with associated hematocolpos. (From Baramkita: *J Reprod Med* 29:376, 1984.)

The initial treatment for an ovarian cyst is observation with analgesics as needed for pain. The majority of follicular cysts resolve spontaneously within 4 to 8 weeks of initial diagnosis. Hemorrhagic cysts, if self-contained, gradually resorb without further management. Oral contraceptive therapy is sometimes employed to remove any influence that pituitary gonadotrophins may have on the persistence or recurrence of an ovarian cyst.[5] Surgical therapy is recommended for cystic masses larger than 8 cm or for those from 5 to 8 cm that have been observed for longer than 8 weeks in menstruating women without any evidence of regression. A ruptured hemorrhagic cyst may require admission for serial hematocrits or, with hemoperitoneum, surgical intervention with cystectomy. Women with a complex adnexal mass and severe pain or an acute abdomen should be evaluated surgically for torsion. An adnexus that has remained viable despite torsion can be untwisted at the time of surgery. A cystectomy is performed and the ovary is stabilized with suture to prevent recurrence. In torsion with vascular compromise and infarction, salpingo-oophorectomy is required.

An endometrioma may be treated with analgesics and hormonal therapy for suppression of endometriosis. Medications that can be employed include oral contraceptives, depomedroxyprogesterone acetate, danocrine, and GnRH agonists. Each of these medications has potential side effects but may produce relief of symptoms. With persistent or severe pain, operative laparoscopy or laparotomy may be employed. Conservative operative therapy includes removal of endometriomas, cautery or excision of endometrial implants, and lysis of adhesions. More aggressive management might include removal of one or both ovaries. The extent of therapy depends on the severity of symptoms and the patient's desire for future childbearing.

In women who present with pelvic inflammatory disease and tuboovarian abscesses, intravenous antibiotic therapy is indicated. The Centers for Disease Control and Prevention have recommended two regimens stressing the polymicrobial etiology of acute pelvic infections and addressing the need for coverage of *C. trachomatis* and some penicillin-resistant *N. gonorrhoeae* (Table 41-1).[6] In women with *C. trachomatis,* a regimen using doxycycline is preferred, with a 14-day course required to completely eradicate this organism. Clindamycin, however, is felt to provide better penetration into an abscess cavity. Therefore, the combination of clindamycin and gentamicin is considered the gold standard for treatment of tuboovarian abscesses. Ampicillin is often added to treat enterococcus. Aztreonam is a potential substitute for the aminoglycosides to avoid renal toxicity when renal disease is present (2 g IVq8h). In women with pelvic inflammatory disease and an intrauterine device (IUD) present, the IUD should be removed after antibiotics have begun. If abscesses do not respond to intravenous antibiotics within 48 to 72 hours, drainage is indicated. Women with cultures positive for *N. gonorrhoeae* or *C. trachomatis* should also inform their sexual partners to seek treatment. Recurrent acute pelvic inflammatory disease is experienced

Table 41-1

INPATIENT TREATMENT FOR PELVIC INFLAMMATORY DISEASE

Regimen A[a]
  Cefoxitin 2g IV q6h

or

Cefotetan 2 g IV q6h
            PLUS
Doxycycline 100 mg IV or PO q12h

Regimen B[a]
  Clindamycin 900 mg IV q8h

and

Gentamicin 2 mg/kg loading dose, followed by 1.5 mg/kg q8h maintenance dose

[a]Each regimen should be continued for 48 h after the patient has shown clinical improvement, after which doxycycline 100 mg PO b.i.d. (after regimen A or B) or clindamycin 450 mg PO q.i.d. (alternative choice for regimen B) should be continued for a total of 14 days' therapy.

by approximately 25 percent women. The risk of ectopic pregnancy, infertility, and chronic pelvic pain are increased, even in "successfully" treated women.

DIVERTICULITIS

Women with acute diverticulitis generally require hospitalization for bowel rest, intravenous fluids, and broad-spectrum antibiotics. "Triple therapy" (e.g., ampicillin, gentamycin, and metronidazole) remains the gold standard in the unstable septic patient, although newer single-agent antibiotics (ampicillin/sulbactam, Impipenum/cilastatin or ticarcillin clavulanate) may be employed for more stable patients with local peritoneal signs. Recurrent attacks may prompt surgical resection. Severe attacks with peritoneal signs, suspected abscess, or perforation require intravenous antibiotics and surgical drainage or resection. A diverting colostomy and resection may be performed acutely, with reanastomosis accomplished at a second operation.

COLORECTAL CANCER

In colorectal cancer, total resection of the tumor is the optimal management. Tumor-related symptoms of gastrointestinal bleeding or obstruction may require immediate management that may result in a less radical procedure. Therefore, when possible, a complete preoperative workup for extent of disease and presence of metastases should be performed. This includes a chest radiograph, liver function studies, plasma CEA level, and complete colonoscopy. After resection, women should be followed for 5 years with semiannual exams, repeat CEA levels (which have been shown to be very sensitive for tumor recurrence), and periodic endoscopic or radiographic surveillance of the large bowel. Radiation therapy is commonly used after resection in cancers that penetrate the serosa or involve regional lymph nodes. This therapy reduces the risk of local recurrence but does not appear to prolong survival. Chemotherapy has had only marginal benefit with advanced cancers.

LYMPHOMA

Therapeutic options for the management of lymphomas are based on histologic subtype and, less frequently, stage. Therefore, tissue biopsy of sufficient quantity to determine pathologic and immunologic subtype is of primary importance. Other studies commonly employed to evaluate extent of disease include a complete blood count, chemistries, liver function studies, serum protein electrophoresis, chest radiograph, CT of the abdomen and pelvis, and bone marrow biopsy. Surgical staging is *not* routine in non-Hodgkin lymphoma and is controversial in Hodgkin lymphoma. Radiotherapy may cure over 80 percent of patients with localized Hodgkin lymphoma and chemotherapy over 50 percent of cases with disseminated disease. Non-Hodgkin lymphoma

may similarly be treated with radiation and chemotherapy but with less promising results. Women with disease resistant to conventional or salvage regimens may be given high-dose chemotherapy or combined chemotherapy and radiation therapy with bone marrow transplantation.

References

1. Leibsohn S, d'Ablaing G, Mishell DR Jr, et al: Leiomyosarcoma in a series of hysterectomies performed for presumed uterine leiomyomas. *Am J Obstet Gynecol* 162:968, 1990.
2. Hibbard LT: Adnexal torsion. *Am J Obstet Gynecol* 152:456, 1985.
3. Hager WD, Eschenback DA, Spence MR, et al: Criteria for diagnosis and grading of salpingitis. *Obstet Gynecol* 61:113, 1983.
4. Friedman AJ, Hoffman DI, Comite F, et al: Treatment of leiomyomata uteri with leuprolide acetate depot: A double-blind, placebo-controlled, multicenter study. *Obstet Gynecol* 77:720, 1991.
5. Steinkampf MP, Hammond KR, Blackwell RE: Hormonal treatment of functional ovarian cysts: A randomized prospective study. *Fertil Steril* 54:775, 1990.Centers for Disease Control and Prevention: 1993 Sexually transmitted diseases: Treatment guidelines. *MMWR* 42:75, 1993.
6. Centers for Disease Control and Prevention: 1993 Sexually transmitted diseases: Treat ment guidelines. *MMWR* 42:75, 1993.

Chapter 42

SEXUALLY TRANSMITTED DISEASES

Sebastian Faro

Sexually transmitted diseases (STDs) constitute one of the largest groups of infectious diseases that are worldwide in their distribution. No sexually active individuals are immune from infection if they place themselves at risk by indiscriminately participating in sexual intercourse. Transmission of sexual diseases is best controlled through prevention. The most logical approach to prevention is one of education, a process that requires the involvement not only of health care providers but also of members of the community, e.g., teachers, parents, etc.

Treatment programs directed against acute infection, to eradicate the offending organism(s), are already in place. New antimicrobials continue to be developed. They now have a broader spectrum of activity, are longer-acting, and remain in the tissue for longer periods. However, without meaningful educational programs, individuals will continue to place themselves at risk for infection. The goals of any treatment program are not solely the eradication of the offending organism but also the prevention of sequelae, which may have far-reaching adverse effects. These could even include damage to the fallopian tubes, which may place the individual at risk for an ectopic pregnancy or result in infertility.[1]

Physicians and nurse practitioners as well as other health care providers should become familiar with the epidemiology of these infections; in turn, they should be able to determine which individuals are at risk for contracting an STD. It is important to remember that it is not only the individual's behavior that places her at risk for contracting an STD but also that the behavior of her partner may also affect her health. Within every community there is likely to be a pool of individuals who are infected and serve as reservoirs for the dissemination of STDs. Some of these individuals do not seek treatment because they are asymptomatic, and others are treated but become reinfected. Hence, the STD pool maintains its stability. Individuals who come in contact with anyone in this STD pool serve as vectors, disseminating disease to unsuspecting partners with whom they have had sexual contact. If an infected individual travels to other areas of the United States or the world and engages in sexual intercourse, the disease can be transmitted still further.

DIAGNOSIS AND MANAGEMENT OF SEXUALLY TRANSMITTED DISEASES

The initial step in the management of any STD is to obtain a detailed history to determine the degree of risk and the types of infection(s) to which the individual has most likely been exposed. The initial interview does not have to be long. Typically, women who may have an STD usually seek medical attention for one of three reasons: lower abdominal pain, irregular vaginal bleeding, or discharge, or fear that they have contracted an STD. They commonly think that they have either vaginal candidiasis or bacterial vaginosis, neither of which is an STD. However, it is important to remember that vaginal trichomoniasis is a sexually transmitted disease, and its presence indicates that the patient may also harbor other STDs or bacterial vaginosis.

The interview should begin by determining the duration of the symptoms. Questions may be posed as follows:

1. When did the symptoms first begin?
2. Have you had a fever?
3. Have you had nausea and/or vomiting?
4. Have you noticed a change in your vaginal discharge with regard to color, odor, and amount?
5. Have you had irregular uterine bleeding prior to this episode?
6. Are you sexually active?
7. How old were you when you first engaged in sexual intercourse?
8. How many sexual partners have you had in your lifetime?
9. How many sexual partners have you had in the past year?
10. How many sexual partners have you had in the last 3 months?
11. How many sexual partners do you currently have?
12. Do you suspect that your current partner(s) is having sex with other individuals?
13. Do you suspect your current or past partner(s) of being bisexual?
14. Have you ever had gonorrhea, chlamydial infection, herpes, syphilis, human papillomavirus, human immunodeficiency virus (HIV) infection, or hepatitis?
15. Have you ever been exposed to anyone with an STD?
16. Have you ever been told you had pelvic inflammatory disease (PID)?
17. Have you ever been treated for an STD?

Questions such as those listed here will also determine the individual's risk of contracting an STD. Once the interview has been concluded, the patient should be prepared for the examination, which should begin with a detailed inspection of the vulva, vestibule, vagina, and cervix. Things to look for include lesions such as ulcers, blisters, excoriations, pustules, rashes, and areas of swelling with cellulitis. A vaginal examination includes determining the status of the vaginal ecosystem. The cervical examination should include the detection of endocervical mucopus, the presence of endocervical epithelial hypertrophy, and whether or not the endocervical epithelium bleeds easily. Specimens for the culture or detection of *Neisseria gonorrhoeae* and *Chlamydia trachomatis* should also be obtained. The examination concludes with a bimanual palpation and motion of the cervix, uterus, and adnexa.

SYPHILIS

The etiologic agent of syphilis is *Treponema pallidum.* Transmission is via contact of mucosal surfaces, predominantly through sexual intercourse. Asexual transmission can occur, however, by kissing an individual with an oral lesion, through perinatal acquisition, or via a blood transfusion. The disease has three stages:

1. Primary. May last up to 3 months.
2. Secondary. Begins approximately 3 to 6 weeks after the primary chancre appears, is highly infectious.
3. Latent phase.
   a. Early latent phase. Seropositive but asymptomatic. Up to one year in duration, it is highly infectious.
   b. Late latent phase. More than one year in duration; pregnant women may transmit the infection in utero up to 4 years into this period.
4. Tertiary (late syphilis). Includes benign tertiary syphilis and involvement of the cardiovascular and central nervous systems.

PRIMARY SYPHILIS

Primary syphilis is characterized by the presence of an asymptomatic chancre, usually solitary with bright-red margins that are raised with an indurated base. Secondary infection may alter the appearance of the chancre in that the base may be covered with a gray or yellow scab. Typically, chancres are found on the vulva, labia, vaginal walls, and cervix, but they may actually occur at any site of inoculation. Inguinal lymphadenopathy tends to be present and is usually bilateral.[2]

Diagnosis is made either by dark-field microscopy or serology. Dark-field microscopy can be used on lesions associated with secondary syphilis—e.g., chancre, maculopapular skin rash, and condylomata lata. Serology should be obtained on all patients suspected of having syphilis and will be positive 3 weeks after the appearance of the primary chancre. In most cases a lesion will not be noted. However, in all cases of suspected contact with an individual known to have syphilis, serologic testing should be performed. If the initial serology is negative, the test should be repeated within 1 month. The initial tests are nonspecific screening tests, the rapid plasma reagin (RPR), which is the most commonly employed test; the venereal disease research laboratory (VDRL) test, or the automated reagin test.[3] If the nonspecific test is positive, then a fluorescent treponemal antibody absorbed (FTA-ABS) test or microhemagglutination assay for antibodies to *T. pallidum* (MHA-TP) is performed. The FTA-ABS and MHA-TP are highly specific and tend to remain positive for life. Therefore, this test is of value only in those individuals who have not already had syphilis.[4,5]

In early primary syphilis, 30 percent of infected individuals will have a nonreactive nontreponemal test on their first visit. If these individuals are suspect, then the test should be repeated in 1 week, 1 month, and 3 months. Individuals with a negative test at 3 months can be considered noninfected. Individuals with secondary syphilis usually have a titer >1 : 16. But people known to have had a negative titer in the previous year should be considered to have early latent syphilis. If this information is not known, the individual should be considered to have late latent syphilis and should be evaluated for neurosyphilis. It should be noted that approximately 20 percent of the individuals with latent syphilis will have negative serology when a nontreponemal test is employed. These individuals should have a spinal tap, and if the VDRL is positive, a diagnosis can be made. However, a negative cerebrospinal fluid (CSF) VDRL does not rule out the possibility of neurosyphilis. A CSF with increased lymphocytes (>5 mm^3) and elevated total protein (≥ 45 mg/dL) are highly suggestive of central nervous system disease.[6]

The nonspecific nontreponemal screening tests are also used to follow the efficacy of treatment for both primary and secondary disease. The VDRL or RPR should be obtained 3 to 4 months following therapy, and there should be a fourfold decline in titer. By 6 to 8 months, there should be an eightfold decline.[6,7] Patients with early syphilis who are successfully treated will have a negative serology after 1 year, whereas individuals treated for latent syphilis will have a slower rate of decline in titer.[8] Approximately 50 percent will have a low titer after 2 years following treatment. A fourfold rise in titer signals reinfection.

False-positive nontreponemal tests may occur following a viral infection, other bacterial infections, fever, recent immunization, and other treponemal infections. Patients with early human immunodeficiency virus (HIV) infection may yield a false-positive test for syphilis. Individuals with an autoimmune disease, narcotic addiction, or chronic bacterial infection may also yield a false positive RPR, VDRL, or automated reagin test (ART). Although specific tests for *T. pallidum,* the FTA-ABS, or MHA-TP remain positive for life, however, there is approximately a 1 percent false-positive rate.[7–10]

Diagnosis

The differential diagnosis should include the following:

Herpes simplex
Chancroid
Lymphogranuloma venereum
Granuloma inguinale
Traumatic lesion
Furuncles
Drug eruptions
Bechet disease
Carcinoma

Treatment

Treatment[11] of primary syphilis is with benzathine penicillin G, 2.4 million units intramuscularly in a single dose.

Patients allergic to penicillin who are not pregnant are given tetracycline 500 mg PO q.i.d. for 14 days, or doxycycline 100 mg PO b.i.d. for 14 days. Patients who are pregnant should be hospitalized for desensitization.[11]

SECONDARY SYPHILIS

Early secondary syphilis is characterized by a variety of clinical manifestations: chancre, condylomata lata, maculopapular rash, inguinal lymphadenopathy, and alopecia. However, the individual may also be asymptomatic, and this type of syphilis is likely to be found in the pregnant patient. She is likely to transmit the infection transplacentally, even during the asymptomatic phase.

Diagnosis in women, especially during pregnancy, is made using serologic evidence. The patient may present with chancres or a rash that appears pale red in color and is distributed over the entire body, including the palms of the hands and soles of the feet. The condylomatous lesions are waxy and usually involve the vulva and perirectal area. This lesion, like all lesions of secondary syphilis, is highly infectious. The patient may present with malaise, myalgias, headache, and sore throat—a typical flulike syndrome. The patient may also develop asymptomatic splenomegaly that may present as hepatitis. Additionally, alopecia may occur spontaneously.

Diagnosis

The differential diagnosis includes the following:

Rubella
Measles
Drug rashes
Erythema multiforme
Early Kaposi sarcoma
Condylomata acuminata

Treatment

Treatment[11] of early secondary syphilis (<1 year) is with benzathine penicillin G 2.4 million units intramuscularly in a single dose.

Late secondary syphilis (≥ 1 year) is treated with benzathine penicillin G 7.2 million units total, administered in three doses of 2.4 million units intramuscularly each, weekly for 3 weeks.

The Jarisch-Herxheimer reaction may occur within a few hours of the administration of the penicillin. It is characterized by fever as well as skin and mucosal lesions. The exact mechanism is not known, but it is thought that the reaction is linked either to a release of endotoxin or the production of antibodies due to the rapid release of antigens. Pregnant patients treated for syphilis should be monitored for several hours (up to 12), as intrauterine death has been reported following treatment and the occurrence of the Jarisch-Herxheimer reaction.[12,13]

HERPES SIMPLEX

It is estimated that there are 55 million people in the United States afflicted with genital herpes. Genital infection is most commonly due to herpes simplex type 2, whereas oral and ocular herpetic disease is the result of infection with type 1.

Primary infection commonly presents as disseminated disease covering the vulva with numerous lesions. Manifestations of genital infection are usually preceded by systemic prodromal symptoms—e.g., fever, malaise, and myalgias. Some individuals also develop headache, thus presenting a symptom complex resembling a flulike syndrome. Vulvar infection begins with the appearance of multiple small blister-like lesions or vesicles. These are painful to touch and spontaneously become unroofed, leaving behind small or even pinpoint defects or ulcers. Vesicles of close proximity may coalesce to form a large ulcer that may be mistaken for a chancre. Individuals with primary herpes often develop bilateral inguinal lymphadenopathy, severe dysuria, and urinary retention. The vulva may also become significantly edematous and erythematous.

There is a subset of patients who may not have experienced a primary episode of genital herpes but have antibodies to herpes simplex. When these individuals experience their first episode of genital herpes, they do not develop numerous lesions covering the external genitalia. Typically, they develop several lesions that are painful but do not develop either vulvar edema or urinary retention. These individuals usually complain of dysuria.

DIAGNOSIS

The disease is usually diagnosed on the basis of clinical findings. However, the diagnosis should be confirmed by either culture and identification of the virus, antigen detection, immunofluorescence, or enzyme-linked immunosorbent assay (ELISA).[14,15] A diagnosis of genital herpes simplex should not be made without good supportive information (e.g., a positive culture), since it will have a significant impact upon the patient's personal relationships and the delivery of children. The cost for identification of herpes should not be prohibitive and should be in the range of $50. Although the clinical presentation of genital herpes simplex is distinctive, it can easily be mistaken for other diseases.

Clinically, primary genital herpes presents with a large number of blisters or vesicles symmetrically distributed over the vulva. The lesions associated with recurrent infection are usually localized in clusters (typically a single cluster). There may be only a single lesion, and the recurrence is usually in the same area. The patient with recurrent disease characteristically experiences a prodrome at the site where the lesion will appear, e.g., itching, burning, pain, and tingling.

If culture and isolation of the virus are to be undertaken, the vesicle or blister should be aspirated or unroofed and the fluid present used to inoculate tissue cultures. If an ulcer is present, the base should be swabbed and this specimen used for inoculating a tissue culture for the detection of herpes simplex virus. If the ulcer is covered with a purulent exudate, a secondary infection is present and the exudate must be removed in order to take a specimen for culture. If the base of the ulcer appears red and clean, it will be suitable for use to obtain virus. This can be achieved by rubbing the base vigorously with a sterile cotton- or Dacron-tipped swab and inoculating tissue culture vials.

A tentative diagnosis can be established by directly staining the aspirated fluid or scrapings with either the Tzanck test or the Giemsa, Wright-Giemsa, or Papanicolaou stains.[16,17] However, this is not a very sensitive technique and will only detect approximately 50 percent of the cases. Other detection methods, which have greater sensitivity and specificity, include immunofluorescence and ELISA.

Herpes simplex infection may present as any of the following:

Labial lesions (cold sore, fever blisters)
Oral lesions
Pharyngitis
Gastrointestinal lesions
Pneumonia
Hepatitis
Herpetic whitlow
Keratitis
Eczema herpeticum
Encephalitis
Genital lesions
Disseminated infection
Newborn infection

TREATMENT

Primary herpetic infection is treated with acyclovir 200 mg PO five times a day for 10 days[11] or valacyclovir 500 mg PO b.i.d. for 10 days.

Recurrent herpetic infection is treated with acyclovir according to one of the following regimens:

200 mg PO five times a day for 5 days[11]
400 mg PO t.i.d. for 5 days[11]
800 mg PO b.i.d. for 5 days[11]

Recurrent herpetic infection may also be treated with valacyclovir 500 mg PO b.i.d. for 7 days or famciclovir 125 mg PO b.i.d. for 5 days.

Disseminated herpetic infection is treated with acyclovir 5 to 10 mg/kg of body weight administered intravenously every 8 h until clinical resolution is obtained.[11]

For suppressive therapy, one may give acyclovir in one of the following regimens:

400 mg PO b.i.d. for 1 year[11]
200 mg PO q.i.d. for 1 year
400 mg PO b.i.d. for 1 year
400 mg PO q.i.d. for 1 year

It would appear that famiciclovir in a dose of 250 to 500 mg administered orally once a day for a year should also be satisfactory for suppressive therapy.

LYMPHOGRANULOMA VENEREUM

The etiologic agent is *C. trachomatis,* serovars L1, L2, and L3; these should not be confused with the serovars responsible for cervicitis, endometritis, and salpingitis. This bacterium is a true parasite because it requires an exogenous source of adenosine triphosphate (ATP), which is derived from the host. It also utilizes amino acids from the host. It has a unique life cycle consisting of two stages: an extracellular stage known as the *infectious stage* and an intracellular stage known as the *metabolic phase.*

The diagnosis of lymphogranuloma venereum (LGV) can be established by clinical findings combined with the use of specific laboratory tests that include the complement fixation test, the microimmunofluorescent test with a titer >1:512, and the isolation of the organism in tissue culture.[18]

Clinically, LGV presents in one of three stages: primary, secondary, and tertiary.

Primary LGV is characterized by the development of an ulcer or chancre, which appears approximately 1 to 3 weeks after inoculation.[19,20] The ulcer, unlike that seen with syphilis, lasts for only a few days and is painful. The lesion may initially develop as a small papule or may appear herpetiform and then be confused with herpes.

Secondary LGV is characterized by the development of unilateral inguinal lymphadenopathy. The femoral lymph nodes may also become involved. Poupart's ligament separates these two groups of lymph nodes, creating the characteristic "groove sign." The lymph nodes may become large and tender and can often be extremely painful. They become soft and are referred to as *buboes.* They may continue to enlarge and rupture spontaneously, with the expression of a thick, purulent exudate.

The patient may develop extragenital lesions with buboe formation. One example is Parinaud's oculoglandular syndrome, which is characterized by the development of conjunctivitis and enlarged maxillary lymph nodes. The infected patient commonly develops systematic dissemination, a fever, and malaise and may also develop pneumonitis, hepatitis, and meningoencephalitis. On rare occasions, the patient may present with a clinical picture of erythema multiforme or erythema nodosum. Another clinical presentation is acute proctocolitis with involvement of the perirectal lymphatics.[21] Clinically, the patient has proctitis, anal pruritus, rectal pain, and tenesmus. The rectal mucosa may become edematous and friable, bleeding easily. Multiple erosions may develop in the mucosa and infection can lead to the development of abscesses. The patient also develops perirectal abscesses and fissures. The perirectal lymphatics become enlarged and obstructed, resembling hemorrhoids. These enlarged, obstructed lymphatics are referred to as *lymphorrhoids.* Further progression of the disease process can lead to the formation of rectovaginal fistulas as well as the development of granulomatous tissue and fibrosis. This leads to rectal stricture formation approximately 3 to 5 cm above the anocutaneous junction. Stricture formation significantly narrows the rectum, giving rise to thin stools, referred to as *pencil stools,* which are characteristic of this stage of LGV.

The lymphatics of the vulva may become involved, giving rise to significant edema. Sclerosing ulcerations may also form and are typically painful. This condition is known as *esthiomene,* tertiary or late-stage LGV; it is characterized by vulvar elephantiasis. Ulcerations of the urethra may occur, disrupting its integrity. This may result in incontinence. Rectovaginal fistulas also develop and strictures may occur in the pelvis along with significant granulation tissue resembling a "frozen pelvis."

DIAGNOSIS

The differential diagnosis includes the following:

Early Inguinal Syndrome
Syphilis
Chancroid
Genital ulcers
Granuloma inguinale
Cat-scratch fever
Filariasis
Incarcerated inguinal hernia
Inguinal lymphadenitis secondary to a septic lesion of the lower extremity

Anorectal Syndrome
Malignancy
Trauma
Tuberculosis
Schistosomiasis
Fungal infection
Parasites

TREATMENT

Treatment[11] is with doxycycline 100 mg PO b.i.d. for 21 days.

Alternative regimens include the following:

Erythromycin 500 mg PO q.i.d. for 21 days (recommended regimen for pregnant patients)
Sulfisoxazole 500 mg PO q.i.d. for 21 days

CHANCROID

The etiologic agent is *Haemophilus ducreyi,* a gram-negative bacillus. The organism is transmitted by mucosal contact with a lesion and should be isolated by culture to establish a diagnosis. The incubation period following contact is 7 days or longer in women. The lesion begins as a papule, develops into a pustule, and then forms a well-circumscribed ulcer.[22] The edges are irregular, undermined, and surrounded by an erythematous halo. The lesion is typically painful, but in women the chancre can be asymptomatic and not easily differentiated from a syphilitic chancre. The patient may develop unilateral inguinal lymphadenopathy, which is often painful. The enlarged lymph node appears erythematous; after 1 to 2 weeks, the center becomes fluctuant and ulcerates.

DIAGNOSIS

The organism can be cultured directly from a lesion and the specimen should be obtained by directly swabbing it. The laboratory should be contacted prior to obtaining the specimen to ensure that proper preparations are made for receiving it. A special medium is required for the growth and isolation of *H. ducreyi,* such as Sheffield's medium or two different types of media.[23,24]

TREATMENT

Treatment[11] consists of any of the following:

Azithromycin 1 g PO in a single dose, or
Erythromycin 500 mg PO b.i.d. for 5 days, or
Amoxicillin/calvulanic acid 250 mg PO b.i.d. for 7 days, or
Ceftriaxone 250 mg IM in a single dose

Alternative therapy may be given with:

Trimethoprim/sulfamethoxazole 160 mg/180 mg PO b.i.d. for 10 days, or
Ciprofloxacin 500 mg PO b.i.d. for 3 days, or
Ofloxacin 400 mg PO b.i.d. for 3 days, or
Spectinomycin 2 g IM once

GRANULOMA INGUINALE

The etiologic agent is *Calymmatobacterium granulomatis,* which belongs to the family Brucellaceae. This disease is also known by the name *donovanosis* because the staining material from a lesion reveals elliptical structures found within mononuclear cells and polymorphonuclear leukocytes, referred to as *Donovan bodies.*[25] Typically, Giemsa and Wright stains are utilized and reveal characteristically stained bacilli within the host cells. The bacteria are deeply stained along the lateral edges and at each end give the organism an image that resembles a safety pin.[26] When stained with Gram reagents, the organism is gram-negative.

The organism is endemic to southern India, western Australia, tropical regions of Africa, Vietnam, Indonesia, Papua New Guinea, and the West Indies. It has also been reported in the southern part of the United States.[27]

Clinically, ulcerative lesions appear on the external genitalia. The lesions are usually multiple, rupture spontaneously, and form round elevated, velvety granulomatous ulcers. They bleed easily and are infectious. As subsequent lesions develop, secondary to autoinoculation, involvement of regional lymph nodes occurs. Scarring of the lymphatics may occur, giving rise to pseudoelephantiasis. Indolent masses may occur in the inguinal area, forming granulomatous lesions in the subcutaneous tissue. This may lead to scarring adjacent to the lymphatics, causing strictures and obstruction resulting in pseudoelephantiasis.

DIAGNOSIS

The diagnosis is made by the identification of Donovan bodies in clinical specimens obtained from a chancre. An immunofluorescent antibody test using Donovan bodies as the antigen has been developed.[28]

Differential Diagnosis
Syphilis
LGV
Chancroid
Anogenital amebiasis

TREATMENT

One of the following may be used:

Clotrimazole 2 tablets PO t.i.d. for 14 days
Tetracycline 500 mg PO q.i.d. for 14 days
Erythromycin 500 mg PO q.i.d. for 14 days

GONORRHEA AND *CHLAMYDIA TRACHOMATIS*

The etiologic agent is *N. gonorrhoeae,* a gram-negative diplococcus typically seen in clinical specimens within polymorphonuclear leukocytes. When this observation is made, the diagnosis can be assumed to be present and treatment initiated. The organism is predominantly transmitted through sexual contact.

Infection of the cervix tends to be asymptomatic, whereas infection of the urethra and Skene's and Bartholin's glands tends to be symptomatic (e.g., purulent discharge, associated cellulitis, swelling, and frequently abscess of the gland). Unlike the case with *C. trachomatis* infection, salpingitis or upper genital tract infection secondary to *N. gonorrhoeae* tends to be symptomatic. It is not uncommon to find these two organisms causing simultaneous infection; therefore, treatment should always be directed against both these bacteria. It has been reported that the two bacteria can be found as coinfecting organisms in 60 to 80 percent of these cases.

Individuals who complain of symptoms of cystitis and are found to be bacteriuric should be evaluated for the possible existence of the urethral syndrome. This can be accomplished by detecting the presence of white blood cells (WBC) in the urine, with a negative culture for typical uropathogens. A swab can be inserted into the urethra and the specimen cultured for *N. gonorrhoeae, C. trachomatis, Mycoplasma hominis,* and *Ureaplasma urealyticum.* This is important, because, except for ofloxacin, antibiotics typically employed to treat cystitis are not effective against the STD organism.

Serovars A through K causes the same types of infections as *N. gonorrhoeae.* However, this organism appears to be more prevalent in certain regions of the United States, while *N. gonorrhoeae* appears to be prevalent in the southern regions. The significant difference between the two STDs is that *C. trachomatis* tends to cause asymptomatic disease and is probably responsible for the greatest number of cases of fallopian tube damage resulting in unsuspected infertility.

Therefore, when patients are screened for any STD, they should be screened for both *C. trachomatis* and *N. gonorrhoeae*. These two organisms are found as coinfecting agents in approximately 60 percent of cases. Treatment should always be directed against the probability that both bacteria are present. Treatment regimens are discussed below, under "Gonorrhea."

Chlamydia trachomatis is diagnosed either by culture, DNA recognition tests, ELISA, or direct fluorescent antibody test. When specimens are collected, they should be taken with a Dacron applicator on a plastic shaft to avoid the potential exposure of toxic substances found in the adhesive used in cotton-tipped applicators. The specimens for culture must either be transported to the laboratory immediately or frozen at $-70°C$ ($-158°F$) until processed. Specimens for either antigen detection or nucleic acid analysis are usually fixed when placed in the specific transport system.

BARTHOLIN'S AND SKENE'S GLAND ABSCESS

Skene's and Bartholin's gland abscesses typically present with a clinical picture of swelling, erythema, and pain. The area overlying the gland may be indurated with no evidence of spontaneous drainage. This is usually due to the fact that the duct draining the gland has become occluded and thus blocked. The gland continues to expand, causing the tissue and skin overlying the abscess to become inflamed and indurated and eventually to thin out. This is an important process because it is at this stage that surgical intervention, coupled with medical therapy, is likely to be successful. Facultative and obligate anaerobic bacteria are commonly found to be involved in a Bartholin's and Skene's gland abscess.

Prior to initiating surgical management of a Bartholin's or Skene's gland abscess, a sterile needle should be inserted into the mass and the fluid that is aspirated sent for Gram staining. The needle should be left in place as a guide to the exact location and depth at which the abscess should be incised. The incision should be approximately 0.5 to 1 cm in length, just long enough to admit the Word catheter. The balloon of the Word catheter should be filled with sterile normal saline, and it should be left in place and allowed to become dislodged spontaneously. It is necessary for the catheter to remain in place for six weeks, thus allowing the incision to reepithelize, forming a new canal.

The Gram stain can be extremely helpful in allowing the physician to choose appropriate antibiotic therapy. For example, the following Gram-stain results may be found:

- Gram-negative intracellular diplocci = probably *N. gonorrhoeae*
- Gram-negative bacilli, morphologically similar = probably facultative anaerobic bacteria, e.g., *Escherichia coli*

- Gram-negative rods, pleomorphic = probably *Prevotella* or *Bacteroides*
- Gram-negative rods, fusiform = *Fusobacterium*
- Gram-negative and Gram-positive bacteria = polymicrobial infection, most likely involving facultative and obligate anaerobic bacteria
- Gram-positive cocci = *Streptococcus agalactiae* or *Staphylococcus aureus*
- Gram stain reveals WBC but no bacteria = should suspect *C. trachomatis* or *M. hominis*

The characteristics of the aspirate fluid can be of assistance in establishing a diagnosis. The presence of a purulent fluid would indicate an abscess. Cloudy serous fluid with the presence of WBCs but no bacteria suggest *Mycoplasma*. Clear serous fluid with no detectable bacteria or WBCs indicates a cyst. Bloody fluid would suggest trauma or malignancy.

An alternative to using a Word catheter is to marsupialize the gland. This can be accomplished by anesthetizing the area with 1% lidocaine (Xylocaine) via infiltration of the area as well as placing a pudendal block. An elliptical incision should be made over the vermilion border, excising a strip of tissue that is sent to the pathologist for histologic evaluation. Once the gland is entered, it should be irrigated with sterile normal saline until all purulent material has been removed. The physician should also ensure that no areas of loculated pus remain. The edges of the abscess and the dermis should be sutured together with simple interrupted stitches (marsupialization). The gland should then be packed with gauze, which is left in place until removed within 48 h. Packing prevents the gland from becoming secondarily infected and/or collapsing and scarring shut. If the gland is not packed, it will collapse and create a closed compartment that can easily become reinfected. If, after the initial 48 h, the cavity is dry (not producing an exudate) and the inflammatory response has resolved, the gland does not have to be repacked.

Skene's gland abscess can be managed in a fashion similar to that described above for Bartholin's gland abscess. Aspirating its contents, incising, irrigating, and packing with gauze is all that may be needed. In incising a Skene's gland, care should be taken not to enter the urethra and disrupting its integrity.

CERVICITIS

Gonococcal cervicitis is typically asymptomatic but may present with subtle signs of infection. The patient may note a sudden onset of postcoital bleeding or dyspareunia. Examination may reveal the presence of endocervical mucopus or hypertrophy of the endocervical epithelium.[29] Gentle palpation of the endocervix with a sterile cotton- or Dacron-tipped applicator may precipitate brisk bleeding. Palpation and motion of the cervix may result in patient complaints of tenderness or pain. Specimens from the endocervix should be obtained with a Dacron-tipped applicator for the isolation of *N. gonorrhoeae* and *C. trachomatis*.

ENDOMETRITIS

Endometritis usually presents as mild lower abdominal pain or cramping. All patients in the reproductive age group with a complaint of lower abdominal pain should receive a pregnancy test even if they are using contraception or have had a tubal ligation. Frequently, these complaints are overlooked and the patient has no indication of infection. The patient may also relate that she began by having breakthrough bleeding, even though she has been taking the same oral contraceptive pill for years. Individuals not taking the oral contraceptive pill may report the recent onset of irregular uterine bleeding. Specimens should be obtained by utilizing an endometrial sampling device, such as the Pipelle.[30] The biopsy should be divided into two specimens. One should be placed in an anaerobic transport medium and taken to the microbiology laboratory immediately for processing for the cultivation, isolation, and identification of facultative and obligate anaerobic bacteria. The other portion should be sent for histologic evaluation, particularly seeking plasma cells. The presence of plasma cells indicates that the patient may indeed have an upper genital tract infection.

SALPINGITIS

Salpingitis due to gonococcal infection tends to be symptomatic, in contrast to chlamydial infection which tends to be asymptomatic.[31] The patient complains of lower abdominal pain, which may range from mild to severe. She may or may not be febrile, have nausea, and show signs of peritonitis. In fact, the patient with a mild infection may be asymptomatic and is likely to develop damage to the fallopian tubes unknowingly.[32,33] There are no clinical symptoms or laboratory tests that are pathognomonic of PID.

It is important to determine if the individual who is suspected or known to be infected can be treated as an outpatient or if she requires hospitalization. Individuals who do not have nausea, signs of peritonitis, and/or fever ≥38°C (100.4°F) can be treated as outpatients. These women must be reevaluated within 72 h to determine if their response to therapy is appropriate. Individuals not showing signs of improvement should be admitted to the hospital for further evaluation and possible laparoscopy. Salpingitis is discussed further in Chap. 44.

TREATMENT OF GONOCOCCAL AND CHLAMYDIAL INFECTIONS

Treatment[11] is guided by the principle that one must always administer an antibiotic regimen that is effective against both *N. gonorrhoeae* and *C. trachomatis*. If the patient is suspected of having her disease for more than 7 days, an antibiotic therapy that is effective against not only the STD but also against aerobic, facultative, and obligate anaerobic bacteria should probably be initiated.

Urethritis and Cervicitis

Neisseria gonorrhoeae
The following antibiotics are administered in a *single dose:*

Ceftriaxone 125 mg IM, or
Cefixime 400 mg PO, or
Ciprofloxacin 500 mg PO, or
Ofloxacin 400 mg PO

Alternative treatment regimens:
Doxycycline 100 mg PO b.i.d. for 7 days

The following are administered in a single dose intramuscularly:
Spectinomycin 2 g, or
Ceftizoxime 500 mg, or
Cefotaxime 500 mg, or
Cefotetan 1 g, or
Cefoxitin 2 g

The following are administered *orally in a single dose:*
Cefuroxime axetil 1 g, or
Cefpodoxime proxetil 200 mg, or
Enoxacin 400 mg, or
Lomefloxacin 400 mg, or
Norfloxacin 800 mg

Chlamydia trachomatis
The following are administered orally:
Doxycycline 100 mg b.i.d. for 7 days

Alternatives:
Azithromycin 1 g in a single dose, or
Ofloxacin 300 mg b.i.d. for 7 days, or
Erythromycin base 500 mg q.i.d. for 7 days, or
Amoxicillin 500 mg t.i.d. for 7 days

If gonococcal cervicitis is documented, 25–50% of patients will be coinfected with chlamydia.[34] As such, a presumptive diagnosis of chlamydial infection should be made and the patient treated unless a documented negative chlamydia test is confirmed. Sexual partners of these women should be referred for treatment.

Endometritis

Since this is a polymicrobial infection, a broad-spectrum antibiotic must be employed. In addition, the patient should also be considered to have involvement of the fallopian tubes even though this may not appear to be the case on bimanual pelvic examination.

The following oral regimens are effective against *N. gonorrhoeae*, *C. trachomatis*, and *gram-positive* and *gram-negative* aerobic, facultative, and obligate anaerobic bacteria:

Amoxicillin/clavulanic acid 500 mg t.i.d. for 7 days

Metronidazole 500 mg t.i.d., pus ofloxacin 300 mg b.i.d. for 7 days

Clindamycin 300 mg t.i.d. plus ofloxacin 300 mg b.i.d. for 7 days

Salpingitis (see Chap. 44)

TRICHOMONIASIS

Trichomoniasis is caused by the flagellated protozoan *Trichomonas vaginalis.* The organism's life cycle is unknown. Transmission is predominantly via sexual intercourse. Although the organism may apparently exist in a dormant state, it is not known whether there is a resistant cystic state that enables it to survive unfavorable conditions. Resistant strains have been reported, but their presence is not as significant as poor patient compliance with medication regimens, reinfection, and poor absorption of medication via the gastrointestinal tract. (See Chap. 43 for more indepth discussion.)

DIAGNOSIS

The diagnosis is typically established by identifying the organism on microscopic examination of the patient's vaginal discharge. The organism can also be identified on Pap smear and by nucleic acid testing (currently under investigation). It can also be easily isolated from the vaginal fluid and cultured on Diamond's media.

TREATMENT

Metronidazole is the agent of choice and there is truly no other effective antimicrobial agent available in the United States. It may be taken orally in either of the following dosages:

2 g in a single dose[11]

500 mg b.i.d. for 7 days[11]

Successful treatment depends upon patient compliance and the simultaneous treatment of her partner, who should also wear a condom during sexual intercourse until it has been documented that the condition is resolved. This practice should be followed when any STD treatment is undertaken.

Metronidazole should not be administered to pregnant patients in the first trimester, but it can be administered in the second and third trimesters.

In the event of treatment failure:

1. Do not treat with metronidazole gel.
2. Treat with metronidazole 500 mg b.i.d. or t.i.d. PO for 7 days.
3. If the above regimen fails and the patient has been compliant in taking her medication and has not been having sexual intercourse or is utilizing a condom, the following are recommended:
   a. Metronidazole 500 mg t.i.d. PO for 7 days plus a 500-mg intravaginal metronidazole suppository at bedtime for 10 days, or
   b. 500 mg metronidazole IV q6h for 7 days
4. The patient must refrain from sexual intercourse through the treatment period.
5. One week after completing therapy, a follow-up examination should be performed, including
   a. Microscopic examination of the vaginal discharge
   b. Culture of the vaginal discharge for detection of *T. vaginalis,* especially if the organism has not been detected microscopically
   c. pH determination of the vaginal discharge (a healthy vaginal ecosystem has a pH of 3.8 to 4.1)
6. If the above regimen is unsuccessful, the patient should be referred to a physician with a special interest in vaginal infections.

BACTERIAL VAGINOSIS

Bacterial vaginosis (BV) is not considered to be an STD but can be considered as a condition that is associated with sexual intercourse. The frequency of recurrence of this condition does appear to be related to the frequency of sexual intercourse. It should be viewed not as an infection or disease but as a disturbance in the vaginal microecosystem (see Chap. 43). The significance of BV is that it may be a precursor to postoperative infection, preterm labor, premature rupture of amniotic membranes, and preterm birth.[35] Therefore, until its relationship to these entities can be established with a degree of certainty, BV should be sought and, when identified, treated.

DIAGNOSIS

Clinically, BV is relatively easy to diagnose using the microscope, as signs and symptoms alone are not reliable. The condition can be identified by (1) determining the pH of the vaginal discharge, (2) performing a "whiff test," and (3) performing a microscopic examination of the vaginal discharge. These are accomplished by obtaining a portion of the vaginal discharge by wiping the lateral vaginal wall with a cotton-tipped swab and placing a drop or two on a glass slide. One to two drops of concentrated potassium hydroxide (KOH) are then added and mixed in thoroughly. Finally, the mixture is sniffed to determine whether it has a fishlike odor. In addition, a specimen of the vaginal discharge obtained from the lateral vaginal wall may be mixed with $\cong 2$ mL of normal saline and stirred vigorously. This will dilute the vaginal discharge, allowing for a more meticulous microscopic examination. One to two drops are placed on a glass slide and covered with a glass coverslip. The preparation is then examined under 40× magnification. Microscopically, BV is characterized by

Clue cells
Numerous individually free-floating bacteria
The absence of a dominant bacterial morphotype
The noticeable absence of WBCs

The *diagnosis* of BV is established by at least three of the following

- a pH >4.5
- a positive whiff test
- Adherent, white, nonfloccular homogeneous discharge
- Presence of clue cells

The presence of a dominant bacterial morphotype or abnormal numbers of WBCs suggests another diagnosis (e.g., *Trichomonas vaginitis*).

A healthy vaginal ecosystem is characterized by

A pH between 3.8 and 4.2
A negative whiff test
Squamous epithelial cells without adherent bacteria
The cytoplasmic membrane and nucleus of the squamous epithelial cells, which are easily identified and not obscured by adherent bacteria
Large bacillary forms are the dominant morphotype; this represents lactobacilli.

TREATMENT

1. Clindamycin intravaginal cream (2%), one applicator full each night for 1 week. This preparation is oil-based and may weaken latex condoms, diaphragms, or cervical caps[11]
2. Metronidazole intravaginal gel (0.75%) b.i.d. for 5 days[11]
3. Clindamycin 300 mg PO b.i.d. for 7 days[11]
4. Metronidazole 2 g PO in a single dose[11] (may be associated with higher recurrence rates)
5. Metronidazole 500 mg b.i.d. for 7 days[11]

References

1. Faro S: Quinolones for the treatment of *Neisseria gonorrhoeae* and *Chlamydia trachomatis*. *Infect Dis Obstet Gynecol* 1:108, 1993.
2. Csonka GW, Oates JK: Syphilis, in Csonka GW, Oates JK (eds): *Sexually Transmitted Diseases*. Philadelphia: Baillière Tindall, 1990, pp 227–276.
3. March RW, Stiles GE: The reagin screen test: A new reagin card test for syphilis. *Sex Transm Dis* 7:66, 1980.
4. Hunter EF, Mckinney RM, Maddison SE, Cruce DD: Double staining procedure for fluorescent treponemal antibody-absorption (FTA-ABS) test. *Br J Vener Dis* 55:105, 1979.
5. Coffey EM, Braford LL, Naritomi LS, Wood RM: Evaluation of the qualitative and automated quantitative microhemagglutination assay for antibodies to *Treponema pallidum*. *Appl Microbiol* 24:26, 1972.
6. Lukehart SA, Hook EW, Baker-Zander SA, et al: Invasion of the central nervous system by *Treponema pallidum*: Implications for diagnosis and therapy. *Ann Intern Med* 109:855, 1988.
7. Jaffe HW, Larsen SA, Jones OG, Dans PE: Hemagglutination tests for syphilis antibody. *Am J Clin Pathol* 78:230, 1978.
8. Goldman JN, Lantz MA: FTA-ABS and VDRL slide test reactivity in a population of nuns. *JAMA* 217:53, 1971.
9. Buchanan CS, Haserick JR: FTA-ABS test in pregnancy: A probable false-positive reaction. *Arch Dermatol* 102:322, 1970.
10. Kraus SJ, Haserick JR, Lantz MA: Fluorescent treponemal antibody-absorption test reactions in lupus erythematosus. *N Engl J Med* 282:1287, 1970.
11. Centers for Disease Control and Prevention: Sexually transmitted diseases—Treatment guidelines. *MMWR* 42:RR-14, 1993.
12. Negussie Y, Remick DG, DeForge LE, et al: Detection of plasma tumor necrosis factor, interleukins 6 and 8 during the Jarisch-Herxheimer reaction of relapsing fever. *J Exp Med* 175:1207, 1992.
13. Fekade D, Knox K, Hussein K, et al: Prevention of Jarisch-Herxheimer reaction by treatment with antibodies against tumor necrosis factor α. *N Engl J Med* 335:311, 1996.
14. Yolken RH: Enzyme immunoassays for the detection of infectious antigens in body fluids: Current limitations and future prospects. *Rev Infect Dis* 146:35, 1982.
15. Vestergaard BF, Jensen O: Diagnosis and typing of herpes simplex virus in clinical specimens by the enzyme-linked immunosorbent assay (ELISA), in Nahmias AJ, Dowdle WR, Schniazi RF (eds): *The Human Herpesviruses*. New York: Elsevier–North Holland, 1981, pp 343–349.
16. Naib ZM, Nahmias AJ, Josey WE: Cytology and histopathology of cervical herpes simplex infection. *Cancer* 19:1026, 1966.
17. Naib ZM: *Exfoliative Cytology*. 2d ed. Boston: Little, Brown, 1976, pp 493–499.
18. Wang SP: A simplified method for immunological typing of trachoma–inclusion conjunctivitis–lymphogranuloma venereum organism. *Infect Immun* 7:356, 1973.
19. Abrams AJ: Lymphogranuloma venereum. *JAMA* 205:59, 1968.
20. Coutts WE: Lymphogranuloma venereum: A general review. *WHO Bull* 2:545, 1950.
21. Dan M, Rotmench HH, Eylan E, et al: A case of lymphogranuloma venereum of 20 years duration: Isolation of *Chlamydia trachomatis* from perianal tissue. *Br J Vener Dis* 56:344, 1980.
22. Hammond GW, Slutchuk V, Scatliff J, et al: Epidemi-

ology, clinical, laboratory and therapeutic features of an urban outbreak of chancroid in North America. *Rev Infect Dis* 1:867, 1980.

23. Hafiz S, Kinghorn GR, McEntegart MG: Sheffield medium for *Haemophilus ducreyi. Br J Vener Dis* 60:196, 1984.

24. Nsanze H, Plummer FA, Magwa A, et al: Comparison of media for the primary isolation of *Haemophilus ducreyi. Sex Trans Dis* 11:6, 1984.

25. Kuberski T: Granuloma inguinale (donovanosis). *Sex Trans Dis* 7:26, 1980.

26. Rosen T, Tschen JA, Ramsell W, et al: Granuloma inguinale. *J Am Acad Dermatol* 11:433, 1984.

27. Sehgal VN, Shyamprasad AL, Bechar PC: The histopathological diagnosis of donovanosis. *Br J Vener Dis* 60:45, 1984.

28. Westrom L, Joesoef J, Reynolds G, et al: Pelvic inflammatory disease and fertility. *Sex Trans Dis* 19:185, 1992.

29. Brunham RC, Paavonen J, Stevens CE, et al: Mucopurulent cervicitis: The ignored counterpart in women of urethritis in men. *N Engl J Med* 311:1, 1984.

30. Martens MG, Faro S, Hammill HA, et al: Transcervical uterine cultures with a new endometrial suction curette: A comparison of three sampling methods in postpartum endometritis. *Obstet Gynecol* 74:273, 1989.

31. Sweet RL, Blankfort-Doyle M, Robbie MO, Schater J: The occurrence of chlamydia and gonococcal salpingitis during the menstrual cycle. *JAMA* 255:2062, 1986.

32. Westrom L: Effect of acute pelvic inflammatory disease on fertility. *Am J Obstet Gynecol* 121:707, 1975.

33. Westrom L, Joesoef J, Reynolds G, et al: Pelvic inflammatory disease and infertility. *Sex Trans Dis* 19:185, 1992.

34. Centers for Disease Control and Prevention: Recommendations for the prevention and management of *Chlamydia trachomatis* infections. *MMWR* 42(RR-12), 1993.

35. Amsel R, Totten PA, Spiegel C, et al: Non-specific vaginitis: Diagnostic criteria and microbiological and epidemiological associations. *Am J Med* 74:14, 1983.

Chapter 43

VAGINITIS

Jack D. Sobel

Vaginal symptoms are extremely common; they are responsible for millions of visits annually to gynecologists' offices. Vaginal discharge is among the 25 most common reasons for consulting physicians in private office practice in the United States.[1] It is found in more than 25 percent of women attending sexually transmitted disease (STD) clinics. Not all women with vaginal symptoms have vaginitis; however, approximately 40 percent of those with vaginal symptoms will have some type of vaginitis.

With 40 million individuals uninsured in the United States and a tradition of millions of Americans lacking a regular primary care physician, additional millions of visits annually take place in emergency departments. Such visits are of two varieties, including (1) those women with severe symptoms who are unable to wait the several hours needed to see their practitioners and (2) women with less acute symptoms who utilize these facilities as their primary site of health care delivery.

Readers are referred also to the chapters on STDs (Chap. 42) and vulvar disease (Chap. 39), since there is considerable overlap in symptomatology. Vaginitis is rarely if ever associated with mortality or even with hospitalization; accordingly, there is a marked tendency to trivialize this entity. The most obvious manifestation of this is the practice of diagnosing the cause of vulvovaginal symptoms inaccurately. Accurate diagnosis is the foundation of effective management and empiricism is the realm of the inept.

A major error in medical education has been to equate vulvovaginal symptoms with vaginitis; this is compounded by a tendency to equate vaginitis with infectious vaginitis. Of the infectious causes of vaginitis, three common entities—bacterial vaginosis (BV), vulvovaginal candidiasis (VVC), and trichomoniasis—are responsible for over 90 percent of vaginal infections (Table 43-1). This chapter emphasizes the provision of a rational diagnostic management approach to the symptomatic patient instead of the tradi-

tional approach, found in most textbooks that deal only with candidal vaginitis, bacterial vaginosis, and trichomonal vaginitis. The recent availability of over-the-counter antimycotics has profoundly influenced the differential diagnosis and management of women with vulvovaginal symptoms.

APPROACH TO THE PATIENT WITH VAGINAL SYMPTOMS

Symptoms related to vaginitis include vaginal discharge, pruritis, and a variety of manifestations of inflammation of the vagina, introitus, and vulva, depending upon the extent and severity of the inflammatory reaction (Table 43-2). These symptoms include soreness, irritation, discomfort, dysuria, and dyspareunia. Physicians frequently fail to inquire about the association of these symptoms with sexual activity and thus lose valuable insight into the chronicity and cause of symptoms. Coitus constitutes a nonspecific but useful "stress test" in establishing the presence, site, and extent of vaginal and introital inflammation.

A thorough history should be obtained, including a detailed description of the symptoms and their duration; sexual history, including recent change of sexual partner; past therapy; and response to therapy. Specific details include a description of the vaginal discharge—its color and consistency and, most importantly, the presence or absence of an offensive odor. Although the odor associated with VVC is absent, minimal, or nonoffensive, most women will describe it as unpleasant. However, women with BV or trichomoniasis have little hesitation in mentioning the offensive, embarrassing nature of the discharge, which characteristically increases in severity immediately after unprotected coitus.

Table 43-1

CAUSES OF VAGINITIS IN ADULT WOMEN

Infectious vaginitis
　　Bacterial vaginosis (40–50%)
　　Vulvovaginal candidiasis (20–25%)
　　Trichomonal vaginitis (15–20%)

Less common
　　Atrophic vaginitis with secondary bacterial infection
　　Foreign body with secondary infection
　　Desquamative inflammatory vaginitis (clindamycin-responsive)
　　Streptococcal vaginitis (group A)
　　Ulcerative vaginitis associated with *Staphylococcus aureus* and toxic shock syndrome
　　Idiopathic vulvovaginal ulceration associated with HIV

Noninfectious vaginitis
　　Chemical/irritant
　　Allergic, hypersensitivity, and contact dermatitis (lichen simplex)
　　Traumatic
　　Atrophic vaginitis
　　Postpuerperal atrophic vaginitis
　　Desquamative inflammatory vaginitis (glucocorticoid-responsive)
　　Erosive lichen planus
　　Collagen vascular disease, Behçet's syndrome, pemphigus syndromes
　　Idiopathic

Physical examination includes careful inspection and palpation (with a cotton swab) of the vulva as well as the vaginal vestibule. The latter area is frequently ignored; as a result, the diagnosis of focal vulvitis, or vestibulitis, is frequently missed. Inspection with a vaginal speculum includes examination of the vaginal mucosa for erythema, petechiae, ulceration, edema, atrophy, and adherent discharge. The pooled vaginal secretions are also assessed with regard to color, consistency, and volume. Finally, as mentioned previously, no vaginal examination is complete without evaluation of the cervix and bimanual digital pelvic examination.

Vaginal discharge can also be caused by mucopurulent cervicitis (MPC) and endometritis; therefore, it is essential to evaluate the cervix in all patients with vulvovaginal complaints. Caused by *Chlamydia trachomatis* and *Neisseria gonorrhoeae*, MPC is characterized by a yellow endocervical exudate and confirmed by the simple identification of yellow exudate on a white cotton-tipped swab specimen of endocervical secretions. The cervix is friable, edematous,

and bleeds easily on physical contact. Mucopurulent cervicitis must be differentiated from cervicitis caused by herpes simplex virus (HSV), vaginitis, and ectropion of the cervix (ectopy). The last is a normal finding without a mucopurulent exudate, although ectopy is associated with increased numbers of polymorphonuclear leukocytes (PMNs) in the vaginal discharge as determined by microscopy (See Chap.35 and color Plate 1).

After inspection, the middle third of the vagina is swabbed to obtain a valid specimen of secretions suitable for rapid pH estimation. Thereafter, swabs of mucosal secretions are obtained for saline and 10% potassium hydroxide (KOH) microscopic examination. Bacterial and fungal cultures are not required on a routine basis and are indicated only in selected cases. An additional swab is obtained for the immediate performance of a 10% KOH amine elaboration test (whiff test). In the presence of suspected cervicitis, cervical specimens should also be obtained for identification of *C. trachomatis, N. gonorrhoeae,* and HSV.

The saline microscopy examination has many purposes, including identification of clue cells, trichomonads, yeast or hyphae, and estimation of whether PMNs are present and/or increased. Most investigators consider a ratio of PMNs to epithelial cells of one or less as within normal limits. Likewise, exfoliated vaginal epithelial cells are studied in order to identify an increase in basal or parabasal cells, which may indicate a relative estrogen deficiency or reflect a "desquamating" inflammatory reaction in the wall of the vagina. The final useful component of saline microscopy includes examination of the vaginal flora, particularly as evident in the intercellular spaces. The normal appearance of the vaginal flora consists of rodlike organisms that are unclumped. This description is preserved in VVC, but it dramatically changes in both trichomoniasis and BV, in which the normal flora is lost and replaced by larger numbers of coccobacillary microorganisms that are often clumped. Gram-stain examination of vaginal secretions, although a useful permanent research and epidemiologic tool, is not required on a routine basis and adds little to a good saline wet-mount examination. Given the low sensitivity of the saline examination in detecting *Candida* species, a 10% KOH microscopic examination should always be performed, even if the saline wet mount identifies other causes of vaginitis, because mixed infections are common.

In the majority of symptomatic women, a thorough history, careful physical examination, and the aforementioned rapid laboratory tests should provide an immediate and reliable clinical diagnosis. In a small percentage of women, the diagnosis will be deferred pending the availability, within a few days, of results of additional studies, especially cultures. Each of the previously described tests has a variable sensitivity and specificity depending on the specific clinical entity in question, and each test is discussed below. Nevertheless, as outlined in Table 43-2, an accurate reliable diagnosis can be reached within a few minutes utilizing the stated guidelines. The fact that the patient may be seen under emer-

Table 43-2

DIAGNOSTIC FEATURES OF INFECTIOUS VAGINITIS

	Normal	Candidal Vaginitis	Bacterial Vaginosis	Trichomonas Vaginitis
Symptoms	None or physiologic leukorrhea	Vulvar pruritus, soreness, increased discharge, dysuria, dyspareunia	Malodorous moderate discharge	Profuse purulent discharge, offensive odor, pruritus, and dyspareunia
Discharge				
Amount	Variable, scant to moderate	Scant to moderate	Moderate	Profuse
Color	Clear or white	White	White/gray	Yellow
Consistency	Floccular nonhomogeneous	Clumped but variable	Homogeneous, uniformly coating walls	Homogeneous
"Bubbles"	Absent	Absent	Present	Present
Appearance of vulva and vagina	Normal	Introital and vulvar erythema, edema and occasional pustules, vaginal erythma	No inflammation	Erythema and swelling of vulvar and vaginal epithelium ("strawberry cervix")
pH of vaginal fluid	<4.5	<4.5	>4.5	5–6.0
Amine test (10% KOH)	Negative	Negative	Positive	Occasionally positive
Saline microscopy	Normal epithelial cell Lactobacilli predominate	Normal flora, blastospores (yeast), 40–50% pseudohyphae	Clue cells, coccobacillary flora predominates, absence of leukocytes, motile curved rods	PMNs+++ Motile trichomonads (80–90%), no clue cells, abnormal flora
10% KOH microscopy	Negative	Positive (60–90%)	Negative (except in mixed infections)	Negative

gency circumstances in no way nullifies this principle. Physicians should recognize that diagnostic algorithms in vaginitis are designed to facilitate the diagnosis of BV, VVC, or trichomoniasis, whereas the vaginal symptoms of many women will not be due to the three commonest causes of infectious vaginitis. When no specific etiological agent has been identified, physicians should not feel obliged to prescribe antimicrobial agents routinely. If no diagnosis has been forthcoming, a variety of effective, nonspecific palliative measures can be prescribed. Nevertheless practitioners prefer to rely on the clinical response to empirically selected antimicrobial therapy and polypharmacy, exploiting the safety and potency of most therapeutic agents and the relatively narrow differential diagnosis. Common pitfalls in diagnosis and management are listed in Table 43-3.

INFECTIOUS VAGINITIS

BACTERIAL VAGINOSIS

EPIDEMIOLOGY

Bacterial vaginosis is the most common cause of vaginitis in women of childbearing age. It has been diagnosed in 17 to 19 percent of women seeking gynecologic care in family practice or student health care settings. The prevalence increases considerably in symptomatic women in STD clinics, reaching 24 to 37 percent. Bacterial vaginosis has been observed in 16 to 29 percent of pregnant women, the low-

Table 43-3

SOME PITFALLS IN THE DIAGNOSIS AND TREATMENT OF VAGINITIS: CAUSES OF TREATMENT FAILURE

Failure to see and examine patient (telephone diagnosis)

Assuming diagnosis in previous attack is same as in present episode

Patient interviewed but not examined

Patient manually examined but no speculum inserted

Speculum examination but no laboratory tests performed

Failure to examine introitus and missing diagnosis of vestibulitis

Limiting differential diagnosis to BV, VVC, and trichomoniasis

Assuming that positive culture for *Gardnerella vaginalis* implies presence of BV

Treating *Escherichia coli,* enterococcus, and so forth (normal flora) as pathogens

Relying on Pap smear to make diagnosis

Use of "shotgun" polypharmacy

Selecting therapy on the basis of "odds and statistics"

Use of topical glucocorticoids for all vulvar symptoms

Failure to recognize that topical therapy may exacerbate symptoms

est figures being found among private patients and the highest in STD and university clinics.

Gardnerella vaginalis has been found in 10 to 31 percent of virgin adolescent girls but is found significantly more frequently among sexually active women, reaching a prevalence in some at-risk populations of 50 to 60 percent.

Evaluation of epidemiologic factors has revealed few clues as to the cause of BV. Use of an intrauterine device and douching were found to be more common among women with BV. It is significantly more common in African Americans and sexually active women, including lesbians.

PATHOGENESIS

Bacterial vaginosis is the result of a massive overgrowth of mixed flora, including peptostreptococci, *Bacteroides* sp., *G. vaginalis, Mobiluncus* sp., and genital mycoplasmas.[8] There is little inflammation, and the disorder represents a disturbance of the vaginal microbial ecosystem rather than a true infection of tissues. The overgrowth of mixed flora is associated with a loss of the normal *Lactobacillus*-dominated vaginal flora. It is apparent that no single recognized bacterial species is responsible for BV. Experimental studies in human volunteers and animal studies indicate that inocula-

tion of the vagina with individual species of bacteria associated with BV (e.g., *G. vaginalis*) rarely results in BV. The role of sexual transmission, however, remains controversial. In support of the role of sexual transmission is the higher prevalence of BV among sexually active young women than among sexually inexperienced women and the observation that the BV-associated microorganisms are more frequently isolated from the urethras of male partners of women with BV.

The cause for the massive overgrowth of anaerobes (*Gardnerella, Mycoplasma,* and *Mobiluncus* sp.) is unknown. Theories include increased substrate availability, increased pH, and loss of the restraining effects of the normally dominant *Lactobacillus* flora that act to inhibit the aforementioned bacteria. Moreover, Eschenbach et al. have reported that, although women without BV are colonized by H_2O_2-producing strains of lactobacilli, women with BV have reduced overall population numbers of lactobacilli, and the lactobacilli species present lack the ability to produce H_2O_2.[7] The H_2O_2 produced by lactobacilli may inhibit the pathogens associated with BV, either directly by the toxicity of H_2O_2 or as a result of the production of H_2O_2-halide complex catalyzed by natural cervical peroxidase.

Accompanying the bacterial overgrowth in BV is the increased production of amines by anaerobes, facilitated by microbial decarboxylases. Amines in the presence of increased vaginal pH volatilize to produce the typical abnormal fishy odor, which is also produced when 10% KOH is added to vaginal secretions. The aromatic amines responsible for the characteristic odor were originally thought to be putrescine and cadaverine; however, trimethylamine is the dominant abnormal amine in BV. It is likely that bacterial polyamines produced together with the organic acids found in the vagina in BV (acetic and succinic acids) are cytotoxic, resulting in exfoliation of vaginal epithelial cells and creating the vaginal discharge. *Gardnerella vaginalis* attaches avidly to exfoliated epithelial cells, especially at the alkaline pH found in BV. The adherence of *Garnerella* organisms results in the formation of the pathognomonic clue cells.

CLINICAL FEATURES

As many as 50 percent of women with BV may be asymptomatic. The cardinal symptom is that of vaginal malodor, often described as fishy and frequently manifesting after unprotected coitus. An abnormal vaginal discharge, which is infrequently profuse, is usually described. Pruritus, dysuria, abdominal pain, and dyspareunia are *not* manifestations of BV. Examination reveals a nonviscous, grayish-white adherent discharge, often visible on the labia and introital area. Apart from the discharge, no other abnormalities are apparent on examination.

Bacterial vaginosis has been considered to be a diagnosis that is primarily of nuisance value. However, there is now considerable evidence that BV may have serious obstetric and gynecologic complications, including asymptomatic BV diagnosed by Gram stain. Obstetric complications include chorioamnionitis, preterm labor, prematurity, and postpartum fever.[9] Gynecologic sequelae are postabortion fever, posthysterectomy fever, cuff infection, and chronic mast-cell endometritis. More recently, association is reported of untreated BV with cervical inflammation and low-grade dysplasia.

DIAGNOSIS

As with all forms of vaginitis, signs and symptoms are unreliable in establishing the diagnosis of BV. The clinical diagnosis can be made reliably in the presence of at least three of the following objective criteria: (1) adherent, white, nonfloccular homogenous discharge; (2) positive amine test, with release of fishy odor on addition of 10% KOH to vaginal secretions; (3) vaginal pH >4.5; and (4) presence of clue cells on light microscopy. These clinical signs are simple and reliable, and testing is easy to perform. Of the four cardinal clinical signs, abnormal discharge has the least specificity. The presence of clue cells is the single most reliable predictor of BV. Clue cells are exfoliated vaginal squamous epithelial cells covered with *G. vaginalis,* giving the cells a granular or stippled appearance with characteristic loss of clear cell borders. At least 20 percent of observed epithelial cells should be clue cells if they are to be of diagnostic significance. Occasionally, clue cells consisting exclusively of curved gram-negative rods belonging to *Mobiluncus* sp. can be demonstrated. The offensive fishy odor may be apparent during the physical examination or may become apparent only during the amine test. Several investigators consider the positive amine test the least sensitive of the four clinical tests, especially compared with the Gram stain. Of the various signs, the pH of the vaginal fluid has the greatest sensitivity but the lowest specificity. A pH of >4.7 increases the specificity of BV diagnosis.

The wet-mount examination is critical, not only because it allows detection of clue cells and exclusion of trichomoniasis but because the diagnosis of BV is supported by the absence of PMNs and the characteristic appearance of the background bacterial flora with the dominance of the coccobacillary organisms. Similar information may also be obtained with the use of Gram stain. This test has a sensitivity of 93 percent and a specificity of 70 percent.

Finally, although cultures for *G. vaginalis* are positive in almost all cases of BV, *G. vaginalis* may be detected in 50 to 60 percent of women who do not meet the diagnostic criteria for BV. Accordingly, vaginal culture has no role in the diagnosis of BV.

TREATMENT

Poor efficacy has been observed with triple sulfa creams, erythromycin, tetracycline, acetic acid gel, and povidone-iodine vaginal douches.

Moderate cure rates only have been obtained with ampicillin (mean, 66 percent) and amoxicillin. The most successful oral therapy remains oral metronidazole. Most studies using multiple divided-dose regimens of 800 to 1200 mg/day for 1 week achieved clinical cure rates in excess of 90 percent immediately and of approximately 80 percent at 4 weeks. The usual treatment is metronidazole 500 mg po b.i.d. for 7 days. Although single-dose therapy with 2 g metronidazole achieves comparable immediate clinical response rates, higher recurrence rates have been reported. The beneficial effect of metronidazole results predominantly from its anti-anaerobic activity and because *G. vaginalis* is susceptible to the hydroxymetabolites of metronidazole. Although *Mycoplasma hominis* is resistant to metronidazole, the organisms are usually not detected at follow-up visits of successfully treated patients. Similarly, *Mobiluncus curtisii* is resistant to metronidazole but usually disappears after therapy.

Topical therapy with 2% clindamycin once daily for 7 days or metronidazole gel 0.75% administered twice daily for 5 days has been shown to be as effective as oral metronidazole, without any of the latter's side effects. Thus the practitioner has several therapeutic options, and the topical regimens are particularly useful in pregnancy as well as for women who are allergic or cannot tolerate oral metronidazole.

In the past, asymptomatic BV was generally not treated, especially since patients often improve spontaneously over several months. However, the growing evidence linking asymptomatic BV with numerous obstetric and gynecologic upper tract complications has brought a reassessment of this policy, especially with additional convenient topical therapies. Asymptomatic BV should be treated prior to pregnancy, in women with cervical abnormalities, and prior to elective gynecologic surgery. Treatment of asymptomatic BV in pregnancy remains controversial pending the outcome of studies proving that treatment reduces preterm delivery.

Treatment of male sexual partners remains controversial despite indirect evidence of sexual transmission. No study has documented reduced recurrence rates of BV in women whose partners have been treated with a variety of regimens, including metronidazole. Accordingly, most clinicians do not routinely treat male partners.

Within 3 months after successful clinical therapy over 7 days with metronidazole, approximately 30 percent of patients who respond initially experience a recurrence of identical signs and symptoms. Recurrence rates in as many as 80 percent of patients within 9 months have been reported. The reasons for recurrence are unclear; they include the possibility of reinfection, but recurrence more likely reflects vaginal relapse with failure to eradicate the offending organisms at the same time that the normally protective *Lactobacillus*-dominant vaginal flora fails to reestablish itself. Management of acute BV symptoms during relapse once more includes oral or vaginal metronidazole or topical clindamycin, usually prescribed for a longer treatment period of 10 to 14 days. Maintenance antibiotic regimens have largely been disappointing and new approaches including exogenous *Lactobacillus* recolonization using selected bacteria-containing suppositories are being studied.

TRICHOMONIASIS

EPIDEMIOLOGY

Studies estimate that 2 to 3 million American women contract trichomoniasis annually, with a worldwide distribution of approximately 180 million annual cases of trichomonal vaginitis. The prevalence of trichomoniasis correlates with the overall level of sexual activity of the specific group of women under study. Thus, trichomoniasis has been diagnosed in about 5 percent of women in family-planning clinics, 13 to 25 percent of women attending gynecology clinics, 50 to 75 percent of prostitutes, and 7 to 35 percent of women in STD clinics. In many countries, recent epidemiologic surveys indicate a decline in the prevalence of trichomoniasis.

PATHOPHYSIOLOGY

Sexual transmission is undoubtedly the dominant method of introduction of *Trichomonas vaginalis* into the vagina. The organisms is usually identified in 30 to 40 percent of male sexual partners of infected women, with identification of urethral isolates rapidly decreasing over a period of days. A prevalence of 70 percent was found among men who had had sexual contact with infected women within the previous 48 h. Trichomoniasis can be documented in at least 85 percent of female partners of infected men. Several studies have demonstrated an increased cure rate in women after treatment of their male sexual partners. There is also a high prevalence of gonorrhea in women with trichomoniasis, and both infections are significantly associated with use of nonbarrier methods of contraception. Oral contraceptives may decrease the prevalence of trichomoniasis; moreover, spermicidal agents such as nonoxynol 9 reduce transmission.

Repeated trichomonal infections are common; therefore, clinically significant protective immunity does not appear to occur. Nevertheless, an immune response to *Trichomonas* does develop, as indicated by low titers of serum antibody. The latter response is insufficient to permit diagnostic use of serology. Local antitrichomonal IgA has been detected in vaginal secretions, but its protective role is ill defined. Delayed hypersensitivity in natural infection can also be demonstrated, but similarly, a protective function is not apparent. The predominate host-defense response is provided by the numerous PMNs, which respond to chemotactic substances released by trichomonads and without ingesting trichomonads are capable of killing *T. vaginalis*. The exact mechanisms by which *T. vaginalis* induces disease remains to be determined. It is thought that *T. vaginalis* destroys epithelial cells by direct cell contact and cytoxicity. Within the vagina, only areas covered by squamous but not columnar epithelium are involved. The urethra and Skene's glands are infected in the majority of patients, and organisms are occasionally isolated from bladder urine.

CLINICAL FEATURES

Trichomonas infection in women ranges from an asymptomatic carrier state to severe, acute inflammatory disease. Approximately one third of asymptomatic infected women became symptomatic within 6 months.

Vaginal discharge is reported by 50 to 70 percent of women diagnosed with trichomoniasis; however, the discharge is not always described as malodorous.[5,6] Pruritus occurs in 25 to 50 percent of patients and is often severe. As many as half of infected women admit to some degree of dyspareunia. Other infrequent symptoms include dysuria and, rarely, frequency of micturition. Lower abdominal pain has been described in fewer than 10 percent of patients and should alert the physician to the possibility of concomitant salpingitis due to other organisms. Symptoms of acute trichomoniasis often appear during or immediately after menstruation. The incubation period has been estimated to range from 3 to 28 days, although this is controversial.

Physical findings represent a spectrum depending on the severity of disease. Vulvar findings may be absent but are typically characterized in severe cases by diffuse erythema (10 to 33 percent) and a profuse vaginal discharge. Edema of the labia may occasionally be present in severe cases. Although the typical discharge of trichomoniasis is often described as being yellow-green and frothy, such a typical discharge is seen in only a minority of patients. The discharge is gray in about 75 percent; likewise, frothiness is seen in a minority of patients and is more commonly seen in BV.

The vaginal walls are typically erythematous and in severe cases may be granular in appearance. Punctate hemorrhages (colpitis macularis) of the cervix may result in a strawberry-like appearance that, although apparent to the naked eye in only about 1 to 2 percent of patients, is present in 45 percent on colposcopy.

The clinical course of trichomoniasis in pregnancy is identical to that seen in the nonpregnant state, and untreated trichomoniasis is associated with premature rupture of membranes and prematurity. Trichomoniasis is also reported to facilitate the transmission of human immunodeficiency virus (HIV).

DIAGNOSIS

None of the clinical features of *Trichomonas* vaginitis are sufficiently specific to allow a reliable diagnosis of trichomonal infection based on signs and symptoms alone.[5,6] Definitive diagnosis requires the demonstration of the organism. Vaginal pH is markedly elevated, almost always above 5.0 and not infrequently above 6.0. On saline microscopy, an increase in PMNs is almost invariably present, although absence of PMNs does not exclude trichomoniasis. The ovoid parasites are slightly larger than PMNs and are best recognized by their mobility. The wet mount is positive in only 40 to 80 percent of cases. Gram stain is of little value because of its inability to differentiate PMNs and nonmotile trichomonads, and use of Giemsa, acridine orange, and other stains has no advantage over saline preparation. Although trichomonads are often seen on Pap smears, this method has a sensitivity of only 60 to 70 percent as compared with saline preparation microscopy, and false-positive results are not infrequently reported.

Several culture-medium methods are available and probably equivalent. Cultures should be incubated anaerobically, and growth is usually detected within 48 h. Culture is now recognized as the most sensitive method for detecting the presence of trichomonads (95 percent sensitivity) and should be considered in patients with vaginitis in whom there is a markedly elevated pH, PMN excess, absence of motile trichomonads, and clue cells. Several new rapid diagnostic kits using DNA probes are under investigation.

TREATMENT

The cornerstone of therapy remains the 5-nitroimidazole group of drugs—metronidazole, tinidazole, and ornidazole—which are all of similar efficacy. Only metronidazole is available in the United States. Oral therapy, as opposed to topical vaginal therapy, is generally preferred, primarily because of the frequency of infection of the urethra and periurethral glands, which provide sources for endogenous reinfection.

Treatment consists of oral metronidazole, 500 mg b.i.d. for 7 days, with a cure rate of 95 percent. Comparable results, however, have also been obtained with a single oral dose of 2 g, achieving cure rates in the range of 82 to 88 percent. The latter cure rate increases to >90 percent when sexual partners are treated simultaneously. The advantages of single-dose therapy include better patient compliance, lower total dose, a shorter period of alcohol avoidance, and possibly decreased subsequent candidal vaginitis. A disadvantage of single-dose therapy is the need to insist on simultaneous treatment of sexual partners.

The 5-nitroimidazoles are not in themselves trichomonacidal, but low-redox proteins reduce the nitro group, resulting in the formation of highly cytotoxic products within the organisms. Aerobic conditions interfere with this reduction process and decrease the anti-anaerobic activity of the 5-nitroimidazoles. Most strains of T. vaginalis are highly susceptible to metronidazole with minimal inhibitory concentrations of 1 μg/mL.

Patients not responding to an initial course often respond to an additional standard course of 7-day therapy. Some patients are refractory to repeated courses of therapy even when compliance is assured and sexual partners are known to have been treated. If reinfection is excluded, these rare patients may have strains of T. vaginalis genuinely resistant to metronidazole. The isolates can be shown in vitro to have metronidazole resistance. Increased doses of metronidazole and longer duration of therapy are necessary to cure these

refractory patients. The patients should be given maximal tolerated doses of oral metronidazole of 2 to 4 g/day for 10 to 14 days. Rarely, high-dose intravenous metronidazole in dosages as high as 2 to 4 g daily may be necessary, with careful monitoring for drug toxicity.

Considerable success has been observed in treating resistant infections with oral tinidazole; however, the drug is not readily available and the optimal dose to be used is unknown. Most investigators use high-dose tinidazole 1 to 4 g/day daily for 14 days. Rare patients not responding to nitroimidazoles can be treated with topical paramomycin.

Side effects of metronidazole include an unpleasant metallic taste. Other common side effects include nausea (10 percent), transient neutropenia (7.5 percent), and a disulfiram-like effect when alcohol is ingested. Caution should be observed when 5-nitroimidazoles are used in patients taking warfarin. Long-term and high-dose therapy increases the risk of neutropenia and peripheral neuropathy. In experimental studies, metronidazole has been shown to be mutagenic for certain bacteria, indicating a carcinogenic potential, although cohort studies have not established an increase in cancer morbidity. Thus, the risk to humans of short-term low-dose metronidazole treatment is extremely small. Superinfection with Candida is by no means uncommon.

Treatment of trichomoniasis in pregnancy is unsatisfactory. Metronidazole readily crosses the placenta, and because of concern for teratogenicity, some consider it prudent to avoid its use in the first trimester of pregnancy. More recently, investigators have become more comfortable using metronidazole throughout pregnancy. Topical clotrimazole and povidone-iodine jelly may offer some benefit, although sound evidence for their efficacy is lacking.

VULVOVAGINAL CANDIDIASIS

EPIDEMIOLOGY

There are no reliable figures defining the incidence of VVC in the United States, mainly because VVC is not reportable. Data from Great Britain reveal a sharp increase in the incidence of VVC. In the United States, Candida is now the second commonest cause of vaginal infections.

It is estimated that 75 percent of women experience at least one episode of VVC during their childbearing years, and approximately 40 to 50 percent of them experience a second attack.[2] A small subpopulation of women, probably less than 5 percent of the adult female population, suffers from repeated, recurrent, often intractable episodes of candidal vaginitis.

Point-prevalence studies indicate that Candida may be isolated from the genital tract of approximately 20 percent of asymptomatic, healthy women of childbearing age. The natural history of asymptomatic colonization is unknown, although both animal and human studies suggest that vaginal carriage may continue for several months and perhaps

Table 43-4

FACTORS ASSOCIATED WITH INCREASED ASYMPTOMATIC VAGINAL COLONIZATION WITH *CANDIDA* AND CANDIDAL VAGINITIS

Genetic
   Blood-group antigen/secretor status

Acquired
   Pregnancy
   Uncontrolled diabetes mellitus
   Corticosteroids/immunosuppressives
   Antimicrobial therapy (systemic, topical)
   HIV infection
   Behavioral (sexual)
      Oral contraceptives
      Intrauterine device
      Nonoxynol 9 spermicide
      High-risk sexual behavior
      Frequent visits to STD clinics
      Receptive oral-genital sex
      Coital frequency(?)

years. Several factors are associated with increased rates of asymptomatic vaginal colonization with *Candida,* including pregnancy (30 to 40 percent), use of oral contraceptives, uncontrolled diabetes mellitus, and frequent visits to STD clinics (Table 43-4). The rarity of candidal isolation in premenarchial girls, the lower prevalence of candidal vaginitis after menopause, and the possible association of this condition with hormone replacement therapy (HRT) emphasize the hormonal dependence of VVC.

PATHOGENESIS

The Organism

Between 85 and 90 percent of yeasts isolated from the vagina are *Candida albicans* strains. The remainder represent other species, the commonest being *C. glabrata* and *C. tropicalis.* Non-*albicans Candida* sp. are capable of inducing vaginitis and are often more resistant to conventional therapy. Although more than two hundred strains of *C. albicans* have been identified by typing, there is no evidence of strain tropism selecting for strains with a predilection to colonize the vagina or to cause vaginitis. Recent surveys indicate an increase in VVC due to non-*albicans Candida* sp., particularly *C. glabrata.*

For candidal organisms to colonize the vaginal mucosa, they must first adhere to the vaginal epithelial cells. *Can-dida albicans* adheres in significantly higher number to vaginal epithelial cells than do non-*albicans Candida* sp. This may explain the relative infrequency of the latter strains in vaginitis. There is considerable person-to-person variation in terms of vaginal cell receptivity to candidal organisms in adherence assays. Nevertheless, vaginal cells from women with recurrent VVC do not show increased in vitro cell avidity or affinity kinetics for *Candida.*

Germination of *Candida* enhances colonization and facilitates tissue invasion. Factors that enhance or facilitate germination—e.g., estrogen therapy and pregnancy—tend to precipitate symptomatic vaginitis, whereas measures that inhibit germination—e.g., bacterial flora and local mucosal cell–mediated immunity—may prevent acute vaginitis in women who are asymptomatic carriers of yeast.

Candidal organisms gain access to the vaginal lumen and secretions predominantly from the adjacent perianal area. This finding is borne out by several epidemiologic and typing studies. Candidal vaginitis is seen predominantly in women of childbearing age, and only in the minority of cases can a precipitating factor be identified to explain the transformation from asymptomatic carriage to symptomatic vaginitis in individual patients.

Host Factors

During pregnancy, the vagina is more susceptible to vaginal infection, resulting in a higher incidence of vaginal colonization and vaginitis and lower cure rates. The clinical attack rate is maximal in the third trimester, and symptomatic recurrences are also more common throughout pregnancy. The high levels of reproductive hormones, by providing a higher glycogen content in the vaginal environment, provide an excellent carbon source for the growth and germination of *Candida.* A more likely mechanism is that estrogens enhance the avidity of vaginal epithelial cells for *Candida* adherence, and a yeast cytosol receptor or binding system for female reproductive hormones has been documented. These hormones also enhance yeast mycelial formation. Several studies have shown increased vaginal colonization rates with *Candida* after the use of estrogen oral contraceptives. Vaginal colonization with *Candida* is more frequent in diabetic women, and uncontrolled diabetes predisposes to symptomatic vaginitis. Glucose tolerance tests have been recommended for women with recurrent VVC; however, the yield is low, and testing is not justified in otherwise healthy premenopausal women.

Symptomatic VVC is frequently observed during or after courses of systemic antibiotics. Although no antimicrobial agent is free of this complication, broad-spectrum antibiotics such as tetracycline, ampicillin, and cephalosporins are mainly responsible and are thought to act by eliminating the normally protective vaginal bacterial flora. The natural flora provides a colonization-resistance mechanism and prevents germination of *Candida. Lactobacillus* sp. have been singled out as providing this protective function. *Lactobacil-*

lus-Candida interaction includes competition for nutrients, stearic interference with the adherence of Candida, and elaboration of bacteriocins that inhibit yeast proliferation and germination.

Other factors that contribute to the increased incidence of candidal vaginitis include the use of tight, poorly ventilated clothing and nylon underclothing, which increases perineal moisture and temperature. Chemical contact, local allergy, and hypersensitivity reactions may also predispose to symptomatic vaginitis (see "Other Noninfectious Vaginitis," below).

During the phase of asymptomatic carriage, candidal organisms exist predominantly in the nonfilamentous form and are found in relatively low numbers. There is a delicate equilibrium among Candida, the resident protective bacterial flora, and other local vaginal defense mechanisms. Symptomatic vaginitis develops in the presence of factors that enhance candidal virulence factors or as a result of loss of local defense mechanisms.

Candida may cause cell damage and resulting inflammation by direct hyphal invasion of epithelial tissue. It is possible that proteases and other hydrolytic enzymes facilitate cell penetration, with resultant inflammation, mucosal swelling, erythema, and exfoliation of vaginal epithelial cells. The characteristic nonhomogenous vaginal discharge consists of a conglomerate of hyphal elements and exfoliated nonviable epithelial cells with few PMNs. Candida may also induce symptoms by hypersensitivity or allergic reaction, particularly in women with idiopathic recurrent VVC (see "Other Noninfectious Vaginitis," below).

Oral and vaginal thrush correlates well with depressed cell-mediated immunity in debilitated or immunosuppressed patients. This is particularly evident in patients with chronic mucocutaneous candidiasis and acquired immunodeficiency syndrome.

PATHOGENESIS OF RECURRENT AND CHRONIC CANDIDAL VAGINITIS

Careful evaluation of women with recurrent vulvovaginal candidiasis (RVVC) usually fails to reveal any precipitating or causal mechanism. These desperate women avoid antibiotics, oral contraceptives, tight-fitting clothing, and hormone therapy and have normal glucose tolerance tests. In the past investigators attributed frequent episodes to repeated fungal reinoculation of the vagina from a persistent intestinal source or to sexual transmission.

The intestinal reservoir theory is based on the report of recovery of Candida on rectal culture in almost 100 percent of women with VVC. Typing of simultaneously obtained vaginal and rectal isolates almost invariably reveals identical strains. This theory has been criticized in the past few years because of lower concordance between rectal and vaginal cultures in patients with RVVC. Moreover, long-term therapy with oral nonabsorbable nystatin is not effective in preventing recurrences.

Although sexual transmission of candidal organisms undoubtedly occurs via vaginal intercourse and orogenital contact, the role of sexual reintroduction of yeast as a cause of RVVC is doubtful, as RVVC frequently occurs in celibate women and only the minority of male partners of women with RVVC are colonized with Candida. Most studies aimed at treating male partners have not reduced the frequency of recurrent episodes of vaginitis.

Vaginal relapse implies that incomplete eradication or clearance of Candida from the vagina occurs after antimycotic therapy. Organisms persist in small numbers in the vagina and result in continued carriage of the organisms, and when host environmental conditions permit, the colonizing organisms increase in number and undergo mycelial transformation, resulting in a new clinical episode.

Whether recurrence is due to vaginal reinfection or relapse, it is apparent that women with RVVC differ from those with infrequent episodes by virtue of their inability to tolerate the small numbers of Candida reintroduced or persisting in the vagina. On the basis of typing of organisms, women with recurrent and infrequent infection have the same distribution frequency of organisms as do women without symptoms.

Host factors responsible for the frequent episodes are not clearly delineated, and more than one mechanism may be operative. There is no evidence of complement, phagocytic cells, or immunoglobulin deficiency in these patients, and RVVC is rarely due to drug resistance. Current theories about the pathogenesis of RVVC include qualitative and quantitative deficiency in the normal protective vaginal bacterial flora and an acquired, often transient antigen-specific deficiency in T-lymphocyte function that similarly permits unchecked yeast proliferation and germination.[3] Another theory is that of an acquired acute hypersensitivity reaction to Candida antigen that is accompanied by elevated vaginal titers of Candida antigen-specific IgE. This theory has a clinical basis in that patients with RVVC often present with severe vulvar manifestations (rash, erythema, swelling, and pruritus) with minimal exudative vaginal changes, little discharge, and lower titers of organisms. Allergic responses to Candida have been reported to involve the male genitalia immediately after coitus with a Candida-infected woman and are characterized by the acute onset of erythema, edema, severe prutius, and irritation of the penis. As yet, only a minority of women with RVVC have been shown to have elevated Candida-specific vaginal IgE. Limited studies using Candida antigen desensitization have been found to be helpful in reducing the frequency of recurrent episodes of vaginitis.

Women who are HIV-seropositive have higher vaginal colonization rates than do seronegative women, but the attack rate of symptomatic VVC appears similar. Reports of chronic, severe RVVC have been given much media attention but remain largely unsubstantiated. In the absence of other risk factors for HIV, RVVC is not an indication for HIV testing.

CLINICAL MANIFESTATIONS

The most frequent symptom is vulvar pruritus, since vaginal discharge is not invariably present and is frequently minimal. Although described as typically cottage cheese–like in character, the discharge may vary from watery to homogenously thick. Vaginal soreness and irritation, vulvar burning, dyspareunia, and external dysuria are commonly present. If present, odor is minimal and nonoffensive. Examination frequently reveals erythema and swelling of the labia and vulva, often with discrete pustulopapular peripheral lesions. The cervix is normal, and vaginal mucosal erythema with adherent whitish discharge is present. Characteristically, symptoms are exacerbated in the week before the onset of menses, with some relief upon the onset of menstrual flow.

DIAGNOSIS

The relative lack of specificity of symptoms and signs precludes a diagnosis that is based only on history and physical examination. Most patients with symptomatic VVC may be readily diagnosed on the basis of simple microscopic examination of vaginal secretions (see Fig. 43-1). A wet mount

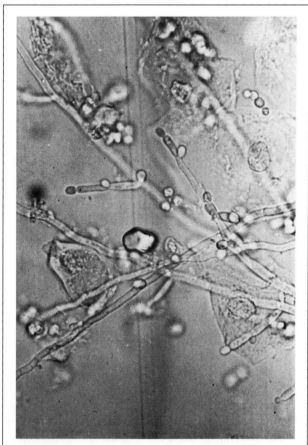

Figure 43-1

Hyphal elements of *C. albicans* seen on high power magnification during saline microscopy. Patient had florid candidal vaginitis.

or saline preparation has a sensitivity of 40 to 60 percent. The 10% KOH preparation is even more sensitive in diagnosing the presence of germinated yeast. A normal vaginal pH (4.0 to 4.5) is found in candidal vaginitis; the finding of a pH in excess of 4.5 should suggest the possibility of BV, trichomoniasis, or a mixed infection.

Although routine fungal cultures are unnecessary, vaginal culture should be performed in the presence of negative microscopy. The Pap smear is unreliable, being positive in only about 25 percent of cases. There is no reliable serologic technique for the diagnosis of symptomatic candidal vaginitis.

TREATMENT

Topical Agents for Acute Candidal Vaginitis

Antimycotics are available for local use as creams, lotions, aerosol sprays, vaginal tablets, suppositories, and coated tampons. There is little to suggest that formulation of the topical antimycotic influences clinical efficacy; in most cases, the patient's preference should dictate which vehicle is used to deliver the local therapy. Extensive vulvar inflammation dictates local application of antifungal cream. Antifungal agents that have been used in the topical treatment of candidal vaginitis are listed in Table 43-5.

Nystatin creams and vaginal suppositories have been used extensively for almost three decades. The average mycologic cure rate of 7- and 14-day courses is approximately 75 to 80 percent. Azole derivatives appear to achieve slightly higher clinical mycologic cure rates than do the polyenes (nystatin), approximately 85 to 90 percent. Although many studies have compared the clinical efficacy of the various azoles, there is little evidence that any one azole agent is superior to others.

Topical azoles are remarkably free of local and systemic side effects; nevertheless, the initial application of topical agents is not infrequently accompanied by local burning and discomfort.

There has been a major trend toward shorter treatment courses with progressively higher antifungal doses, culminating in highly effective single-dose topical regimens. Although short-course regimens are effective for mild and moderate vaginitis, cure rates for severe and complicated vaginitis are lower.

Oral systemic azoles are now available for the treatment of VVC, including ketoconazole 500 mg b.i.d. for 5 days, itraconazole 200 mg daily for 3 days (or 200-mg b.i.d. single-day regimen), and finally fluconazole 150 mg in a single dose.[4] All the oral regimens achieve clinical cure rates in excess of 80 percent; however, only fluconazole is approved for use for VVC in the United States. Oral regimens are generally preferred by women because of their convenience and lack of local side effects. None of the systemic regimens should be prescribed during pregnancy and, as with all oral agents, the potential for systemic side effects and toxicity exists. In particular, hepatotoxicity with ketoconazole precludes its widespread use in VVC.

Table 43-5

THERAPY FOR VAGINAL CANDIDIASIS— TOPICAL AGENTS

Drug	Formulation	Dosage Regimen
*Butoconazole	2% cream	5 g/day for 3 days
*Clotrimazole	1% cream	5 g/day for 7–14 days
	100 mg vaginal tablet	1 tablet per day for 7 days
	100 mg vaginal tablet	2 tablets per day for 3 days
	500 mg vaginal tablet	1 tablet (single dose)
*Miconazole	2% cream	5 g/day for 7 days
	100 mg vaginal suppository	1 suppository per day for 7 days
	200 mg vaginal suppository	1 suppository per day for 3 days
	1200 mg vaginal suppository	1 suppository (single dose)
Econazole	150 mg vaginal tablet	1 tablet per day for 3 days
Fenticonazole	2% cream	5 g/day for 7 days
*Tioconazole	2% cream	5 g/day for 3 days
	6.5% cream	5 g (single dose)
Terconazole	0.4% cream	5 g/day for 7 days
	0.8% cream	5 g/day for 3 days
	80 mg vaginal suppository	80 mg/day for 3 days
Nystatin	100,000-U vaginal tablet	1 tablet/day for 14 days

*Available over the counter (OTC).

Table 43-6

CLASSIFICATION OF VULVOVAGINAL CANDIDIASIS

Uncomplicated	Complicated
Candida albicans +	Non-*albicans Candida* spp.
	Resistant *C. albicans* (rare)
	or
Infrequent episodes +	History of recurrent VVC
	or
Vaginitis mild to moderate +	Severe VVC
	or
Normal host	Abnormal host (e.g., uncontrolled diabetic, pregnant, immunocompromised)

A useful guide to selecting antifungals for VVC is provided in Table 43-6. Vulvovaginal candidiasis is classified as uncomplicated or complicated on the basis of the likelihood of achieving clinical and mycologic cure with short-course therapy. Uncomplicated VVC represents by far the most common form of vaginitis seen, is caused by highly sensitive *C. albicans,* and—provided that the severity is mild to moderate—patients respond well to all topical or oral antimycotics including single-dose therapy. In contrast, patients with complicated VVC have either an organism, host factor, or severity of infection that dictates more intensive and prolonged therapy lasting 7 to 14 days. Most non-*albicans Candida* infections respond to conventional topical or oral antifungals provided that they are administered long enough. Vaginitis caused by *C. glabrata* often fails to respond to azoles and may require treatment with vaginal capsules of boric acid 600 mg/day for 14 days.

Treatment of Recurrent Vulvovaginal Candidiasis

The management of women with RVVC aims at control rather than cure. The clinician should first confirm the diagnosis of RVVC. Uncontrolled diabetes must be controlled if there is to be any chance of clinical success. Similarly, the use of corticosteroids, other immunosuppressive agents, and hormones such as estrogen should be discontinued when possible. Unfortunately, in the majority of women with RVVC, no underlying or predisposing factor can be identified.

Recurrent VVC requires long-term maintenance with a suppressive prophylactic regimen. Several studies have confirmed the success of maintenance regimens in reducing the frequency of symptomatic episodes of VVC during long-term prophylactic therapy. Because of the chronicity of therapy, the convenience of oral treatment is apparent, and the best suppressive prophylaxis has been achieved with weekly fluconazole orally at a dose of 100 mg. An effective topical prophylactic regimen consists of weekly vaginal suppositories of clotrimazole 500 mg. Treatment of male partners of women with RVVC is rarely of benefit.

ATROPHIC VAGINITIS

It is important to distinguish between the symptomatic patient with an inflamed atrophic vagina and the patient with simple atrophy who has no symptoms other than dryness and no specific inflammation. Clinically significant atrophic vaginitis is actually quite rare, and the majority of women with an atrophic vagina are asymptomatic. Because of reduced endogenous estrogen, the epithelium becomes thin and lacking in glycogen, which contributes to a reduction in lactic acid production and an increase in vaginal pH. This change in the environment encourages the overgrowth of nonacidophilic coliform organisms and the disappearance of *Lactobacillus* sp. Despite these major but usually gradual changes, symptoms are usually absent, especially in the absence of coitus.

Typical symptoms include vaginal soreness, dyspareunia, and occasional spotting or discharge. Burning is a frequent complaint and is often precipitated by intercourse. The vaginal mucosa is thin, with diffuse redness, occasional petechiae, or ecchymoses with few or no vaginal folds. Vulvar atrophy may also be present; discharge, if present, may be bloodlike, thick, or watery, and the pH of the vaginal secretions ranges from 5.5 to 7.0. The wet smear frequently shows increased PMNs associated with small, round epithelial cells. The latter parabasal cells represent immature squamous cells that have not been exposed to sufficient estrogen. The *Lactobacillus*-dominated flora is replaced by a mixed flora of gram-negative rods. Bacteriologic cultures in these patients are not unnecessary but can be misleading.

The treatment of atrophic vaginitis consists primarily of topical vaginal estrogen, especially in the absence of systemic symptoms. Nightly use of half or all the contents of an applicator for 1 to 2 weeks is usually sufficient to alleviate the atrophic vaginitis. Oral treatment with usual doses of estrogen replacement therapy (e.g., 0.625 mg of conjugated estrogen) is also effective.

OTHER NONINFECTIOUS VAGINITIS

Women frequently present with chronic or acute vulvovaginal symptoms due to noninfectious etiologies. Symptoms are indistinguishable from those of infectious syndromes but are most commonly confused with acute candidal vaginitis, as these patients present with pruritus, irritation, burning, soreness, and variable discharge. Noninfectious causes have been poorly studied and their true prevalence is largely unknown. Such causes include (1) irritants, physical (e.g., minipads) or chemical (e.g., spermicides, povidone-iodine, topical antimycotics, soaps and perfumes, etc.); (2) allergens, responsible for immunologic acute and chronic hypersensitivity reactions including contact dermatitis (e.g., latex condoms, antimycotic creams). There is an endless list of topical factors responsible for local inflammatory reactions and symptoms and many more have yet to be defined. Depending on the site of contact, symptoms may be vaginal or vulvar. Not infrequently, a noninfectious mechanism may coexist with an infectious process or may follow upon it.

A noninfectious cause should be considered in patients when the three common infectious causes are excluded and

in the presence of a normal vaginal pH, normal saline, KOH microscopy, and, ultimately, by a negative yeast culture. Unfortunately, given the anticipated 20 percent colonization rate in normal, asymptomatic patients, a positive yeast culture will occasionally reflect the presence of an innocent bystander and not the putative cause of the vulvovaginal symptoms. The only logical way of establishing the role of *Candida* in this context is to treat with an oral antifungal agent and assess the clinical response.

Once a local chemical, irritant, or allergic reaction is suspected, the practitioner is required to initiate a detailed inquiry into possible causal factors. Offending agents or behaviors should be eliminated wherever possible. In addition, patients should generally be advised to avoid chemical irritants and allergens (e.g., soaps, detergents, etc.). The immediate management of severe vulvovaginal symptoms of noninfectious etiology remains a challenge and does not consist of topical corticosteroids, which are rarely the solution; moreover, high-potency steroid creams frequently cause intense burning. Avoidance of the offending agent, if identified, will usually result in improvement or resolution of the symptoms. Local relief measures include sodium bicarbonate sitzbaths, or oral antihistamines.

Some investigators have described a syndrome of hyperacidity of the vagina due to overgrowth of lactobacilli. Rebound increase in the *Lactobacillus*-dominant vaginal flora occurs after completion of topical antimycotics, which may suppress population numbers of healthy resident flora. This proposed syndrome of cytolytic vaginosis is characterized clinically by vulvovaginal burning, irritation, soreness, and dyspareunia and is usually incorrectly diagnosed as VVC. The finding of large numbers of lactobacilli on wet mount together with extensive cytolysis of squamous epithelial cells is said to confirm the diagnosis. Recommended therapy for cytolytic vaginosis is daily alkaline douching using sodium bicarbonate to elevate the low vaginal pH and suppress growth of lactobacilli.

ALGORITHMS IN THE MANAGEMENT OF ACUTE VAGINITIS

Several algorithms have recently been published based entirely on symptoms, without performing a physical examination or any laboratory tests. These algorithms, although useful in the developing world where lack of medical care precludes accurate diagnosis, are to be condemned and not applied in the United States. All courses of management should avoid guesswork and empiricism. Figures 43-2 and 43-3 outline a rational approach to the management of women with symptomatic vulvovaginal disease. These pathways are not empiric but based upon easily measurable objective findings (e.g., pH and microscopy of vaginal secretions).

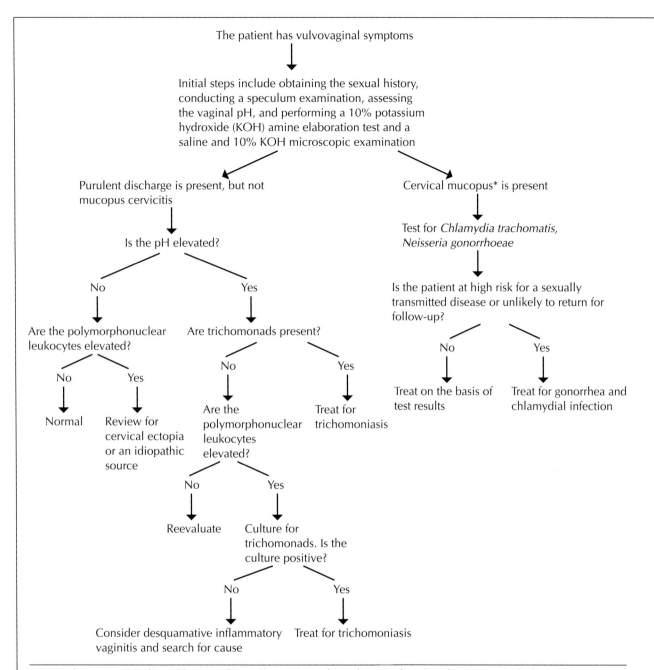

Figure 43-2

The algorithm summarizes initial management of a patient with vulvovaginal symptoms that include either purulent vaginal discharge or the presence of cervical mucopus. Mixed infections are possible.

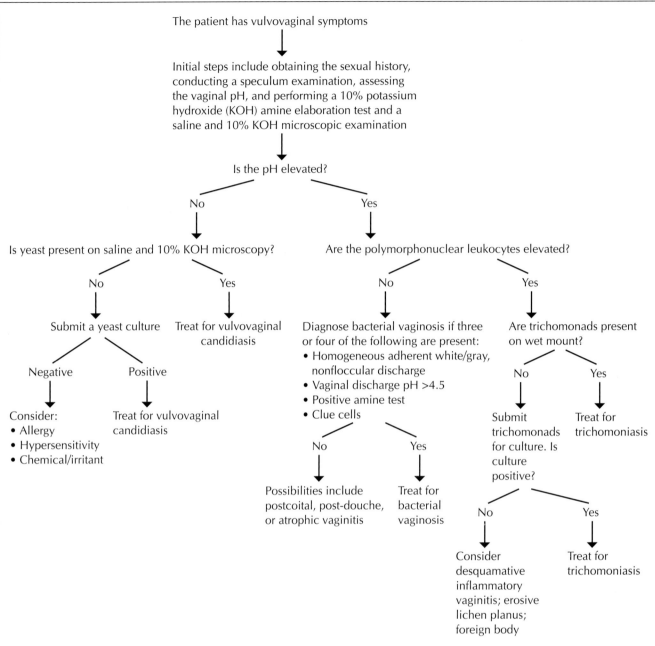

Figure 43-3

The algorithm summarizes initial management of a patient with vulvovaginal symptoms that *do not* include either purulent vaginal discharge or the presence of cervical mucopus. Mixed infections are possible.

References

1. Kent HL: Epidemiology of vaginitis. *Am J Obstet Gynecol* 165(4 pt 2):1168, 1991.
2. Sobel JD: Candidal vulvovaginitis. *Clin Obstet Gynecol* 36:153, 1993.
3. Fidel PL Jr, Lynch ME, Redondo-Lopez V, et al: Systemic cell-mediated immune reactivity in women with recurrent vulvovaginal candidiasis. *J Infect Dis* 168:1458, 1993.
4. Sobel JD, Brooker D, Stein GE, et al: Single oral dose fluconazole compared with clotrimazole topical therapy of *Candida* vaginitis: Fluconazole Vaginitis Study Group. *Am J Obstet Gynecol* 172:1263, 1955.
5. Spence MR, Hollander DH, Smith J, et al: The clinical

and laboratory diagnosis of *Trichomonas vaginalis* infection. *Sex Transm Dis* 7:168, 1980.

6. Wolner-Hanssen P, Krieger JN, Stevens CE, et al: Clinical manifestations of vaginal trichomoniasis. *JAMA* 261:571, 1989.

7. Eschenbach DA, Davick PR, Williams BL, et al: Prevalence of hydrogen peroxide producing *Lactobacillus* species in normal women and women with bacterial vaginosis. *J Clin Microbiol* 27:251, 1989.

8. Hill GB: Microbiology of bacterial vaginosis. *Am J Obstet Gynecol* 169:450, 1969.

9. Hillier SL, Krohn MA, Cassen E, et al: The role of bacterial vaginosis and vaginal bacteria in amniotic fluid infection in women in preterm labor with intact fetal membranes. *Clin Infect Dis* 20(suppl 2):276, 1995.

Chapter 44

PELVIC INFLAMMATORY DISEASE AND TUBOOVARIAN ABSCESS

Mark D. Pearlman

Judith Tintinalli

PELVIC INFLAMMATORY DISEASE

Pelvic inflammatory disease (PID) is the clinical syndrome resulting from infection of the female upper genital tract and can include any combination of endometritis, salpingitis, pelvic peritonitis, or tuboovarian abscess.[1]

Pelvic inflammatory disease is the most frequent cause of hospitalization for gynecologic disorders in reproductive-age women. According to the National Hospital Discharge Survey (1988–1990), the average annual hospitalization rate for women aged 15 to 44 for pelvic inflammatory disease was 49.3 per 10,000 (range, 31.4 to 48.6 for ages 15 to 19 and 25 to 29, respectively). When hospitalization rates were stratified by races other than white, the average annual hospitalization rate was 75.5 per 10,000 women (range, 58.3 to 88.3 for ages 15 to 19 and 25 to 29, respectively). More than

40 percent of women diagnosed with PID are between the ages of 15 and 24, and over half are nulliparous. Of all women hospitalized with PID, about one-third had a surgical procedure during the admission, and in one-third of those having surgery, the procedure was a hysterectomy.[2] Of women hospitalized with chronic PID, 90 percent underwent an operation during that admission.[3] Other consequences of PID include recurrent infection, formation of pelvic adhesions, development of tuboovarian abscess (TOA), chronic pelvic pain, infertility, and ectopic pregnancy (Table 44-1). The estimated annual cost for PID ranges from $800 million to $3 billion in the United States.

PATHOPHYSIOLOGY/MICROBIOLOGY

The commonest mechanism of infection is a sexually acquired organism (e.g., *Chlamydia trachomatis* or *Neisseria*

Table 44-1

COMMON SEQUELAE OF PELVIC INFLAMMATORY DISEASE

Sequelae	Approximate Incidence after a Single Episode of PID
Infertility	20–25%
Chronic pelvic pain/dyspareunia	15–20%
Ectopic pregnancy	6–10%
Tuboovarian abscess	2–5% (of patients hospitalized for PID)
Need for surgery	15%
Any of the above	≥25%

gonorrhoeae), leading to the ascending spread of microorganisms from the vagina and endocervix to the normally sterile upper reproductive tract. Other much less common mechanisms include spread from adjacent infection, such as appendicitis or diverticulitis; hematogenous dissemination from a distant focus, such as in tuberculosis; and transuterine spread, as from iatrogenic instrumentation (dilatation and curettage or abortion) or the placement of an intrauterine device. Bacteria attach to the ciliated tubal epithelium and invade the tubal muscularis. An intense inflammatory reaction results in the adherence of tubal surfaces, with occlusion of the lumen, destruction of the cilia and microvilli on the mucosal surface of the lumen, or the formation of blind pouches, all of which can predispose to ectopic pregnancy. Pyosalpinx or tuboovarian abscess may form, and rupture of the abscess can result in intraperitoneal dissemination of infection.[4]

Although most cases of PID are polymicrobial, it has no typical microbiologic profile. Aerobic and anaerobic bacteria—such as streptococci, staphylococci, *Gardnerella vaginalis,* peptostreptococci, *Bacteroides* sp., *Escherichia coli, N. gonorrhoeae, C. trachomatis,* and genital mycoplasmas—have all been cultured from the genital tracts of women with documented PID.[4] In about half of the cases of PID, *N. gonorrhoeae* and *C. trachomatis* are isolated from the upper genital tract, with a variety of nongonococcal/nonchlamydial organisms isolated in 60 to 85 percent.[5] *Chlamydia* and *N. gonorrhoeae* are the primary pathogens of the endocervix and cause a mucopurulent endocervicitis. The endocervical canal and its mucous plug are thought to provide a mechanical barrier, protecting the endometrium and upper genital tract from the vaginal flora. The most likely mechanism of disease development is through cervical infection with chlamydial or gonococcal organisms, which interfere with these barriers and permit ascending infection from a variety of pathogenic and endogenous vaginal flora.[6]

A relationship exists between the onset of PID and the time of menses, such that two-thirds to three-quarters of women with PID present during or just after their menses. This relationship may be due to the fact that normal menses bring about changes in the cervical mucus permitting passage of organisms to the upper genital tract.

DIAGNOSIS

The clinical diagnosis of PID can be difficult. Its presentation and severity vary widely, and there is no single historical, physical, or laboratory finding that is both sensitive and specific for PID.[7] Common historical findings in women with laparoscopically confirmed PID include lower abdominal pain (94 percent), subjective increase in vaginal discharge (55 percent), history of fever and/or chills (41 percent), irregular bleeding (35 percent), and urinary or GI symptoms (19 and 10 percent, respectively). Objective findings in this same group of women have included adnexal tenderness in 97 percent, visually abnormal vaginal discharge in 64 percent, and fever in one-third.[8] However, many women with these findings were subsequently shown to have other pathology (e.g., appendicitis, endometriosis, ruptured ovarian cysts, or normal pelvis), demonstrating the nonspecificity or poor positive predictive value of clinical diagnosis. In fact, 20 to 25 percent of women given a diagnosis of PID will have a normal pelvis on laparoscopic examination. A list of other disease processes with similar symptoms is given in Table 44-2.

The accurate clinical diagnosis of PID is often dependent upon and improved by evaluating the epidemiologic characteristics and clinical setting of the patient. Women presenting with signs and symptoms of PID who are sexually

Table 44-2

DIFFERENTIAL DIAGNOSIS OF ACUTE PELVIC INFLAMMATORY DISEASE

Adnexal torsion with or without neoplasm
Appendicitis
Diverticulitis
Ectopic pregnancy
Endometriosis
Gastroenteritis
Lower genital tract infection (cervicitis)
Normal pelvis (20–25%)
Ruptured ovarian cyst (mittelschmerz, hemorrhagic corpus luteum)
Septic abortion
Urinary tract pathology (pyelonephritis, low ureteral calculus)

active, are in their teens, are attending an STD clinic, have a prior history of PID, or belong to a socioeconomic group with a high incidence of gonorrhea or chlamydia infections are more likely to have PID as opposed to women who do not have these characteristics.[1] Other factors associated with PID include douching, bacterial vaginosis, recent IUD insertion or uterine manipulation (e.g., dilatation and curettage) and presentation during or following the bleeding phase of the menstrual cycle.[9] A list of risk factors for PID is given in Table 44-3.

The accurate diagnosis of PID on the basis of clinical signs and symptoms is a challenging task since the positive predictive value of clinical diagnosis is only slightly better than two-thirds, using laparoscopy as the standard.[8] The Centers for Disease Control and Prevention (CDC) developed guidelines for the diagnosis of PID in 1993.[1] Because a delay in the diagnosis of PID can result in substantial tubal damage, an effort was made to make these diagnostic criteria as sensitive as possible. These criteria (Table 44-4) were established knowing that the specificity and hence positive predictive value of the diagnostic criteria would not be as high as more rigorous criteria. Simply put, the use of these criteria will likely overdiagnose PID, resulting in an effort to treat as many women as possible who actually have PID. Recognizing this, one must be aware of the social implications of this diagnosis, which is likely to be inaccurate one-third of the time. Counseling patients (couples) about the imprecision of diagnosis is a good policy. Although prior PID is a risk factor for future episodes of PID, caution should be exercised in simply rediagnosing PID each time a woman presents again with lower abdominal pain, as recurrent pelvic pain can have many other causes (e.g., endometriosis, adenomyosis, ovarian cysts). Of course, should cervical specimens for *N. gonorrhoeae* or *C. trachomatis* return positive, the definite sexually acquired nature of this infection must be discussed to prevent further spread. It is important to inform women diagnosed with PID of the possibility of

Table 44-4

CRITERIA FOR THE DIAGNOSIS OF PELVIC INFLAMMATORY DISEASE

Minimal criteria (all three must be present in the absence of an established cause other than PID)
Lower abdominal tenderness
Adnexal tenderness
Cervical motion tenderness

Additional criteria (improve specificity)
Temperature >38°C (100.9°F)
Abnormal cervical or vaginal discharge
Elevated erythrocyte sedimentation rate
Elevated C-reactive protein
Cervical culture positive for *N. gonorrorhea* or *C. trachomatis*

Elaborate criteria
Endometritis on endometrial biopsy
Tuboovarian abscess on sonography or other radiologic test
Demonstration of disease by laparoscopy

Source: Adapted from Centers for Disease Control and Prevention,[1] with permission.

a sexually transmitted disease (STD), the need for treatment or testing of sexual partners, and the need for condom use if sexual activity occurs before laboratory results return. It is also important to recommend screening for other STDs in these women [e.g., human immunodeficiency virus (HIV), syphilis, hepatitis B]. Women who are HIV-positive are more likely to fail antimicrobial therapy and to require operative intervention.[10]

The physical examination of women with PID can be quite variable. Fever is likely to be present in only one-third of these women. Unless a ruptured TOA is present (rare), vital signs are usually stable, with only a mild tachycardia being common. The lower abdomen is virtually always tender, ranging from mild to severe. The finding of peritoneal signs (involuntary guarding, rebound tenderness) may simply reflect purulent material in the peritoneal cavity from an otherwise uncomplicated PID but should raise some suspicion about a more complicated process, such as a ruptured appendicitis or a tuboovarian mass. The presence of fever and lower abdominal tenderness, and signs of peritoneal irritation in a woman with unstable vital signs (tachycardia, hypotension, tachypnea), should raise the specter of a ruptured TOA—a true surgical emergency.

On speculum examination, an inflamed cervix with mucopurulent discharge supports the diagnosis, but its absence does not eliminate the possibility of PID. Adnexal tenderness (usually bilateral) and cervical motion tenderness are almost always present, but in varying degrees of severity. Physical

Table 44-3

RISK FACTORS FOR PELVIC INFLAMMATORY DISEASE

- Prior episodes of PID
- Multiple sexual patterns (more than two partners in the past 30 days)
- Exposure to gonorrhea or chlamydial infection
- Recent IUD insertion (within 4 months) or IUD use with multiple sexual partners
- Sexually active adolescents
- Douching

evaluation of cervical motion tenderness (CMT) should be performed with care, as it can be elicited in women without pelvic pathology if excessive lateral displacement is used. In patients with PID, CMT results from stretching of the inflamed parametrial structures, including the fallopian tube as well as the broad ligament and its contents. Gentle, limited lateral movement of the cervix (2 to 3 cm) is sufficient to elicit CMT if it is present. Adequate examination of the adnexal structures is frequently compromised by tenderness. If the examination is inadequate because of tenderness or if a mass is palpable, pelvic ultrasound should be obtained (see "Imaging Studies," below). Although the clinical criteria for diagnosing PID are listed in Table 44-4, the gold standard for the diagnosis of PID is laparoscopy with demonstration of tubal edema, erythema, and purulent exudate. Laparoscopy is usually reserved for women with an uncertain diagnosis, particularly if there is concern over a need for surgical intervention (e.g., differentiating PID from appendicitis or adnexal torsion).

Routine laboratory studies are not necessary (except cervical cultures for gonorrhea and chlamydia) for the diagnosis of PID; however, their use can help to improve the specificity (hence positive predictive value) of the diagnosis. Cultures (or other methods of identification) of *N. gonorrhoeae* and *Chlamydia* from the cervix should be routinely performed. Determination of the white blood cell (WBC) count, sedimentation rate, or level of C-reactive protein may be helpful in supporting the diagnosis.[11] Pregnancy should be excluded using a sensitive pregnancy test. Screening for other STDs including HIV, syphilis, and hepatitis B is appropriate. Screening for other, more uncommon STDs may also be performed if clinical signs and symptoms are present (see Chap. 42). These women are also more likely to have Pap smear abnormalities. Pap smears, if not obtained within the prior year, should either be performed or the patient should be referred for follow-up.

TREATMENT

Treatment can be accomplished as an inpatient or outpatient, depending on the clinical status of the patient. Tables 44-5, 44-6, and 44-7 list the CDC's guidelines for hospitalization as well as inpatient and outpatient treatment regimens. There is no single antimicrobial agent that both provides adequate antibiotic coverage and has been evaluated sufficiently in this setting. Some practitioners consider providing empiric treatment of the patient's sexual partner(s) for both gonorrhea and chlamydial infection, whether or not cultures from the partner have been obtained and whether or not they are positive. An algorithm for the diagnosis and management of PID is shown in Fig. 44-1.

Women with an intrauterine device and suspected PID may recover from the initial infection with the IUD remaining in place, but such women are at high risk for recurrence. Therefore, most experts advise removal of an IUD in the presence of PID. If the IUD is to be removed, intravenous antibiotics should be administered before IUD removal to prevent bacteremia or septic shock.[12]

Table 44-5

INDICATIONS FOR HOSPITALIZATION FOR PELVIC INFLAMMATORY DISEASE

1. Uncertain diagnosis, especially if appendicitis or ectopic pregnancy is in the differential diagnosis
2. Pelvic abscess
3. Concomitant pregnancy
4. Adolescence
5. HIV-positive status or acquired immunodeficiency syndrome
6. Clinical toxicity or persistent nausea and vomiting
7. Inability to manage outpatient therapy
8. Failure to respond to outpatient management
9. Inability to provide follow-up within 72 h

Source: Adapted from Centers for Disease Control and Prevention,[1] with permission.

INDICATIONS FOR SPECIALTY CONSULTATION AND FOLLOW-UP

Any of the indications for hospitalization (Table 44-5) should initiate a consultation with a practitioner familiar with the inpatient management of PID. When the diagnosis

---

Table 44-6

RECOMMENDATIONS FOR INPATIENT THERAPY

Regimen A[a]
  Cefoxitin 2g IV q6h
  OR
  Cefotetan 2 g IV q12h
  PLUS
  Doxycycline 100 mg IV or PO q12h

Regimen B[b]
  Clindamycin 900 mg IV q8h
  AND
  Gentamicin 2 mg/kg loading dose, followed by 1.5 mg/kg IV q8h

[a]This regimen should be continued for at least 48 h, and improvement is expected within 3 to 5 days. After termination of intravenous therapy, doxycycline should be continued at a dose of 100 mg PO b.i.d. to total 14 days of treatment.
[b]Preferred for tuboovarian abscess.
Source: Adapted from Centers for Disease Control and Prevention,[1] with permission.

<table>
<tr><td colspan="1">

Table 44-7

OUTPATIENT TREATMENT OF PELVIC
INFLAMMATORY DISEASE[a]

</td></tr>
</table>

Regimen A
  Cefoxitin 2 g IM plus 1 g probenecid concurrently PO
  OR
  Ceftriaxone 250 mg IM
  AND
  Doxycycline 100 mg PO b.i.d. for 14 days

Regimen B
  Ofloxacin 400 mg PO b.i.d. for 14 days
  AND EITHER
  Clindamycin 450 mg PO q.i.d. for 14 days
        OR
  Metronidazole 500 mg PO b.i.d. for 14 days

[a]Follow up in 72 h.
Source: Adapted from Centers for Disease Control and Prevention,[1]
with permission.

is not certain and there is a reasonable possibility of the need for surgical intervention (e.g., lower abdominal tenderness and signs of peritoneal irritation), consultation with a gynecologist or surgeon is appropriate. If outpatient therapy is chosen, follow-up must be arranged within 72 hours to assess adequate response to therapy. Inability to arrange follow-up is an indication for hospitalization. Finally, patients must be informed of their gonorrheal and chlamydial culture results and state or county health departments should also be informed of positive cultures, as required by local ordinance.

TUBOOVARIAN ABSCESS

Tuboovarian abscess (TOA) occurs in approximately 5 percent of women hospitalized for PID, though estimates of up to one-third of hospitalized women with PID have been reported. Interestingly, 30 to 40 percent of women diagnosed with TOA will have no preceding diagnosis of PID and may present with a variety of findings, including an asymptomatic pelvic mass.

Women presenting with symptomatic TOA have a constellation of findings similar to those of PID. Therefore, lower abdominal pain, cervical motion tenderness, adnexal tenderness, and the presence of an inflammatory adnexal mass is the most predictable combination of findings. However, pelvic tenderness may preclude the performance of an adequate exam, and reliance on imaging techniques, partic-

ularly ultrasound, becomes important in establishing the diagnosis. In a large series of patients with TOA, a history of fever and chills was present in half, whereas abnormal vaginal discharge, nausea, and abnormal bleeding were found in 25 percent or fewer.[13] On physical examination, only two-thirds of women have documented fever, and a similar frequency of leukocytosis was seen. Therefore, one cannot rely on absence of fever or leukocytosis to rule out a TOA.

PATHOPHYSIOLOGY/MICROBIOLOGY

The basic cause of TOA is similar to that of PID—cervicitis, followed by an ascending migration of bacteria from the lower genital tract, resulting in tubal infection with erythema, edema, and the production of purulent fluid. Though the process is usually initiated by way of an STD, genital tract or colon malignancy and diverticulitis are important causes of TOAs in menopausal women. As a TOA develops, a progression from an aerobic to anaerobic environment occurs, with a concomitant change in bacterial species. As such, primary infecting organisms, which are typically facultative anaerobes (*Escherichia coli,* streptococci), are gradually replaced by obligate anaerobic organisms (e.g., *Bacteroides* sp., *Prevotella* sp., peptostreptococci) as the abscess cavity develops over several days. Although many of these organisms originate in the lower genital tract, some may originate in the bowel, migrating across the inflamed bowel wall. Both the small and large bowels can be primarily involved as part of the abscess wall. While *N. gonorrhoeae* and *C. trachomatis* can frequently be isolated from the cervix of women with TOA, it is unusual to isolate either organism from the abscess cavity itself (<5 percent). *Actinomyces* may also be isolated from the abscess, particularly in women with IUDs.

IMAGING STUDIES

Ultrasound is the primary imaging procedure used in the diagnosis of adnexal masses, including inflammatory complexes. While alternative modalities like computed tomography (CT), magnetic resonance imaging, and radionuclide scanning can also demonstrate TOAs, their expense, radiation exposure, or general inability to produce fine resolution make them less desirable as primary imaging procedures. Ultrasound is helpful for primary diagnosis as well as a useful method of following response to therapy through serial exams. The characteristic appearance of a TOA on ultrasound is a thick-walled, multiseptate mass that has layered sediment or debris in the most dependent portion (Fig. 44-2). Similar findings can be seen on CT.

TREATMENT

Rupture of a TOA is a true surgical emergency. Hemodynamic stabilization and initial administration of a broad

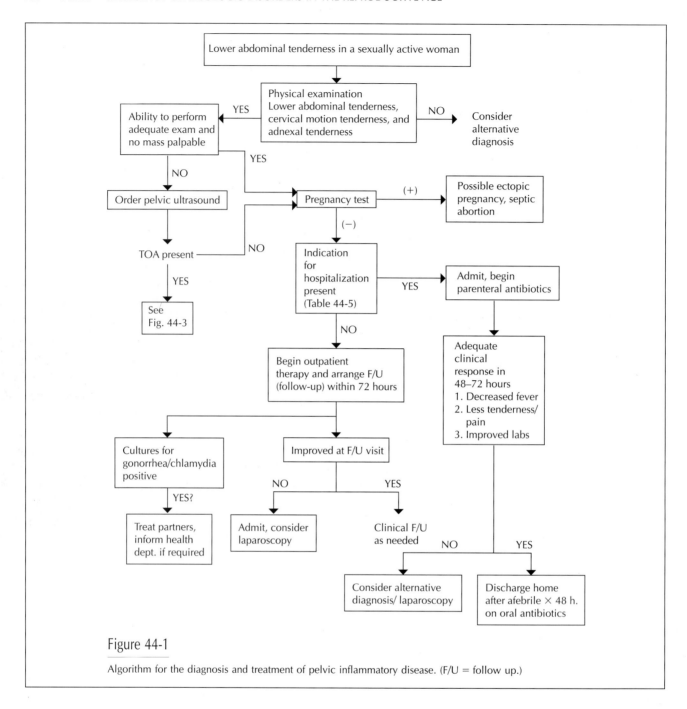

Figure 44-1

Algorithm for the diagnosis and treatment of pelvic inflammatory disease. (F/U = follow up.)

spectrum antibiotic followed by prompt surgical intervention with removal of the involved pelvic organs is necessary. Delay in diagnosis and surgical management results in increased mortality. Untreated, mortality rates of up to 100 percent have been reported.

Unlike abscesses elsewhere in the body, many unruptured TOAs can be successfully managed with antibiotics alone without the need for drainage or surgical removal.[5,13] The use of antibiotics without surgery or drainage is associated with a 60 to 80 percent likelihood of clinical improvement and hospital discharge. One of the key factors in obtaining an adequate response to antibiotics is the utilization of agents

with a sufficiently wide antimicrobial spectrum to cover the bacteria typically seen in TOAs (Table 44-6). Landers and Sweet demonstrated an 81 percent response rate (175 of 217) with the use of clindamycin and gentamicin.[13] In a similar population, the same investigators reported that use of antibiotics with poor anaerobic coverage (e.g., penicillin and gentamicin) resulted in a failure rate of two-thirds! However, long-term success of antibiotics without surgery is less than the quoted 60 to 80 percent, as some of these initial responders (perhaps 20 to 30 percent) will eventually require an operation because of continued or recurrent pain. *Bacteroides fragilis*, a common isolate, has shown increasing re-

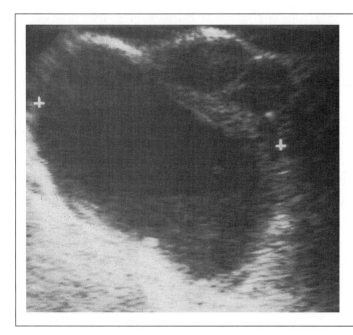

Figure 44-2

Ultrasound of tuboovarian abscess demonstrating thick-walled, multiseptate adnexal abscess with dependent layering of inflammatory debris. (From Sweet RL, Gibbs RS: *Infectious Diseases of the Female Genital Tract,* 3d ed. Baltimore: Williams & Wilkins, 1996, with permission.)

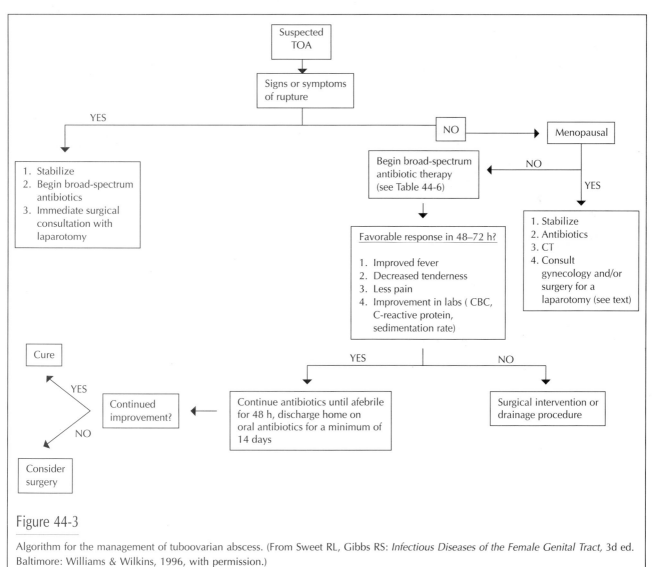

Figure 44-3

Algorithm for the management of tuboovarian abscess. (From Sweet RL, Gibbs RS: *Infectious Diseases of the Female Genital Tract,* 3d ed. Baltimore: Williams & Wilkins, 1996, with permission.)

sistance to clindamycin in the last 5 to 10 years, and metronidazole-containing regimens (e.g., ampicillin, metronidazole, and gentamicin) or broad-spectrum single agents with good anaerobic coverage (e.g., ampicillin/sulbactam) are being used with comparable success to clindamycin-containing regimens reported in the 1980s, albeit with a more limited experience.[5]

Clinical response to antibiotic therapy is usually demonstrated in 48 to 72 hours, with reduction in fever, pain, abdominal tenderness, and laboratory markers of inflammation (e.g., WBC count, C-reactive protein, sedimentation rate). Failures are more commonly seen in TOAs more than 8 cm in diameter or when there is bilateral adnexal involvement.

Failure of TOA to respond to initial medical management indicates a need for surgical intervention. A variety of treatment modalities—ranging from drainage procedures under imaging guidance to hysterectomy with bilateral salpingo-oophorectomy—have been successfully used. While there are some reports of successful series of ultrasound- or CT-guided drainage,[14] in general the experience is limited, and clear recommendations for patient selection are lacking. Total abdominal hysterectomy with bilateral salpingo-oophorectomy results in the highest rate of successful resolution of symptoms but is less desirable in some women, as it leaves them menopausal and infertile. Unilateral involvement has been treated successfully with unilateral adnexectomy. An algorithm for management of TOA is shown in Fig. 44-3. Tuboovarian abscess in the menopausal age group represents a special circumstance, since there is a significant association between TOAs and gastrointestinal or genitourinary malignancy[15,16] (colon, endometrial, cervical, and ovarian cancer). Diverticular abscess is also seen as a cause of TOAs in this group of women. Because of the high incidence of malignancy, stabilization, antibiotics, and gynecology or other surgical referral is recommended in menopausal women with a pelvic abscess.

References

1. Centers for Disease Control and Prevention: 1993 Sexually transmitted disease treatment guidelines. *MMWR* 42:44, 1993.

2. Velebil P, Wingo P, Zhisen X, et al: Rate of hospitalization for gynecologic disorders among reproductive age women in the United States. *Obstet Gynecol* 86:764, 1995.

3. Rolfs RT, Galaid EL, Zaida AA: Pelvic inflammatory disease: Trends in hospitalization and office visits, 1979 through 1988. *Am J Obstet Gynecol* 166:983, 1992.

4. Rice P, Schachter J: Pathogenesis of pelvic inflammatory disease. *JAMA* 266:2587, 1991.

5. Sweet RL: Pelvic inflammatory disease and infertility in women. *Infect Dis Clin North Am* 1:199, 1987.

6. Pastorek JG: Pelvic inflammatory disease and tubo-ovarian abscess. *Obstet Gynecol Clin North Am* 16:347, 1989.

7. Kahn J, Walker C, Washington AE, et al: Diagnosing pelvic inflammatory disease. *JAMA* 266:2594, 1991.

8. Jacobsen L, Westrom L: Objectivized diagnosis of acute pelvic inflammatory disease. *Am J Obstet Gynecol* 105:1088, 1969.

9. Washington AE, Aral SO, Wolner-Hanssen PW, et al: Assessing risk for pelvic inflammatory disease and its sequelae. *JAMA* 266:2581, 1991.

10. Korn AP, Landers DV, Green JR, Sweet RL: Pelvic inflammatory disease in HIV infected women. *Obstet Gynecol* 82:765, 1993.

11. Piepert JF, Boardman L, Hogan JW, et al. Laboratory evaluation of acute upper genital tract infection. *Obstet Gynecol* 87:730, 1996.

12. Peterson HB, Walker CK, Kahn JG, et al: Pelvic inflammatory disease. *JAMA* 266:2605, 1991.

13. Landers DV, Sweet RL:Tubo-ovarian abscess: Contemporary approach to management. *Rev Infect Dis* 5(S):876, 1983.

14. Aboulghar MA, Mansour RT, Serour GI: Ultrasonographically guided transvaginal aspirations of tuboovarian abscess and pyosalpinges: An optional treatment for acute pelvic inflammatory disease. *Am J Obstet Gynecol* 172:1501, 1995.

15. Hoffman M, Molpus K, Roberts WS, et al: Tuboovarian abscess in postmenopausal women. *J Reprod Med* 35:525, 1990.

16. Barton DP, Fiorica JV, Hoffman MS, et al: Cervical cancer and tuboovarian abscesses: A report of three cases. *J Reprod Med* 38:561, 1993.

Chapter 45

COMPLICATIONS OF GYNECOLOGIC PROCEDURES

William W. Hurd

Jean A. Hurteau

Gynecologic procedures are among the most common surgical procedures performed in the United States today. In the past, all major surgical procedures were followed by close hospital observation until complete recovery was assured. Today, in part because of fiscal considerations, patients are often sent home within 12 to 24 h of major surgery. The unavoidable result is the increased presentation of postoperative complications to the emergency department (ED) that, only a generation ago, would have rarely been seen outside a hospital ward. In contrast to the hospital setting, where trained observers can often detect and treat a complication at its earliest stage, a patient may not return for evaluation until the complication has progressed significantly. The result is that complications seen in the ED may be much further advanced than those seen in an inpatient setting.

After any gynecologic procedure, a progressive resolution of symptoms during the first postoperative week is to be expected. With abdominal procedures, slow return to completely normal bowel function may take several days. For any procedure, pain may be perceived as slightly worse on the day following the procedure, but it should only improve after this point. Likewise, the incision should appear healthy and should become almost painless within the first week.

Patients should be clearly counseled on the natural postoperative course of events, and any deviation from this course should lead the patient to call. A natural tendency may be to reassure the patient that her postoperative discomfort is within the normal range. However, delay of appropriate care can often compound the effects of complications and may potentially be fatal. If a patient who calls cannot be assured with absolute certainty that she is not experiencing surgical complications, the patient should be advised to come in for an evaluation by a practitioner experienced in recognizing them.

PATHOPHYSIOLOGY

Gynecologic surgery, whether approached abdominally or vaginally, carries a risk of postoperative complications in the range of 1 to 4 percent.[1,2] In general, these complications may involve the abdominal incision, the urinary tract, or intraabdominal processes. Because of the unique nature of both laparoscopic and vaginal surgery, the seriousness of the complication may have no relationship to the size (or even presence) of an abdominal incision.

Complications related to abdominal incisions may result from operative procedures involving either laparotomy or laparoscopy. Wound infections are among the most common complications after laparotomy, but they are relatively infrequent with laparoscopy. In either case, infection will most commonly develop within 3 to 5 days of surgery, with erythema and tenderness along all or part of the incision. This complication is most commonly related to bacterial contamination of the wound at the time of surgery or colonization shortly after surgery by skin flora. It is extremely important to determine the extent of the infection, since superficial infections are safely treated in an outpatient setting, whereas extensive cellulitis and necrotizing fasciitis are almost always treated in an inpatient setting.

With laparoscopy, wound infections are relatively uncommon. However, laparoscopy more commonly results in the formation of a hematoma beneath the incision site. This is because laparoscopic trocar insertion can result in occult injury to vessels in the abdominal wall with, in some cases, little external bleeding. This problem is much more likely to arise when large trocars ($\geq$10 mm in diameter) are placed lateral to the midline. In most cases, problems of this nature appear within hours of surgery.

Incisional drainage may sometimes be encountered after laparotomy or laparoscopy. When significant drainage originates from an incision immediately above the symphysis, bladder injury should always be suspected, as this may be the first indication of such a problem. Bladder injury may be more common in cases where the patient has undergone a previous laparotomy that has resulted in displacement of the bladder above the symphysis. Bowel injuries may occasionally present as incisional drainage from a enterocutaneous fistula. A wound dehiscence can also present as a serosanguinous discharge; thus the integrity of the fascia should be verified. Finally, a seroma, or collection of serous fluid in the subcutaneous area, which may occur as part of the normal healing process, may present as wound discharge. However, the possibility of a more serious underlying condition should always be ruled out before making this diagnosis.

Abdominal pain may be the most common presenting symptom after gynecologic surgery. In some cases, this pain may represent an incisional complication. A special case may be entrapped incisional hernias that occur after laparoscopy. Herniation is rare at the site where the laparoscope is placed through the umbilicus. However, bowel herniation has been reported to occur when large trocars ($\geq$10 mm) are used in locations lateral to the midline. Apparently, this is not related to herniation through a fascial defect but rather to entrapment of bowel that has herniated through the peritoneum into the preperitoneal space. This appears to be a different process from that of an incisional hernia occurring after laparotomy, where a palpable bulge is the most common presenting symptom and entrapment is uncommon. After laparoscopy, herniation may present as severe abdominal pain accompanied by signs of bowel obstruction. Although incisional hernias should always be considered as a possible cause of abdominal pain after laparoscopic surgery, they are relatively infrequent. Thus, other intraabdominal processes should also be considered.

Abdominal pain may be related to problems involving the urinary tract. A common complaint within the first 24 h after laparoscopy is urinary retention. Even if no surgery has been performed around the bladder, some patients find it difficult to void immediately after receiving general anesthesia for surgery.[3] Whether this is an anesthetic effect or the result of the inability to bear down because of incisional pain is questionable. Whatever the cause, increasing lower abdominal discomfort associated with a midline mass should suggest this easily treatable possibility.

Occasionally postoperative abdominal pain may result from a urinary tract infection (UTI). Prior to most gynecologic procedures, most patients are catheterized to minimize the risk of bladder injury during trocar placement. For laparoscopy, an indwelling catheter is not commonly used. For laparotomy, an indwelling bladder catheter is used in most cases. In either case, catheterization is associated with the risk of UTI, regardless of the sterile precautions taken. The result can be symptomatic cystitis or pyelonephritis that may not manifest until days after the original surgery.

Although incisional or urinary tract problems can result in postoperative abdominal pain, this symptom may represent a more serious intraabdominal complication. When extensive intraabdominal surgery has been performed by laparotomy, by laparoscopy, or via the vagina, the risk of a major complication is increased. Intraabdominal hemorrhage, while not the most common complication, is probably the most serious.

Postoperative hemorrhage is a risk after any gynecologic surgery, which usually manifests within 24 h of surgery. In rare cases, hemorrhage may take several days to become apparent. From an ED perspective, this complication may be of increased importance after operative laparoscopy, since laparoscopic procedures are almost always performed on an outpatient basis. Blood usually causes peritoneal irritation; thus most patients will present with abdominal pain with or without signs of hemodynamic compromise. In other patients, dizziness or syncope may be the earliest signs of a significant intraabdominal hemorrhage. Abdominal distention is a late finding consistent with massive intraabdominal hemorrhage.

Infection at the site of surgery is the most common complication following hysterectomy or vaginal procedures.[1] The risk may be especially high in patients who had a postoperative fever that resolved with or without antibiotic treatment. These patients may have indolent infections that manifest as a pelvic abscess or cellulitis at the vaginal cuff after hysterectomy. The presenting symptom may be pain and fever, abnormal vaginal discharge, or abdominal distention caused by hypoactive intestines (often termed *functional ileus*) related to bowel irritation. Presentation of this problem to the ED may be more common when patients are discharged within 24 h of surgery after laparoscopically assisted vaginal hysterectomy or vaginal hysterectomy, since the first signs of infection may appear after the patient has been discharged. After vaginal hysterectomy, no special precautions are needed for a speculum examination. Vaginal cuff disruption is rare and impossible to cause by exam.

Ureteral injury is another complication that may be seen after hysterectomy or any surgery requiring dissection or ligation of side-wall vessels, such as removal of an adnexus. It has also been reported after fulgurization of endometriosis on the pelvic side wall. Ureteral injuries—including complete ligation, transection, partial resection, or thermal injuries—will usually manifest within hours to days of surgery. With shorter periods of hospitalization after surgery, this may be more commonly diagnosed in an outpatient. Complete obstruction will usually result in severe flank pain, whereas transection may manifest as the symptoms of intraabdominal irritation caused by urine leakage. Transperitoneal thermal injuries resulting from fulgurization of endometriosis may be similar to those after transection, but the appearance of symptoms may be delayed for several days until tissue necrosis occurs.

A potentially catastrophic complication of gynecologic surgery is bowel injury. During laparotomy, this is usually recognized immediately and repaired because there is more complete visualization. During laparoscopic or vaginal surgery, bowel injuries may be more difficult to recognize and thus may go undiagnosed until secondary symptoms develop. The potential for this problem to go unrecognized is increased by the brief hospitalizations associated with these procedures.

With vaginal hysterectomy, the peritoneal cavity is never completely visualized. Bowel injuries may result from blunt lysis of unseen adhesion between the reproductive organs and bowel or by the inadvertent inclusion of a section of bowel in a uterine pedicle above the view of the operator. Bowel injuries of this nature will often manifest with peritonitis or signs of bowel obstruction several days after surgery.

Laparoscopic surgery may result in injuries to either the small or large intestine by several mechanisms. An unrecognized bowel injury may occur at the time of trocar insertion. Thermal bowel injuries may also occur during laparoscopy, since power sources such as electrocautery and laser are commonly used during these procedures. Major bowel injuries usually become obvious during surgery. However, because of the limited field of view, some major bowel injuries and many smaller ones may not be seen during surgery. These injuries usually manifest themselves 1 to 3 days after surgery, well after the patient has been released following these primarily outpatient procedures.

Perforations of the large intestines usually present as an intraabdominal infectious process within the first 24 h after surgery because of the resulting bacterial contamination of the peritoneal cavity. Thermal injury of the colon may characteristically be delayed in presentation for 1 to 5 days or more, until bowel wall necrosis results in intraperitoneal infection. Injuries of the small intestines are often more subtle in presentation. Apparently normal postoperative discomfort may progress to signs of peritonitis with eventual abdominal distention as the sterile contents of the small intestine leak from the bowel. Because of the lack of signs of infection in many cases, this diagnosis may be more difficult to make.

Another presentation of complications following gynecologic surgery is vaginal bleeding or discharge. After hysterectomy, a minimal amount of bleeding commonly occurs within the first 2 to 3 weeks as the sutures at the top of the vagina (the cuff) dissolve and loosen, exposing healing tissue that can ooze. During the first few days after hysterectomy, profuse vaginal bleeding may occur if a suture has loosened from a vascular pedicle. After a cone biopsy of the cervix, where the center of the cervix is removed and hemostasis is obtained by a combination of cauterization and suturing, bleeding within the first week occurs in up to 14 percent of patients. After vaginal reconstructive surgery, bleeding may be the only sign of a vaginal hematoma that can form underneath the repair.

Significant vaginal discharge, especially associated with fever or pain, may indicate infection at the site of the surgery. After minor gynecologic surgery, such as dilatation and curettage or laparoscopic tubal surgery, endometritis or cervicitis may manifest as a purulent discharge associated with pelvic tenderness. After hysterectomy, a similar presentation may represent localized cuff cellulitis or a cuff abscess. Less commonly after hysterectomy, a bowel or bladder injury with resultant fistula formation may present as vaginal discharge.

DIAGNOSIS AND DIFFERENTIAL DIAGNOSIS

INCISIONAL PAIN

In general, the diagnosis of infection or hematoma is made by inspection and palpation of the incision. Localized erythema and induration suggest a superficial infection. Fluctuance indicates a possible subcutaneous abscess. A deeper mass suggests a subfascial hematoma or abscess, although bowel herniation should also be considered (Fig. 45-1).

If cellulitis is present, the extent of the infection must be determined accurately. One of the most important differential diagnoses to make in this situation is that of necrotizing fasciitis. This rare complication may present similar to a wound abscess; however, erythema and induration with ecchymosis may be relatively more widespread and the wound is usually extremely painful. Fascial and subcutaneous necrosis may manifest as a relative lack of resistance to probing of these tissue planes. Late signs of necrotizing fasciitis are tissue crepitus and decreased sensation at the incision site. This surgical emergency requires immediate hospitalization with high-dose antibiotics and surgical debridement in an effort to treat this condition effectively, as it is associated with a 20 to 30 percent mortality rate.[4]

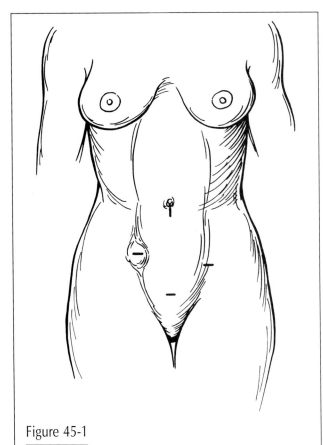

Figure 45-1

The differential diagnosis for a bulging mass underlying a surgical incision after laparoscopy should include hematoma, abscess, and bowel herniation.

Incisional drainage of clear fluid can be the sign of something as innocuous as a subcutaneous seroma. However, it must be verified that this is not the symptom of something more serious, such as a wound dehiscence or injury of bladder or bowel. Initial evaluation should be probing of the wound with a sterile, cotton-tipped applicator to verify that the fascial layer is intact. If the wound drainage is significant in quantity or resembles urine, a dilute solution of indigo carmine or methylene blue can be placed into the bladder via an indwelling catheter to check for bladder injuries. Bowel injuries that present as wound drainage are usually associated with hypoactive bowel function. However, if bowel contents drain only transcutaneously and do not spill intraperitoneally, diffuse abdominal signs may be absent. Oral charcoal has been used as a simple method to determine the presence of an enterocutaneous fistula of the small bowel.

ABDOMINAL PAIN

Abdominal pain, probably the most common presenting symptom to the ED after gynecologic surgery, can be of mul-

tiple etiologies. One common cause in the first 24 h postoperatively is urinary retention. Severe pain with a midline mass in a woman who has not voided recently suggests this diagnosis. A more common condition that may manifest postoperatively is UTI, either cystitis or pyelonephritis. With cystitis, suprapubic tenderness with or without urgency or frequency may be the presenting symptom. With pyelonephritis, costovertebral angle tenderness, usually associated with fever and leukocytosis, may be accompanied by abdominal pain or other symptoms of cystitis. Urinalysis (UA) will usually reveal bacteriuria, pyuria, leukocyte esterase activity, and occasionally hematuria.

The rest of the problems that may cause postoperative abdominal pain originate intraabdominally and may be difficult to differentiate. Intraabdominal hemorrhage may present with peritoneal signs and is verified by a decreased hemoglobin. However, usually some degree of hemodynamic instability will also be apparent, ranging from tachycardia and orthostatic hypotension to hypovolemic shock.

Operative site infection may also present with peritoneal signs associated with fever and leukocytosis. Although generalized peritonitis may be present, discrete tenderness to deep palpation over the site of surgery may be more common.

Abdominal pain may also result from a bladder or ureteral injury. Intraabdominal leakage of urine will result in peritoneal signs and leukocytosis. Fever is usually not present unless the injury has resulted in the development of a concomitant urinary tract infection. In contrast, occlusion of the ureter will result in flank pain without any peritoneal signs. On urinalysis, hematuria alone is suggestive of a urinary tract injury. Hematuria with bacteriuria and pyuria may indicate either injury with a superimposed infection or, more commonly, infection alone. Conversely, the absence of hematuria can be seen in the complete occlusion of a ureter.

Bowel problems usually present as signs of obstruction, such as nausea, vomiting, and abdominal distention. When bowel herniation at a laparoscopic trocar site leads to mechanical obstruction, there may be tenderness and a mass at the incision as well. With perforating injuries of the colon, signs of bowel obstruction are usually associated with peritonitis, functional bowel obstruction, and possibly signs of sepsis. In contrast, perforating injuries of the small intestines may be associated with functional bowel obstruction because of chemical irritation, but signs of infection are less common.

VAGINAL SYMPTOMS

Vaginal bleeding or discharge may occur after minor vaginal surgery or hysterectomy. Bleeding is the most common symptom. After cone biopsy of the cervix, approximately 14 percent of patients will have significant enough bleeding within the first 10 days to seek medical attention.[5] Speculum examination will usually reveal a discrete bleeding site on the cervix.

After uterine curettage or hysteroscopy, subsequent heavy bleeding originating from the uterine cavity is uncommon. However, after hysterectomy performed either vaginally or abdominally, vaginal bleeding may occasionally occur within the first week. In the presence of bright red vaginal bleeding, inspection of the highly vascular vaginal apex where the cervix has been excised may reveal an active bleeding site. If dark, sanguinous discharge is coming from the vaginal cuff, this may be the manifestation of a cuff hematoma that is draining vaginally.

Vaginal drainage of purulent discharge indicates infection of the surgical site. After minor gynecologic surgery, cervicitis may present as inflammation and cervical discharge associated with cervical tenderness. Endometritis and parametritis may appear similar but is associated with uterine or ovarian tenderness as well. Advanced cases of parametritis may result in more generalized peritoneal signs as well as fever and chills.

After hysterectomy, significant malodorous discharge usually indicates an infection at the vaginal cuff. Cuff cellulitis is characterized by induration and tenderness at the vaginal apex. A cuff abscess will, in addition, have a discrete mass at the apex that is either palpable or visible by ultrasound (Fig. 45-2). Both of these conditions are usually associated with fever and leukocytosis.

When vaginal discharge after hysterectomy is atypical, a fistula between the vagina and either the bladder or bowel should be considered. A vesicovaginal fistula is associated with leaking of clear fluid (urine) vaginally that the patient cannot control. This condition is usually associated with recurrent urinary tract infections. An entero-vaginal fistula is associated with the passage of intestinal contents, which may vary depending on the level of the fistula. A fistula involving the rectosigmoid is associated with passage of malodorous fecal material. In contrast, a fistula involving the small intestines will be associated with significant vaginal and vulvar inflammation, resulting from the irritating nature of the small bowel contents.

LABORATORY TESTS

In almost every case in which a woman presents to the ED after gynecologic surgery, a complete blood count (CBC) and UA will be helpful. Leukocytosis or anemia may be one of the earliest signs of several postoperative complications, as noted above. The UA will help to detect urinary tract injuries or infections, both of which are common problems after gynecologic procedures. Although hematuria as an isolated finding suggests a urinary tract injury, hematuria with pyuria and bacteriuria may represent either a UTI or a urinary tract injury with a superimposed infection.

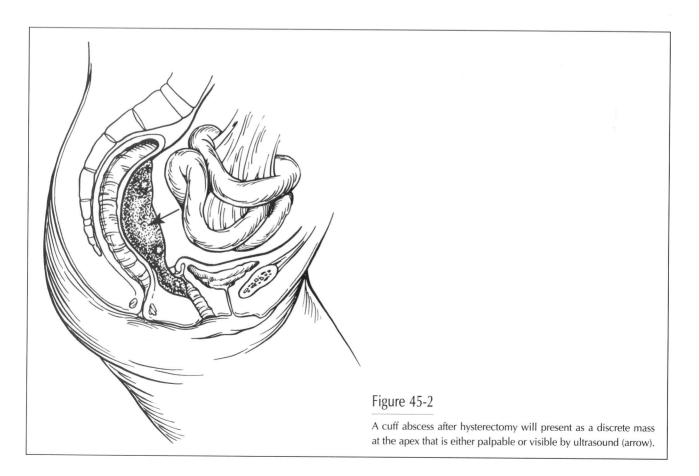

Figure 45-2

A cuff abscess after hysterectomy will present as a discrete mass at the apex that is either palpable or visible by ultrasound (arrow).

Radiologic examinations are often helpful. If an intraabdominal process is suspected, flat and upright abdominal examinations that include the diaphragm are helpful. Free air under the diaphragm more than 2 days after laparoscopy or more than a week after open abdominal surgery is suggestive of a bowel injury. Although "air" under the diaphragm can be seen the same day as laparoscopy because of the gas used for insufflation of the peritoneal cavity, the carbon dioxide that is used for this purpose is quickly absorbed. If any air is seen under the diaphragm more than 48 h after laparoscopy, bowel perforation must be strongly considered.

Pelvic ultrasound can also be very helpful in the presence of a fever or pain after hysterectomy. The presence of a loculated fluid collection in this case is suggestive of a cuff abscess, which may be drained transvaginally. In some cases, computed tomography may be necessary to locate abscesses distant from the vaginal cuff.

TREATMENT

Relatively few postoperative complications will be treated in the ED without gynecologic consultation (Fig. 45-3). Many serious complications first appear with very subtle findings that can mimic normal postoperative discomfort. The most common problems that can be treated without gynecologic consultation are superficial wound infections and urinary tract problems after injury has been ruled out.

Superficial wound infections are examined carefully to rule out deep tissue involvement and then gently explored to determine if an abscess or fascial defect exists. If an abscess is discovered but the fascia is intact, the wound should be opened completely, thoroughly irrigated, and packed with iodoform gauze. If the surrounding inflammation is limited and the patient does not appear toxic, she may be treated as an outpatient with daily dressing changes. Systemic antibiotics are often given but may be of limited benefit in a well-localized wound infection. If there is any indication of a fascial defect or a surrounding cellulitis or fasciitis, gynecologic evaluation is required for possible inpatient therapy with appropriate antibiotic coverage and surgical treatment.

Vaginal bleeding after cervical cone biopsy can often be effectively treated in the ED. In the presence of a discrete bleeding site, hemostasis can usually be obtained by suturing the site. If more widespread oozing is present, packing the operative site with a hemostatic material such as oxidized cellulose may be effective.

Many urinary tract problems that occur after gynecologic surgery can also be treated effectively in the ED. Urinary retention after laparoscopy is treated by draining the bladder with a catheter. If the UA is completely normal, the patient can be observed until she voids spontaneously. If the postvoid residual is low (i.e., less than 100 mL), she can be sent home with instructions to return if further problems with voiding arise.

However, if the residual is higher than 100 mL, she should be sent home with an indwelling catheter connected to a collection bag for follow-up the following day. This problem almost always resolves spontaneously within 24 h. Medications that may contribute to urinary retention, such as narcotics, may need to be discontinued until normal bladder function resumes.

In the absence of hematuria or significant abdominal tenderness, cystitis and pyelonephritis can also be treated appropriately in the ED. However, in the presence of flank tenderness after pelvic surgery, intravenous pyelography or renal ultrasonography should be performed to investigate the possibility of ureteral injury or obstruction. In the presence of hematuria or any intraabdominal symptoms, gynecologic evaluation may be required.

DISCHARGE INSTRUCTIONS AND FOLLOW-UP INTERVAL

For any postoperative problem treated in the ED, close follow-up is extremely important. Telephone or clinical consultation with the operating gynecologist should always be obtained. What appears to be a relatively minor problem may be the first symptom of a potentially serious postoperative complication. Follow-up within 24 to 48 h is appropriate in most cases, usually with the operating gynecologist. Wound infection, urinary retention, and urinary tract infection should respond quickly with appropriate treatment. If the symptoms do not resolve or are worsening, the possibility of a more serious complication must be considered.

INDICATIONS FOR SPECIALTY CONSULTATION AND HOSPITALIZATION

Because of the risk of serious postoperative complications, the vast majority of postoperative complications will require gynecologic evaluation in the ED. Even after diagnosis and treatment of a relatively minor problem, close follow-up by the operating gynecologist is important. Complications after gynecologic surgery are inevitable. However, failure to recognize the complication or inappropriate treatment or follow-up can significantly compound the problem.

If there is any concern that a wound infection is more than superficial, gynecologic evaluation is required to rule out dehiscence, cellulitis, or fasciitis. If an apparent UTI is associated with hematuria or signs and symptoms of an intraabdominal process, gynecologic evaluation is warranted to rule out ureteral or bladder injury. In the presence of localized abdominal pain or more widespread peritonitis, gynecologic evaluation is always required.

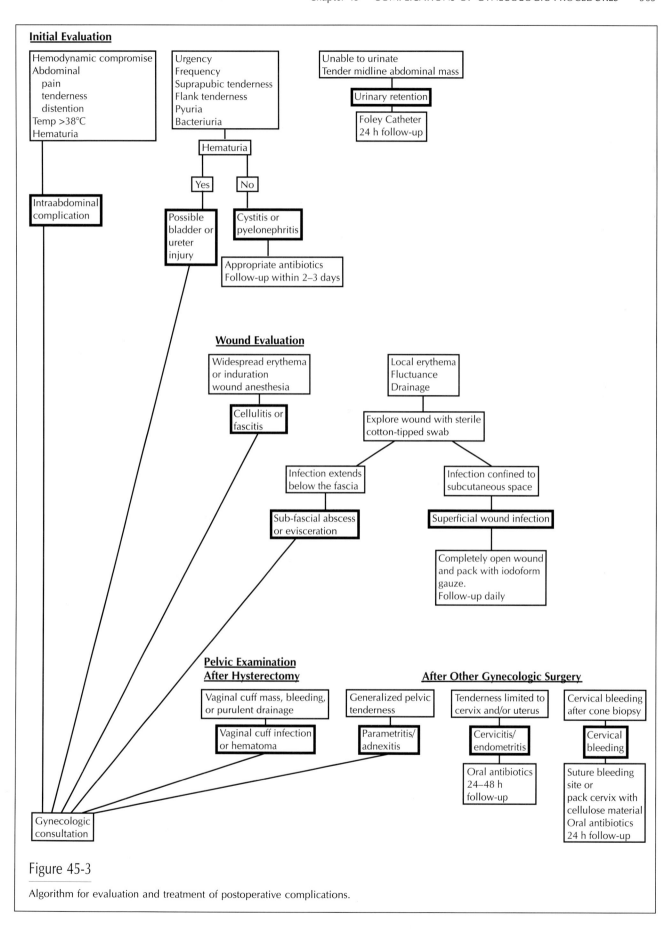

Initial Evaluation

Hemodynamic compromise
Abdominal
  pain
  tenderness
  distention
Temp >38°C
Hematuria

Intraabdominal
complication

Urgency
Frequency
Suprapubic tenderness
Flank tenderness
Pyuria
Bacteriuria

Hematuria

Yes   No

Possible
bladder or
ureter
injury

Cystitis or
pyelonephritis

Appropriate antibiotics
Follow-up within 2–3 days

Unable to urinate
Tender midline abdominal mass

Urinary retention

Foley Catheter
24 h follow-up

Wound Evaluation

Widespread erythema
or induration
wound anesthesia

Cellulitis or
fascitis

Local erythema
Fluctuance
Drainage

Explore wound with sterile
cotton-tipped swab

Infection extends
below the fascia

Sub-fascial abscess
or evisceration

Infection confined to
subcutaneous space

Superficial wound infection

Completely open wound
and pack with iodoform
gauze.
Follow-up daily

**Pelvic Examination
After Hysterectomy**

Vaginal cuff mass, bleeding,
or purulent drainage

Vaginal cuff infection
or hematoma

After Other Gynecologic Surgery

Generalized pelvic
tenderness

Parametritis/
adnexitis

Tenderness limited to
cervix and/or uterus

Cervicitis/
endometritis

Oral antibiotics
24–48 h
follow-up

Cervical bleeding
after cone biopsy

Cervical
bleeding

Suture bleeding
site or
pack cervix with
cellulose material
Oral antibiotics
24 h follow-up

Gynecologic
consultation

Figure 45-3

Algorithm for evaluation and treatment of postoperative complications.

In the case of significant vaginal bleeding after gyneco-logic surgery, gynecologic evaluation is usually required. When significant vaginal discharge indicates a post-opera-tive infection, the need for gynecologic evaluation is deter-mined by the type of surgery and the degree of infection.

After minor surgery, mild infections confined to the cervix and uterus (i.e., without abdominal manifestations) can of-ten be treated with oral antibiotics. However, if infection is accompanied by temperature elevation or leukocytosis after minor surgery, or in the presence of any sign of infection after hysterectomy, gynecologic consultation is usually re-quired.

PROCEDURES

EXPLORATION AND PACKING OF INFECTED WOUNDS

The patient is placed in a supine position and the area of the wound is prepped and draped. A sterile, cotton-tipped ap-plicator is used to gently probe along the incision until the wound is entered. If purulent discharge is encountered, the wound is opened gently along its entire course if possible. The base of the wound is probed for defects in the fascial layer. If none are encountered, the entire wound is copiously irrigated with a solution of half normal saline and half hy-drogen peroxide (5% solution).

After appropriate irrigation, the wound should appear clean and the edges slightly bloody. If the wound is sur-rounded by necrotic tissue, it should be lightly dressed and the gynecologist called to evaluate the wound for possible surgical debridement. If the wound appears to be surrounded by viable tissue, it should be packed with gauze to the level of the skin. A large dressing is then placed over the pack-ing. The patient is instructed to return for follow-up at fre-quent intervals until the base of the wound shows signs of granulation.

EVALUATION FOR BLADDER INJURIES WITH INDIGO CARMINE

In the presence of a copious amount of watery discharge af-ter gynecologic surgery from either a suprapubic incision or from the vagina, the possibility of a bladder injury should be investigated by dyeing the urine blue. One simple tech-nique is to use a balloon catheter to place a dilute solution of indigo carmine or methylene blue in normal saline (2 mL in 200 mL of normal saline) directly into the bladder. If a gauze pad placed over the wound is dyed blue within 10 to 20 min, bladder involvement is verified. For a vaginal dis-charge after hysterectomy, a tampon can be placed into the vagina and removed after 20 to 30 min. A blue stain on the tampon indicates bladder involvement. An alternate ap-proach is to inject 5 mL of indigo carmine intravenously. Methylene blue should not be given intravenously because of the risk of hemolytic anemia associated with this drug.

References

1. Harris WJ: Early complications of abdominal and vagi-nal hysterectomy. *Obstet Gynecol Surv* 50:795, 1995.
2. Mintz M: Risks and prophylaxis in laparoscopy: A sur-vey of 100,000 cases. *J Reprod Med* 18:269, 1977.
3. Frazee RC, Thames T, Appel M, et al: Laparoscopic cholecystectomy: A multicenter study. *J Laparoendosc Surg* 1:157, 1991.
4. File TM Jr, Tan JS: Treatment of skin and soft-tissue in-fections. *Am J Surg* 169:27S, 1995.
5. Larsson G, Gullberg B, Grundsell H: A comparison of complications of laser and cold knife conization. *Obstet Gynecol* 62:213, 1983.

Chapter 46

SEXUAL ASSAULT

Andrew J. Satin
Nancy F. Petit

Sexual assault is defined as any sexual act performed by one person on another without that person's consent. This may occur as the result of force, the threat of force, or the inability to give consent. Although any person regardless of age, race, or cultural background may be a victim, this chapter focuses on sexual assault of adult women. Sexual assault in the pediatric age group is covered in Chap. 32. Sexual assault is the fastest-growing violent crime in America, accounting for 6 percent of all violent crimes. In fact, statistics generated by the U.S. Justice Department demonstrate that the rate has increased from 17 per 100,000 women in 1960 to 73 per 100,000 in 1987[1]. Furthermore, this figure is a severe underestimate because victims may not report assault because of embarrassment, feelings of guilt, fear of court appearances or retribution, or even apprehension and reluctance to let health care providers do a physical exam.

Rape is defined as the act of forced vulvar penetration by a penis, object, or body part without the victim's consent. Ejaculation may or may not occur. Rape is only one category of sexual assault. Other variants of sexual assault include spousal rape, date rape, and statutory rape. Spousal assault is forced coitus or sexual acts within a marital relationship without the consent of the partner. Fifty-three percent of cases of domestic violence involve marital rape. Date rape implies forced intercourse without mutual consent. Statutory rape is intercourse with a female below a specified age or with impaired mental capacity regardless of whether or not she gives consent. Physical injury has been found to occur in approximately 40 percent of rape victims. Approximately 1 percent of victims require hospitalization and major operative repair. Finally, it has been estimated that 1 in 1000 injuries associated with sexual assault are so severe as to be fatal.

Victims of sexual assault may suffer psychological or emotional sequelae. Rape-trauma syndrome may be present for years after an incident. The syndrome presents in two phases. The acute or disorganized phase may last for weeks. It is characterized by a distortion or paralysis of coping mechanisms. The victim may appear to be numb, in disbelief, labile, anxious, or weak. She may feel guilty, humiliated, or fearful. Signs of the syndrome may include generalized body pains, eating or sleeping disturbances, and physical or emotional complaints. Physical complaints are often gynecologic, such as vaginal drainage, vaginal or vulvar pruritus, dysmenorrhea, dyspareunia, and rectal pain. The delayed or organizational phase may present with nightmares, flashbacks, phobias, and gynecologic complaints. The delayed phase may occur months or years after the event.

Health care providers caring for victims of sexual assault have both medical and legal responsibilities (Table 46-1). In this regard, they should be aware of the laws in their local jurisdiction. All emergency or gynecologic departments caring for victims of assault should have very specific guidelines for the evaluation of an assault victim and procedures for obtaining and transferring evidence to the proper authorities. Medical responsibilities include obtaining an assault history, treating physical injuries, culturing and treating infections, offering therapy to prevent unwanted conception, offering prophylaxis and surveillance for infectious diseases, and arranging follow-up care and counseling. Legal responsibilities include obtaining an accurate record of events, documenting injuries, collecting samples to be used as evidence of sexual contact, determining use of force or identity of the perpetrator, and reporting findings and transferring samples and evidence to the appropriate au-

The opinions expressed are those of the authors and not necessarily those of the United States Air Force, Navy, or Department of Defense.

Table 46-1

RESPONSIBILITIES OF HEALTH CARE PROVIDERS IN EVALUATION OF SEXUAL ASSAULT

Medical responsibilities
  Treat physical injuries
  Prevent sexually transmitted diseases
  Prevent unwanted pregnancy
  Provide counseling
  Arrange follow-up for physical and psychological injuries
Legal responsibilities
  Obtain accurate history
  Collect evidence and present to police according to law

---

thorities utilizing the proper chain of custody. It is important to remember that sexual assault is a legal matter and not a medical diagnosis. The physician should be empathetic but express no conclusions, opinions, or diagnoses to the victim or others, nor should these be written into the record.

MEDICAL EVALUATION

Informed consent must be obtained before beginning the history and at each phase of the physical examination. This not only fulfills the legal obligation for consent but also helps the victim regain a sense of control. By granting consent, the victim can decide to what extent she will accept assistance and cooperate in the forensic gathering of evidence. An explanation of each step of the examination is further helpful in allowing the victim to gain control over her person. The patient should be reassured of her safety, that she is not to blame, and will not be left alone. During the history and physical examination, a chaperone should be present, providing support and reassurance to the victim as well as helping her to feel less vulnerable. The physician should be empathetic and should involve the patient in treatment decisions. A female clinician is not necessary and may not be preferable. In many instances, an empathetic, nonthreatening male practitioner can help the patient retain control of her interpersonal skills. After acute injuries are diagnosed and stabilized, the assault-specific history and physical examination should commence.

This must include an accurate and detailed account of events, including the date and time of the assault, the gender of the perpetrators and their number, as well as the type of assault and penetration. The presence of weapons or types of physical violence used during the assault should be ad-

dressed. In addition, the patient should be asked about all activities that occurred subsequent to the assault, i.e., bathing, urinating, changing clothes, etc., in a nonjudgmental way. A thorough gynecologic history is also a key feature of the sexual assault evaluation. Questions concerning menstrual and contraceptive history, current contraceptive use, the date and time of the patient's last voluntary sexual experience, and a history of previous gynecologic infections or sexually transmitted diseases should be asked.

Treatment centers should have sexual assault evaluation kits (otherwise known as rape kits or physical evidence recovery kits) or protocols to assure completeness and the proper chain of custody. An assault kit assists the clinician in the collection of evidentiary specimens. A typical sexual assault collection kit involves 14 steps (Table 46-2). Furthermore, most kits contain preprinted history and examination forms. Examples of those used in Dallas County, Texas, are shown in Figs. 46-1 through 46-4. Occasionally, patients may refuse use of the assault kit. They should be reassured that the emergency department medical record will still be available should they change their minds later and decide to prosecute.

Step 1 includes recording of administrative information: the name of the victim, time and date of emergency department admission, police report number, and next of kin. This intake processing is done in private if possible.

Step 2 involves obtaining informed consent from the victim authorizing the collection and release of information to legal authorities and to a counseling center following the exam. Consent for the taking of photographs as a means of documenting injuries is also obtained at this time.

Step 3 involves a detailed medical, gynecologic, and assault history. Although the patient must not be forced to an-

---

Table 46-2

STEPS IN THE EVALUATION OF SEXUAL ASSAULT

1. Administrative information
2. Informed consent for exam
3. Detailed history
4. Collection of foreign material and clothing
5. Detailed physical exam
6. Debris collection
7. Pubic hair combings
8. Pulled pubic hairs
9. Vaginal, rectal, and oral swabs and smears
10. Pulled head hairs
11. Saliva and blood samples
12. Anatomic drawings
13. Treatment for sexually transmitted diseases
14. Prevention of unwanted pregnancy

STEP 1—MEDICAL REPORT

Name of patient: _____   Law enforcement information:

Admitted to emergency room: Officer with patient _____

    Date _____   Badge No. _____

    Time _____ am-pm   Police case No. _____

EOR No. _____   Police agency _____

**STEP 2—AUTHORIZATION FOR COLLECTION OF EVIDENCE AND RELEASE
        OF INFORMATION**

I hereby authorize Memorial Hospital and _____
to collect any blood, urine, tissue or other specimen needed and to supply copies of ALL
medical reports including any laboratory reports, immediately upon completion, to the
Police Dept. and the Office of the District Attorney having jurisdiction. This authorization
includes photography for the purpose of documentation.

        Signature of person examined _____

                Address _____ City _____

Date _____   Parent or Guardian _____

Witness _____   Address _____ City _____

NURSE: Rape Crisis Center Service:

        Offered   YES ☐   NO ☐

        Patient declined   YES ☐   NO ☐

        Rape Crisis Center called YES ☐   NO ☐

Figure 46-1

The first two steps of the assault evaluation used in Dallas County, Texas, include background information and informed consent for the exam.

swer questions she is uncomfortable answering, specific questions regarding penile penetration of the vulva, mouth, and anus should be asked. Whether or not a patient douched, bathed, urinated, or defecated since the assault is determined. The use of alcohol, drugs, or any means of force, fear, or collusion is detailed. The forms provided in the assault kit serve as a guides. Any additional pertinent history should be annotated in the form of progress notes and added to the kit.

Step 4 is the collection of foreign material, outer clothing, and underpants. Some kits include a separate bag for underpants. If the victim is not wearing the clothes worn at the time of assault, only the underpants are collected. If she is wearing the same clothes, they are collected as well. The victim stands on the center of a paper sheet included in the kit and carefully disrobes. Each item is placed in a separate bag, labeled, and sealed. Clothes should not be shaken, as microscopic evidence may thus be lost. If the victim is unable to remove her own clothes, care must be taken not to cut through existing holes or stains in victim's clothing. After the disrobing process is completed, the paper sheet is carefully folded, placed in a sealed envelope, and labeled. The emergency department should provide appropriate clothing (e.g., a scrub suit) for the victim before discharge if necessary.

Step 5 constitutes the detailed physical examination. This includes a description of the victim's general appearance, emotional status, clothing stains, bruises, scratches, lacerations, and bite marks. All injuries should be noted on anatomic drawings (Figs. 46-3 and 46-4). If the patient's permission was previously obtained, photographs may be taken to document physical injuries. If the victim is still wearing the original clothing, which is torn or otherwise damaged, photographs of that should also be obtained. The pelvic ex-

STEP 3—HISTORY

1. Date of assault: _____ Time of assault: _____ am-pm

2. Age: _____ Race: _____

3. Gravidity: _____ Parity: _____

4. Age of menarche (if appropriate): _____

5. Date of last menses: _____

6. Last menses normal: YES ☐   NO ☐   If no, describe: _____

_____
Patient's Name or Stamp

7. Patient known to be pregnant: YES ☐   NO ☐
   If yes, gestational age: _____ weeks

8. Current mode of contraception (prior to alleged assault): _____

9. Coitus in the 72 hours prior to alleged assault?   YES ☐   NO ☐
   If yes, most recent Date _____ Time _____
   Condom Used?   YES ☐   NO ☐

10. Douching practiced: YES ☐   NO ☐   Most recent _____

11. During alleged assault
    Did penis penetrate:

Vulva:	Yes ☐	No ☐	Unknown ☐
Mouth:	Yes ☐	No ☐	Unknown ☐
Anus:	Yes ☐	No ☐	Unknown ☐

    Did assailant wear condom?   Yes ☐   No ☐   Unknown ☐
    Did assailant put his mouth on victim's genitals? Yes ☐   No ☐   Unknown ☐

12. Since alleged assault has patient:

Douched	Yes ☐	No ☐	Unknown ☐
Bathed or showered	Yes ☐	No ☐	Unknown ☐
Urinated	Yes ☐	No ☐	Unknown ☐

13. Has patient knowledge of:

any present illness	Yes ☐	No ☐	_____
any present medication	Yes ☐	No ☐	_____
any drug allergy (esp. penicillin)	Yes ☐	No ☐	_____

14. In 24 hours prior to alleged assault, did patient use alcohol or drugs, or was she forced to take drugs?
    Yes ☐   No ☐
    Is drug and/or alcohol testing requested?   Yes ☐   No ☐

> Note: If toxicologic analysis is required, blood should be taken in two 10-mL green-topped
> vacutainers and placed in sexual assault kit.

If yes, indicate drug and/or alcohol; date, time and amount of ingestion; frequency of use; duration of use; usual amount of intake.

_____

_____

_____

_____

_____

_____   _____
Date   Examiner's Signature

Figure 46-2

The history related to assault includes gynecologic and assault-specific questions.

PHYSICAL EXAMINATION

Patient's Name or Stamp

A) Patient's B.P.: _____   Pulse: _____   Temp: _____

B) Patient's general appearance: _____

C) Patient's emotional status: _____

D) Clothing stains: _____

Bruises?	Yes ☐	No ☐
Scratches?	Yes ☐	No ☐
Lacerations?	Yes ☐	No ☐
Bitemarks?	Yes ☐	No ☐

If yes, collect saliva from bitemark with a distilled water moistened swab, photograph and note all injuries on anatomical drawing below:

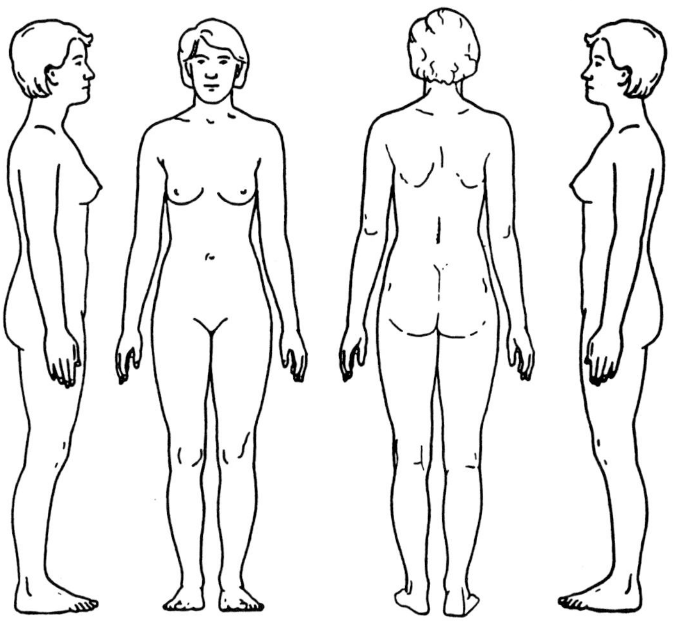

_____   _____
Date   Examiner's Signature

Figure 46-3

Documentation of the physical exam should include details regarding areas of injury, noted on an anatomic chart.

amination should be performed in a private room with a chaperone present. Many providers reserve this portion of the examination to the very end in order to minimize both discomfort and embarrassment to the patient. The examination should be performed by someone competent and comfortable in performing gynecologic exams, especially because legal involvement might be necessary later. Medical students should not perform the examination and interns and junior residents should be supervised. Sexual assault response teams, such as the one in San Diego, California, utilize highly trained nurse practitioners for the examination.

An examination table that allows the patient to be in the dorsal lithotomy position and a proper light source are necessary (Tables 46-3 and 46-4). The speculum must not be

Patient's Name or Stamp

PELVIC EXAMINATION (use a non-lubricated speculum)

Vulva:	Normal ☐		
	Abnormal ☐	Describe: _____
Perineal:	Normal ☐		
	Abnormal ☐	Describe: _____
Hymen:	Normal ☐		
	Abnormal ☐	Describe: _____
Vagina:	Normal ☐		
	Abnormal ☐	Describe: _____
Cervix:	Normal ☐		
	Abnormal ☐	Describe: _____
Uterus:	Normal ☐		
	Abnormal ☐	Describe: _____
Adnexa:	Normal ☐		
	Abnormal ☐	Describe: _____
Recto-vaginal:	Normal ☐		
	Abnormal ☐	Describe: _____
	Not Done ☐		

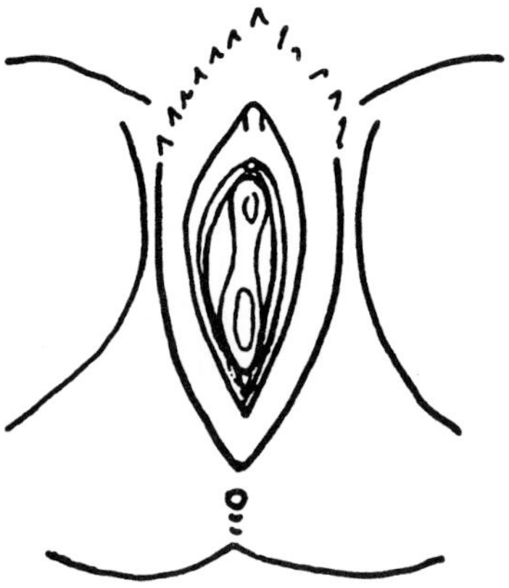

A) Where intercourse is reported,
   were spermatozoa observed in the: Vaginal Vault: YES ☐   NO ☐
                                       Rectum: YES ☐   NO ☐

B) Were these motile?   Vagina: YES ☐   NO ☐
                                       Rectum: YES ☐   NO ☐

C) Where intercourse is reported more than 24 hours prior to examination,
   were spermatozoa observed in cervical mucous?   YES ☐   NO ☐

NOTE: DISCARD PIPET AND SLIDES AFTER EXAMINATION FOR SPERMATOZOA.

_____   _____
Date   Examiner's Signature

Figure 46-4

The pelvic exam should be very detailed. A chart with anatomic figures aids in documenting trauma. The presence of sperm and their motility should be noted.

Table 46-3

EQUIPMENT NEEDED FOR PHYSICAL EVALUATION OF THE ASSAULT VICTIM

Gynecologic exam table
Light source
Speculum (nonlubricated)
Comb
Swabs
Cultures (*Neisseria gonorrhoeae, Chlamydia, Mycoplasma*)
Glass slides
Nail scraper or clipper

lubricated so as not to interfere with the sensitivity of cultures or smears. Warm water can be used on the speculum to make the examination more comfortable. A detailed description of physical evidence collection is given below.

The relevant anatomy of the female genital tract is reviewed in Fig. 46-5. Physical evidence is often absent in cases of assault. In an effort to increase the sensitivity of the physical examination to obtain evidence, toluidine blue may be applied to the vulva. Toluidine blue is a nuclear stain commonly used in gynecologic practice to detect vulvar cancer. Since normal vulvar skin contains no nuclei, it will not bind the dye. Lacerations that expose the deeper dermis, however, will bind it. This technique is limited to the vulva, and dye will not be taken up in areas of injury that are superficial or are beginning to reepithelialize. The colposcope is essentially a magnifying glass designed to evaluate cervical intraepithelial neoplasia. Gross inspection of the perineum, introitus, hymen, vaginal mucosa, and cervix may be repeated using a colposcope at ×15 magnification. A green filter on the colposcope may aid in the identification of ejaculate (Fig. 46-6).[2] Most colposcopes are equipped with a camera to facilitate documentation.

Step 6 is debris collection. Foreign debris includes dirt, leaves, fibers from the assailant's clothing, and hair. These

Table 46-4

EQUIPMENT THAT MAY AID IN PHYSICAL EVALUATION

Wood's UV light
Toluidine blue
Colposcope

are individually placed on clean paper and sealed in envelopes included in the kit and individually labeled. Foreign debris such as dried semen, blood, and saliva is collected by moistening swabs with saline and swabbing the area. It is important to let the swabs dry thoroughly before placing them in evidence envelopes. Fingernail scrapings should be collected, particularly when the victim has grabbed or scratched her assailant. A Wood's (ultraviolet) lamp may be helpful in identifying foreign material under the fingernail. The victim's hand is placed over clean paper, and a fingernail scraper or clipper is then used and the debris allowed to fall on the paper, which is sealed in an envelope and labeled. Nails broken during the struggle with the assailant should be clipped and collected, taking care to avoid damaging the broken edges.

Step 7, pubic hair combings, is done to obtain pubic hairs shed by the assailant during the assault. A clean piece of paper is placed under the victim's buttocks and, using a comb provided in the kit, pubic hair is combed downward so that loose hairs or debris falls onto the paper. If the victim prefers, it is perfectly acceptable for her to do this herself. The comb is then placed on the paper and sealed in the envelope along with any debris collected.

Step 8, the pulling of pubic hairs, is necessary to distinguish the hair of the victim from that of the assailant. Approximately 15 hairs must be pulled and not cut.[3] The examiner, using a gloved hand, should pull down with gentle steady traction, thereby removing hair at the end of the growth phase and minimizing patient discomfort.

Step 9 involves the collection of vaginal, rectal, and oral swabs, which will subsequently be analyzed for the presence of sperm and seminal plasma (acid phosphatase). These samples need be collected only if the assault involved the vaginal, rectal, or oral cavities, respectively. Two swabs—which are not moistened, stained, or chemically fixed—are used to rub the area in question. They are then air-dried and placed in individual collection sleeves and envelopes. In addition, the examiner performs a saline wet mount of the vaginal secretions to look for the immediate presence of motile or nonmotile sperm.

Step 10 involves pulling head hairs from the victim in order to compare them with hair found at the crime scene or on the alleged assailant. Approximately 15 hairs are pulled from various sites on the scalp and placed in a labeled evidence envelope.

Step 11 involves taking saliva and blood samples from the victim, thereby obtaining her secretor status (some women do not secrete blood-type antigen), blood type, and DNA profile. Many kits provide filter paper that is placed in the victim's mouth for the saliva sample; it is then air-dried and stored in a breathable bag. Standard tubes may be used for the blood samples.

Step 12 consists of checking the forms included in the assault kit, including the anatomic drawings, for completeness. A copy is sealed in the kit along with the evidence and samples collected. These are then transferred to law enforcement

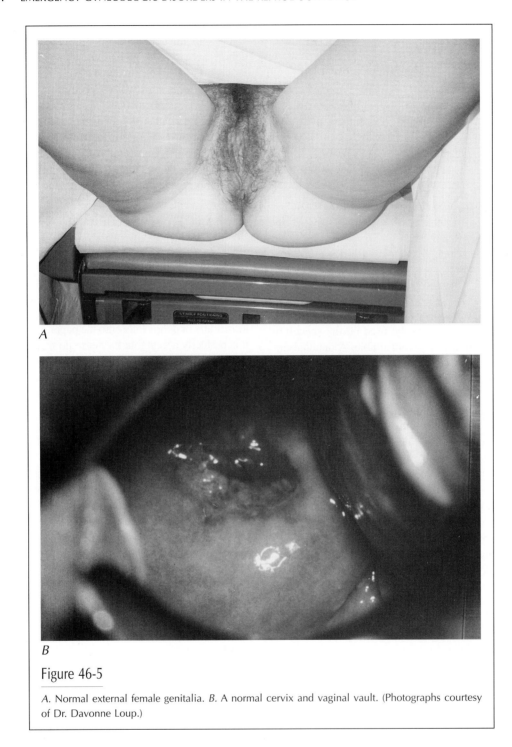

Figure 46-5

A. Normal external female genitalia. *B*. A normal cervix and vaginal vault. (Photographs courtesy of Dr. Davonne Loup.)

authorities according to the proper chain of custody established in the area.

Step 13 is the provision of prophylactic antibiotics for STDs. Approximately 5 to 10 percent of sexual assault victims may acquire a sexually transmitted disease. Since many of these women are lost to follow-up, it is important to offer prophylactic antibiotics to prevent sexually transmitted diseases. Prior to prescribing, baseline Venereal Disease Research Laboratory or rapid plasma reagin (RPR) results can

be obtained. The cost-effectiveness of obtaining such cultures at evaluation has been challenged, since the patient will be treated anyway and cultures must be taken at follow-up to make sure that treatment has been effective. Baseline testing for human immunodeficiency virus (HIV) should be done only where proper counseling and follow-up can be assured. This is difficult in the emergency department, where so many sexual assault victims are lost to follow-up. However, the American College of Obstetricians and Gynecolo-

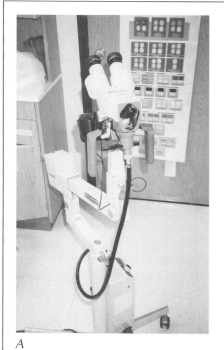
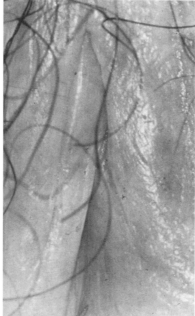
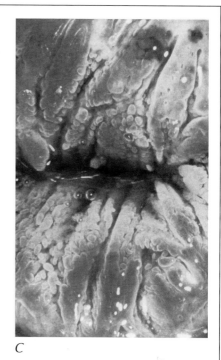

A   B   C

Figure 46-6

A colposcope *(A)* and a colposcopic view of the vulva *(B)*, and cervix. *(C)*. (Photographs courtesy of Dr. Davonne Loup.)

gists'[1] recommends obtaining baseline cultures and serology.

Serologic and culture specimens are sent to the hospital laboratory; they become part of the medical record and are not

Table 46-5

PROPHYLACTIC ANTIBACTERIAL REGIMENS FOR THE PREVENTION OF SEXUALLY TRANSMITTED DISEASES IN THE VICTIM OF SEXUAL ASSAULT

Ceftriaxone 250 mg IM in a single dose
    or
Spectinomycin 2 g IM
    followed by either
Doxycycline[a] 100 mg PO b.i.d. for 7 days
    or
Erythromycin 500 mg PO q.i.d. for 7 days
    or
Azithromycin 1 g PO in a single dose

[a]Doxycycline should not be used during pregnancy.
Source: Adapted from Centers for Disease Control and Prevention: Sexually transmitted diseases—Treatment guidelines. *MMWR* 42:RR-14, 1993.

placed in the evidence collection kit. Appropriate antibiotic regimens to cover the prevention of gonorrhea, chylamydia, and syphilis are listed in Table 46-5. Recently, azithromycin 1 g orally has been used in lieu of doxycycline or erythromycin because of its efficacy and ease of administration.

The risk from anal or vaginal intercourse with an HIV-infected partner is similar to that associated with parenteral exposure with an HIV-contaminated needle (0.0032). Postexposure prophylaxis in the setting of needle exposure is estimated to decrease the odds of HIV infection by 79 percent.[4] While the exact risk from an HIV-infected assailant in a rape is unknown, it is probably at least that of consensual sexual exposure, particularly if ejaculation occurs. Postexposure prophylaxis can be offered to the sexual assault victim. Treatment should be the same as for occupational exposure to HIV.[5] The current recommendations are zidovudine (200 mg, 3 times a day for 4 weeks) and lamivudine (150 mg, 2 times a day for 4 weeks). Postexposure prophylaxis should be provided to all patients, but only with their informed consent. It is important to remember that in addition to medical prevention of sexually transmitted diseases, tetanus toxoid 0.5 mg intramuscularly should be prescribed as indicated, and antibiotics may be necessary for the treatment of lacerations or injuries associated with the assault.

Step 14 is postcoital pregnancy prevention.

The patient's gynecologic and menstrual history, use of birth control, and pregnancy status should be assessed and

Table 46-6

PRESCRIPTIVE EQUIVALENTS FOR THE YUZPE METHOD OF EMERGENCY CONTRACEPTION[a]

Trade Name	Formulation	Number of Pills Taken with Each Dose
Ovral	0.05 mg of ethinyl estradiol 0.50 mg of norgestrel	2
Lo-Ovral	0.03 mg of ethinyl estradiol 0.30 mg of norgestrel	4
Nordette	0.03 mg of ethinyl estradiol 0.15 mg of levonorgestrel	4
Levlen	0.03 mg of ethinyl estradiol 0.15 mg of levonorgestrel	4
Triphasil	(Yellow pills only) 0.03 mg of ethinyl estradiol 0.125 mg of levonorgestrel	4
Tri-Levlen	(Yellow pills only) 0.03 mg of ethinyl estradiol 0.125 mg of levonorgestrel	4

[a]Treatment consists of two doses taken 12 h apart. Use of an antiemetic before taking the medication will lessen the risk of nausea, a common side effect.
Source: The American College of Obstetricians and Gynecologists: Emergency oral contraception. *ACOG Practice Patterns*, number 3, December 1996, with permission.

documented. Approximately 2 to 4 percent of sexual assault victims not using birth control become pregnant as a result of rape.[1] If the patient is at risk for pregnancy secondary to assault (as signified by a negative result on an HCG test) she should be offered medical therapy (the "morning-after" pill) to prevent pregnancy (Table 46-6). Two oral contraceptive pills with 50 μg of ethinyl estradiol followed by two more pills 12 h later is a commonly used pregnancy prophylaxis regimen. This regimen has a 1 percent failure rate if used within 72 h of the assault. An antiemetic, such as trimethobenzamide (Tigan) or promethazine (Phenergan) should also be prescribed, since nausea is common and can be quite severe. If the patient declines pregnancy prophylaxis, some clinicians recommend weekly pregnancy tests until the onset of menses.[6] If the patient is already pregnant, pregnancy should not hinder evaluation, collection of evidence, or prevention of sexually transmitted diseases.[7] The 14 steps outlined above are intended to serve as a guide. It is important for practitioners who perform assault evaluations to be familiar with the protocol approved in their institution.

DISCHARGE INSTRUCTIONS AND FOLLOW-UP

Upon completion of the medical evaluation of the sexual assault victim, collection of evidence, administration of indicated immediate treatments, and completion of the stepwise protocol, follow-up plans should be discussed. Follow-up should deal with both the physical and psychological needs of the patient. The victim should be invited to express her anxieties and should state her understanding of what has happened and what will occur. Serologic tests for hepatitis B and syphilis (RPR or VDRL) and cultures for *Neisseria gonorrhoeae* and *Chlamydia* should be performed by 4 weeks after assault.[8] Tests for HIV should be obtained as a baseline and repeated at 6 months. Providers trained to handle rape-trauma victims should be consulted and follow-up arranged prior to patient discharge. All follow-up appointments, discharge instructions, information regarding the signs and symptoms associated with acute medical and psychological ailments, as well as phone numbers through which the patient can access timely medical care should be written down and given to the victim. An emergency point of contact should be established in the event of acute psychological decompensation prior to the follow-up appointment. Ideally, the patient should be seen within 2 to 3 and 4 to 6 weeks for psychological and medical evaluation, respectively.

References

1. American College of Obstetricians and Gynecologists: *Sexual Assault.* ACOG technical bulletin no. 101. Washington, DC: American College of Obstetricians and Gynecologists, 1987.
2. Slaughter L, Brown CRV: Colposcopy to establish physical findings in rape victims. *Am J Obstet Gynecol* 166:83, 1992.
3. Young WW, Bracten AC, Goddard MA, et al: Sexual assault: Review of a national model protocol for forensic and medical evaluation. *Obstet Gynecol* 80:878, 1992.
4. Katz MH, Gerberding JL. Sounding board: Post exposure treatment of people exposed to the human immunodeficiency virus through sexual contact or injection-drug use. *N Engl J Med* 336:1097, 1997.
5. Case control study of HIV seroconversion in health care workers after percutaneous exposure to HIV infected blood—France, United Kingdom, United States, January 1988–August 1994, *MMWR* 44:929, 1995.
6. Dupre AR, Hampton HL, Morrison H, Meeks GR: Sexual assault. *Obstet Gynecol Surv* 48:640, 1993.
7. Satin AJ, Hemsell DL, Stone IC, et al: Sexual assault in pregnancy. *Obstet Gynecol* 77:710, 1991.
8. Jenny C, Hooton TB, Bouels A, et al: Sexually transmitted diseases in victims of rape. *N Engl J Med* 322:713, 1990.

Chapter 47

PARTNER VIOLENCE

Elizabeth Shadigian

Although in the past the term *domestic violence* has been used to describe violence within marital relationships, a new awareness of the pervasiveness of the problem of violence in a variety of other significant relationships allows for the more generic terms *partner violence, partner abuse,* or *woman abuse* to be used more accurately. These terms encompass dating violence, abuse within marital relationships, and victimization in cohabitation. The majority of victims of domestic violence are women,[1] so throughout this chapter the victim/survivor is called *she,* while the perpetrator is referred to as *he.* The literature is now growing on same-sex relationship violence, which may often be doubly stigmatizing in labeling a person as both "battered" and "gay" in a still mostly homophobic society.[2] This chapter will focus on physical assault against women as well as the common occurrence of sexual assault within violent relationships, both of which are crimes of power and control. Sexual assault is also covered in Chap. 46.

Partner violence is the leading cause of all injuries to women.[3] Failure of medical providers to identify women in violent, ongoing relationships allows this violence to continue, usually escalating over time and sometimes ending in the death of the woman. If violence could be screened for by an inexpensive laboratory test, it should probably be drawn on all women annually. Although such a test does not exist, simple questioning can be developed and used in a medical context to screen for partner violence and sexual assault. It is estimated that the direct dollar costs for providing medical care to the victims of partner violence is approximately $1.8 billion per year,[4] not including lost work days, decreased productivity, and loss of young individuals from the workplace because of death or disability.[5] Therefore, many physician organizations, including the American Medical Association, the American College of Obstetricians and Gynecologists, and the American College of Emergency Physicians, have advocated that all health care providers screen and identify women who are the victims of partner violence and initiate interventions for victimized women.[6,7,7a] When a woman is identified as a victim of partner violence, this woman's situation should be considered urgent or even emergent, depending on the individual details. It may be compared to diagnosing a hypertensive crisis or making the diagnosis of preeclampsia—intervention may make a large difference in the outcome for the patient or possibly the patient and her child or children. Prompt intervention may save the woman's life and possibly her children's while also reducing morbidity.

Thus, learning to effectively identify victims of partner violence is the cornerstone of any initiation of interventions for victims. Partner violence should be on the list of differential diagnoses for all women seeking care in emergency departments, because 12 percent of women presenting for any reason are current victims.[8] In addition, all women should be screened at least annually for partner violence, because the prevalence is approximately 20 percent in primary care settings.[9]

EPIDEMIOLOGY

Women in the United States are more likely to have been injured, raped, or murdered by a male partner than by all other types of assailants.[3] From national surveys, experts estimate that 4 million women annually experience severe or life-threatening assaults from a male partner in the United States.[10,11] Physical assault includes but is not limited to hitting, punching, kicking, shoving, choking, assault with a weapon, holding, tying down or restraining, leaving a person in a dangerous place, and refusal to offer aid to the sick or injured.[6] Sexual assault is usually considered separately but is another form of physical assault.

Between 14 and 25 percent of married women have been forced to have intercourse at least once during their marriages. Additionally, more than twice as many women report being sexually assaulted by husbands as by strangers.[12,13] Approximately 2000 women are murdered by their current or former male partners each year in the United States. Two-thirds of these women had been physically assaulted before they were murdered.[13,14] Sheltered homeless and low-income housed mothers have a higher lifetime prevalence of severe physical and sexual assault—over 90 and 80 percent, respectively. Over 7 percent of all adult Americans have been homeless at some time during their lives, placing a greater percentage of women at particularly high risk for assault if they have ever been homeless.[15]

On the basis of data from emergency departments, the incidence of acute partner violence is about 12 percent, while the lifetime prevalence of partner assault for women in the emergency department setting is over 50 percent.[8] One in seven women utilizing primary care settings have a history of partner abuse.[9]

BARRIERS AND SCREENING

"Until you have sat on the floor and begged for someone to leave you alone, you just can't understand."—victim of domestic violence at The House of Ruth, Baltimore, Maryland, 1994, from the videotape *Take a Stand.*

Part of the problem with having health care providers, especially physicians, ask about partner violence is their lack of training in medical school, residency, and continuing medical education, as well as the denial that many bring to the subject. Another factor that contributes to physicians' limitations in dealing with battering is that violence does not fit the medical model. Partner abuse has generally not been a diagnosis given to a victim. If a woman's experience is reduced to medical facts while her feelings are not acknowledged, medical staff inadvertently re-create an abusive dynamic between themselves and their patients.[16]

Health care providers need to look at their own life experiences honestly before they can ask their patients about abuse. Were they abused as children or in an adult relationship? Have they been sexually assaulted? Have they been perpetrators or do they find it hard to imagine that violence exists? The providers need not share this with their patients but do need to evaluate themselves to see what personal biases may hinder their ability to care for victims of abuse. In addition, confronting violence in the lives of patients may stimulate awareness among those providers who themselves have been abused.[17]

Several approaches may be necessary to elicit a history of abuse. Before being asked any questions about violence, the woman must be alone or at least without any adults other than the health care provider in the room. In the section of the history concerning habits or social background, after other personal issues such as cigarette smoking, alcohol and drug use, nutrition, and exercise have been asked, screening questions can be placed that address violence against women. The examiner may, for example, ask "Have you ever been in a relationship where you have been kicked, hit, shoved, or choked?" and "As a child or as an adult, have you ever been sexually assaulted—raped or inappropriately touched sexually?"—questions that are likely to elicit a history of violence (see Table 47-1). Other useful questions may be better placed in the past medical history or elsewhere. For example, asking about depression and alcoholism in family members, or how discipline was used in her current or childhood home, can give clues to abuse. Not all victims will answer screening questions truthfully at first, but they may do so later in the evaluation or at a subsequent visit if the provider is seen as nonjudgmental and genuinely caring.[18]

Table 47-1

QUESTIONS FOR ELICITING AN ABUSE HISTORY BY CATEGORY

Social History or Habits Section	Past Medical History	Follow-up Questions
Have you ever been hit, slapped, shoved, choked, beaten, or restrained?	As a child, were you even beaten?	Are you in danger from a current or past partner?
Have you ever been raped or inappropriately touched sexually?	When you were a child, did anyone touch you sexually?	Have you even been forced to have sex with your partner?
Was your first sexual experienced forced or by choice?	How was/is anger handled in your home?	Are you afraid of your partner or anyone else?
		Is your life in danger?
		Do you have an escape plan?

Source: Modified from Shadigian,[18] Sasseti,[20] and Courtios.[26]

Focusing on victim attributes that might predict violence before it occurs has not been useful. The only such potential risk marker identifying a potential victim of physical assault is a history of having witnessed parental violence as a child. The partner's characteristics are better predictors of violence against a woman than are any characteristics of her own. The most influential risk factor for abuse is being female, which should be understood to mean that the victimization of women is the outcome of unacceptable male behavior.[19]

Although it is not possible to predict who will be abused, several subgroups with higher prevalence rates of partner violence have been identified (see Table 47-2). Asking screening questions (see Table 47-1) may not guarantee an accurate history at an initial visit but it does set a tone of caring and a willingness to discuss the subject at a later date. When a woman reveals her victimization, the listener, by remaining nonjudgmental and relaxed, will encourage her to continue seeking help. Offering access to resources about partner violence without being asked sends the strong although unspoken message that the patient's safety is important to her care provider.[20] Public restrooms in medical facilities should post, and new patient information packets should include, information about partner abuse. Also, asking all people, male or female, about sexual orientation as well as about abuse will prevent same-sex violence from being overlooked and other important health care issues to be addressed.[18]

CURRENT ASSAULTIVE RELATIONSHIP

Figure 47-1 emphasizes that partner violence screening should occur at least yearly, usually at annual exams. Other key screening opportunities include visits to the emergency department for urgent care visits, for prenatal care, upon hospital admission for surgery or any other treatment, and when a patient is found to have suspicious injuries such as fractures, head injuries, choking, loss of consciousness, and soft tissue injuries. Women with frequent, vague, or recurrent generalized symptoms; those with complaints consistent with depression, anxiety disorders, or chronic fatigue; and women who seek shelter in the emergency department (ED) by bringing in children for physical exams that turn out not to correlate with the stated complaints should also be screened by using questions as described above (see Table 47-1).

If a woman is in a current battering relationship, several steps should be quickly taken to ensure her safety, especially if she is presenting just after an assault. A safety and legal assessment should be performed (see Fig. 47-2) while, with the woman's permission, local domestic/partner violence advocates are called. A thorough medical assessment (see Fig. 47-3) and dangerousness assessment (see Table 47-3) with attention to a number of risk factors for homicide should also be carried out. In addition to this, any involved children should be assessed for child abuse (approximately 50 percent will also be abused). Facilitated referrals to women's shelters should be made and safety planning reviewed (see Table 47-4).

If the woman presenting for care divulges that she is a prior victim of partner violence, she should be screened for ongoing stalking and referred to counseling as warranted by the current situation. The emergency department may be the first place where a woman is exposed to health care, so helping her see herself as a victim of partner violence, understand the severity of the violence and the possibility of its escalation, and explore safety and treatment options are vital.[21] If it is unclear that a woman is a victim—if she is unwilling to talk or talk openly—then the woman should be believed but offered services anyway. Sharing with a woman that she has risk factors for severe abuse or homicide may help her feel more comfortable discussing her situation with the health care provider.

A safety and legal assessment (see Fig. 47-2) must be performed to make sure that the woman and her health care providers are safe during the rest of the assessment. Perpetrators may attack the woman and/or health care providers when adequate security measures (such as visible safety officers) are lacking and when information on a victim's

---

Table 47-2

SUBGROUPS WITH HIGHER PREVALENCE RATES OF PARTNER VIOLENCE

Women with disabilities—physical or mental[40]

Women who abuse drugs or alcohol[23]

Mothers currently or ever homeless[15]

Low-income-housed mothers[15]

Adolescent women/teens[29]

Pregnant women entering prenatal care in the third trimester[27]

Women with unintended pregnancies[31]

Women who were victims of child sexual abuse[13]

Women whose children are physically or sexually abused[13]

Women who, as children, have witnessed parental violence[19]

Women with partners who never leave their sides and/or answer questions for them

Women who are isolated from family and/or friends

Women whose partners have a history of criminal assaults (especially against other women)

Women recently separated or divorced

Women whose partners stalk them after they try to leave

Women whose partners kill or abuse pets

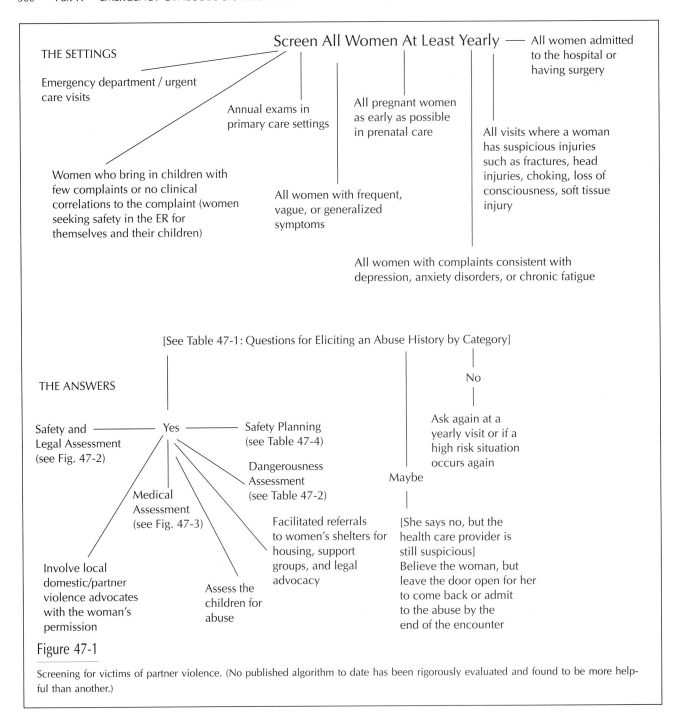

Figure 47-1

Screening for victims of partner violence. (No published algorithm to date has been rigorously evaluated and found to be more helpful than another.)

location is divulged to the perpetrator. In concert, a legal assessment ensures that the police will be contacted when appropriate. If the situation involves the abuse of children, the dependent elderly, the disabled, or a deadly weapon, or if local laws mandate reporting, the health care provider must contact law enforcement officials.

A thorough medical assessment is outlined in Fig. 47-3. The cornerstones of an effective medical assessment remain (1) a comprehensive, sensitive history where a woman is believed and (2) a detailed head-to-toe physical examination, both including appropriate documentation (that is accurate

and legible). Written documentation should be accompanied by body maps and appropriate photographs (see Table 47-5) taken by health care or law enforcement professionals with proper training in safeguarding the chain of evidence. Managing follow-up with health care providers at 48 h and again in 1 week to further document change in soft tissue injuries, review safety planning, explain test results, and answer remaining questions is essential. Physical, psychological, and somatic consequences of violence against women as well as physical examination issues are reviewed below. Referring a woman for additional counseling (cou-

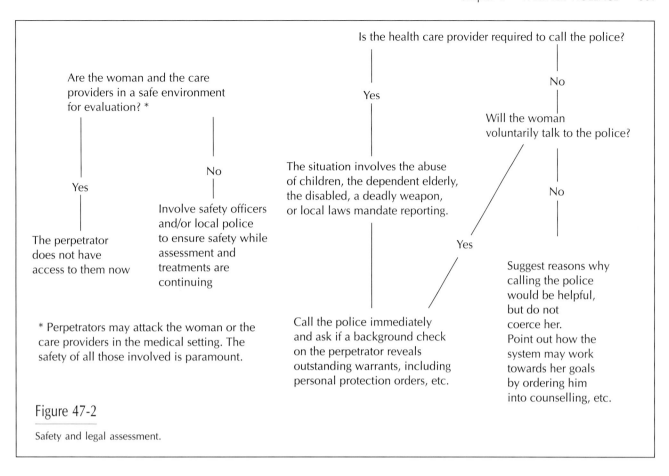

Figure 47-2

Safety and legal assessment.

ples counseling is not recommended) and treatment can be very healing because it implies that the physician acknowledges the problem of abuse and its frequent connection with many physical and psychological symptoms.[3,6,13] A list of "don'ts" for health care providers is provided in Table 47-6, which range from medical issues to avoiding self-blame if she does not leave the relationship.

Ideally, an on-call or in-house partner violence team would be present in every institution. This team could be composed of health care providers (physicians, nurse practitioners, physician assistants, and nurses) along with social workers, psychologists, and community partner violence advocates and experts. Despite its obvious advantages, most health care facilities do not have such a team. Finally, a dangerousness assessment should also be performed as part of each partner violence evaluation by the health care provider or by someone on the on-call team (see "Dangerousness Assessment," below).

PHYSICAL, PSYCHOLOGICAL, AND SOMATIC CONSEQUENCES OF VIOLENCE AGAINST WOMEN

Victimized women perceive their health status less favorably, experience more symptomatology, and report higher levels of smoking and failure to use seat belts.[22] Medical utilization increases when a woman is victimized[21] and may be another tacit sign that abuse has occurred. This utilization is greatest during the second year following victimization, and the severity of abuse was the most powerful predictor of yearly visits and outpatient medical costs.[22]

MANIFESTATIONS OF ABUSE

Physical injury patterns of abuse include lacerations and contusions of the trunk and breasts (bathing-suit pattern), face and head (including past injuries in various stages of healing), old vulvar and rectal scarring, and old or new fractures. Later complications of victimization include gastrointestinal, joint, chest, back, abdominal, and pelvic pain, a choking sensation, and headaches.[21] Depression, generalized anxiety, and suicidal ideation are more common among victims of violence. The prevalence of substance abuse and the battered-woman syndrome are also high.[3,6,21] Substance abuse does not cause battering; instead, correlations between substance use and battering should be considered as coping mechanisms.[23] The battered woman syndrome is akin to posttraumatic stress disorder, which involves an extreme traumatic stressor (actual threatened death or serious injury) and symptoms of intrusion, denial, dissociation, increased arousal, and difficulty sleeping.[13]

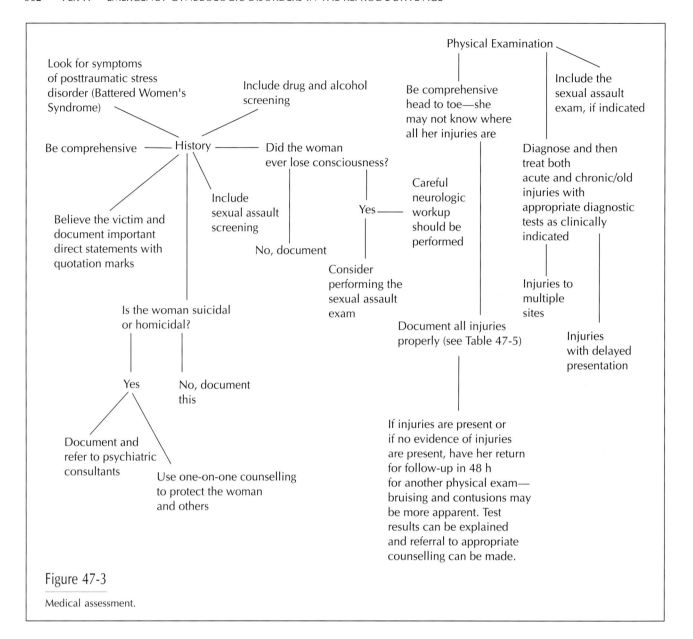

Figure 47-3

Medical assessment.

Behaviorally, a victim of abuse may appear evasive, jumpy, nervous, embarrassed, or passive.[24] She may have a partner who is constantly at her side and who answers questions directed to her.[6] The partner may be the perpetrator, and she needs time alone with her care provider so that an accurate history can be elicited. Many times an excuse of going to the rest room can allow for private time without arousing the partner's suspicions. During that time, questions should be asked about her own background and current safety. Questions about her children's safety are also important, because in half of the families where the woman is assaulted, the children are also being abused. Children are also traumatized by witnessing violence.[6,18]

SEXUAL ASSAULT IN VIOLENT RELATIONSHIPS

Sexual assault frequently occurs within battering relationships. Between 14 and 25 percent of married women report forced sexual intercourse.[12,24] Many women find it even more difficult to report sexual assault within relationships because of a perceived stigma. When asking about marital/partner rape, the word *rape* should be avoided. Instead, asking if a woman has ever been "forced to have sex" when she did not want to is more likely to elicit accurate information. Additionally, sexual violence is least likely to be reported if questions are

Table 47-3

RISK FACTORS FOR HOMICIDE

Gun access or ownership
Use of weapon in prior abusive episodes
Threats with weapons
Threats to kill
Serious injuries prior to abusive episodes
Threats of suicide
Drug or alcohol abuse
Sexually assaulting the partner
Extreme obsessiveness, jealousy, or dominance
History or parental abuse of the man
Recent separation
Escalation of the frequency and severity of assaults

Source: From Campbell,[14] with permission.

phrased insensitively, because women fear humiliation, the risk of not being believed, and being devalued for having participated. Some women may have been acculturated into believing that a forced sexual relationship is a husband's right.[13]

Sexual abuse in violent relationships ranges from performing sexual acts against a woman's will (or when she is not fully conscious), and assaulting her genitals or hurting her physically, including using weapons or other objects orally, vaginally, or anally. A wide range of injuries may be seen, from vulvar and rectal bruising to serious injuries and scarring. Additionally, sexually degrading names may be used or contraception may be withheld.[21] Knowing that a large number of battered women also experience sexual violence may help in guiding the physical exam and may necessitate offering the sexual assault exam (forensic medical sexual assault exam). Sexually assaulted women are at higher risk for being the victim of homicide and for killing their abusive partners.[14] Posttraumatic stress disorder, suicide attempts, and depression are each seen in one-third of all sexually assaulted women.[25]

Table 47-4

SAFETY PLANNING: SAFEGUARDS, DOCUMENTS, AND ESSENTIALS

Safeguards	Documents	Essentials
Formulate an escape plan before danger arises so friends/family may help	Checkbook and savings account books	Suitcase with clothes and toiletries
Children should be able to dial 911 or call the police and be aware of the safety plan, so they can also escape	Birth certificates for the woman and all children	Emergency cash
Have ready: telephone numbers for the police, victim advocate hotlines, and shelters (these may need to be hidden)	Financial records (rent receipts, utility bills, pay stubs)	Medications
Let neighbors know about the violence so they can call the police if they hear a disturbance	Driver's license	Keys
A code phrase to use with a friend that means call the police—"I need a can of soup"	Titles and/or deeds	Special toy for each child
	Insurance papers	Eyeglasses or contacts
	Social security cards	Prescriptions
	School and/or health records	Transportation
	Passports	(These essentials should be left with a friend for quick access)
	Work permits	
	Green cards	
	Civil action papers	
	Address book	
	Welfare records	
	Unemployment records	

Source: Modified from Shadigian,[18] Sasseti,[20] Buel.[34]

Table 47-5

DOCUMENTATION OF INJURIES

1. Include detailed written descriptions
2. Use body maps to localize injuries
3. Photographs should be used and should
    A. Be taken before altering the appearance of injuries, if possible
    B. Use both color and black and white film for bites, but all other injuries should have color film
    C. Use a color bar if possible
    D. Be taken from a distance and up close with at least two photos of each injury and more than one angle
    E. Use a coin or ruler to help assess injury size
    F. Document the location of each injury
    G. Include the date, victim's name, and an identifying item such as her registration number or face in each photo
    H. Include the photographer's name and others also present

Source: American Medical Association,[41] with permission.

Table 47-6

DON'TS FOR CARE PROVIDERS

Don't routinely prescribe tranquilizers (they do not help and may be used for suicide attempts)

Don't coerce a woman (you may be putting her at increased risk and revictimizing her)

Don't blame yourself if she does not leave immediately (leaving is a process that rarely takes one attempt)

Don't refer her to couples counseling (it is not effective and may delay her leaving and thus her safety)

Don't forget to have her make follow-up appointments (medical and trained psychological follow-up is essential)

Don't forget to screen for drug use, alcoholism, and other addictions (they are more prevalent in assaulted women)

Don't minimize the situation (it may become lethal)

Don't forget to screen for suicidal or homicidal ideation (she may see no other way out)

Don't forget to ask about sexual assault (she may need the sexual assault exam)

Don't ask, "Are you abused?" (most women cannot see themselves as abused, especially at first)

PHYSICAL EXAM ISSUES

A survivor of violence may be hesitant to have a physical examination for a variety of reasons. Fear of being "found out" by the health care provider as a victim of violence because of embarrassment or shame may play a role. Some victims are fearful that the perpetrator will find out that someone else knows and place her at risk for escalating violence. The fear of pain during the examination is also a concern for some women, especially if the victim has been sexually abused. Increased awareness of the pervasiveness of sexual assault in relationships will allow care providers to be sensitive to women who identify themselves as sexual assault victims at the time of screening as well as those who have not labeled themselves that way but are sexual assault victims.[18]

In some cases, fear of the physical examination can be overcome by explaining what will happen during the physical examination and why it is necessary as well as asking the woman for permission to perform the examination. Asking for permission is essential so that the woman does not feel revictimized by her health care provider, especially when photos are also being taken. These issues are only intensified when sexual assault has occurred and a breast and pelvic examination will be performed.[18]

Allowing her to touch the speculum and help during a breast exam, offering a mirror so that she can see, allowing her to say "stop" during the exam, and respecting the request by really stopping, will help put a woman at ease. Maintaining eye contact, performing the bimanual exam at the woman's side, and keeping the head of the table at a 45° angle will all be helpful adjuncts.[18,26] All care providers should have a chaperone present during the examination as an advocate for the woman, regardless of the gender of the health care provider.[18]

PREGNANCY

The prevalence of partner abuse toward pregnant women ranges from 8 to 17 percent.[27] Although some studies have suggested that violence may worsen in severity[28] and frequency[29] during pregnancy, most survey data have failed to substantiate this. Instead, national data suggest that women under 25 years of age who are pregnant are more likely to be victims of partner abuse.[29] In other words, pregnancy does not protect young women from high rates of violence.

Abused women are twice as likely to initiate prenatal care in the third trimester, possibly because of forced avoidance by the perpetrator.[27] Battered women are also two to four times more likely to give birth to a low–birth weight infant than are nonbattered women.[30] If the pregnancy is unintended, a fourfold increased risk for partner violence is present.[31] In addition, physical assault during pregnancy is associated with a twofold risk of preterm labor and chorioamnionitis.[32] Direct effects of the physical violence on the pregnancy include abruptio placentae; rupture of the uterus, liver, or spleen; and maternal pelvic and fetal fractures.[33]

Pregnancy may be one of the only times that an abused woman is allowed to seek medical attention. Pregnancy is also a unique time because a woman realizes that she has new responsibilities to another person, her unborn baby. Pointing out that her children have a 50 percent chance of also becoming victimized by the perpetrator may also help a pregnant woman decide to leave.

THE TRAP OF ABUSE AND INTERVENTION

The trap of abuse can happen to women of any socioeconomic status, age, level of education, or race.[20,26] Abuse in any form is a way of exerting power and control. Partner violence is not only a punch or a kick but a way of dominating another person physically, emotionally, financially, and sexually.

The attachment of assaulted women to their partners is already well established before their partners become violent. At least 75 percent of women in battering relationships were not assaulted until after they made a commitment to the relationship.[13] Abuse usually begins with minor physical contacts and escalates and becomes chronic over time through intimidation, isolation, and emotional and economic abuse. Some perpetrators may seem remorseful after a battering incident, but many are not. Perpetrators tend to choose the place, time, and intensity of an assault and feel that it is their right to batter their partners. Until recently male violence against women has been historically sanctioned in most cultures throughout the world and has been seen as a manifestation of gender inequality.[13]

Instead of asking women why they stay in an abusive relationship (which imposes judgment upon the victim instead of the perpetrator), it is more helpful to evaluate the relationship itself. Economics, cultural and religious beliefs, fear of disapproval of family and friends, concern about losing their children, psychological factors, the legal system, and fear of retaliation by the violent partner may all play a role in the decision to stay in or leave an abusive relationship. Many women rely on their partner's income and may fear homelessness for themselves and their children if they were to leave. Psychological demoralization may lead to low self-esteem which may become another barrier to leaving. Homicide rates are highest during the process of leaving a violent relationship, so fear of increasing violence in the short term may also keep a woman in a violent relationship, particularly if the legal system is perceived as ineffective.[34]

Victimization is an "overwhelming assault" on a woman's "world of meaning."[35] A survivor of abuse may stop believing that the world is a secure place where meaning and order exist. She may find it hard to believe that she is a worthy person.[36] Feelings of self-blame, loss of control, and vulnerability may persist.[13,36]

DANGEROUSNESS ASSESSMENT

Predictions of severe partner assault and homicide aid practitioners in their attempts to help women understand the seriousness of their situation. The generally smaller size and lesser strength of women explain why serious consequences occur when acts of violence are aimed by men at women. The three risk factors in the perpetrator for severe assault are generalized aggression, alcohol abuse, and abuse by parents. The severe batterer is generally also violent outside the home. Alcohol may contribute to the severity of the assault but is not a causative factor. Finally, men who were the victims of childhood abuse are more likely to be perpetrators of severe partner assault. The abuse by partners may also be related to generalized aggression and alcohol abuse.[37]

The clinician has a "duty to warn" battered women of the extent of dangerousness and risk of homicide. However, the intuition or clinical judgment of the care provider has not been a good predictor of dangerousness. Several instruments have been developed to assess danger to women in abusive relationships. The clinical prediction of the severity of dangerousness is essential and may be made by weighing several risk factors for homicide (see Table 47-3). This list should be used as a tool for educating the battered woman about the seriousness of her situation. However, the prediction of partner homicide is difficult due to its rarity.[14]

By reviewing a battered woman's situation in detail, she may be helped to plan a course of action more effectively by seeing the danger that she is in. One way to help a woman is by asking the following questions:

1. When and what was the first, most recent, and most serious assault?
2. Are the severity and frequency changing?
3. Is stalking involved?
4. Has the abuser threatened to kill the woman, her children, or himself?

If incidents are getting more frequent or more severe and several risk factors for homicide are present, the woman should be considered at high risk for homicide. Whether a woman is currently living with the abuser is unimportant, because the homicide risk is still present (if it is not higher). Possible courses of action need to be addressed more vociferously if the woman is at higher risk for homicide. Health care providers have an ethical and legal mandate to assess dangerousness accurately.[14]

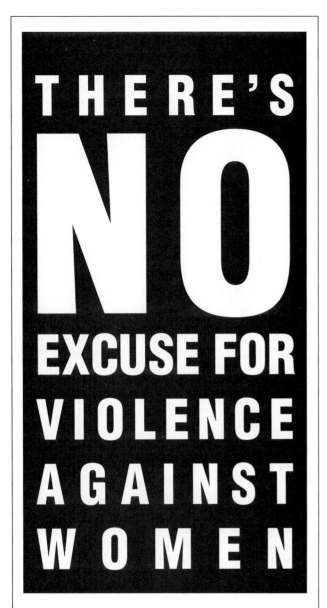

Figure 47-4

Public messages on billboards, buses, and elsewhere help to demonstrate a coordinated approach to stopping violence against women. (From the Ann Arbor Mayor's Task Force on Increasing Safety for Women, Ann Arbor, MI, 1995, with permission.)

LEGAL RESPONSIBILITIES OF HEALTH CARE PROVIDERS

Local laws differ from state to state. Health care providers should familiarize themselves with the laws in their practice area so as to maximize their role in helping victims of violence. In general, domestic violence does not carry a mandatory reporting requirement except in the case of wounds being inflicted with a deadly weapon. The term *deadly weapon*

is open to interpretation. Health care providers are required to report suspected child abuse to the local child protective services agency. In addition, the abuse, neglect, or exploitation of vulnerable adults, including the dependent elderly or those with physical or mental impairment, to adult protective services is a reporting requirement.[38] Finally, assessing the risk of homicide is a legal mandate.[14]

INTEGRATING A COMMUNITY RESPONSE

A coordinated community response (Figs. 47-4 and 47-5) to victims of partner violence teamed with changes among medical institutions and individual practitioners creates the most effective environment for helping the abused woman. An integrated response that encourages identification of abuse with education of the health care staff about partner violence interventions is ideal. This model should include mutually respectful behavior among the staff, faculty, trainees, and victims. Appropriate resource materials need to be developed as well as community resources for battered women and their children, including shelter, legal advocacy, and police involvement. Health care providers should not

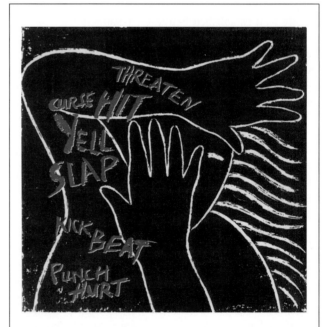

Figure 47-5

"No matter how you say it, it's all abuse." (From Chez RA, Chambliss LR, Dattel BJ, et al., for the ACOG Family Violence Work Group: *Domestic Violence: The Role of the Physician in Identification, Intervention, and Prevention.* Washington, D.C.: American College of Obstetricians and Gynecologists © 1993, with permission.)

work alone; instead, partner violence teams should include members from nursing, social work, psychology, and the community.[39]

CONCLUSION

Any person can be a victim of violence, and any health care provider can learn to identify abuse and offer help. Women are usually the victims of partner assault, a crime overlooked in the past that has far-reaching medical, psychological, and societal consequences. As health care providers learn to identify abusive relationships and facilitate help for victimized women, morbidity and mortality will decrease over time and society as a whole will benefit.

A coordinated community and health care response to violence against women is the mainstay for helping abused women and their families survive and recover from partner violence. These efforts also form the cornerstone for breaking the intergenerational cycle of violence.

References

1. Finkelhor D, Gelles R, Hotaling G, Strauss M: *The Dark Side of Families; Current Family Violence Research.* Beverly Hills, CA: Sage Publications, 1983.
2. Margolies L, Leeder E: Violence at the door: Treatment of lesbian batterers. *Violence Against Women* 1:139, 1995.
3. American Medical Association, Council on Scientific Affairs: Violence against women: Relevance for medical practitioners. *JAMA* 267:3184, 1992.
4. Miller T, Cohen M, Wiersema B: *Crime in the United States: Victim Costs and Consequences.* (Final Report to the National Institutes of Justice.) Washington, DC: The Urban Institute and the National Public Services Research Institute, 1995.
5. Salber P: *Introduction in Improving the Health Care System's Response to Domestic Violence: A Resource Manual for Healthcare Providers.* San Francisco: The Family Violence Prevention Fund, 1995.
6. American Medical Association. *Diagnostic and Treatment Guidelines on Domestic Violence.* Chicago: American Medical Association, 1992.
7. American College of Obstetricians and Gynecologists: *The Obstetrician-Gynecologist and Primary Preventive Health Care.* Washington, DC: ACOG, 1993.
7a. American College of Emergency Physicians Policy Statement. *Emergency Medicine and Domestic Violence.* Dallas, TX: ACEP, 1994.
8. Abbott J, Johnson R, Kozial-McCain I, et al: Domestic violence against women: Incidence and prevalence in an emergency department population. *JAMA* 273:163, 1995.
9. McCauley J, Kern D, Kolodner K, et al: The "battering syndrome": Prevalence and clinical characteristics of domestic violence in primary care internal medicine practices. *Ann Intern Med* 123:737, 1995.
10. Straus M, Gelles R, Steinmetz S: *Behind Closed Doors: A Survey of Family Violence in America.* New York: Doubleday, 1980.
11. Novello A, Rosenberg M, Saltzman L, et al: From the Surgeon General, U.S. Public Health Service. *JAMA* 267:3132, 1992.
12. Bergen RK: Surviving wife rape: How women define and cope with the violence. *Violence Against Women* 1:117, 1995.
13. Koss M, Goodman L, Browne A, et al: *No Safe Haven: Male Violence against Women at Home, at Work, and in the Community.* Washington, DC: American Psychological Association, 1994.
14. Campbell J: Prediction of homicide of and by battered women, in Campbell J (ed): *Assessing Dangerousness: Violence by Sexual Offenders, Batterers, and Child Abusers.* London: Sage Publications, 1995.
15. Bassuk E, Weinreb L, Buckner J, et al: The characteristics and needs of sheltered homeless and low-income housed mothers. *JAMA* 276:640, 1996.
16. Warshaw C: Limitations of the medical model in the care of battered women. *Gender and Society* 4:506, 1989.
17. Sugg N, Inui T: Primary care physicians' response to domestic violence: Opening Pandora's box. *JAMA* 267:3157, 1992.
18. Shadigian E: Domestic violence: Identification and management for the clinician. *Comp Ther* 22:424, 1996.
19. Hotaling B, Sugarman D: An analysis of risk markers in husband to wife violence: The current state of knowledge. *Violence and Victims* 1:101, 1986.
20. Sasseti M: Domestic violence. *Primary Care* 20:289, 1993.
21. Koss M, Heslet L: Somatic consequences of violence against women. *Arch Fam Med* 1:53, 1992.
22. Koss M, Koss P, Woodruff W: Deleterious effects of criminal victimization on women's health and medical utilization. *Arch Intern Med* 151:342, 1991.
23. Warshaw C: Identification, assessment and intervention with victims of domestic violence, in *Improving the Health Care System's Response to Domestic Violence: A Resource Manual for Healthcare Providers.* San Francisco: The Family Violence Prevention Fund, 1995.
24. Billy B: Life patterns and emergency care of battered women. *J Emerg Nurs* 9:251, 1983.
25. National Victims Center: *Rape in America: A Report to the Nation.* Arlington, VA: Author, 1992.
26. Courtios C: Adult survivors of sexual abuse. *Primary Care* 20:433, 1993.
27. McFarlane J, Parker B, Soeken K, Bullock L: Assessing for abuse during pregnancy. *JAMA* 267:3176, 1992.
28. McFarlane J: Abuse during pregnancy: The horror and the hope. *AWHONN Clinical Issues* 4:350, 1993.

29. Gelles R: Violence and pregnancy: Are pregnant women at greater risk of abuse? *J Marriage Family* 50:841, 1988.

30. Bullock L, McFarlane J: The birth-weight/battering connection. *Am J Nursing* 89:1153, 1989.

31. Gazmararian J, Adams M, Saltzmann L, et al and the PRAMS Working Group: The relationship between pregnancy intendedness and physical violence in mothers of newborns. *Obstet Gynecol* 85:1031, 1995.

32. Berenson A, Wieman C, Wilkenson G, et al: Perinatal morbidity associated with violence experienced by pregnant women. *Am J Obstet Gynecol* 170:1760, 1994.

33. Newberger E, Barkan S, Lieberman E, et al: Abuse of pregnant women and adverse birth outcome. *JAMA* 267:2370, 1992.

34. Buel S: Family violence: Practical recommendations for physicians and the medical community. *Women's Health Issues* 5:158, 1995.

35. Conte J: The effects of sexual abuse on children: Results of a research project. *Ann NY Acad Sci* 528:311, 1988.

36. Janoff-Bulman R, Frieze I: A theoretical perspective for understanding reactions to victimization. *J Social Issues* 39:1, 1983.

37. Saunders D: Prediction of wife assault, in Campbell J (ed): *Assessing Dangerousness: Violence by Sexual Offenders, Batterers, and Child Abusers.* London: Sage Publications, 1995.

38. Michigan State Medical Society Forum on Family Violence: *Reach Out: Intervening in Partner Abuse.* East Lansing, MI: 1993.

39. Warshaw C: Establishing an appropriate response to domestic violence in your practice institution and community, in *Improving the Health Care System's Response to Domestic Violence: A Resource Manual for Healthcare Providers.* San Francisco: The Family Violence Prevention Fund, 1995.

40. Chenowith L: Violence and women with disabilities. *Violence Against Women* 2:391, 1996.

41. American Medical Association: Diagnostic and treatment guidelines on child physical abuse and neglect. *Arch Fam Med* 1:187, 1992.

Chapter 48

CONTRACEPTIVE PROBLEMS

Margaret R. Punch

Contraceptive use in one form or another is widespread among women of childbearing age. Although it is recognized that condoms provide the best protection against human immunodeficiency virus (HIV) and sexually transmitted diseases, oral contraceptives and female sterilization remain the most popular forms of birth control in the United States today. Many issues factor into an individual's or couple's decision regarding choice of contraceptive. These include but are not limited to efficacy, safety, convenience, cost, and the potential for noncontraceptive benefits.

Complications from contraceptive use can range from minor side effects due to hormonal or mechanical factors to serious illness, such as myocardial infarction. While a major complication will necessitate discontinuing a method, minor side effects or complications can often be treated and the method continued. Because the complication risks vary from method to method, they are discussed below by method. Contraception used by women generally falls into one of four categories: hormonal methods, barrier methods, intrauterine devices, and sterilization. Methods such as periodic abstinence or withdrawal are not considered, since the main risk they carry is that of unintended pregnancy.

The final section of the chapter is a review of emergency or postcoital contraception. This is sometimes referred to as the "morning-after" pill. It has been recognized for a long time as an option in the setting of sexual assault, broken condoms, misplaced diaphragms, and failure to use a chosen method. It has recently been more widely publicized, and it received Food and Drug Administration approval in 1997.

COMPLICATIONS OF HORMONAL CONTRACEPTIVES

As a group, hormonal contraceptives include oral, injectable, and implantable means of contraception. Because the complications and side effects vary with the method, they are described separately. Oral contraceptives include both progestin-only pills (minipills) and pills that contain estrogens and progestins in fixed or variable combinations. Hormonal contraception may also be prescribed for its noncontraceptive benefits, including cycle control; relief of dysmenorrhea, menorrhagia, and acne; and reduction of premenstrual symptoms.

COMPLICATIONS OF COMBINED ORAL CONTRACEPTIVES

Birth control pills are used by millions of women in the United States each year. When taken properly, they can provide reliable contraception, menstrual cycle control, relief of dysmenorrhea, and a variety of other noncontraceptive benefits. Currently, over thirty oral contraceptives are commercially available for prescription use. Combined oral contraceptives each contain an estrogenic agent and a progestational agent. The estrogen is either ethinyl estradiol or mestranol. Available progestins include norethindrone, norethindrone acetate, ethynodiol diacetate, norgestrel, levonorgestrel, norethynodrel, desogestrel, and norgestimate. The ratio of the estrogen and progestin may be fixed (monophasic) or may vary across the cycle (biphasic or triphasic). Active medication is taken for 21 days followed by a week of placebo (28-day pack) or simply not taking any pills for the last seven days of the cycle (21-day pack). Menstrual flow typically will occur during the week when no active medication is taken. In some instances, a woman may receive a prescription for the active pills to be taken in a continuous fashion, to avoid having menses.

PATHOPHYSIOLOGY

Oral contraception is effective because of the inhibition of ovulation that results from suppression of follicle-stimulating hormone (FSH) and luteinizing hormone (LH). Progestins also result in thickening of cervical mucus, which may inhibit sperm transit. Changes also occur in the endometrium, which would inhibit implantation if ovulation and fertilization were to occur. With careful patient selection, serious complications of oral contraceptives should be minimized. Patients at risk for cardiovascular disease, thromboembolism, and cerebrovascular disease should not be given combined oral contraceptives. It is generally recommended that cigarette smokers over the age of 35 not be placed on combined oral contraception because of unacceptably increased risk for serious complications.

Medications that enhance hepatic glucocorticoid metabolism may decrease the effectiveness of combination oral contraceptives.[1,2] These are summarized in Table 48-1.

DIAGNOSIS AND DIFFERENTIAL DIAGNOSIS

The most common "complications" of oral contraception are side effects, which are often mild and transient and occur at the initiation of therapy. These are summarized in Table 48-2; they include bleeding abnormalities, nausea, acne, weight gain, breast tenderness, and transient mild increases in blood pressure. These effects can generally be managed

expectantly, with improvement in several cycles of continued use of oral contraception.

Oral contraceptive use may accelerate the development of gallbladder disease in women at risk for it.

Table 48-3 lists serious complications of oral contraceptive use that would necessitate discontinuation of oral contraception and institution of appropriate treatment. There may be instances where a significant bleeding episode develops in the oral contraceptive user. If a patient has been taking oral contraceptives for some time and acutely develops complications such as abnormal bleeding, depression, or migraine headaches, the oral contraceptives should not be assumed to be the causative agent and alternative explanations should be investigated. Evaluation of abnormal bleeding should include a search for fibroids, endometrial polyps, cervical cancer, and severe cervicitis.

Table 48-2

COMMON EARLY SIDE EFFECTS OF ORAL CONTRACEPTIVE USE

Breakthrough bleeding
Breast tenderness
Nausea
Changes in acne
Weight gain
Transient mild increase in blood pressure

Table 48-1

MEDICATIONS THAT MAY DECREASE ORAL CONTRACEPTIVE EFFECTIVENESS[a]

Phenobarbital
Phenytoin
Carbamazepine
Primidone
Ethosuximide
Rifampin
Griseofulvin

[a]For long-term use consider a higher-dose oral contraceptive or alternative means of contraception.

Table 48-3

INDICATIONS TO DISCONTINUE ORAL CONTRACEPTIVES IMMEDIATELY

Deep venous thrombosis
Pulmonary embolism
Myocardial infarction
Stroke or transient ischemic attack
Retinal vein thrombosis
Worsening or onset of migraine headaches
Liver carcinoma or hepatoma
Breast cancer
Severe depression temporally related to OC use
Pregnancy

TREATMENT

Nausea may respond to switching to a nighttime dosing schedule. At times improvement may occur with a lower-dose estrogen pill.

Breast tenderness is also usually transient; in some instances switching to a lower dose estrogen may result in improvement.

The management of bleeding complications in oral contraceptive users is summarized in Table 48-4. Birth control pill usage may be associated with increased risk of chlamydial cervicitis because of the increased prominence of the cervical ectropion. In patients at risk for sexually transmitted disease, this should be investigated.

In cases of breakthrough bleeding when it is thought that a short course of estrogen supplementation is necessary, this can be managed with estradiol (e.g., Estrace 1 mg) or conjugated estrogens (e.g., Premarin 0.625 mg) on a daily basis from the time of spotting onset until the placebo portion of the oral contraceptive pack is reached. Patients should be counseled that their menstrual flow may increase with this intervention. Often, repeated treatment is not necessary.

Significant hemorrhage on oral contraception requires prompt diagnostic and treatment intervention. A dilatation

Table 48-5

MANAGEMENT OF MISSED ORAL CONTRACEPTION DOSES

Number of Missed Pills	"Catch-Up" Dosing Schedule	Alternative Method Necessary
One pill	Take missed pill immediately	No
Two pills	One every 12 h till caught up	Yes
Three pills	Stop for menses then begin new pack	Yes
More than three pills	Stop for menses then begin new pack	Yes

and curettage may be necessary or treatment with intravenous estrogen may be required. This should be undertaken only in consultation with a provider familiar with these treatments.

A management scheme for missed doses is provided in Table 48-5. Patients should be encouraged to stay on a consistent dosing schedule, but it is not uncommon for pills to be forgotten on occasion. If two or more pills are missed, patients should be advised to use a backup method of birth control until they have been back on active hormone-containing pills for 7 days. If pills are missed during the fourth week of a 28-day pill pack, no intervention is necessary, as these do not contain active hormones.

DISCHARGE INSTRUCTIONS AND FOLLOW-UP INTERVAL

Whenever a patient is advised to discontinue her chosen method of contraception, education should be provided regarding reliable alternatives.

If a patient is advised to continue with her oral contraceptives to observe for symptom resolution, she should be told to make follow-up arrangements with a provider who would be able to change her oral contraceptive appropriately if that becomes necessary.

Serious side effects will require admission and treatment by physicians skilled in the management of these conditions. Bleeding resulting in anemia should be promptly evaluated by a specialist.

PROGESTIN-ONLY CONTRACEPTIVE COMPLICATIONS

There are currently three types of progestin-only contraception available in the United States. The first is the pro-

Table 48-4

MANAGEMENT OF BLEEDING COMPLICATIONS ON ORAL CONTRACEPTIVES

Problem	Management
First three to four cycles of OC use	
Breakthrough bleeding	Expectant management
Amenorrhea	Pregnancy test
	If not pregnant: expectant management
	If pregnant: discontinue OC
Beyond three to four cycles of OC use	
Breakthrough bleeding	Evaluate for other causes
	Chlamydia
	Cervicitis
	Polyps
	Consider short-term estrogen supplementation or changing OC
Amenorrhea	Pregnancy test
	If not pregnant
	Reassurance or change OC
	Consider single cycle of estrogen supplementation
	If pregnant
	Discontinue OC

gestin-only birth control pill, often called the "minipill." The progestin-only pills contain norethindrone or levonorgestrel and are taken in a continuous fashion (i.e., no placebo days). The Norplant System (Wyeth-Ayerst) is currently the only implanted subdermal delivery system available for continuous release of levonorgestrel. Once in place, it can provide reliable, coitus-independent contraception for 5 years. Depot medroxyprogestrone acetate (Depo-Provera, Upjohn and Pharmacia) is an injectable long-acting form of progestin-only contraception. Intramuscular injections of 150 mg are given every 12 weeks. Progestin-only contraception is often considered for women who have contraindications to estrogen, including those with seizure disorders, congenital heart disease, sickle cell anemia, and a history of thromboembolic disease, or older women who smoke. Progestin-only contraception is also often recommended for women who are breast-feeding because it does not seem to diminish milk supply, as do combined oral contraceptives.

PATHOPHYSIOLOGY

The effectiveness of progestin-only oral contraception results from changes in the cervical mucus and the endometrium, which inhibit sperm penetration and endometrial receptivity to implantation. It is less reliable at suppressing ovulation than combination oral contraceptives or other progestin-only contraceptives. If ovulation persists, menstrual bleeding will remain regular and failure rates may be higher. However, it is not uncommon for patients to develop irregular menses while taking this form of oral contraception. Patients should be advised to take their pills at about the same time each day in order to provide continuous effect on the cervical mucus and sperm penetration.

The effectiveness of the levonorgestrel implants results from continuous low-dose diffusion of levonorgestrel from six inert Silastic capsules. Although effective levels of release persist for 5 years, there is some decrease in levonorgestrel release over the first 18 to 24 months. Changes in the cervical mucus and endometrium will take place, as with the minipill, but ovulation is more likely to be suppressed. Menstrual bleeding patterns can range from regular menses to irregular menses to complete amenorrhea. Because of the continuous suppressive effect of progestins on the endometrium, it is not uncommon to have periods of persistent spotting, but it is unusual to have prolonged heavy bleeding. Failure rates are higher in patients with regular menses and may be increased in patients who weigh over 154 lb. Levonorgestrel implant capsules are flexible, and it is unlikely that they would be damaged by trauma to the arm unless they were lacerated.

Depot medroxyprogesterone acetate is the most effective of all the progestin-only contraceptives in suppressing ovulation. Levels of FSH and LH are suppressed, with inhibition of the LH surge. Atrophy of the endometrium and thickening of the cervical mucus also occur. Menstrual changes are very pronounced in users of depot medroxyprogesterone acetate, and amenorrhea after 1 year is as common as 50 per-

cent. Although injections are recommended every 12 weeks, contraceptive effectiveness probably lasts reliably up to 14 weeks.

Levonorgestrel metabolism is enhanced by medications that induce hepatic enzymes. Levonorgestrel implants and levonorgestrel minipills should be avoided by women who take the medications listed in Table 48-6. If a levonorgestrel implant user is begun on one of these medications, alternative contraception should be recommended.

COMPLICATIONS OF PROGESTIN-ONLY ORAL CONTRACEPTIVES

DIAGNOSIS AND DIFFERENTIAL DIAGNOSIS

Progestin-only oral contraceptives are more likely to fail than combination oral contraceptives, levonorgestrel implants, or depot medroxyprogesterone acetate. They also provide less protection against ectopic pregnancy, although ectopic pregnancy rates are not increased among women using this method as compared with pregnancy rates among noncontracepting women. Menstrual irregularity is common, but sudden changes in bleeding patterns should be investigated promptly and should include evaluation for pregnancy.

Contraceptive efficacy may be compromised if progestin-only oral contraceptives are not taken on a fairly rigid dosing schedule. Breakthrough bleeding may also be more likely to result if doses are missed or delayed.

Acne may be increased among patients using minipills or implants containing levonorgestrel. This results from decreases in sex-hormone-binding globulin and the increased free glucocorticoid levels of levonorgestrel and testosterone.

There may be slightly increased risk of functional ovarian cysts in progestin-only users compared to combined oral contraceptive users. Functional cysts are often asymptomatic and found only at the time of routine pelvic examination. Symptoms, if present, would include lower abdominal pain or pressure.

Table 48-6

MEDICATIONS THAT ENHANCE LEVONORGESTREL METABOLISM[a]

Carbamazepine
Primidone
Phenytoin
Phenylbutazone
Phenobarbital
Rifampin

---

[a]Avoid use of levonorgestrel implants or levonorgestrel-only oral contraceptives because these are associated with higher pregnancy rates.

TREATMENT

If a patient complains of bleeding irregularities that are not associated with pregnancy and are not causing anemia, she may be reassured that this is common and that no intervention is required. Some patients will find this unacceptable and request a change to an alternative form of contraception.

If a dose of progestin-only oral contraception is taken more than 3 h late (27 h or more following the previous dose), the woman should be advised to use a backup method for 48 h following resumption of medication.

Acne may be treated conservatively while the contraceptive is continued, but it may also lead the user to choose to discontinue this method of contraception.

Ovarian cysts that are felt to be functional can be managed expectantly. Resolution will usually occur within two to three cycles. If severe pain occurs in the setting of an ovarian cyst, rupture or torsion should be considered and a specialist consulted for immediate evaluation and possible intervention.

DISCHARGE INSTRUCTIONS AND FOLLOW-UP INTERVAL

Women with bleeding abnormalities due to the method of contraception and no other apparent pathology should be advised to keep a bleeding calendar and return to the prescribing provider for follow-up in one to three cycles.

If an ovarian cyst is identified that is presumed to be functional, follow-up should occur in two to three cycles. Patients with mildly symptomatic cysts should be followed up within 1 week for reexamination. Patients should be advised to return for acute exacerbation of pain, the development of nausea or vomiting, or fever.

Serious side effects are unlikely on progestin-only oral contraceptives. Presumed rupture or torsion of an ovarian cyst will require evaluation and treatment by physicians skilled in the management of these conditions.

COMPLICATIONS OF DEPOT MEDROXYPROGESTERONE ACETATE CONTRACEPTION

DIAGNOSIS AND DIFFERENTIAL DIAGNOSIS

Serious side effects of depot medroxyprogesterone acetate are rare. In rare instances, allergic or anaphylactic reaction may occur. Reactions noted to occur with depot medroxyprogesterone acetate include headaches, nervousness, decreased libido, breast discomfort, and depression. Weight gain is also often noted; in a small percentage patients, this may be significant. Depot medroxyprogesterone acetate is more effective than the progestin-only oral contraceptives or levonorgestrel implants at suppressing ovulation, and the incidence of functional cysts does not seem to be increased.

Menstrual changes are very common with continued use of depot medroxyprogesterone acetate. Amenorrhea is not harmful in the face of continuous progestin dosing, and patients should be informed of this. Sudden amenorrhea or symptoms of pregnancy should be investigated with sensitive pregnancy tests. Persistent spotting or light bleeding may respond to a short course of estrogen supplementation with a cycle of oral estrogen or combined oral contraceptive. Amenorrhea becomes more common over time with continued use of depot medroxyprogesterone acetate, and most instances of mild, persistent bleeding do not require intervention. Some patients may request discontinuation of the method for bleeding reasons. They should be advised that menstrual patterns may not normalize for some time. They may be switched to oral contraceptives or other contraceptive measures at any time.

TREATMENT

Because depot medroxyprogesterone acetate is a long-acting injection, it is not possible to remove its effect once an injection is given. If side effects such as headaches or depression occur, appropriate therapy should be instituted immediately. Anaphylaxis requires prompt, aggressive intervention. Allergic reactions should be closely monitored because of the long-acting nature of the injections.

DISCHARGE INSTRUCTIONS AND FOLLOW-UP INTERVAL

Women receiving depot medroxyprogesterone acetate injections should have appointments for injections every 12 weeks. They should be advised to inform their provider of any medical illnesses or interventions that have occurred between visits. Maintaining a bleeding calendar is very helpful for the evaluation of bleeding patterns. It may also help the patient to see whether a trend toward decreased bleeding is occurring.

COMPLICATIONS OF LEVONORGESTREL IMPLANTS

COMPLICATIONS OF INSERTION AND REMOVAL

Diagnosis and Differential Diagnosis

The first series of complications of levonorgestrel implants to consider are those that result from insertion of the capsules. The insertion process involves placement of the six capsules into a subdermal location using a trocar. The skin is cleaned (as in preoperative preparation) and a local anesthetic is employed. The insertion site is closed either with a reinforced tape or a suture and a pressure dressing is applied. Moderate bruising is common following insertion. Local swelling may also be pronounced. Table 48-7 summarizes complications that may follow insertion and provides treatment recommendations.

Levonorgestrel implant removal is technically more difficult than levonorgestrel implant insertion. Using aseptic

Table 48-7

COMPLICATIONS OF LEVONORGESTREL IMPLANT INSERTION

Complication	Management
Bruising at insertion site	Expectant management
Infection at insertion site	Antibiotics appropriate for skin flora (e.g., cephalexin, ciprofloxacin)
	Removal if infection persists
Expulsion of one or more capsules	Replacement with new capsule(s)
	Alternative method until replacement
Pain or itching	Expectant management

technique and local anesthetic beneath the tips of the capsules, the capsules are removed from a small incision using a combination of blunt and sharp dissection. Capsules that have been in place for some time are usually surrounded by a tissue sheath that must be opened in order to remove the capsule. At times, improper insertion technique or capsule movement postinsertion will result in capsule locations that will require more than one incision to facilitate removal, but multiple incisions should be avoided whenever possible. If removal is very difficult, edema and bruising develop to further hinder the removal process. A second visit may be required to complete capsule removal following resolution of edema and bruising. Occasionally, ultrasound can be used to assist in localization and removal.

Treatment

Expulsion of a capsule may be difficult to determine when postinsertion bruising and swelling are prominent. Waiting 1 to 2 weeks will usually make counting of subdermal capsules easier. If a patient has possession of an expelled capsule, one may wait for the swelling and bruising to resolve and then insert a replacement capsule in the same location. It is advisable to observe for cellulitis and treat if necessary with antibiotics appropriate for skin flora (e.g., cephalexin or ciprofloxacin).

Insertion or removal of levonorgestrel implants should *not* be undertaken by providers who are unfamiliar with these procedures. Incorrectly inserted capsules are very difficult to remove. It would be unusual to require emergency removal of levonorgestrel implants, and if a provider is not available who is skilled at the procedure, it should not be attempted. Marked bruising, edema, and difficulty in removing all six capsules are more likely to be encountered by someone unfamiliar with removal techniques.

Discharge Instructions and Follow-up Interval

Alternative means of contraception should be recommended to the patient if it is not certain that six active capsules are in place. Patients treated for infection should expect initial improvement within 48 h. They should be given instructions to follow up with an experienced levonorgestrel implant provider if improvement does not occur, because removal of the capsules would then be indicated.

COMPLICATIONS OF THE LEVONORGESTREL METHOD

Diagnosis and Differential Diagnosis

Menstrual changes are common in users of levonorgestrel implants. Careful patient selection and education prior to insertion will minimize unscheduled follow-up or termination of the method due to dissatisfaction with bleeding patterns. Regular bleeding in the first year of implantation occurs in only about one-third of levonorgestrel implants users. In subsequent years, the rates of regular bleeding increase to 55 to 67 percent. Bleeding abnormalities are attributed to anovulation in some users and the effect of continuous levonorgestrel on the endometrium. Failure rates may be higher in women with regular menses, but pregnancy can occur in women with irregular bleeding patterns. Although the number of days of bleeding may be increased in levonorgestrel implant users, especially in the first year of use, blood loss is usually scant and anemia rarely develops.

Other side effects of levonorgestrel implant use are listed in Table 48-8. Adnexal enlargement may occur as a result of functional ovarian cyst formation. This will usually resolve without intervention.

Pregnancy can occur in users of levonorgestrel implants. If insertion is performed after day 7 of the menstrual cycle, pregnancy is more likely to occur during the insertion cycle. Cumulative pregnancy rates are 0.2 per 100 in the first year and 3.9 per 100 over 5 years of use. Failure rates are higher in women with regular menses and may be increased

Table 48-8

ADVERSE REACTIONS TO LEVONORGESTREL IMPLANTS

Headache	Nervousness
Nausea	Dizziness
Adnexal enlargement	Dermatitis
Acne	Change of appetite
Mastalgia	Weight gain
Hirsutism	Hypertrichosis
Scalp-hair loss	

in those weighing over 154 lb. The incidence of ectopic pregnancy is decreased to 1.3 per 1000 women-years as compared with noncontraceptors, with an incidence of 2.7 to 3.0 per 1000 women-years.

Treatment

Treatment for abnormal bleeding during levonorgestrel implant use is not always needed. If the patient is not anemic and she can be reassured that menstrual irregularity is common, no intervention may be required. If the patient is seen during the first year of use, she should be advised that the incidence of bleeding problems decreases after the first year. If the patient finds the abnormal bleeding unacceptable, consideration may be given to treating the bleeding rather than resorting to removal of the capsules. Diaz et al. reported several different treatment options for women with prolonged bleeding episodes.[3] A prolonged bleeding run was defined as 8 or more consecutive days of bleeding or spotting, and this occurred in half of levonorgestrel implant users within the first year following insertion. Treatment arms included placebo, levonorgestrel 0.03 mg twice a day for 20 days, ethinyl estradiol 0.05 mg daily for 20 days, and ibuprofen 800 mg three times a day for 20 days. Results of the study show that all three active regimens decreased the total number of bleeding and spotting days compared to placebo during the first year. The greatest effect seemed to occur with the ethinyl estradiol–treated group, but it should be kept in mind when prescribing intervention that some patients are using levonorgestrel implants because of contraindications to estrogen. If ethinyl estradiol is not available in the clinical setting, a single cycle of a combined oral contraceptive may also be effective in decreasing bleeding. The patient should be cautioned to expect a menstrual period following a cycle of estrogen supplementation.

Other medical side effects of levonorgestrel implants can often be managed conservatively or expectantly. Approximately 6 percent of levonorgestrel implant users will request removal in the first year of use because of nonbleeding abnormalities. Levonorgestrel implants have not been associated with an increase in the incidence of birth defects, but they should be removed immediately in patients desiring to continue a pregnancy.

Discharge Instructions and Follow-up Interval

Patients treated for abnormal bleeding should be advised to keep a menstrual calendar or diary. They should be encouraged to keep a record of whether bleeding is heavy or light or consists of spotting. They should follow up with a levonorgestrel implant provider 1 to 3 months following an evaluation or treatment for abnormal bleeding.

Patients with other side effects should also be advised to follow up with their providers to assess for symptoms resolution or implant removal if symptoms are significant.

COMPLICATIONS OF BARRIER CONTRACEPTIVES AND SPERMICIDES

Currently available barrier contraceptives include both male and female condoms, the diaphragm, and the cervical cap. Except for the female condom, all barrier methods are recommended to be used in conjunction with spermicide, so their complications and risks are considered together. Barrier contraceptive efficacy is a result of mechanical obstruction to the path of sperm into the uterus. Two spermicidal agents are contained in commercially available products. Nonoxynol-9 is the most commonly used, but some preparations contain the spermicide Octoxynol. Spermicides function as surfactant-like agents that destroy sperm cell membranes.

PATHOPHYSIOLOGY

Barrier contraceptives require use around the time of intercourse. They are recommended to be placed on the penis or in the vagina prior to any penile-vaginal contact. Condoms remain in place only until intercourse is completed and then should be removed. The diaphragm and cervical cap are recommended to be left in the vagina a minimum of 6 h following intercourse but should not be left in place more than 24 h for the diaphragm or 48 h for the cervical cap. The presence of a foreign body and spermicide in the vagina may result in alterations in the vaginal mucosa and normal vaginal flora. A variety of complications may arise from the use of barrier contraception. These are generally minor and are easily diagnosed and treated. They are summarized in Table 48-9.

DIAGNOSIS AND DIFFERENTIAL DIAGNOSIS

Vaginal irritation is the most common complication associated with barrier contraceptive use, especially when sper-

Table 48-9

COMPLICATIONS OF BARRIER CONTRACEPIVES AND SPERMICIDES

Complication	Treatment
Displacement or breakage	Postcoital contraception
Urinary tract infection	Single-dose antibiotic
Bacterial vaginosis	Metronidazole PO or Metrogel per vagina
Vaginal trauma or irritation	Change spermicide, check fit of diaphragm or cap
Toxic shock syndrome	Admission and treatment
Allergic reaction to spermicide or latex	Discontinuation of method

micide is used. Included in the differential diagnosis is local irritation, vaginal infection, and allergy to spermicide or latex. Although it is true that barrier methods decrease the likelihood of sexually transmitted diseases, these should be considered when a woman presents with symptoms. Careful speculum examination of the vaginal side walls should be performed in conjunction with a saline preparation and potassium hydroxide preparation and endocervical cultures. Bimanual examination should help to localize the area of discomfort to the vagina, bladder, or pelvis. Urinalysis and culture should be performed whenever urinary tract infection (UTI) is considered. The diaphragm is more likely to be associated with UTI than the cervical cap.

The risk of nonmenstrual toxic shock syndrome is low, but it is slightly increased in users of the diaphragm and cervical cap. In a study that included the contraceptive sponge, which is no longer commercially available, it was estimated that 2.25 cases of nonmenstrual toxic shock may occur for every 100,000 women using barrier methods. Toxic shock is caused by toxins from *Staphylococcus aureus;* symptoms include high fever, vomiting, diarrhea, dizziness, weakness, myalgia, and sunburn-like rash. See Chap. 49 for discussion of toxic shock syndrome.

TREATMENT

Vaginal irritation will usually resolve without any intervention following several days of abstinence. Patients should be cautioned that if irritation is recurrent, they should consider another form of contraception. Specific infections should be treated as they would be in any setting. Whenever a woman is advised to discontinue the method of contraception she has been using, she should be given specific suggestions for alternative means of birth control.

DISCHARGE INSTRUCTIONS AND FOLLOW-UP INTERVAL

Patients who are treated for vaginal or urinary infections should expect improvement within 48 h and seek further evaluation if this does not occur. Recurrent urinary tract infections in diaphragm users may be decreased by instructing the patient to void immediately following intercourse. In some instances postcoital antibiotic prophylaxis may be given with single postcoital doses of antibiotics such as trimethoprim-sulfamethoxazole, nitrofurantoin, or cephalexin.

COMPLICATIONS OF IUD USE

INTRODUCTION

There are currently two intrauterine devices (IUDs) available for insertion in the United States. The Para Gard or Copper T 380A (Gyno Pharma, Inc., Somerville, NJ) is a polyethyl-

ene device with copper wire wrapped around the vertical stem and parts of each horizontal arm. Both the device and the copper are radiopaque. It is approved for continuous use without replacement for 10 years. The Progestasert (Alza Corporation, Palo Alto, CA) is a "T" shaped ethylene vinyl acetate copolymer with a reservoir of progesterone and barium sulfate (radiopaque) on the vertical stem. A slow release of progesterone occurs following insertion; however, the reservoir is not long-lasting and this IUD must be removed and replaced annually. Both of these IUDs contain monofilament tails. Other styles of IUD are available in other countries, and not all of these utilize strings or tails.

PATHOPHYSIOLOGY

The contraceptive effectiveness of IUDs is not entirely understood, but a number of mechanisms of action work together to provide a highly effective, coitus-independent means of contraception. These devices were originally thought to act primarily by preventing implantation due to endometrial influences. Currently it is recognized that fertilization is also prevented by changes in cervical mucus, preventing sperm passage, and local factors that inhibit sperm capacitation and survival. Pregnancy rates in IUD users are low, and ectopic pregnancy rates are approximately half those of women using no contraception.

The IUD is placed through the cervix to a location in the uterine fundus. This method is generally reserved for use in women in monogamous long-standing relationships because of an increased risk of pelvic inflammatory disease (PID) in women with an IUD in place who are at risk for sexually transmitted diseases. The insertion process is also a risk for PID, with PID rates of 10 per 1000 women-years within the first 30 days following insertion. These rates fall to 1 per 1000 women-years after 21 days of IUD use. Perforation is estimated to occur in 1 per 100 insertions; however, these rates may vary from one practitioner to another, depending on level of experience and expertise. Complications related to IUD usage that may cause a woman to seek urgent medical attention include pain and bleeding, infection, pregnancy, and the inability to palpate the IUD string, raising questions about the IUD's location.

LOST IUD STRING

DIAGNOSIS AND DIFFERENTIAL DIAGNOSIS

When a woman presents a report that her IUD string is no longer palpable on vaginal self-examination, several diagnoses must be considered, as summarized in Table 48-10. It may simply be that she has not successfully palpated the string; however, pregnancy, perforation, and expulsion must be considered. Expulsion is most likely to occur during the first month after insertion. Perforation is most likely to occur upon insertion but may not be recognized for some time.

Table 48-10

LOST IUD STRING: DIFFERENTIAL DIAGNOSIS

Patient unable to palpate, but string visible from os on speculum examination

String in endocervix or endometrial cavity, IUD correctly positioned

Expulsion of the device

Perforation of the device through the uterine wall

Pregnancy with device pulled up into uterus

Uterine fibroids with device pulled up into enlarging uterus

Evaluation of the patient with a lost IUD string should begin with a menstrual history and a history of the IUD placement. Expulsion is most likely to occur within the first year following insertion, with the highest rate in the first month. Cumulative expulsion rates are 5 to 6 percent for the first year and 1 to 2 percent per year thereafter for the Copper T 380A. Progesterone IUDs have a 2.7 percent expulsion rate during their 1 year of use. If the menses are delayed in any way or if abnormal bleeding is present, a pregnancy test should be performed immediately. Physical examination of the patient with a lost IUD string should begin with a simple speculum examination. The string may be visible on examination. An IUD will settle into the uterine cavity after placement, and the string may seem shorter than it was originally cut. Similarly, fibroid growth causing uterine enlargement may result in disappearance of the IUD tail from the vagina. If the string is indeed not visible on examination, a search for the IUD's location should ensue. After confirming that the patient is not pregnant, a uterine sound may be used to gently probe the uterine cavity following cleansing of the cervix with a Betadine solution. If present within the cavity, the IUD may be palpable as a gentle bump on the sound. If the IUD is palpable, the patient may be reassured. Alternatively, or if this procedure is not diagnostic, an ultrasound or x-ray (PA and lateral) may be obtained to localize the IUD. A uterine sound or contrast material may be placed in the endometrial canal to try to verify an intrauterine location. If no IUD is visible on x-ray, an unrecognized expulsion is most likely. If the IUD is localized in the abdominal cavity or appears to be partially perforating the uterine wall, consultation should be undertaken for laparoscopic removal or for laparotomy. Resulting PID or bowel obstruction requires immediate consultation.

TREATMENT

No intervention is required if proper IUD location is verified. Expulsion of an IUD is treated by reinsertion of a second device or institution of alternate means of contraception. Partial expulsion, when the device is partly visible through the external cervical os, is treated by removal and either reinsertion of a new IUD or an alternate means of contraception. Removal of an IUD when the string can be grasped is usually easily accomplished with gentle traction (Table 48-11). Patients should be evaluated for pregnancy and infection whenever expulsion occurs.

DISCHARGE INSTRUCTIONS AND FOLLOW-UP INTERVAL

If the IUD is located within the uterine cavity, no special follow-up is required. If expulsion or perforation is diagnosed, alternative forms of contraception should be provided to the patient. The reinsertion of an IUD should be performed only by someone skilled in the procedure.

If the uterine cavity has been instrumented in some way, consideration should be given to a short course of antibiotics to minimize the risk of pelvic infection. Although the use of antibiotics around the time of insertion remains somewhat controversial, a 5- to 7-day course of doxycycline may be prudent in some circumstances, including partial expulsion when the device lies partially in the uterus and partially in the vagina.

Table 48-11

IUD REMOVAL INSTRUCTIONS

String visible
   Insert speculum in vagina
   Cleanse cervix with Betadine or Hibiclens solution
   Grasp string with alligator forceps or ring forceps
   Pull gently with steady pressure
String not visible
   Insert speculum in vagina
   Cleanse cervix with Betadine or Hibiclens solution
   Probe for string in cervical os using alligator forceps
   If still unable to locate string and patient not pregnant:
      probe uterine cavity using alligator forceps, IUD hook, uterine packing forceps or Novak curette
   Grasp IUD with instrument and gently pull through the os
Removal caveats
   Consider placement of a paracervical block with local anesthetic if the patient experiences severe cramping
   Pretreat with antibiotics in cases of PID
   In some instances, cervical dilation may result in easier removal
   If gentle traction does not result in IUD removal, it may be embedded in the uterine wall or partially perforated and require hysteroscopic removal
   Do not attempt removal in a pregnant patient if the string is not visible or easily located in the endocervix

PREGNANCY WITH IUD IN UTERO

DIAGNOSIS AND DIFFERENTIAL DIAGNOSIS

Evaluation of abnormal bleeding or amenorrhea in a woman with an IUD in place should always include a pregnancy test. If the test is positive, evaluation must be undertaken to determine the IUD's location as well as the pregnancy's location and viability. It is estimated that one-third of pregnancies will be due to unrecognized IUD expulsion. When a pregnancy occurs with an IUD in place, there is a 3 to 9 percent chance it is an ectopic pregnancy. For this reason prompt evaluation is indicated with ultrasound and serial β-hCG levels, depending on the presumed gestational age of the pregnancy. Pregnancy with an IUD in place is not associated with an increased risk of birth defects. The IUD will remain outside the amniotic sac and will not affect the fetus in any way other than to increase the chances of miscarriage.

TREATMENT

If the patient has a nonviable pregnancy, the uterus should be emptied, the IUD removed, and a course of doxycycline or ampicillin prescribed. If there is a viable pregnancy within the uterus, the patient should be counseled about increased rates of miscarriage and preterm labor and delivery if the IUD is left in place (Table 48-12). If the IUD string is visible, removal of the IUD will decrease these rates. The string may be grasped with an instrument like a ring forceps or alligator grasper and gently pulled. If the string is not visible, no attempt should be made to remove an intrauterine IUD in a patient who desires to maintain her pregnancy.

DISCHARGE INSTRUCTIONS AND FOLLOW-UP INTERVAL

If a pregnancy occurs with an IUD in the uterine cavity and it is nonviable or electively terminated, antibiotic coverage should be provided with doxycycline or ampicillin. If a preg-

nancy is maintained following IUD removal or with an IUD in situ, the patient should be referred for immediate prenatal care. She should be informed of warning signs of miscarriage and infection. Pregnancy following IUD expulsion carries no apparent increased risk.

INDICATIONS FOR ADMISSION AND SPECIALTY CONSULTATION

Whenever the diagnosis of ectopic pregnancy is a serious consideration, consultation should be undertaken with a provider skilled in the management of ectopic pregnancy. If a nonviable pregnancy is diagnosed in the presence of an IUD, uterine evacuation should be undertaken promptly to minimize the risk of infection.

PELVIC INFLAMMATORY DISEASE

DIAGNOSIS AND DIFFERENTIAL DIAGNOSIS

Much information has been published regarding IUDs and PID. It is now believed that the IUDs currently available are associated with PID only in the first 20 days following insertion (9.7 per 1000). The rate is significantly decreased after the first 20 days (1.4 per 1000). The rates of delayed PID are increased in populations whose behavior puts them at risk for sexually transmitted diseases. For this reason, patients should be counseled prior to insertion, and those who engage in risky behavior should be encouraged to use a barrier method for contraception instead of an IUD.

The symptoms of PID in the presence of an IUD are the same as the symptoms in a woman without an IUD and are outlined in Chap. 44. Other diagnostic consideration include UTI, peritonitis from IUD perforation, appendicitis, or other abdominal disorders.

TREATMENT

Whenever PID is diagnosed in the presence of an IUD, the IUD should be removed (see Table 48-11). The stable patient with mild symptoms may be treated as an outpatient, but severe symptoms require hospitalization immediately. Antibiotic coverage should precede any attempt to remove the IUD. Admission criteria are the same as in any PID circumstances. See Chap. 44 for management of PID.

DISCHARGE INSTRUCTIONS AND FOLLOW-UP INTERVAL

Patients who are deemed suitable for ambulatory treatment should be given strict dosing instruction for the medication being prescribed. They should be seen for 48- to 72-h follow-up to be certain that their symptoms are resolving. Al-

---

Table 48-12

PREGNANCY AND IUD

One-third of IUDs previously expelled (unrecognized)

3–9% ectopic pregnancy

50% spontaneous abortion rate if IUD left in place

25% spontaneous abortion rate if IUD removed

Fourfold increase risk of preterm labor and delivery if IUD left in place

No increased risk of birth defects

ternative means of contraception should be offered following IUD removal.

BLEEDING AND PAIN

DIAGNOSIS AND DIFFERENTIAL DIAGNOSIS

Whenever abnormal bleeding or pain occurs in a woman with an IUD in place, consideration should be given to pelvic infection and pregnancy. Perforation of the uterus and expulsion of the IUD may also be factors in the differential diagnosis. The time of the episode in relation to IUD placement plays a critical role in the differential diagnosis. This is summarized in Tables 48-13 and 48-14. It is not possible to assume that all conditions that arise with an IUD in place are causally related to the IUD. Patients may develop symptomatic endometriosis or other conditions causing pelvic pain. Bleeding abnormalities may result from the growth of uterine polyps or fibroids, cervical cancer, or other pathology unrelated to the IUD. In a perimenopausal patient, it may be difficult to diagnose and manage anovulatory bleeding patterns with an IUD in place.

TREATMENT

Menorrhagia is common following IUD placement. Mild anemia may be treated with iron therapy and dietary adjustment. Nonsteroidal anti-inflammatory agents taken during the menses may also act to decrease menstrual blood loss. In cases where the hemoglobin falls below 9 g/dL or falls more than 2 g/dL, it is advisable to remove the IUD and provide alternative contraception. In situations where the etiology of abnormal bleeding is uncertain, IUD removal may facilitate diagnosis and management.

Pain immediately following insertion may be treated conservatively with acetaminophen or nonsteroidal anti-inflammatory agents. If the pain is severe, perforation should be considered more strongly and investigated. Immediate removal of the IUD may be necessary in the setting of severe pain.

Table 48-13

CAUSES OF ABNORMAL BLEEDING IN IUD USERS

Menorrhagia due to IUD
Cervicitis
Pelvic inflammatory disease
Intrauterine pregnancy
Ectopic pregnancy
Pathology unrelated to IUD

Table 48-14

CAUSES OF PELVIC PAIN IN IUD USERS

Immediately following insertion
    Pain related to cervical dilation
    Perforation of the uterus
    Partial expulsion
Worsening following insertion
    Pelvic inflammatory disease
    Perforation of the uterus
With menses
    Dysmenorrhea, menorrhagia
Delayed following insertion
    Ectopic pregnancy
    Expulsion (often silent)
    Perforation

DISCHARGE INSTRUCTIONS AND FOLLOW-UP INTERVAL

Patients treated conservatively for bleeding or pain complications should be instructed to follow up with their provider within 4 to 6 weeks. They should be instructed to return for immediate follow-up for bleeding of more than one large pad per hour or severe exacerbation of pain.

If an IUD is removed, alternative means of contraception should be provided. In addition, patients should be given strict instructions on when to return for follow-up if their symptoms do not resolve. Bleeding abnormalities due to an IUD should resolve within one menstrual cycle of IUD removal. Persistent abnormal bleeding beyond that point should be reevaluated.

COMPLICATIONS OF STERILIZATION

It is estimated that over 9 million women in the United States rely on permanent female sterilization for contraception. Female sterilization can be performed by a number of techniques, as shown in Table 48-15. Although generally uncomplicated, sterilization can result in both immediate and delayed complications. Immediate complications are generally related to surgical or anesthetic complications. Delayed complications result from subsequent risk of failure and conception with a high risk of ectopic pregnancy.

Table 48-15

FEMALE STERILIZATION TECHNIQUES AND INCISIONS

Setting	Procedure	Incision
Nonpregnant	Minilaparotomy with partial or complete salpingectomy	Suprapubic
	Laparoscopy Electrocautery Bands or clips Partial or complete salpingectomy	Single umbilical trocar site or dual puncture with second suprapubic trocar site
Pregnant/ postpartum	Cesarean section with partial or complete salpingectomy	Cesarean section incision
	Postpartum: partial or complete salpingectomy (performed 1 to 2 days postpartum)	Infraumbilical

ACUTE POSTOPERATIVE COMPLICATIONS OF STERILIZATION

PATHOPHYSIOLOGY

The acute complications of tubal ligation generally fall into three categories: (1) complications related to anesthesia, (2) complications due to laparotomy or laparoscopy, and (3) unrecognized bleeding from tubal injury.

The surgical complications will vary with the type of surgical technique employed. The type of incisions made will provide some clues; however, in the case of laparoscopic complications it is important to know if electrocautery was utilized or if clips or bands were applied to the fallopian tubes. If the patient is uncertain how the sterilization was performed and this information is important, the gynecologist or surgeon who performed the procedure should be contacted. Early diagnosis and management of these complications can minimize their long-term consequences.

DIAGNOSIS AND DIFFERENTIAL DIAGNOSIS

Table 48-16 lists a variety of symptoms that may indicate postoperative complications following sterilization.

Postoperative voiding difficulty may arise for a variety of reasons. Patients are often straight-catheterized prior to laparoscopy or laparotomy in order to minimize the risk of bladder injury while entering the abdomen in a suprapubic location. This may result in urinary urgency and will in-

crease the risk of bladder infection. Urinalysis will help to differentiate between infection and urgency due to irritation without infection. Depending on the type of anesthesia and surgery, urinary retention may also occur. Physical examination would reveal a large mass in the suprapubic region that resolves upon straight catheterization of the bladder. If over 1 L of urine is retained, prolonged drainage with an indwelling catheter is indicated. Surgical bladder injury is usually recognized at the time of surgery but may result from laparotomy or laparoscopy with suprapubic trocar placement. This type of complication is more common in women with previous lower abdominal incisions and previous cesarean sections. Unrecognized bladder injury may result in urinary leakage into the abdominal cavity or through the suprapubic incision.

Incisional bleeding may be a result of subcutaneous or intraabdominal bleeding. The patient who presents acutely in the postoperative period with incisional bleeding should be assessed for hemodynamic stability and hematocrit changes. Physical examination is also useful to determine the source of bleeding by looking for evidence of subcutaneous bruising or intraabdominal distention. Serosanguinous fluid draining from a suprapubic incision in the acute postoperative period should be evaluated with spot creatinine levels to assess for urinary leak from a bladder injury. Delayed drainage is more likely to be a result of a wound seroma, dehiscence, or infection.

Table 48-16

ACUTE COMPLICATIONS OF STERILIZATION

Symptom	Diagnoses
Voiding difficulty	Urinary tract infection Surgical bladder injury Urinary retention
Bleeding from incision	Subcutaneous bleeding Intraabdominal bleeding
Fluid from incision	Bladder injury Wound seroma
Fever	Infection following surgery Wound infection UTI Pneumonia Pelvic infection
Abdominal distention Nausea Vomiting	Ileus Surgical bowel injury Reaction to anesthesia or other medications given
Shoulder pain	Intraabdominal bleeding Distention from laparoscopy gas
Fainting/dizziness	Anesthetic complication Intraabdominal bleeding

Because laparoscopy involves the blind placement of sharp trocars into the abdominal cavity, the most serious complications of intraabdominal injury, including bowel perforation, are most likely to follow this type of sterilization. Although often recognized at the time of surgery, these can also present as postoperative peritonitis. The risk of trocar damage is increased in patients with a history of previous intraabdominal surgery who may have adhesions. In addition, if electrocautery has been utilized to cauterize the fallopian tubes, unrecognized bowel burns may result in delayed perforation and peritonitis.

Any evidence of hypotension should be critically evaluated. In the pregnant state, the mesosalpinx is extremely vascular and tubal ligation may be complicated by bleeding from these vessels. If bleeding from the mesosalpinx is unrecognized at the time of surgery, the patient may present with intraabdominal hemorrhage. Other intraabdominal structures may be damaged and result in bleeding as well. Evaluation of orthostatic blood pressure and serial hematocrit levels will usually yield evidence of significant blood loss. While this bleeding may occasionally stop spontaneously, a second operation is often required.

Because of shared innervation and referred pain, pelvic irritation is often felt as shoulder pain. Shoulder pain following tubal ligation may result from intraabdominal bleeding, bowel contents, irrigation fluid from surgery, or gas instilled in the abdomen for visualization at the time of laparoscopy. If the patient is stable and there is no evidence of visceral injury, this will usually resolve without intervention other than pain medication.

A variety of infectious complications occasionally follow tubal ligation. These include UTI, wound infection, and, rarely, aspiration pneumonia. Pelvic infection may also occasionally occur. Symptoms are similar to those of PID, and diagnosis and management are as described in Chap. 44.

Menstrual history should always be obtained in patients who have symptoms or concerns following sterilization. If the procedure was performed in the luteal phase of the menstrual cycle, ovulation and conception may have occurred in that cycle prior to tubal ligation. Any evaluation of postoperative amenorrhea or abnormal menstrual bleeding should include performance of a sensitive pregnancy test.

TREATMENT

Treatment is directed to the specific diagnosis. Any time a surgical complication is identified, it is important to notify the physician who performed the procedure, if possible. Immediate notification should take place if hemodynamic instability exists or if other complications that require surgical intervention are identified. A gynecologist who performs laparoscopy should be adept in the management of most postoperative complications, but consultation with a general surgeon may be indicated if a bowel injury is identified. Similarly, a urologist may be consulted if a bladder injury has occurred.

If a patient is unable to maintain appropriate oral intake and hydration, she should be admitted and observed for symptom resolution. In addition, if significant diagnostic uncertainty exists about potential serious operative complications, the patient should be admitted and observed.

DISCHARGE INSTRUCTIONS AND FOLLOW-UP INTERVAL

Patients who are managed expectantly should follow up with their surgeon in 24 to 72 h, depending on the complication and its severity.

DELAYED COMPLICATIONS OF STERILIZATION

PATHOPHYSIOLOGY

The major long-term complication associated with tubal ligation is the risk of ectopic pregnancy in the event of sterilization failure. The risk of pregnancy is low following tubal ligation (1.85 per 100 women after 10 years), but the rate of ectopic pregnancy among sterilized women is clearly increased. Fertilization is thought to be possible in the event of fistula formation in the mesosalpinx or recanalization of the fallopian tube. Tubal implantation is common in the event of fertilization because of the sustained tubal damage following any sterilization.

DIAGNOSIS AND DIFFERENTIAL DIAGNOSIS

Any woman presenting with abnormal bleeding, pelvic pain, or new amenorrhea following a permanent sterilization should have a sensitive pregnancy test performed immediately. The differential diagnoses include other causes of these symptoms in nonpregnant, nonsterilized women. Pelvic inflammatory disease is thought to be less common in the sterilized patient because of the decreased likelihood of ascending infection. In those who have a positive pregnancy test, evaluation for ectopic gestation should be started immediately. This includes vital signs, pelvic examination, quantitative levels of beta human gonadotropin (β-hCG), and ultrasound when appropriate. If the woman is not pregnant, other causes of abnormal uterine bleeding should be sought.

DISCHARGE INSTRUCTIONS AND FOLLOW-UP INTERVAL

As with any evaluation for ecoptic pregnancy, the stable patient in whom the location of the pregnancy is not yet certain and who is followed on an outpatient basis should be given strict instructions regarding follow-up evaluation. Follow-up evaluation at a minimum includes 48-h repeat of β-hCG levels. The ultrasound follow-up interval would be dependent upon changes in the β-hCG levels, the woman's symptoms, and the absolute level of β-hCG present. Repeat physical examination and evaluation by a practitioner experienced in the diagnosis and management of ectopic pregnancy should occur within 48 h of the initial evaluation.

POSTCOITAL CONTRACEPTION

Effective means of postcoital or "morning after" contraception have been known for many years; however, lack of physician and patient knowledge have limited their use. The terminology *morning-after pill* is misleading because the treatment may be initiated at any time within 72 h of the unprotected intercourse and also because two doses of several pills are required. The risk of pregnancy following an act of unprotected intercourse is affected by the timing of the woman's cycle, but it is estimated to be between 2 and 4 percent from any single act and as high as 25 to 30 percent at midcycle. The Yuzpe method described below is believed to reduce the risk of pregnancy by at least 75 percent.[4] Alternative, effective methods include postcoital IUD placement, but this should be initiated only by someone skilled in IUD placement and in a setting where there is a low risk for sexually transmitted diseases. Postcoital IUD placement may be effective up to 7 days following the sexual contact.

PATHOPHYSIOLOGY

The prevention of pregnancy most likely results from changes in the endometrium due to the hormonal composition of the oral contraceptives taken in high doses.

DIAGNOSIS AND DIFFERENTIAL DIAGNOSIS

Indications for postcoital contraception include but are not limited to (1) failure of a chosen method of contraception, (2) a broken condom, (3) incorrectly placed or disrupted placement of a diaphragm or cervical cap, (4) failure to use any method of contraception, and (5) sexual assault.

Because many women are unaware of the availability of postcoital contraception, it should be offered to patients when appropriate. It should be kept in mind, however, that not all patients who are candidates for postcoital contraception will desire it (see Table 48-17).

TREATMENT

Emergency Contraception

The Yuzpe method is the most widely studied means of emergency postcoital contraception. The Food and Drug Administration has approved the use of oral contraceptives as described for emergency postcoital contraception. Two tablets each containing 0.5 mg ethinyl estradiol and 0.5 mg DL-norgestrel are taken within 72 h of unprotected intercourse.

Table 48-17

EMERGENCY POSTCOITAL CONTRACEPTION

Unprotected intercourse within 72 h
Desire for emergency contraception
Prescribe two doses 12 h apart of appropriate oral contraceptive
Prescribe antiemetic to be taken 1 h prior to each dose
Counsel to expect menses within 21 days
Counsel regarding future contraception plans if appropriate

The same dose is repeated 12 h later. This combination of medications is contained in the oral contraceptive Ovral. Prescription equivalents are listed in Table 48-18.[5] Care should be taken if triphasic preparations or 28-day pill packs are prescribed to be sure that the patient is carefully instructed about which pills in the pack are to be taken.

Table 48-18

PRESCRIPTIVE EQUIVALENTS FOR THE YUZPE METHOD OF EMERGENCY CONTRACEPTION[a]

Trade Name	Formulation	Number of Pills Taken with Each Dose
Ovral	0.05 mg of ethinyl estradiol 0.50 mg of norgestrel	2
Lo-Ovral	0.03 mg of ethinyl estradiol 0.30 mg of norgestrel	4
Nordette	0.03 mg of ethinyl estradiol 0.15 mg of levonorgestrel	4
Levlen	0.03 mg of ethinyl estradiol 0.15 mg of levonorgestrel	4
Triphasil	(Yellow pills only) 0.03 mg of ethinyl estradiol 0.125 mg of levonorgestrel	4
Tri-Levlen	(Yellow pills only) 0.03 mg of ethinyl estradiol 0.125 mg of levonorgestrel	4

[a]Treatment consists of two doses taken 12 h apart. Use of an antiemetic before taking the medication will lessen the risk of nausea, a common side effect.
Source: The American College of Obstetricians and Gynecologists: Emergency oral contraception. *ACOG Practice Patterns,* number 3, December 1996, with permission.

Nausea will occur in 30 to 66 percent of patients who use postcoital oral contraception. Emesis occurs in 12 to 22 percent of patients. Antiemetic agents may be prescribed prophylactically 1 h prior to each dosage.

DISCHARGE INSTRUCTIONS AND FOLLOW-UP INTERVAL

Menstrual flow should be expected within 21 days after treatment. Patients should be given instructions to obtain pregnancy testing in the event that their menses have not begun after 21 days. If pregnancy occurs, the patient should be made aware that while there is limited information specific to emergency contraception and teratogenicity, numerous studies of conception with regular use of oral contraceptives have failed to show an increased risk of teratogenicity.

Patients should be referred for outpatient contraceptive counseling when appropriate. If an incorrectly placed or dislodged diaphragm or cervical cap was the indication for postcoital contraception, the patient may be instructed to use an alternative form of contraception (usually condoms) until she can see her provider to have her barrier contraceptives size and fit evaluated.

References

1. Back DJ, Bates M, Bowden A, Breckinridge AM, et al: The interaction of phenobarbital and other anticonvulsants with oral contraceptive steroid therapy. *Contraception* 18:472, 1980.
2. Diamond MP, Greene JW, Thompson JM, Van Hooydonk JE, et al: Interaction of anticonvulsants and oral contraceptives in epileptic adolescents. *Contraception* 31:623, 1985.
3. Diaz S, Croxatto HB, Pavez M, et al: Clinical assessment of treatments of prolonged bleeding in users of Norplant implants. *Contraception* 42:97, 1990.
4. Yuzpe AA, Percival Smith R, Rademaker AW: A multicenter clinical investigation employing ethinyl estradiol combined with dl-norgesterel as a postcoital contraceptive agent. *Fertil Steril* 37:508, 1982.
5. The American College of Obstetricians and Gynecologists: Emergency oral contraception. *ACOG Practice Patterns*. Number 3, December 1996.

GENERAL CONTRACEPTIVE REFERENCES

Hatcher RA, Trussell J, Stewart F, et al: *Contraceptive Technology*, 16th rev ed. New York: Irvington Publishers, 1994.

Jones HW, III, Jaffe RB, Cefalo RC, Watson WA Jr (eds). IUDs: A state of the art conference. Supplement to *Obstet Gynecol Surv* 51(suppl):S1–S72, 1996.

Speroff L, Darney PD: *A Clinical Guide for Contraception*, 2d ed. Baltimore: Williams & Wilkins, 1996.

Chapter 49

TOXIC SHOCK SYNDROME

Carl B. Lauter

The toxic shock syndrome (TSS) continues to be a serious and potentially life-threatening medical problem in contemporary clinical practice. The syndrome was first named by Todd et al.[1] in 1978. It has been recognized and reported in medical history to have a link to *Staphylococcus aureus* infection since at least 1927. In the early 1980s, clinical experience with TSS was dominated by the menstrual and tampon-associated cases.[2] Later in the 1980s and 1990s, nonmenstrual cases of TSS were recognized with much greater frequency.[3,4] In addition, a variety of different causes and syndromes of TSS have been described.[5] The reemergence of invasive group A *Streptococcus pyogenes* infections causing a TSS-like illness in patients of all ages has served to remind us of the life-threatening nature of puerperal sepsis with this bacterium.[6]

Toxic shock syndrome is caused by *S. aureus, S. pyogenes* (the group A beta-hemolytic streptococcus) and occasionally other gram-positive coccal organisms: *Streptococcus agalactiae* (the group B beta-hemolytic streptococcus) certain strains of alpha-hemolytic streptococci, and, on rare occasions, strains of coagulase-negative staphylococci. In contrast to septic shock due to gram-negative rods, which usually occurs as a nosocomial infection or in debilitated, elderly, or immunosuppressed patients, TSS most commonly occurs in otherwise healthy outpatients. The manifestations of TSS may actually be different or "atypical" in immunosuppressed patients, such as those with acquired immunodeficiency syndrome (AIDS), than in most patients who have an intact immune system.[7]

Staphylococcal TSS (versus streptococcal TSS) usually occurs predominantly in women (over 80 percent). Over 90 percent of staphylococcal TSS develops in white women between the ages of 15 and 19 years.[8] In the early 1980s, most cases of TSS were linked to the use of superabsorbent tampons.[9] In 1980, the incidence of staphyococcal TSS rose as high as 16 per 100,000 population.[10] In some parts of the United States, rates varied and were as low as 2.4 cases per 100,000 population in that same year.[11]

Epidemiologic studies linked staphylococcal TSS to young, menstruating women with *S. aureus* vaginal colonization and/or infection. Todd et al.[1] originally recognized the role of *S. aureus* vaginal colonization in children with TSS; later, its role in menstrual and nonmenstrual cases of TSS was further clarified. The isolation and subsequent identification of a new staphylococcal enterotoxin, toxic shock syndrome toxin-1 (TSST-1) from over 90 percent of *S. aureus* strains in patients with menstrual TSS further confirmed the etiology of the syndrome.[12]

After the early 1980s, there was a marked decline in the number of cases of staphylococcal TSS, mostly accounted for by a decline in the menstrual cases associated with tampon use, but there was no decline at all in nonmenstrual cases.[5] This led many to speculate that Rely tampons, which had been removed from the market, had, in fact, been a major cofactor in the expression of the tampon-associated syndrome. In some parts of the United States, however, menstrual cases of TSS did not decline.[8] Other factors that may have contributed to the overall decline in menstrual cases of TSS include increased public and medical awareness, more aggressive use of antistaphylococcal antibiotics with even the most minor of symptoms associated with menstruation, and underreporting of cases.[13]

Once menstrual cases became less prevalent, the breadth and scope of nonmenstrual cases of staphylococcal TSS were better appreciated. The literature was filled with case reports of TSS associated with postoperative infections and trauma as well as nasal and wound packs. Primary *S. aureus* infections—such as skin abscesses, postpartum infections, and respiratory infections—were also increasingly reported. The nonmenstrual TSS cases were as common in men as in women, occurred in any and all ages, were less often associated with TSST-1, and were more often associated with staphylococcal enterotoxin B (SEB).[14]

In 1987, Cone et al.[6] described their "clinical and bacteriologic observations of a toxic shock–like syndrome due to *Streptococcus pyogenes*." The medical literature began to document increased numbers of streptococcal TSS infections as well as fulminant, rapidly fatal cases of invasive streptococcal bacteremias, necrotizing fasciitis, myositis, and multiple organ failure.[15]

Streptococcal TSS cases tend to occur sporadically rather than in clusters. The prevalence has been estimated at approximately 10 to 20 cases per 100,000 population. This syndrome was more fully characterized in a series of 20 patients described by Stevens et al.[15] in 1989. Ten isolates of invasive group A beta-hemolytic streptococci (GABS) from this series were available for bacteriologic analysis. M types 1 and 3 were most common. Pyrogenic exotoxin A was produced by 80 percent of the GABS strains. The case fatality rate in this series was 30 percent. In some patients, no site of infection was readily identified at the time of presentation even though the patients progressed rapidly into shock.[15]

PATHOPHYSIOLOGY

The elucidation of toxic shock syndrome's pathogenesis began with the isolation of a protein by Bergdoll et al.[12] from 90 percent of the strains of *S. aureus* that cause the menstrual form of the disease. They called the protein *staphylococcal enterotoxin F*. At about the same time, Schlievart et al. described and purified a protein that they called *pyrogenic exotoxin C*.[16] These two proteins were later proved to be the same, and the causative toxin was then renamed *toxic shock syndrome toxin-1* or TSST-1. Study of the pathogenesis of TSS has led to the delineation of novel aspects of our immune system, the role of cytokines, and the discovery of superantigens, which may have much broader implications in biology and medicine.[17]

The major toxins of *S. aureus* can be divided into three groups: enterotoxins, exfoliative toxins, and TSST-1 (Table 49-1). The enterotoxins are medium-sized proteins, of which there are seven distinct types, that can cause staphylococcal food poisoning and shock in humans and experimental animals.[17] These toxins are very potent. Submicrogram quantities can induce vomiting and diarrhea in 1 to 4 h after ingestion. The exfoliating toxins A and B (EXF-A, EXF-B) that cause the staphylococcal scalded-skin syndrome in children may also cause bullous impetigo in adults as well as

Table 49-1

TOXIN-MEDIATED DISEASES WITH SUPERANTIGEN MECHANISMS IN HUMANS

Condition	Organism	Toxin/ Superantigen
Gastroenteritis	*Staphylococcus aureus*	Enterotoxins SEA SEB SEC-1 SEC-3 SEC-3 SED SEE
Toxic shock syndrome	*Staphylococcus aureus*	TSST-1
Scalded skin syndrome	*Staphylococcus aureus*	Exfoliatin A Exfoliatin B
Scarlet fever with shock	*Streptococcus pyogenes*	Exotoxins SPE-A SPE-B SPE-C
Invasive fulminant infection	*Streptococcus pyogenes*	Exotoxins SPE-A SPE-B SPE-C
Rheumatic fever	*Streptococcus pyogenes*	M protein

in children. Toxic shock syndrome toxin-1 is generally distinguishable from the other toxins both biochemically and by the diseases they each cause.[12,14] There is some overlap, however, as in the causal relationship of one of the enterotoxins (staphylococcal enterotoxin B, or SEB) to nonmenstrual TSS.[14]

The ability of an *S. aureus* strain to produce TSST-1 and SEB is genetically determined, most likely by transposons. Other genetic mechanisms, such as plasmid or bacteriophage mediation, have been sought but not identified. Toxic shock syndrome-1 and other enterotoxin production is maximal when the staphylococci are in the late log and early stationary growth phases.

Specific humoral immunity to TSS is confirmed by identifying the antibody to TSST-1. Acquisition of this antibody is age-related, and the great majority of persons who are over age 30 have measurable quantities. Patients with antibody to TSST-1 are still found to be susceptible to nonmenstrual TSS caused by staphylococcal enterotoxin B or other toxins.[14]

Most patients with TSS-related to menstruation either lack this antibody or have a very low titer. Over 50 percent of recovered patients do not develop anti–TSST-1 antibodies. Absence of a humoral response may explain the recurrent bouts some individuals experience. The lack of specific immunity development to TSST-1 has been correlated with deficiencies of IgG subclasses 2 and 4. Interestingly, TSST-1 has been demonstrated to suppress B-lymphocyte response in vitro.[17]

Patients who are nasal carriers of *S. aureus* strains that produce TSST-1 rarely develop the full-blown disease; they also tend to have the highest titers of corresponding antibody. Perhaps alterations in the local environment are needed for the staphylococci to express their toxins. Extensive studies in menstrual-related TSS suggest that tampon absorbency and chemical composition influence toxin expression. In addition, several environmental factors, when reproduced in vitro, have resulted in increased production of TSST-1. These include an aerobic atmosphere, a neutral pH, high protein, low glucose, low to normal magnesium, and high carbon dioxide content.

Endocrine influences on the immune system may also play a role in susceptibility. Many patients at risk for TSS are in defined hormonal states, most prominently associated with menstruation, the postpartum period, and clinical circumstances in children marked by low levels of sex hormones. Oral contraceptive use appears to be protective. Reversible defects in neutrophil function have been found in some women during menstruation; however, it is uncertain what roles these changes play in the pathophysiology of TSS.

Toxic shock syndrome toxin-1 has been shown to exert profound effects on the immune system.[17,18] It can induce fever, as can interleukin-1 (IL-1), tumor necrosis factor, and certain other mediators of inflammation. The toxin is a potent T-lymphocyte mitogen. In addition, TSST-1 can do the following:

- Stimulate release of interferon-γ
- Suppress neutrophil chemotaxis
- Induce T-suppressor factor, which can inhibit the production of immunoglobulin
- Block the reticuloendothelial system
- Enhance the susceptibility of humans and animals to endotoxin shock

Most recently, the concept of superantigens has been postulated to explain the profound effects on the host associated with exposure to small quantities of toxin in both the staphylococcal and streptococcal clinical syndromes. The term *superantigen* was coined by White et al.[18] in 1989 to describe antigens that can stimulate proliferation of a much larger percentage of T-lymphocytes than can more conventional antigens. Just a few molecules of staphylococcal enterotoxins could trigger significantly more pronounced lym-

phocyte replication than that induced by billions of copies of conventional antigen, such as the influenza virus proteins. Prodigious amounts of cytokines can be stimulated by the toxins. These and other studies suggest that the massive release of mediators may account for many of the profound clinical changes seen in patients with TSS.

Simultaneous binding of TSST-1 and the other staphylococcal enterotoxins to both T-lymphocytes and monocytes has resulted in T-cell proliferation by the superantigen mechanism.[17] It can also cause a rapid outpouring of enormous quantities of lymphokines, particularly IL-2, γ-interferon, and tumor necrosis factor beta (TNF-β), in addition to TNF-α, IL-1, and IL-6.

The pathophysiology of streptococcal TSS resembles that of staphylococcal TSS in that potent enterotoxins, acting as superantigens, are essential in both disorders (Table 49-1). In the initial two cases described by Cone et al.[6] streptococcal pyrogenic exotoxin A (SPE-A) was produced by the infecting strains in the first case and SPE-B in the second case.

In both the TSS variants induced by *S. aureus* and *S. pyogenes,* the pyrogenic exotoxins produce fever and shock, most likely after they stimulate mononuclear cells to release cytokines. Schlievert[19] has demonstrated in vitro and in animal models that these exotoxins also lower the host's threshold for responses to endotoxin. The streptococcal exotoxins (SPE-A, SPE-B) induce the production of TNF-α, IL-1β, and IL-6.

In contrast to staphylococcal TSS, where *S. aureus* bacteremia is uncommon, streptococcal TSS is associated with bacteremia, with *S. pyogenes* in 60 percent of cases.[15] In fact, bacteremia is so rare in staphylococcal TSS that its presence in a TSS-like illness was originally considered an exclusion factor in the early Centers for Disease Control (CDC) case definition.

Streptococcus pyogenes is a remarkably potent pathogen. Other exotoxins such as streptolysin O can also cause release of cytokines from mononuclear cells and may act synergistically, in this regard, with the pyrogenic exotoxins. In addition, cell wall products such as peptidoglycan, teichoic acid, and even killed streptococci can induce inflammatory mediators.[20] Finally, there is evidence in support of the quantitative importance of exotoxin production by "toxic strep." In general, streptococci isolated from patients with TSS produce much more toxin than do isolates from carriers or mild, local infections.

The recently described systemic inflammatory response syndrome (SIRS) can be caused by both infectious and noninfectious stimuli.[21] The term *sepsis* is associated with the presence of infection; therefore, this term would appropriately be applied to the two toxic shock syndromes. Trauma, burns, pancreatitis, drug reactions, and other triggers can also cause SIRS. Cytokine and mediator release seems to be central to the pathophysiology of both the infectious and noninfectious causes of SIRS.[22] The staphylococcal TSS may sometimes be confused with other noninfectious causes of SIRS because of the relatively noninvasive nature of the *S. aureus* strains causing the disease and the prominent rash. This may sometimes lead to delayed recognition and delayed antibiotic therapy.

DIAGNOSIS AND DIFFERENTIAL DIAGNOSIS

Many of the presenting clinical features of both staphylococcal and streptococcal TSS overlap. The features of staphylococcal and streptococcal TSS are described below; the clinical manifestations are summarized in Table 49-2.

STAPHYLOCOCCAL TOXIC SHOCK SYNDROME

Sudden vasomotor collapse in a previously healthy person is a striking and regular feature of toxic shock syndrome.[2] In milder cases, transient hypotension and syncope or near syncope occur. Severe cases are usually marked by a fever

of more than 38.9°C (102°F) and diffuse erythroderma. The involvement of multiple body systems and the exclusion of alternative diagnoses help to establish the clinical diagnosis. Not all features are found in all cases at onset (Fig. 49-1). Some signs and symptoms develop over the first 1 to 3 days. In particular, mucous membrane involvement tends to become most prominent on day 4 or 5 in most patients, and the very characteristic digital desquamation appears at 7 to 14 days. In milder cases, the CDC's strict case definition (Table 49-3) cannot be met, and the diagnosis instead depends on meticulous clinical skill and experience.

Great progress has been made over the past few years in understanding the pathogenesis of some aspects of the systemic dysfunction in TSS. The hypotension is due to at least four factors:

- Decreased systemic vascular resistance
- Systemic leakage of protein-rich fluid from the microcirculation into the interstitium, thereby decreasing intravascular volume
- External depletion of body fluids secondary to vomiting and diarrhea
- Myocardial depression, similar to the myocardial changes seen in septic shock

In many instances these phenomena occur in response to the massive release of cytokines, such as IL-1 and TNF, prompted by the interaction of staphylococcal toxins and the patient's immune system.[17] In fact, many of the changes in the respiratory, musculoskeletal, renal, and genitourinary systems can also be explained by the host's release of cytokine mediators. The neurologic changes, on the other hand, are not as well understood, but cerebral edema has been suggested as a cause of the toxic encephalopathy that is seen clinically.

The skin manifestations cannot be considered parallel to those of septic shock, since rash is uncommon in septic shock. The rash differs from the hemorrhagic changes of meningococcemia and/or disseminated intravascular coagulation. The rash in TSS is a key feature and the best clue in early diagnosis. Usually a blanching, nonpruritic, macular eruption that has a sunburn-like appearance, the rash is easy to overlook or to ascribe to the flushing associated with a high fever. Although in the United States the incidence of TSS seems to be lower in African Americans than in whites, the rash is extremely difficult to see on darker skin in confirmed cases. On the other hand, the mucosal changes in all patients can be dramatic, typically involving the eyes, mouth, and tongue—and, in women, the vagina. The frequently identified "strawberry tongue" is indistinguishable from that of scarlet fever.

Many of the gastrointestinal manifestations of TSS are likely to be direct effects of the staphylococcal toxins as the dramatic secretory diarrhea is not often seen in septic shock. Vomiting usually appears early, while diarrhea often develops 1 to 2 days later.[23] Clinical and histologic changes in the gut mucosa are similar to those seen in association with

---

Table 49-2

CLINICAL MANIFESTATIONS OF STAPHYLOCOCCAL AND STREPTOCOCCAL TOXIC SHOCK SYNDROMES

Manifestation	Staphylococcal	Streptococcal
Age	Primarily 15–35 years	Primarily 20–50 years
Sex	Predominantly women	Either
Predisposing factors	Tampons, surgical wound packing	Cuts, burns, bruises, varicella, alcoholism, the elderly
Severe pain	+	+ + + +
Hypotension	100%	100%
Erythroderma rash	+ + + +	+ +, often localized
Bacteremia	+	+ + +
Renal failure	+ + +	+ + +
Thrombocytopenia	+ + +	+ + +
Tissue necrosis	+	+ + +
Mortality	<3%	30–70%

Key: + = rare
  + + = less common
 + + + = common
+ + + + = very common

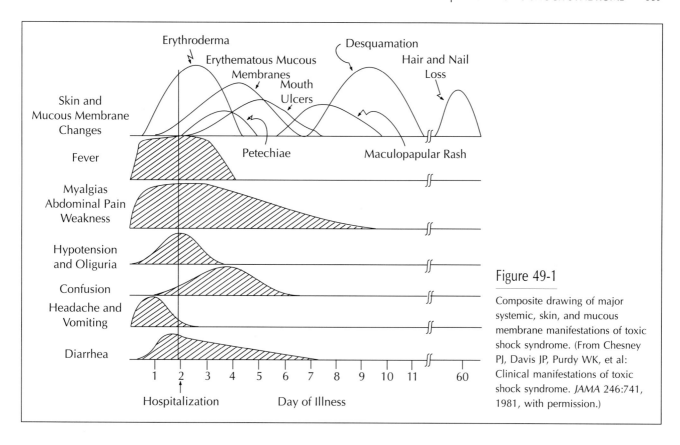

Figure 49-1

Composite drawing of major systemic, skin, and mucous membrane manifestations of toxic shock syndrome. (From Chesney PJ, Davis JP, Purdy WK, et al: Clinical manifestations of toxic shock syndrome. *JAMA* 246:741, 1981, with permission.)

staphylococcal food poisoning, a disease caused by different staphylococcal enterotoxins.

Nonmenstrual cases of TSS span the spectrum of focal and systemic staphylococcal diseases. Postpartum infections, surgical wound infections, infected sites of trauma, the use of barrier contraception, and various skin, soft tissue, and mucosal abscesses have been implicated.[4] Respiratory infections—including sinusitis, infections behind nasal packs, and postinfluenza bronchitis-pneumonias—are a few selected examples.

Several interesting aspects of postpartum TSS deserve special emphasis.[24,25] Both staphylococcal and streptococcal TSS cases have been described in the postpartum period. In most such patients, there has been no evidence of preexisting intrauterine infection and no history of postpartum tampon use. Postpartum intrauterine manipulation is documented in some of the staphlococcal TSS cases. Often these patients present with a septic or "toxic" clinical picture but lack the localizing signs and symptoms of an interauterine infection, such as pain, tenderness, and abnormal vaginal discharge. Fatal cases of *Clostridium sordelli* infection, a TSS-like syndrome, have been described in the postpartum patient with retained gauze sponges.[26]

In addition, the more recent literature has documented the "return" of cases of life-threatening puerperal sepsis caused by GABS.[27,28] In contrast to staphylococcal TSS, which may appear early or late after delivery, streptococcal TSS has a rapid fulminant onset within hours to just a few days post-

partum. Blood cultures are often positive in GABS TSS but rarely so in postpartum staphylococcal TSS. The clinical features of the two syndromes may otherwise be indistinguishable, leading to shock, multiple organ failure, and death if not treated rapidly. In severe cases of staphylococcal TSS, dilatation and curettage is often required, especially when patients do not respond promptly to appropriate antibiotics. In streptococcal TSS, uterine and other pelvic-organ necrosis has often required emergency total abdominal hysterectomy.[27,28]

Another fascinating aspect of postpartum TSS is the occasional description of congenital TSS in infants born to mothers with postpartum TSS.[29] Mahieu et al.[30] described such a neonate born to a mother with streptococcal TSS. At presentation, this infant lacked antibodies against streptococcal pyrogenic exotoxins. He responded to treatment with intravenous immune globulin, which was later demonstrated to contain neutralizing antibodies against all three streptococcal pyrogenic exotoxins. Others had previously reported staphylococcal TSS in mother-infant pairs, with suspected intrapartum transmission of the *S. aureus* infection.[29]

Toxic shock syndrome toxin-1 has been identified in over 90 percent of patients with menstrual TSS but in only about 50 percent of those who have the nonmenstrual type. A recent reevaluation of this observation has confirmed that staphylococcal enterotoxin B is often found in nonmenstrual patients who are negative for TSST-1.[14] Staphylococcal enterotoxin A is often found to coexist with TSST-1, but

Table 49-3

CENTERS FOR DISEASE CONTROL AND PREVENTION CASE DEFINITION OF TOXIC SHOCK SYNDROME

1. Fever: temperature ≥38.9°C (102°F)
2. Rash: diffuse macular erythroderma
3. Desquamation: 1–2 weeks after onset of illness, particularly of palms and soles
4. Hypotension: systolic blood pressure ≤ 90mmHg, orthostatic drop in diastolic ≥ 15 mmHg; orthostatic syncope of dizziness
5. Involvement of three or more of the organ systems
   Gastrointestinal: vomiting or diarrhea at onset of illness
   Muscular: severe myalgia or twice-normal CPK
   Mucous membranes: vaginal, oropharyngeal, or conjunctival hyperemia
   Renal: twice-normal BUN or creatinine or pyuria (>5 WBC/hpf)
   Hepatic: twice-normal bilirubin or transaminases
   Hematologic: platelets < 100,000/mm³
6. Central nervous system: disorientation or alterations in consciousness without focal neurologic signs when fever and hypotension are absent
7. Negative results on following tests, if obtained:
   Blood, throat, or cerebrospinal fluid cultures (blood culture may be positive for *Staphylococcus aureus*)
   Serologic tests for Rocky Mountain spotted fever, leptospirosis, or measles

Key: CPK = creatine phosphokinase; BUN = serum urea nitrogen; WBC = white blood cells; hpf = high-power field.

---

staphylococcal enterotoxin B is almost never found in this association. Some 62 percent of the reported cases of the nonmenstrual condition were found to be caused by staphylococci that produced enterotoxin B.[14]

Unfortunately, because of the perception of TSS as a "tampon disease," patients and many physicians do not think of the diagnosis in men as often or as quickly as they otherwise might. This diagnostic bias is real and has been studied and described in detail.[13] The CDC case definition specifically avoids menstruation and/or tampons as a marker (Table 49-3).

When patients with staphylococcal TSS are first evaluated, they may express a wide range of symptoms and signs, depending upon the day of illness and particularly the toxin load. In some patients, the syndrome is so mild that it is only suspected retrospectively 7 to 14 days after recovery from an apparent febrile gastroenteritis with otherwise inexplicable desquamation of the fingers and toes. In more severe cases, high fever, tachycardia, tachypnea, and hypotension are already present at the time of first examination. The rash must be carefully sought by examining the patient's skin and mucous membranes in a well-lighted room or direct sunlight if possible. Some patients never develop the typical rash of TSS.

STREPTOCOCCAL TOXIC SHOCK SYNDROME

In contrast, patients with *streptococcal TSS* often present with severe or even excruciating pain of abrupt onset.[31] This pain can be dramatic and quite puzzling to both the patient and the physician, since it often precedes the development of local tenderness and/or physical signs of inflammation. The pain usually begins in an extremity, but it can occur in the head, chest, or abdomen, mimicking such other disorders as sinusitis, myocardial infarction, pericarditis, peritonitis, and pelvic inflammatory disease, respectively.

About 20 percent of patients with streptococcal TSS may first appear with symptoms that suggest a febrile gastroenteritis or an influenza-like illness.[15] Fever, myalgias, nausea, vomiting, and diarrhea are not rare in such patients, and they may suspect food poisoning or other gastroenteritides. The onset of the illness may be very subtle in such patients and fulminant in others.

A fever often as high as 40.5 to 41°C (105 to 106°F) is usually the first sign at the onset of streptococcal TSS.[15] Other common clinical features include confusion (50 percent) and soft tissue infection (80 percent). About 70 percent of the patients with focal soft tissue infection will develop necrotizing soft tissue infection, heralded by the appearance of vesicles, bullae, and ultimately necrosis. The ensuing necrotizing fasciitis and/or myositis will require emergent surgical exploration for diagnosis and debridement. Delayed diagnosis and surgery may lead to amputation and death. Among the 20 percent without soft tissue localization, a number of other clinical syndromes have been observed, including endophthalmitis, peritonitis, myocarditis, and the otherwise unexplained sepsis-like syndrome, previously mentioned, known as SIRS.[15,31]

Only about 10 percent of patients with streptococcal TSS develop a diffuse faint rash.[31] Localized erythema overlying the site of focal cellulitis is more common. This absence of a generalized diffuse erythema is in distinct contrast to staphylococcal TSS, where over 80 percent of patients will develop a rash. Nearly half of patients with streptococcal TSS are normotensive at presentation.[15] However, most will manifest a significant drop in blood pressure over the 4 to 8 h of observation.

A case definition of streptococcal TSS proposed by the Working Group on Severe Streptococcal Infections was published in 1993 (Table 49-4).[32] An updated (Table 49-5) classification of streptococcal infections was outlined in the same article. In an accompanying article, Hoge et al.[33] presented a retrospective analysis of 128 cases of severe streptococcal infections reviewed from the medical records of 10 hospitals in Pima County, Arizona. These authors found Na-

Table 49-4

PROPOSED CASE DEFINITION FOR THE STREPTOCOCCAL TOXIC SHOCK SYNDROME[a]

I. Isolation of group A streptococci (*Streptococcus pyogenes*)
  A. From a nomally sterile site (e.g., blood, cerebrospinal, pleural, or peritoneal fluid, tissue biopsy, surgical wound, etc.)
  B. From a nonsterile site (e.g., throat, sputum, vagina, superficial skin lesion, etc.)
II. Clinical signs of severity
  A. Hypotension systolic blood pressure ≤90 mmHg in adults or < fifth percentile for age in children
  and
  B. ≥2 of the following signs
    1. Renal impairment: creatinine ≥177 μmol/L (≥2 mg/dL) for adults or greater than or equal to twice the upper limit of normal for age. In patients with preexisting renal disease, a ≥ twofold elevation over the baseline level
    2. Coagulopathy: platelets ≤100 × 10^9/L (≤100,000/mm^3) or disseminated intravascular coagulation defined by prolonged clotting times, low fibrinogen level, and the presence of fibrin degradation products
    3. Liver involvement: alanine aminotransferase (SGOT), aspartate aminotransferase (SGPT), or total bilirubin levels greater than or equal to twice the upper limit of normal for age. In patients with preexisting liver disease, a ≥ twofold elevation over the baseline level
    4. Adult respiratory distress syndrome defined by acute onset of diffuse pulmonary infiltrates and hypoxemia in the absence of cardiac failure, or evidence of diffuse capillary leak manifested by acute onset of generalized edema, or pleural or peritoneal effusions with hypoalbuminemia
    5. A generalized erythematous macular rash that may desquamate
    6. Soft-tissue necrosis, including necrotizing fasciitis or myositis, or gangrene

[a]An illness fulfilling criteria IA and II (A and B) can be defined as a *definite* case. An illness fulfilling criteria IB and II (A and B) can be defined as a *probable* case if no other etiology for the illness is identified.
Source: The Working Group on Severe Streptococcal Infections,[32] with permission.

tive Americans to have a tenfold higher frequency of streptococcal infections than other groups. Advanced age, age under 5 years, hypotension, and multiple organ failure were significantly associated with mortality. Toxic shock syndrome occurred in 8 percent of these patients. The patients with TSS tended to be younger than the non-TSS cases (median age 15 versus 54 years) and less likely to have underlying medical disorders.

The differential diagnosis of invasive streptococcal infection and/or TSS includes staphylococcal TSS, gram-negative septic shock, and other causes of SIRS (Table 49-6). In the patients with focal infections, uncomplicated streptococcal cellulitis must be distinguished from the necrotizing syndromes, fasciitis and myositis due to GABS, as well as other causes of serious destructive soft tissue infections (e.g., clostridial gas gangrene, clostridial cellulitis, and *Vibrio vulnificus* infections in patients recently exposed to sea life or to the ocean or saltwater). Some of the common conditions that can be confused with focal forms of streptococcal TSS

Table 49-5

CLASSIFICATION OF GROUP A STREPTOCOCCAL INFECTION[a]

I. Streptococcal toxic shock syndrome (streptococcal TSS): Defined by criteria in Table 49-4
II. Other invasive infections: Defined by isolation of group A streptococci from a *nomally sterile site* in patients not meeting criteria for streptococcal TSS
  A. Bacteremia with no identified focus
  B. Focal infections with or without bacteremia. Includes meningitis, pneumonia, peritonitis, puerperal sepsis, osteomyelitis, septic arthritis, necrotizing fasciitis, surgical wound infections, erysipeas, and cellulitis
III. Scarlet fever: Defined by a scarfatina rash with evidence of group A streptococcal infection, most commonly pharyngotonsillitis
IV. Noninvasive infections: defined by the isolation of group A streptococci from a nonsterile site
  A. Mucous membrane: includes pharyngitis, tonsillitis, otitis media, sinusitis, vaginitis
  B. Cutaneous: includes impetigo
V. Nonsuppurative sequelae: Defined by specific clinical findings with evidence of a recent group A streptococcal infection
  A. Acute rheumatic fever
  B. Acute glomerulonephritis

[a]Examples of conditions in each category are not inclusive.
Source: The Working Group on Severe Streptococcal Infections,[32] with permission.

Table 49-6

DIFFERENTIAL DIAGNOSIS OF THE TOXIC SHOCK SYNDROMES

Toxin-mediated infections
   Staphylococcal scalded skin syndrome
   Scarlet fever
   Gastroenteritis, staph-toxin food poisoning
Localized infections with abdominal pain and shock
   Urinary tract infections
   Pelvic inflammatory disease
   Septic abortion
   Gastroenteritis, with rapid volume depletion
Multisystem infections
   Septic shock with localized infection (meningococcus,
      gonococcus, pneumococcus, *Haemophilus influenzae*
      type b)
   Leptospirosis
   Rubeola, atypical measles
   Rocky Mountain spotted fever, other rickettsias, *Ehrlichia*
   Other viral syndromes (adenoviruses or enteroviruses)
   Legionnaire's disease
   Toxoplasmosis, cytomegalovirus
Multisystem illness, possibly infectious
   Kawasaki syndrome in children and teenagers
Noninfectious diseases
   Systemic lupus erythematosus
   Acute rheumatic fever
   Drug-related eruption (erythema multiforme, Stevens-
      Johnson syndrome), systemic vasculitis
   Juvenile rheumatoid arthritis

are outlined in Table 49-7. The subject of necrotizing soft tissue infections has recently been concisely reviewed.[34]

LABORATORY TESTS

Confirmation of the diagnosis of staphylococcal and streptococcal TSS requires the microbiologic identification of the responsible organism. In addition, an array of hematologic and chemical tests are useful in defining certain characteristic laboratory profiles. Identifying significant metabolic derangements and organ system toxicities allows specific supportive measures to be instituted.

STAPHYLOCOCCAL TOXIC SHOCK SYNDROME

In staphylococcal TSS, the dramatic laboratory tests have been carefully recorded and studied serially.[23] The complete blood count is very useful. Mild anemia evolves quickly and probably has several causes. Leukocytosis is universal and often includes immature forms (band forms, or "left shift"), and toxic neutrophilic changes are usually present. In milder cases, a reduction in platelets is an isolated finding, but a decreased platelet count is part of a generalized disseminated intravascular coagulation (DIC) syndrome in some severe cases. A prolonged prothrombin time (PT), partial thromboplastin time (PTT), and decreased serum fibrinogen will be seen if severe DIC is present. Eosinophils may increase later in the course, sometimes creating diagnostic confusion between an allergic reaction to antibiotics and TSS itself.

Liver, pancreatic, and skeletal muscle enzymes may rise quite significantly in many patients. Creatine phosphokinase levels are less commonly elevated in staphylococcal TSS than in streptococcal TSS; they may be in the tens of thousands in a few patients, but myocardial involvement has rarely been documented.

Electrolyte abnormalities are also very common and include hypokalemia, hyponatremia, hypocalcemia, hypophosphatemia, and hypomagnesia.[23] Hypocalcemia is almost universal, is not proportional to mild hypoalbuminemia, and is not explained by the occasional episodes of pancreatitis, renal dysfunction, or hypomagnesia. It is not due to hypotension or toxic shock alone. The changes are similar to those seen in septic shock but do not occur in otherwise uncomplicated cardiogenic shock. Calcium depression, which can be profound, lasts for 5 to 7 days. The clinical severity of the TSS seems to determine the degree of serum calcium depression.[35,36]

Elevations of plasma calcitonin and, to a lesser degree, parathyroid hormone have been noted. These changes are not related to renal impairment and are also seen in septic shock but not in cardiogenic shock. Toxic shock syndrome toxin-1 and other staphylococcal toxins may have a direct effect on calcitonin release.

A positive culture for *S. aureus* from an obviously involved focus (e.g., vagina, tampon materials, an infected postoperative wound, or traumatic injury site) supports the clinical diagnosis. In many patients, the site of infection may be subtle; some of these toxic staphylococcal strains are apparently weakly invasive, eliciting little to no local inflammatory reaction. A high clinical index of suspicion is required. Wounds that are not obviously infected should nevertheless be opened and a culture obtained.

Staphylococcus epidermidis and other coagulase-negative staphylococci have been isolated in pure culture from patients with otherwise classical TSS. In some of these case studies, such strains have been reported to carry genes related to *S. aureus* enterotoxins B and C. Despite the inability to identify specific enterotoxin production from these coagulase-negative staphylococci, whole killed bacteria are able to elicit a profile of cytokine release in a dose-dependent fashion similar to that seen in laboratory studies of the more classical *S. aureus* enterotoxins.

Table 49-7

DIFFERENTIAL DIAGNOSIS OF LIFE-THREATENING SKIN AND SOFT TISSUE INFECTIONS

Conditions	Erysipelas	Streptococcal Gangrene (Fasciitis, Myositis)	Synergistic Gangrene	Clostridial Gas Gangrene (Myonecrosis)	Clostridial Cellulitis (Anaerobic Cellulitis)	Infected Vascular Gangrene
Predisposing conditions	Previous respiratory infection, ↓ drainage	DM, myxedema w/o abd. surgery, varicella, NSAID, use, spontaneous	Surgery, draining sinus, DM, trauma	Local trauma, DM, surgery	Local trauma, surgery, DM	Arterial insufficiency
History of injury	Often not	Almost always	Yes	Yes	Yes	Yes
Incubation	1–3 days	3–4 days	1–4 days to 14 days	1–2 days	>3 days	≫5 days
Onset	Gradual	Very rapid	Slow or rapid	Extremely rapid	Gradual	Gradual
Site of diseases	Skin	Subcutaneous tissue and/or muscle	Subcutaneous and fascia	Muscle	Subcutaneous tissue	Full thickness of skin
Toxemia	Nil to moderate	Severe, shock	Delayed, severe	Very severe	Nil or slight	Nil to minimal
Skin color and sensation	Red, raised tender	Dark red, anesthetic	Red to black, tender	Bronze, tender	Whitish to red, tender	Discolored, often black and dessicated, anesthetic
Fever	Present	High	Minimal to moderate	Moderate to high	Low-grade	Unusual
Pain in extremity	Often and severe	Variable, often severe	Variable	Severe	Variable	Variable, often absent
Swelling	Slight	Tense, coppery	Tense	Tense, white	Slight	Often marked
Crepitation	No	No/slight	Variable	Some	Marked	Present
Gram stain of exudate	No exudate	Gram-positive cocci in chains	Mixed flora: 1) strep & staph 2) anaerobes, aerobes-GNR	Few gram-positive rods often without spores	Many positive rods spores often seen (variable)	Mixed flora, especially gram-negative rods, anaerobes
Appearance of exudate	None	Profuse, seropurulent	Miniprofuse "dishwater"	Profuse, serous, or blood-stained	Slight	Often dry
Odor of exudate	None	None to "sour"	Putrid	Variable, slight, foul or sweet-smelling	Putrid	Fetid
Muscle	No	Edema, ±	Edema, none to ±	Marked	No	Dead
CT scan or MRI	Superficial edema	Subcutaneous and/or muscle changes	Subcutaneous changes	"Combing" of muscles	Subcutaneous changes	Full-thickness changes, often including bone

↓ = minimal

DM = diabetes mellitus

GNR = gram negative rods

± = may or may not be present

≫ = much greater

613

The demonstration of TSST-1 or other staphylococcal enterotoxin production in the laboratory would confirm that a specific strain of staphylococcus was, in fact, the cause of the syndrome. As noted earlier, patients who are susceptible to staphylococcal TSS are lacking in the specific antibody to the TSST-1, or in the case of non-menstrual TSS, to SEB or other staphylococcal enterotoxins. Testing patients for antitoxin antibodies, as well as testing specific staphylococcal isolates for toxin production is not readily available outside of the research laboratory.

STREPTOCOCCAL TOXIC SHOCK SYNDROME

Laboratory testing in streptococcal TSS is also very important.[15] As in staphylococcal TSS, the complete blood count is very useful. Despite a profoundly "septic" clinical picture, the white blood cell count may be normal or only slightly elevated. Since there is always, however, an extreme increase in immature forms (left shift), a differential white blood cell count is mandatory. Similarly, red blood cell and platelet changes mimic those seen in staphylococcal TSS.

Electrolyte changes can also be profound. Hypocalcemia and, to a lesser degree, hypoalbuminemia are routinely seen and persist for almost the entire acute phase of the illness. Renal abnormalities—including abnormalities in the urine sediment, as well as elevations in the BUN and creatinine—occur in over 80 percent of patients. Creatinine phosphokinase (CPK) levels are elevated in most patients, in contrast to the case in staphylococcal TSS. These rises in CPK can be massive and prolonged in duration. They reflect the severe tissue injury in the underlying fascia and muscles and should be considered a major clue to the diagnosis in an otherwise apparently uncomplicated cellulitis.[15,31,32]

Laboratory abnormalities will identify disease in a number of organ systems and thus will not only unmask the systemic aspects of the syndrome but also assist in meeting the currently accepted case definition. In addition to the laboratory abnormalities already mentioned, changes in the common electrolytes, liver function tests, and tests of coagulation are often abnormal.

The growth of GABS, *S. pyogenes,* from blood cultures or another sterile site is essential to the diagnosis. In contrast to staphylococcal TSS, where bacteremia is exceedingly rare, over 60 percent of patients with streptococcal TSS may be bacteremic. Specimens to be tested for individual strains of *S. pyogenes* for "toxigenic" properties are often sent to the specialized reference or research laboratory. The association between other beta (non–group A) streptococci, alpha-hemolytic streptococcal infection, and TSS-like illnesses can only be suspected clinically at present.

RADIOGRAPHY

Radiologic studies can support and enhance the diagnosis of streptococcal TSS, particularly when the differential diagnosis involves other forms of spreading soft tissue infections. The plain radiograph will not show soft tissue gas in patients with streptococcal fasciitis or myositis, in contrast to the findings in clostridial gas gangrene and the various mixed aerobic-anaerobic soft tissue infections, such as those seen commonly in the feet of diabetics (Table 49-7). On the other hand, computed tomography (CT) or MRI may demonstrate profound soft tissue changes in the fascia and/or muscles.[37] This may assist in the diagnosis of what might otherwise appear to be puzzling cases of atypical and severe cellulitis prior to the development of shock and organ failure. Early surgical consultation is necessary in these cases to reduce morbidity and mortality.

In patients who present with the recently described disorder involving recalcitrant erythematous desquamation (RED), toxigenic *S. aureus* strains have been isolated from blood, subcutaneous tissue, and other focal sites.[7,38] In contrast to that of patients with the more usual TSS, the course of those with RED is subacute, lasting from 32 to 77 days. To date, this entity has been described only in patients with acquired immunodeficiency syndrome (AIDS). Laboratory tests for human immunodeficiency virus-1 (HIV-1) infection would be indicated in patients who have such an illness. Finally, since invasive streptococcal infection may complicate varicella, viral and serologic identification of this predisposing infection may assist in the prevention of secondary cases.

TREATMENT

The most important components of managing TSS (Fig. 49-2) are a high index of suspicion and early recognition as the process unfolds. In this regard, presentations considered atypical are the most challenging. These include suspicious findings in men, children and nonmenstruating women; it is also important to recognize the streptococcal form of the disease.

Initial steps involve admitting the patient to the intensive care unit, if necessary, and instituting appropriate hemodynamic monitoring. This may mean inserting a Swan-Ganz catheter along with an arterial line and Foley catheter to allow accurate measurement of urine output. Fluid and electrolyte management should be vigorous and meticulous. Cardiorespiratory support with mechanical ventilation and vasoactive amines may be needed. Some severely affected patients require as much as 20 L of normal saline or Ringer's lactate in the first 24 hours.

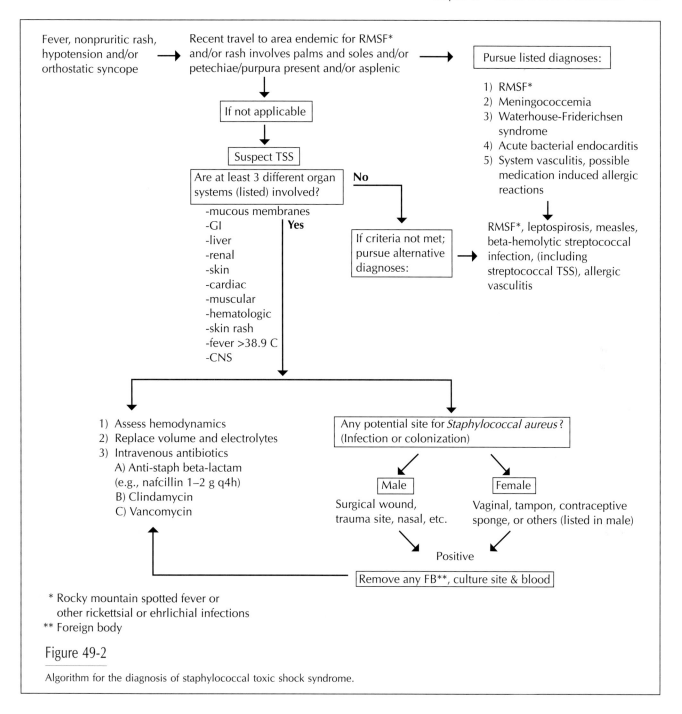

Figure 49-2

Algorithm for the diagnosis of staphylococcal toxic shock syndrome.

At the same time, sources of staphylococcal or streptococcal infection must be searched for assiduously, abscesses should be drained, and wounds need to be explored even if they do not look obviously infected. Any packing must be removed and fasciitis, myositis, or gangrenous areas should be promptly and extensively debrided in an operating room setting.

Antibiotic therapy is mandatory. Early experience confirmed that antistaphylococcal antibiotic treatment prevents relapse of menstrual-related TSS. Most experts feel strongly that acute morbidity and mortality are also significantly in-

fluenced by antibiotic treatment.[23] The antibiotics of choice for staphylococcal TSS are the antistaphylococcal beta-lactams. Nafcillin sodium or oxacillin sodium can be given in large doses intravenously—for example, 2 g q4h in adults, but smaller doses usually suffice. First-generation cephalosporins, such as cefazolin sodium, 1 g IV q6–8h, are also very effective. The fixed drug combination of ampicillin-sulbactam has appreciable antistaphylococcal, as well as antistreptococcal activity. It is not considered effective against methicillin-resistant staphylococci. Ampicillin-sulbactam is an attractive initial antibiotic choice in patients in whom mixed aerobic-anaerobic infections or gas gangrene is part of the differential diagnosis. The usual dose of intravenous ampicillin-sulbactam in severely ill adults without significant renal dysfunction should be 3.0 g q6h.

Although the prevalence of methicillin-resistant *S. aureus* infection has increased dramatically in the past two decades, TSS-producing strains have rarely been encountered. Nonetheless, in certain high-risk clinical settings—i.e., with intravenous drug abusers and in hospital acquired infections—initial treatment with intravenous vancomycin, using pharmacokinetic dosing guidelines, is recommended.

Vancomycin (usually 1 g IV q12h) or clindamycin, 900 mg (for the average-sized adult) q8h are appropriate alternatives to the antistaphylococcal beta-lactams in penicillin-allergic patients. Clindamycin may have a unique role in TSS. Laboratory studies have shown that, independent of its antibiotic activity, it can turn off toxin production in the staphylococci. A 5- to 7-day course of antibiotics is reasonable. Longer treatment may be required in recalcitrant cases, especially when an infectious focus cannot be found or is not amenable to drainage. In the sickest patients, especially those with multiple catheters and mechanical ventilation, continuous vigilance should be maintained for nosocomial, ICU-associated superinfections.

Many textbooks continue to recommend penicillin G, 1 to 2 million units intravenously every 4 h for severe streptococcal infections. However, accumulating laboratory data,[39] animal studies, and anecdotal clinical reports provide compelling testimony that favors clindamycin in toxic streptococcal infections. The killing of group A beta-hemolytic streptococci in the laboratory by penicillin is highly inoculum-dependent.[41] No such inoculum effect occurs with clindamycin.[40,43] The inoculum or load of GABS in the blood and tissues of patients with invasive and toxic GABS infections can be very high. This lack of an inoculum effect coupled with the ability of clindamycin to turn off the microorganisms' ability to produce toxins may partly explain its observed clinical superiority. Clindamycin also facilitates phagocytosis by inhibiting M-protein synthesis and has a prolonged postantibiotic effect. Penicillin remains effective for clostridial soft tissue infections.

More controversial forms of therapy include the use of corticosteroids and intravenous immunoglobulins. Animal studies and two human studies[42,43] support the administration of corticosteroids if begun as early as possible—no later than the third day of illness of staphylococcal TSS. Since most patients lack anti–TSST-1 antibody and some may be incapable of developing protective antibody, passive immunization with intravenous immunoglobulin seems rational. Commercial intravenous immune globulin preparations in the United States and Europe contain appreciable quantities of neutralizing antibody to TSST-1. At least two animal studies support this approach, but no controlled studies have been performed.[43]

Commercial intravenous immune globulin preparations in the United States and Europe also may contain (some brands, some lots) appreciable quantities of neutralizing antibodies against the streptococcal enterotoxins. Isolated case studies have described impressive improvements in patients with streptococcal TSS.[30] In one large, uncontrolled study of 15 patients, the mortality was 13 percent in patients given intravenous immune globulin. The expected mortality, based on historic controls, was 66 percent.[44]

The role of the surgeon in the management of both staphylococcal and streptococcal TSS must not be forgotten. For staphylococcal TSS, prompt drainage of any suspected foci will improve outcome and allow culture identification of the culprit organism. Location of the organism at the site is particularly important in staphylococcal TSS, since blood cultures are almost never positive.

In streptococcal TSS, prompt biopsy and exploration of any suspected soft tissue site of infection is mandatory. Frozen-section specimens should be Gram stained while the patient is in the operating suite. Extensive fascia and muscle debridement may be required. In patients who have a late diagnosis, amputation of the involved extremity may be lifesaving. If the infection and areas of tissue necrosis have developed in or spread to nonresectable areas, the prognosis is much worse.

DISCHARGE INSTRUCTIONS, FOLLOW-UP INTERVALS

Once the acute stage of staphylococcal TSS subsides, recovery in most patients is rapid and complete. Patients should be advised that desquamation of the skin, especially at the tips of the fingers and toes, will develop in 7 to 21 days and is of no clinical concern. Desquamation of the skin is very characteristic of TSS.[23] Other toxin-mediated diseases such as scarlet fever and streptococcal TSS are also followed by similar desquamation. Kawasaki disease, a condition felt by some investigators also to be caused by a variant TSS-like toxin, is also characterized by such desquamation of the distal extremity. Some patients will also develop loss of their hair and/or nails.[23] These latter changes may not be specific to TSS, since similar effects are seen in survivors of other severe illnesses. However, patients should be warned of these possible effects and assured that normal nail and hair regrowth is usually accomplished within 6 months.

In those patients with the most severe illnesses or who have had late diagnosis or treatment, organ damage such as renal failure may require dialysis therapy until renal function returns. In rare instances, permanent renal failure has been documented. Rarely have any of the other organ toxicities been permanent.

Outpatient follow-up is an important part of medical management. Women with menstrual-related disease are advised to avoid the use of superabsorbent tampons. Those who continue to be vaginal carriers of *S. aureus* should be given oral antistaphylococcal antibiotics to prevent recurrent TSS with subsequent menstrual periods. The determination of humoral immunity to TSST-1 might be useful in selected patients with menstrual-related syndromes but would be of limited value in nonmenstrual cases because this toxin is not the usual cause.

In contrast to that of staphylococcal TSS, the recovery phase of streptococcal TSS may be very protracted. In particular, patients whose manifestations include necrotizing fasciitis and/or myositis will often face additional weeks of repeated surgical debridement. Skin grafting, plastic surgery repair, and sometimes the amputation of gangrenous extremities may be required. Months of physical therapy and rehabilitation are often needed to return such patients to full and useful lives. Repeated operations, the risk of secondary infections, and ongoing psychological trauma may haunt these patients for months and sometimes years. Counseling is often necessary.

The specific follow-up intervals after discharge will vary widely according to the real or anticipated short- and long-term problems outlined above. As a general rule, a first outpatient visit 7 to 10 days after discharge is appropriate. This serves as a convenient mechanism to discuss ongoing management, if needed, and to answer any additional questions and concerns.

Recently, new information provided by the only large-scale prospective clinical study of toxic and invasive streptococcal infections has confirmed earlier clinical impressions[45,46] that secondary cases can and do occur in close contacts and family members. During 1992 and 1993, a total of 323 cases of invasive GABS were identified and studied in Ontario, Canada.[47] In this series, 14 percent of cases were nosocomial and 4 percent occurred in nursing home residents, often in association with disease outbreaks. Invasive disease occurred in two household contacts. These represented an estimated risk of 3.2 cases per 1000 household contacts. This risk is approximately the same as the risk associated with exposure to sporadic cases of meningococcal infection. The authors suggest that chemoprophylaxis would appear to be indicated. However, there is no scientifically derived information, at present, on how to apply this knowledge to patient care.

INDICATIONS FOR HOSPITAL ADMISSION AND SPECIALTY CONSULTATION

From the foregoing discussion, it would appear likely that all patients suspected to have either form of TSS should be admitted to the hospital. As is usually the case when "new" illnesses are first described, the most severe and dramatic examples tend to define the diagnostic and therapeutic guidelines; so too has our experience with TSS evolved. Even early in the 1980s, mild forms of staphylococcal TSS were recognized. The introduction of orthostatic dizziness and mild hypotension into the CDC case definition was done to allow the inclusion of otherwise classical cases that were milder and where shock never developed. Some tampon-using women have presented themselves for evaluation because of the development of desquamation of their palms and soles. Additional history has revealed an acute febrile gastroenteritis with high fever, a flushed appearance, and orthostatic dizziness that had occurred 2 weeks earlier, at the time of a menstrual period. These symptoms had improved spontaneously soon after cessation of the menses, removal of a tampon, and/or "incidental" antistaphylococcal antibiotic use.

Initial reports estimated a 10 percent mortality in staphylococcal TSS related to menstruation. Most recent experience reports 2.5 to 3.0 percent mortality in all cases of the staphylococcal type. Streptococcal TSS is more dangerous. Multiple organ failure occurs more often and the estimated mortality rate is 30 percent and much higher in selected groups, such as the elderly.

Examples of milder forms of streptococcal TSS are easily recognized and separated from other GABS infections that are neither invasive nor toxic. It certainly remains reasonable to initiate appropriate antibiotic therapy (e.g., cephalexin 250 mg PO q6h) in outpatients with presumed streptococcal cellulitis or other focally evident skin and soft tissue infections as long as they are otherwise well.

Patients with high fever, chills or rigors, mental confusion or any mental status change, orthostatic symptoms, vomiting, and/or diarrhea should be carefully and rapidly assessed for evidence of staphylococcal and/or streptococcal TSS. The differential diagnosis outlined earlier (Table 49-6) should be reviewed in an emergency department setting.

Specialty consultation will rarely be required in patients with straightforward menstrual-related staphylococcal TSS unless they present late and are already in advanced stages of shock. The obstetrician-gynecologist may be needed to assist in the care of pregnant patients and those with postpartum TSS. General as well as, at times, specialty surgeons may play a major role in identifying and surgically eliminating foci of *S. aureus* infection. In patients with severe shock, respiratory and hemodynamic instability, and/or multiorgan damage, specialists in critical care medicine should be consulted if they are available. Nephrologist consultation will be indicated for those patients with renal failure. Specialists in infectious diseases may be helpful in the evaluation if there is diagnostic confusion and in the management of patients with allergies to antibiotics.

In patients with streptococcal TSS, general and later plastic-reconstructive surgical comanagement is frequently required on an emergent basis. Specialty care in physical medicine and rehabilitation may also be required after the infectious and toxic symptoms have been controlled. Patients with both forms of TSS may suffer with severe psychological sequelae, similar to the posttraumatic stress syndrome. Psychiatric consultation and comanagement will be of benefit in such situations.

References

1. Todd J, Fishaut M, Kapral F, et al: Toxic shock syndrome associated with phage group I staphylococci. *Lancet* 2:116, 1978.
2. Shands KN, Schmidt GP, Dan BB, et al: Toxic shock syndrome in menstruating women. *N Engl J Med* 303:1436, 1980.
3. Reingold AL, Hargrett NT, Dan BB, et al: Non-menstrual toxic shock syndrome: A review of 130 cases. *Ann Intern Med* 96:871, 1982.
4. Garbe PL, Arko RJ, Reingold AL, et al: *Staphylococcus aureus* isolates from patients with non-menstrual toxic shock syndrome. *JAMA* 253:2538, 1985.
5. Jacobson JA, Kasworm E, Daly JA: Risk of developing toxic shock syndrome associated with toxic shock syndrome toxin-1 following nongenital staphylococcal infection. *Rev Infect Dis* 11:S8, 1989.
6. Cone LA, Woodard DR, Schlievert PM, et al: Clinical and bacteriologic observations of a toxic shock-like syndrome due to *streptococcus pyogenes*. *N Engl J Med* 317:146, 1987.
7. Cone LA, Woodard DR, Byrd RG, et al: A recalcitrant erythematous desquamating disorder associated with toxin-producing staphylococci in patients with AIDS. *J Infect Dis* 165:638, 1992.
8. Osterholm MT, Davis JP, Gibson RW, et al: Tri-state toxic shock syndrome study I: Epidemiologic findings. *J Infect Dis* 145:431, 1982.
9. Schlech WF, Shands KN, Reingold AL, et al: Risk factors for the development of toxic shock syndrome: Association with a tampon brand. *JAMA* 248:835, 1982.
10. Todd JK, Wiesenthal AM, Ressman M, et al: Toxic shock syndrome: II. Estimated occurrence in Colorado as influenced by case ascertainment methods. *Am J Epidemiol* 122:857, 1985.
11. Petitti DB, Reingold AL, Chin J: The incidence of toxic shock syndrome in northern California: 1972–1983. *JAMA* 255:368, 1986.
12. Bergdoll MS, Crass BA, Reiser RN, et al: A new staphylococcal exotoxin, enterotoxin F, associated with toxic shock syndrome *Staphylococcus aureus* isolates. *Lancet* 1:1017, 1981.
13. Harvey M, Horwitz RI, Feinstein AR: Diagnostic bias and toxic shock syndrome. *Am J Med* 76:351, 1984.
14. Lee VTP, Chang AH, Chow AW: Detection of staphylococcal enterotoxin B among toxic shock syndrome (TSS) and non-TSS associated *Staphylococcus aureus* isolates. *J Infect Dis* 166:911, 1992.
15. Stevens DL, Tanner MH, Winship J, et al: Severe group A streptococcal infections associated with a toxic shock–like syndrome and scarlet fever toxin A. *N Engl J Med* 321:1, 1989.
16. Schlievert PM, Shands KN, Dah BB, et al: Identification and characterization of an exotoxin from *Staphylococcus aureus* associated with toxic shock syndrome. *J Infect Dis* 143:509, 1981.
17. Marrack P, Kappler J: The staphylococcal enterotoxins and their relatives. *Science* 248:705, 1990.
18. White J, Herman A, Pullen AM, et al: The Vβ-specific superantigen staphylococcal enterotoxin B: Stimulation of mature T cells and clonal deletion in mature mice. *Cell* 56:27, 1989.
19. Schlievert PM: Role of superantigens in human disease. *J Infect Dis* 167:997, 1993.
20. Muller-Alouf H, Alouf JE, Gerlach D, et al: Comparative study of cytokine release by human peripheral blood mononuclear cells stimulated with *Streptococcus pyogenes* superantigenic erythrogenic toxins, heat-killed streptococci, and lipopolysaccharide. *Infect Immun* 62:4915, 1994.
21. Bone RC: Sepsis, sepsis syndrome and the systemic inflammatory response syndrome (SIRS)—Gulliver in Laputa. *JAMA* 273:155, 1992.
22. Casey LC, Balk RA, Bone RC: Plasma cytokine and endotoxin levels correlate with survival in patients with the sepsis syndrome. *Ann Intern Med* 119:771, 1993.
23. Chesney PJ: Clinical aspects and spectrum of illness of toxic shock syndrome: Overview. *Rev Infect Dis* 11:S1, 1989.
24. Whitfield JW, Valenti WM, Magnussen R: Toxic shock syndrome in the puerperium. *JAMA* 246:1806, 1981.
25. Lauter CB, Tom WB: Spiking fever and rash in a postpartum patient (postpartum toxic shock). *Hosp Pract* 17:163, 1982.
26. McGregor JA, Soper DE, Lovell G, Todd JK: Maternal deaths associated with *Clostridium sordelli* infection. *Am J Obstet Gynecol* 161:987, 1989.
27. Silver RM, Heddleston LN, McGregor JA, et al: Life-threatening puerperal infection due to group A streptococci. *Obstet Gynecol* 79:894, 1992.
28. Nathan L, Peters MT, Ahmed AM, et al: The return of life-threatening puerperal sepsis caused by group A streptococci. *Obstet Gynecol* 169:571, 1993.
29. Chow AW, Whittmann BK, Bartlett KH, et al: Variant postpartum toxic shock syndrome with probable intrapartum transmission to the neonate. *Am J Obstet Gynecol* 148:1074, 1984.
30. Mahieu CM, Holm SE Goossens HJ, et al: Congenital streptococcal toxic shock syndrome with absence of antibodies against streptococcal pyrogenic exotoxins. *J Pediatr* 127:987, 1995.
31. Wolf JE, Rabinowitz LG: Streptococcal toxic shock–like syndrome. *Arch Dermatol* 131:73, 1995.
32. The Working Group on Severe Streptococcal Infec-

tions: Defining the group A streptococcal toxic shock syndrome. *JAMA* 269:390, 1993.

33. Hoge CS, Schwartz B, Talkington DF, et al: The changing epidemiology of invasive group A streptococcal infections and the emergence of the streptococcal toxic shock–like syndrome. *JAMA* 269:384, 1993.

34. Sapico FL: Commentary: Necrotizing soft tissue infections. *Infect Dis Clin Pract* 2:330, 1993.

35. Chesney RW, McCarron DM, Haddad JG, et al: Pathogenic mechanisms of the hypocalcemia of staphylococcal toxic shock syndrome. *J Lab Clin Med* 101:576, 1983.

36. Winokur R, Ospina L, Lauter CB: Hypocalcemia in toxic shock syndrome. *Rev Infect Dis II* (Suppl) 5:329, 1989.

37. Kaldijian L, Andriole VT: Necrotizing fasciitis: Use of computed tomography for noninvasive diagnosis. *Infect Dis Clin Pract* 2:325, 1993.

38. Dondorp AM, Veenstra J, vanderPoll T, et al: Activation of the cytokine network in a patient with AIDS and the recalcitrant erythematous desquamating disorder. *Clin Infect Dis* 18:942, 1994.

39. Dickgiesser N, Wallach U: Toxic shock syndrome toxin-1 (TSST-1): Influence of its production by subinhibitory antibiotic concentrations. *Infect Immunol* 15: 351, 1996.

40. Stevens DL, Sizhuang Y, Bryant AE: Penicillin-binding protein expression at different growth stages determines penicillin efficacy in vitro and in vivo: An explanation for the inoculum effect. *J Infect Dis* 167:1401, 1993.

41. Peterson PK, Schlievert PM, Conroy W, et al: Protection against staphylococcal pyrogenic exotoxin type C—enhanced endotoxin lethality with methylprednisolone and IgG. *J Infect Dis* 147:358, 1983.

42. Todd JK, Ressman M, Caston SA, et al: Corticosteroid therapy for patients with toxic shock syndrome. *JAMA* 252:3399,1984.

43. Barry W, Hudgins L, Donta ST, et al: Intravenous immunoglobulin therapy for toxic shock syndrome. *JAMA* 267:3315, 1992.

44. Lamothe F, D'Amico P, Ghosn P, et al: Clinical usefulness of intravenous immunoglobulins in invasive group A streptococcal infections: Case report and review. *Clin Infect Dis* 21:1469, 1995.

45. Schwartz B, Elliott JA, Butler JD, et al: Clusters of invasive group A streptococcal infections in family, hospital and nursing home settings. *Clin Infect Dis* 15:277, 1992.

46. Valenzuela TD, Hooten TM, Kaplan EL, et al: Transmission of "toxic strep" syndrome from an infected child to a firefighter during CPR. *Ann Emerg Med* 20:90, 1991.

47. Davies HD, McGeer A, Schwartz B, et al: Invasive group A streptococcal infections in Ontario, Canada. *N Engl J Med* 335:547, 1996.

PART V

EMERGENCY GYNECOLOGIC DISORDERS IN OLDER WOMEN

Chapter 50

MENOPAUSE

Mark D. Pearlman

EPIDEMIOLOGY OF AGING

The current world population is 5 billion, with a projected doubling in size over the next 30 years. In the United States, the older population has been growing at a rate faster than the younger population since 1960, and it is estimated that 20 percent of the population will be over the age of 60 by the year 2050. The U.S. Census Bureau estimates that between 1990 and 2050, the number of women over the age of 55 will increase from 28.7 to 45.9 million. By the year 2000, there will be an estimated 700 million women over the age of 45 in the world. In the western world, the average woman lives until about age 80, as compared with men, who live, on average, to age 73. If a woman reaches the menopause, actuarial analysis suggests that she will live another 33 years; that is, about 40 percent of her life will occur after the menopause. Within the older population, the average age is increasing. As an illustration, comparing the growth in different older age groups from 1900 to 1984, there has been a 7-fold increase of individuals between the ages of 65 to 74, an 11-fold increase in the 75-to-84 year old group, and a 21-fold increase in individuals over the age of 85.

DEFINITION AND PHYSIOLOGY OF MENOPAUSE

Menopause is defined as the period during which the menses cease permanently; this cessation is usually certain after 12 months of amenorrhea. The climacteric is a broader concept, depicting the endocrine, somatic and psychic changes when a regularly menstruating woman undergoes transition to menopause. Perimenopause is that period when menstrual irregularity begins, preceding the onset of menopause; it lasts about 4 years. In the United States, the average age for the menopause is 51.

Menopause is ultimately the result of a depletion in oocytes and the hormone-producing cells that surround them. It can be a result of surgery (surgical menopause), chemotherapy or other agents toxic to the oocyte, or a natural attrition of oocytes from ovulation (natural menopause). In natural menopause, the cessation of ovarian hormone production is gradual and alterations in gonadal function can occur for a decade prior to the stopping of menstruation. The premenopausal ovary produces more than ten hormones that are important in the process of normal menstruation. Estrogen and progesterone are the two most prominent of these. Their cyclic secretion during the normal menstrual period are illustrated in Fig. 50-1. With the gradual decline in the number of ovarian follicles in the ovary during the perimenopause, the production of estrogen and progesterone decrease. A decrease in the production of glycoprotein *inhibin*, produced by the ovary, results in the loss of negative feedback on the pituitary gland's production of follicular stimulating hormone (FSH); as a result, there is a rise in FSH. An elevated serum FSH (>30 IU/L), along with a decreased estradiol (≤20 pg/mL) is clinical evidence of ovarian failure, and these tests are often used to confirm the onset of menopause. Eventually, there is a 10- to 20-fold increase in FSH (> 100 IU/L), reaching a maximum value 2 to 3 years after the onset of menopause. Luteinizing hormone will reach a level three times normal, but more slowly, lagging behind FSH. After menopause, the follicular cells of the ovary no longer produce any appreciable amount of estradiol, but the surrounding stroma continues to produce androgen, mostly androstenedione. Much of the estrogen circulating in the postmenopausal woman is in the form of estrone, a result of peripheral conversion of androstenedione, produced in the ovaries. Circulating estradiol levels after

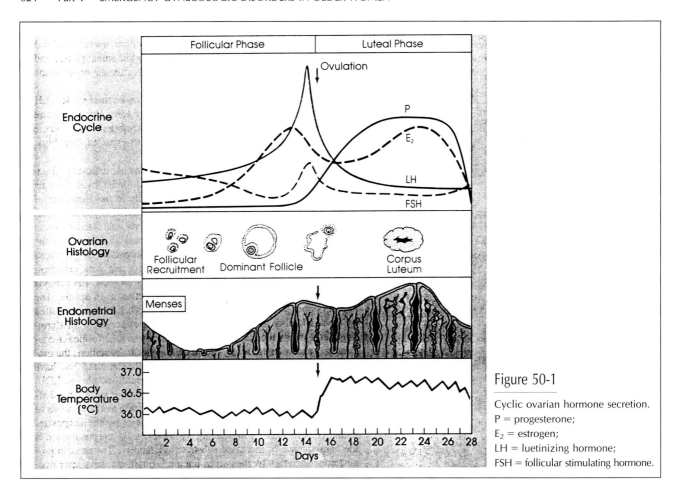

Figure 50-1

Cyclic ovarian hormone secretion.
P = progesterone;
E$_2$ = estrogen;
LH = luetinizing hormone;
FSH = follicular stimulating hormone.

menopause are in the range of 10 to 20 pg/mL; most of it resulting from peripheral conversion of estrone to estradiol. Peripheral conversion typically occurs in adipose tissue; therefore women with excess adipose are more likely to have higher levels of unopposed circulating estrogen, placing them at higher risk for the development of endometrial carcinoma. Therefore, problems in women during the menopause result from either estrogen deprivation, estrogen excess (obese women), or complications of attempts to replace estrogen/progesterone (hormone replacement therapy, or HRT). The clinical presentation of these problems and their management follow. In the woman of reproductive age, the cyclic production of estrogen by the ovaries, followed by progesterone, and the subsequent cessation of progesterone production results in the normal, periodic withdrawal of menstrual bleeding. This sequence can vary if, as is commonly the case, ovulation does not occur.

ABNORMAL BLEEDING IN THE OLDER WOMAN

For most women, there is a period of abnormal, irregular menstrual bleeding that precedes the cessation of menses by 3 to 4 years and up to a decade in some cases. The bleed-

ing pattern associated with these changes in ovarian function include menstrual intervals of varying length, most typically characterized by a time of "skipping and missing" periods, though other patterns of abnormal bleeding are also seen (see Table 50-1). The different menstrual pattern during this time results from changes in hormone production by the perimenopausal ovary. For example, anovulation becomes more frequent in women in their forties, with lengthening of the menstrual cycles commonly to 5 to 6 weeks. Shortened follicular phases can also occur, with a shorter than expected menstrual interval. The clinician faced with a woman presenting with abnormal bleeding in this age group is still obligated to rule out pregnancy and neoplasia. A careful history and physical examination, menstrual calendar, and judicious use of laboratory testing, ultrasound, and endometrial biopsy or dilatation and curettage will establish the cause of abnormal bleeding in virtually all cases (Table 50-1). Frequently symptoms associated with the menopause (e.g., hot flashes) also occur during this time of perimenopause and can be an important historical clue to determine the cause of abnormal bleeding.

PERI- AND POSTMENOPAUSAL BLEEDING

Dysfunctional uterine bleeding is a common event in women as they approach the menopause. Understandably,

Table 50-1

TESTS FREQUENTLY USED TO DETERMINE THE CAUSE OF ABNORMAL BLEEDING IN THE PERIMENOPAUSAL WOMAN

Test	Cause of Bleeding					
	Perimenopause	Neoplasia	Fibroid	Adenomyosis	Polyp	Pregnancy Related
History						
Associated hot flashes	Yes	No	No	No	No	No
Increased cramping	No	Sometimes	Sometimes	Yes	No	Sometimes
Bleeding pattern						
Skips and misses	Yes	Possible	No	No	No	—
Amenorrhea	Yes	No	No	No	No	Yes
Regular but shorter interval	Yes	No	No	No	No	No
Regular but heavy	No	No	Yes	Yes	Yes	No
Irregular	Yes	Possible	No	No	Yes	Yes
Physical exam						
Enlarged uterus	No	Sometimes	Yes	Yes	No	Yes
Enlarged and tender uterus	No	No	No	Yes	No	Possible
Ultrasound						
Enlarged uterus	No	No	Yes	Yes	No	Yes
Enlarged uterus with intrauterine mass	No	Yes	Sometimes	No	Yes	Yes
Lab Tests						
FSH	Elevated	Normal	Normal	Normal	Normal	Normal
CBC	Usually normal	Normal/low	Normal/low	Normal/low	Normal/low	Normal/low
HCG	Negative	Negative	Negative	Negative	Negative	Positive

Key: FSH = follicular stimulating hormone; CBC = complete blood count; HCG = human chorionic gonadotropin.

concerns of endometrial carcinoma are real, though neoplasms are infrequent among women who present with postmenopausal bleeding (Table 50-2). Among 249 women with benign causes of postmenopausal bleeding, atrophic vaginitis was the most common (52 percent), followed by cervical polyps (26 percent), leiomyoma (10 percent), and endometrial hyperplasia (5 percent). A variety of other causes were found less than 1 percent of the time, including cervical erosion, trichomoniasis, hematuria, trauma, vaginal endometriosis, hemorrhoids, candidal vaginitis, Bartholin gland abscess, vulvar warts, and urethral caruncle.[1]

Extrauterine causes of postmenopausal bleeding include cervical bleeding (cervical polyps, trauma, or neoplasia),

Table 50-2

ENDOMETRIAL CAUSES OF POSTMENOPAUSAL BLEEDING

	Percent
Normal endometrium/atrophic endometrium	80
Endometrial hyperplasia	15
Endometrial polyps	3
Endometrial carcinoma	2

vaginal bleeding (vaginal lacerations due to trauma, or vaginal neoplasia), or vulvar/perineal causes (neoplasia, atrophy, or trauma). Occasionally, nongenital causes of bleeding will present with "vaginal bleeding" (e.g., rectal bleeding due to hemorrhoids or hemorrhagic cystitis).

The initial evaluation of the patient with peri- or postmenopausal bleeding should include a careful history, comprising data on the last menstrual period, the recent pattern of bleeding, history of abnormal Pap smears, timing of most recent Pap smear, recent operative procedures, blood dyscrasias, and medication use (especially hormone replacement therapy). Patients who are on hormone replacement therapy frequently have abnormal patterns of bleeding, particularly if their regimen was initiated within the preceding few months. Physical examination should include careful inspection of the rectum, perineum, vulva, urethra, vagina, and cervix. If all of these areas appear normal, it is reasonable to assume that the bleeding is uterine in origin. Evaluation of all postmenopausal bleeding of uterine origin should include sampling of the endometrium. The use of a disposable endometrial biopsy instrument is well tolerated; the results are accurate and the procedure can be readily performed in the outpatient setting. Dilatation and curettage should be reserved for those women who either do not tolerate the endometrial biopsy or those in whom it cannot be successfully completed due to cervical stenosis.

The necessity for endometrial biopsy is rarely an emergency and the procedure can be reasonably deferred to the office setting. The procedure is typically performed with minimal or no cervical dilatation. After placement of an appropriate-sized speculum, the cervix is cleaned with an antiseptic solution and the catheter passed through the endocervix into the endometrial cavity. Often, a single toothed tenaculum is placed at the 12 o'clock position in order to pass the plastic cannula successfully. The endometrial cavity is thoroughly curetted by withdrawing the plunger and rotating the instrument while curetting the endometrial cavity with a back and forth motion. The instrument is then withdrawn and the contents are placed in formalin for processing and pathologic diagnosis. If necessary, two or three passes can be made to empty the endometrial cavity. The procedure is usually well tolerated, with minimal cramping. Occasionally, a prostaglandin inhibitor can be prescribed to control any cramping that may occur. If a tenaculum is used and there is bleeding at the tenaculum site, application of silver nitrate is typically all that is necessary to control it.

Extremely heavy vaginal bleeding is rarely encountered in the postmenopausal woman; when seen, it is usually due to erosive cervical neoplasia. Heavy perimenopausal uterine bleeding is, however, occasionally encountered, and gynecologic consultation is then indicated. The use of intravenous conjugated estrogen, 25 mg every 3 hours, has been shown to be successful in slowing or stopping heavy uterine bleeding in the woman of reproductive age, but it has not been evaluated in the treatment of heavy post-

menopausal bleeding.[2] Usually, dilation and curettage with or without hysteroscopy is necessary. Interventional radiology with catheterization of the internal iliac vessels and thrombosis is also successful in this setting and is discussed in Chap. 55.

Management of the patient with postmenopausal bleeding is clearly dependent on diagnosis. In the woman with perimenopausal bleeding who is without organic disease, the use of medroxyprogesterone acetate, 10 mg for 10 days each month, is appropriate if proliferative or hyperplastic endometrium (without atypia) is present. Withdrawal bleeds should be expected after the 10-day therapy. Alternatively, if contraception is required in the perimenopausal woman, the use of low-dose oral contraceptives in the nonsmoker without other contraindications to oral contraceptive use is both appropriate and safe.

SYMPTOMS OF THE MENOPAUSE

Decreasing circulating estrogen levels are the cause of the characteristic hot flash or flush of menopause. Presumably, changes in estrogen levels result in alterations in thermoregulation by the hypothalamus. Sudden changes in estrogen levels (e.g., surgical menopause) result in more severe and sustained hot flashes. Fifty percent of women experience hot flashes with the onset of menopause. However, 30 percent will experience hot flashes during the perimenopausal period. The incidence of hot flashes decreases over time after the cessation of menses, such that only 20 percent of women report hot flashes 4 years after menopause.[3]

The hot flash is an event that results in an uncomfortable sensation of warmth, often accompanied by a noticeable redness in the face, neck, and upper chest and is sometimes accompanied by profuse perspiration. They occur more frequently at night, during times of stress, and in a warm environment. While the hot flash is the most common complaint during menopause, it has no attendant intrinsic health risk. Hot flashes are very effectively treated by estrogen. Double-blind, placebo-controlled trials demonstrate that most women with hot flashes will successfully have diminution or eradication of these symptoms.[4] Conjugated estrogens, 0.625 mg, estrone sulfate 0.625 mg, estradiol 1 mg orally, and 0.05 mg estradiol transdermally are all effective in treating hot flashes. Higher doses (up to 1.25 mg conjugated estrogen) are occasionally necessary to eradicate hot flashes. In women with a contraindication to estrogen use, oral medroxyprogesterone acetate in a dosage of 20 mg daily is effective.[5] Megestrol acetate 20 mg twice daily is also effective.[6] Other agents have been effective in the treatment of hot flushes, including clonidine, 0.10 mg orally every day or 0.25 mg transdermal patch (which delivers 0.1 mg) placed once a week.

ATROPHIC CHANGES OF THE GENITAL TRACT

Loss of estrogen support of the vagina and vulva can lead to distressing vulvovaginal symptoms. Atrophic changes in the vagina can, in part, result in loss of support of the bladder (cystocele), rectum (rectocele), or cul-de-sac (enterocele). These entities are covered in detail in Chap. 51. Atrophic vaginitis resulting in pruritus, burning, discomfort, dyspareunia, and bleeding may also occur. Estrogen replacement therapy is effective in the treatment of atrophic vaginitis. While therapy can be initiated with topical (i.e., vaginal) estrogen, thickening of the vagina may result in irregular absorption. In the long term, atrophic vaginitis is best managed with oral or transdermal estrogen replacement. In addition, the systemic benefits from estrogen replacement therapy are gained by systemic, not topical administration. The trigone of the bladder and proximal urethra are also estrogen-sensitive tissues, and estrogen deprivation associated with the menopause can cause symptoms of urinary urge incontinence, dysuria, nocturia, and urinary frequency. Urinary tract infection should be ruled out prior to attributing urinary problems to estrogen deficiency. Urinary symptoms due to hypoestrogenism are frequently treated successfully with oral or transdermal estrogen therapy in the same doses used for the treatment of hot flashes.

OTHER SYMPTOMS

Cognitive function can be improved with estrogen replacement therapy. Improved performance on memory tests has been reported by different investigators.[7,8] Senile dementia (Alzheimer disease) was recently reported to be less prevalent in women who received estrogen replacement therapy compared with a similar population who did not receive estrogen. Also, cognitive function is improved in women with Alzheimer disease who receive estrogen compared with those who do not receive estrogen.[9]

Headaches are common in pre- and postmenopausal women, and most migraine headaches improve or disappear at the time of menopause. Tension headaches are typically unchanged.[10]

Anxiety, irritability, depression, and fatigue are frequently said to increase following the menopause. However, numerous investigators have suggested that women who develop psychiatric symptoms at the time of menopause are not directly estrogen-related, and the causal relationship of many of these symptoms to low estrogen levels is uncertain. Certain investigators have suggested, however, that replacement with estrogen can improve sleep patterns by decreasing hot flashes and may result in an improvement in mood and a decrease in emotional liability.[4] One study has suggested that estrogen replacement therapy may reduce the prevalence of depression by modifying beta-endorphin and beta-lipotrophin levels.[11]

LONG-TERM SEQUELAE OF THE MENOPAUSE

OSTEOPOROSIS

Bone fractures are common reasons for presentation to the emergency department by older women. By age 60, one-quarter of white and Asian women who are not on estrogen replacement therapy will have spinal compression fractures. Furthermore, one in five white women will develop hip fracture by age 80 if they are not using estrogen replacement therapy. Each year in the United States, there are one-half million non-hip fractures (100,000 distal radius fractures, the rest being mostly thoracic vertebral fractures) and 300,000 hip fractures. Nearly one in six women who develop a hip fracture after the age of 80 will die within 6 months; as a result, femoral neck fractures are the 12th leading cause of death among women. Direct and indirect costs of complications of osteoporosis exceed $6 billion annually.

Estrogen is vitally important in maintaining the calcification of bone, particularly trabecular bone. Cortical bone loss is not as pronounced; therefore, fractures of the vertebral spine and distal radius occur at a younger age than do femoral fractures. There are a variety of risk factors for the development of postmenopausal osteporosis, including cigarette smoking, diabetes mellitus, hyperthyroidism, Cushing's disease, family history of osteoporosis, and low body weight.

After menopause, urinary excretion of calcium increases and there is less inhibition of parathyroid hormone on bone resorption which leads to increased bone loss. This appears to be directly linked to the decline in estrogen levels. The use of estrogen can clearly maintain the mineral content of the bone (Fig. 50-2). From an outcome standpoint, vertebral and hip fractures are decreased among women using estrogen as compared with women not using this hormone.[12] Furthermore, estrogen replacement therapy results in reduced long-term mortality among women using estrogen.[13] While dietary calcium supplementation alone does not prevent postmenopausal bone loss completely, inadequate calcium supplementation will result in bone loss. Twelve hundred to 1500 mg of calcium daily appears to be sufficient to prevent osteoporosis in postmenopausal women using estrogen. The use of exercise in the premenopausal years can increase bone density but has not been demonstrated to decrease postmenopausal bone fractures. However, when a moderate exercise program is combined with estrogen replacement therapy, bone loss in the forearm is decreased.[14] As exercise has been demonstrated to be beneficial to overall health, postmenopausal women should be encourage to exercise.

In terms of therapy, the minimum dose demonstrated to be effective in preventing postmenopausal bone loss is conjugated estrogen 0.625 mg. This is comparable to 0.5 mg micronized estradiol, 0.625 mg esterone sulfate, or trans-

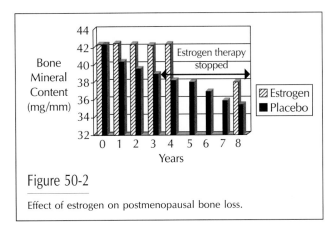

Figure 50-2

Effect of estrogen on postmenopausal bone loss.

dermal administration of 0.05 mg of estradiol. In women who have contraindications to estrogen use, who have osteoporosis, or who desire preventative maintenance, the bisphosphonate alendronate can suppress resorption of bone. The recommended dose is 5 mg for prophylaxis, and 10 mg as treatment for osteoporosis; and it is indicated both for treatment of osteoporosis or prevention of osteoporosis in women who have contraindications to estrogen use or desire not to use hormones. Recognize that alendronate and the other bisphosphonates do not provide any cardiovascular protection, will not reduce hot flashes, or offer any of the other benefits of estrogen.

CARDIOVASCULAR DISEASE AND STROKE

Women who use estrogen or estrogen and progestin therapy postmenopausally reduce their likelihood of myocardial infarction approximately 50 percent.[15] This reduction has been demonstrated to significantly lower cardiovascular mortality compared to nonusers. The relative risk of death from cardiovascular disease is 0.34 (95 percent confidence interval, 0.12 to 0.81); interestingly, both smokers and women with existing cardiovascular disease demonstrate a reduction in mortality.[16] One of the largest studies of estrogen and cardiovascular disease to date involves a cohort of nearly 60,000 women. This prospective study of the effect of estrogen on postmenopausal major cardiovascular disease demonstrated a risk of 0.60 in estrogen users as compared with nonusers.[17]

The risk of stroke in postmenopausal estrogen users versus nonusers is significantly reduced, particularly in women over the age of 75. In one study, the incidence of stroke was reduced by 30 percent, whereas morbidity was reduced by 65 percent.[18] However, this experience is not universal. For example, in the Nurses' Health Study, the risk of postmenopausal stroke was not reduced in estrogen users.[17] However, it is noted that most of the women in this study were under the age of 70 and that stroke more commonly occurs in older women. The protective effect of estrogens with regard to cardiovascular disease as well as cerebrovas-

cular disease does not appear to be reduced by the addition of progestins.

ADVERSE EFFECTS OF HORMONE REPLACEMENT THERAPY

Concerns regarding hormone replacement therapy can be divided into three major categories: neoplastic risk (especially breast and endometrial), thrombogenic risk (particularly in women with a history of thrombotic disease), and existing contraindications to estrogen use.

One of the greatest deterrents to the use of estrogen replacement therapy is concern regarding neoplasia, particularly breast cancer. The risk of breast cancer in postmenopausal women using long-term estrogen therapy has been summarized in several metaanalyses. While these summaries of numerous studies show conflicting results, most do demonstrate a small but statistically significant increased risk of breast cancer. For example, Colditz et al. demonstrated that the risk of breast cancer was significantly increased among women who were currently using estrogen alone (relative risk 1.32, with 95 percent confidence intervals of 1.14 to 1.54), or estrogen plus progestin (relative risk 1.41, 95 percent confidence interval 1.15 to 1.74) as compared with postmenopausal women who had never used hormones.[19] In a metaanalysis combining 37 studies, Sillero-Arenas and colleagues demonstrated a small but statistically significant relative risk of 1.06.[20] The risk for breast cancer has not been demonstrated in all studies. For example, a case-controlled study demonstrated no increase risk in long-term users of estrogen replacement therapy for 20 years or more (relative risk, 1.0).[21] Similarly, a case-control study of 3000 women with breast cancer did not demonstrate any change in the risk of breast cancer with estrogen or estrogen and progestin therapy. This lack of risk was seen in short-term, medium duration, and long-term users of hormone replacement therapy.[22]

Numerous studies of risk for endometrial cancer have demonstrated that if progestins are administered to women using estrogen replacement therapy, there is no significant risk of endometrial cancer. However, women on unopposed estrogen replacement therapy (i.e., estrogen use without progestin) demonstrate a relative risk of 2.3 compared with those who have never used estrogen.[23] Of interest, endometrial cancer that does develop in estrogen users is nearly always well differentiated, with good prognosis.[23] The addition of progestins to estrogen has been shown to prevent the increased risk of endometrial hyperplasia associated with estrogen alone. This reduction in endometrial hyperplasia and carcinoma is demonstrated whether progestins are administered continuously (daily) or cyclically (10 to 14 days each month). Women who are on unopposed estrogen and who still have a uterus should either have progestins added or have an evaluation of the endometrium either through endometrial biopsy or sonographic visualization of the endometrium. Women on unopposed estrogen with postmenopausal bleeding should be assumed to have neoplastic disease until proven otherwise. Appropriate sampling of the endometrium or referral is indicated in this latter circumstance.

Neoplastic risk in estrogen replacement users has not been demonstrated in other organ systems. There appears to be no increased risk of colon cancer, ovarian cancer, cervical cancer, or pancreatic cancer in women receiving hormone replacement therapy. Controversy continues regarding administration of estrogens to women who have a history of breast or endometrial cancer. Unfortunately, randomized, controlled trials have not been done to demonstrate whether estrogen or progestin administration can be used in these women. Retrospective and case series have suggested that these hormones can be used in selected women who are without evidence of residual disease after a variable period of observation. The American College of Obstetrics and Gynecology recently made the following statement. "Because estrogen replacement therapy has well documented health benefits including prevention of osteoporosis, some clinicians may consider it for women who appear to be free from disease."[24]

Contraindications to estrogen therapy do exist and include the presence of active breast or endometrial cancer, active thrombophlebitis, undiagnosed abnormal uterine bleeding, active liver disease, and a prior history of thromboembolic disease associated with exogenous estrogen administration. Women who have a history of thromboembolic disease not associated with estrogen use may be at increased risk for recurrent thrombogenic events. However, a clear cause-and-effect relation has not been established, and the use of hormone replacement therapy in these women should be individualized based on individual circumstances (e.g., severe hot flashes, existing osteoporosis, high risk for myocardial infarction.)[1,2]

Hormone replacement therapy is commonly used and is associated with an overall increased life expectancy. However, complications occasionally do occur, rarely requiring discontinuation or modification of use.

References

1. Dewhurst J: Postmenopausal bleeding from benign causes. *Clin Obstet Gynecol* 26:769, 1983

2. DeVoregr, Ownes O, Case N: Use of intravenous premarin in the treatment of dysfunction uterine bleeding. A double blind randomized controlled study. *Obstet Gynecol* 59:285, 1982.

3. McKinley SM, Brambilla DJ, Posner JG: The normal menopause transition. *Maturitas* 14:103, 1992.

4. Coope, Wiklund I, Karlberg J, Mattson LA: Quality of life of postmenopausal women on a regimen of transdermal estradiol therapy: A double blind placebo controlled study. *Am J Obstet Gynecol* 168:824, 1993.

5. Schiff I, Tulchinsky D, Cramer D, Ryan KJ: Oral medroxyprogesterone in the treatment of post-menopausal symptoms. *JAMA* 224:1443, 1982.

6. Loprinzi CL, Michalaklak JC, Quella SK, et al: Megestrol acetate for the prevention of hot flushes. *N Engl J Med* 331:347, 1994.

7. Robinson D, Friedman L, Marcus R, et al: Estrogen replacement therapy and memory in older women. *J Am Geriatr Soc* 42:919, 1994.

8. Kampen DL, Sherwin BB: Estrogen use and verbal memory in healthy postmenopausal women. *Obstet Gynecol* 83:979, 1994.

9. Paganini-Hill A, Henderson VW: Estrogen deficiency and risk of Alzheimer's disease in women. *Am J Epidemiol* 140:256, 1994.

10. Neri I, Granella F, Nappi R, et al: Characteristics of headaches at menopause: A clinico-epidemiologic study. *Maturitas* 17:31, 1993.

11. Genazzani AR, Petraglia F, Facchinetti F, et al: Steroid replacement treatment increases beta endorphin and beta lipotrophin plasma levels in postmenopausal women. *Gynecol Obstet Invest* 294:1261, 1988.

12. Ettinger B, Jenant HK, Cann CE: Long term estrogen replacement therapy prevents bone loss and fractures. *Ann Intern Med* 102:319, 1985.

13. Ettinger B, Friedman GD, Bush T, Quesenberry CP Jr: Reduced mortality associated with long-term postmenopausal estrogen therapy. *Obstet Gynecol* 87:6, 1996.

14. Prince RL, Smith M, Dick IM, et al: Prevention of postmenopausal osteoprosis: A comparative study of exercise, calcium supplementation, and hormone replacement therapy. *N Engl J Med* 325:1189. 1991.

15. Grodstein F, Stampfer MJ: The epidemiology of coronary heart disease in estrogen replacement therapy in postmenopausal women. *Prog Cardiovasc Dis* 38:199, 1995.

16. Bush TL, Barrett-Connor E, Cowan LD, et al: Cardiovascular mortality in non-contraceptive use of estrogens in women, results from the lipid research clinics program follow-up study. *Journal Circ* 75:1102, 1987.

17. Grodstein, Stampfer MJ, Manson JE, et al: Postmenopausal estrogen and progestin use and the risk of cardiovascular disease. *N Engl J Med* 335:453, 1996.

18. Finucane FF, Madans JH, Bush TL, et al: Decreased risk of stroke among postmenopausal hormone users: Results from a national cohort. *Arch Intern Med* 153:73, 1993.

19. Colditz GA, Hankinson SE, Hunter DJ, et al: The use of estrogens and progestins and the risk of breast cancer in postmenopausal women. *N Engl J Med* 332:1589, 1995.

20. Sillero-Areanas M, Delgado-Rodriguez M, Rodigues-Canteras R, et al: Menopausal hormone replacement therapy in breast cancer: A metaanalysis. *Obstet Gynecol* 79:286, 1992.

21. Standford JL, Weiss NS, Voigt LF, et al: Combined estrogen and progestin hormone replacement therapy in relation to the risk of breast cancer in middle age women. *JAMA* 274:137, 1995.

22. Newcomb PA, Longnecker MP, Mittendorf J, et al: Long term hormone replacement therapy and risk of breast cancer in postmenopausal women. *Am J Epidemiol* 142:788, 1995.

23. Grady D, Gebretsadik T, Kerlikowske K, et al: Hormone replacement and the endometrial cancer risk: A metaanalysis. *Obstet Gynecol* 85:304, 1995.

24. American College of Obstetricians and Gynecologists: Committee opinion, no. 135—Estrogen replacement therapy in women with previously treated breast cancer. April 1994.

Chapter 51

GENITAL PROLAPSE

Kris Strohbehn

Genital prolapse is not often an emergency condition, but one that develops over many years. Nonetheless, the patient may identify her chronic condition as an acute event when protrusion is first observed (Fig. 51-1). Because genital prolapse resembles a mass, the patient or her family may mistake a protrusion for cancer. The extreme concern related to prolapse may impel her to the emergency department for evaluation. Additionally, many women who undergo corrective surgery for genital prolapse are at risk for postoperative complications for which they may seek emergent care. Two other conditions, hemorrhoids and rectal prolapse, may also lead to emergent evaluation of a protruding mass near the genital area. All of these conditions are reviewed in this chapter.

The term *genital prolapse* is synonymous with *pelvic organ prolapse* or *pelvic support disorder*. It encompasses a range of anatomic defects that have different symptoms depending upon the location of the defect. Although rarely an emergent condition itself, there are occasional sequelae to genital prolapse that require acute attention (Table 51-1). In addition to these rare emergencies, other complications may arise as a result of therapy for prolapse. These complications can occur after surgery (Table 51-2) and following conservative therapies, such as the use of pessaries (Table 51-3).

The exact prevalence of genital prolapse is unknown. The best information available in the literature regarding prolapse is the data on indications for hysterectomies. In these studies, the incidence of uterovaginal prolapse can be assessed for those patients with prolapse severe enough to require surgery. In the United States, approximately 15 percent of hysterectomies are performed for uterine prolapse.[1] This translates to an incidence of approximately 40 hysterectomies per 100,000 women per year for prolapse. In addition, approximately 176 anterior or posterior repairs are performed annually for cystoceles and rectoceles in the United States per 100,000 total population.[2] While these numbers provide an estimate of the prevalence of genital prolapse, there are many women who are likely to be less forthcoming about problems of prolapse or who decline surgical repair. Thus, the true incidence of prolapse is probably much higher than what we can abstract from surgical data.

PATHOPHYSIOLOGY

GENITAL PROLAPSE

Anatomically, the urogenital hiatus of a woman's pelvis is an opening in the pelvic floor. The urethra, vagina, and rectum traverse this space, allowing outlet for the uterus, birth canal, urine, and stool, and an inlet for coital function. Normally, the coordinated effects of the pudendal and pelvic nerves, levator ani muscle, and connective tissue maintain support of the visceral structures of the pelvis. These support mechanisms usually function well despite maximal stresses during childbirth, which may cause extreme stretching or breakage of these structures as the fetal head passes through the urogenital hiatus via the vagina. Recent observations with detailed scientific study using electromyography and nerve conduction studies confirm that pudendal nerve damage occurs in a significant percentage of women undergoing vaginal delivery.[3,4] An important concept regarding the damage occurring at childbirth is that multiple acute events occur during labor that lead to chronic denervation and secondary muscle atrophy. The ultimate result is breakdown of the last supportive structure, the connective tissue (Fig. 51-2).

Besides previous vaginal birth, other factors associated with an increased risk for genital prolapse include increasing parity, obesity, a history of hard physical labor, inherent connective tissue disorders,[5] and a history of a previous urinary incontinence procedure to suspend the bladder.[6] Other factors that have been hypothesized to predispose to devel-

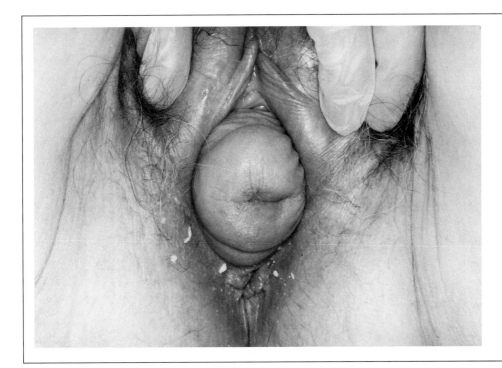

Figure 51-1

Uterine prolapse. The cervix is prolapsing through the vaginal introitus. (Photograph, copyright John O.L. Delancey, M.D., University of Michigan.)

oping prolapse include chronic constipation and conditions that lead to increased intraabdominal pressures, such as chronic bronchitis.

HEMORRHOIDS

Hemorrhoids are extremely common, with more than 1 million Americans being affected yearly.[7] It has been estimated that 35 to 50 percent of the population will be afflicted with hemorrhoids at some time in their lives. Hemorrhoids cause anorectal symptoms, including painless rectal bleeding, pain, anal discharge, and pruritus. Hemorrhoids can also become engorged or may prolapse through the anus, causing a mass to be identified at the anal canal. One recent study[8] has

pointed to obesity and chronic diarrhea as risk factors for developing hemorrhoids. The idea that constipation is a primary cause of hemorrhoids is probably a misconception. Nonetheless, constipation can aggravate the symptoms of hemorrhoids once they are present. Hemorrhoids also occur frequently among pregnant and postpartum women, especially those undergoing vaginal delivery.

Previous theories suggested that both internal and external hemorrhoids were varicosities resulting from deficient venous tone. Instead, current concepts suggest that hemorrhoids result from prolapse of normal vascular cushions of the anus. The three submucosal vascular cushions are located at the right posterior, right anterior, and left lateral positions (Fig. 51-3B) of the anorectum. These cushions are composed of a plexus of superior (internal) hemorrhoidal veins and venules, connective tissue, and smooth muscle. The cushions are located above the dentate (anorectal) line,

Table 51-1

EMERGENT CONDITIONS CAUSED BY GENITAL PROLAPSE

Incarceration of prolapsed organ
Acute urinary retention
Renal insufficiency due to bladder outlet obstruction (rare)
Erosions of the vaginal wall causing profuse vaginal bleeding
Rectovaginal or vesicovaginal fistula caused by deep erosions
  or retained pessary

Table 51-2

ACUTE POSTOPERATIVE COMPLICATIONS

Urinary retention
Urinary tract infections
Bleeding from the repair site
Pelvic or vaginal cuff cellulitis or abscess
Constipation or fecal impaction
Evisceration of bowel through posthysterectomy vaginal cuff

Table 51-3

COMPLICATIONS FROM A PESSARY

Bleeding from chronic irritation and resultant erosions
Acute urinary retention (especially in the first 24 h following insertion)
New-onset urinary incontinence
Erosion of pessary into bladder or rectum
Purulent discharge and severe vaginitis from chronic retained pessary
Allergic reaction to pessary

where they prevent trauma to the mucosa at the anal sphincter. The dentate line is the junction of columnar epithelium of endodermal origin and the squamous epithelium of ectodermal origin (Fig. 51-3A). Along with the coordinated effects of the puborectalis muscle and the internal and external anal sphincter muscles, the vascular cushions help maintain fecal continence.

Internal hemorrhoids always originate above the dentate line. As described above, these hemorrhoids, rather than being caused by a dilation of venules, are due to the prolapse of one or more of the cushions beyond the dentate line due to the gradual breakdown of the connective tissue supports. The prolapse of the cushions may then result in dilation, engorgement, and bleeding of the venules of the superior hemorrhoidal plexus. Because the superior hemorrhoidal veins drain into the portal venous system via the superior rectal and inferior mesenteric veins, portal hypertension was previously regarded as a risk factor for hemorrhoids. Despite this anatomic association, portal hypertension has not been proved to be such a risk factor. During pregnancy, the increased venous pressure from obstruction by the enlarged uterus has been implicated in increased hemorrhoids. Instead, it is more likely that connective tissues in the vascular cushions are weakened and break down during pregnancy.

External hemorrhoids always occur distal to the dentate line. The inferior (external) hemorrhoidal veins are located distal to the dentate line and anastomose with the superior hemorrhoidal veins. The inferior hemorrhoidal veins drain into the pudendal and iliac veins. External hemorrhoids are usually caused by extravasation and subepithelial hemorrhage from the inferior hemorrhoidal veins and resultant hematoma formation. Occasionally, a true thrombus can form within the inferior hemorrhoidal veins.

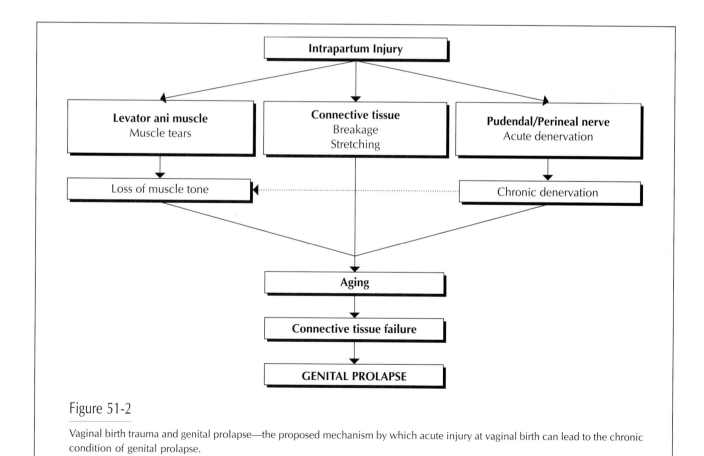

Figure 51-2

Vaginal birth trauma and genital prolapse—the proposed mechanism by which acute injury at vaginal birth can lead to the chronic condition of genital prolapse.

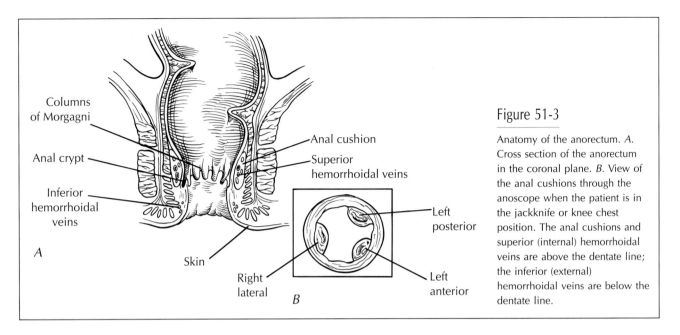

Figure 51-3

Anatomy of the anorectum. *A.* Cross section of the anorectum in the coronal plane. *B.* View of the anal cushions through the anoscope when the patient is in the jackknife or knee chest position. The anal cushions and superior (internal) hemorrhoidal veins are above the dentate line; the inferior (external) hemorrhoidal veins are below the dentate line.

RECTAL PROLAPSE

Rectal prolapse, also called *rectal procidentia,* is a relatively rare disorder caused by a defect in the support of the rectum and sigmoid colon. It is more common among young children and women than among men. Although rectal prolapse is sometimes found concomitant with genital prolapse, it is thought to have a different pathophysiology. Rectal prolapse may be the result of abnormal bowel habits and chronic straining with defecation, which lead to loss of the posterior rectosigmoid attachments. Rectal prolapse may be divided into three categories: (1) prolapse of rectal mucosa only, also called *partial rectal prolapse;* (2) prolapse of all layers of the rectum; and (3) intussusception of the upper rectum into and through the lower rectum, such that it protrudes through the anus. Partial prolapse is quite common in children, usually those less than 2 years old, because of loose attachments of the rectal mucosa to the submucosa, laxity of the anal sphincter, and straining with bowel movements. The latter two types of rectal prolapse are more common among the elderly, especially women, and may result in protrusion of as much as 10 to 15 cm of rectum beyond the anus.

DIAGNOSIS AND DIFFERENTIAL DIAGNOSIS

GENITAL PROLAPSE

Patients with genital prolapse often find their symptoms embarrassing and difficult to discuss. The patient may not associate symptoms of urinary or fecal incontinence or difficulty with sexual intercourse with the symptoms of protrusion through the vagina. It is important to ask open-ended questions about these specific problems, as they will rarely be spontaneously volunteered by an embarrassed patient (e.g., "Have you been having any bladder or bowel problems?").

SYMPTOMS AND DIFFERENTIAL DIAGNOSIS

Symptoms associated with genital prolapse are dependent upon the compartment of the vagina that has lost support. Nonetheless, there are some symptoms that can be applied to all types of prolapse. Most patients with genital prolapse report a sensation of pressure in the pelvis or a bulge protruding from the vaginal introitus. The chronicity of the protrusion may be unrecognized and the patient may believe that the prolapse occurred acutely. Since standing increases intraabdominal pressure, most patients report that problems with prolapse are worse in the upright position. With careful questioning, many patients will report difficulty with normal voiding, defecation, and coitus as well as chronic low back pain when standing. Other common symptoms include postmenopausal or intermenstrual bleeding, usually due to mucosal erosions from chronic exposure of the vaginal or cervical mucosa.

The symptoms of genital prolapse depend upon which supports of the vagina and pelvis have been lost (Fig. 51-4). The symptoms of all these types of support include a protrusion through the vagina, especially with standing, or other causes of increased intraabdominal pressure. Accompanying symptoms can be divided into those associated with loss of support at the apex of the vagina and cervix, the anterior wall, and the posterior vaginal wall. Quite frequently, the patient has loss of support at more than one location in the vagina and thus may have symptoms associated with more than one location. *Uterine prolapse,* also called *uterine procidentia* or

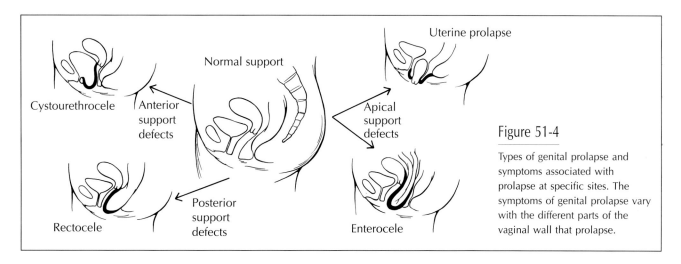

Uterine prolapse

Normal support

Cystourethrocele   Anterior
support
defects

Apical
support
defects

Figure 51-4

Types of genital prolapse and symptoms associated with prolapse at specific sites. The symptoms of genital prolapse vary with the different parts of the vaginal wall that prolapse.

Rectocele

Posterior
support
defects

Enterocele

uterovaginal prolapse, is defined as loss of support at the vaginal apex and cervix. An *enterocele* is a herniation of bowel into the rectovaginal space, which frequently accompanies loss of support at the vaginal apex. If the patient has previously undergone a hysterectomy, loss of support at the vaginal apex is termed *vaginal vault eversion,* which is almost always accompanied by an enterocele. A *cystocele* describes defects of the anterior vaginal wall, because the bladder accompanies the prolapsed anterior vaginal wall. The term *cystourethrocele* implies descent of both the urethra and bladder neck due to loss of anterior support. A cystocele produces symptoms of difficulty with voiding and recurrent urinary tract infections. A cystourethrocele will commonly result in urinary incontinence. A *rectocele* occurs when the rectum protrudes into the posterior vaginal wall and produces symptoms of difficulty with defecation. A rectocele is quite different from *rectal prolapse,* in which the rectal mucosa or the entire rectal wall everts through the anal canal due to intussusception of the rectum. Finally, a *separated perineal body* (not shown in Fig. 51-4) implies loss of perineal support due to disruption of the central tendon of the perineum. This type of defect can also involve loss of the anterior integrity of the internal and/or external anal sphincter muscle and may be seen acutely following dihiscence of an episiotomy repair.

The differential diagnosis for prolapse of these different sites is discussed below. Table 51-4 lists a summary of the differential diagnoses for genital prolapse based upon the presenting symptoms.

Cystocele and Cystourethrocele

Besides a protrusion from the vagina, other symptoms specific to a cystocele include incomplete emptying of the bladder and recurrent urinary tract infections. Some patients must elevate the bulge digitally in order to void. The cystocele may kink the urethra, resulting in bladder obstruction, urinary retention, and, very rarely, uremia and renal failure. Conversely, if support of the urethra at the bladder neck is lost, the patient will commonly present with symptoms of *stress urinary incontinence* (SUI). Patients with SUI usually report leakage of urine only with activity and not when they are asleep or recumbent. This urine leakage occurs with a cough, laugh, or sneeze, in contrast with *urge incontinence,* which is due to involuntary contraction of the detrusor muscle of the bladder. Patients with urge incontinence usually have leakage unrelated to activity. Urge incontinence may be exacerbated by the sound of water or bladder irritants such as caffeine, alcohol, or tobacco.

Included in the differential diagnosis of a cystocele or urethrocele is a suburethral diverticulum. Suburethral diverticula, or outpouchings of urethral mucosa, arise from the upper two-thirds of the posterior urethral wall. Patients with a urethral diverticulum usually present with recurrent urinary tract infections, leakage of small amounts of urine immediately after voiding, and tenderness along the undersurface of the urethra. Occasionally, an abscess or calculus can develop in a urethral diverticulum. An abscess in this location should *not* be drained in the emergency department without consultation of a urologist or gynecologist specializing in lower urinary tract problems, because a urethrovaginal fistula would likely result.

Uterine Prolapse, Vaginal Vault Eversion, and Enterocele

The most common symptom of descent of the uterus or the apex of the vagina (vaginal vault eversion) is a bulge protruding through the vagina. However, the patient may complain only of low back pain due to the stretching of the cardinal/uterosacral complex and referred pain from the T10-T12 innervation of the uterus via pelvic nerves. Back pain usually occurs with standing and worsens throughout the day. Defects of the vaginal apex and cervix are rarely isolated defects. These defects are usually accompanied by anterior and posterior defects, so bladder and rectal symptoms are common. A rare symptom for the patient with an enterocele is narrow-caliber stools and inability to evacuate

Table 51-4

DIFFERENTIAL DIAGNOSES FOR SPECIFIC SYMPTOMS OF GENITAL PROLAPSE

Symptom or Physical Sign	Differential Diagnosis
Protruding genital mass	Genital prolapse (uterine prolapse, vaginal vault prolapse, cystocele, rectocele, enterocele)
	Evisceration of bowel through vaginal apex (always after hysterectomy)
	Cancer of the cervix, uterus, vagina, bladder, or rectum
	Abscess or cyst (Bartholin gland, inclusion cyst, Wolffian remnant cyst)
	Hematoma
	Rectal prolapse
	Hemorrhoid
Urinary hesitancy, urinary retention, or elevated postvoid residual	Large cystocele with kinking of the urethra
	Urinary tract infection
	Urethral or bladder tumor causing outlet obstruction
	Central or peripheral neuropathy
Bleeding erosions from vagina or cervix	Chronic prolapse with secondary mucosal injury
	Cancer of the vagina, cervix, uterus
	Chancre, chancroid, herpes, or other infectious cause
	Trauma
Urinary incontinence	Cystourethrocele
	Intrinsic sphincter deficiency of the urethra
	Detrusor instability (urge incontinence)
	Fecal impaction
	Vesicovaginal fistula
Difficulty with defecation or incontinence of flatus or stool	Rectocele
	Enterocele
	Internal anal sphincter and/or external anal sphincter deficiency
	Fecal impaction
	Rectovaginal fistula

the rectum. These patients usually strain excessively during defecation, and the harder they strain, the more the enterocele occludes the rectum. The enterocele occludes the rectum because the anterior rectal wall is compressed dorsally by the enterocele against the posterior rectal wall. More commonly, an enterocele protrudes ventrally, causing symptoms of a bulge or protrusion of the posterior vaginal wall into the vaginal lumen.

Incarceration of a prolapse is extremely rare. If present, it would usually involve uterine procidentia with incarceration of the uterus or vaginal vault eversion and enterocele with incarceration of small bowel. These patients may develop symptoms of bowel obstruction, including nausea, vomiting, and abdominal pain.

Rectocele

A rectocele protrudes at the posterior vaginal wall. Like other types of genital prolapse, it presents with symptoms of a pro-

trusion through the vaginal introitus. Other common symptoms include incomplete defecation and the need to splint or manually support the perineum in order to defecate. It is important to define what the patient means by constipation. Many women with a rectocele will complain of constipation, but when asked to explain, they report regular, soft, daily bowel movements. Their difficulty is usually a problem with defecation because they are unable to empty the rectum once it is filled with stool, even if the stool is soft.

Separated Perineal Body

A separated perineal body frequently occurs simultaneously with a rectocele and may therefore present with similar symptoms. Occasionally, a separated external anal sphincter muscle is found with a separated perineal body. Therefore, it is important to ask the patient about any symptoms of incontinence of stool, diarrhea, or flatus. More commonly, the patient complains of a gaping vagina and vaginal laxity noted by the patient or her partner during intercourse, especially in the postpartum period.

PHYSICAL EXAMINATION

In general, the diagnosis of genital prolapse can be made by physical examination. The patient should void before being evaluated. Initial inspection of the vaginal introitus, with the labia slightly separated, should be performed without a speculum. To identify the prolapse, the examination is performed at rest and then with straining or coughing, so that increased intraabdominal pressure forces the prolapse through the introitus. If the patient states that the protrusion exists only in the standing position, it may be useful to reexamine the patient standing. The prolapse can usually be reduced manually with gentle digital pressure applied at the center of the prolapsed structure. Use of a lubricant may ease the reduction. A speculum is then gently introduced to further inspect the vagina and, if present, the cervix. Emptying the bladder with a transurethral catheter may also aid in reducing the prolapse. Before the bladder is drained with a catheter, the patient should be asked to attempt to void so that a postvoid residual (PVR) can be measured (see "Laboratory Tests," below).

To determine the anatomic location of the defect, it is often helpful to examine the patient with a single blade of a speculum that has been separated. The posterior blade of the speculum is inserted and the posterior wall of the vagina is depressed (Fig. 51-5). The anterior vaginal wall and urethra are then inspected for laxity and protrusion of a cystocele while the patient performs a Valsalva maneuver or coughs. If a cystocele is present, one should advance the speculum blade to the vaginal apex. If the protrusion (cystocele) disappears, there is likely to be a problem of apical support, such as a vaginal vault eversion, uterine prolapse, or enterocele rather than solely a loss of anterior vaginal wall support. The single speculum blade is then reinserted and used to elevate the anterior vaginal wall. If there is a protrusion at the posterior vaginal wall, this suggests a rectocele or enterocele. Again, the tip of the speculum blade is advanced to the vaginal apex, and if the protrusion disappears, this suggests an apical support defect as opposed to an isolated posterior vaginal wall defect.

After inspection, a bimanual pelvic examination is performed and should focus on excluding a pelvic mass. If the bladder feels enlarged, it may be useful to empty the bladder with a catheter and repeat the bimanual examination. A rectovaginal examination will often help identify an enterocele produced by small bowel prolapsed into the rectovaginal space. An enterocele is suspected when a soft mass is palpated between the rectal and vaginal fingers, separating the vagina from the rectum during a Valsalva maneuver.

Cancer of the cervix, vagina, uterine corpus, or vulva is in the differential diagnosis for patients with prolapse. Thus, it is important to examine the entire surface of the vagina and cervix if present. The mucosal surfaces of the vagina and cervix should be rugated or smooth and without ulceration or polypoid masses. If either is present, then cancer must be considered and an appropriate referral made for biopsy. Chronic exposure of prolapsed mucosa to air and external pressure commonly causes benign erosions and ulceration (Fig. 51-6). This distorts the normal surface anatomy and can make the diagnosis of prolapse more difficult.

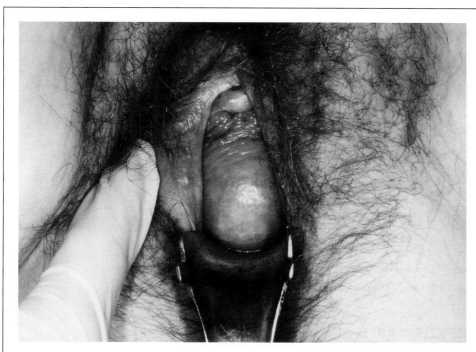

Figure 51-5

Examination of a cystocele. Examination of the anterior vaginal wall can be performed by supporting the posterior vaginal wall with the posterior half of a divided speculum. (Photograph, copyright John O.L. DeLancey, M.D., University of Michigan.)

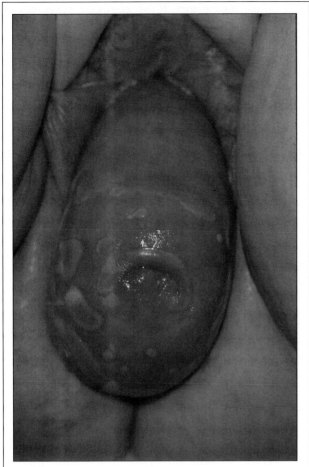

Figure 51-6

Complete uterine procidentia with severe erosions of the vaginal epithelium. Erosions of the vagina or cervix may cause bleeding; an underlying carcinoma should be excluded.

GRADING

A common grading system for genital prolapse is listed in Table 51-5.[9] Each compartment (cystocele, rectocele, vaginal apex or cervix, enterocele) is graded by its leading part in relation to the hymen. This system is quite useful in that the reference landmarks (the hymen or its remnants) for grading the leading part of the prolapse are easy to identify. The major limitation with this grading scheme is its assumption that the examiner knows what part is prolapsed. A new grading scheme has recently been proposed for acceptance by the International Continence Society, the Society of Gynecologic Surgeons, and the American Uro-Gynecologic Society.[10] This scheme is somewhat more complex, as it is based on specific measurements of the vaginal profile, and it is probably less useful for the purpose of evaluating emergency patients with prolapse.

HEMORRHOIDS

SYMPTOMS AND DIFFERENTIAL DIAGNOSIS

Common symptoms of hemorrhoids include anal pruritus, painless rectal bleeding, protruding anal mass, or pain. Rectal bleeding or pain are the symptoms that would be most likely to lead a patient to seek emergent care. Bright red bleeding per rectum usually occurs from internal hemorrhoids and often presents with a complaint of "dripping" into the toilet during or after defecation. Although the bleeding can be brisk, it is usually self-limited. Thus if anemia is present, other sources of bleeding must be considered. Other common symptoms of internal hemorrhoids include prolapse and mucous discharge. Occasionally, prolapsed internal hemorrhoids can become strangulated, causing edema and thrombus in both the superior and inferior hemorrhoidal veins. Strangulated (thrombosed) hemorrhoids can be quite painful.

External hemorrhoids are the more common cause of anal pain, swelling, and difficulty with hygiene. Pain at the anal canal that is not attributable to external hemorrhoids is most likely due to an anal fissure, perirectal abscess, or fistula in ano. Skin tags, the remnants from external hemorrhoids, frequently cause problems with proper hygiene after defecation.

PHYSICAL EXAMINATION

To examine a patient for hemorrhoids, she can be placed in the Sims lateral, knee-chest, dorsal lithotomy, or jackknife position. If any procedures are anticipated and a proctoscopic examination table is available, the jackknife position is most useful. External hemorrhoids are usually palpable and can be visualized by separating the buttocks gently (Fig. 51-7).

Prolapse of the anal cushions and internal hemorrhoids (Fig. 51-8) is best seen by inspection with the patient straining in the squatting position, as if on the toilet. Internal hemorrhoids are not usually palpable, but a digital examination should be performed to exclude other masses of the

Table 51-5		
GRADING OF GENITAL PROLAPSE		
Grade	**Level of Prolapse with Straining**	
1	Halfway to the hymen	
2	To the hymen	
3	Halfway outside the hymen ($\leq$4 cm beyond the hymen)	
4	Complete prolapse (>4 cm beyond hymen)	

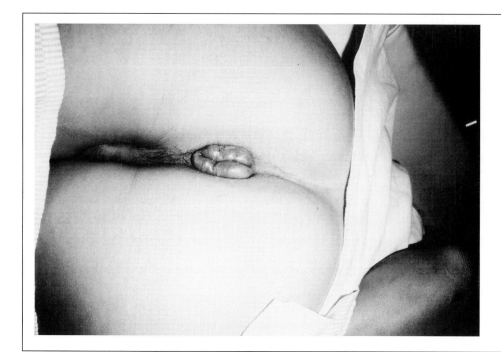

Figure 51-7

External hemorrhoids. Usually tender, they are caused by vessel extravasation and resultant subcutaneous hematoma rather than thrombus within a vessel. (Photograph, courtesy of Richard Burney, M.D., University of Michigan.)

lower rectum or anal canal and to assess the tone of the anal sphincter. An anoscopic examination can be performed to diagnose internal hemorrhoids that have not prolapsed below the dentate line (Table 51-6), or to identify fissures, fistula in ano, or masses of the anorectum. The anoscope is lubricated with examination jelly and the patient asked to bear down slightly on introduction of the anoscope. The anoscope is introduced to its proximal limit, the obturator is removed, and the anoscope is slowly withdrawn with inspection of all sides of the anal canal being performed.

The differential diagnosis for hemorrhoids includes all other potential sources of anorectal bleeding, including tumors of the rectum and sigmoid. Therefore, anyone over 40 years old with rectal bleeding should be referred for a sigmoidoscopy; if over 50 years old, the patient should have an evaluation of the entire colon with a colonoscopy or barium enema. As bowel preparation is often needed, the emergency department is not usually a proper setting to complete this examination. Occasionally, if acute evaluation of rectal bleeding is necessary, rigid sigmoidoscopy can be performed. A spontaneous or induced bowel movement 1 to 2 hours before the examination is ideal.

GRADING

The classification of internal hemorrhoids is presented in Table 51-6.

RECTAL PROLAPSE

SYMPTOMS AND DIFFERENTIAL DIAGNOSIS

Common symptoms of rectal prolapse include an inability to evacuate the rectum completely with defecation, a mucous discharge, and discomfort during defecation. Over 50 percent of patients with significant rectal prolapse have some element of fecal incontinence. The differential diagnosis of rectal prolapse should include prolapsed internal hemorrhoids and rectal intussusception secondary to intraluminal tumors.

PHYSICAL EXAMINATION

When a patient with overt rectal prolapse is being examined, definite rings of the circumferential rectal mucosal folds

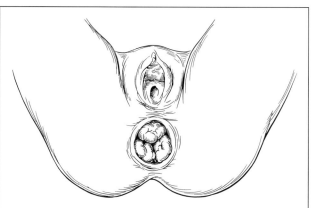

Figure 51-8

Prolapsed internal hemorrhoids. These do not usually cause pain but rather painless vaginal bleeding. Second-degree internal hemorrhoids can often be seen with the patient straining in the squatting position.

Table 51-6

CLASSIFICATION OF INTERNAL HEMORRHOIDS

Degree	Physical Signs/Anatomic Changes	Symptoms
First	Anal cushions pass below dentate line with straining	Painless rectal bleeding
Second	Anal cushions prolapse through the anus with straining but reduce spontaneously	Bleeding, discharge, discomfort
Third	Anal cushions prolapse through the anus but require manual replacement	Bleeding, discharge, perianal pruritis/irritation, discomfort
Fourth	Prolapse stays out at all times	Bleeding, discharge, irritation

should be visible (Fig. 51-9) and a distinct sulcus should be evident between the mucosa of the rectum and that of the anus. Prolapsed internal hemorrhoids are in the differential diagnosis for rectal prolapse, and the two conditions may occur together. If internal hemorrhoids are prolapsed with rectal mucosa only, a distinct sulcus is not seen.[11] The mucosa should be inspected to look for tumors, bleeding sites, or evidence of strangulation with necrotic tissue. If the prolapse cannot be reduced, it is considered incarcerated and requires immediate surgical consultation. As in examining for the detection of third- or fourth-degree internal hemorrhoids (Table 51-6), the most effective way to make the diagnosis of rectal prolapse is to have the patient strain while on the toilet. Rectal tumors are also in the differential diagnosis for rectal prolapse.

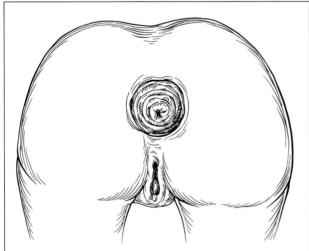

Figure 51-9

Rectal prolapse. This is also seen best in the squatting position with the patient straining; distinct mucosal rings of the rectal mucosa confirm the diagnosis.

LABORATORY TESTS

GENITAL PROLAPSE

Genital prolapse can usually be diagnosed on the basis of physical examination alone and rarely requires any acute laboratory testing. If acute urinary retention is suspected, a postvoid residual should be checked using a catheter. A postvoid residual is usually considered normal if it is less than 60 to 100 mL. If the postvoid residual is greater than 500 mL, a transurethral catheter should be left in place until the patient can be followed by a specialist. If the postvoid residual is 100 to 500 mL, a catheter need not be left in place but a timely referral should be made. Serum electrolytes, creatinine, and blood urea nitrogen levels should be obtained if uremia is suspected. If acute or chronic cystitis is suspected, a urinalysis and culture can be obtained from the catheterized specimen. If severe bleeding has occurred secondary to erosions on the vagina, a hemoglobin level or hematocrit should be checked. If infection is suspected, a white blood cell count is indicated. If small bowel obstruction due to an incarcerated prolapse is suspected, an abdominal flat plate and upright radiograph may be helpful but is unnecessary otherwise.

HEMORRHOIDS

Anemia secondary to bleeding from hemorrhoids is extremely rare. In one recent series of individuals with hemorrhoids, the incidence of anemia with a hemoglobin of less than 11.5 g/dL was 0.5 per 100,000 total population per year.[12] If severe bleeding is present, a hemoglobin level or hematocrit should be obtained. If anemia is found, other sources should be considered, such as rectal or colonic tumors or coagulopathies. Other laboratory evaluation for hemorrhoids is of limited benefit. Radiologic or colonoscopic evaluation to exclude rectal tumors can usually be performed on an outpatient basis.

RECTAL PROLAPSE

Strangulation of the bowel rarely occurs with rectal prolapse. In this circumstance evaluation should include similar diagnostic evaluation to that of bowel obstruction, including abdominal flat plate and upright roentgenograms as well as a complete blood count, serum electrolytes, blood urea nitrogen, and creatinine. Like patients with incarcerated genital prolapse, patients with rectal prolapse are often malnourished and infirm; they generally have multiple medical problems. If immediate surgical correction is required, an assessment of baseline nutrition and cardiopulmonary status may be desired by the surgeon. In the acute setting, other tests would be of limited use in evaluating the patient with rectal prolapse. Prior to surgical treatment of rectal prolapse, a barium enema can help to make sure that no rectal neoplasms or strictures have initiated the prolapse.

TREATMENT

GENITAL PROLAPSE

Problems of genital prolapse rarely cause immediate danger to the patient. After reassurance is provided, the patient can be given an appropriate referral to a gynecologist for further evaluation and treatment. Treatment options for prolapse include conservative treatment with a vaginal pessary or surgical repair. Estrogen cream will often help thicken the mucosa of a postmenopausal patient's atrophic vagina and help to prevent further erosions. This treatment can be helpful as an adjunctive therapy to improve the tissue integrity for pessary use or in preparation for surgery. A typical dose is 2 to 4 g (one-half to one applicator full) once daily. Long-term use (more than 1 month) should be discussed with a gynecologist. If the patient still has a uterus and has an undiagnosed source of vaginal bleeding, estrogen should not be used until the source of the bleeding is determined. Furthermore, long term use of estrogen will require the addition of a progestational agent if the uterus is still present. Surgical resuspension of the vaginal vault succeeds in 85 to 95 percent of cases (with variable time intervals reported for follow-up), whether it is performed vaginally or abdominally. Surgical treatment of urinary incontinence can approach 5-year success rates of 85 percent. Many nonoperative therapies can also significantly improve continence status, such as pelvic muscle (Kegel) exercises, behavioral treatment, and pessaries.

Treatment of specific emergency conditions associated with prolapse is discussed below.

Incarcerated Prolapse

If a genital prolapse cannot be reduced by gentle digital reduction, catheterization of the bladder should be performed, as mentioned above. In attempting to empty the bladder, it is important to remember that the axis of the urethra may be considered altered when the bladder is prolapsed. The axis of the urethra may be perpendicular to rather than parallel with the floor when the patient is in the lithotomy position. It may be necessary to elevate the prolapse gently with several fingers to empty the bladder adequately during catheterization because the dependent portion of a prolapsed bladder may be below the level of the urethra. Care should be taken during elevation and manipulation of the prolapse because edema and strangulation may considerably weaken the tissues and increase the risk of perforation into the bladder, rectum, or intraperitoneal cavity. Occasionally, mild sedation and analgesics will allow reduction of a prolapse that is difficult to replace. If these measures are not successful, immediate consultation with a gynecologist should be obtained. Other factors preventing reduction of the prolapse should be considered in this situation, such as bladder calculi, bladder or rectal tumors, or a pelvic mass.[13] Often, patients with incarcerated prolapse have neglected routine gynecologic care and may be at higher risk for gynecologic cancers. Careful assessment of the cervix and biopsy of ulcerations should be performed to exclude carcinoma.

Strangulation and necrosis of small intestine is rare but has been reported with incarcerated genital prolapse. If intestinal obstruction is suspected by symptoms, then abdominal flat plate and upright roentgenograms may be useful further management. If intestinal obstruction and necrosis are not present, conservative measures may be considered by placing the patient in the Trendelenburg position, with local care to the prolapse. If this is unsuccessful, reduction under sedation or regional or general anesthesia should be attempted. Once the prolapse is successfully reduced, a saline-soaked vaginal pack can be placed to try to reduce the edema, but it should not be left in place for more than 48 to 72 hours without being changed. Once the edema and inflammation from incarceration have been resolved, surgical repair should be considered to prevent recurrence.

Urinary Retention

Using sterile technique, transurethral catheterization should be performed to empty the bladder. If there is a large postvoid residual ($\geq$500 mL), the patient should have an indwelling catheter placed and be referred to a specialist for further evaluation.

Bleeding

Bleeding from erosions of the mucosal surface can usually be stopped by applying pressure; however, this should be done cautiously if the tissues appear friable or necrotic, as it may then worsen the bleeding and result in further damage. Occasionally, applications of silver nitrate or ferric subsulfate (Monsel's) solution is necessary for hemostasis.

HEMORRHOIDS

Internal hemorrhoids, especially of first and second degree (Table 51-6), are often successfully treated with conservative measures. Initial management of internal hemorrhoids should include bulk agents to decrease the trauma caused by hard stools as well as the efforts needed to defecate. This can be accomplished by increasing fiber intake or with supplements such as psyllium seed preparations (e.g., Metamucil) or high-fiber cereals (at least 8 ounces daily). The patient should drink plenty of water with the fiber. Topical medications such as glucocorticoids and antiinflammatory suppositories or creams have had limited success in clinical trials; however, many individuals find relief with them. These therapies are most successful for first- and second-degree internal hemorrhoids, but they may improve the higher-degree hemorrhoids as well. Other treatment options include rubber-band ligation of the prolapsed cushion, laser therapy, cryotherapy, and sclerotherapy.

The most common urgent complaint for external hemorrhoids is pain from thrombosed external hemorrhoids. Surgical excision of the clot and the overlying skin can be performed under local anesthesia (Fig. 51-10). As described below, it is important to excise the entire area of thrombosis and overlying skin rather than simply performing inci-

sion and evacuating clot. Excision is recommended only in the first 72 hours after thrombosis occurs. Thereafter, local care to the area is more effective and the pain will usually resolve without excision.

Strangulated or gangrenous hemorrhoids can occur when there is massive prolapse of the internal hemorrhoids, with resultant edema and thrombosis of both internal and external hemorrhoidal veins. Immediate reduction is indicated in this circumstance. The prolapse can be reduced by massage after injection of hyaluronidase, 0.25% bupivicaine, and 1:200,000 epinephrine. After the prolapse is reduced, the edema resolves and the internal hemorrhoids can be excised or ligated and the external thrombi excised.[14] Surgical consultation would usually be warranted for managing this condition.

Excision of thrombosed external hemorrhoids (Fig. 51-10) can easily be accomplished in the emergency setting. As noted above, this is most successful within the first 72 hours after the onset of pain. Following this time interval, the pain from excision is likely to exceed the pain from the thrombus. The patient is placed in the jackknife position and the thrombosed area prepped with an iodine or other antiseptic solution. Local infiltration with 0.25 to 0.5 percent bupivicaine with 1:200,000 epinephrine is performed using a small-gauge needle (25- or preferably 30-gauge). The skin overlying the thrombus is grasped at its external apex, distal to the anal canal. An elliptical incision is then made around the entire thrombus and the skin and thrombus are excised. The excision line should not cross the dentate line, as this increases the risks of anal stricture formation. The base of excision should include all thrombi,

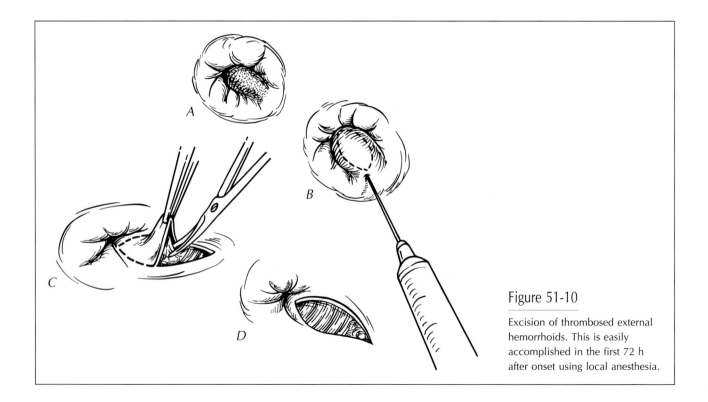

Figure 51-10

Excision of thrombosed external hemorrhoids. This is easily accomplished in the first 72 h after onset using local anesthesia.

but care should be taken to avoid injury to the underlying sphincter muscle. The incision is left open. Electrocautery or ferrous subsulfate (Monsel's) solution can be used for hemostasis. If necessary to control hemostasis, a small packing can be placed, but it should be removed within 24 h to minimize the risk of infection. A gauze pad is used to cover the site lightly. Sitzbaths in warm water should be initiated two to three times daily, beginning on the day following excision. Follow-up examination should be scheduled within 2 weeks.

RECTAL PROLAPSE

In general, therapy for rectal prolapse is nonemergent. Among the pediatric population, rectal prolapse is usually self-limiting, since only the mucosa is prolapsed. Teaching the child to avoid straining during defecation is useful. In the adult population, prolapsed rectal tissue occasionally becomes incarcerated. In this circumstance, immediate surgical consultation is warranted. Nonsurgical methods to reduce the prolapse that have been reported included application of ice packs and local injection of dilute epinephrine and hyaluronidase to reduce the edema. Attempts at reduction under anesthesia may succeed by providing relaxation of the pelvic floor muscles. Recently, a small series of eight cases of transperineal repair of incarcerated prolapse were reported on that were treated with 75 percent success.[15] The transperineal approach avoids abdominal resection with diverting colostomy. This may be particularly desirable in an infirm population that will be more likely to have complications with a laparotomy. If a rectal prolapse is reducible, a timely referral to a general or colorectal surgeon should be established. Rarely, evisceration of the small bowel can occur through the wall of the rectum if strangulation has been prolonged. This too requires emergent surgical consultation and operation.

POSTOPERATIVE COMPLICATIONS

Postoperative complications from surgical repair of these conditions may be more likely to result in an emergent visit than the initial presenting problem, since these problems are often evaluated and managed in the outpatient clinic setting. For this reason, a separate review is offered of the more common surgical complications in the repair of these problems.

Complications following surgery for genital prolapse via transabdominal or transvaginal approaches include urinary retention, acute cystitis, and wound infection or hematoma at the vaginal wall (including vaginal cuff cellulitis), abdominal incision site, or in the retropubic space of Retzius. In addition, a vesicovaginal or ureterovaginal fistula may result in constant leakage. Finally, evisceration of small bowel, tube, or ovary can occasionally occur through the vaginal apex after hysterectomy. Specific evaluation and treatment of these complications are discussed below. Other postoperative complications are covered in Chapter 45.

URINARY RETENTION

Acute urinary retention usually manifests itself as acute lower abdominal pain with inability to void and sometimes constant dribbling. It should be managed with transurethral catheterization. As mentioned above, if a postvoid residual is elevated, (>500 cc), an indwelling catheter should be left in place and the patient instructed to follow up with her surgeon.

ACUTE CYSTITIS

Postoperative management for genital prolapse surgery often requires prolonged catheter use because of postoperative urinary retention after resuspension of the bladder neck or due to pain after posterior colporrhaphy. Bladder overdistention may be prevented with an indwelling suprapubic catheter, a transurethral catheter, or by intermittent self-catheterization. Acute cystitis is a common complication of catheter use. Patients with acute cystitis present with dysuria, hesitancy, urinary frequency, or urgency. The patient will often be on a prophylactic antibiotic once daily. The diagnosis of acute cystitis can be made with urinalysis and culture, preferably obtained from a catheterized specimen. Antibiotic therapy should be initiated in the symptomatic patient if the urinalysis is not contaminated and confirms leukocytes (>5 leukocytes per high power field). Typically, this will consist of trimethoprim/sulfamethoxazole (Bactrim DS) b.i.d. for 3 days, a first-generation cephalosporin (e.g., cephalexin 500 mg b.i.d. for 7 days), or a fluoroquinolone (e.g., norfloxacin 400 mg b.i.d. for 3 days). If the patient is already on antibiotic prophylaxis, the choice of a therapeutic antibiotic should be changed to include coverage of potentially resistant organisms.

WOUND INFECTION, HEMATOMA, OR ABSCESS

Wound hematomas and abscesses frequently require surgical or radiologically guided drainage, and the surgeon who performed the initial procedure should be consulted if possible. If cellulitis is surrounding a wound infection or if the patient is septic, antibiotics with anaerobic, gram-negative and gram-positive coverage should be administered. If the tissues have a dusky appearance, are exquisitely tender, and display ecchymoses, then necrotizing fasciitis should be considered.

NECROTIZING FASCIITIS

Necrotizing fasciitis is an infection usually limited to the tissues above the deep fascia, but it is polymicrobial, with both anaerobic and aerobic bacteria. Broad-spectrum antibiotics (e.g., penicillin, gentamicin, and clindamycin) should be initiated. Because of its rapid spread and high mortality, immediate surgical consultation should be obtained for radical debridement.[15]

RECTOVAGINAL FISTULA

While fistula formation is an uncommon complication of prolapse surgery, the result can be devastating to the patient. A rectovaginal or enterovaginal fistula should be suspected postoperatively if there is a history of stool or gas passage per vagina or a copious foul-smelling discharge with severe vaginal irritation. The diagnosis of a fistula is usually made on physical examination. Examination should include a careful inspection of the entire posterior vaginal wall and apex while supporting the anterior vaginal wall with a separated speculum blade. A digital rectal examination should be performed while inspecting the posterior vaginal wall. A fistula can be confirmed with a radiologic fistulogram, barium enema, or small bowel follow-through, depending upon its location. If a fistula is discovered, the patient should be started on a low-residue diet and appropriate referral made to the primary surgeon, with consideration of consultation with a colorectal surgeon. Zinc oxide or other occlusive agents can be used to protect the skin of the posterior fourchette until surgical repair can be initiated. Sometimes a large balloon (30 to 60 mL) catheter can be successfully retained intravaginally after insufflation to collect the drainage and reduce irritation to the skin until repair can be completed. If this is attempted, the indwelling tip of the catheter should be cut off to drain more of the fistulous fluids.

VESICOVAGINAL OR URETEROVAGINAL FISTULA

A vesicovaginal or uterovaginal fistula should be suspected when copious and continuous watery discharge is present. The apex and anterior vaginal wall should be inspected carefully. To establish the diagnosis of a vesicovaginal fistula, a tampon or cotton balls can be inserted into the vagina and methylene blue instilled into the bladder via a transurethral catheter. If blue dye stains the tampon at the proximal vagina, this confirms a vesicovaginal fistula. In this case, an indwelling transurethral catheter should be placed and the patient referred back to her surgeon or to a urologist or gynecologist trained in the repair of genitourinary fistulas. If this test is negative but a genitourinary fistula is still suspected, a similar test can be performed with a tampon in the vagina and the administration of intravenous indigo carmine dye or 400 mg of oral pyridium. Blue dye staining the tampon after intravenous indigo carmine injection or orange staining after pyridium confirms the diagnosis of a ureterovaginal fistula. A ureterovaginal fistula requires consultation with a urologist for possible retrograde stent placement, immediate reoperation, or temporary renal shunting with nephrostomy tubes.

POSTHYSTERECTOMY EVISCERATION AT THE VAGINAL APEX

The diagnosis of evisceration at the vaginal cuff is usually self evident on examination, with small bowel protruding through the cuff. It is a rare complication but usually presents within 8 weeks after hysterectomy or resuspension of the vaginal vault. Immediate surgical repair is usually indicated. As the bowel can be strangulated in this circumstance, a general surgeon may need to be consulted in addition to the primary gynecologic surgeon.

PROLAPSED FALLOPIAN TUBE OR OVARY

Prolapse of the fallopian tube or ovary through the vaginal cuff can occur uncommonly after vaginal surgery. This complication usually causes symptoms of dyspareunia, postcoital bleeding, or a watery vaginal discharge. If there is bleeding from the vaginal apex from a prolapsed fallopian tube, this can be treated with application of ferrous subsulfate (Monsel's solution) or silver nitrate. Although rare, tumors of the vaginal apex are in the differential diagnosis, and referral for a confirmatory biopsy and treatment should be obtained with the primary gynecologic surgeon within 1 to 2 weeks.

HEMORRHOIDS

In one large series, the most common complications after surgical repair of hemorrhoids included urinary retention (17.1 percent), urinary tract infection (3.3 percent), major secondary bleeding (2.4 percent), and fecal impaction (2.4 percent).[7] Urinary retention should be treated with transurethral catherization. Urinary tract infections should be treated with appropriate antibiotic coverage, as described above. Major delayed bleeding should be evaluated with a rigid sigmoidoscopy examination and possible religation or electrocautery. Prior to religation or electrocautery, injection at the bleeding site with 1% lidocaine with 1:200,000 epinephrine has been found to control the bleeding in most circumstances.[14] Fecal impaction is usually resolved with enema therapy and/or digital disimpaction. External hemorrhoidal thromboses have been described as a complication in 0.5 percent of patients undergoing rubber-band ligation of internal hemorrhoid ligation. Excision of external hemorrhoidal thrombosis should be performed (Fig. 51-10) if identified within 72 hours of the onset of pain. Postoperative thrombosed internal hemorrhoids should not be excised in an emergency department setting. Sepsis, and even death, have been described after rubber-band ligation of hemorrhoids. Hospitalization and prompt broad-spectrum antibiotic coverage should be initiated in patients with persistent postoperative pain and suspected sepsis.[14]

RECTAL PROLAPSE

Postoperative complications of surgical repairs for rectal prolapse include postoperative wound infection, dehiscence of anastomosis of bowel with resultant intraperitoneal viscus leak, stricture with bowel obstruction, or fecal impaction. The management of wound infections and fecal impaction would be similar to that described for genital prolapse and hemorrhoids, above. If an anastomotic leak or bowel obstruction is suspected, immediate surgical consultation is warranted.

DISCHARGE INSTRUCTIONS AND FOLLOW-UP INTERVAL

GENITAL PROLAPSE

Patients with uncomplicated genital prolapse can follow up with a gynecologist within 4 to 6 weeks to confirm the diagnosis and review their treatment options. If urinary retention requiring catheterization is present, the patient should have follow-up within 48 to 72 h. If ulcerations are present because of chronic irritation of the prolapsed mucosa, a more prompt referral should be made so that carcinoma of the cervix or vagina can be excluded. If a prolapse is incarcerated but is successfully reduced, packing the vagina with a saline-soaked vaginal pack should be considered and the patient instructed to follow up with a gynecologist in 48 to 72 h for pack removal and evaluation for surgical repair.

HEMORRHOIDS

First- and second-degree hemorrhoids are more likely to resolve with conservative measures and can often be managed by the patient's primary-care physician. Because carcinoma of the rectum is in the differential diagnosis, referral for sigmoidoscopy should be established especially if the patient is over 40 years of age. If the patient is over 50, she should undergo evaluation of the entire colon with colonoscopy or a barium enema. If external hemorrhoids are excised, the patient should be instructed to follow up within 2 weeks with a physician who is capable of evaluating the excision site as well as performing anoscopy and sigmoidoscopy.

RECTAL PROLAPSE

Since conservative measures will rarely cure rectal prolapse in adults, a timely outpatient referral to a colorectal or general surgeon is appropriate for adult rectal prolapse. The patient should be instructed to begin a high-fiber diet and to take a psyllium seed preparation (1 to 2 teaspoons two to three times daily). The patient should be instructed to return immediately if she has severe pain and/or bleeding or if the prolapse cannot be reduced before she is able to see a surgeon. If an incarcerated prolapse is successfully reduced, follow-up with a surgeon should be established within 48 to 72 h.

INDICATIONS FOR SPECIALTY CONSULTATION AND HOSPITALIZATION

GENITAL PROLAPSE

Rarely does genital prolapse require acute specialty consultation unless the examining physician is uncertain of the diagnosis. The patient should be reassured and referral for outpatient management established. In general, genital prolapse is managed by gynecologists, although some family practitioners, generalists, and nurse practitioners have excellent training in the nonsurgical management of genital prolapse (e.g., using pessaries). In many tertiary care settings and larger communities, there may be a gynecologist who specializes in female urinary incontinence, genital prolapse, and pelvic reconstructive surgery. Many urologists are trained in female urinary incontinence as well, although many are less familiar with the repair of genital prolapse. Specific indications for immediate specialty consultation include incarcerated genital prolapse, or evisceration of small bowel through the vagina. Indications for hospitalization would be the same, in addition to renal failure from outlet obstruction of the bladder. Patients with ulcerations of the vagina or cervix, a vesicovaginal or enterovaginal fistula, or urinary retention should be referred in a timely fashion.

HEMORRHOIDS

Specialty consultation for hemorrhoids is also rarely necessary in the acute setting. Exceptions to this include patients with strangulated, thrombosed internal and external hemorrhoids, major postoperative bleeding, or in the rare situation of a patient with severe anemia and active hemorrhage from their hemorrhoids. Outpatient follow-up should be established with the patient's primary-care provider. If high-grade (third- or fourth-degree) internal hemorrhoids exist, referral to a physician who is highly experienced in the treatment of hemorrhoids should be considered. Inpatient hospitalization may be necessary for postoperative complications of sepsis following rubber-band ligation or other surgical repairs for hemorrhoids or if control of acute hemorrhage is necessary.

RECTAL PROLAPSE

Incarcerated rectal prolapse should be referred to a general or colorectal surgeon, as should complications following repair of rectal prolapse, including a leaking anastomosis, sepsis, or bowel obstruction. If the prolapse is easily reduced, then a timely referral should be made to a surgeon.

References

1. Carlson KJ, Nichols DH Schiff I: Indications for hysterectomy. *N Engl J Med* 328:856, 1993.
2. Graves EJ: National Hospital Discharge Survey: Annual Summary, 1993. National Center for Health Statistics. *Vital Health Stat* 13:45, 1995.
3. Allen RE, Hosker GL, Smith RB, Warrel DW: Pelvic floor damage and childbirth: A neurophysiologic study. *Br J Obstet Gynaecol* 97:770, 1990.
4. Sultan AH, Kamm MA, Hudson CN: Pudendal nerve damage during labour: Prospective study before and after childbirth. *Br J Obstet Gynaecol* 101:22, 1994.
5. Spernol R, Bernashek G, Schaller A: Enstehunsursachen des Descenzus. *Geburtshilfe Frauenheilk* 43:33, 1983.
6. Wiskind AK, Creighton SM, Stanton SL: The incidence of genital prolapse after the Burch colposuspension. *Am J Obstet Gynecol* 167:406, 1992.
7. Bleday R, Pena JP, Rothenberger DA, et al: Symptomatic hemorrhoids: Current incidence and complications of operative therapy. *Dis Colon Rectum* 35:477, 1992.
8. Johanson JF, Sonnenberg A: Constipation is not a risk factor for hemorrhoids: A case-control study of potential etiologic factors. *Am J Gastroenterol* 89:1981, 1994.
9. Baden WF, Walker T: Fundamentals, symptoms, and classification, in Baden WF, Walker T (eds): *Surgical Repair of Vaginal Defects.* Philadelphia: Lippincott, 1992, pp 9–24.
10. Bump RC, Mattiason A; Bo K, et al: The standardization of terminology of female pelvic organ prolapse and pelvic floor dysfunction. *Am J Obstet Gynecol* 175:10, 1996.
11. Nivatvongs S: Anorectal diseases, in Phillips SF, Pemberton JH, Shorter RG (eds): *The Large Intestine: Physiology, Pathophysiology and Disease.* New York: Raven Press, 1991, pp 775–832.
12. Kluiber RM, Wolff BG: Evaluation of anemia caused by hemorrhoidal bleeding. *Dis Colon Rectum* 37:1006, 1994.
13. DeLancey JOL: Uterovaginal prolapse that is difficult or impossible to reduce, in Nichols DH, DeLancey JOL (eds): *Clinical Problems, Injuries and Complications of Gynecologic and Obstetric Surgery,* 3d ed. Baltimore: Williams & Wilkins, 1995, pp 147–151.
14. Salvati EP, Eisenstat TE: Hemorrhoidal disease, in Zuidema GD, Condon RE (eds): *Shackleford's Surgery of the Alimentary Tract,* 4th ed. Philadelphia: Saunders, 1996, pp 330–343.
15. Ramanujam PS, Venkatesh KS: Management of acute incarcerated rectal prolapse. *Dis Colon Rectum* 35:1154, 1992.
16. Mead PB: Postoperative infections, in Thompson JD, Rock JA (eds): *TeLinde's Operative Gynecology,* 7th ed. Philadelphia: Lippincott, 1992, pp 195–208.

Additional Reading

Burstein M: Managing anorectal emergencies. *Can Fam Physician* 39:1782, 1993.

Keighley MRB: Rectal prolapse, in Keighley MRB, Williams NS (eds): *Surgery of the Anus, Rectum and Colon.* Philadelphia: Saunders, 1993, pp 639–674.

Prager E: Common ailments of the anorectal region, in Block GE, Moosa AR (eds): *Operative Colorectal Surgery.* Philadelphia: Saunders, 1994, pp 389–415.

Pfenninger JL, Surrell J: Nonsurgical options for internal hemorrhoids. *Am Fam Physician* 52:821, 1995.

Williams NS: Haemorrhoidal diseases, in Keighley MRB, Williams NS (eds): *Surgery of the Anus, Rectum and Colon.* Philadelphia: Saunders, 1993, pp 295–363.

PART VI

ULTRASONOGRAPHY

Chapter 52

ULTRASONOGRAPHY IN PREGNANCY

Christine H. Comstock

In pregnancy there are two patients—the mother and her fetus. Before the advent of medical ultrasound, the physician could examine only one patient directly, resorting to indirect means of evaluating the second. Ultrasound has revolutionized obstetrics because it allows us to examine the "other patient."

WHAT IS ULTRASOUND?

Ultrasound means "beyond (audible) sound"—that is, frequencies above 20,000 Hz (cycles per second). Ultrasound frequencies as used in obstetrics are extremely high—usually 3,500,000 Hz or 3.5 to 7 mHz. Consequently, this ultrasound is not audible to either the fetus or the mother.

Ultrasound is generated by passing an electric current through a special crystal (piezoelectric) causing the crystal to expand; as the face of the crystal expands, molecules in front of it are pushed away, starting a sound wave. The sound travels into the mother's body and is reflected back to the transducer when it encounters the dividing line between two substances of different acoustic impedance; the greater the difference in acoustic impedance, the greater the amount of reflection. The transducer, which is both the sending and listening device, is deformed by the returning sound, setting up an electric current in the piezoelectric crystal and reversing the process used in producing sound initially. This current is transformed into a signal, which is displayed on the ultrasound monitor. The piezoelectric crystals in the ultrasound transducer are very delicate. If dropped, they break, and if broken, the transducer usually cannot be repaired—a new one must be purchased. Hence, care must be taken in the handling and storage of transducers.

FREQUENCIES OF TRANSDUCERS

Transducers send different frequencies of sound; there are, for example, 2.5-, 3.0-, 3.5-, and 5.0-mHz transducers and so on. The rule of thumb is that the higher the frequency, the better the resolution but the poorer the penetration. Consequently, a 5-mHz transducer would be selected for a thin woman and a 2.5- or 3-mHz transducer would be used for a heavy woman or for a term pregnancy where depth of penetration was needed. If a patient is extremely obese, it may not be possible to get much useful information even with an abdominal or transvaginal transducer, as fat (subcutaneous or omental) is very reflective of sound.

TYPES OF TRANSDUCERS

The shape of the image is determined by the type of transducer, which, in turn, depends on the array pattern of the piezoelectric crystals. If they are lined up in a row, the transducer is termed *linear*. If they are lined up in a curve, it is called *curvilinear*. If they are arranged and the beam is steered so that the image is pie-shaped, the transducer is called a *sector* transducer.

A real advance occurred with the design of long, narrow transducers that could be inserted into the vagina (Fig. 52-1). Thus the pelvic contents could be visualized while the sound beam did not penetrate the skin, muscle, or fat of the anterior abdominal wall; a full bladder was not needed and gas in the bowel was not a problem. A protective covering is needed before the transducer is inserted. Latex gloves do not provide enough protection; however, unlubricated condoms of good quality are adequate. The transducer

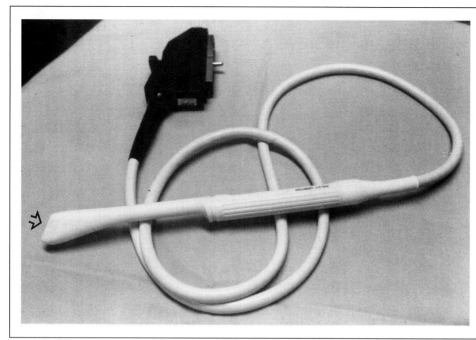

Figure 52-1

Transvaginal transducer. The transducer face (*arrow*) is linear. A special covering must be used before this is inserted into the vagina.

must be mechanically cleansed with soap and water afterward and then soaked in a solution such as Sporocidin or whatever is recommended by the institution and manufacturer. The solution must be one that does not cause separation of the special rubber covering of the transducer face. The device should be soaked for not less than 10 minutes and not more than several hours. In addition, the concentration of the soaking solution must be monitored and fresh solution mixed up every few weeks.

BLADDER FILLING

Sound travels best through water and worst through air. That is, almost all sound continues forward in water (as in the case of sonar, with which submarines are detected) but travels slowly in air and is quickly reflected at interfaces of air and anything else because of large differences in acoustic impedance. This is why the bladder must be filled in pelvic ultrasound—it displaced air-filled bowel upward and provides a window of water through which sound can travel into the pelvis. Pregnant patients must drink enough fluid to allow visualization of the cervix and the lower edge of the placenta. Early in gestation, the adnexa and the top of the uterus should be visible. Why not just do vaginal ultrasonography instead of having patients drink water? Often, structures more than 8 to 10 cm from the tip of the transvaginal transducer are out of range, since these transducers are of the 5- to 7-mHz range. Thus, they are designed for imaging small structures such as yolk sacs but do not have deep penetration. If there is a possibility that a patient will need to have surgery, she does not need to drink water—not

voiding until the scan is usually sufficient. Foley catheters should not be placed unless requested by the department doing the scanning.

TYPES OF DISPLAY

B-mode is the type of display we are accustomed to. It has width and depth and resembles a slice of anatomy. When B-mode images are refreshed very frequently (resembling a movie) we call this a *real time* display. The other type of display used frequently is M-mode, which shows reflected echoes along one line over time. This is usually used to determine amount and frequency of motion, as in the fetal heart.

DOPPLER

The Doppler principle states that the frequency of sound reflected off a moving object will change from the original transmitted frequency in an amount proportional to the speed of that moving object. That is, if an object is not moving, there will be no change in the frequency of reflected sound; but if an object, such as blood, is moving, the frequency of returning sound will be changed in proportion to the object's velocity. Note the word *velocity*. Doppler ultrasound does not measure flow. We may know that cars are traveling at 65 mph along a highway (velocity), but unless we know how many lanes there are, we do not know how many cars are passing at any moment (flow). This change in velocity between sound sent into the body and reflected back is usually under 20,000 Hz and is, therefore, discernible by the human ear. When amplified, it can be heard with a simple instrument held to the uterine wall (as in hand-held electronic auscultating devices or uterine monitors), either to detect heart tones or to continuously monitor the fetus. The "continuous" variety of Doppler used in these simple devices measures movement along the entire path into the abdomen, which is important to know when auscultating for viability. "Continuous" Doppler is not specific for a certain point within the abdomen such as a fetal heart or vessel.

HOW TO ORDER AN EXAM

Often a clinician will not provide clinical information to the imaging department in the hopes of letting someone else make a "fresh decision" and not be "prejudiced." However, no other physician would see a patient without a history, because this helps to guide thinking in the right direction; the same is true for ultrasound. If a patient has had bleeding, the ultrasound examiner might do a careful transvaginal scan to exclude a placenta previa or look at the adnexa if she has pain. If neither the cervix nor ovaries can be seen abdomi-

nally, however, this type of scan would not normally be done as part of an ultrasound survey.

THE FIRST 20 WEEKS OF PREGNANCY

NORMAL DEVELOPMENT

An intrauterine sac is first apparent on ultrasound with a transvaginal transducer at about 5 weeks (Fig. 52-2) or when the beta human chorionic gonadotropin (β-hCG) is at about 1000 mIU/mL (third international standard). On an abdominal scan, this may not be visible until the β-hCG is about 6000 mIU/mL. Next appears a doughnut-shaped structure called the yolk sac (Fig. 52-3). At about 5½ weeks, a faint flickering can be seen along one of the surfaces of the yolk sac; this means that the embryonic heart tube has started to contract. This motion may be detected only with low "persistence"—a canceling of the smoothing added to most machines to make the picture pleasing.

Next, an embryonic pole appears—1 to 2 mm if transvaginal scanning is being used (Fig. 52-3). Tables correlate

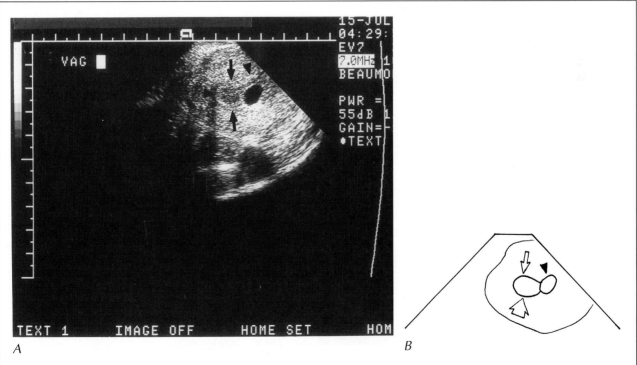

A

B

Figure 52-2

An early gestational sac appears as a black circle *(arrowhead)*. Note that it is eccentrically placed in relation to the uterine cavity *(arrows)*. This is an important point in differentiating a true gestational sac from a pseudosac of an ectopic pregnancy, which is centrally placed.

this to gestational age. This is usually the most reliable way to establish gestational age, as there is little variation in size for each gestation week. That is, all fetuses of 3 mm are 6 weeks in age, with a variation of only ±3 days. By the time the pole measures 4 to 5 mm (6 to 6.5 weeks), it will be visible by transabdominal scanning on most patients. From 6.5 to 11 weeks, fetal age will be measured by a crown-rump length (Fig. 52-4).

If no sac can be seen even when the β-hCG is at 1000 mIU/mL or higher, the following possibilities should be considered: the patient has more than two sacs (e.g., triplets)[1] or the sac is outside the uterus (ectopic pregnancy), or the patient has had an intrauterine pregnancy (IUP) that she has passed or which has been resorbed (Table 52-1). If there has been no bleeding, the latter is unlikely. If the patient has had any assisted reproduction, the first possibility is likely. A history of previous ectopic pregnancy suggests the second. Examination of the cul-de-sac and adnexa will often determine the diagnosis. An intrauterine sac can be imitated by a pseudogestational sac, which is merely fluid, or a decidual reaction with the endometrium.

ECTOPIC PREGNANCY

This term means that a pregnancy is outside of the uterus—in a fallopian tube, ovary, the cervix, or free in the abdomen. *It is imperative that every women presenting in an emergency situation be considered pregnant until proven otherwise. As a corollary to this statement, it is imperative that every woman of reproductive age presenting in an emergency department with any complaints whatsoever be suspected of having an ectopic pregnancy until a pregnancy test can be shown to be negative or an intrauterine pregnancy is confirmed.*

Ultrasound has played a large role, along with increasingly sensitive tests for hCG, in decreasing the rate of death in ectopic pregnancy.[2,3] With a combination of these two modalities, it is possible to detect most ectopics *when a high index of suspicion is maintained* (see Fig. 3-2).

The ultrasound examination of the problematic early pregnancy is the most difficult in pelvic ultrasound and one that should be entrusted to the most experienced person available; it is not an exam to be left to someone who does not have considerable experience in this diagnosis, as the stakes are too high. A case has been made that it is possible to triage patients by allowing relatively inexperienced physicians to identify heart motion in an intrauterine pregnancy, therefore "excluding" ectopic pregnancy.[4] In the patient without a history of assisted reproduction, tubular disease, tubal surgery, use of an intrauterine device (IUD), or severe pain, this is probably a valid pathway.

The incidence of heterotopic pregnancies (simultaneous intrauterine pregnancy and ectopic pregnancy) has increased markedly with the advent of assisted reproduction (the use of ovulation induction, in vitro fertilization, or zygote im-

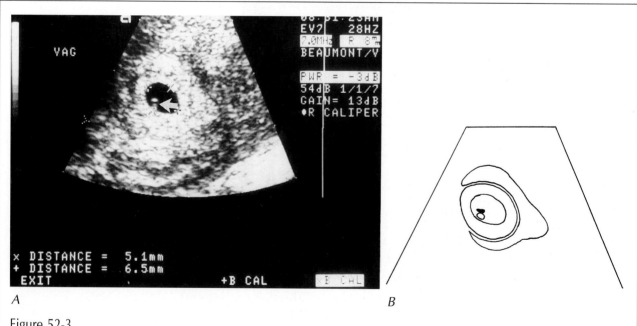

Figure 52-3

Yolk sac. This can be detected by ultrasound at about 5½ weeks (menstrual dates). It is a round, doughnut-shaped structure (*arrow*), on the surface of which the embryo will appear (*white "dash" just above tip of arrow*).

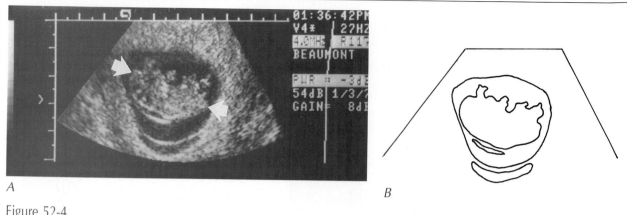

Figure 52-4

Crown-rump length. From the time the embryo can be seen by ultrasound to 11 weeks (menstrual dates). It is measured from the head to rump (*arrows*).

plantation, etc.) and of more widespread tubular disease. Although deaths from ectopic pregnancy have markedly decreased, heterotopic pregnancies are still a cause of maternal death because the intrauterine pregnancy is identified but the ectopic gestation is missed.

The primary use of ultrasound is to positively identify an intrauterine pregnancy. If none can be definitely identified, experienced examiners will then attempt to identify the ovaries (Fig. 52-5) and look for extraovarian masses; these are often difficult to find because they are hidden by bowel, are very small, or are of an acoustic impedance so similar to that of the uterus or ovaries that they cannot be distinguished from those structures. Special ultrasound settings are needed to identify fetal heart motion in extraovarian masses. Another finding typical of an ectopic pregnancy is echogenic cul-de-sac fluid. Occasionally the diagnosis cannot be made at the first examination and the patient will need to return for a second exam.

Unless there is a heterotopic pregnancy (uterus and ectopic), the uterine cavity will not contain a gestational sac.

However, in some ectopics, a pseudogestational sac (a collection of fluid surrounded by by uterine lining which mimics a gestational sac) will be seen; these can be notoriously difficult to distinguish from an intrauterine sac (Fig. 52-6). Often there will be echogenic fluid in the pelvis—small particles can be seen swirling around within the fluid, making it most likely to be blood.[5] A mass separate from the ovaries can usually be detected by an experienced examiner. Sometimes this appears to be solid and in other instances it may contain just a visible sac within a mass ("bagel sign") (Fig. 52-7). In still others an actual embryo with a heartbeat will be seen (Fig. 52-8). The latter is obviously absolutely diagnostic of an ectopic pregnancy. A major difficulty is that the ectopic mass can be hidden behind swirling loops of bowel or can be of such similar acoustic impedance as the ovaries or uterus or in such close approximation to them that it cannot be distinguished as a separate mass. An extraovarian mass and an empty uterus are together very sensitive signs for an ectopic pregnancy.

Occasionally a sac will be seen in the uterus but will be very eccentric in location. This appearance raises the possibility of an *interstitial* pregnancy (sometimes erroneously termed a *cornual pregnancy*), a pregnancy which implants in the part of the tube that travels through the myometrium into the cavity. It is very important to make the distinction between an eccentric intrauterine pregnancy and an interstitial pregnancy because the latter is notorious for the amount of bleeding that occurs upon rupture. The problem becomes one of determining if this is an ectopic pregnancy in the proximal tube or in the interstitium.[6] In any case, interstitial pregnancies can easily be missed unless the top of the uterus is examined with meticulous care by an experienced examiner. An ectopic pregnancy can also occur within an ovary (Fig. 52-9). The diagnostic challenge is to then distinguish between this and a corpus luteum cyst or other ovarian mass. A preg-

---

Table 52-1

IMPLICATIONS OF ABSENT GESTATIONAL SAC

No sac on transvaginal ultrasound with βhCG > 1,000 mIU/mL:

- Intrauterine pregnancy <5 weeks with triplets or more
- Ectopic pregnancy
- Failing intrauterine pregnancy >5 weeks

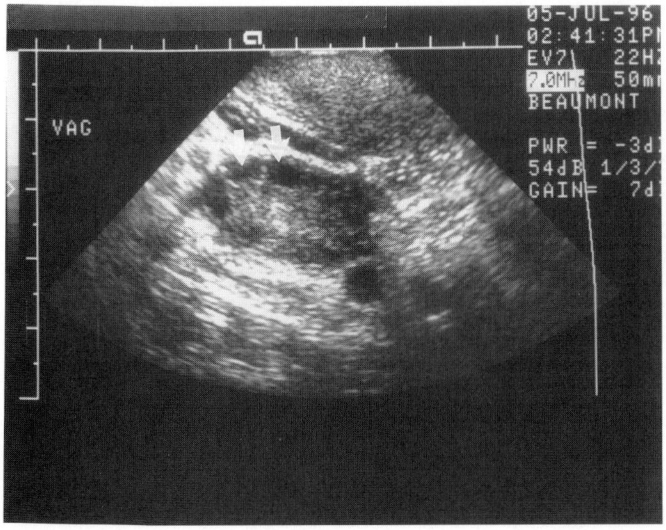

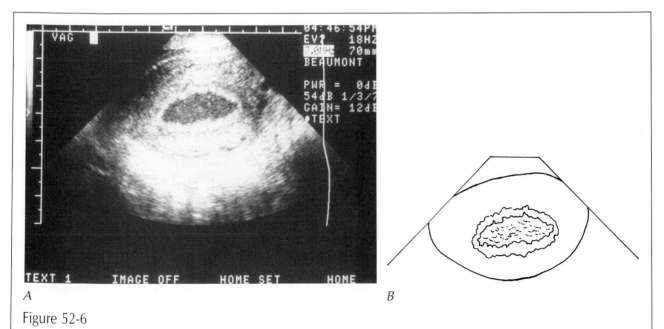

Figure 52-5

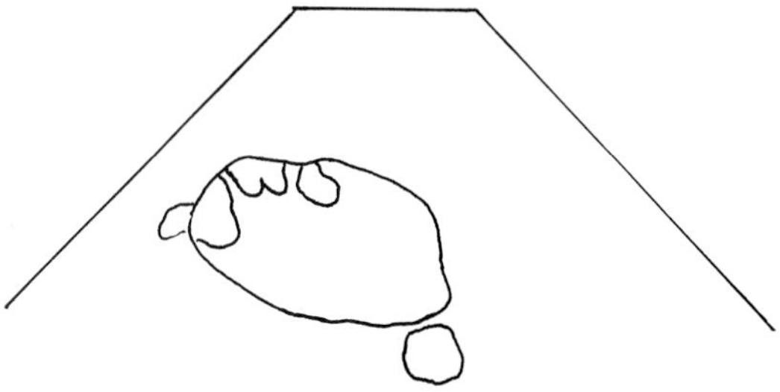

Normal ovary. The ovary is oval with small follicles (*arrows*) arrayed around the outer rim.

Figure 52-6

A pseudogestational sac. This sac has a definite border similar to the one found in a true gestational sac. However, note that it is centrally located and contains debris. Compare to Fig. 52-2.

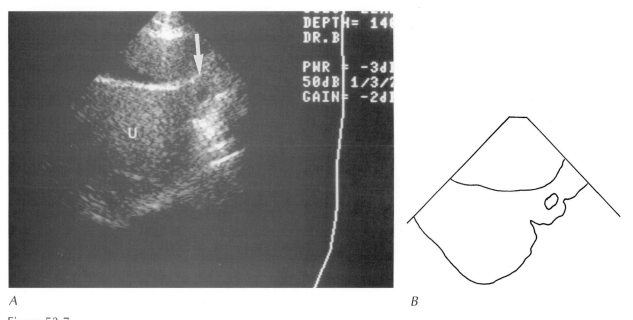

A   *B*

Figure 52-7

Ectopic pregnancy. An extrauterine mass containing a small gestational sac ("bagel sign") (*arrow*) lies to the right of the top of the uterus (u).

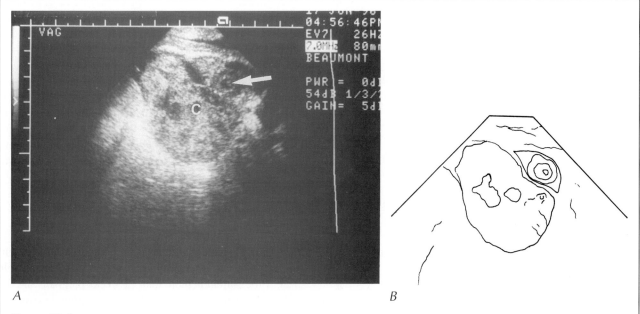

A   *B*

Figure 52-8

Ectopic pregnancy. A mass containing a gestational sac and small embryo (*arrow*) lies to the right of an intraperitoneal clot (c). Since a heartbeat could be seen in the embryo, this was absolutely diagnostic of an ectopic pregnancy.

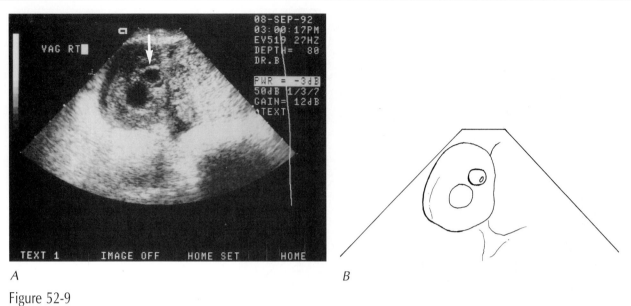

Figure 52-9

Ovarian ectopic. The sac with the definitive white line around it (*arrow*) proved to be an ovarian ectopic. The diagnosis was made by laparoscopy after a tentative diagnosis of ectopic was made by clinical and ultrasound evidence.

nancy may also implant in the cervix. This type is known for the amount of bleeding that occurs when it is disturbed.

FAILING INTRAUTERINE PREGNANCY

Frequently a sac implants in the uterus and then fails to produce an embryo or the embryo fails to grow. The popular term for the latter is *miscarriage,* more correctly termed *demise of an intrauterine pregnancy (IUP)* or *failed IUP.* The placenta may grow for a while and the β-hCG level may go up, but eventually the placenta degenerates and the β-hCG level goes down. The patient may have experienced no change, but usually, upon close questioning, she will report pelvic discomfort, spotting, or "not feeling pregnant." To make a diagnosis of no heart motion, persistence (smoothing) must be lowered. A slow fetal heartbeat has a very poor prognosis. The best prognosis is with a fetal heartbeat of 110 beats per minute or more.

Often an embryo or yolk sac will altogether fail to appear on ultrasound. The common term for this is *blighted ovum,* but this is just one more type of failed intrauterine pregnancy. In some pregnancies, growth is stopped before the embryo appears or when it is less than 1 mm in length, but more often an embryo has formed and then died and been resorbed, so that when a first or second scan is done, only a sac is visible. History or previous scans separate this from lagging dates and very early IUPs.

HYDATIDIFORM MOLE

When the uterus appears to be occupied only by placenta and there is no fetus, the patient may have a mole. In this entity, the placenta appears very heterogeneous, with many lucent areas interspersed by brighter areas (Fig. 52-10). This is a reflection off the surfaces of the vesicles of the mole. In the older literature, it was referred to as a "snowstorm." The appearance of gray-scale imaging showing many more gradations of detail has made that term obsolete. This appearance can be imitated by a degenerating placenta in the demise of an intrauterine pregnancy; occasionally the fetus is resorbed first and the placenta becomes very heterogeneous in appearance. The actual diagnosis can be determined only by pathologic examination. The ovaries sometimes contain theca lutein cysts, which result from stimulation from the large amount of hCG produced by the mole (Fig. 52-11).

Occasionally, part of the placenta appears normal and part resembles a mole and an abnormal fetus is present; this is termed a *partial mole* and is usually a result of *triploidy,* in which there are three sets of each chromosome. These fetuses usually have very small abdomens and abnormal central nervous systems and extremities. They almost never reach term.

INCARCERATION OF THE UTERUS

Occasionally a patient with an early pregnancy will present with acute urinary retention and abdominal pain (Table 52-2). If the patient is more than 11 weeks pregnant and the fundus is still in the pelvis with nothing palpable over the symphysis, it is possible that she has an incarcerated uterus. In this entity, a sharply retroflexed uterus does not straighten out and rise into the abdomen; instead, the fundus becomes wedged on the sacrum, forcing the cervix up against the symphysis and compressing the urethra between the fundus

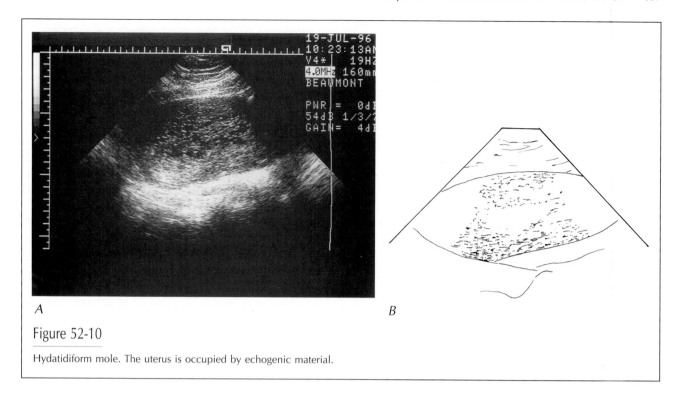

A   *B*

Figure 52-10

Hydatidiform mole. The uterus is occupied by echogenic material.

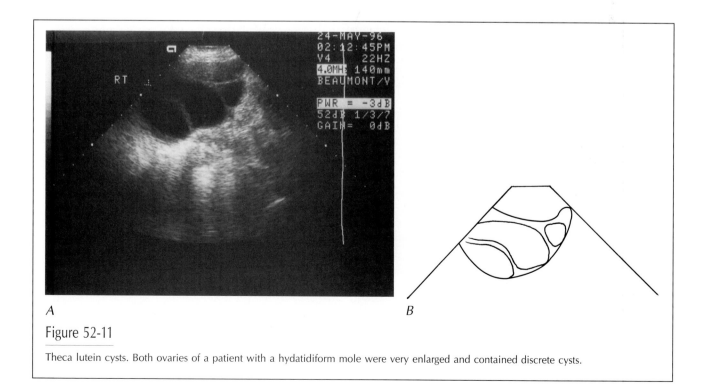

A   *B*

Figure 52-11

Theca lutein cysts. Both ovaries of a patient with a hydatidiform mole were very enlarged and contained discrete cysts.

Table 52-2

PELVIC PAIN IN EARLY PREGNANCY

Failing IUP (contractions)
Ectopic pregnancy
Ovarian cyst—torsion, rupture, pressure
Incarceration of the uterus
Stretching of the round ligament
Ureteral stones
Appendicitis

and symphysis. This entity is seen in patients with very "tipped" or retroflexed uteri and is even more likely in patients with uterine malformations such as uterine didelphia. This diagnosis can be made clinically and confirmed by ultrasound, which shows the fundus wedged in the pelvis and the cervix immediately under the symphysis (Fig. 52-12).

DETERMINING FETAL AGE

At 11 weeks it becomes possible to measure the width of the head, which is known as the biparietal diameter (BPD) (Fig. 52-13). The mandible, maxilla, cranium, spine, and long bones are calcified enough to provide strong reflections of sound back to the transducer, allowing measurement of calcified bones such as the femur (Fig. 52-14). These measurements are more accurate than crown-rump length (CRL) at this age, because the fetus is curling and uncurling, making a CRL measurement variable. Measurements at 11 to 20 weeks of gestation will provide a very accurate estimate of dates, with only a slightly greater variation (± 1 week) than CRL performed at 6 to 11 weeks. In addition, it is now possible to identify some major organs: the bladder and stomach are seen as dark (echolucent) areas within the fetus. Besides measurements intended to determine gestational age or growth (if dates are firm), nuchal thickness is measured to provide a screen for Down and Turner syndromes. The placenta is homogeneous at this point and fluid is plentiful. If the placenta is heterogeneous or there is little fluid, referral to an obstetrician should be made. Although some organs can be seen at the 11- to 12-week range, it is not until 17 weeks that enough of the organs can be seen to also provide an accurate anatomic screen. The checklist for this screen is available from the American Institute of Ultrasound in Medicine (AIUM). Individuals specially trained in this work and certified by the American Registry of Diagnostic Medical Sonographers (RDMS) should be able to screen the fetus accurately. They must be supervised by a physician experienced in this work.

FETAL VIABILITY

Doppler or real-time ultrasound can be used to establish heart motion if heart tones cannot be auscultated with a

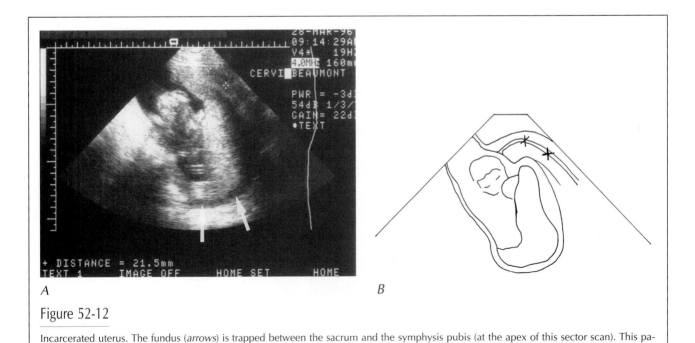

A   *B*

Figure 52-12

Incarcerated uterus. The fundus (*arrows*) is trapped between the sacrum and the symphysis pubis (at the apex of this sector scan). This patient presented with acute urinary retention because the urethra (*above cross hairs on cervix*) was compressed between the symphysis and cervix.

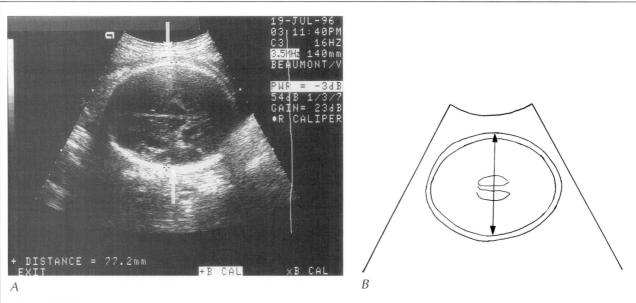

Figure 52-13

Biparietal diameter. The measurement across the widest part of the fetal head in this axial (transverse) scan (*arrows*) is a reliable measure of gestational age from 11 weeks upward.

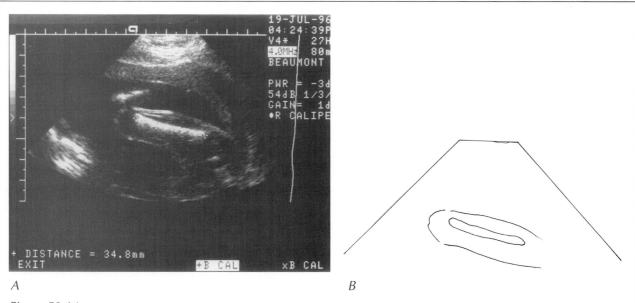

Figure 52-14

Femur length. The measurement of the calcified part of the femur from metaphysis to lesser trochanter is also a reliable measurement of gestational age.

stethoscope. Auscultation is the first line of inquiry, however. The small portable electronic listening devices that use ultrasound rely on the Doppler principle, as discussed above. These types of devices detect all reflected sound along the path into the mother's abdomen; therefore, although they may detect the sound reflected off of the fetal heart valves (fetal heart rate), they may also detect the mother's heart rate, since the beam can reflect off the mother's vessels instead of the baby's. For that reason, the maternal heart rate or pulse should be palpated at the same time.

Example: Heart tones cannot be heard by stethoscope, so a Doppler device is used on a mother with a fever. A rate of 120 is obtained. However, palpation of the mother's pulse shows that it is also 120 beats per minute. A real-time ultrasound scan shows that there is no motion of the fetal heart (the baby is dead—sound was being reflected from the maternal vessels).

Example: A patient with known lupus has ausculted fetal heart tones of 80. Since the mother's pulse is 80, it is not clear if the fetus is alive. Real-time scanning shows fetal heart motion with a ventricular rate of 80. However, the atrial rate is 140 to 160. This fetus has complete heart block, which occurs in some mothers with lupus in the late second trimester.

Example: Heart tones of 120 beats per minute are auscultated on each of twins. However, on real-time ultrasound, only one twin has heart motion—the other is dead. Why were heart tones heard in two different places? The ultrasound Doppler beam was directed at the heart of the live fetus from two different directions.

THE SECOND 20 WEEKS OF PREGNANCY

BLEEDING IN LATER PREGNANCY

Bleeding in the first half of pregnancy is usually a variation of normal or related to failure of the pregnancy (Table 52-3). In the late second and all of the third trimester placental causes are more common.

PLACENTA PREVIA

The placenta frequently lies over the internal os in the first and second trimesters of pregnancy, but as the lower uterine segment elongates in the second and third trimesters, the edge becomes farther and farther from the uterine os. If it still covers the internal os in the third trimester, this is termed "placenta previa" (Fig. 52-15). If the margin of the placenta comes just up to but not over the internal os, this is termed a *marginal previa.*

If the placenta is centrally implanted so that its center is somewhere overlying the internal os, abdominal ultrasound

Table 52-3
BLEEDING IN THE THIRD TRIMESTER
Placenta previa
Abruptio placentae
Vasa previa
Low-lying placenta
Polyp

is quite accurate. However, if the edge of the placenta appears to be just up to or over the internal os on abdominal scan, it is useful to perform a vaginal scan. Bladder filling so influences the appearance of the lower uterine segment that vaginal scanning not only gives better definition but obviates the need for a full bladder. Often what appeared to be placenta overlying the os is not, and what appeared not to be over the os is, in actuality, over it. Transvaginal scanning will not cause additional bleeding when properly done, since usually only 2.5 to 5 cm. of the probe are inserted and its tip is nowhere near the internal os.

LOW-LYING PLACENTA

In the third trimester, if the edge of the placenta is within 2 cm of the internal os but its edge is not up to the os itself, this is termed a *low-lying* placenta. Although it is not a placenta previa, some bleeding may occur since the lower edge is not well attached.

ABRUPTIO PLACENTAE

If a patient has had a scan by a reliable source and is known not to have a placenta previa, it is not necessary to obtain a scan to exclude abruption, since this is a clinical diagnosis made when a patient known not to have a previa has pain, bleeding, and uterine contractions. These patients should have continuous fetal monitoring and should not be sent to be scanned elsewhere unless the value of the clinical information provided will outweigh the risk of sending the patient away from a monitored bed. An abruption may appear as a collection of fluid behind the placenta or at its edge, but usually the scan is entirely normal. Occasionally a patient will have unusual pain or contractions, the source of which cannot be identified, and she will be found to have an abruption on ultrasound. In these cases in which the clinical picture is not diagnostic, ultrasound may be of value.

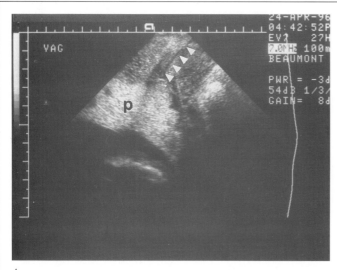

A

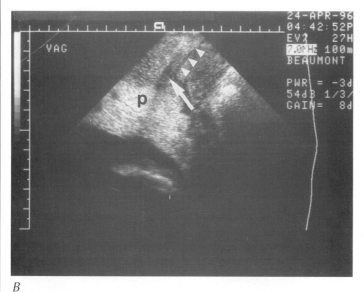

B

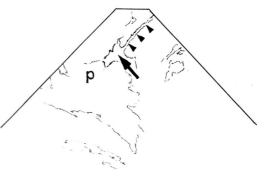

Figure 52-15

A. Placenta previa (abdominal scan). The placenta (p) covers the internal os (*arrowheads*). *B.* Placenta previa (vaginal scan). The placenta (p) covers the internal os (*lowest arrowhead*). Endocervical canal (*arrowheads*).

VASA PREVIA

When fetal blood vessels cross the cervix and membranes rupture, those vessels may tear, allowing the fetus to quickly exsanguinate. Vasa previa is sometimes but not always detected by ultrasound. Its detection depends upon the identi-fication of vessels crossing the internal os (something which generally requires color ultrasound) or the identification of the condition which produces vasa previa—either an extra lobe of the placenta (succenturiate) or a velamentous insertion of the cord.[7] The vessels lead from one lobe of the placenta to the other or from the cord, which is inserted into the membranes (velamentous) to the placenta (Fig. 52-16).

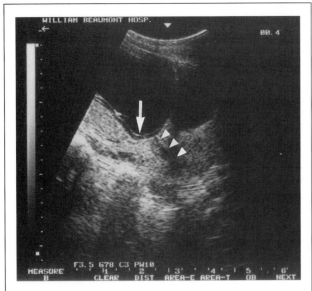

Figure 52-16

Vasa previa. A vessel (*arrow*) traverses the area of the internal os (*cervical canal—arrowheads*) from placenta to a succenturiate lobe. Rupture of this vessel could result in rapid fetal loss.

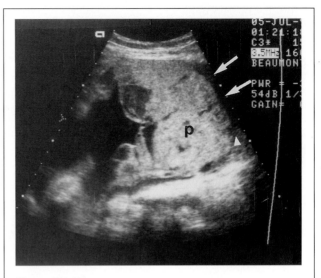

Figure 52-17

Placenta accreta. The internal os (*arrowhead*) is covered by placenta (p). It contains many more lakes (*clear spaces*) than usual. The normal clear space (*arrows*) between the placenta and uterus does not extend upward.

PLACENTA ACCRETA

Occasionally the normal separation of the placenta and uterine wall is not present and the cells of the placenta actually grow into the myometrium (Fig. 52-17) and even through it (percreta) and occasionally into the bladder (Fig. 52-18). At delivery, the uterus cannot contract and continuous uncontrollable bleeding may result, necessitating cesarean hysterectomy. Although the latter may not be avoided, it is sometimes possible, if the condition is identified beforehand, to plan for the appropriate blood replacement and cardiovascular support.

There are some clues on ultrasound that may strongly suggest placenta accreta.[8] There is almost always a placenta previa. In a patient with a previous cesarean section, the normal clear space between the placenta and uterine wall should be identified. If this is absent, there may be a placenta accreta. Numerous clear spaces in the placenta and increased blood flow also suggest it. The loss of the bladder wall definition suggests that the placenta may have grown through the bladder wall.

ABDOMINAL PREGNANCY

Occasionally a pregnancy develops outside the uterus. Its placenta implants on the bowel, abdominal wall, or mesentery. Clues are a relative lack of amniotic fluid, unusual lie (persistent transverse, for example), and no uterine wall seen under the surface of the placenta.[9] These pregnancies can reach term.

FIBROIDS

Fibroids are benign overgrowths of uterine muscle that can be located in the submucosal or subserosal areas or in the

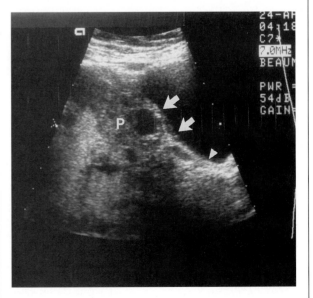

Figure 52-18

Placenta percreta. The normal smooth white line of the bladder wall (*arrowhead*) is interrupted (*arrows*) by placenta (p), which has grown through it.

wall of the uterus (intramural) (Fig. 52-19) or may be on a pedicle either within the cavity or outside of the uterus. Not all fibroids increase in size in pregnancy. If they do, however, they are susceptible to infarction due to an insufficient blood supply. This causes exquisite site tenderness and considerable pain. The most frequent time for infarction is at 16 to 20 weeks.

THE OVARY IN PREGNANCY

As the uterus enlarges, the ovaries, which are not closely applied to the pelvic side wall but rather tethered by the broad ligament, rise into the abdomen like sandbags attached to a hot-air balloon. This is one of the reasons why the entire abdomen should be scanned in dealing with a pregnancy; the appendix and ovaries can be located at a very high point.

FETAL SIZE AND WEIGHT

Fetal weight can be determined by measuring the size of the head, femur, and abdomen (Fig. 52-20) and using one of several formulas to determine weight.[10] Actual fetal length cannot be determined. The accuracy of these estimates depends upon several factors—primary among which is the accuracy of the measurements of the femur, abdomen, and head. There are many instances in which these cannot be accurately obtained. The abdominal measurement is particularly difficult to obtain when the fetus is lying against the abdominal wall, is large, or there is little fluid. The estimates are more accurate in the lower weight categories and become less accurate, particularly in the 4000-g range and above.

All fetuses have similar growth patterns in early pregnancy. It is only later that they express their genetic variability (family, racial), influence of environment (social, economic status, and smoking), and influence of medical factors such as glucose intolerance and hypertension. As we mentioned earlier, CRL is used to express the size of a fetus until 11 weeks. Crown-rump length is quite accurate and can establish dates to within ±4 days. At 11 weeks and beyond, the usual measurements of head, femur, and abdomen are used. At this point, up to about 20 weeks, fetal size predicts gestational age ±1 week. Later, as fetal variability increases, measurements are less accurate in predicting gestational age: 20 to 30 weeks, ±1.5 weeks to ±3 weeks at term. Consequently, it is important to determine gestational age before 20 weeks.

Another important feature of evaluating size is the relation of the abdomen size to head size. When a fetus is exposed to increased glucose in its bloodstream, it responds with an increase in insulin and converts glucose to glycogen, which is then stored in the fetal liver. Since the fetal abdomen is mostly occupied by the liver, the abdominal girth increases inappropriately. The abdomen will be disproportionately enlarged compared to the head. Conversely, if the fetus is not receiving the appropriate nutrients, the glycogen stores in the normal liver will shrink and the liver will shrink in size. The abdomen then becomes disproportionately small when compared to the head. If this restriction of nutrients continues for a long time and to a marked degree, eventually the brain stops growing and head size becomes small.

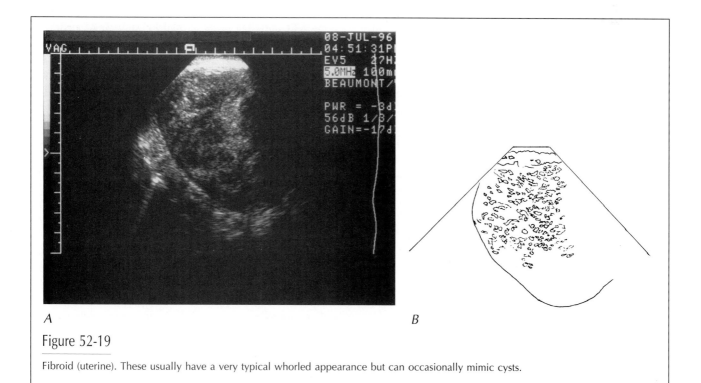

A   *B*

Figure 52-19

Fibroid (uterine). These usually have a very typical whorled appearance but can occasionally mimic cysts.

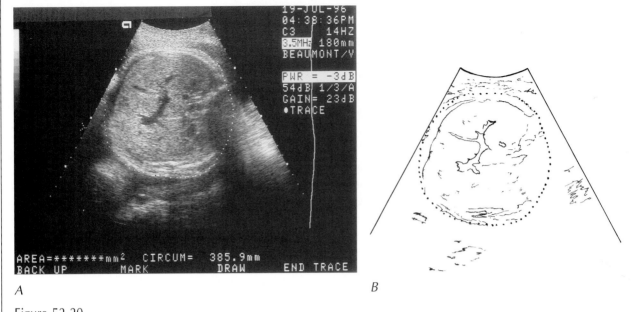

A

B

Figure 52-20

Abdominal circumference. This measurement is traced around the skin of the fetal abdomen scanned transversely at a certain level. It reflects gestational age, liver size, and subcutaneous fat.

If dates are very firm and gestational age is known without a doubt, small fetal size suggests growth restriction.

Example: A mother with known menstrual dates of 9 weeks comes for ultrasound. She has a regular 28-day cycle and has not been on oral contraceptives. Crown-rump length is measured and correlates with 7 weeks (+4 days). Comment: Size is lagging. A chorionic villous sampling shows that this fetus has trisomy 18. Fetuses with trisomy 18 can lag in size from early in gestation. Size will increase at an inappropriate rate but along a suboptimal percentile.

Example: A mother with established dates comes in for a scan. She is at 30 weeks of gestation, but the scan shows a very large abdomen for dates (greater than the 95th percentile) and increased amniotic fluid. Estimated weight is increased for dates. Comment: this mother has an abnormal glucose tolerance and has just been started on insulin. Her baby is showing the effects of increased glucose with enlargement of the liver. For some reason large fetuses of diabetic mothers often have mild to moderate increases in amniotic fluid.

GROWTH

Growth estimation depends upon a comparison of known size at a previous gestational age and an estimation of whether size has increased at an appropriate rate. If a fetus has been growing along the 80th percentile and suddenly drops down in size to the 10th percentile for weight with an abdomen below the 10th percentile, it is showing signs of growth restriction.

TWINS

Ultrasound is very important in identifying multiple pregnancies and following growth, because in these instances the tape measure fails us and does not reflect what is occurring in the uterus. Twins normally follow along singleton growth curves until the middle of the third trimester, at which point some will show lag in the growth of abdominal girth.[11] In the older literature, there was frequent mention of growth discordance or a size difference between twins. This has given way to an evaluation of each twin's growth potential and growth between exams (Fig. 52-21). In fraternal (dichorionic twins), particularly of different sexes, there may be significant size differences at each point, but neither should drop below the 10th percentile in weight at any time. Besides evaluation of the growth of twins, it is imperative to establish amnionicity as early as possible; at the first exam, amnionicity should be established without a doubt. That is, the dividing membrane should be documented (Fig. 52-22). If no dividing membrane is seen on an exam by a very experienced scanner and there is no great disparity of size, the twins are probably *monoamniotic* and the pregnancy will need special care and plans in attempt to deliver before cord entanglement occurs.

If twins are of different sexes, they must be dichorionic and are, therefore, not at risk for twin-twin transfusion syndrome (but, of course, they are at risk for all the other problems of multiples). However, if they share a placenta and are of the same sex, they may be monochorionic. These twins may develop twin-twin transfusion syndrome in which blood

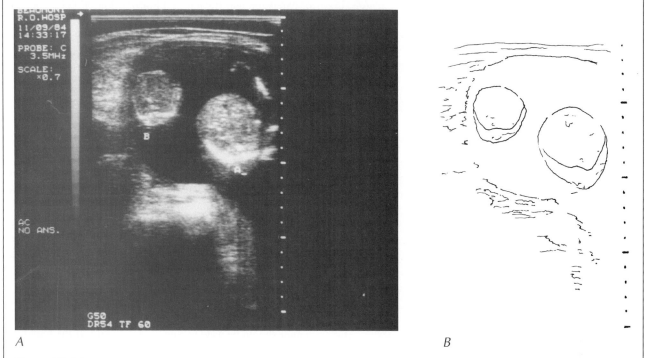

A   *B*

Figure 52-21

Growth restriction of one twin. Transverse scans through both abdomens show that twin B is markedly smaller than twin A (which has grown at a normal rate).

from one goes to the other across a connecting vessel in the placenta. There is usually one growth-retarded twin with no fluid around it, which is the donor, and a recipient that is normal in size or large, often with hydrops and sometimes with increased fluid. There is some treatment available for these pregnancies. It is important to identify the problem as early as possible. Sometimes the placentas appear to be one but are actually just fused. Placental tissue between these placentas will indicate that they are actually dichorionic (Fig. 52-22).

If twins are facing each other and are in the same presentation (e.g., vertex-vertex), it is important to make sure they are completely separated. Conjoined twins are an obstetric as well as a pediatric problem (Fig. 52-23).

BIOPHYSICAL PROFILE

This is a test with a total of 10 possible points that combines a nonstress test (2 points) and certain ultrasound observations (8 points). The ultrasound portion is similar to the evaluation done on newborns (Apgar score). A score of 10 is a perfect one: the following are given 2 points each—a reactive nonstress test, fetal breathing for 30 seconds or more, two or more fetal movements, a pocket of amniotic fluid of 2 cm or more in two directions, and fetal tone (as judged by a clenched fist

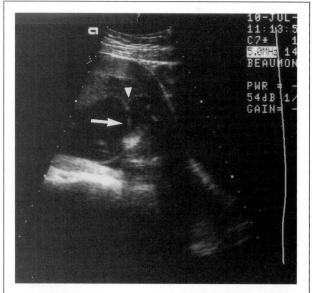

Figure 52-22

Twins—dividing membrane (*arrow*). This should be documented early, since management will be changed if it is not present. In monochorionic (identical) twins, it will contain two layers; in dichorionic ones, four layers. A placental peak (*arrowhead*) reliably establishes dichorionicity in this pregnancy.

Table 52-4

FETAL HEART RATES AND THEIR MEANING

Slow
   Heart block (lupus or structural defects)
   Physiologic slowing
   Maternal pulse
   Fetal hypoxia

Irregular[a]
   Premature atrial contractions
   Premature ventricular contractions
   Atrial tachycardia with irregular conduction
   Heart block with irregular conduction

Fast
   Maternal fever or hypothyroidism
   210–300 beats per minute: supraventricular tachycardia
   300–400 beats per minute: atrial flutter
   Fetal hypoxia

[a]The key to fetal arrhythmias is to measure separately both the atrial and ventricular rate (Fig. 52-25). If they are equal, there is no heart block.

or extension and flexion of a limb)[12] (Fig. 52-24). There are many variations to the original test just described—most of them relate to the amount of fluid.[12] A biophysical profile is used in the following instances: before a nonstress test is deemed reliable as a stand-alone entity, on multiples, and when the nonstress test is nonreassuring or nonreactive.

FETAL CARDIAC ARRHYTHMIAS

Both auscultation with a stethoscope and Doppler devices detect the fetal *ventricular* cardiac rate (Table 52-4). Does a heart rate of 80 beats per minute mean that the fetus is in distress? Not necessarily. If a slow heart rate is heard with a Doppler device, stethoscope auscultation will often detect the true fetal rate and show that the slow rate detected with Doppler was that of the mother's aorta. The reason for this is that anything in the path of the ultrasound beam will be reflected back to the transducer, including the maternal aorta. If a normal rate cannot be detected, real-time ultrasound should be used to find the fetal heart. If the fetal heart is truly beating at 80 beats per minute, there may be normal slowing and speeding up of the fetal heart when the mother is in the recumbent position before 30 weeks. Turning the mother on her side or supporting the transducer's weight

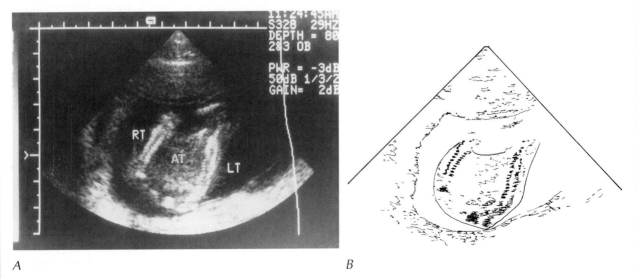

A

B

Figure 52-23

Conjoined twins. The spines of these conjoined twins are echogenic (*white*). They are facing each other and joined by a common abdomen and thorax (AT).

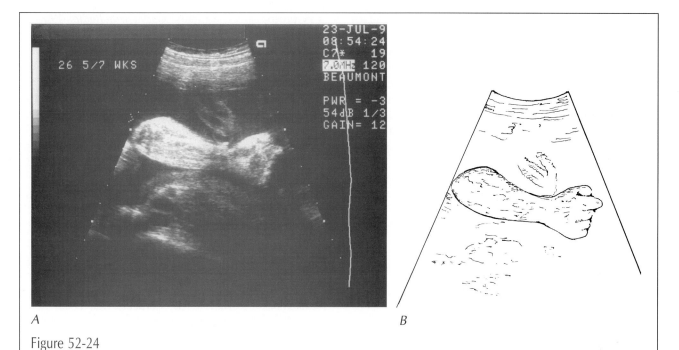

A   B

Figure 52-24

Arm with clenched fist (*to the right*). This indicated good fetal tone and would be given 2 points on a biophysical profile.

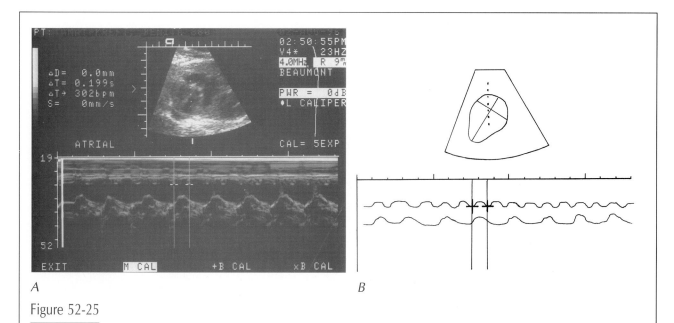

A   B

Figure 52-25

A B-mode image of the fetal heart lies at the top. The dotted lines through it define the line along which the M-mode (*bottom*) image will be produced. The M-mode shows rapid motion (302 beats per minute) of the atrial wall (one cycle is between the cursors) and a ventricular rate of 150 beats per minute. This is supraventricular tachycardia with a 2:1 block. It may be auscultated as an irregular heartbeat as the degree of block changes.

with the operator's hand will usually result in a rapid return to normal sinus rhythm. An alternative possibility is that there is fetal heart block due to antibodies to the fetal conducting system, as found in lupus, or to disruption of the conduction system by severe structural anomalies. Heart block can be distinguished by M-mode scanning—the atrial rate will be normal but the ventricular rate will be disparate and invariably slower (Fig. 52-25). Fetal bradycardia is usually constant or disappears and returns with the next contraction. A rate over 200 beats per minute may reflect supraventricular tachycardia, in which the atrium is beating at that rate: the ventricular rate may be the same or, if the heart has trouble conducting from the atrium to the ventricle at this fast rate, some beats may be dropped and a slow or irregular ventricular rate will be heard.

References

1. Keith SC, London SN, Weitzman GA, et al: Serial transvaginal ultrasound scans and β-human chorionic gonadotropin levels in early singleton and multiple pregnancies. *Fertil Steril* 59:1007, 1993.
2. Cacciatore B: Can the status of tubal pregnancy be predicted with transvaginal sonography? A prospective comparison of sonographic, surgical, and serum hCG findings. *Genitourin Radiol* 177:481, 1990.
3. Frates MC, Laing FC: Sonographic evaluation of ectopic pregnancy: An update. *AJR* 165:251, 1995.
4. Braffman BH, Coleman BG, Ramchandani P, et al: Emergency department screening for ectopic pregnancy: A prospective U.S. study. *Genitourin Radiol* 190:797, 1994.
5. Nyberg DA, Hughes MP, Mack LA, Wang KY: Extrauterine findings of ectopic pregnancy at transvaginal US: Importance of echogenic fluid. *Radiology* 178:823, 1991.
6. Ackerman TE, Levi CS, Dashefsky SM, et al: Interstitial line: Sonographic finding in interstitial (cornual) ectopic pregnancy. *Radiology* 189:83, 1993.
7. Gianupoulo SJ, Carver T, Tomich PG, et al: Diagnosis of vasa previa with ultrasonography. *Obstet Gynecol* 769:488, 1987.
8. Finberg HJ, Williams JW: Placenta accreta: Prospective sonographic diagnosis in patients with placenta previa and prior cesarean section. *J Ultrasound Med* 11:333, 1992.
9. Hallatt JG, Grove JA: Abdominal pregnancy: a study of twenty-one consecutive cases. *Am J Obstet Gynecol* 152:444, 1985.
10. Hadlock FP, Harrist RB, Carpenter RJ, et al: Sonographic estimation of fetal weight. *Radiology* 150:535, 1984.
11. Yarkoni S, Reece EA, Holford T, et al: Estimated fetal weight in the evaluation of growth in twin gestations: A prospective longitudinal study. *Obstet Gynecol* 69:636, 1987.
12. Manning FA, Platt LD, Sipos L: Antepartum fetal evaluation: Development of a fetal biophysical profile score. *Am J Obstet Gynecol* 136:787, 1980.
13. Vintzileos AM, Campbell WA, Nochimson DJ, Weinbaum PJ: The use and misuse of the fetal biophysical profile. *Am J Obstet Gynecol* 156:527, 1987.

Chapter 53

ULTRASONOGRAPHY OF GYNECOLOGIC DISORDERS

Christine H. Comstock

An emergency setting in gynecology almost always involves pain or profuse bleeding. Before working up a patient for the usual causes of pelvic pain, it must be remembered that *a woman of reproductive age is pregnant until proved otherwise* (despite a history of regular menses, tubal ligation, or even of "no intercourse ever, at all"). There are many causes of pelvic pain in the pregnant woman, the most threatening of which is an ectopic pregnancy. As in the pregnant patient, in the nonpregnant woman the differential diagnosis revolves around all the organs of the pelvis—not just the uterus and ovaries but also the bowel and urinary system.

Ultrasound is not a substitute for a pelvic exam; the patient should not be sent for an ultrasound examination as a delaying technique. A thorough history and physical exam, including a pelvic exam, will help interpret the results of the pelvic ultrasound. Has the patient had a history of endometriosis? Renal stones? Has the patient ever menstruated at all? Has she ever had an ultrasound exam of the pelvis, and, if so, what did it show?

Ultrasound of a pelvic mass may be nonspecific unless the mass has very unique ultrasound characteristics. Benign masses have thin exterior walls, no septa or thin, smooth septa and little if any solid material within them. Doppler of contained or supplying arteries can aid in the differentiation of benign and malignant masses but is by no means foolproof. It is based upon the fact that there is little resistance to flow in tumor vessels because they contain no smooth muscles in their walls. There are some artifacts and

pitfalls in pelvic ultrasound that can lead to the discovery of a normal pelvis at laparotomy or laparoscopy. The usual problem is that bowel can simulate or hide a mass. In addition, in some institutions, only a pelvic scan is performed when ultrasound of the pelvis is ordered. With a proper history and physical, it may be appropriate to extend that exam to the appendix, kidneys, and lower ureters and even the gallbladder.

The pelvic scan is not complete unless the uterus, ovaries, and cul-de-sac are visualized. This is usually accomplished first with a partially filled bladder and abdominal scan and then, when necessary, by a transvaginal scan (after emptying the bladder). As in all imaging, "the most commonly missed abnormality is the second"; an ovarian mass or enlarged uterus may not be the reason for the patient's pain.

INTRAUTERINE DEVICES

There are occasions when an ultrasound examination is necessary to find an intrauterine device (IUD). Usually this occurs when the string is not visible. Because IUDs are reflective, they can usually be located with ultrasound (Fig. 53-1), unless they are outside the uterus. Whether or not they are entirely in the uterine cavity or partially embedded in the uterine wall can often be determined by ultrasound. If they are not visible in the uterus, a plain film of the pelvis will reveal whether or not the IUD is in the body at all or has been expelled.

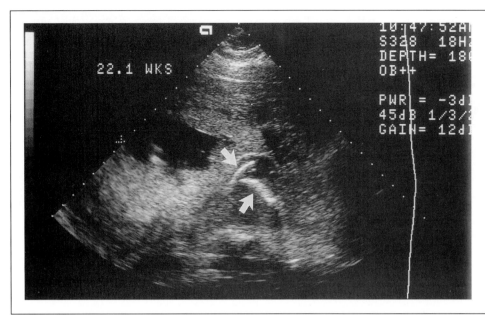

Figure 53-1

Intrauterine device. A copper 7 IUD (*arrows*) lies below an intrauterine pregnancy (the cervix lies to the right).

FUNCTIONAL CYSTS

The term *functional cysts* refers to enlarged follicles or corpora luteii. The ultrasound appearance is usually that of a cyst completely filled with clear or nonechoic fluid (Fig. 53-2). On the other hand, bleeding into this cyst may produce some solid material, which can then mimic cysts of different origin. These cysts have smooth, thin walls with few if any internal septations. Pain occurs when they are very large, have internal bleeding, have ruptured, or have caused torsion of the ovary. Considerable bleeding can occur upon rupture.

OVARIAN REMNANT

Occasionally, when an ovary is removed, a microscopic part of it is left behind, particularly if there were intraabdominal adhesions. This tiny piece of ovary, often invisible to the human eye, can produce functional cysts and resulting pain

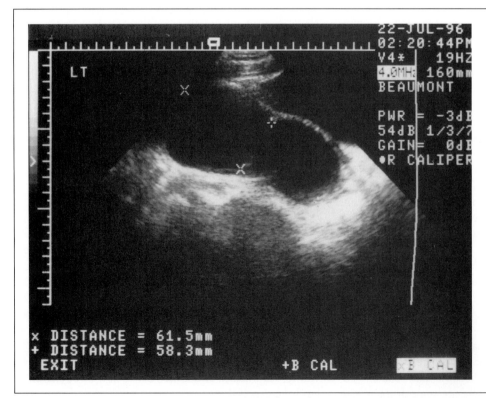

Figure 53-2

Functional cysts. Two follicular cysts are shown here. Note the lack of internal material or septations.

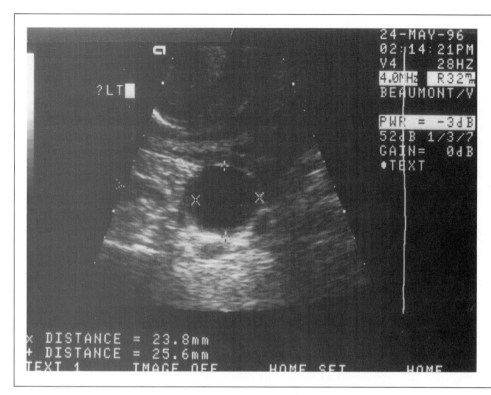

Figure 53-3

Ovarian remnant. A functional cyst has formed in a microscopic ovarian remnant left behind after removal of an ovary.

(Fig. 53-3). These can produce a confusing clinical picture in the patient who claims to have had an oophorectomy.

MUCINOUS CYSTADENOMAS

These benign masses are the largest of the ovarian neoplasms. They can grow so large that they occupy part of the abdomen, making the patient look pregnant. They are filled with a mucinous material that produces an ultrasound picture of many small white dots (Fig. 53-4). They have little if any solid material within.

SEROUS CYSTADENOMAS

These contain serous fluid and are generally not as large as mucinous cystadenomas. The more septations they have, the thicker the wall, and the more solid material they contain, the more likely it is that they are malignant (serous cystadenocarcinoma).

ENDOMETRIOMAS

These ovarian masses are lined with endometrium-like tissue (uterine gland tissue) and contain old blood, hence the name *chocolate cysts*. They are found in patients with a history of endometriosis. Their ultrasound appearance is quite variable, but normally they appear almost semisolid with considerable echoic material within them (Fig. 53-5).

DERMOIDS

Other than functional cysts, these are the most common ovarian masses in the younger woman. They contain elements of fat, cartilage, teeth, and hair, which give a very characteristic appearance: hair and fat provide a strong acoustic interface that strongly reflects sound (Fig. 53-6). Fat may layer out on surrounding fluid. Calcified areas produce a complete sound shadow behind them by reflecting sound completely. Dermoids may be the cause of ovarian torsion in younger women—a condition that produces severe pain and occasionally an acute abdomen. The contained teeth can be seen on a plain film of the pelvis. Occasionally these tumors are a part of a complex ovarian mass. Figure 53-7 illustrates why it can be so difficult to determine pathology by ultrasound.

UTERINE/VAGINAL ANOMALIES

Rarely, there can be a blind horn of a uterus that acts like an endometrioma. The patient experiences severe pain during menses. A careful ultrasound examination will show that the mass is separate from the ovary on that side. Alternatively, there may be a high vaginal septum that impedes the exit of menstrual flow or normal mucus, causing the uterus to become larger and larger. Again, physical examination and history are key, since an ultrasound examination may be confusing. Fibroids may be single or multiple and are usually easily identified by ultrasound (see Fig. 52-19).

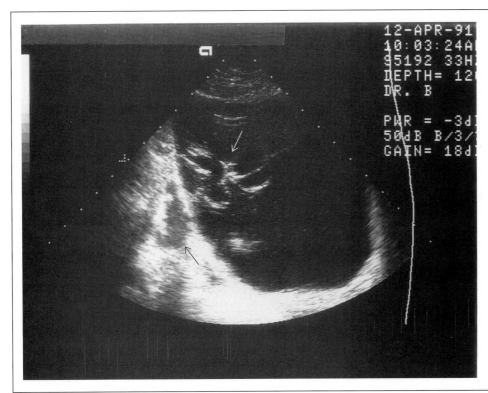

Figure 53-4

Mucinous cystadema. This large mass (*black arrow*) contains faintly echogenic material and "daughter cysts" (*white arrow*).

NONGYNECOLOGIC CAUSE OF PELVIC PAIN

Conditions such as appendicitis, diverticulitis, or a ureterovesical stone may cause acute pelvic pain, simulating pain from a gynecologic source. Again careful bimanual and abdominal examinations will usually point to the correct diagnosis. If the bimanual examination is unrevealing, a pelvic ultrasound may be of help. Its first use is to show a normal uterus and ovaries and no free intraperitoneal fluid. After looking at the uterus and ovaries, it is useful to determine if there is unilateral hy-

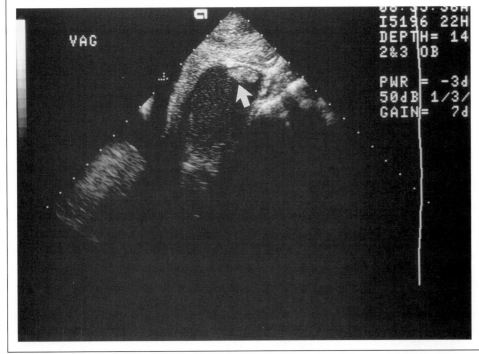

Figure 53-5

Endometrioma. The content (old blood) is quite echogenic, giving a "salt and pepper" appearance. There is a small amount of solid material (*arrow*).

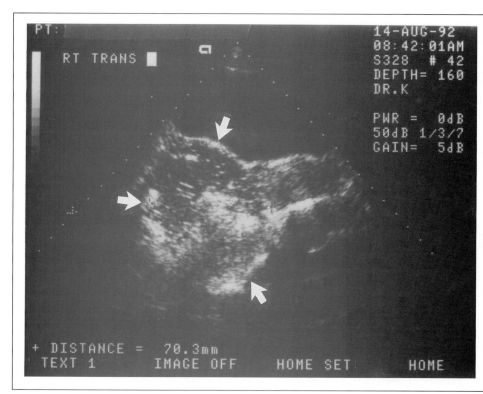

Figure 53-6

Dermoid. A mass of fat and hair produce heterogeneously echogenic areas in this dermoid (*arrows*).

dronephrosis. If the pain is in the midline or to the right of midline, an attempt should be made to visualize the appendix. When the appendix is inflamed and swollen, its wall is thickened and echoic areas may be seen within it (air or a fecalith) (Fig. 53-8*A* and *B*). Diverticulitis may produce a mass as well, but again, it will be separate from the ovaries. It is important to inspect an ultrasound report for identification of the ovaries and to ask whether a mass could be definitely seen to be separate from the ovaries.

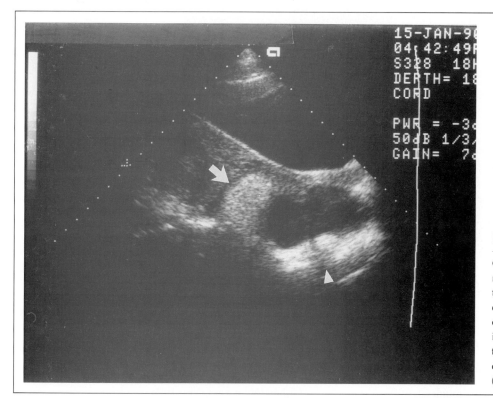

Figure 53-7

Combination of benign ovarian masses. This case demonstrates that it may be impossible to determine the nature of an ovarian mass by ultrasound. This is a combination of a cystic teratoma (*arrow*), serous cystadenoma, and teratoma (arrowhead).

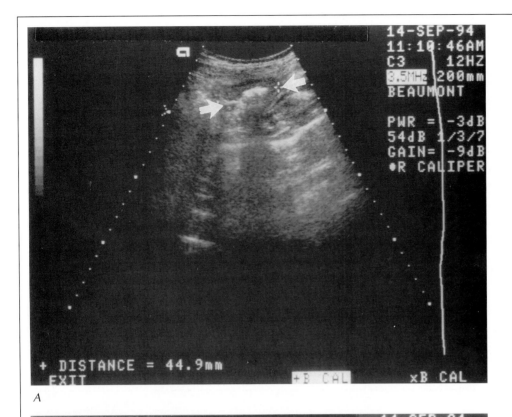

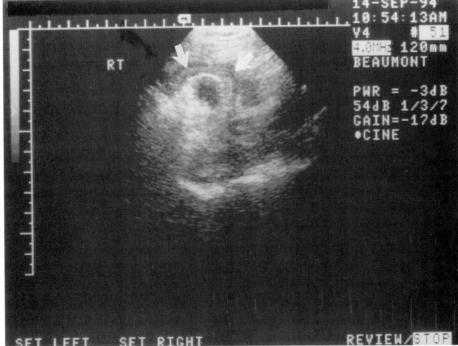

Figure 53-8

Appendicitis. *A.* The length of the appendix is bracketed by arrows. Note the linear echo within the appendix. *B.* The appendix wall (*arrows*) is thickened and the interior contains an echogenic ring. This appearance can be mimicked by an inflamed fallopian tube.

Suggested Readings

Sabbagha RE: *Diagnostic Ultrasound Applied to Obstetrics and Gynecology.* Philadelphia: Lippincott, 1994.

Shirkhoda A, Madrazo B: *Pelvic Ultrasound.* Baltimore: Williams & Wilkins, 1993.

Rumack C, Wilson S, Charboneau JW: *Diagnostic Ultrasound.* St Louis: Mosby–Year Book, 1991.

Callen P: *Ultrasonography in Obstetrics and Gynecology.* Philadelphia: Saunders, 1994.

PART VII

GYNECOLOGIC ONCOLOGY

Chapter 54

PAIN MANAGEMENT IN THE GYNECOLOGIC ONCOLOGY PATIENT

Catherine Christen

James A. Roberts

The general public has come to equate the diagnosis of cancer with the development of pain.[1] A recent survey of women diagnosed with gynecologic cancer[2] has revealed that while 56 percent feared dying, even more (63 percent) were afraid of pain. The presence and management of pain were found to be the two greatest concerns of women who were facing gynecologic cancer. These fears are not unfounded, as it has been estimated by the World Health Organization that 25 percent of all patients with cancer will experience unrelieved pain.[3] Therefore it should not be surprising that many of these women end up in the emergency setting requesting relief. All too often, this relief is all that the physician is able to provide.

While the presence of *chronic* pain from cancer may not be considered an emergency in the usual sense, its has been shown to increase the risk of suicide.[4] One only need to look at the cases of highly publicized physician-assisted suicides in terminally ill women with pain to see the emergent nature of this condition. The fact that many of these women could have had their pain controlled with oral analgesics[5] makes this situation all the more concerning. A report from 54 Eastern Cooperative Oncology Group centers[6] revealed that the problem of poor pain control is often the result of failure on the part of the treating physician to understand the nature and treatment of cancer pain. They also found that uncontrolled pain was more common in their female patients.

The best approach to the management of cancer pain is through an established multidisciplinary pain service. However, all too often it falls to the emergency department physician to address this *chronic* condition when it becomes an *acute* problem. This chapter is provided as a guide for the emergency department physician to use when these women present for care.

OBSTACLES TO ADEQUATE PAIN CONTROL

Before pain treatment can be initiated, several obstacles must be overcome by both patient and physician. The most significant of these is both parties' fear of addiction. The major emphasis of the "War on Drugs" has been a public relations effort to show the adverse effects of drug use. This picture of addiction is very vivid in the minds of most women who present for pain relief. Such a patient must be informed that addiction is possible, but that it should be viewed as no more evil than a diabetic's *addiction* to insulin or her own *addiction* to air! In each of these cases, the addiction is to a chemical that is necessary for the individual to function normally. The use of these drugs will not induce the drug-seeking behavior seen in those with physical pain who are addicted to drugs.

Physicians are also affected by the concern about addiction.[7,8] This concern arises in the same way as it does in their patients but also stems from their experience in treating women with addiction problems. Again, drugs must be viewed as playing an important part of patient care just as any other nonaddicting medication would be. In addition, through review of the actions of state medical boards, one sees another concern physicians have about the use of pain medication—i.e., most disciplinary actions taken by these boards are drug-related. Therefore, many physicians are concerned that if they provide the pain medication their patients need, they will find themselves at the center of a disciplinary action. They often lack the necessary training and/or role models to help them deal with this concern.[9] State medical boards have, in fact, taken disciplinary action for appropriate dispensing of narcotics for oncology patients. The development of standardized pain-management guidelines should help physicians to overcome these concerns.[10] Finally, many states, as a part of their antidrug programs, have developed special prescription forms for the dispensing of most pain medications. While these help to protect the general public from illicit drugs, they become an additional barrier to obtaining needed medication for those in pain. It is mandatory that anyone who cares for these women, including emergency department physicians, have these prescription forms.

The final obstacle to pain control is the patient's difficulty in communicating. Nearly 40 percent of women with gynecologic cancer express a concern about communicating with their physicians.[2] This communication problem, coupled with the concern about addiction, often stands in the way of pain management. Thus, it is incumbent upon the physician to question every woman with a cancer diagnosis about pain control, no matter what her presenting complaint may be. In addition, she must be made to feel comfortable about expressing the need for such aid.

PATHOPHYSIOLOGY OF PAIN

Portenoy[11] has suggested that the pathophysiology of pain can be viewed in two broad categories: nociceptive, or that pain which is caused by direct organ damage, and neuropathic (nonnociceptive), or pain resulting from nervous system dysfunction. Women battling gynecologic cancer can present with either or both forms of pain.

In most cases, the pain gynecologic cancer patients present with is of the nociceptive type. Women with squamous cell carcinoma of the lower genital tract can experience severe, deep pain when the disease invades the pelvic bones or a dull, throbbing pain with invasion to the soft tissue of the pelvis. In cases where more distant spread has occurred, back pain may occur in the face of paraaortic lymph node invasion or point pain may present at the site of bony invasion. In those women with epithelial ovarian cancer or uterine adenocarcinoma, the pain can spread throughout the abdominal cavity. In these cases, it results from the interaction of the disease with the abdominal organs. This is generally a colicky or deep gnawing pain. Pain medications are useful for all these types of pain except for the colicky pain caused by intestinal obstruction.

Neuropathic pain can often be seen in women who have received cytotoxic therapy. The most common regimen for ovarian cancer is a combination of cisplatin (Platinol) and paclitaxel (Taxol). Both of these drugs can induce significant peripheral neuropathies, which are manifest by symptoms of burning pain or uncomfortable numbness. The remaining gynecologic cancers are treated with these and other neurotoxic drugs, which lead women to present to the emergency department with complaints of pain. This discomfort is no less significant than that caused by nociceptive pain, and it requires the same immediate attention.

PAIN ASSESSMENT

A thorough history of the patient's pain must be obtained in order to treat it adequately.[12] Many cancer patients have more than one site of pain, and each site must be assessed individually. Careful physical and neurological examinations must be performed in order to evaluate pain fully. Palliative and provocative factors for pain should be reviewed; these include activities and interventions that make the pain better and worse. The quality of pain should be described by the patient, who should be asked if the pain is sharp, throbbing, burning or tingling, dull, or achy. It is important to have patients locate their pain and to determine if the pain radiates, because radiation of pain can be an indicator of neuropathic damage. The severity of pain, qualitatively measured with the use of visual analogue scales as judged by the patient, are often helpful in measuring the degree of pain control once pain-control treatment has been implemented. These scales can be used quantitatively to assess pain in an individual patient, but they are less useful in comparing patient groups due because of the subjectivity of the measure. Several different types of visual analogue scales can be used. One scale asks patients to rate their pain from zero to ten, with zero being no pain and ten being the worst pain imaginable. Another scale has patients mark on a 100-mm line where they rate their pain. Some scales use color intensity (with red for the most severe pain) and others use faces with smiles and frowns when patients are not able to relate to numerical scales. Temporal factors, such as time of day, are useful to ascertain if there is a variation of pain throughout the day. Interference with daily activities due to pain should be assessed. The patient's psychological state should be evaluated, because anxiety and depression can be significant factors in the cancer patient's experience of pain. Prior history of chronic pain syndromes and drug or alcohol abuse should be elucidated, because this may influence how medications are handled. Finally, response to previous and current analgesic therapies should be determined in order to prescribe therapies more effectively.

PAIN MANAGEMENT

Pain should be managed early, with institution of appropriate therapy. Pain therapy must be individualized and discussed fully with the patient. The World Health Organization (WHO) has devised a stepwise approach to the titration of analgesic therapy on the basis of severity of pain (see Fig. 54-1).[13] The concepts of the WHO approach are as follows: use oral therapy; administer therapy around the clock in a stepwise fashion, using more potent therapies for more severe pain; and individualized therapy for each patient. The first step in this approach to analgesic therapy is the use of acetaminophen, aspirin, or other nonsteroidal anti-inflammatory drugs (NSAIDs) for the relief of mild to moderate pain. These drugs can also be used adjuvantly to enhance pain control with opioids. When pain persists or increases, the second step is to add moderately potent opioids, such as codeine or oxycodone to the first-step therapy (acetaminophen or NSAIDs) to provide additive analgesia. Patients who have moderate to severe pain at presentation to the emergency department or pain that continues to persist despite the administration of moderately potent opioids should be managed by using more potent opioids, such as morphine, or higher dosages of the moderately potent opioids.

When drug therapy is inadequate to control pain, other measures—such as parenteral, epidural, or intrathecal infusion of opioids—nerve blocks, surgical procedures, radiation therapy, and/or antineoplastic therapy, should be considered.

ACETAMINOPHEN

Medications such as acetaminophen (Tylenol) have commonly been used to enhance the effectiveness and quality of pain relief of opioid analgesics. Acetaminophen, a metabolite of phenacetin, has both analgesic and antipyretic effects. It has few adverse effects when taken in appropriate dosages; however, with excessive dosing (greater than 4 g/day), it can cause hepatotoxicity[14,15] or nephropathy.[16] In addition, ethanol intake and fasting appear to increase the risk of these long-term effects.[14] Acetaminophen alone or in combination with opioids can be useful in managing postoperative pain after discharge from the hospital. Daily ingestion of some of the opioid/acetaminophen drug combinations (e.g., Tylenol with codeine) can exceed the maximal daily dose of acetaminophen; therefore, these fixed-dose opioid/acetaminophen combinations are not appropriate for the management of cancer pain except as breakthrough pain medications in conjunction with other opioids.

NONSTEROIDAL ANTI-INFLAMMATORY DRUGS

The NSAIDs are helpful in managing not only postoperative pain but also bone pain in cancer patients. Naproxen (Naprosyn), indomethacin (Indocin), and diclofenac (Voltaren) are also useful in the management of neoplastic fevers in cancer patients.[17–20] Only small doses of naproxen (250 mg two or three times daily), indomethacin (25 mg three times daily), or diclofenac (25 mg three times daily) are necessary to achieve this effect. Recommended dosages of NSAIDs for pain management are listed in Table 54-1.

The NSAIDs are thought to exert their anti-inflammatory effect through inhibition of prostaglandin synthesis, although other mechanisms have been proposed to be involved as well. In debilitated cancer patients, use of NSAIDs is not without risk because of their adverse effects profiles (see Table 54-2). The most worrisome adverse effects in cancer patients include

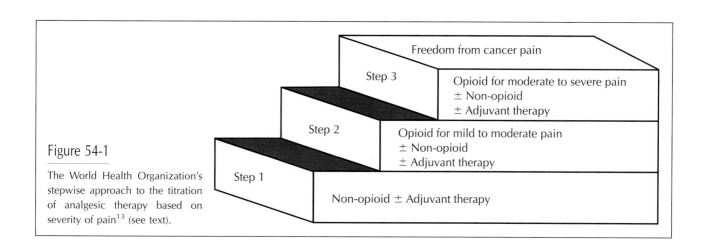

Figure 54-1

The World Health Organization's stepwise approach to the titration of analgesic therapy based on severity of pain[13] (see text).

Freedom from cancer pain

Step 3 — Opioid for moderate to severe pain ± Non-opioid ± Adjuvant therapy

Step 2 — Opioid for mild to moderate pain ± Non-opioid ± Adjuvant therapy

Step 1 — Non-opioid ± Adjuvant therapy

Table 54-1

SELECTED NONOPIOID ANALGESICS: ANALGESIC DOSAGE

Drug	Proprietary Names	Analgesic Dose, mg (avg.)	Dose Interval, H	Daily Adult Dose, mg (max.)	Dosage Units	Comments
Acetaminophen	Tylenol	500–1000 PO	4–6	4000	Tablets: 325 mg, 500 mg Oral liquid: 160 mg/5 mL Rectal suppositories: 325 mg, 650 mg	
Salicylates						
Aspirin	Numerous	650–975 PO	4–6	4000 or 65 mg/kg per day	Tablets: 325 mg Rectal suppositories: 325 mg, 650 mg	Do not use in children <12; enteric-coated tablets decrease GI upset
Choline magnesium trisalicylate	Trilisate	1000–1500 PO	6–12	1500–2500	Tablets: 500 mg, 750 mg, 1000 mg Oral liquid: 500 mg/5 mL	
NSAIDs Proprionic acids						
Ibuprofen	Numerous	400–600 PO	4–6	3200	Tablet and liquid forms	
Ketoprofen	Orudis-KT[a] Actron[a] Orudis, Oruvail SR	25–50 PO 200 (SR) PO[b]	6 12	300	OTC[a] tablets: 12.5 mg Tablets: 25 mg, 50 mg, 75 mg SR[b] capsules: 100 mg, 150 mg, 200 mg	
Naproxen	Naprosyn, generics	500 PO initial 250–375 PO subsequent	8–12	1250	Tablets: 250 mg, 375 mg, 500 mg Oral liquid: 125 mg/5 mL	
Naproxen sodium	Anaprox, Aleve[a]	550 PO initial, 275–550 PO subsequent	8–12	1375	OTC tablets: 200 mg Tablets: 275 mg, 550 mg	
Oxaprozin	Daypro	600 PO	12–24	1800	Tablets: 600 mg	
Nabumetone	Relafen	1000 PO	12–24	2000	Tablets: 500 mg 750 mg	GI-sparing, but expensive
Indoleacetic acids						
Indomethacin	Indocin, generics	25–50 PO	8–12	150	Capsules: 25 mg, 50 mg SR[b] capsule: 75 mg Rectal suppositories: 50 mg	
Sulindac	Clinoril	150–200 PO	12	400	Tablets: 150 mg, 200 mg	
Pyrrolacetic acids						
Ketorolac	Toradol, generics	15 mg IM/IV elderly (≥65) or weight ≤50 kg; 30 mg IM/IV adults age <65 or weight >50 kg; 10 mg PO	6	60 mg IM/IV elderly (≥65) or weight ≤50 kg; 120 mg IM/IV adults age <65 or weight >50 kg; 40 mg PO	Injection: 15 mg, 30 mg, 60 mg Tablets: 10 mg	All forms limited to <5 days therapy; oral form must be used only subsequent to parenteral therapy
Oxicams						
Piroxicam	Feldene, generics	10–20 PO	24	20 mg	Capsules: 10 mg, 20 mg	More photo-sensitivity and rashes

[a]Products available without prescription, over the counter.
[b]Sustained release.
Source: McEvoy[59] and Olin et al.,[60] with permission.

Table 54-2

COMMON ADVERSE EFFECTS OF NON-OPIOID ANTI-INFLAMMATORY DRUGS

Adverse Drug Effect	Comment
Central nervous system	
Dizziness/drowsiness	More common in elderly; prevent by using lower NSAID doses.
Headache	Headache more common with indomethacin.
Aseptic meningitis	Aseptic meningitis has been reported mostly in patients with connective tissue disease commonest with ibuprofen. Symptoms reversible with NSAID discontinuation.
Gastrointestinal	
Gastrointestinal bleeding	Use lower doses in elderly.
	Mucosal barrier breakdown due to inhibition of prostaglandin synthesis.
Nausea/vomiting	Incidence of nausea: 3–9%/vomiting <1–3%
Constipation	Incidence 3–9%
Abdominal pain	Incidence 3–9%; more frequent with nabumetone and ketorolac.
Dyspepsia	Incidence 3–9%; more frequent with ketoprofen and nabumetone.
Diarrhea	Incidence 3–9%; more frequent with meclofenamate and nabumetone. NSAIDs can exacerbate inflammatory bowel disease.
Hepatotoxicity	Up to 15% incidence. Can be dose-related for some NSAIDs and salicylates or possibly a drug hypersensitivity reaction.
Nephrotoxicity	More common in elderly, from prostaglandin inhibition or idiosyncratic reaction.
Dermatologic	
Rashes	Often due to hypersensitivity reaction
Photosensitivity	More common with naproxen and piroxicam.
Hematologic	
Platelets	Aspirin: Irreversible inhibition of platelet function; discontinue 1 week prior to invasive procedures.
	Other NSAIDs: Reversible inhibition of platelet function; discontinue 1–2 days prior to invasive procedures.
Hypersensitivity reactions	Asthma or anaphylaxis; due to susceptibility to prostaglandin synthesis inhibition.

Source: McEvoy[59] and Olin et al.,[60] with permission.

enhanced bleeding potential (due to inhibition of platelet function), renal dysfunction, and formation of gastrointestinal ulcers. The NSAIDs should be used at lower dosages in elderly patients due to the greater risk of adverse effects in this population. Also, NSAIDs can interact with other concurrent therapies, especially cardiovascular medications, because of their ability to inhibit prostaglandin synthesis. A list of some of the more significant drug interactions is given in Table 54-3.

OPIOID THERAPIES

Opioids must be used in effective dosages in order to manage cancer pain adequately (see Tables 54-4 and 54-5). Morphine is the standard of comparison for the potency of opioids, and it is the least costly. Typically, the moderately potent opioids, such as codeine and oxycodone, are used initially, with the more potent opioids—such as morphine, hydromorphone, and methadone—being reserved for severe pain. The duration of effect must be considered in prescribing opioids, as many of the immediate-release formulations are effective over a 3- to 4-hour period only. Sustained-release preparations of morphine (MS Contin and Oramorph-SR) and oxycodone (Oxycontin) or longer-acting agents, such as methadone (Dolophine), can be administered every 8 to 12 hours. Increased opioid dosages over time may be necessary because of the development of opioid tolerance or increasing pain due to further extension of disease.

Prior to conversion to oral therapy, parenteral administration of opioids is often necessary to obtain pain control in the emergency department or inpatient setting. After pain control is obtained, conversion to oral therapy is often possible. If attempts to manage pain with oral therapy fail, other routes of opioid administration should be tried. Transdermal

Table 54-3

COMMON DRUG INTERACTIONS WITH NONSTEROIDAL OR NONOPIOID ANTI-INFLAMMATORY DRUGS

Interacting Drug	Possible Effect
Anticoagulants	Prolongs prothrombin time.
Cardiovascular agents ACE inhibitors Beta blockers Digoxin Loop diuretics Thiazide diuretics	Alteration of sodium homeostasis; fluid retention; loss of blood pressure control.
Cyclosporine	Nephrotoxicity.
Lithium	Increased serum lithium levels.
Methotrexate	Decreased renal tubular secretion of methotrexate, resulting in increased serum methotrexate levels.
Phenytoin	Increased serum phenytoin levels.
Probenecid	Decreased renal clearance of some NSAIDs.

Source: McEvoy[59] and Hansten et al.,[61] with permission.

fentanyl (Duragesic) is much more expensive than oral opioids. Therefore, fentanyl patches should be used only in patients who are unable to tolerate or control pain with oral opioid therapy. Fentanyl transdermal patches are, however, much less costly than intravenous or subcutaneous infusion of opioids. The recommended doses to convert patients from oral or parenteral opioids to transdermal fentanyl are listed in Table 54-6. These dose conversions are based on the assumption that fentanyl is 50 to 100 times more potent than parenteral morphine and 200 to 300 times more potent than oral morphine.[21,22] Fentanyl patches are changed every 72 hours and supplemental doses of opioids may be required during initial dose titration and for episodes of breakthrough pain. There is a lag time after application of the patch until plasma levels of fentanyl are available because a skin reservoir of the drug develops. Although steady-state plasma levels of fentanyl are not reached until after 3 or 4 days, the degree of analgesia and sedation can usually be assessed 24 hours after the patch has been applied in order to titrate the fentanyl dose upward or downward. Elderly patients appear to absorb a greater amount of transdermal fentanyl and/or to clear the drug more slowly, and dosing in the elderly should be more conservative so as to avoid excessive nausea and vomiting, decreased respiratory rate, and other ad-

verse effects.[23] Transdermal fentanyl shares all of the typical adverse effects of oral and parenteral opioids, requiring measures to prevent constipation and other opioid side effects.

Prevention of opioid side effects is important in order to maximize analgesia (see Table 54-7). Many cancer patients have chronic constipation due to decreased fluid and food intake, tumor involvement with the gastrointestinal tract, lack of mobility, or medications, including opioids, vincristine, and anticholinergic drugs. All patients receiving opioids should be on a regimen to prevent constipation. Tolerance usually develops to the sedating effects of the opioids; however, methylphenidate (Ritalin) may be necessary to improve cognitive function while maximizing the opioid doses needed for analgesia. Methylphenidate has been used successfully in cancer patients to prevent excessive sedation as well as to improve analgesia and the depression associated with cancer.[24–26] Methylphenidate can cause insomnia, hallucinations, and paranoid-aggressive reactions; therefore, the drug should be administered in small doses of 2.5 to 5 mg in the morning and at noon, and the dosage should be increased slowly. The greater portion of the daily methylphenidate dose should be administered in the morning to avoid insomnia at night.

Intraspinal opiate administration which allows for the direct delivery of small amounts of narcotics, may be one of the most exciting developments in cancer pain control, as it greatly decreases the systemic effects of these drugs. At the same time, the effects are dependent on the continuous administration of drug; therefore, women who experience unacceptable results can alter the rate of drug administration (either up or down) in order to eliminate these unwanted side effects. The use of implantable devices has increased the acceptance and safety of these procedures.[58] The single disadvantage of this approach is the fairly rapid development of drug resistance. While this can be addressed by increasing the rate of administration or dosage of the drug, it can result in periods of poor pain control, particularly in those women who have implanted pumps that can be filled only weekly. Therefore it may be necessary to prescribe an additional medication to control this breakthrough pain.

ADJUVANT MEDICATIONS

CORTICOSTEROIDS

In addition to their anti-inflammatory effects in pain management, dexamethasone (Decadron) and prednisone have been useful in managing edema due to brain metastasis and radiation therapy directed to the head and spinal cord. While corticosteroids exert their anti-inflammatory effect through the inhibition of prostaglandin synthesis and other immunosuppressive mechanisms, these drugs may be useful in patients unable to tolerate NSAIDs because they appear not to cause renal dysfunction. Dexamethasone also has excellent antiemetic activity and is useful as a premedication for chemotherapy as well as for managing delayed nausea and

Table 54-4

ORAL OPIOID ANALGESICS COMMONLY USED FOR MODERATE PAIN

	Proprietary Names	Dosing Forms	Initial Adult Dose	Comments
Codeine	Codeine Tylenol No. 2, 3, 4	15-mg, 30-mg, 60-mg tablets Acetaminophen 325 mg/ codeine 15–60 mg	30–60 mg codeine	Often combined with acetaminophen
Hydrocodone	Vicodin Vicodin ES	Acetaminophen 50–750 mg/hydrocodone 5–7.5 mg	5 mg hydrocodone	
Oxycodone	Roxicodone Tylox, Percocet	5-mg tablets; 1-mg/mL liquid Acetaminophen 325–500 mg/oxycodone 5 mg	5–10 oxycodone	
Meperidine	Demerol	50-mg tablets	50 mg	Poor oral absorption (20%) and short duration of analgesia
Pentazocine	Talwin-NX	Pentazocine 50 mg/ naloxone 0.5 mg tablets	50 mg pentazocine	Not recommended; naloxone added to formulation to prevent abuse
Propoxyphene	Darvon Darvocet-N-100	65-mg capsules Acetaminophen 650 mg/ propoxyphene napsylate 100 mg tablets	65–130 mg 1–2 tablets	

*a*Moderately expensive to expensive.
Source: Reisine and Pasternak,[21] Management of Cancer Pain Guideline Panel,[22] American Pain Society,[62] with permission.

vomiting after chemotherapy. Because corticosteroids are immunosuppressive, these drugs can increase the risk of infection in cancer patients, in addition to their multitude of well-known long-term adverse effects.

BIPHOSPHONATES AND STRONTIUM-89

Biphosphonate medications, such as pamidronate (Aredia), have significantly improved the outcome of hypercalcemia and pain due to bony metastasis in normocalcemic cancer patients.[27] Patients tolerate the treatment well except for a 24 percent incidence of drug fever (within the first 24 hours of infusion) and a 12 percent incidence of asymptomatic hypocalcemia. Glover et al. evaluated several different dosing regimens of pamidronate in 61 breast cancer outpatients with painful bony metastasis.[28] These authors found that after 3 months, regimens of pamidronate 60 mg every 4 weeks, 60 mg every 2 weeks, and 90 mg every 4 weeks all resulted in a significant reduction of bone pain by the sixth week of

treatment. Radiographic changes consistent with bone healing of lytic lesions were also found in 25 percent of patients.

Strontium-89 chloride (Metastron), a radioisotope that is incorporated into bone and radiates bone directly, is approved for palliation of cancer pain in patients with widespread bony metastases. Most evaluations have been undertaken in patients with prostatic or breast cancer.[29,30] Strontium 89 relieved pain in 47 to 60 percent of patients, with a duration of response of 3 to 7 months.[29,30] Strontium 89 has significant bone marrow toxicity, especially thrombocytopenia, with nadirs occurring about 6 weeks after treatment;[31] therefore, patients should be carefully evaluated prior to treatment. If treatment with Strontium 89 is being considered, referral to experts in nuclear medicine is required.

BENZODIAZEPINES

Benzodiazepines, such as alprazolam (Xanax), lorazepam (Ativan), and diazepam (Valium), can be very useful in man-

Table 54-5

OPIOID ANALGESICS COMMONLY USED FOR SEVERE PAIN

Drug	Proprietary Name	Oral Equianalgesic Dose, mg	Parenteral Equianalgesic Dose, mg	Initial Oral Dose	Precautions/ Contraindications
Morphine	Roxanol, MS-IR	20–30	10	30 mg PO every 3–4 h 10 mg IM/IV every 3–4 h	Respiratory depression. Use with caution in hepatic disease.
Morphine SR	MS Contin,[a] Oramorph-SR[a]	20–30	Not applicable	30 mg PO every 8–12 h; equal to intake of immediate-release morphine	Sustained-release preparations release drug over 8–12 h.
Hydromorphone	Dilaudid	7.5	1.5	4 mg PO every 3 h 1–2 mg IV every 2 h	
Oxycodone	Generic oxycodone Oxycontin-SR[a] Oxycodone/ acetaminophen: Tylox, Percocet	5–10	Not applicable	5–10 mg PO every 3–4 h	
Methadone	Dolophine	20	10	20 mg PO every 6–8 h 10 IV every 6–8 h	Accumulates with repetitive dosing (days 2–5). Good for chronic pain, but not for acute pain.
Levorphanol	Levo-Dromoran[a]	4	2	4 mg PO q 6–8 h 2 mg IM q 6–8 h	CNS reactions can be problematic.
Fetanyl	Duragesic[a] transdermal patches	100 μg/h	0.1	Individualize dose based on intake of opioid medications. In opioid-naive patients, start at 25 μg/h. Change patch every 72 hours.	Wait 24 h to evaluate response. Fever increases release rate of drug. Use breakthrough pain medications.
Meperidine	Demerol	300	1–2 mg/kg	Not recommended (*see* Table 54-4)	Avoid in patients with impaired renal function and in those receiving MAOIs.

[a]Moderately expensive to expensive.
Source: Reisine and Pasternak,[21] Management of Cancer Pain Guideline Panel,[22] American Pain Society,[62] with permission.

Table 54-6

CONVERSION OF MORPHINE TO TRANSDERMAL FENTANYL

Parenteral Morphine,[a] 24-h intake, mg/day $\mu g/h$	Oral Morphine, 24-h intake, mg/day	Transdermal Fentanyl,[b]
up to 65	45–134	25
66–112	135–224	50
113–157	225–314	75
158–202	315–404	100
203–247	405–494	125
248–292	495–584	150
293–337	585–674	175
338–382	675–764	200

[a]Based on conversion ratio of 1:2 for parenteral to oral morphine.
[b]Fentanyl 25 $\mu g/h$ should be used in opioid-naive patients.
Sources: Reisine and Pasternak[21] and Janssen Pharmaceutica,[64]

aging anxiety and muscle spasms in cancer patients. Often, family pressures and concern about the future may cause significant anxiety and insomnia in cancer patients with pain, which can worsen their pain. Small doses of benzodiazepines can relieve anxiety and muscle spasms and thereby reduce pain.

ANTIDEPRESSANT MEDICATIONS

Antidepressant medications are effective in the management of neuropathic pain in patients with both normal and depressed moods. Antidepressant medications have been evaluated in several chronic pain populations—including those with headache, diabetic and postherapetic neuropathies, and rheumatic and back pain. However, there are few evaluations in the literature of antidepressant medications for the management of cancer pain.

The mechanism of action of tricyclic antidepressants (TCAs) and other antidepressants is not thought to be mediated by their antidepressant activity because of a much faster onset of action of pain relief than that of their antidepressant effect. The TCAs inhibit presynaptic reuptake of serotonin and norepinephrine—neurotransmitters required to modulate the endogenous pain-suppressing system. They also block histamine receptors, interact with opioid receptors, and have a membrane-stabilizing effect similar to that of quinidine.[32] Amitriptyline[33] (Elavil), imipramine[34,35] (Tofranil), doxepin[36,37] (Sinequan), desipramine[36,38] (Norpramin) and nortriptyline[39] (Aventyl or Pamelor), have all been used in the management of neuropathic pain. Other antidepressant medications have been used less frequently, including paroxetine[40,41] (Paxil) and trazodone[22] (Desyrel).

Amitriptyline has been evaluated more fully for chronic pain than the other antidepressants; however, because of its anticholinergic and cardiovascular effects, this drug may not be tolerated by many debilitated cancer patients. Doxepin and nortriptyline are safer antidepressants in patients with cardiovascular disease because they have fewer anticholinergic effects. The dosage of antidepressants required for analgesia is usually less than that required for treatment of depression.[42] Plasma concentrations of TCAs needed to achieve neuropathic pain relief are also much lower than those required for antidepressant activity.[43] If a patient is clinically depressed in addition to being in pain, the antidepressant dosage may be titrated up to that required for the treatment of depression (see Table 54-8). It is recommended that the dosage of antidepressants be titrated slowly, starting with the smallest dose and increasing the dose as often as every 3 days. Because of the sedating effects of these drugs, it is recommended that the entire dose or the greater portion of it be given at bedtime.

ANTICONVULSANT MEDICATIONS

Anticonvulsant medications have also been used for the management of neuropathic pain and are generally utilized after a trial of antidepressant medications. The mechanism of these medications is incompletely understood; however, effects on the descending pathways of the spinothalmic tract have been proposed. These drugs have significant adverse-reaction profiles and potential for drug interactions.

Carbamazepine (Tegretol) has been used for the management of trigeminal neuralgia and neuropathic pain.[44,45] The mechanism of pain relief is thought to be related to their ability to block sodium channels in nerve cells. Carbamazepine is typically started at doses of 200 mg twice daily, with an increase in dose based on therapeutic efficacy and plasma levels. Plasma concentrations should be measured to ensure that toxic levels are avoided. The maximum trough level should be <12 $\mu g/mL$. The adverse-reaction profile of carbamazepine includes central nervous system effects, rashes, and leukopenia.

Phenytoin (Dilantin) is infrequently used for the management of neuropathic pain[46,47] because of its adverse-effects profile and potential for drug interactions with other medications. Due to the its nonlinear pharmacokinetics, phenytoin must be gradually titrated for relief of pain. The usual starting dose of phenytoin is 100 mg two or three times daily, with assessment of phenytoin plasma levels to ensure that they remain below 20 $\mu g/mL$ to avoid toxicity.

Gabapentin (Neurontin) is indicated for adjunctive therapy in the management of partial seizures with and without secondary generalization in adults with epilepsy. Because gabapentin is very well tolerated, many practitioners are using it for the management of neuropathic pain despite the lack of controlled trials. There have been a few anecdotal reports of gabapentin's effectiveness in the management of neuropathic pain, including reflex sympathetic dystrophy,[48] postherpetic neuralgia,[49] migraine headaches,[50] radiation

Table 54-7

PREVENTION AND MANAGEMENT OF OPIOID ADVERSE EFFECTS

Adverse Drug Effect	Prevention	Management

Constipation	Increased activity and exercise
	Increased fluid and fiber dietary intake
	Stool softeners
	   Docusate sodium (Colace)
	   Psyllium (Metamucil)
	Stimulant laxatives
	   Bisacodyl (Dulcolax)
	   Milk of magnesia
	   Senna (Senokot)
		Stimulant laxatives
		   Milk of magnesia
		   Bisacodyl (Dulcolax)
		Enemas

Sedation	Tolerance occurs over time	Change opioid
		Decrease opioid dose and increase dosing frequency (maintain same daily dose if pain is well-controlled).
		CNS stimulant medications:
		   Methylphenidate (Ritalin) 2.5–10 mg every morning and noon (Start with low doses and titrate up)
		   Caffeine (tea, coffee, soft drinks, etc.)

Nausea/vomiting	Tolerance occurs over time	Determine cause of nausea/vomiting (opioid or physiological)
		Change opioid
		Decrease opioid dose and increase dosing frequency
		Antiemetics
		   Prochlorperazine 10 mg PO/IV, 25 mg PR
		   Thiethylperazine 10 mg PO/IM

Pruritus	Tolerance occurs over time	Antihistamines
		   Diphenhydramine (Benadryl) 25–50 mg PO IV
		   Hydroxyzine (Atarax) 25–50 mg PO/IM
		Change opioid

Respiratory depression	Use of low opioid doses Caution with concurrent use of benzodiazepines and tranquilizers	Naloxone 0.1 mg IV, repeat as needed
Urinary retention	Use of low opoid doses	Change opoid
Hypersensitivity reactions	Reactions are very rare	Change to a different class of opioids Morphine derivatives: morphine, codeine, oxycodone, hydromorphone Meperidine derivatives: meperidine and fentanyl Methadone derivatives: methadone, propoxyphene

Cardiovascular effects
  Orthostatic hypotension
  Peripheral vasodilation
	Use of low opioid doses
	Maintain good hydration
		Hydration with IV fluid

Table 54-8

ANTIDEPRESSANT MEDICATIONS COMMONLY USED FOR CANCER AND CHRONIC PAIN

Drug	Proprietary Names	Usual Starting Dose, mg/day	Usual Analgesic Dose, mg/day	Effective Antidepressant Dose, mg/day	Maximum Dose	Dosage Units	Comments
Amitriptyline[32,42,65-67]	Elavil	10–25	25–75 PO	50–150 PO 10–40 IM	300 mg/day PO	10-mg, 25-mg, 50-mg, 75-mg, 100-mg tablets; 10-mg/mL injection (IM)	Anticholinergic side effects. Avoid in cardiovascular disease or glaucoma.
Nortriptyline[39,42]	Pamelor, Aventyl	25	25–100	75–100 PO	100 mg/day PO	10-mg, 25-mg, 50-mg capsules; 10-mg/mL oral liquid	Metabolite of amitriptyline. Fewer anticholinergic effects and less sedating.
Imipramine[34,35,42]	Tofranil	10–25	25–75	50–150 PO 25–100 IM	200 mg PO 100 mg/day IM	10-mg, 25-mg, 50-mg tablets; 12.5-mg/mL injection	Anticholinergic side effects.
Desipramine[38,42,50,67]	Norpramin	25–50	25–100	100–200 PO	300 mg/day PO	25-mg, 50-mg tablets	Metabolite of imipramine.
Doxepin[23,637,42]	Sinequan	10–25	25–75	75–150 PO	300 mg/day PO	10-mg, 25-mg, 50-mg capsules; 10-mg/mL oral liquid	Well tolerated in the elderly. Fewer anticholinergic side effects.
Trazodone[33]	Desyrel	25–50	75–225	150–400 PO	400 mg/day PO	50-mg, 100-mg tablets	Good hypnotic effects
Paroxetine[40,41]	Paxil	10		10–50 PO	50 mg/day PO	20-mg, 30-mg tablets	

myelopathy,[51] and other peripheral neuropathies. These reports indicate that the effective dose of gabapentin is often lower than the dose required for seizure control. The usual starting dose of gabapentin for neuropathic pain is 300 mg once daily, then twice daily the following day, and then three times daily. Gabapentin is cleared renally; therefore, it is recommended that doses not exceeding 600 mg/day be used for patients with creatinine clearances ranging from 30 to 60 mL/min, 300 mg/day for patients with clearances ranging from 15 to 30 mL/min, 300 mg every other day for patients with clearances less than 15 mL/min, and 200 to 300 mg after every hemodialysis session for patients with end-stage renal disease.[52] The adverse-effects profile of gabapentin includes central nervous system reactions such as dizziness, paresthesias, decreased or increased reflexes, hypertension, bruising, and visual changes.

INDICATIONS FOR ADMISSION AND SPECIALTY CONSULTATION

In most cases, the women presenting with acute pain can be treated with one of the regimens listed above and discharged to their homes. However, acute control may not always be achieved, particularly in those women who have experienced long-standing pain. In these cases a hospital admission may be required and larger doses of pain medication administered. This requires close supervision by the health care team. In these cost-conscious times, many see this as an unnecessary use of hospital resources, but it will likely eliminate several return trips to the emergency department, which would use even more resources. In addition, the improvement in patient quality of life resulting from improved pain control should be considered a fair return for the cost incurred. Last, this admission may allow the introduction of a multidisciplinary pain service into the woman's care. This group—made up of oncologists, pain specialists, nurses, social workers, physiatrists, physical therapists, psychologists, psychiatrists, community healthcare providers, clergy, and hospice workers—can provide the most effective management of cancer pain.[53]

There are certain instances where consultation is required. These occur when women present with pain that is symptomatic of a condition requiring surgical correction. In the case of gynecologic cancers, these are generally obstructive processes, gastrointestinal or urinary. It is very common for a woman with ovarian cancer to develop intestinal obstructions. The pain resulting from these can be relieved with medication, but this simply masks the condition. The pain will return, in some cases with more intensity, when the effects of the medicine have worn off. These conditions require suction decompression or operative intervention to decompress the distended bowel. Any cancer arising in the pelvis can adversely affect the urinary tract, with resulting obstructive symptoms. As with bowel obstructions, these require decompression rather than pain medication. In all of these cases, a consultation with a gynecologic oncologist or surgical specialist familiar with gynecologic cancer must be obtained and hospital admission is likely.

NONPHARMACOLOGIC TREATMENT

With the development of so many pain-controlling chemicals, the demand for nonpharmacologic procedures has decreased greatly. However, there are some women who do not achieve adequate control with any of the many agents available. These women require consultation from a pain team with expertise in nonpharmacologic techniques.

Neurostimulation techniques have been around for many years. The most commonly used technique is the *transcutaneous electrical nerve stimulation* (TENS), comprising small, battery-operated units including electrodes that are applied to the area of discomfort. They have been shown to provide good short-term benefit, but their effectiveness can decrease quickly. Their benefit can be augmented by incorporating the use of psychotropic drugs and NSAIDs. This system can be used for *dorsal column stimulation* by applying the electrical stimulation to the dorsal columns of the spinal cord. This positioning increases A-fiber input, which will inhibit marginal cells in lamina 1 while stimulating the cerebral endorphin system. Again, a short-term benefit is seen in most (up to 80 percent), but long-term improvement is limited to as few as 30 percent. In those who experience good relief with this approach, both the electrodes and the generator can be implanted for patient convenience. This form of pain control is most appropriate for neuropathic pain.

Severe somatic or visceral pain can be approached with *deep brain stimulation*. This technique involves electrical stimulation of the medial thalamus and midbrain reticular formation via stereotaxically placed electrodes. These are attached to a radiofrequency generator, which is activated for 20 min two to three times per day. This stimulation activates the enkephalins and endorphins, which produce opiate-like analgesia.

The most basic and direct approaches to the relief of cancer pain may be those that involve the surgical or chemical *transection* of the nerves carrying the pain. These approaches include neurosurgical procedures, neurolytic blocks, intraspinal opiate techniques, and local anesthetic regional blocks.

Neurosurgical procedures—which include hypophysectomy, sympathectomy, dorsal rhizotomy, dorsal root entry zone lesions, and cordotomy—have a long track record for successful pain control. Improvement in these techniques have resulted in the development of percutaneous approaches for many ablative procedures.[54] However, careful patient selection is required before any woman is offered one of these procedures. Those who have a life expectancy of less than 3 months should not be considered. In addition, the refinement of pharmacologic and intraspinal opiate administration has greatly reduced the demand for neurosurgical interventions. At the same time, Loeser[55] has found that the ill effects of these procedures are so frequent that for every woman who benefits from them there are likely to be two who experience no improvement or are made worse as a result of increased pain or neurologic deficit. Some of the causes for this may be related to the fact that few neurosurgeons have sufficient experience in performing these procedures.

While the neurosurgical procedures have become less common, the neurolytic blocks have enjoyed widespread use. With experience, an anesthesiologist can become very skilled in the administration of blocks to the subarachnoid/epidural region, lumbar sympathetic nerve, sacral root, or superior hypogastric plexus, which will offer relief to those women suffering from cancer-related pain.[56] Neurolytic blocks can also be placed[57] under computed tomography guidance. The most common agents used in these procedures are ammonium sulfate, phenol, and ethyl alcohol. It must be remembered that, just as with the neurosurgical procedures, these techniques can lead to worsening of the pain or the development of side effects, which may be viewed as more concerning than the original pain. Once again, patient selection is of major importance in the successful use of these procedures.

The pain due to bony metastases that is not controlled by systemic drug therapy can be palliated with radiation treatment. Consultation with a radiation oncologist is helpful to determine how best to approach these patients.

DISCHARGE INSTRUCTIONS AND FOLLOW-UP

It is important to make sure that patients are prescribed an adequate supply of medication to last until the next clinic visit so as to avoid problems with refills. Schedule II controlled substances cannot be refilled and may require special prescription forms in some states. Most pharmacies will not accept telephone prescriptions for controlled substances. Patients should be informed of potential side effects of these medications, as well as measures to manage side effects.

References

1. Levin DN, Cleeland CS, Dar R: Public attitudes toward cancer pain. *Cancer* 56:2337, 1985.
2. Roberts JA, Brown D, Elkins TE, Larson D: Influences on gynecologic cancer patients' preferences in end-of-life decisions. *Am J Obstet Gynecol.* In press.
3. Portenory RK: Cancer pain: Epidemiology and syndromes. *Cancer* 63:2298, 1989.
4. Breitbart W: Suicide, in Holland J, Rowland J (eds): *Handbook of Psychooncology.* New York: Oxford University Press, 1990, pp 291–299.
5. Ventafridda V, Tamburini M, Caraceni A, et al: A validation study of the WHO method for cancer pain relief. *Cancer* 59:850, 1987.
6. Cleeland CS, Gonin R, Hatfield AK, et al: Pain and its treatment in outpatients with metastatic cancer. *N Engl J Med* 330:592, 1994.
7. Hill CS, Fields HL (eds): *Drug Treatment of Cancer Pain in a Drug-Oriented Society: Advances in Pain Research and Therapy.* Vol 11. New York: Raven Press, 1990.
8. Friedman D: Perspectives on the medical use of drugs of abuse. *J Pain Symptom Mgt* 5(suppl):S2, 1990.
9. von Roenn JH, Cleeland CS, Gonin R, et al: Physician attitudes and practice in cancer pain management: A survey from the eastern cooperative oncology group. *Ann Intern Med* 119:121, 1993.
10. Acute Pain Management Guideline Panel: *Acute Pain Management: Operative and Medical Procedures and Trauma: Clinical Practice Guideline.* AHCPR Pub no 92-0032. Rockville, Md: Agency for Health Care Policy and Research, Public Health Service, U.S. Department of Health and Human Services, 1992.
11. Portenoy RK: Mechanisms of clinical pain: observations and speculations. *Neurol Clin* 7:207, 1989.
12. Foley KM: Supportive care and the quality of life of the cancer patient: Management of cancer pain, in DeVita VT, Hellman S, Rosenberg SA (eds): *Cancer: Principles and Practice of Oncology,* 4th ed. Philadelphia: Lippincott, 1993, pp 2417–2448.
13. World Health Organization: *Cancer Pain Relief and Palliative care. Report of a WHO Expert Committee* (World Health Organization Technical Report Series, 804). Geneva: World Health Organization, 1990, pp 1–75.
14. Whitcomb DC, Block GD: Association of acetaminophen hepatoxicity with fasting and ethanol use. *JAMA* 272:1845, 1994.
15. Bonkowsky H: Chronic hepatic inflammation and fibrosis due to low dose of paracetamol. *Lancet* 1:1016, 1978.
16. Perneger TV, Whelton PK, Klag MJ: Risk of kidney failure associated with the use of acetaminophen, aspirin, and non-steroidal antiinflammatory drugs. *N Engl J Med* 331:1675, 1994.
17. Chang JC, Gross HM: Utility of naproxen in the differential diagnosis of fever of undetermined origin in patients with cancer. *Am J Med* 76:597, 1984.
18. Romeu J, Chadha N, Fukilman O et al: Indomethacin therapy in symptomatic hepatic neoplasms. *Am J Gastroenterol* 77:655, 1982.
19. Chang JC, Gross HM: Neoplastic fever responds to the treatment of an adequate dose of naproxen. *J Clin Oncol* 3:552, 1985.

20. Tsavaris N, Zinelis A, Karabelis A, et al: A randomized trial of the effect of three non-steroid anti-inflammatory agents in ameliorating cancer-induced fever. *J Intern Med* 228:451, 1990.

21. Reisine T, Pasternak G: Opioid analgesics and antagonists, in Hardman JG, Limbird LE, Molinoff PB, et al (eds): *Goodman & Gilman's The Pharmacological Basis of Therapeutics,* 9th ed. New York: McGraw-Hill, 1996, pp 521–555.

22. Management of Cancer Pain Guideline Panel: *Clinical Practice Guideline: Management of Cancer Pain.* Rockville, MD: U.S. Department of Health and Human Services, 1994.

23. Holdsworth MT, Forman WB, Killilea TA, et al: Transdermal fentanyl disposition in elderly subjects. *Gerontology* 40:32, 1994.

24. Fernandez F, Adams F, Holmes VF, et al: Methylphenidate for depressive disorders in cancer patients: An alternative to standard antidepressants. *Psychosomatics* 28:455, 1987.

25. Bruera E, Miller MJ, Macmillan K, et al: Neuropsychological effects of methylphenidate in patients receiving a continuous infusion of narcotics for cancer pain. *Pain* 48:163, 1992.

26. Bruera E, Chadwick S, Brenneis C, et al: Methylphenidate associated with narcotics for the treatment of cancer pain. *Cancer Treat Rep* 71:67, 1987.

27. Averbuch SD: New biphosphonates in the treatment of bone metastases. *Cancer* 72:3443, 1993.

28. Glover D, Lipton A, Keller A, et al: Intravenous pamidronate disodium treatment of bone metastases in patients with breast cancer: A dose-seeking study. *Cancer* 74:2949, 1994.

29. Robinson RG: Strontium-89: Precursor targeted therapy for pain relief of blastic metastatic disease. *Cancer* 72:3433, 1993.

30. Berna L, Carrio I, Alonso C, et al: Bone pain palliation with strontium-89 in breast cancer patients with bone metastases and refractory bone pain. *Eur J Nucl Med* 22:1101, 1995.

31. Lee CK, Aeppli DM, Unger J, et al: Strontium-89 chloride (Metastron) for palliative treatment of bony metastases: The University of Minnesota experience. *Am J Clin Oncol* 19:102, 1996.

32. Sindrup SH, Brosen K, Gram LF: The mechanism of action of antidepressants in pain treatment: Controlled cross-over studies in diabetic neuropathy. *Clin Neuropharmacol* 15(suppl 1):380A, 1992.

33. Ventafridda V, Bonezzi C, Caraceni A, et al: Antidepressants for cancer pain and other painful syndromes with deafferentation component: Comparison of amitriptyline and trazodone. *Ital J Neurol Sci* 8:579, 1987.

34. Sindrup SH, Ejlertsen B, Froland A, et al: Imipramine treatment in diabetic neuropathy: Relief of subjective symptoms without changes in peripheral and autonomic nerve function. *Eur J Clin Pharmacol* 37:151, 1989.

35. Kvinesdal B, Molin J, Froland A, et al: Imipramine treatment of diabetic neuropathy. *JAMA* 251:1727, 1984.

36. Ward N, Bokan JA, Phillips M, et al: Antidepressants in concomitant chronic back pain and depression: Doxepin and desipramine compared. *J Clin Psychiatry* 45(3 sec 2):54, 1984.

37. Hameroff SR, Weiss JL, Lerman JC, et al: Doxepin's effects on chronic pain and depression: A controlled study. *J Clin Psychiatry* 45(3 pt 2):47, 1984.

38. Kishore-Kumar R, Max MB, Schafer SC, et al: Desipramine relieves post-herpetic neuralgia. *Clin Pharmacol Ther* 47:305, 1990.

39. Panerai AE, Monza G, Movilia P, et al: A randomized within-patient, cross-over, placebo-controlled trial on the efficacy and tolerability of the tricyclic antidepressants chlorimipramine and nortriptyline in central pain. *Acta Neurol Scand* 82:34, 1990.

40. Sindrup SH, Grodum E, Gram LF, et al: Concentration-response relationship in paroxetine treatment of diabetic neuropathy symptoms: A patient-blinded dose-escalation study. *Ther Drug Monit* 13:408, 1991.

41. Sindrup SH, Gram LF, Brosen K, et al: The selective serotonin reuptake inhibitor paroxetine is effective in the treatment of diabetic neuropathy symptoms. *Pain* 42:135, 1990.

42. Godfrey RG: A guide to the understanding and use of tricyclic antidepressants in the overall management of fibromyalgia and other chronic pain syndromes. *Arch Intern Med* 156:1047, 1996.

43. Sindrup SH, Gram LF, Skjold T, et al: Concentration-response relationship in imipramine treatment of diabetic neuropathy symptoms. *Clin Pharmacol Ther* 47:509, 1990.

44. Tomson T, Ekbom K: Trigeminal neuralgia: time course of pain in relation to carbamazepine dosing. *Cephalalagia* 1:91, 1981.

45. Tanelian DL, Brose WG: Neuropathic pain can be relieved by drugs that are use-dependent sodium channel blockers: Lidocaine, carbamazepine, and mexiletine. *Anesthesiology* 74:949, 1991.

46. Yajnik S, Singh GP, Singh G, Kumar M: Phenytoin as a coanalgesic in cancer pain. *J Pain Symptom Mgt* 7:209, 1992.

47. Swerdlow M, Cundill JG: Anticonvulsant drugs used in the treatment of lancinating pain, a comparison. *Anaesthesia* 36:1129, 1981.

48. Mellick GA, Mellick LB: Gabapentin in the management of reflex sympathetic dystrophy. *J Pain Symptom Mgt* 10:265, 1995.

49. Segal AZ, Rordorf G: Gabapentin as a novel treatment for post herpetic neuralgia (letter). *Neurology* 46:1175, 1996.

50. Mathew NT, Lucker C: Gabapentin in migraine prophylaxis: A preliminary open label study (abstr). *Neurology* 46:A169, 1996.

51. Cheville A, Narcessian E, Elliot K: Neuropathic pain in radiation myelopathy: A case report (abstr). 14th Annual Scientific Meeting of American Pain Society, 1995.

52. Parke-Davis. *Neurontin product information.* Morris Plains, NJ: Parke-Davis, 1994.

53. NIH Consensus Development Conference Statement: The integrated approach to the management of pain. 6: 1986.

54. Sanders M. Zuurmond W: Safety of unilateral and bilateral percutaneous cervical cordotomy in 80 terminally ill cancer patients. *J Clin Oncol* 13:1509, 1995.

55. Loeser JD: Ablative neurosurgical procedures, in Bonica JJ (ed): *The Management of Pain.* Philadelphia: Lea & Febiger, 1990, pp 2040–2043.

56. de Leon-Casasola OA, Kent E, Lema MJ: Neurolytic superior hypogastric plexus block for chronic pelvic pain associate with cancer. *Pain* 54:145, 1993.

57. Orlandini G: Selection of patients undergoing neurolytic superior hypogastric plexus block. *Pain* 56:121, 1994.

58. de Jong PC, Kansen PJ: A comparison of epidural catheters with or without subcutaneous injection ports for treatment of cancer pain. *Anesth Analg* 78:94, 1994.

59. McEvoy GH: *American Hospital Formulary Service Drug Information.* Bethesda, MD: American Society of Health-System Pharmacists, 1996.

60. Olin BR, et al: *Facts and Comparisons.* St. Louis: Facts and Comparisons, 1996.

61. Hansten PD, Horn JR, Koda-Kimble MA, Young LY: *Drug Interactions and Updates.* Vancouver: Applied Therapeutics, 1993.

62. American Pain Society: *Principles of Analgesic Use in the Treatment of Acute Pain and Cancer Pain.* 3d ed. Skokie, IL: American Pain Society, 1993.

63. *1996 Drug Topics Red Book:* Montvale, NJ: Medical Economics Co, 1996.

64. Janssen Pharmaceutica: Duragesic package insert. Titusville, NJ: Janssen Pharmaceutica, 1994.

65. Max MB, Culnane M, Shafer SC, et al: Amitriptyline relieves diabetic neuropathy in patients with normal or depressed mood. *Neurology* 37:589, 1987.

66. McQuay HJ, Carroll D, Glynn CJ: Dose-response for analgesic effect of amitriptyline in chronic pain. *Anaesthesia* 48:281, 1993.

67. Max MB, Lynch SA, Muir J, et al: Effects of desipramine, amitriptyline, and fluoxetine on pain in diabetic neuropathy. *N Engl J Med* 326:1250, 1992.

Chapter 55

GYNECOLOGIC MALIGNANCIES AND COMPLICATIONS OF THEIR MANAGEMENT

R. Kevin Reynolds

Gynecologic malignancies as a group account for 13 percent of all cancers in women. Only breast, lung, and colorectal tumors cause more cancer-related deaths than gynecologic cancers.

Complications attributable to gynecologic malignancies can be divided into several categories. In the first category, symptoms, signs, and syndromes such as bleeding, nausea and vomiting, obstructive uropathy, and paraneoplastic syndromes are often due to the natural history of gynecologic tumors themselves. A brief overview of each type of gynecologic malignancy and its associated natural history will serve as an introduction to the most likely complications encountered.

The second category includes treatment-related complications involving treatment modalities such as surgery, chemotherapy, and radiation therapy. Surgical complications generally occur in the perioperative period and include injury to bowel and urologic systems as well as thromboembolic and bleeding complications. Chemotherapy-related problems include febrile neutropenia, stomatitis, neuropathy, nausea and vomiting, and extravasation injury, among others. Radiation-associated problems include injury to gastrointestinal and genitourinary tracts as well as the possibility of secondary malignancy affecting survivors of therapy years after completion of treatment.

TYPES, INCIDENCE, AND NATURAL HISTORY OF GYNECOLOGIC MALIGNANCIES

ENDOMETRIAL CARCINOMA

Endometrial cancer is the most common gynecologic neoplasm, with an incidence of 32,800 cases resulting in 5900 deaths per year in the United States.[1] About 2.5 to 3 percent of all women will develop endometrial cancer in their lifetimes. The average age at time of incidence is 58 years. Most endometrial cancers are endometrioid adenocarcinomas (75 to 85 percent), many of which will contain areas of squamous differentiation that do not appear to affect the natural history of the tumors. Less common histologic types include the aggressive uterine papillary serous tumors and clear cell carcinomas, accounting for 7 and 4 percent of cases, respectively.

Obesity is a risk factor for development of endometrial cancers. Women who are 20 to 50 lb overweight have a relative risk of 3 compared to women of normal weight, while women who are more than 50 lb overweight are 10 times more likely to develop endometrial cancer. Production of the weak estrogen estrone by adipose cells is thought to lead to development of hyperplastic endometrium, which can, in turn, progress to invasive endometrial cancer. Several other risk factors for endometrial cancer are related to noncyclic or prolonged estrogen stimulation, such as late menopause, the nulligravid state, and unopposed estrogen replacement therapy. Tamoxifen, a weak estrogen analogue used to treat many breast cancers, also increases the risk of endometrial cancer.

Ninety percent of women with endometrial cancer will present with postmenopausal or abnormal vaginal bleeding. The bleeding is rarely heavy enough to be hemodynamically significant. Of all women who present with postmenopausal bleeding, only 15 percent will be found to have endometrial cancer. The likelihood that postmenopausal bleeding indicates the presence of endometrial cancer rises as a function of age. Fewer than 1 percent of women with postmenopausal bleeding who are less than 50 years of age have endometrial cancer, whereas 60 percent of women with postmenopausal bleeding who are more than 80 years old will be found to have endometrial cancer.[2] Persistent vaginal discharge is another common presenting symptom of this disease.

The diagnosis of endometrial cancer is generally obtained via an endometrial biopsy, although if the specimen is nondiagnostic, fractional dilatation and curettage may be warranted. Ultrasonographic measurement of the endometrial stripe thickness may be a useful adjunct for evaluation of postmenopausal bleeding in women when endometrial biopsy is not possible. An endometrial stripe thickness of 5 or more mm is indicative of a higher risk of endometrial cancer.[3] Most cases of endometrial cancer are detected while still at stage I. Staging is surgical and requires that pelvic washing for cytology and sampling of both pelvic and paraaortic lymph nodes be performed at the time of hysterectomy and bilateral salpingo-oophorectomy. Women with low-risk disease (stages IA and IB—myometrial invasion less than one third, grade 1 or 2) do not require postoperative adjuvant therapy and have an expected 5-year survival rate of 85 to 94 percent. Intermediate-risk tumors (stages IB and IC—invasion into the middle or outer third of the myometrium, grade 1 or 2) will often receive postoperative radiation therapy, although this is controversial. Most women with high-risk tumors (stage IC—invasion into outer third of myometrium, or grade 3; or advanced stages with adnexal or lymph node involvement) receive pelvic and possibly paraaortic radiation therapy. Distant metastases are generally treated with investigational chemotherapy protocols because of poor survival using available drugs (only 30 percent response with cisplatin and doxorubicin).

When endometrial cancer recurs, the vagina and pelvis are the most common sites (50 percent), but 25 percent will recur in the lungs. Patients with recurrence may present with vaginal bleeding, uremia due to ureteral or urethral obstruction, pain due to nerve compression, or respiratory symptoms. If they have been previously radiated, they may present with complications associated with radiation injury.

OVARIAN CANCER

There are 26,600 new cases of ovarian cancer each year in the United States, resulting in 14,500 deaths per year. Ovarian cancer is more deadly than all other gynecologic cancers combined.[1] A woman with no family history of ovarian, breast, or colon cancer has a 1.4 percent lifetime risk of developing ovarian cancer. A family history of cancers of the above types increase the risk of developing ovarian cancer. The magnitude of this risk is based on the number and relationship of the affected relatives as well as the identified pedigree. Ovarian cancer can be divided into three major histologic categories: epithelial tumors, germ-cell tumors, and sex-cord stromal tumors. Each histologic type has a very different natural history.

EPITHELIAL TUMORS

The most common type of ovarian cancer is the epithelial variety, which accounts for 80 to 90 percent of ovarian cancers and can be divided into invasive cancer (85 percent) and low-malignant-potential or "borderline" tumors (15 percent). The peak incidence of invasive tumors is between the ages of 55 and 64. Peak incidence for borderline tumors is 10 to 15 years earlier. The invasive tumors are aggressive, and up to 75 percent have metastasized prior to detection, whereas borderline tumors are confined to the ovary (stage I) at the time of diagnosis in up to 80 percent of cases.[4] Unlike germ-cell and sex-cord stromal tumors, epithelial tumors frequently involve both ovaries, making conservative surgery impractical for all but a few cases of early-stage low-malignant-potential tumors. The standard of care has been defined by the National Institutes of Health (NIH) consensus development conference.[5] Initial treatment of invasive and borderline epithelial tumors should include abdominal hysterectomy, bilateral salpingo-oophorectomy, surgical staging, and aggressive attempts to complete cytoreductive surgery. Women with well-differentiated invasive epithelial tumor confined to the internal portions of one or both ovaries (stages IA-1 and IB-1) do not require adjuvant therapy. All women with grade 3 invasive tumors, surface involvement of ovaries (stage IC), or extraovarian metastases (greater than stage I) should receive postoperative chemotherapy. The best currently available chemotherapy regimen for invasive tumors is a combination of cisplatin and paclitaxel. Although the response rate to chemotherapy is excellent, the 5-year survival rate for women with spread of invasive disease in the abdominal cavity (stage III) is only 15 percent. Adjuvant therapy has not been shown to result in improved survival for borderline tumors, but survival is excellent for patients where all of the macroscopic tumor volume is removed.

Ovarian neoplasm is most likely to recur in the abdomen or retroperitoneum. Recurrence is often associated with nausea and vomiting, symptomatic ascites, pelvic and abdominal masses, and obstructions of the small or large bowel.

The tumors occasionally erode into the vagina or erupt through the umbilicus and cause bleeding or discharge. Malignant pleural effusions large enough to cause respiratory compromise occasionally occur, usually in women with ascites. Patients with ovarian cancer are subject to the complications associated with chemotherapy.

GERM-CELL TUMORS

Germ-cell tumors account for 3 to 5 percent of all ovarian cancers and are almost always found in adolescents or women under the age 30. The different cell types of germ-cell tumors include dysgerminomas, endodermal sinus tumors, embryonal carcinomas, immature teratomas, and mixed germ-cell tumors. Most of these tumors, with the occasional exception of dysgerminoma, are unilateral, and the majority are detected while they are confined to the ovary (stage I).[6] Fifty percent of women with dysgenetic gonads eventually develop germ-cell tumors, but only 5 percent of all women with germ-cell tumors will have dysgenetic gonads. The majority of the cases appear to arise sporadically. Presenting symptoms and signs often include pain, sometimes due to torsion or rupture, both of which result in an acute abdomen and are emergencies requiring surgical intervention. A mass will usually be palpable, and tumor markers specific to germ-cell tumors will often be elevated. These include alpha-fetoprotein (endodermal sinus tumors), lactate dehydrogenase, and placental alkaline phosphatase (dysgerminoma), as well as human chorionic gonadotropin (embryonal carcinoma and mixed germ-cell tumors). Immature teratomas are not associated with elevation of a tumor marker. Germ-cell tumors are surgically staged, usually including unilateral salpingo-oophorectomy, lymphadenectomy, omentectomy, and peritoneal biopsies. Postoperative adjuvant therapy varies by tumor type and stage but generally includes chemotherapy with either bleomycin, etoposide, and cisplatin (BEP) or vincristine, dactinomycin, and cyclophosphamide (VAC). Survival for women with germ-cell tumors is generally very good, ranging up to 95 percent, even with advanced-stage lesions. Fertility is generally spared as long as adequate surgical staging is performed, followed by appropriate chemotherapy. Complications associated with these tumors include acute abdomen from torsion or rupture of an enlarged ovary, bowel obstruction in cases of advanced or recurrent disease, and chemotherapy-related complications to be outlined later in this chapter.

SEX-CORD STROMAL TUMORS

Sex-cord stromal tumors are derived from the hormonally active ovarian stroma and account for up to 5 percent of all ovarian cancers.[6] Sertoli-Leydig tumors, which produce androgens often resulting in masculinization, occur at a mean age of 25 years. Granulosa-cell tumors produce estrogens that can lead to the development of endometrial hyperplasia or carcinoma and can occasionally produce androgens leading to masculinization. The average age of incidence of granulosa tumors is 53 years. As with germ-cell tumors, these tumors are unilateral more than 90 percent of the time and are detected while still confined to the ovary (stage I) in 85 percent of cases. Sex-cord stromal tumors are usually staged with unilateral salpingo-oophorectomy in reproductive-age women or hysterectomy with bilateral salpingo-oophorectomy in women no longer wishing to remain fertile. All patients should undergo lymphadenectomy, omentectomy, and peritoneal biopsies. Postoperative adjuvant therapy varies by tumor type and stage but generally includes chemotherapy with either bleomycin, etoposide, and cisplatin (BEP) or cisplatin, vinblastine, and bleomycin (PVB). Survival for women with sex-cord stromal tumors approaches 90 percent, although late recurrence of granulosa-cell tumors causes the 10-year survival rate to drop to 68 percent.

Sex-cord stromal tumors may undergo torsion or rupture, leading to symptoms of peritonitis or acute abdomen. Recurrent or advanced-stage disease may impinge on bowel, leading to obstruction.

CERVICAL CANCER

The incidence of cervical cancer has fallen dramatically in recent decades due to effective screening and treatment of preinvasive lesions. The current incidence of cervical cancer is 15,800 cases per year, which results in 4800 deaths annually in the United States.[1] The average age of women at the time of diagnosis is 54 years. Most cervical cancers are of squamous histology, but 5 to 10 percent are adenocarcinomas. Squamous cervical carcinoma most commonly arises as a result of human papillomavirus (HPV) infection, and HPV DNA is demonstrable in more than 90 percent of these cancers. Cofactors such as smoking and immunodeficiency [human immunodeficiency virus (HIV), glucocorticoids, cyclosporine, and other immunosuppressant drugs] greatly increase cancer risk in HPV-infected individuals. Other risk factors for this disease include early age at first coitus and multiple sexual partners. Cervical adenocarcinomas, which are clinically similar to cervical squamous cancers, contain HPV DNA in only about 30 percent of cases.

Presenting symptoms of cervical cancer include postmenopausal bleeding (46 percent), polymenorrhea or metrorrhagia (20 percent), postcoital bleeding (10 percent), vaginal discharge (9 percent), and pain (6 percent).[2] Physical examination will demonstrate a cervical mass, often friable, which tends to spread by direct extension to the pelvic side wall via the broad ligament causing an adnexal thickness. Lymphatic spread is common, typically involving first the obturator nodes and then the pelvic and paraaortic nodes. Disease confined to the cervix or with minimal spread to the surrounding vagina (stages IB and IIA) can be treated with either radical hysterectomy and pelvic lymphadenectomy or pelvic radiotherapy. Spread of the disease into the supporting cardinal and uterosacral ligaments (stage II) requires treatment with radiation therapy. Most cervical cancers are detected while still confined to the cervix. Treatment of stage I lesions with either radical hysterectomy or radiation results in 5-year survival of 90 percent. When cervical cancer recurs, vaginal apex and pelvic side-wall sites are most common. Radiation is recommended for patients with recurrences after previous surgery. Pelvic exenteration (extirpation of all pelvic viscera including the uterus, vagina, bladder, and rectum, followed by extensive reconstruction) is indicated for selected cases of recurrence after previous radiation therapy and may result in long-term salvage of up to 60 percent.

Untreated cervical cancers are friable and prone to significant bleeding. Large cervical tumors, both untreated and recurrent, may obstruct the ureters, resulting in uremia. Radiation therapy for treatment of cervical cancer is intensive and results in significant long-term morbidity for 5 percent of patients. Complication rates are higher for patients radiated after previously undergoing radical pelvic surgery, with urinary tract fistulas reported in 27 percent of cases. Patients undergoing pelvic exenteration have a high rate of morbidity, including deep venous thrombosis (DVT), bowel obstruction, and pyelonephritis as well as hyperchloremic acidosis associated with urinary conduits. If tumors extend to the pelvic side wall or if patients are treated with both surgery and radiation, chronic lymphedema of the lower extremities may occur.

VULVAR CANCER

Cancer of the vulva is relatively uncommon, accounting for only 3 percent of gynecologic malignancies and less than 1 percent of cancers in women. The mean age of women developing vulvar cancer is 65, although a bimodal age distribution with an increasing number of cases occurring in younger women has recently been identified. In younger women, the tumors are usually associated with HPV and share other risk factors with cervical cancer. In older women, HPV is much less likely to be found in the tumors. Other risk factors include smoking, caffeine, chemical exposure (benzene, aniline dyes), and prior chronic granulomatous infections (granuloma inguinale, lymphogranuloma venereum). About 85 to 90 percent of vulvar cancers are squamous carcinomas. The second most common histology is malignant melanoma (6 percent). Most women with vulvar carcinoma present with a perceived mass (45 percent) or pruritus (45 percent), and less commonly, with pain (23 percent) or ulceration (13 percent). Vulvar carcinoma is treated surgically, with radical subtotal vulvectomy the method of choice for squamous lesions 2 cm or less in diameter. If the depth of the lesion exceeds 1 mm, inguinal lymphadenectomy is performed. Melanoma lesions are treated with wide local excision, but lymphadenectomy is controversial. Survival is 91 per-

cent at 5 years for patients with stage I squamous lesions treated in this fashion and 95 percent if the nodes are negative.

Recurrence of vulvar cancer may be local, or it may involve inguinal or pelvic nodes or distant sites, including the lung. Complications associated with vulvar carcinoma include bleeding at the site of tumor and lymphedema associated with lymphadenectomy, particularly if radiation therapy is utilized in women with positive nodes. Areas affected by lymphedema are prone to develop cellulitis and deep venous thrombosis. Bone metastases, which occur infrequently, may promote hypercalcemia, pain, and pathologic fractures. Pulmonary metastases often demonstrate lymphangitic spread on chest radiographs and may lead to respiratory symptoms.

VAGINAL CANCER

Cancer of the vagina represents 1 to 2 percent of all gynecologic cancers and less than 1 percent of all cancers in women. Childhood tumors include sarcoma botryoides (embryonal rhabdomyosarcoma) and germ-cell tumors resembling those in the ovary. A vaginal tumor occurring predominantly in adolescence is the clear-cell carcinoma associated with in utero diethylstilbestrol (DES) exposure. However, since this drug has been administered rarely in the United States since 1971, most of these women are now adults. In adults, 80 percent of vaginal carcinomas are of squamous histology, occurring at a mean age of 60 to 65 years. Vaginal adenocarcinoma (14 percent) and melanoma are less common (6 percent). Vaginal bleeding and discharge are the most common symptoms, occurring in 70 percent of cases. Vaginal carcinoma spreads by direct extension and if untreated may eventually invade rectal or bladder mucosa.

Childhood tumors respond well to multimodal therapy, including chemotherapy (vincristine, dactinomycin, cyclophosphamide) with either surgery or radiation. Clear-cell carcinoma in DES-exposed women and squamous-cell carcinoma in older women is usually treated with radiation therapy, although radical hysterectomy and vaginectomy are sometimes utilized. On a stage-for-stage basis, survival for vaginal cancer is worse than for cervical and vulvar squamous carcinomas. Stage I lesions treated with radiation result in 77 percent 5-year survival. Survival for melanoma is much lower, averaging only 15 to 20 percent.

Complications that might be expected with vaginal cancer patients include bleeding, rectovaginal and vesicovaginal fistulas, and complications of radiation.

FALLOPIAN TUBE CANCER

Fallopian tube cancer is rare and is often mistaken for ovarian cancer because of its similar gross and histologic appearance, patterns of spread, and natural history.

GYNECOLOGIC SARCOMAS

Gynecologic sarcomas are uncommon. The predominant site for gynecologic sarcomas is the uterus, where smooth muscle tumors of the myometrium and sarcomas arising in endometrial stroma develop. Uterine sarcomas account for about 3 percent of all uterine tumors, whereas the remainder are endometrial carcinomas. Uterine sarcomas usually occur after menopause and are diagnosed prior to hysterectomy in less than 20 percent of cases. The most common presenting symptom is vaginal bleeding; physical findings include uterine enlargement and, occasionally, prolapse of an intrauterine mass through the cervix and into the vagina. Sarcomas arise rarely in the ovary, cervix, vulva, and vagina.

The usual treatment for uterine sarcoma is hysterectomy. Adjuvant chemotherapy has not been found to be effective for prevention of recurrence. Metastatic lesions are often treated with doxorubicin or ifosfamide. Adjuvant radiation therapy decreases pelvic recurrence but does not appear to improve survival except for cases of malignant mixed Müllerian tumors (MMMT). Unfortunately, the survival rate is poor for virtually all gynecologic sarcomas, even when no evidence of metastasis is evident at the time of initial diagnosis. Common sites of recurrence include the pelvis and lungs. These tumors are often vascular, and hemorrhage may occur.

GESTATIONAL TROPHOBLASTIC DISEASE

Gestational trophoblastic disease is a neoplasm arising in the trophoblastic cells of the placenta and develops in about 1 of every 1700 pregnancies in North America. The noninvasive form of this disease is the hydatidiform mole, which can be divided into complete and partial types. Complete moles are more common, accounting for 85 percent of hydatidiform moles. A fetus does not develop in complete moles, and the placenta is replaced by hydropic tissue forming vesicles. More than 90 percent of complete moles have a 46XX genotype containing only paternally derived chromosomes. Partial moles are nearly always triploid, containing 69 chromosomes, two-thirds of which are paternal in origin. A malformed, nonviable fetus is often present, and the placenta is hydropic but has less prominent vesicles in comparison with complete moles. About 10 to 15 percent of women with hydatidiform moles will develop gestational trophoblastic disease after initial treatment, and metastases occur in 4 percent of cases. Moles and invasive forms of gestational trophoblastic disease are composed of trophoblasts that produce and release human chorionic gonadotropin (hCG). The biological action of hCG causes stimulation of the ovarian stroma and thyroid gland. High levels of hCG may result in ovarian hyperstimulation and cyst formation in up to 50 percent of cases in addition to clinically evident hyperthyroidism in 7 percent of cases.

Measurement of hCG provides a sensitive and specific tumor marker that is helpful for monitoring treatment.

Symptoms include first- or second-trimester bleeding in 75 to 95 percent and hyperemesis in 26 percent of cases. Physical findings include excessive uterine size in association with 50 percent of complete moles. Obstetric ultrasound is indicated and demonstrates a heterogenous placenta without a fetus. The placenta has many lucent areas interspersed with brighter areas; the latter are a reflection off the surfaces of the vesicles of the mole (see Fig. 52-10). In contrast, ultrasound examination of a partial mole reveals a small-for-dates fetus, usually with multiple anomalies, and a hydropic placenta.

Treatment of molar pregnancy begins with suction curettage, which should be performed by an experienced individual because of the risk of intraoperative hemorrhage, uterine perforation, and trophoblastic embolization to the lungs. Because of the risk of hemorrhage, this should not be performed in an emergency department setting. After evacuation, if the hCG level falls normally, no additional treatment is likely to be needed. About 10 to 15 percent of patients will develop persistent or invasive disease, evidenced by a plateau or rise of the hCG level. These cases will require chemotherapy. Fortunately, even metastatic disease is highly responsive to chemotherapy, resulting in long-term survival for more than 90 percent of patients. In most cases, fertility is spared and subsequent pregnancy is possible.

A complication commonly attributed to gestational trophoblastic disease is bleeding due to the friable, vascular, necrotic nature of the tumor. Metastatic lesions in the lung and liver may cause significant injury at each site, while brain metastases are considered an oncologic emergency because of the potential for intracranial hemorrhage. Pulmonary metastases may lead to respiratory symptoms and hemoptysis. Trophoblastic embolization, which may occur spontaneously or as a result of uterine evacuation, results in a rapid onset of respiratory distress, resembling amniotic fluid embolus. Complications due to chemotherapy and other treatment-related complications occur in some patients.

SYMPTOMS, SIGNS, AND SYNDROMES

GENITAL TRACT BLEEDING

Bleeding associated with gynecologic malignancies may be acute or chronic; it may begin at any pelvic site; and it may be associated with a number of etiologies. A friable or necrotic tumor may spontaneously develop bleeding from ulcerations, or it may fracture when it is traumatized during coitus or pelvic examination. Tumors may erode into the ileac or femoral vessels, causing massive hemorrhage. Adnexal masses may rupture, leading to hemoperitoneum.

Treatment modalities such as chemotherapy and radiation therapy may themselves contribute to bleeding complications. For example, chemotherapy-associated thrombocytopenia or radiation-associated hemorrhagic cystitis and hemorrhagic enteritis result in acute and chronic blood loss.

Approach to the gynecologic patient who is known or suspected to be bleeding always begins with assessment of the basics: airway, breathing, and circulation. Indications of significant acute blood loss include tachycardia, orthostatic blood pressure changes, oliguria, lethargy, dizziness, and other manifestations of shock. If hemodynamic instability and hypovolemia are diagnosed, a large-bore intravenous line should be started and crystalloids infused. Blood should be drawn for complete counts and crossmatch. Careful examination is then performed to locate the site and extent of genital tract bleeding.

For bleeding originating on the accessible surfaces of the genital tract, including the vulva, vagina, and cervix, the site of bleeding should be compressed. For persistent venous oozing and small arterial bleeders, topical application of silver nitrate using commercially available applicator sticks will generally suffice. Another useful topical astringent is Monsel's solution, a commercially available ferric subsulfate solution, which is prepared by allowing the solution to evaporate until it reaches a pastelike consistency. The solution is kept in a tightly capped container until needed. When applied topically, Monsel's solution adheres to the site of bleeding, resulting in excellent hemostasis. Both silver nitrate and Monsel's solution are safe to use on mucosal surfaces in the vagina and rectum. If the oozing is not controlled with topical astringents alone, application of absorbable hemostat material such as gelatin sponges (Gelfoam), collagen sponges (Instat), or oxidized cellulose fabric (Surgicel) held with pressure to the site of bleeding will promote clot formation. The absorbable hemostats are left in place once bleeding has subsided. If the site of bleeding is vaginal or cervical, application of a topical astringent or absorbable hemostat may be followed by vaginal packing. Packing material should be a long, continuous strip of sterile gauze rather than cotton balls or gauze squares. This facilitates removal and prevents packing material from being inadvertently left in the vagina. If packing is successful in attaining hemostasis, it should be removed the following day to minimize risk of infection. When the vagina is tightly packed, voiding will be difficult or impossible: a urinary catheter should be inserted and the patient should be confined to bed to prevent dislodgement of the pack. Other less commonly used topical hemostatic agents include hemostatic sprays such as topical thrombin (Thrombogen) and fibrin glue. Fibrin glue is made by simultaneously spraying equal volumes of cryoprecipitate (12 mL/U) and bovine thrombin (1000 U/mL) onto the bleeding site.[7] The hemostatic sprays work best if the surface is as dry as possible; their efficacy is limited when brisk bleeding is present.

Focal bleeding sites may occasionally be accessible for suture placement or ligation. Suture material should be tied with great care, because tumor is generally friable and can easily tear, potentially worsening the bleeding.

The differential diagnosis for uterine bleeding is complex, including pregnancy, hormonal disturbance, endometrial hyperplasia, and cancer. Any volume of postmenopausal bleeding, even if scant, in addition to hemorrhage at any age, requires evaluation before treatment. Once pregnancy has been ruled out (in the premenopausal patient), diagnostic endometrial biopsy can be performed and treatment appropriately selected based upon the result. A formal dilatation and curettage procedure may have both therapeutic and diagnostic benefit for patients with heavier bleeding. Consultation with a gynecologist is indicated prior to performing endometrial biopsy or therapeutic curettage.

For tumors not previously treated, initiation of appropriate therapy, such as radiation therapy or surgical resection, may alleviate bleeding and prevent future bleeding episodes. High-dose fractionation of radiation therapy will palliate bleeding that is expected to persist but may compromise curability of the lesion and increase long-term gastrointestinal and genitourinary complications. If recurrent tumor is the source of bleeding, then, in addition to hemostatic interventions, consultation with the oncologist regarding code status, palliation, and quality-of-life issues should be addressed.

Vulvar cancer metastatic to inguinal lymph nodes occasionally erodes into the femoral vessels, and pelvic tumors—including cervical, vaginal, and uterine sarcomas—will occasionally breach the iliac vessels along the pelvic side wall. The ensuing bleeding ranges from slow, chronic bleeding to catastrophic hemorrhage. Brisk arterial bleeding in friable tumor tissue is unlikely to respond to the hemostatic measures described above. Electrocautery and argon beam coagulation may allow control of smaller vessels. Hemorrhage not controllable by other means may be controlled via transcatheter angiographic embolization of the artery or arteries entering the tumor. Small vessels may be selectively occluded using pledgets of Gelfoam and larger vessels with a coil spring (Gianturco spring) wrapped with Dacron.[8,9] If embolization is to be considered, early consultation with the radiologist is indicated. Success rates for control of hemorrhage approach 75 percent. Complications include ischemic injury distal to the occluded artery and migration of the embolus in addition to radiocontrast-associated allergic reactions and nephrotoxicity.[10]

PELVIC CYSTS, MASSES, AND ASCITES

Patients will occasionally present with abdominal distention and discomfort. Associated symptoms may include early satiety, anorexia, weight loss, nausea, vomiting, narrowing of the fecal stream, diarrhea, urinary frequency, urinary incontinence, dyspnea, and orthopnea. Complete physical examination should include both pelvic and rectal examination. Physical findings may indicate the presence of pelvic or abdominal masses and ascites. Many patients with ascites will also have pleural effusions. Initial diagnostic studies that may be of benefit include pelvic ultrasound, chest radiograph, and blood tests, including complete blood count, electrolytes, blood urea nitrogen, and creatinine.

The differential diagnosis should be divided to include patients with a new diagnosis of pelvic mass and ascites versus those with a past history of gynecologic malignancy. Newly detected ovarian masses, even very large ones, may be benign. It is known that both benign and malignant ovarian neoplasms can induce ascites and pleural effusions. Large masses or ascites will compress the abdominal viscera and the diaphragm, resulting in symptoms, and large ovarian tumors will occasionally undergo torsion, causing acute onset of cramps and pain. Ovarian neoplasms may also be prone to rupture and hemorrhage—spontaneously as in the case of germ-cell tumors in adolescents or in response to trauma.

If patients with masses or ascites and no prior cancer diagnosis present with peritoneal signs—including rebound and percussion tenderness, hypoactive bowel sounds, guarding or other signs of acute abdomen—the possibility of torsion, ruptured adnexal mass, or bowel perforation must be entertained. A pelvic mass in this setting should not be deliberately punctured with a needle to aspirate fluid or cells, since this may iatrogenically upstage an ovarian malignancy and possibly worsen prognosis.[11] Careful aspiration of ascitic fluid with a paracentesis procedure may relieve symptoms of abdominal and thoracic pressure and allow a cytologic diagnosis to be made. Ultrasound guidance of the paracentesis procedure minimizes the risk of perforating the bowel lumen and rupturing confined ovarian cysts. Large volumes of ascites can be removed from patients with ovarian cancer without significant complications of hypovolemia due to rapid fluid shifts. Patients presenting with a history of recent trauma or those in whom hemoperitoneum is suspected are candidates for diagnostic peritoneal lavage in the emergency department or laparoscopy in the operating room. Consultation with a gynecologist, gynecologic oncologist, or surgeon is indicated. If a large pleural effusion is present, thoracentesis will aid in relieving dyspnea as well as confirming the possible presence of malignant cells in the effusion.

GASTROINTESTINAL COMPLICATIONS

BOWEL OBSTRUCTION

Patients with an established history of gynecologic malignancy will not infrequently present with progressive enlargement of masses or ascites. Ovarian cancer, uterine papillary serous tumors, and fallopian tube cancers are especially prone to this pattern of spread, and bowel obstruction is the end point of the natural history of these tumors. Bowel obstruction in this setting may be either mechanical, typically at multiple sites, or may involve tumor ileus, a functional obstruction that occurs when tumor encasement or nerve plexus dysfunction results in a bowel segment that is no longer capable of peristalsis.

Symptoms suggestive of bowel obstruction include persistent nausea and vomiting, progressive abdominal distention, colicky abdominal discomfort, and cessation or narrowing of bowel movements. On physical examination, the abdomen will often be distended and tympanitic. Bowel sounds may be high-pitched and hyperactive, with tinkles and rushes. Flat and upright radiographs of the abdomen are of use in confirming the diagnosis. Dilated loops of small or large bowel may be seen, and the presence of multiple air-fluid levels suggests either ileus or obstruction of the small bowel. Massive dilation of the colon, where the cecal diameter is greater than 10 cm, indicates impending rupture if decompression is not carried out promptly. Surgical or gynecologic oncology consultation is indicated.

Palliative surgery may result in temporary restoration of bowel patency, but the likelihood of success for this surgery is only 51 percent and the median duration of survival with successful surgery is 87 days. Prognostic factors that indicate inability to palliate surgically include ascites of greater than 3 L, palpable pelvic and abdominal mass, multiple sites of obstruction, and preoperative weight loss of more than 9 kg.[12] If surgery is not feasible, outpatient palliative management of terminal bowel obstruction is facilitated by placement of a gastrostomy tube for drainage. These tubes are more comfortable for patients than nasogastric tubes and may be placed either surgically in the operating room or percutaneously in the ultrasound suite or under endoscopic guidance.[13,14]

If a bowel obstruction is bypassed, malabsorption of nutrients, vitamins, and bile salts may occur depending on which portions of the bowel are bypassed and on the length of remaining functional bowel.[15] Bypass or resection of the ileum is not as well tolerated as are resections of the jejunum or colon. Bile salts and vitamin B_{12} are selectively absorbed in the terminal ileum: loss of this segment may result in incomplete fat absorption, steatorrhea, and megaloblastic anemia. Poor absorption of fats decreases absorptions of fat-soluble vitamins such as vitamins A and K, which may lead to night blindness and coagulopathies, respectively. Calcium may become sequestered in the unabsorbed fats, resulting in hypocalcemia and bone loss. If the functional length of the small bowel is very short (i.e., less than 100 cm), the patient may not be able to absorb sufficient water and nutrients to survive without parenteral replacement therapy. If short bowel syndrome is suspected, nutritional consultation is indicated.

GASTROINTESTINAL FISTULA

Tumor-related bowel encasement or obstruction may lead to fistula formation. Possible sites of fistulous drainage include the abdominal wall, vagina, uterus, and bladder. Intraperitoneal leaks of enteric contents also occur, leading to abscess formation and peritonitis. If the fistula is difficult to confirm, oral administration of charcoal (50 g in aqueous solution) will demonstrate communication with the intestinal tract by passage of charcoal-stained fluid from the suspected fistula site. A suspected fistula may also be confirmed by an upper gastrointestinal series or barium enema. Alternatively, injection of radiopaque contrast into the fistulous opening ("fistulogram") may aid in determining the course of the fistulous tract. Treatment options depend on the status of the gynecologic malignancy and the performance status of the patient. Patients with short life expectancy may receive palliative treatment, while those with long life expectancy may receive definitive treatment. For patients who are to be treated but who are poor operative risks, bowel rest with total parenteral nutrition and somatostatin treatment to decrease enteric secretions leads to spontaneous closure in up to 82 percent within 14 days of initiating therapy.[16] Patients with no evidence of persistent malignancy can be candidates for definitive resection and repair if bowel rest is not successful.

URINARY TRACT COMPLICATIONS

OBSTRUCTIVE UROPATHY

Ureteral obstruction often occurs with progression of cervical cancer and can develop with many other pelvic malignancies when recurrence or progression occurs. Radiation therapy may induce dense scar tissue capable of obstructing the ureters in 2.5 percent of cases, but most ureteral obstructions are due to recurrence of tumor.[17] Cystoscopic placement of ureteral stents is generally not successful with tumor or radiation-induced obstruction.

Patients presenting with acute renal failure due to ureteral obstruction may be fluid overloaded and may develop metabolic acidosis, hyperkalemia, hyperphosphatemia, and hyperuricemia. If blood urea nitrogen (BUN) and creatinine are markedly elevated, mental status changes or convulsions as well as nausea and vomiting will occur. Uremic pericarditis, causing an audible pericardial friction rub, may also occur.

In the presence of pelvic tumor and with laboratory results demonstrating acute renal failure, renal ultrasound is useful for confirmation of obstruction. Prerenal (e.g., congestive heart failure, hypovolemia, hypotension) and renal causes (e.g., allergic or drug induced nephritis, glomerulonephritis, vasculitis) of acute renal failure must be considered in the differential diagnosis. Intravenous pyelography or computed tomography with intravenous administration of radiocontrast are discouraged in this setting because of increased risk of further nephrotoxicity.

The placement of a percutaneous nephrostomy tube under ultrasound guidance allows urinary diversion when distal ureteral obstruction is present. If obstruction developed due to previously untreated cervical cancer, percutaneous nephrostomy followed by primary radiation therapy results in resolution of the cancer in 33 percent of patients; but if obstruction occurs due to recurrent tumor, then percutaneous nephrostomy prolongs median survival by only 51 days, with no long-term survival observed.[18] Because of this poor prognosis, if recurrent tumor is present, discussion between the patient and her oncologist regarding intervention versus palliative care is indicated. The most favorable group for the placement of a percutaneous nephrostomy tube are those with no evidence of disease whose obstructions resulted from stricture related to treatment (i.e., radiation).

If percutaneous nephrostomy tubes are placed or if ureteral stents can be inserted, copious postobstructive diuresis follows. The resultant polyuria may lead to dehydration, hypokalemia, and hyponatremia. Careful fluid and electrolyte replacement is necessary until renal function recovers, usually in 5 days or less.

GENITOURINARY FISTULA

A vesicovaginal or ureterovaginal fistula may develop at the site of untreated or recurrent tumor. In addition, treatment-related complications may result in fistula formation in 1 percent of patients treated with radical pelvic surgery or in 2.6 percent of patients treated with radiation.[19] The symptom most suggestive of urinary tract fistula is continuous urinary leakage. Examination of the vagina may identify the site of leakage, but small tracts are difficult to identify. A useful clinical test to demonstrate a vesicovaginal fistula is to place a tampon in the vagina followed by filling of the bladder with methylene blue. The tampon is removed after 10–15 min and blue stain on the tampon confirms the presence of a vesicovaginal fistula. Ureterovaginal fistulas will not stain the tampon. If a ureterovaginal fistula is suspected, another tampon is placed and one ampule of indigo carmine dye is injected intravenously. The tampon should be removed after 1 h; the presence of dye indicates a ureterovaginal fistula.

Treatment of bladder and ureteral fistulas will depend on the presence or absence of tumor at the site, whether the patient has been previously radiated or had surgery, and the presence of infection or inflammation in the surrounding tissues. If a fistula is identified, consultation with a urologist or gynecologic oncologist is necessary.

LYMPHEDEMA

Chronic mild lymphedema of the lower extremities develops in half of all patients who have undergone inguinal lymphadenectomy and is uncommon after pelvic lymphadenectomy.[20] Radiation therapy of the pelvis is also associated with mild pedal lymphedema. Treatments combining radical surgery and radiation therapy are much more likely to cause symptomatic lymphedema. The differential diagnosis should include deep venous thrombosis, especially if unilateral edema is noted. A duplex Doppler study of venous flow can rule out the likely presence of a thrombus. Lymphedema is treated symptomatically with elevation and support stockings. Severe cases may benefit by treatment with a pneumatic compression device.

DISTANT METASTASIS

Most metastatic lesions arising from gynecologic malignancies are within the peritoneal cavity or retroperitoneal lymph nodes, leading to ascites and bowel obstruction, as discussed earlier in this chapter. Metastases outside the abdomen may be detected in pleural effusions, often seen with ovarian cancer and malignant uterine papillary serous tumors. Lesions in the lung parenchyma are often seen with gestational trophoblastic disease and gynecologic sarcomas, occasionally with endometrial carcinoma, and rarely with cervical and vulvar carcinomas. Intracranial metastases are most likely to occur with gestational trophoblastic disease (10 percent of metastases) but are uncommon with other gynecologic malignancies. Bone metastases are late findings with cervical, vaginal, and vulvar squamous cell carcinomas and may result in hypercalcemia due to bone destruction and resorption. If limited in number, osteolytic metastases may be palliated, with resultant reduction of calcium levels and pain by use of radiation therapy to the metastatic sites. Medical management of hypercalcemia is discussed later in the chapter.

PARANEOPLASTIC SYNDROMES

Paraneoplastic syndromes are defined as clinical effects caused by a cancer at sites distant from the tumor or its metastases.[21] Many gynecologic tumors are known to produce hormones and humoral factors which can cause paraneoplastic syndromes and associated complications. The paraneoplastic effects may be subdivided into endocrine syndromes attributed to hormone and paraendocrine effects, nervous system disorders, connective tissue disorders, hematologic disorders, cutaneous syndromes, and nephrotic syndrome.[22]

Ectopic human chorionic gonadotropin (hCG), most frequently produced by ovarian germ-cell tumors and rarely by ovarian epithelial tumors, may result in stimulation of sex steroid production by ovarian stromal cells. Syncytiotrophoblasts in gestational trophoblastic disease actively produce chorionic gonadotropin, occasionally at levels many fold higher than peak concentrations attained during normal pregnancy. This may lead to development of theca lutein cysts, which are physiologic ovarian cysts. These can become large enough to rupture and hemorrhage or undergo torsion, leading to an acute abdomen. In addition, the hCG molecule is a weak thyroid-stimulating hormone (TSH) analogue, the marked elevation of which in gestational tro-

phoblastic disease may cause a hyperthyroid state.[22] Another type of thyroid-like endocrine function by ovarian tumors arise in struma ovarii, which are benign germ-cell tumors (i.e., mature teratomas) containing functional ectopic thyroid tissue. These tumors occasionally secrete enough thyroxine to cause hyperthyroid symptoms. Carcinoid tumors have been reported to arise uncommonly in the ovary and rarely in the cervix (two cases). Unlike carcinoid tumors of gastrointestinal origin, symptoms of an ovarian and cervical carcinoid syndrome occur in the absence of metastatic disease. This is attributable to the venous drainage of the ovary, which bypasses the liver, whereas peptides released by gastrointestinal carcinoid tumors are removed upon passage through the hepatic circulation. Other uncommon cases of ectopic hormone production by gynecologic tumors include gastrin-producing mucinous ovarian tumors causing Zollinger-Ellison syndrome and cortisol production by ovarian steroid cell tumors or cervical small-cell carcinomas causing Cushing syndrome. Insulin, prolactin, and renin-producing tumors of the ovary have rarely been reported. Rare cases of syndrome of inappropriate antidiuretic hormone (SIADH) have been reported with cervical and epithelial ovarian tumors.

Hypercalcemia is noted with a variety of gynecologic tumors. Potential mechanisms of hypercalcemia include ectopic parathyroid hormone (PTH) and PTH-related peptide production, induction of osteoclast-activating factor, production of vitamin D analogues, and lytic lesions of bone due to bone metastases.[21,22] The latter is the only nonparaneoplastic mechanism of this group and has been previously discussed. The acute need for management of hypercalcemia is dependent on whether or not the patient is symptomatic. An immediate but short-term decrease of serum calcium levels is attainable using a combination of vigorous intravenous hydration and diuresis with furosemide. Intermediate duration of response, lasting up to 3 weeks, is obtained using the bisphosphonate class of drugs or mithramycin. Long-term reduction of elevated calcium levels requires effective treatment of the tumor.

Neurologic paraneoplastic syndromes have been reported in up to 16 percent of ovarian epithelial cancers. The most common of these is subacute cerebellar degeneration, which results in irreversible progressive ataxia, which may precede the clinical appearance of neoplasm by more than a year.[22] The syndrome is caused by development of antibodies to Purkinje cells. Other antibody-mediated neurologic paraneoplastic syndromes are considerably rarer. These include retinal degeneration, encephalomyelitis, amyotrophic lateral sclerosis, Guillain-Barré syndrome, and myasthenia gravis.

A fairly common cause of dermatomyositis is ovarian cancer, which may account for 12 percent of reported cases.[22] The symptoms of progressive weakness, sometimes accompanied by skin changes or elevated muscle enzymes, may precede clinical development of tumor by up to 2 years. Symptoms typically resolve with treatment of the neoplasm. Tumors rarely associated with dermatomyositis include cervical, endometrial, and vaginal cancers. Other rheumatic and connective tissue disorders associated with unusual cases of ovarian cancer include polyarteritis, palmar fasciitis, rheumatoid arthritis, scleroderma, and systemic lupus erythematosus.

Hematologic paraneoplastic syndromes include autoimmune hemolytic anemia associated with epithelial, germ-cell, and sex-cord stromal tumors of the ovary as well as with disseminated intravascular coagulation (DIC), which is detected in more than 70 percent of ovarian epithelial tumors. In this setting, however, DIC is rarely manifest clinically and is detectable only on coagulation studies. Hypercoagulable states are common and occasionally manifest as nonbacterial thrombotic endocarditis, microangiopathic hemolytic anemia, cerebrovascular accidents, deep venous thrombosis, pulmonary emboli, and migratory thrombophlebitis.

A common variety of paraneoplastic dermatopathy includes acanthosis nigricans, a velvety pigmented lesion usually found in intertriginous areas of the axilla, neck and groin.[21] Ovarian, endometrial, and cervical cancers have been reported as uncommon causes of acanthosis nigricans.

About 5 percent of patients with nephrotic syndrome will have underlying malignancies, which are only rarely of gynecologic origin. Ovarian epithelial carcinoma and gestational trophoblastic disease have been reported to manifest nephrotic syndrome.

THROMBOEMBOLIC COMPLICATIONS

Gynecologic tumors have long been associated with increased risk of thromboembolic complications. Half of all postoperative thrombi are detected within 48 h of surgery, and only 1 percent of patients develop symptomatic thromboembolic disease after discharge from the hospital postoperatively.[23,24] Risk factors for postoperative thromboembolic complications include pelvic surgery, age greater than 40, history of leg edema or varicosities, non-Caucasian race, prior radiation therapy or history of deep venous thrombosis, obesity and/or estrogen excess, in addition to duration of surgery exceeding 30 min. Patients over age 40 with surgery longer than 30 min having any other single risk factor will form deep venous thrombosis in 2 to 10 percent of cases and fatal pulmonary emboli will occur in up to 0.7 percent. If any additional risk factors are identified, risk of deep venous thrombosis is 10 to 20 percent and of fatal pulmonary emboli 1 to 5 percent. Overall, 7.8 percent of gynecologic oncology patients will develop symptomatic thromboembolic disease postoperatively.[25] Many nonsurgical gynecologic oncology patients are subject to the same risks.

When symptoms and signs suggestive of thrombus develop—including swelling, pain, Homan's sign, palpable venous cords—appropriate diagnostic tests include venogram, venous duplex Doppler flow study, or impedance phlebography. The latter two methods are noninvasive and do not expose patients to either radiation or contrast material. Pul-

---

Table 55-1

CALCULATION OF THE ALVEOLAR-ARTERIAL GRADIENT

$$P_{(A-a)O_2} = F_{IO_2} \times (P_B - P_{H_2O}) - (Pa_{CO_2} \times 1.2) - Pa_{O_2}$$

Where F_{IO_2} = inspired concentration of oxygen, percent

P_B = barometric pressure in millimeters of mercury

P_{H_2O} = 47 mmHg, vapor pressure of water

Pa_{CO_2} = arterial partial pressure of carbon dioxide in millimeters of mercury

Pa_{O_2} = arterial partial pressure of oxygen in millimeters of mercury

Normal < 15 mmHg

Age-adjusted normal = 2.5 mmHg + 0.25 × (age in years)

Wide gradient, especially if < 80 mmHg, suggests pulmonary embolus or shunt

---

monary embolus should be suspected if the patient complains of sudden dyspnea or if tachypnea, wheezing, hypoxemia, hypotension, tachycardia, or mental status changes are noted. Diagnosis can be aided by measurement of an increased alveolar-arterial gradient [$P_{(A-a)O_2}$] of partial pressure of oxygen (see Table 55-1). A ventilation/perfusion scan will often confirm the diagnosis but may not be interpretable in cases of pleural effusion or pneumonia. The most accurate but also most invasive and morbid test is the pulmonary angiogram. Angiography is generally indicated if clinical suspicion of pulmonary embolism is high and ventilation/perfusion scan is intermediate probability because of problems such as effusion or pneumonia. Angiography may allow anticoagulation to be avoided in patients at high risk for bleeding—e.g., friable tumor in the pelvis. Once deep venous thrombosis or pulmonary embolus is diagnosed, treatment consists of anticoagulation with heparin followed by conversion to warfarin (Coumadin). Duration of anticoagulation therapy is dependent on the clinical response of the patient as well as whether or not the underlying cause persists. For most patients, 3 months of anticoagulation is probably sufficient. Patients with persistent tumor may require permanent anticoagulation.

TREATMENT-ASSOCIATED COMPLICATIONS

SURGICAL COMPLICATIONS

Most surgical complications are encountered either during surgery or prior to discharge from the hospital. Delayed complications include infection and deep venous thrombosis as well as genitourinary and gastrointestinal fistulas. These topics are discussed elsewhere in this chapter.

CHEMOTHERAPY COMPLICATIONS

Patients with ovarian cancer, gestational trophoblastic disease, and fallopian tube cancer are usually treated with chemotherapy as primary therapy. Other tumors, such as gynecologic sarcoma and endometrial, cervical, vaginal, and vulvar cancers are treated with chemotherapy only if distant metastases are present at the time of diagnosis, tumor persists after surgical resection, or disease recurs after primary therapy. Table 55-2 lists the chemotherapeutic agents most commonly used for the treatment of gynecologic malignancies.

HEMATOLOGIC TOXICITY

The rapid proliferation of stem cells in bone marrow predisposes them to toxicity in the presence of cytotoxic chemotherapy drugs, resulting in reversible neutropenia, thrombocytopenia, and anemia.

Neutropenia and Fevers

Many chemotherapy drugs cause neutropenia, the severity and duration of which are dependent on a number of factors including dose, schedule, multidrug regimens, extent of prior treatment, and performance status of the patient. Chemo-

therapy nadirs typically occur between the seventh and fourteenth day after treatment, although carboplatin has a nadir that lasts from the 18th to the 25th day. The definition of neutropenia varies, but the World Health Organization (WHO) definition includes neutrophil counts as 1999 to 1500/mm^3 for grade 1, 1499 to 1000/mm^3 for grade 2, 999 to 500/mm^3 for grade 3, and less than 500/mm^3 for grade 4. The patient's risk of developing serious infection while neutropenic is dependent on several variables, including neutrophil count, duration of neutropenia, status of the cellular and humoral immune system, nutrition, and physical defense barriers. The endogenous bacteria, fungi, and viruses carried by the patient are the source of most neutropenic infections. Serious infections occur in 10 percent of patients with grade 3 neutropenia lasting less than 1 week, rising to 19 percent for grade 4 toxicity of similar duration and 50 percent or more for neutrophil counts of less than 100/mm^3 lasting for more than a week.[26]

In cases of febrile neutropenia, 60 to 70 percent of patients will not have an identifiable source of infection.[27] When sites of infection can be identified, oral cavity and lung infections occurred most frequently (19 percent each), followed by skin and soft tissue in 14 percent, urinary tract in 11 percent, anorectum in 9 percent, and bacteremia in 7 percent.[28] Common gram-positive organisms isolated in cases of neutropenic fever include *Staphylococcus aureus* and *Staphylococcus epidermidis* (both associated with vascular access devices); *Streptococcus pneumoniae, Streptococcus pyogenes, Streptococcus viridans,* and *Enterococcus faecalis.*[29] Gram-negative isolates commonly include *Escherichia coli, Klebsiella* species, and

---

Table 55-2

CHEMOTHERAPEUTIC AGENTS USED IN GYNECOLOGIC ONCOLOGY

Tumor	Drug
Ovarian cancer Epithelial Fallopian tube cancer	Primary: cisplatin (Platinol), **or** carboplatin (Paraplatin), **with** paclitaxel (Taxol), **or** cyclophosphamide (Cytoxan) Secondary: ifosfamide (IFEX), altretamine (Hexalen), doxorubicin (Adriamycin), etoposide (VePesid), melphalan (Alkeran), or topotecan (Hycamptin)

Ovarian cancer
  Germ cell
  Sex cord stromal
	Primary: cisplatin, etoposide, **and** bleomycin (Blenoxane)
	Secondary: vincristine (Oncovin), dactinomycin (Cosmegen), **and** cyclophosphamide, **or** vinblastine (Velban)

Gestational trophoblastic disease	Primary: methotrexate, **or** dactinomycin Secondary: etoposide, cyclophosphamide, vincristine, cisplatin
Cervical, vulvar, and vaginal cancer	Cisplatin, carboplatin, ifosfamide, 5-fluorouracil, bleomycin, mitomycin C (Mutamycin), doxorubicin
Endometrial cancer	Cisplatin, carboplatin, doxorubicin, paclitaxel
Gynecologic sarcoma	Ifosfamide, etoposide, doxorubicin, dacarbazine

Pseudomonas aeruginosa. Fungal organisms such as *Candida* species and *Aspergillus* are less common than bacterial pathogens but are more likely to be isolated if neutropenia persists for more than a week or if the patient is diabetic or has a vascular access device. Candidal infection of the oral mucosa does not imply systemic infection but may lead to disseminated infection if mucosal integrity is damaged. Viral infections likely to be encountered include recrudescence of herpes simplex and herpes zoster lesions. Cytomegalovirus infections occur less frequently.

Asymptomatic neutropenia does not require intervention or antibiotic prophylaxis. Any fever of 38°C (100.4°F) lasting for 2 h or more while the patient is neutropenic (grade 3 or 4) is an indication for evaluation and treatment.[29] Patients should be instructed to contact their physician if they experience chills, swelling, rash, cough, urinary frequency, sore throat, diarrhea, or new onset of pain. Occasionally, a patient will report having a fever at home, only to be found afebrile upon evaluation. This does not obviate the requirement for careful evaluation and treatment. Initial evaluation includes careful history and physical examination. A complete blood count and peripheral blood cultures should be obtained, and if a venous access device is present, each lumen should be cultured separately. Urine culture completes the routine laboratory work. A chest radiograph should also be obtained. Inflammatory oropharyngeal lesions should be cultured, and if diarrhea is present, evaluation for *Clostridium difficile* is indicated. If the patient shows any evidence of hemodynamic instability, she should be admitted to an intensive care unit and broad-spectrum antibiotics administered. Aggressive fluid support and invasive monitoring are initiated as needed. Granulocyte colony-stimulating factor (filgrastim, Neupogen) is useful for treatment of the seriously ill neutropenic patient, especially if the neutrophil count is less than 100/mm^3 or if the expected duration of neutropenia exceeds 5 days.[30]

Stable patients may be admitted to the ward, where empiric antibiotic therapy is initiated. Antibiotics should not be delayed while awaiting laboratory results if the patient is likely to be neutropenic. The Infectious Diseases Society of America has published consensus recommendations for treatment which include use of an antipseudomonal beta-lactam antibiotic and an aminoglycoside as the first-choice regimen (e.g., ticarcillin/clavulanic acid and gentamicin or piperacillin and tobramycin).[29] If renal impairment is documented or if nephrotoxic chemotherapy drugs such as cisplatin are being used, substitution of the aminoglycoside with a second beta-lactam antibiotic or single-agent therapy with a broad-spectrum carbapenem (imipenem/cilistatin) is acceptable. If *Staphylococcus* species are suspected, add vancomycin to the regimen. If the patient remains febrile after 72 h, particularly if evidence of progressive infection is present, antibiotics should be changed. If a source is identified, antibiotics should be adjusted in accordance with antibiotic sensitivities.

If the patient remains febrile for 7 days, empiric antifungal coverage with amphotericin B, ketoconazole, or fluconazole should be initiated.[29] Administration of amphotericin B requires great care in patients who have received or will receive nephrotoxic chemotherapy. Herpes simplex infections respond to treatment with acyclovir, and varicella zoster infections respond to famciclovir. Cytomegalovirus infections are treated with ganciclovir. Antibiotics may be discontinued when the patient is afebrile and the neutrophil count is greater than 1000/mm^3, although some authors suggest completing 7 days of treatment.[27,29,31] Routine use of filgrastim is costly and should be reserved for patients with neutrophil counts of less than 100/mm^3 or those with anticipated nadirs in excess of 5 days.

Selected low-risk patients with febrile neutropenia (stable, compliant, accompanied by a responsible party, and in close proximity to medical care) have been treated in outpatient settings, but usually in the context of research protocols.

Thrombocytopenia

Chemotherapy-induced thrombocytopenia increases the risk of bleeding moderately if the platelet count falls below 50,000/mm^3; the risk becomes more serious when the platelet count falls below 20,000/mm^3. Spontaneous, potentially fatal hemorrhage in the central nervous system, gastrointestinal tract, respiratory tract, and tumor sites occurs when fewer than 10,000/mm^3 platelets are in circulation.[28] Thrombocytopenia due to chemotherapy is transient, with nadirs typically occurring between the seventh and tenth days following treatment. Platelet nadirs are later and more protracted following carboplatin (14 to 18 days) and mitomycin C (28 to 35 days).

When a patient is thrombocytopenic, risk factors for bleeding should be minimized by having her avoid all preventable physical trauma as well as medications that inhibit platelet function or blood clotting (e.g., aspirin and other nonsteroidal anti-inflammatory agents, heparin, and warfarin). Stool, urine, and emesis should be tested for occult blood. If clinical suspicion of bleeding is present, intravenous access should be obtained and blood products crossmatched. Platelet transfusion is indicated if the patient is bleeding and the platelet count is <50,000/mm^3, or if a nonelective surgical procedure must be performed and the platelet count is <50,000/mm^3. Maintenance of platelets in excess of 50,000 to 100,000/mm^3 is desired in these settings. Prophylactic transfusion of platelets is indicated if the platelet count falls below 10,000 to 20,000/mm^3 in the asymptomatic patient, although several studies indicate that counts as low as 5000/mm^3 may be safely observed in some circumstances.[32]

A unit of platelets will typically increase the platelet count by 5000 to 10,000/mm^3 in the absence of antiplatelet antibodies or active bleeding. Six units of platelets are usually administered when transfusion is indicated. Posttransfusion platelet counts should be ordered 1 h and 24 h after transfusion. A lower-than-expected rise in the platelet count (less than 3000/mm^3 per unit) indicates the presence of antiplatelet antibodies. Sensitization is common if a patient has previously been transfused with red cells or platelets. Subsequent platelet transfusions for the sensitized patient require consultation with the blood bank: use of HLA-matched or single-donor platelets may be warranted. Pretreatment with acetaminophen and diphenhydramine minimizes the common symptoms of chills and hives.

Anemia

Anemia occurring during chemotherapy may arise as a direct result of the marrow toxicity of the drugs used, and typically occurs 60 to 90 days after initiation of treatment due to the 120-day life span of red blood cells. The differential diagnosis in this population usually includes iron deficiency, folate and vitamin B_{12} deficiency, hemolysis, and losses attributable to bleeding. In an asymptomatic patient, hemoglobin greater than 8 to 9 g/dL generally requires no intervention. If the patient is symptomatic related to her anemia with reports of fatigue, dizziness, and dyspnea on exertion or is noted to be tachycardic or to have orthostatic changes in vital signs, transfusion with packed red blood cells is indicated. Patients with preexisting cardiovascular or chronic lung diseases may require hemoglobin to be maintained at a higher concentration.

Use of the cytokine epoetin (Procrit), a synthetic variant of erythropoietin, is controversial but may be indicated for management of chemotherapy-associated anemia if measured erythropoietin levels are less than 200 mU/mL. The starting dose for epoetin administration is 150 U/kg subcutaneously three times weekly. Reevaluation of the need for continued therapy is performed after 4 to 8 weeks of treatment. An advantage of epoetin use is a reduced likelihood of transfusion, but drawbacks include hypertension and high cost.

NAUSEA AND VOMITING

Many chemotherapy drugs and regimens provoke nausea and vomiting. Complex reflex pathways are responsible for this process. Enterochromaffin cells in the intestine release serotonin in response to toxic stimuli, which in turn binds to vagal $5HT_3$ receptors and in the chemoreceptor trigger zone (CTZ). The neurologic "emesis center" is located in the medulla near the CTZ and receives input from the CTZ, intestinal afferents, midbrain, limbic system, and vestibular system.[33] Stimulation of $5HT_3$ receptors leads to a coordinated reflex that expels the gastric contents. Chemotherapy drugs used for the treatment of gynecologic malignancies have variable emetic potential, as listed in Table 55-3. For most chemotherapy drugs, nausea and vomiting is more likely in the first 24 h after treatment, although cisplatin-induced nausea frequently lasts for 4 days or more.

A number of drugs are available for the treatment of chemotherapy-induced nausea and vomiting. Antiemetic drugs are compared in Table 55-4. Young women are more predisposed to extrapyramidal effects with phenothiazines. These can be treated with diphenhydramine or by switching to a different class of antiemetic such as trimethobenzamide. Addition of lorazepam may potentiate the action of these regimens. If patients experience refractory delayed nausea, treatment may include dexamethasone (2 mg PO t.i.d. for 3 days), possibly combined with an oral serotonin antagonist such as granesetron (1 mg PO b.i.d. for 3 days) or ondansetron (8 mg PO t.i.d. for 3 days).

Prolonged nausea and vomiting can easily lead to dehydration, electrolyte disturbance, and mucosal irritation or ulceration. Careful assessment for evidence of dehydration and laboratory evaluation of electrolytes should be performed prior to allowing discharge of the patient. If the patient is not able to maintain adequate oral intake despite antiemetic therapy, admission to the hospital for intravenous hydration and parenteral antiemetic therapy is warranted.

STOMATITIS

Patients undergoing chemotherapy for gynecologic malignancies will develop stomatitis (mucositis) in up to 40 per-

---

Table 55-3

EMETOGENIC POTENTIAL OF CHEMOTHERAPY DRUGS

Highly Emetogenic, %	Moderately Emetogenic, %	Minimally Emetogenic, %
Cisplatin (>90)	Altretamine (30–60)	Bleomycin (10–30)
Dacarbazine (>90)	Doxorubicin (30–60)	5-Fluorouracil (10–30)
Carboplatin (60–90)	Etoposide (30–60)	Methotrexate (10–30)
Cyclophosphamide (60–90)	Ifosfamide (30–60)	Vinblastine (10–30)
Dactinomycin (60–90)	Topotecan (30–60)	Vincristine (<10)
		Paclitaxel (<10)

Source: Ref. 33.

Table 55-4

ANTIEMETIC DRUGS USED WITH CHEMOTHERAPY REGIMENS

Drug	Dose	Mechanism	Toxicity
Serotonin antagonist Ondansetron (Zofran)	24–32 mg IV 15 min prior to chemotherapy; or 8 mg PO t.i.d. for 3 days after	Blocks 5HT$_3$ receptors on vagus and in CTZ[a]	Mild headache, dry mouth, sedation, diarrhea, constipation
Granesetron (Kytril)	10 μg/kg IV 15 min prior to chemotherapy; or 1–2 mg PO b.i.d. for 3 days		
Phenothiazines Prochlorperazine (Compazine)	10 mg PO, IM, or IV q4h, 15 mg spansules PO q12h, or 25 mg PR q6h	Blocks dopamine receptors in CTZ and central cholinergic receptors; increases lower esophageal tone	Extrapyramidal symptoms (EPS), sedation, anticholinergic effects, hypotension
Thiethylperazine (Torecan)	10 mg PO, IM, or PR q4h		
Chlorperazine (Thorazine)	10–25 mg PO q4–6h, or 25–50 mg PR q6–8h		
Metoclopramide (Reglan)	1–3 mg/kg IV q2–3h, up to six doses, or 10–20 mg PO q4h	Blocks dopamine receptors, 5HT$_3$ receptors (at high doses); increases lower esophageal tone and increases GI motility via 5HT$_4$ receptors	EPS, sedation, anxiety, and agitation
Corticosteroids Dexamethasone (Decadron)	Acute nausea: 10–20 mg PO or IV q4h Delayed nausea: 2 mg PO t.i.d. for 3 days	Not understood; may be due to prostaglandin inhibition and euphoric effect	Insomnia, mood swing, cataracts, insulin resistance, adrenal suppression
Antihistamines Diphenhydramine (Benadryl)	25–50 mg PO or IV q6h	Blocks central cholinergic receptors	Sedation, anticholinergic effects
Trimethobenzamide (Tigan)	250 mg PO q.i.d. or 200 mg PR q.i.d.	Uncertain; probably acts on CTZ	Sedation. Reye syndrome (rare)
Benzodiazepines Lorazepam (Ativan)	0.5–2 mg PO or IV q6h	Anxiolytic, sedative, amnesia	Sedation, paradoxical reactions
Cannabinoids Dronabinol (Marinol)	5 mg/m^2 PO q4h	Cortical inhibition of medullary activity; inhibition of prostaglandin synthesis	Chemical dependence, sedation, dysphoria, dry mouth, tachycardia, hypotension

[a]CTZ = chemoreceptor trigger zone.

cent of cases. The oral mucosa is vulnerable to chemotherapy due to rapid proliferation of cells, resulting in atrophy, ulceration, inflammation, and infection. Severity of stomatitis is quantified using the WHO grading criteria: grade 1 lesions are painless, grade 2 lesions are painful but do not prevent eating, grade 3 lesions are sufficiently painful to prevent eating, and grade 4 lesions require parenteral or enteral nutritional support. Chemotherapy drugs most often associated with stomatitis include methotrexate, dactinomycin, doxorubicin, and bleomycin. Less frequent occurrence is noted with etoposide and vinblastine. Patients with stomatitis are at risk for systemic bacterial and fungal infections if the integrity of the mucosal surface is disrupted.

Table 55-5

REGIMENS FOR TREATMENT OF SYMPTOMATIC STOMATITIS ATTRIBUTED TO CHEMOTHERAPY

Equal volumes of diphenhydramine syrup (not elixir due to alcohol content) and either Mylanta or Kaopectate	10 mL PO, swish and expectorate or swallow q.i.d.
Diphenhydramine syrup (50 mL), and Mylanta (50 mL), and Viscous lidocaine 2% (50 mL)	15 mL PO, swish and expectorate or swallow q.i.d.
Viscous lidocaine 2% (100 mg/5 mL)	15 mL PO, swish and expectorate or swallow q.i.d., not to exceed 120 mL/day due to neurotoxicity
Sucralfate suspension (1g/ 15 mL)	15 mL PO, swish and expectorate or swallow q.i.d.

Source: Ref. 34.

Preventive strategies include meticulous oral hygiene and rinses with salt-and-soda mouthwash (1 tbsp salt and 1 tbsp sodium bicarbonate per liter of water, swished and expectorated q.i.d.).[34] If symptoms develop, examination should determine the sites and extent of the stomatitis. Symptomatic relief in mild cases (grade 1) can be obtained using ice chips and artificial saliva products (Salivart, Xerolube, Oralbalance Gel). Moderately painful stomatitis (grades 2 and 3) may be palliated using analgesic washes, which are listed in Table 55-5. Thrush occurs following 5 percent of chemotherapy treatments for gynecologic malignancies. If evidence of thrush is present, treatment with oral nystatin suspension (5 mL of 100,000 U/mL solution, swish and swallow q.i.d.) or clotrimazole troches (10 mg dissolved orally five times daily) is generally sufficient. Bacterial infections are best treated with systemic antibiotics appropriate for the organism identified. Viral stomatitis with herpes simplex can be ameliorated with oral or intravenous acyclovir (200 mg PO 5 times per day or 250 mg/m^2 IV t.i.d.).[34]

URINARY TRACT TOXICITY

Nephrotoxicity, hematuria, and electrolyte disturbances may occur as a result of chemotherapy. Risk factors for renal toxicity include type of chemotherapy drug, dose and schedule, adequacy of prehydration before chemotherapy, age, nutritional status, preexisting renal dysfunction, and administration of other nephrotoxic drugs. Use of potentially nephrotoxic drugs such as aminoglycosides, amphotericin B, nonsteroidal anti-inflammatory drugs, and diuretics such as furosemide should be avoided whenever possible for patients undergoing nephrotoxic chemotherapy.

Cisplatin is the most common cause of nephrotoxicity, but methotrexate, ifosfamide, and mitomycin C are also capable of causing significant renal damage. Prevention is dependent on vigorous intravenous hydration of patients before, during, and after treatment. Patients receiving cisplatin generally receive mannitol to encourage diuresis. The U.S. Food and Drug Administration has recently approved the drug amifostine (Ethyol) for prevention of cumulative renal toxicity associated with repeated administration of cisplatin in patients with advanced ovarian cancer. It is not indicated for treatment of preexisting or acute nephrotoxicity. Patients undergoing high-dose methotrexate therapy should have their urine alkalinized during infusion with intravenous sodium bicarbonate sufficient to alkalinize the urine to a pH of 7 or greater. This prevents precipitation of methotrexate in the renal tubules. Patients who are discharged after chemotherapy with inadequate antiemetic regimens will occasionally develop refractory nausea and vomiting. The resulting state of dehydration exacerbates renal toxicity. Electrolyte disturbances including hypomagnesemia and hypokalemia are common with cisplatin regimens; these are thought to be due to acute tubular necrosis (ATN) and dysfunction of the loop of Henle. Many electrolytes are wasted, especially divalent cations. Cyclophosphamide has been associated with the syndrome of inappropriate antidiuretic hormone secretion (SIADH), which may result in oliguria and hyponatremia.

Evaluation of Renal Damage

Evaluation of patients with possible nephrotoxicity should include urinalysis and measurement of urine specific gravity, in addition to blood urea nitrogen, creatinine, and creatinine clearance using the Cockcroft and Gault equation.

$$\text{Creatinine clearance} = [(140 - \text{age}) \times (0.85) \times (\text{weight in kilograms})]/(72 \times \text{serum creatinine})$$

Creatinine clearance <50 mL/min is rarely a cause for concern. Patients treated with cisplatin will not infrequently have a creatinine clearance in the range of 30 to 50 mL/min. If this is a stable value, it is still not too concerning, but the trend must be watched. If the creatinine clearance reaches <30 mL/min, cisplatin (CDDP) is usually stopped. Other drugs should be dosed according to decreased clearance.

If SIADH is suspected, fractional excretion of sodium (FE$_{Na}$) should be measured using the following formula:

$$\text{FE}_{Na} = [U_{Na} \times P_{Cr}/(P_{Na} \times U_{Cr})] \times 100$$

Where U_{Na} = urine sodium, meq/L
        P_{Cr} = plasma creatinine, mg/dL
        P_{Na} = plasma sodium, meq/L
        U_{Cr} = urine creatinine, mg/dL

Normal FE_{Na} is below 1 percent. If FE_{Na} is greater than 1 percent, the diagnosis of SIADH is supported.

Patients presenting with nausea and vomiting may benefit from aggressive rehydration to minimize nephrotoxicity. They should have electrolytes appropriately replaced when deficiencies are identified. If SIADH is diagnosed, admission for careful fluid restriction and electrolyte repletion is indicated.

Hemorrhagic cystitis is common with ifosfamide and relatively uncommon with cyclophosphamide (below 10 percent). Vigorous hydration and, for ifosfamide treatment, prophylaxis with the uroprotector drug mesna minimize the risk. If gross hematuria occurs, chemotherapy should be discontinued, intravenous hydration continued, and continuous bladder irrigation with saline instituted. Persistence of bleeding warrants early consultation with the oncologist.

NEUROPATHY

A number of neurologic toxicities have been reported with chemotherapy agents. Both central nervous system and peripheral nerves can be affected, with peripheral neuropathy the most common among gynecologic oncology patients. Development of peripheral neuropathy, in addition to being related to the chemotherapy drug administered, is schedule-dependent and more prevalent in patients with diabetes, alcohol abuse histories, and nutritional deficiencies.[35] Unlike hematologic toxicity, peripheral neuropathy is permanent in nearly 75 percent of the affected patients. Mild neuropathy is observed and does not require alteration of the chemotherapy regimen, but severe or progressive neuropathy requires discontinuation of the neurotoxic drug.

Up to 50 percent of patients treated with cisplatin report sensory peripheral neuropathy, resulting in loss of proprioception in mild cases; in severe cases, pain, loss of deep tendon reflexes, sensory ataxia, and loss of touch perception can occur. Onset of platinum-associated neuropathy is related to cumulative doses of 300 mg/m^2 or more. Paclitaxel and carboplatin cause similar sensory neuropathies, but of lesser intensity. No pharmacologic cure for neuropathy exists, but treatment with tricyclic antidepressants such as amitriptyline may alleviate dysesthesia and the symptom of "restless legs." Mixed sensory and motor neuropathy is associated with vincristine, which can cause a peroneal nerve palsy associated with "foot drop" as well as vagal nerve dysfunction leading to constipation and abdominal pain.

Tinnitus and ototoxicity resulting in high-frequency hearing loss are common with cisplatin, while optic neuropathy is rare. Vincristine, vinblastine, and 5-fluorouracil have been associated with cranial neuropathy in sporadic cases. Cerebellar syndromes associated with imbalance and ataxia have been reported with altretamine and 5-fluorouracil. Encephalopathies, ranging from confusion to seizures and coma, have been reported with many drugs and are associated with dose schedule, protein binding (increased risk with low albumin levels), renal and hepatic function, and concomitant cranial radiation therapy. Ifosfamide, altretamine, cisplatin, cyclophosphamide, 5-fluorouracil, and methotrexate encephalopathies have also occurred.

Patients presenting with acute encephalopathic symptoms should be stabilized, an intravenous line started, and blood drawn for a complete blood count, electrolytes, and renal and hepatic function tests. Consultation should be obtained with the patient's oncologist.

PULMONARY FIBROSIS

Pulmonary injuries attributable to chemotherapy may present clinically as pneumonitis/fibrosis, hypersensitivity pneumonitis, and noncardiogenic pulmonary edema. The drug most commonly associated with pulmonary toxicity is bleomycin, which induces pulmonary fibrosis. Mitomycin C and methotrexate have also been reported to cause pulmonary fibrosis with gradual onset. This usually occurs when the cumulative dose is high. Patients may present with nonproductive cough, fatigue, and weight loss. Auscultation of the chest will generally detect crackles. Measurement of the diffusion capacity of carbon monoxide (DL_{CO}) via pulmonary function testing is sensitive, but nonspecific, as a predictor of early fibrosis. Chest radiographs show no change until significant damage has occurred, resulting in an interstitial infiltrate pattern. Treatment requires discontinuation of chemotherapy to prevent further damage, although pulmonary fibrosis is not reversible. Some reports support glucocorticoid administration as empiric therapy, although this is controversial.

Pulmonary hypersensitivity can occur as an acute reaction during or immediately after treatment. It is often rapid in onset and can occur with the first treatment, resulting in chills, wheezing, dyspnea, and cough. Hypersensitivity reactions are most likely to occur after treatment with bleomycin and methotrexate. Treatment with steroids is indicated and chances for recovery are good.

CARDIOMYOPATHY

Congestive heart failure associated with irreversible cardiomyopathy is related to doxorubicin treatment, and the risk is proportionate to cumulative dose. The incidence of cardiomyopathy is less than 5 percent if the cumulative dose is less than 450 mg/m^2 and rises to 30 percent at doses in excess of 600 mg/m^2. Both high-dose cyclophosphamide and

5-fluorouracil have also been reported to cause cardiac injury. Mediastinal radiation, preexisting heart disease, high peak plasma levels, age over 70, and combination chemotherapy all appear to increase risk. Early detection of congestive heart failure is possible by comparing serial radionuclide angiography studies or echocardiograms. If the left ventricular ejection fraction declines by more than 10 percent, treatment should be discontinued. If symptoms of congestive heart failure occur, medical optimization of cardiac function is attempted.

Doxorubicin and paclitaxel occasionally cause transient arrhythmia during infusion. Paclitaxel frequently causes bradycardia, which is asymptomatic unless preexisting problems such as conduction defects exist. Complete heart block has been reported under these conditions.

ALLERGIC REACTIONS

Approximately 5 percent of patients will express an allergic response to chemotherapy drugs. Mild allergic reactions do not require discontinuation of the chemotherapy regimen. Allergic reactions in response to paclitaxel are frequent, to the extent that all patients are treated with dexamethasone (20 mg PO 12 and 6 h before treatment), diphenhydramine (50 mg IV 30 min prior to treatment), and cimetidine (300 mg IV 30 min prior to treatment). Occasionally, delayed allergic reactions to paclitaxel may result in cutaneous flushing, urticaria, bronchospasm, and stridor as well as hypotension. This usually happens during the first 2 or 3 days. After 3 days, most of the drug has been cleared from the system. After initial evaluation and stabilization, patients should be treated with dexamethasone, diphenhydramine, and cimetidine, as before treatment. Use of a bronchodilator or epinephrine may be necessary if bronchospasm is clinically significant.

VASCULAR ACCESS DEVICES

Blood clots, accumulation of fibrin sheath, and intraluminal debris may cause occlusion of implanted venous access ports. If a port is accessed but does not allow infusion or aspiration of fluids, occlusion should be suspected. Dissolution of clot and fibrin sheath may be accomplished by injection of urokinase (5000 IU/mL, 1-mL volume) followed by aspiration after 1 h. The process may be repeated once if needed. If catheter occlusion has occurred due to precipitation of a medication, consultation with the pharmacist regarding safe solvents to dissolve the precipitate is indicated.

EXTRAVASATION INJURY

Extravasation, or leakage of an intravenously administered chemotherapy drug into perivascular tissues, may cause symptoms ranging from local irritation to necrosis of tis-

Table 55-6

CHEMOTHERAPY DRUGS CAPABLE OF CAUSING INJURY IF EXTRAVASATED

Severe Vesicants, DNA-Bound, Long-Term Injury	Mild Vesicants, not DNA-Bound, Short-Term Injury
Dactinomycin	Cisplatin
Doxorubicin	Etoposide
Mitomycin	5-Fluorouracil
	Paclitaxel
	Vinblastine
	Vincristine

Source: Refs. 36–38.

sue. Vesicants are chemotherapy agents that cause severe local tissue injury if extravasation occurs. Extravasation of drugs that do not bind DNA results in immediate local tissue injury, after which the drugs are quickly metabolized and cleared from the site of injury, allowing healing to occur. Vesicants that bind DNA will cause both immediate and long-term damage to local tissues, resulting in chronic, progressive ulceration. If extravasation of DNA-bound drugs occurs near hand or antecubital intravenous sites, the resulting tissue damage may lead to the loss of function of the extensor tendons or the joint, respectively. Table 55-6 lists chemotherapy drugs that are considered to be vesicants used for the treatment of gynecologic malignancies. Symptoms suggesting extravasation may occur immediately or several days to weeks later; they include pain, burning, erythema, swelling, and induration—followed by ulceration and necrosis, depending on the type and amount of drug extravasated.

The best treatment for extravasation injury is prevention. Safe practice involves administering vesicant drugs through recently placed, freely flowing peripheral intravenous catheters placed away from the dorsum of the hand and antecubital fossa. Central venous lines and venous access ports provide reliable long-term vascular access. If extravasation is suspected, drug infusion should be stopped immediately and aspiration of extravasated fluids should be attempted. Depending on the type of vesicant involved, antidotes or treatments to minimize tissue damage may be prescribed,[36–38] as shown in Table 55-7. Early consultation with a plastic surgeon should be initiated if pain, erythema, or swelling persist. Wide debridement and skin grafting may be necessary, particularly if ulceration or necrosis occurs.

Table 55-7

TREATMENT FOR EXTRAVASATION OF VESICANT CHEMOTHERAPEUTIC AGENTS

Drug	Treatment
Dactinomycin	Ice pack, 30 minutes q.i.d. for 72 h, elevate extremity
	Sodium thiosulfate 10%, 4 mL + 6 mL water, inject 5–6 mL subcutaneously at IV site
Doxorubicin	Ice pack, 30 min q.i.d. for 72 h, elevate extremity
	Sodium bicarbonate, 1 mEq/mL, inject 5 mL subcutaneously at IV site
	Hydrocortisone 50 mg/mL, inject 1–2 mL subcutaneously at IV site
	Dimethylsulfoxide (DMSO) 99%, apply topically q6h for 12 days
Mitomycin	Ice pack, 30 min q.i.d. for 72 h, elevate extremity
	Dimethylsulfoxide (DMSO) 99%, apply topically q6h for 12 days
Vincristine or vinblastine	Warm compresses, 30 min q.i.d. for 24 h
	Do *not* use ice pack, as it may worsen toxicity
Etoposide	Hyaluronidase, 150 U/mL, inject 1–6 mL SQ at IV site
Cisplatin Dacarbazine 5-Fluorouracil Paclitaxel	None known

Source: Refs. 36–38.

COMPLICATIONS OF RADIATION THERAPY

ACUTE VERSUS CHRONIC

Complications associated with radiation therapy may be acute, occurring during or immediately after treatment, or chronic, resulting in complications years or decades after treatment. Acute toxicities include diarrhea, nausea with vomiting, and myelosuppression. These symptoms can usually be successfully controlled using antiemetics such as prochlorperazine, constipating drugs such as diphenoxylate hydrochloride with atropine sulfate (Lomotil) or loperamide (Imodium), and avoidance of high-fiber foods. Ongoing research suggests that glutamine-rich diets or treatment with sucralfate may significantly reduce radiation-induced diarrhea. Occasionally, interruption of treatment is necessary to allow symptoms to subside, but this may compromise chances for control of the tumor. Once treatment has been completed, most symptoms subside over several weeks. Complications of chronic radiation arise primarily as a result of progressive endarteritis.

GASTROINTESTINAL COMPLICATIONS

In some patients, chronic diarrhea may persist for years after radiation. The incidence of chronic diarrhea may range between 3 and 40 percent, depending on the volume of small bowel radiated and total radiation dose. Cramping and diarrheal symptoms are often exacerbated by fiber-containing foods. Diarrhea associated with radiation-induced vasculopathy may result in malabsorption of nutrients and vitamins. Most significant bowel complications occur within the first 2 years after completion of radiation therapy. The incidence of severe gastrointestinal complications has been reported to be as high as 10 to 15 percent in patients treated for advanced-stage cervical cancers, in which high-dose radiation treatment is necessary. Small bowel complications include strictures, perforation, and formation of fistulas and occur in about 5 percent of patients who have undergone pelvic radiation.[39] Complications affecting the large bowel include obstruction, perforation, fistula formation, and hematochezia.[40] Fistula formation is much more likely in patients who have undergone hysterectomy after radiation treatment. A fistula will not heal spontaneously in radiated tissue. Radiation proctitis may result in clinically significant hematochezia requiring serial transfusions. Diagnosis should be confirmed by colonoscopy in order to rule out recurrent cancer or other causes. Treatment should be coordinated between the oncologist and gastroenterologist. Control of bleeding has been attained using steroid retention enemas, colonoscopically directed coagulation, estrogen therapy, and intrarectal formalin application.[41] Severe bleeding occasionally requires diverting colostomy or bowel resection.

UROLOGIC COMPLICATIONS

Chronic urologic symptoms such as urgency and incontinence occur in up to 26 percent of patients after pelvic radiotherapy. The risk of severe urologic complications—including stricture, fistula formation, and hemorrhagic cystitis—is 1 percent during the first 3 years after treatment and increases at a rate of 0.25 percent per year thereafter.[19] Ureteral stricture may result in loss of function of either or both kidneys. Development of obstructive uropathy should always be considered suspicious for recurrent disease before being attributed to radiation toxicity. A fistulous tract may develop between ureter, bladder or urethra, and vagina or gastrointestinal tract. Formation of a fistula is much more likely in patients who undergo hysterectomy after radiation.

Spontaneous closure of genitourinary fistulas will not occur in radiated tissue. Diagnosis of a genitourinary fistula has been discussed earlier.

Hemorrhagic cystitis as a result of radiation occurs in about 6.5 percent of patients after pelvic radiation. The majority of these cases are mild, but 18 percent are severe enough to warrant hospitalization and transfusion.[42] Initial diagnosis requires cystoscopy, generally performed by a urologist or gynecologic oncologist. The treatment for mild hemorrhagic cystitis is bladder irrigation with saline or water. In severe cases, continuous irrigation with alum and bolus irrigation with silver nitrate, formalin, or prostaglandin $F_{2\alpha}$, as well as systemic administration of conjugated estrogens, have been reported to be successful in 80 to 90 percent of cases. Severe hemorrhagic cystitis recurs despite treatment in one-third of cases and occasionally requires a urinary diversion procedure to alleviate blood loss.

SECONDARY MALIGNANCIES

Although radiation therapy may result in the successful treatment of many malignancies, the ionizing radiation also affects surrounding normal tissues. The resultant mutation of somatic genetic material promotes carcinogenesis, generally years after treatment. Little is known about the prediction of this risk or the prevention of carcinogenesis after radiation therapy.

References

1. Wingo PA, Tong T, Bolden S: Cancer statistics, 1995. *CA* 45:8, 1995.
2. Morrow CP, Curtin JP, Townsend DE: *Synopsis of Gynecologic Oncology,* 4th ed. New York: Churchill Livingstone, 1993.
3. Granberg S, Wikland M, Karlsson B, et al: Endometrial thickness as measured by endovaginal ultrasonography for identifying endometrial abnormality. *Am J Obstet Gynecol* 164:47, 1991.
4. Ozols RF, Rubin SC, Dembo AJ, et al: Epithelial ovarian cancer, in Hoskins WJ, Perez CA, Young RC (eds): *Principles and Practice of Gynecologic Oncology.* Philadelphia: Lippincott,1992.
5. National Institutes of Health Consensus Development Conference Statement. Ovarian cancer: Screening, treatment, and follow-up. *Gynecol Oncol* 55:S4, 1994.
6. Williams SD, Gershenson DM, Horowitz CJ, et al: Ovarian germ cell and stromal tumors, in Hoskins WJ, Perez CA, Young RC (eds): *Principles and Practice of Gynecologic Oncology.* Philadelphia: Lippincott-Raven, 1997.
7. Malviya VK, Deppe G: Control of intraoperative hemorrhage in gynecology with the use of fibrin glue. *Obstet Gynecol* 73:284, 1989.
8. Horowitz IR, Abbas FM, Mitchell S, et al: Selective ar-

terial embolization to control pelvic hemorrhage in the oncology patient. *Proc Annu Mtg Am Soc Clin Oncol* 10:A614, 1991.
9. Pisco JM, Martins JM, Correia MG: Internal iliac artery: Embolization to control hemorrhage from pelvic neoplasms. *Radiology* 172:337, 1989.
10. Rosenthal DM, Colapinto R: Angiographic arterial embolization in the management of postoperative vaginal hemorrhage. *Am J Obstet Gynecol* 151:227, 1985.
11. Trimbos JB, Hacker NF: The case against aspirating ovarian cysts. *Cancer* 72:828, 1993.
12. Jong P, Sturgeon J, Jamieson CG: Benefit of palliative surgery for bowel obstruction in advanced ovarian cancer. *Can J Surg* 38:454, 1995.
13. Hopkins MP, Roberts JA, Morley GW: Outpatient management of small bowel obstruction in terminal ovarian cancer. *J Reprod Med* 32:827, 1987.
14. Marks WH, Perkal MF, Schwartz PE: Percutaneous endoscopic gastrostomy for gastric decompression in metastatic gynecologic malignancies. *Surg Gynecol Obstet* 177:573, 1993.
15. Cowan GSM, Luther RW, Sykes TR: Short bowel syndrome: Causes and clinical consequences. *Nutr Support Svc* 4:25, 1984.
16. DiCostanzo J, Cano N, Martin J, et al: Treatment of external gastrointestinal fistulas by a combination of total parenteral nutrition and somatostatin. *J Parenteral Enteral Nutr* 11:465, 1987.
17. McIntyre JF, Eifel PJ, Levenback C, et al: Ureteral stricture as a late complication of radiotherapy for stage IB carcinoma of the uterine cervix. *Cancer* 75:836, 1995.
18. Chan S, Robinson AC, Johnson RJ: Percutaneous nephrostomy: Its value in obstructive uropathy complicating carcinoma of the cervix. *Clin Oncol* 2:156, 1990.
19. Eifel PJ, Levenback C, Wharton JT, et al: Time course and incidence of late complications in patients treated with radiation therapy for FIGO stage IB carcinoma of the uterine cervix. *Int J Radiat Biol Phys* 32:1289, 1995.
20. Delgado G, Smith J: *Management of Complications in Gynecologic Oncology.* New York: Wiley, 1982.
21. Agarwala SS: Paraneoplastic syndromes. *Med Clin North Am* 80:173, 1996.
22. Clement PB, Young RH, Scully RE: Clinical syndromes associated with tumors of the female genital tract. *Semin Diagn Pathol* 8:204, 1991.
23. Clarke-Pearson DL, DeLong ER, Synan IS, et al: Variables associated with postoperative deep venous thrombosis: A prospective study of 411 gynecology patients and creation of a prognostic model. *Obstet Gynecol* 69:146, 1987.
24. Clarke-Pearson DL, Synan IS, Coleman RE, et al: The natural history of postoperative venous thromboemboli in gynecologic oncology: A prospective study of 382 patients. *Am J Obstet Gynecol* 148:1051, 1984.
25. Clarke-Pearson DL, Jelovsek FR, Creasman WT: Thromboembolism complicating surgery for cervical and

uterine malignancy: Incidence, risk factors, and prophylaxis. *Obstet Gynecol* 61:87, 1983.

26. Bodey GP, Buckley M, Sathe YS, et al: Quantitative relationships between circulating leukocytes and infection in patients with acute leukemia. *Ann Intern Med* 64:328, 1966.

27. Pizzo PA: Management of fever in patients with cancer and treatment-induced neutropenia. *N Engl J Med* 328:1323,1993.

28. Fischer DS, Knobf MT, Durivage HJ: *The Cancer Chemotherapy Handbook,* 4th ed. St Louis: Mosby, 1993.

29. Hughes WT, Armstrong D, Bodey GP, et al: Guidelines for the use of antimicrobial agents in neutropenic patients with unexplained fever: From the Infectious Diseases Society of America. *J Infect Dis* 161:381, 1990.

30. Miller LL (ed): American Society of Clinical Oncology recommendations for the use of hematopoietic colony stimulating factors: Evidence-based, clinical practice guidelines. *J Clin Oncol* 12:2471, 1994.

31. Curtin JP: Management of the neutropenic patient, in Rubin SC (ed): *Chemotherapy of Gynecologic Cancers.* Philadelphia: Lippincott-Raven, 1996.

32. Morgan MA: Use of blood products and hematologic growth factors, in Rubin SC (ed): *Chemotherapy of Gynecologic Cancers.* Philadelphia: Lippincott-Raven, 1996.

33. Perez EA, Hesketh PJ, Gandara DR: Serotonin antagonists in the management of cisplatin-induced emesis. *Semin Oncol* 18:73, 1991.

34. Himmelberg C, Christen C: Management of stomatitis. *Michigan Drug Lett* 8:1, 1989.

35. Forman A: Peripheral neuropathy in cancer patients: Incidence, features, and pathophysiology. *Oncology* 4:59, 1990.

36. Henssen JA: Protocol for treatment of vesicant antineoplastic extravasation. *Hosp Pharm* 24:705, 1989.

37. Fish LS: Prevention and treatment of extravasation of antineoplastic agents. *Hosp Pharm Hot Line* 3(5):1, 1990.

38. Rudolph R, Larson DL: Etiology and treatment of chemotherapeutic agent extravasation injuries: A review. *J Clin Oncol* 5:1116, 1987.

39. Letschert JG: The prevention of radiation induced small bowel complications. *Eur J Cancer* 31A:1361, 1995.

40. Mann WJ: Surgical management of radiation enteropathy. *Surg Clin North Am* 71:977, 1991.

41. Biswal BM, Lal P, Rath GK, et al: Intrarectal formalin application, an effective treatment for grade III hemorrhagic radiation proctitis. *Radiother Oncol* 35:212, 1995.

42. Levenback C, Eifel PJ, Burke TW, et al: Hemorrhagic cystitis following radiotherapy for stage IB cancer of the cervix. *Gynecol Oncol* 55:206, 1994.

APPENDIXES

RAPID GUIDE TO DRUG USE DURING PREGNANCY*

Table A1-1

THERAPEUTIC AGENTS COMMONLY USED IN EMERGENCY SETTINGS WITH KNOWN ADVERSE EFFECTS IN HUMAN PREGNANCY

Drug	Effect
ACE inhibitors	Renal failure, oligohydramnios
Aminoglycosides	Ototoxicity
Androgenic steroids	Masculinize female fetus
Anticonvulsants	Dysmorphic syndrome, anomalies
Antithyroid agents	Fetal goiter
Aspirin	Bleeding, antepartum and postpartum
Cytotoxic agents, i.e., methotrexate	Multiple anomalies
Isotretinoin	Hydrocephalus, deafness, anomalies
Lithium	Congenital heart disease (Ebstein anomaly)
Methotrexate	Anomalies
Nonsteroidal anti-inflammatory drugs (prolonged use after 32 weeks)	Oligohydramnios, constriction of fetal ductus arteriosus
Tetracycline (after first trimester)	Discoloration of deciduous teeth, inhibits bone growth
Thalidomide	Phocomelia
Warfarin	Embryopathy—nasal hypoplasia, optic atrophy

Table A1-2

DRUGS CONTRAINDICATED DURING BREAST-FEEDING

Amphetamines	Ergotamine
Aspirin (high doses)	Lithium
Bromocriptine (Parlodel)	Radiopharmaceuticals
Cytotoxic agents	

Source: American Academy of Pediatrics,[90] with permission.

Table A1-3

DRUGS WHOSE EFFECTS ON NURSING INFANTS IS UNKNOWN BUT MAY BE OF CONCERN

Metronidazole (Flagyl)	Antidepressant drugs
Psychotropic drugs	Antipsychotic drugs
Antianxiety drugs	

Source: American Academy of Pediatrics,[90] with permission.

Table A1-4

DRUGS POTENTIALLY AFFECTING MILK SUPPLY

Decongestants
Diuretics
Combination oral contraceptives

Table A1-5

DRUGS USUALLY CONSIDERED COMPATIBLE WITH BREAST-FEEDING

Analgesics	Antihypertensives
Antiasthmatics	Antithyroid agents
Antibiotics	Corticosteroids
Anticoagulants	Digoxin
Anticonvulsants	Narcotics
Antiemetics	Oral contraceptives
Antihistamines	Sedatives

Source: American Academy of Pediatrics,[90] with permission.

*See Chap. 16 for more detailed information.

A2

IMAGING SAFETY DURING PREGNANCY

Mitchell M. Goodsitt

Emmanuel G. Christodoulou

When a pregnant woman undergoes a diagnostic x-ray procedure, possible deleterious effects to the fetus are a logical concern. Fortunately, recent analyses have shown that, in nearly all cases, the x-ray doses for clinical radiographs are below those at which statistically significant increases in fetal abnormalities arise.[1] This appendix covers the units used for x-ray exposure and dose, lists fetal doses for many common procedures, discusses the risks of radiation to the fetus, gives recommendations concerning alternative imaging modalities such as ultrasound and magnetic resonance imaging, and provides an example of a policy to follow when a pregnant or potentially pregnant patient presents for a possible x-ray procedure.

THE THREE RS: ROENTGEN, RAD, AND REM

X-rays are a form of electromagnetic radiation, similar to visible light, ultraviolet light, microwaves, and radio waves. The primary distinguishing feature of x-ray photons is that they have much higher energies and can therefore ionize matter. Ionizing radiation is commonly quantified in three ways: *exposure, dose,* and *relative effective dose.* The unit of x-ray exposure, the *roentgen* (R), is a specific amount of ions or charge per unit mass (or volume) of air. Skin surface exposures are often provided in units of roentgen or milliroentgen (mR), where 1 mR equals 1/1000 R (Table A2-1).

The *dose* is the amount of energy deposited by the x-rays in our tissues and is measured in *rads* (radiation absorbed dose). One rad is equal to 0.01 joule per kilogram of tissue. At diagnostic x-ray energies, 1 rad is roughly equal to 1 R.

In addition to x-rays, we are exposed to other types of ionizing radiation, such as alpha particles from the decay of radon gas. In contrast to x-rays, which can penetrate our bodies, alpha particles are completely absorbed by less than 1 mm of soft tissue (actually, by just a few hundredths of a millimeter).[2] Consequently, the energy deposition and damage are more localized resulting in greater biological effect. The relative biological effect or *relative effective dose* of the different types of ionizing radiation is accounted for in the quantity termed the *dose equivalent.* The unit for dose equivalent is the *rem.* For diagnostic x-rays, 1 rem equals 1 rad. The rem is also used as the unit for effective dose equivalent[3] and effective dose,[4] both of which account for the effects of partial body irradiation and radiosensitivity of specific organs.

In summary, *for diagnostic x-rays, 1 R of exposure is equal to approximately 1 rad of absorbed dose in soft tissue, which is equal to approximately 1 rem dose equivalent.*

Recently, the SI or system international set of units has been established. The SI unit for dose is the *gray* (Gy). One gray is equal to 1 joule (J) of absorbed energy per kilogram of tissue; hence, 1 Gy is equal to 100 rads. The SI unit for dose equivalent, effective dose equivalent, and effective dose is the *sievert* (Sv), and 1 Sv is equal to 100 rem.

Table A2-1

MEASURES OF RADIATION

Measure	Definition	Unit	SI Unit
Exposure	Ions produced per kilogram of air	Roentgen (R)[a]	Coulomb/kg[a]
Dose	Energy absorbed per kilogram of tissue	Rad (rad)[b]	Gray (Gy)[b]
Dose equivalent	Energy absorbed per kilogram of tissue corrected for biological effect	Rem (rem)[c]	Sievert (Sv)[c]

[a] $1 R = 2.58 \times 10^{-4}$ C/kg
[b] $1 Gy = 100$ rad
[c] $1 Sv = 100$ rem
kg = kilogram
C = coulomb

RISKS OF IONIZATION

The primary risk of ionization is damage to the DNA in our cells. Depending upon the extent, location, and timing of the x-ray exposure, the DNA damage may be repaired, or it may result in cell death, rapid cell growth (cancer), abnormal growth (birth defects) in the fetus, and/or genetic mutation. The majority of the damage to DNA from x-ray exposure arises indirectly from interactions with free radicals produced when the x-rays ionize water molecules in our bodies. These free radicals are electrically neutral hydrogen atoms and hydroxylmolecules that have an unpaired electron in the outermost shell and are chemically very reactive. In order to become stable, they rapidly acquire or share electrons with nearby molecules, in the process breaking chemical bonds within those molecules. Furthermore, free radicals can interact with themselves and other molecules to produce toxins such as hydrogen peroxide. Compared with chemical agents, ionizing radiation is particularly effective at damaging DNA because of the ability of ionizing radiation to produce chemical bond breakages and lesions in the various components of DNA, all within a very small region.[5]

DOSE TO THE FETUS FROM COMMON DIAGNOSTIC X-RAY PROCEDURES

The x-ray dose to the fetus depends upon a number of factors including the skin surface exposure to the mother, the effective energy of the x-ray beam, the size of the x-ray field, the depth of the fetus, and the size of the patient. Even when the fetus is not located within the x-ray field, it can still receive an x-ray dose due to scattered x-rays within the mother's body. Abdominal shielding can reduce external scatter of radiation and resultant fetal dose, and is advised when the patient is pregnant. However, shielding has little effect on fetal dose once the beam has entered the body (internal scatter). In that case, in addition to the above factors, the dose depends on the distance between the x-ray field and the fetus.[6–14] One of the most useful references for calculating internal scatter is the *Handbook of Selected Tissue Doses for Projections Common in Diagnostic Radiology*[8] published by the Food and Drug Administration (FDA). The organ doses in this pamphlet are based on calculations made with a sophisticated computer simulation method known as the Monte Carlo method. Normalized organ dose (dose divided by free-in-air exposure at the skin surface position) tables are provided for various x-ray beam qualities.

FETAL DOSES FROM RADIOGRAPHIC EXAMINATIONS

We measured the free-in-air exposures and beam qualities for many common radiographic (film) procedures that women undergo in the emergency department and used the normalized organ dose tables[8] to estimate fetal dose. That dose is actually the dose to the uterus and is valid for fetuses up to the age of 2 months. Beyond 2 months, because of the increased uterine size, other methods must be employed. Table A2-2 lists the estimated doses to the uterus for the various types of examinations. The doses in Table A2-2 represent values for an average-sized patient. The doses are directly proportional to the tube current exposure time product (mAs) employed, and they are fairly strongly dependent upon the x-ray beam's half-value layer (HVL). As long as the HVL, or effective energy, for a particular examination is similar to the one listed, the dose to the conceptus of a specific average-sized patient can be estimated by simply multiplying the dose in the final column of Table A2-2 by the ratio of the actual mAs to the mAs

ESTIMATED FETAL DOSES FOR COMMON RADIOGRAPHIC EXAMINATIONS

Examination	kVp	mAs	HVL, mmAl	SID, cm	Field Size at Film, cm-cm	Average Patient Thickness, cm	Exposure in Air at Skin Surface mR	Dose to the Uterus (Fetus) per Film, mrad
Chest AP/PA	125	5	5.4	183	35x43	22	36	0.2
Chest lateral	125	20	5.4	183	35x43	32	162	0.3
Chest (portable)	90	2.5	3.0	122	35x43	22	19	0.0
Abdomen AP	70	40	3.0	102	35x43	20	400	138.0
Abdomen decub.	70	80	3.0	102	35x43	20	800	39.0
Abdomen (portable/grid)	70	64	2.3	102	35x43	20	521	135.0
Pelvis AP	75	40	3.2	102	35x43	20	457	171.0
Pelvis (portable/grid)	76	40	2.4	102	35x43	20	343	95.0
C-spine AP	75	8	3.2	102	24x30	13	77	0.0
C-spine lateral	70	10	3.0	102	24x30	17	75	0.0
C-spine lateral/grid	75	16	3.2	102	24x30	17	169	0.0
C-spine AP (portable/grid)	70	12	3.0	102	24x30	13	77	0.0
C-spine oblique	65	10	2.8	102	24x30	13	71	0.0
C-spine odontoid	75	25	3.2	102	24x30	13	238	0.0
T-spine AP	75	32	3.2	102	35x43	22	386	0.4
T-spine lateral	80	32	3.4	102	35x43	32	603	0.3
L-spine AP	75	40	3.2	102	35x43	20	457	150.0
L-spine lateral	85	64	3.6	102	35x43	32	1371	64.0
IVP	65	30	2.8	102	24x30	20	306	78.0
Hip AP	75	32	3.2	102	24x30	20	365	95.0
Hip lateral	75	32	3.2	102	24x30	18	346	15.0
Femur AP	75	12	3.2	102	18x43	20	137	1.0
Femur lateral	75	10	3.2	102	18x43	20	114	0.3
Shoulder AP	70	8	3.0	102	24x30	17	73	0.0
Humerus AP	60	2	2.5	102	18x43	17	14	0.0
Orbits AP	70	50	3.0	102	24x30	18	474	0.0
Orbits lateral	70	7	3.0	102	24x30	18	66	0.0
Skull AP	70	40	3.0	102	24x30	18	379	0.0
Skull lateral	70	10	3.0	102	24x30	18	95	0.0
Skull townes	70	64	3.0	102	24x30	18	606	0.0
Skull waters	70	40	3.0	102	24x30	18	379	0.0
Zygoma axial	70	6	3.0	102	24x30	18	57	0.0
Soft tissue neck AP	70	10	3.0	102	24x30	13	83	0.0
Soft tissue neck lateral	100	2	4.4	102	24x30	17	38	0.0
Nuclear Medicine Studies								
Thyroid scan								270*[†]
Bone, brain, renal, cardiovascular scan								<500*[19]
Pulmonary Ventilation/perfusion scan								~50*[19]

*Per study

[†]Husak V, Wiedermann M: Radiation absorbed dose estimates to the embryo from some nuclear medicine procedures. *Eur J Nucl Med* 5:205, 1980.

Key: kVp = peak kilovoltage (x-ray tube potential)

mAs = milliampere•seconds (x-ray tube current exposure time product)

HVL = half-value-layer (thickness of aluminum necessary to reduce x-ray intensity by a factor of 2)

SID = source-to-image distance (x-ray tube to film distance)

in the table. If the HVL of a particular x-ray unit differs from that listed in Table A2-2 by more than 0.2, the actual dose may differ by more than 20 percent. Under those circumstances, we recommend using the organ dose versus HVL data in the original FDA publication[8] to obtain a more accurate dose estimate. The normalized organ doses are not applicable to individuals whose anthropometric characteristics differ significantly from the reference (average) patient. Hence, the fetal doses listed in the last column of Table A2-2 are not as accurate in very thin or obese patients. Finally, if an average-sized patient has multiple examinations, the total dose to the conceptus is computed by simply summing the doses from each individual examination.

FETAL DOSES FROM COMPUTED TOMOGRAPHY EXAMINATIONS

Computed tomography (CT) examinations usually involve higher radiation doses than other radiographic examinations. For an examination of the pelvic region, the conceptus dose will be in the vicinity of 2000 mrad (20 mGy). The dose depends on the position of the conceptus with respect to the part of the patient's body that is scanned, the beam quality, the examination technique used, and the patient's size and contour.

One of the methods for estimating fetal doses from CT examinations was developed by Mini et al.[15] This group used thermoluminescent dosimeters (TLDs) to measure doses at 70 locations inside an anthropomorphic phantom that was scanned using standard CT examination protocols. They determined the typical location and size of several organs of interest in that phantom from CT images of previously examined patients. The dose to the fetus was assumed to be equal to the mean dose to the uterus. In addition, Mini et al. established conversion factors that relate measured free-in-air dose (kerma) to organ dose at the rotation axis of any CT scanner. One of the simplest methods to estimate fetal dose from a CT examination is to measure the free-in-air dose for the technique employed and multiply by the appropriate conversion factor. Table A2-3 shows the conversion factors (F) for radiation doses to the uterus for whole-area CT examination of the thorax, abdomen, and pelvis. Our calculated doses to the uterus for the GE 9800 CT scanner at our institution and those calculated by Mini et al. for their Siemens Somatom Plus CT scanner are listed in Table A2-4.

Notice that the dose values for the two CT scanners are very similar. Also, the doses quoted by Mini et al. include the dose for the scout (localization) view, whereas ours do not. The doses to the conceptus for the scout views are quite small (<1 mrad, 3 mrad, and 31 mrad for the thorax, abdomen, and pelvis regions respectively).[15]

When a more accurate assessment of the fetal dose from a CT examination is required, a method developed by Felmlee et al.[16] may be used. This method is especially useful when more detailed information is available concerning the

Table A2-3
CONVERSION FACTORS (F)* FOR RADIATION DOSES TO THE UTERUS FOR COMPUTED TOMOGRAPHY EXAMINATIONS OF THREE REGIONS

Thorax	Abdomen	Pelvis
7	40	441

Source: Mini et al.,[15] with permission.
*mrad to uterus/rad free-in-air kerma at center of gantry

exact locations of the CT slices and/or when slice thicknesses other than the 10 mm assumed by Mini et al. are employed.

Felmlee et al. measured fetal doses in an adult anthropomorphic phantom. For these measurements, they used four CT scanners (Picker 1200, Siemens DRH, GE 9800, and GE 8800), four kilovoltages (100, 120, 130, and 140 kVp), and three radiation scan thicknesses (2, 5, and 10 mm). The fetal dose estimates are based on the CT dose index (CTDI) measured using a pencil ionization chamber (10 cm long, 3 cm^3) at the center position of a 16-cm-diameter cylindrical acrylic phantom.

Other methods for computing fetal doses that have appeared in the literature include those of Panzer and Zankl,[17] who calculated doses with a Monte Carlo method using a "female mathematical reference phantom," and Wagner et al.,[18] who measured doses along the central axis and surface of two abdominal phantoms that simulated the female pelvis and derived formulas for computing fetal dose for specific CT scanners from the mAs, number of sections over the conceptus, and total number of sections.

FETAL DOSES FROM FLUOROSCOPY EXAMINATIONS

In general, fluoroscopy examinations, especially those that are long and involved, result in the highest patient doses in radiology departments. The typical skin surface exposure rate is about 2000 mR/min. The dose to the conceptus from such studies can be computed using the normalized-organ-dose tables for corresponding radiographic techniques.[8] To use these tables, one must account for the closer x-ray focus-to-patient distance employed in conventional (x-ray tube under table) fluoroscopy. Usually, this distance is about 46 cm for fluoroscopy units, as compared with about 74 cm for radiography units. Assuming these distances, that the thickness of the mother's body is approximately 20 cm, and that the uterus is located 8 cm from the front surface for the anteroposterior (AP) projection and 12 cm from the rear sur-

Table A2-4

MEAN DOSE TO THE UTERUS (CONCEPTUS)

	Examination Site		
CT Scanner	Thorax	Abdomen	Pelvis
Siemens Somatom Plus (Mini et al.)	**16 mrad** 120 kVp 150 mAs 10 mm	**150 mrad** 120 kVP 210 mAs 10 mm	**1930 mrad** 120 kVP 340 mAs 10 mm
GE 9800 (University of Michigan)	**23 mrad** 120 kVp 200 mAs 10 mm	**186 mrad** 120 kVp 280 mAs 10 mm	**2050 mrad** 120 kVp 280 mAs 10 mm

Key: mrad = millirad
kVp = peak kilovoltage
mAs = milliampere•second
mm = millimeter
Source: Mini et al.,[15] with permission.

face for the posteroanterior (PA) projection,[7] one can estimate that the normalized organ doses (mrad/R free-in-air skin surface exposure) for AP fluoroscopy are about 0.89 times those for AP radiography, and those for PA fluoroscopy are about 0.85 times those for PA radiography. For example, the normalized dose to the uterus (conceptus) for AP fluoroscopy of the abdomen, assuming an x-ray spectrum with a HVL of 4 mm of A1 (aluminum), would be 0.89 times the normalized dose from AP radiography (442 mrad/R[8]), i.e., 393 mrad per 1 R entrance exposure. If a woman undergoes a fluoroscopic procedure that lasts 2 to 3 min and receives a typical free-in-air skin surface exposure of 2 R/min, her total skin surface exposure is 4 to 6 R, and the estimated dose to the fetus is 3930 mrad (3.93 cGy).

If a pregnant woman undergoes an upper gastrointestinal fluoroscopic examination, in particular an examination using barium as the contrast agent, the dose to the fetus can be estimated using data from another FDA publication.[9] Some examples of normalized doses to the uterus for such examinations are listed in Table A2-5.

We have chosen not to list the normalized dose to the uterus for many upper GI examinations such as LPO (left posterior oblique) and RAO (right anterior oblique) projections of the upper, middle, and lower esophagus because those doses are very low (<0.1 mrad). Furthermore, the doses listed in the table are considerably less than those for the lower GI tract and abdomen, where the fetus is directly exposed. In particular, using the same fluoroscopy factors as those used above to estimate the conceptus dose for a fluoroscopy examination of the abdomen, (4 mm HVL and 10R entrance exposure), one would estimate a conceptus dose of only 10 mrad (0.01 cGy) for an RAO barium study of the stomach. This is about 400 times less than the dose we estimated for a lower abdomen study.

In estimating the dose from fluoroscopy studies, one must consider the fact that the skin surface exposure varies dramatically with patient thickness and fluoroscopic image field of view. In general, higher skin surface exposures are required for thicker patients and smaller fields of view. An increase in patient thickness by only 1 in. typically results in

Table A2-5

DOSE TO THE UTERUS (mrad) PER 1 R FREE-IN-AIR SKIN ENTRANCE EXPOSURE

	HVL (mmAl)	
Examination	4.0	5.0
Gastroesophageal junction, LPO	0.2	0.2
Stomach, LPO	2.0	2.0
Duodenum, LPO	1.0	0.9
Gastroesophageal junction, RAO	0.3	0.4
Stomach, RAO	1.0	2.0
Duodenum, RAO	1.0	1.0

Key: mmAl = millimeters of aluminum
LPO = left posterior oblique
RAO = right anterior oblique

a two-times increase of the skin surface exposure, and changing the field of view from 12 to 6 in. often results in a four-times increase of the exposure. Federal regulations limit the maximum free-in-air skin surface exposure to 10 R/min under normal operation and 20 R/min under optional high-dose-level operation.

DOSE TO THE FETUS FROM COMMON NUCLEAR MEDICINE PROCEDURES

Radioactive isotopes are used in nuclear medicine primarily to image internal organs and to evaluate various physiologic functions and secondarily for therapeutic purposes.[2] During a nuclear medicine study, a chemical agent labeled with a radioactive isotope is introduced into the patient's body and selectively accumulated in the region of interest. For example, radioactive isotopes of iodine accumulate in the thyroid. Iodine is also used to treat hyperthyroidism.

During pregnancy, the ventilation-perfusion study is very commonly performed for detecting pulmonary embolism. Macroaggregated albumin labeled with technetium 99m (^{99m}Tc), one of the radioactive isotopes used most often in diagnostic procedures, is used for the perfusion portion and inhaled xenon 127 (^{127}Xe) or xenon 133 (^{133}Xe) is used for the ventilation portion. The dose to the fetus from such a study is approximately 50 mrad (0.05 cGy).[19] The dose to the fetus during bone, cardiovascular, brain, and renal imaging procedures with ^{99m}Tc is less than 500 mrad (0.5 cGy).[20, 21]

Radioactive iodine readily crosses the placenta and can affect the fetal thyroid, especially when used after 10 to 12 weeks of pregnancy. If a diagnostic procedure of the thyroid is deemed necessary, iodine 123 (^{123}I) or ^{99m}Tc should be used instead of iodine 131 (^{131}I) because ^{131}I results in a much higher dose per unit activity to the fetal thyroid. It is highly recommended that therapeutic use of radioactive iodine in the mother be delayed until after the delivery of the baby.[22]

RISKS TO THE EMBRYO AND FETUS FROM EXPOSURE TO IONIZING RADIATION

Some of the most recent information concerning the risks to the embryo and fetus from exposure to ionizing radiation is contained in the National Council on Radiation Protection (NCRP) commentary number 9, which was published in May 1994[23]; much of what follows is based on the material in that commentary. In general, the risks to the embryo and fetus can be classified into two categories: those due to deterministic effects and those due to stochastic effects.

DETERMINISTIC EFFECTS

Deterministic effects are those believed to occur only at x-ray doses above certain thresholds. The probabilities of these effects are strongly related to the stage of pregnancy at which the embryo/fetus is exposed.

All of the effects described above have been observed after fetal doses of 100 rads (1 Gy) or more. It is believed that these effects have thresholds below which no effect occurs and above which the chance of harm increases as the radiation dose increases. The exact values of the thresholds are not known. However, studies to date indicate that for acute exposures of the whole body of the conceptus, the thresholds for malformations and growth retardation may be in the range of 10 to 20 rads (0.1 to 0.2 Gy); for mental retardation, 10 to 20 rads (0.1-0.2 Gy) or as high as 40 rads (0.4 Gy) if Down syndrome cases are excluded; and for small head size, as low as 5 rads (0.05 Gy).

EXPOSURE DURING FIRST 2 WEEKS OF PREGNANCY

The predominant deterministic effect due to exposure during the first 2 weeks of pregnancy is resorption of the embryo.

EXPOSURE DURING WEEKS 2 TO 8

The second to eighth week postconception is the period of organogenesis. Significant x-ray exposure during this period may result in teratogenesis (birth defects). Examples include gross malformation and growth retardation, the latter of which can occur both at term and later at adulthood. Neuropathology and small head size may also occur as a result of significant exposures during weeks 2 to 8.

EXPOSURES DURING WEEKS 8 TO 15

The embryo has developed into a fetus at about the seventh to eighth week, and neurologic development occurs during the next 7 weeks. Significant x-ray exposure at this time (between weeks 8 and 15) may result in mental retardation, small head size, and decreased IQ. Other possible but less likely effects due to significant exposure during this period include growth retardation as an adult and sterility. Even less likely but still possible are cataracts, neuropathology, and growth retardation at term.

EXPOSURES BEYOND WEEK 15

Most of the deterministic effects mentioned above are either not observed or observed much less frequently when the fetus receives significant radiation dose beyond 15 weeks postconception. Mental retardation has been observed as a result of significant exposure during the 8th to 25th weeks but not beyond. Other effects that have been observed because of exposure after week 15 include sterility and growth retardation as an adult. Less likely effects that have been demonstrated are cataracts, neuropathology, and growth retardation at term.

RISKS OF DETERMINISTIC EFFECTS IN PERSPECTIVE

To better comprehend the actual risks involved with exposure of the conceptus to doses at or above a threshold, consider the case of mental retardation. When the fetus receives an unusually high dose of 100 rads (1 Gy) during the 8th to 15th weeks postconception, the frequency of severe mental retardation is 43 percent.[22] This is 100 times greater than the 0.4 percent frequency of severe mental retardation due to natural causes.[24] On the other hand, if the fetus were to receive a dose of 10 rads (0.1 Gy), which is closer to the threshold, the frequency of severe mental retardation is about 4 percent. While it is true that this frequency is 10 times that due to natural causes, one must also consider that there is about a 96 percent chance that the person will not be severely mentally retarded subsequent to receiving such a dose in utero. Furthermore, had the x-ray dose been received 16 to 25 weeks after conception, the relative risk of severe mental retardation would have been at least 4 times less.

Another example is small head size. The natural incidence is about 4 percent.[25] A whole-body dose of 10 rads (0.1 Gy) to a fetus 4 to 7 weeks after conception increases the incidence to about 9 percent (a 91 percent chance of not having a small head size).[26] If this dose is received 9 to 11 weeks postconception, the risk of small head size increases to about 13 percent (an 87 percent chance of not having a small head size).[26] The exact thresholds and risks are still a matter of debate, and the values cited above are not to be taken as absolutes but as reasonable estimates that may be revised with further studies.

STOCHASTIC EFFECTS

Stochastic effects have no threshold. They occur at random with a probability that increases with radiation dose. Interestingly, the severity of the effect is unrelated to dose, indicating that radiation triggers a disease process "whose ultimate course is determined by other factors in the individual."[5] The most prevalent stochastic effects are induction of cancer and genetic mutations in future generations. The probabilities of these effects are quite low. In fact, the most recent analyses of Japanese A-bomb survivors who were exposed in utero show no significant increase in rates of childhood or adult cancer.[27,28] Furthermore, radiation-induced genetic effects have not been observed in the births of the Japanese A-bomb survivors. Because of the uncertainties involved in estimating risks, experts believe it is reasonable to assume that "the embryo or fetus is as susceptible to the carcinogenic effects of radiation as the young

child... viz. 10×10^{-2} Sv^{-1}" and that "the embryo, fetus and nursing child are as sensitive to induction of hereditary effects as the adult... viz. 1×10^{-2} Sv^{-1}."[23]

RISKS OF STOCHASTIC EFFECTS IN PERSPECTIVE

To put the risks of stochastic effects in perspective, consider the increase in the probability that a fetus exposed to 10 rem (0.1 Sv) will develop cancer in his or her lifetime. This increase is about 0.01. If this increase is added to the normal probability of developing cancer during one's lifetime, which is 0.20, the overall risk increases from 20 to 21 percent, which is relatively insignificant.

BIOLOGICAL RISKS ASSOCIATED WITH NONIONIZING IMAGING MODALITIES

Although the risks to the fetus are relatively small from the ionization produced in diagnostic examinations with ionizing radiation, it is possible to avoid those risks entirely by employing a nonionizing imaging modality such as ultrasound or MRI. These alternative modalities (in particular, ultrasound) have been found to be relatively free of risk. The risks of ultrasound and MRI are described below.

RISKS OF ULTRASOUND EXAMINATIONS

Although no ultrasonically induced adverse bioeffects have been reported during the approximately four decades that ultrasonography has been used clinically, at sufficiently high exposure levels, ultrasound has been demonstrated to produce changes in living systems.

Ultrasonography involves the transmission of high-frequency pressure waves into the body and the reception of echoes (reflections and scatter) from interfaces and regions characterized by variations in compressibility and/or mass density. The interaction of the ultrasonic waves with tissues can produce heating and/or cavitation.

Heating results from the absorption of ultrasound energy by tissues. The absorption is highly dependent upon the tissue type and ultrasonic frequency. For example, fluids such as amniotic fluid, blood, and urine absorb almost no ultrasound energy. Soft tissues attenuate (absorb and scatter) a typical (5-MHz) ultrasound beam by about 50 percent for every centimeter traveled (e.g., intensity ~50 percent after 1 cm, ~25 percent after 2 cm, etc.). Cartilage is more absorbing than soft tissue, and bone is the most absorbing tissue. Fetal bone absorption depends upon the degree of ossification. Ultrasonic absorption and scatter increase in all tissues as the ultrasonic frequency is increased (e.g., greater absorption for 5 MHz than 3.5 MHz). In scanning a pregnant woman, one of the potential concerns is significant temperature rises at or near the fetal bone due to its high absorption coefficient. Indeed, if one neglects the pulsed nature of ultrasound employed in imaging and the cooling effects of local blood flow and assumes an ultrasound power level near the maximum employed clinically, temperature rises of about 4°C (7.2°F) are possible.[29] This is very close to the temperature rise of 5°C (9°F) that has been associated with cell killing. The low duty factor of the pulsed beam (pulses "on" about 0.5 to 1.0 percent of the time) and the local blood flow make such temperature rises extremely unlikely.

Cavitation is a general term used to describe the generation, growth, oscillation and possible collapse of microbubbles in tissues.[29] The generation of new microbubbles and growth of existing microbubbles is due to the negative pressure (rarefaction) part of the ultrasound wave. Cavitation is unlikely to produce a significant adverse biological effect unless the cavitation is widespread over an organ or tissue. To date, we have no evidence that diagnostic ultrasound examinations have resulted in cavitation in humans.[29]

In the interest of keeping the ultrasound exposure to the patient as low as reasonably achievable, manufacturers are now incorporating in diagnostic ultrasound equipment real-time display of indexes related to the potential for bioeffects. Establishment of these indexes is the result of a joint effort by the National Equipment Manufacturers Association (NEMA), the FDA, and the American Institute of Ultrasound in Medicine (AIUM).[30] Two types of indexes may be displayed: a thermal index (TI), which is related to potential temperature increase, and a mechanical index (MI), which is related to potential cavitation. Both types are relative. For example, a thermal index of 2 does not indicate a temperature rise of 2°C. Rather, it indicates a temperature rise twice as great as that for a thermal index of 1. Furthermore, the fact that an index is displayed does not mean that temperature rise or cavitation is actually occurring. Many other factors such as tissue types, intervening layers of absorbing or nonabsorbing tissues, ultrasound beam faces and tissue perfusion may alter the bioeffects.

In terms of official recommendations, the AIUM, in March 1993, approved the following Official Statement on the clinical safety of Diagnostic Ultrasound[31]:

Diagnostic ultrasound has been in use since the late 1950s. Given its known benefits and recognized efficacy for medical diagnosis, including use during human pregnancy, American Institute of Ultrasound in Medicine herein addresses the clinical safety of such use: No confirmed biological effects on patients or instrument operators caused by exposure at intensities typical of present diagnostic ultrasound instruments have ever been reported. Although the possibility exists that such biological effects may be identified in the future, current data indicate that the benefits to patients of the prudent use of diagnostic ultrasound outweigh the risks, if any, that may be present.

RISKS OF MAGNETIC RESONANCE IMAGING EXAMINATIONS

In magnetic resonance imaging, the human body is placed in a strong static magnetic field and exposed to radiofrequency fields as well as static and rapidly switching magnetic field gradients. The purpose of all these is to image the distribution of hydrogen in the body and the rates at which hydrogen atoms perturbed by radiofrequency (rf) pulses at specific locations return to equilibrium (T1 and T2 relaxation times).

The predominant sources of possible bioeffects from MRI are (1) the static magnetic field of the MRI system, (2) the gradient magnetic fields, (3) the rf electromagnetic fields, (4) the combination of the three different electromagnetic fields, and (5) the imaging contrast agents. Effects 1 through 3 have been reviewed comprehensively by Hendee and Ritenour.[5]

The primary effect of the static field is the induction of electrical potentials in the body. These result from blood (a conductor) moving through the magnetic field. The induced potentials are quite small (on the order of millivolts) and do not have any known adverse effects. To ensure that the effects from the static fields are minimal, the FDA has established guidelines that restrict the intensity of the static magnetic fields to less than or equal to 2.0 teslas.

Time-varying gradient fields on the order of 2 teslas per second (T/s) are fairly typical in today's images. Such fields induce currents of about 10 to 30 mA/m^2 in the body. Chronic exposure to currents of this magnitude can result in changes in cell function including variations in cell growth rate, respiration and metabolism, immune response, and gene expression. However, patient exposure to time-varying fields in MRI is of an acute nature, and scan duration is orders of magnitude less than that which has been associated with the above-mentioned effects. The FDA guidelines require time varying fields to be less than or equal to 3 T/s.

The rf pulses of energy to which the patient is exposed during the "transmit" portion of the imaging cycle can cause heating of tissue. The rf pulses induce electrical currents in the tissues, and the resistance of the tissues to these currents result in the transfer of the energy of the currents to heat with an associated temperature rise. While temperature rises of about 5°C (9°F) above body core temperature are known to cause cell killing, typical temperature elevation with clinical MRI is significantly below this.

It has been shown that some intravenous MRI contrast agents cross the placenta and circulate through the fetus several times as it swallows and excretes the amniotic fluid. The rates of clearance of these contrast agents from the amniotic fluid and the fetal circulation are unknown. Therefore some authors recommend[32] against administering any MRI contrast agents to pregnant patients until more data become available.

The issue of the possible adverse bioeffects on pregnant women of the MRI environment is reviewed extensively in a recent book by Shellock and Kanal.[32] They state that there are two facts that make it nearly impossible to prove the safety of

MRI for pregnant women: (1) the many possible combinations of the multiple risk factors associated with the MRI environment and (2) the relatively high spontaneous abortion rate in humans (>30 percent) during the first trimester of pregnancy.

Shellock and Kanal reviewed the literature related to MRI procedures and pregnancy over a period of 20 years (1973–1993). They point out that the evidence regarding the bioeffects of the electromagnetic fields used in the MRI procedures, particularly on developing organisms, is contradictory. At present, there is no conclusive evidence regarding any deleterious effects that MRI may have on the developing fetus. It is well known, though, that cells undergoing division are more susceptible to damage. Also, a number of mechanisms exist with which the electromagnetic radiation used in MRI could be hazardous to the developing fetus. Therefore, until further investigations prove otherwise they recommend[32] that MRI be used with caution during pregnancy, especially during the first trimester.

In terms of official recommendations, the *Policies, Guidelines, and Recommendations for MR Imaging Safety and Patient Management* issued by the Safety Committee of the Society for Magnetic Resonance Imaging[33] states:

MR imaging may be used in pregnant women if other non-ionizing forms of diagnostic imaging are inadequate or if the examination provides important information that would otherwise require exposure to ionizing radiation (e.g., fluoroscopy, CT, etc.). It is recommended that pregnant patients be informed that, to date, there has been no indication that the use of clinical MR imaging during pregnancy has produced deleterious effects. However, as noted by the FDA, the safety of MR imaging during pregnancy has not been proved.

Furthermore, the International Non-Ionizing Radiation Committee of the International Radiation Protection Association has issued a publication entitled *Protection of the Patient Undergoing a Magnetic Resonance Examination*[34] in which the following is stated:

There is no firm evidence that mammalian embryos are sensitive to the magnetic fields encountered in magnetic resonance systems. However, pending the accumulation of more data regarding MR in pregnancy, it is recommended that elective examination of pregnant women should be postponed until after the first trimester. Because ultrasound is the modality of choice for fetal and uterine examination during pregnancy, an MR examination should be limited to cases in which unique diagnostic information can be obtained. Exposure duration should be reduced to the minimum, consistent with obtaining useful diagnostic information.

PREGNANT PATIENT POLICY

It is recommended that all clinics and institutions adopt a policy to follow when a pregnant or potentially pregnant patient presents herself for a possible x-ray procedure. An example of a step-by-step flowchart section of such a policy is shown in Fig. A2-1.

Most of this flowchart should be self-explanatory. With respect to the bottom right box, methods that can be employed to reduce x-ray dose include (1) use of a higher x-ray tube voltage (kVp) technique in both radiography and fluoroscopy, (2) employment of a technique without a grid in both fluoroscopy and radiography, (3) employment of a higher-speed screen-film combination in radiography, (4) operation of fluoroscopy equipment in a pulsed mode at a lower pulse rate if available (e.g., the dose for 7.5 pulses per second is about one-fourth the dose for 30 pulses per second), (5) use of greater TV camera gain in fluoroscopy, and (6) use of larger fields of view in fluoroscopy. All of these methods have disadvantages in terms of reducing image quality. For example, use of higher-kVp techniques, greater fluoroscopic TV camera gain, removal of the scatter-reducing grid, and lower fluoroscopic pulse rates will all result in degraded image contrast, and use of higher-speed screen-film combinations and larger fluoroscopic fields of view will result in degraded spatial resolution. Physicians must decide upon the amount and type of image degradation they are willing to accept before choosing to use one of the dose-reduction techniques.

SUMMARY

This appendix can probably be best summarized by a set of guidelines that was recommended in September of 1995 by the Committee on Obstetric Practice of the American College of Obstetricians and Gynecologists.[35] They state: "The following guidelines for x-ray examination or exposure during pregnancy are suggested:

1. Women should be counseled that x-ray exposure from a single diagnostic procedure does not result in harmful effects. Specifically, exposure to less than 5 rad has not been associated with an increase in fetal anomalies or pregnancy loss.

2. Concern about possible effects of high-dose ionizing radiation exposure should not prevent medically indicated diagnostic x-ray procedures from being performed on the mother. During pregnancy, other imaging procedures not associated with ionizing radiation (e.g., ultrasonography, MRI) should be considered instead of x-rays when possible.

3. Ultrasonography and MRI are not associated with known adverse fetal effects. However, until more information is available, MRI is not recommended for use in the first trimester.

4. Consultation with a radiologist may be helpful in calculating estimated fetal dose when multiple diagnostic x-rays are performed on a pregnant patient.

5. The use of radioactive isotopes of iodine is contraindicated for therapeutic use during pregnancy."

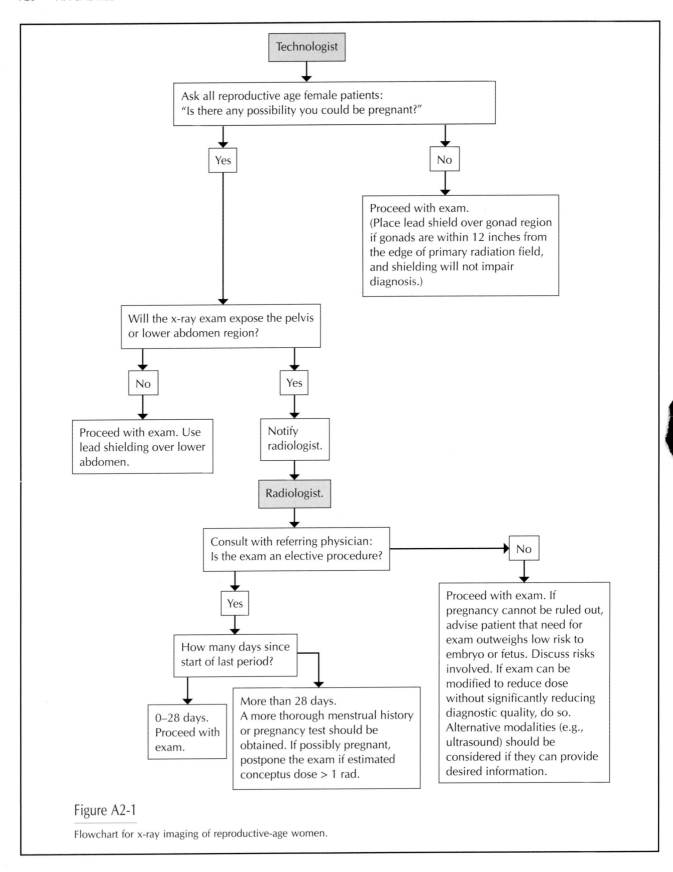

Figure A2-1

Flowchart for x-ray imaging of reproductive-age women.

A3

COLLECTION AND TRANSPORT OF GYNECOLOGIC MICROBIOLOGY SPECIMENS

Carl L. Pierson

GENERAL CONSIDERATIONS REGARDING SPECIMEN COLLECTION AND WORKING WITH THE DIAGNOSTIC LABORATORY

Proper collection and handling of microbiology specimens requires the collector to know which infectious agents may be present in the sample and have some understanding of the procedures that will be used in the microbiology laboratory to detect these agents once the specimen is received. Culture continues to be the principal method used to detect potential pathogens; therefore, when this method is used, the organism must be received in a viable state. As more molecular diagnostic techniques are developed and adapted for clinical laboratory use, the preservation of specific target molecules in the specimen may be more important than maintaining viability and may require that the specimen be placed in a specially designed transport device. These devices frequently are specific for a commercial kit or instru-

ment being used in a laboratory, and a substitute collection device may yield an erroneous test result.

The collector must also be aware of the time it may take a specimen to get from the collection point to the testing laboratory. If the specimen will arrive within 1 to 2 hours, room-temperature transport may be satisfactory; however, if the specimen may set overnight or require prolonged transport, cold storage may be required.

Information provided on the accompanying requisition is usually the only information that the laboratory will receive prior to processing the sample; therefore, the practitioner should carefully complete the requisition and include pertinent clinical information that may assist the technologists. Including a probable diagnosis with the etiologic agent can significantly alter a setup routine. It also allows the technologist to match the requested test with the specimen received for appropriateness. Can the test be done from the sample received? If not, the practitioner should be contacted in a timely manner and specimen requirements discussed so that less time is wasted; there may still be time to take another specimen. When in doubt, it is advisable to contact the

729

laboratory and discuss specimen requirements. This is one of the underused services provided by laboratory personnel, and such contact can prevent a considerable amount of frustration and unnecessary expenditure for all parties. Also, if the exact test desired is not obvious from the requisition, there is usually space available to write in which tests are needed, or to indicate the organism(s) suspected. If the receiving laboratory does not perform the requested test, the specimen should automatically be sent to a certified reference laboratory that does. The Food and Drug Administration (FDA) requires that the actual laboratory performing the test be identified on the issued report.

Most laboratories provide their clients with handbooks that should provide the necessary information and instructions for proper collection and transport of specimens. Having such a handbook available on site can be very helpful and may decrease the frequency of rejected specimens.

INFECTIOUS LESIONS OF THE EXTERNAL GENITALIA

HERPES SIMPLEX VIRUS TYPES 1 AND 2

The most commonly used methods for the laboratory diagnosis of herpetic infections are culture and direct antigen testing. Vesicular or pustular fluid usually contains a high concentration of virus particles that can be collected either with a swab or by needle aspiration. As the lesion ulcerates and then crusts over, the number of viable virions decreases; therefore, samples taken from older lesions may result in a false-negative culture (see Fig. A3-1).

To send a specimen for culture, the skin covering the vesicle should first be cleaned with water or saline, not with alcohol or iodine compounds that may inhibit viral replication. Vesicular fluid can be aspirated with a tuberculin syringe fitted with a 26-gauge needle. Optimally, the fluid should be placed into viral transport medium and sent to the virology laboratory on ice. Alternatively, the aspirated fluid can be pulled into the syringe barrel, the needle removed and discarded appropriately, and the syringe capped and placed in ice for transport. (Syringes with attached needles are considered a biohazard and are no longer accepted in clinical laboratories.) If a swab is to be used, the skin covering the vesicle must be removed and a Dacron swab used to absorb the vesicular fluid. The swab is to be placed immediately into a viral transport device that will maintain the swab in moist condition. The device should be placed on ice for transport to the virology laboratory for culture. Herpes simplex virus can be stored under these conditions for at least 24 h without significant loss of cell culture infectivity. If an ulcer is present, the base should be swabbed with a Dacron swab and the swab placed into viral transport medium.

Direct antigen test methods are rapid (tests can be completed within 1 to 2 h following specimen receipt) and do not require viable virions. Vesicular fluids collected either by aspiration or swab can be tested using rapid enzyme-linked antigen-capture methods.[1] Herpes simplex virus antigens can also be detected directly by harvesting cells from the base of the vesicle with a swab and sending it to the laboratory. The technologist will transfer the cells to a slide for special staining with specific fluoroscein-labeled antibody that can differentiate between HSV types 1 and 2.[2]

Nucleic acid detection methods using specific probes with or without initial amplification are available but are usually not required for the detection of HSV in lesions of the skin

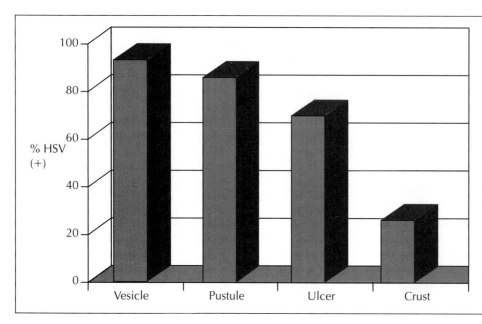

Figure A3-1

Herpes simplex virus culture by stage of lesion. (Modified from Fife KH, Corey L: Herpes simplex virus, in Holmes KK, Mardh PA, Sparling PF, et al. (eds): Sexually Transmitted Diseases, 2d ed. New York: McGraw-Hill, 1990, p. 942, with permission.)

or mucous membranes; they are also considerably more expensive to use.[3]

Histologic stains (Papanicolaou or Tzanck) can be used but are both insensitive and less specific. Solomon et al. found that only 67 percent of vesicular lesions positive by culture were positive by Tzanck stain.[4]

Herpes simplex virus serology is of limited usefulness for initial diagnosis. Blood collected during the course of the infection may contain elevated IgM-class antibodies that may aid in diagnosis. Serology is of little value in diagnosing recurrent HSV infections and currently available tests cannot be relied upon to accurately assess whether the infection was caused by HSV type 1 or 2 due to cross-reactivity as a result of shared antigens.[5] Western blot methods appear to be more specific for this purpose but currently are not widely available.

HUMAN PAPILLOMAVIRUS

The human papillomavirus (HPV) family of viruses are not cultivated in the clinical laboratory and viral antigens may not be detectable in tissues. External genital warts, also known as condyloma acuminata, are one manifestation of HPV which can be readily detected by hybridization assays that use specific nucleotide probes labeled with immunoperoxidases or fluorescent molecules. Assay sensitivity can be enhanced using nucleic acid amplification methods, such as the polymerase chain reaction (PCR).[6,7] Hybridization techniques can also be used to determine the specific HPV type.[8] Cytologic examination for the presence of koilocytes in lesions is also quite specific but insensitive.[9]

Specimens can be collected by biopsy or by scraping the base of the lesion with a scalpel. The tissue should be kept cold and transported to the laboratory in special kit-specific transport fluid. The biopsy can also be frozen and maintained at −70°C (−94°F) during shipment, using dry ice.

SYPHILIS OR SOFT CHANCRE

Treponema pallidum is not cultivated in the clinical laboratory. The laboratory diagnosis of *T. pallidum* in lesions of the skin or mucous membranes is made by direct microscopic examination of serous exudate collected from the base of the suspected lesion. Accumulated exudate should be removed to expose the ulcer base prior to scraping. The base is then gently scraped (e.g., with a scalpel blade) to cause serous fluid to collect within the ulcer base. This fresh exudate should contain viable treponemes. The exudate is then collected and placed directly onto the surface of a glass slide, covered with a cover slip and examined by dark-field microscopy within minutes of collection for detection of characteristic morphology and motility. The organism is quite thin (∼0.2 μm in diameter) and variable in length (6 to 20 μm) with a helical morphology having a wavelength of about 1 μm. Freshly isolated organisms may demonstrate a corkscrew type of motility coupled with an undulating mo-

tion. The scrapings can also be suspended in a tube containing a small amount of saline or nutrient broth available from the laboratory and transported immediately to the laboratory at room temperature for immediate dark-field examination. Extreme care should be taken in handling such samples, since the spirochetes in this state are viable and infectious. A limited number of laboratories have specific fluorescein-conjugated antibody (DFA-TP) that can detect nonviable *T. pallidum* in exudate which has been dried and fixed on a standard microscope slide. This type of specimen can be transported to the laboratory in a clean, dry container at room temperature.

Serology is the method by which most cases of syphilis are diagnosed.[10] Serum is usually screened using one of several nontreponemal tests (e.g., VDRL, RPR, RST, TRUST), which are quite sensitive but somewhat nonspecific in that they measure antilipid antibodies rather than antitreponemal antibodies. Undiluted serum is screened and, if found to be positive, titrated to provide a quantitative result expressed as a dilution ratio—e.g., 1:8. Sera that prove to be positive using nontreponemal tests must be confirmed using a more specific treponemal antibody test (e.g., FTA-abs or MHA-TP), a qualitative test, the results of which are usually expressed as either nonreactive or reactive. Some labs will report the intensity of the fluorescence, e.g., strong (4+) to weak (1+). In the early stages of primary syphilis, the serology tests may be negative, especially the nontreponemal tests. Nontreponemal antibody titers decline with effective treatment and can be used to measure response to therapy, whereas positive treponemal tests usually remain positive for life. Enzyme-linked immunosorbent assay (ELISA) methods that specifically measure IgM are also available but not widely used except for detecting congenital syphilis. Only the Venereal Disease Research Laboratory (VDRL) nontreponemal antibody test is approved for testing cerebrospinal fluid (CSF) for evidence of neurosyphilis. Chapter 42 describes the clinical use of these tests.

CHANCROID OR HARD CHANCRE

Chancroid is caused by *Haemophilus ducreyi*. Chancroid ulcers must be cleaned to reduce the amount of necrotic exudate frequently present. A swab is then used to collect residual exudate from the ulcer base or margin. The laboratory will use the swab to prepare a slide for Gram staining and to inoculate nonselective and selective blood-containing media. *Haemophilus ducreyi* can be difficult to cultivate unless the transport time is very short and the growth medium fresh and free of any inhibitory substances.[11–13] Although most clinical laboratories do not maintain special growth media for *H. ducreyi,* it is advisable to note on the requisition that *H. ducreyi* is suspected, thus alerting the technologist to examine the medium closely for possible growth. Laboratory diagnosis may rest solely on the appearance of the Gram stain where the organisms present as boxlike coccobacillary rods lined up in a parallel (school-of-fish) arrangement.

LYMPHOGRANULOMA VENEREUM

Lymphogranuloma venereum (LGV) is caused by *Chlamydia trachomatis* serotypes L1, 2, or 3. Its prevalence in the United States is very low; most cases are imported. Samples of the ulcer can be obtained by biopsy or swab and transported to the laboratory, preferably in a sucrose phosphate solution, for culture in permissive cell lines (e.g., McCoy or HeLa 229 cells). Calcium alginate–containing swabs may be toxic to Chlamydia and should not be used for collection. The organism forms cytoplasmic inclusions which can be detected using fluorescein isothiocyanate (FITC)-labeled monoclonal antibody. Suppurating inguinal lymph nodes can be aspirated or biopsied and sent as above. Other direct detection methods using DNA probes or antigen-capture ELISA techniques are also available and do not necessitate maintaining the organism in viable condition, but they do require that the specimen be transported in specific transport media for optimal detection.

Serum antibodies are frequently produced in high titer ($\geq 1:64$) as lymphadenitis develops. Serum antibodies can be detected using complement fixation or, more recently, by micro-immunofluorescent (micro-IF) methods.

GRANULOMA INGUINALE OR DONOVANOSIS

Granuloma inguinale is caused by a gram-negative bacillus currently classified as *Calymmatobacterium granulomatis.* This bacterium has been successfully cultivated only in chick chorioallantoic membranes and therefore is not isolated in the clinical laboratory. Diagnosis is based on the appearance of "donovan bodies" in Giemsa- or Wright-stained material collected from the lesions. Lesion biopsies can be submitted in a small amount of saline or formalin if available.

MOLLUSCUM CONTAGIOSUM

Molluscum contagiosum virus is the etiologic agent and it can be cultured; however, this is not attempted in the typical clinical laboratory. The diagnosis is usually made clinically based on the characteristic appearance of the lesion, which presents as a 3- to 5-mm umbilicated, dome-shaped papule. If culture is needed, biopsied tissue should be sent to a special reference laboratory where the characteristic cytopathic effect that occurs in selected cell lines can be recognized.[14] Lesion biopsies should be kept cold in a moist saline environment during transport. No serologic tests are currently available.

BARTHOLINITIS OR INFECTION OF THE GREATER VESTIBULAR GLAND OR DUCT

Since the ducts open onto the inner surface of the labia minora, any organisms colonizing the vaginal mucosa could cause infection of either the duct or the gland. Usually specimens are submitted for detection of *C. trachomatis* or *Neisseria gonorrhoeae,* but other aerobic and anaerobic organisms may be involved.

To collect exudate from the duct, decontaminate the duct orifice with an iodine solution and collect the expressed exudate on a swab. To sample an infected gland, decontaminate the mucosal surface of the area over the gland and aspirate the glandular exudate using a needle and syringe; or the fluid may be collected on a swab at the time of incision and drainage.

Place the swab or aspirate in an anaerobic transport medium and instruct the laboratory to perform a Gram stain and process for *C. trachomatis* and *N. gonorrhoeae* only on exudate from the duct and for *C. trachomatis* and *N. gonorrhoeae* plus aerobic and anaerobic microorganisms on exudate from the gland. Mixed infections are common. Concurrent endocervical specimens should be collected for *C. trachomatis* and *N. gonorrhoeae* to improve diagnostic sensitivity.

INFECTIONS OF THE VAGINA

VAGINITIS/VAGINOSIS

The three most common causes of vaginitis/vaginosis are:

- Mixed aerobic and anaerobic bacteria associated with bacterial vaginosis
- Yeast
- *Trichomonas vaginalis*

Other organisms—e.g., *Staphylococcus aureus* and β-hemolytic streptococci—may cause vaginal infections, especially if foreign bodies are present. Vaginal infections are usually diagnosed by a wet preparation or "hanging drop" microscopic examination (see Tables A3-1 and A3-2).

Bacterial vaginosis is usually diagnosed at the point of care by the appearance, odor, and pH of the discharge.[15,16] Microscopic examination of the discharge usually shows a lack of inflammatory cells and the appearance of "clue cells."[17,18] Clue cells are vaginal epithelial cells covered with small pleomorphic gram-negative bacilli to the point of obscuring the squamous-cell membranes.[19,20] The number of lactobacilli (long, slender gram-positive rods in chains) is usually reduced or absent.[21] Culture of vaginal discharge is discouraged, since vaginosis is thought to be due to an abnormal mixture of anaerobic and aerobic bacteria that frequently colonize healthy vaginal surfaces; therefore, the culture results are nonspecific.

Yeasts, primarily *Candida albicans,* are a frequent cause of vaginitis; symptoms may range from a mild to severe vulvovaginal pruritus or burning. The production of a thick, whitish, often flocculent, vaginal discharge is common. It is rarely necessary to submit specimens to the laboratory to

---

Table A3-1

PREPARATION OF VAGINAL SECRETIONS FOR "WET PREP" EXAMINATION

1. Collect vaginal secretions from middle third of vaginal wall using a swab.
2. Roll swab onto nitrazine paper to obtain pH, then place into test tube with 1–2 mL of saline.
3. Place one drop of fluid from swab onto each end of a clean microscope slide.
4. Add one drop of 10% KOH to one of the two drops on the slide, noting any amine or "fishy" odor.
5. Coverslip both drops, taking care not to intermix the two drops.
6. Examine both drop areas using the low-power objective, noting:
   a. Appearance of epithelial cells (look for "clue cells")
   b. Presence of WBCs
   c. Motile trichomonads
   d. Fungal elements, pseudohyphae (easier to visualize in KOH-treated drop)
   e. Background bacterial morphotypes, e.g., predominant rods, cocci, etc.

---

make the diagnosis[22]; the yeast cells are easily detected microscopically by preparing a wet-mount of vaginal secretions or by Gram stain. However, if no fungal elements are seen, the yeasts can be readily cultured in the laboratory within 1 to 3 days. Identification of species is sometimes helpful (see Chapter 43). Exudate should be collected with a sterile swab and sent to the laboratory in an aerobic transport.

Trichomonas vaginitis may be suspected in a sexually active patient presenting with a thin, profuse, foamy, yellowish or greenish discharge which may be malodorous. Petechial or punctate hemorrhagic lesions may be present on the mucosal surfaces. Culture is usually unnecessary.[23] Exudate can be collected with a swab and mixed in saline and the mixture used to prepare a wet mount that can be examined microscopically. Examination of urine sediment may also demonstrate motile trichomonads. The parasites typically display a twitchy motility due to four anterior flagellae and another attached to a rapidly undulating membrane that runs about halfway down the length of the cell; however, inactive and dying cells resemble and can be confused with polymorphonuclear leukocytes. Significant leukorrhea frequently accompanies *T. vaginalis* vaginal infection.

Culture is a more sensitive method for detecting *T. vaginalis* and may be required when vaginal douches, creams, or jellies have recently been used because these may interfere with recognition of the parasite.[24] The exudate or a swab used to collect exudate can be submitted to the laboratory, which can be used to inoculate a modified Diamond's media. The specimen should reach the laboratory within 2 hours of collection and maintained at room temperature. The culture medium will support the growth of *T. vaginalis* and allow detection of viable parasites in the original exudate usually within 2 to 4 days.

A DNA probe kit (Affirm VP Microbial Identification Test; MicroProbe Corp., Bothell, WA) has recently become available. It specifically detects moderate to high concentrations of either *Candida* spp., *T. vaginalis,* or *Gardnerella vaginalis* from a single specimen within 1 hour.[25] It is an automated procedure designed to be used in an office setting but has been designated by the Clinical Laboratories Improvement Amendment 1988 (CLIA-88) as a moderately complex test requiring ongoing proficiency testing of personnel and maintenance of quality control records.

TOXIC SHOCK SYNDROME

Toxic shock is usually caused by the proliferation of *Staphylococcus aureus* in the vaginal mucosa and production of a potent exotoxin designated TSST-1. A Dacron swab can be used to collect vaginal exudate and sent to a laboratory for culture using an aerobic transport device. The isolated organism can be sent to a reference laboratory that tests for toxigenic isolates.

Recently, *Streptococcus pyogenes* has proved to be responsible for producing a toxic shock–like syndrome.[27] Isolation of *S. pyogenes* from this body site should be reported to the clinician immediately. Clinical management of toxic shock syndrome is covered in Chap. 49.

GROUP B STREPTOCOCCUS OR *STREPTOCOCCUS AGALACTIAE*

Approximately 15 to 20 percent of women are colonized with *S. agalactiae* and remain asymptomatic; therefore, culturing for this organism in normal, nonpregnant women is of little clinical value. However, during pregnancy, urogenital antepartum carriage of *S. agalactiae* may present a significant risk to the fetus during labor and may cause neonatal sepsis, pneumonia, and meningitis as well as postpartum endometritis. Therefore, pre- or intrapartum screening for the presence of this organism or in the vagina or anorectal area is frequently performed.[28]

To screen for *S. agalactiae,* use a single Dacron swab to collect a specimen from the vaginal wall and perirectal area. A speculum should not be used for this collection. For optimal recovery, place the swab directly into a tube of Todd-Hewitt broth containing antimicrobials, usually gentamicin and nalidixic acid, which will inhibit the growth of most other normal flora, and send the specimen to the laboratory for culture. Alternatively, the swab can be placed into an aer-

Table A3-2

DIAGNOSTIC FEATURES OF INFECTIOUS VAGINITIS

	Normal	Candidal Vaginitis	Bacterial Vaginosis	Trichomonas Vaginitis
Symptoms	None or physiologic leukorrhea	Vulvar pruritus, soreness, increased discharge, dysuria, dyspareunia	Malodorous moderate discharge	Profuse purulent discharge, offensive odor, pruritus, and dyspareunia
Discharge				
Amount	Variable, scant to moderate	Scant to moderate	Moderate	Profuse
Color	Clear or white	White	White/gray	Yellow
Consistency	Floccular, nonhomogeneous	Clumped but variable	Homogeneous, uniformly coating walls	Homogeneous
"Bubbles"	Absent	Absent	Present	Present
Appearance of vulva and vagina	Normal	Introital and vulvar erythema, edema and occasional pustules, vaginal erythema	No inflammation	Erythema and swelling of vulvar and vaginal epithelium "strawberry cervix"
pH of vaginal fluid	<4.5	<4.5	>4.7	5–6.0
Amine test (10% KOH)	Negative	Negative	Positive	Occasionally present
Saline microscopy	Normal epithelial cell Lactobacilli predominate	Normal flora, blastopores (yeast), 40–50% pseudohyphae	Clue cells, coccobacillary flora predominates, absence of leukocytes, motile curved rods	Many PMNs Motile trichomonads (80–90%), no clue cells, abnormal flora
10% KOH microscopy	Negative	Positive (60–90%)	Negative (except in mixed infections)	Negative

obic transport medium and submitted for culture, but low numbers of organisms may not be recovered. If viable *S. agalactiae* is present, it usually can be detected within 24 h. This incubation time to detection can be shortened by incubating the selective media for 4 to 6 h and testing for the production of specific group B antigen using one of several direct antigen detection kits available commercially. These kits have also been used to detect *S. agalactiae* directly in vaginal specimens, but their test sensitivity has been uniformly low when few organisms are present or interfering substances are produced and are not used.[29–33]

Urine cultures positive for *S. agalactiae* may indicate heavy vaginal colonization rather than a urinary tract infection and careful collection techniques to eliminate the potential for vaginal contamination of urine must be employed to differentiate between the two.

MYCOPLASMA/UREAPLASMA

Like *S. agalactiae,* both *Mycoplasma hominis* and *Ureaplasma urealyticum* frequently colonize the vagina. They cause no known lower tract disease but may cause urethritis. *Ureaplasma urealyticum* has been implicated as a cause of pelvic inflammatory disease (PID), postpartum fever and neonatal sepsis, meningitis, and pneumonia; nevertheless, its clinical significance remains controversial.[34] Detection of either organism currently requires culture using specific culture media that are unavailable in most clinical laboratories. For optimal recovery, the specimen should be taken by swab, kept moist, and transported rapidly to the laboratory, where it will be used to inoculate selective growth media. Both *M. hominis* and *U. ure-*

alyticum grow rapidly, and results can be available within 1 to 2 days of inoculation.

CERVICITIS

CHLAMYDIA TRACHOMATIS SEROTYPES D THROUGH K

Chlamydia trachomatis is an obligate intracellular gram-negative bacterium that primarily infects columnar and cuboidal epithelial cells found within the endocervix, urethra, and upper genital tract. Infection may be asymptomatic initially, but they eventually cause PID and salpingitis, leading to diverse sequelae, including infertility. Several methods are being employed to detect *C. trachomatis,* including cell culture,[35,36] antigen capture enzyme immunoassay (EIA),[37] direct fluorescent monoclonal antibody,[38,39] DNA probe,[40,41] and nucleic acid amplification techniques such as the PCR, the ligase chain reaction,[42] and transcription-mediated amplification. For optimal detection, the specimen must be collected and transported using collection kits that are compatible with the method of detection. Collecting specimens from both endocervical and urethral sites improves diagnostic sensitivity compared with that achieved by sampling either site alone. Avoid sampling in the presence of lubricants, which may cause false-negative test reactions.

For culture, columnar or transitional endocervical cells containing infectious elementary bodies must be collected using a Dacron swab (avoid calcium alginate swabs) and transported in a preservative-free buffered sucrose phosphate solution.

The remaining detection methods do not require viable organisms but do require the use of special collection and transport materials to preserve either target proteins or nucleic acids. Once the specimen is in the appropriate transport container, it is usually stable for several days—a distinct advantage over culture, when the specimen must be sent to a distant reference laboratory.

Methods that employ amplification techniques can detect specific nucleotide sequences shed in urine as well as endocervical specimens with increased sensitivity.[42] Collection kits are available for both specimen types and specific to the manufacturer of the kit (e.g., Roche Diagnostic Systems, Branchburg, NJ, and Abbott Diagnostics, North Chicago, IL).

NEISSERIA GONORRHOEAE

The endocervix is the optimal site to sample for the diagnosis of *N. gonorrhoeae*. Additional sites to consider are the urethra, anorectum, and oropharynx. The most convenient collection method is by swab through a water-lubricated speculum. Other lubricants may be bactericidal. Excess mucus should be removed prior to collection, since organisms in the mucus are frequently nonviable. Microscopic examination of gram-stained exudate can be useful but it should be followed up by culture. Errors in interpretation are possible, since other organisms with similar morphology may be present (e.g., other *Neisseria* spp., *Moraxella* spp., and *Acinetobacter* spp.). But if intracellular gram-negative diplococci are seen, a presumptive diagnosis of gonorrhea can be made.

Neisseria gonorrhoeae is a relatively fastidious bacterium that frequently dies in transport unless it is maintained on nutrient media in an elevated CO_2 concentration at room temperature.[43] Endocervical specimens collected by swab, especially cotton-tipped swabs, and transported in the typical aerobic transport devices frequently yield false-negative culture results. Dacron or calcium alginate swabs are preferred. The swabs must be maintained in a moist environment at room temperature and used to inoculate supportive growth media within 12 h of collection. Commercial nutrient transport devices such as JEMBEC (Ames Co., Elkhart, IN), and Isocult, Bio-Bag, and Gono-Pak (Becton Dickinson Microbiology Systems, Cockeysville, MD) contain selective growth media such as Thayer-Martin or Martin-Lewis formulations, along with a CO_2-generating tablet that can be activated to maintain a favorable atmosphere. These systems can be incubated on site if transport is to be delayed.

Alternative methods for direct detection of specific antigens and nucleic acid sequences in endocervical and urine specimens are now available; they are quite sensitive and highly specific. These methods are similar to those described above for the direct detection of *C. trachomatis,* and samples are to be collected and transported according to kit instructions using kit-specific materials. Currently these direct, nonculture methods cannot be used if the organism is to be tested for antimicrobial susceptibility.

UPPER GENITAL TRACT INFECTIONS

Upper genital tract infections can be caused by a wide spectrum of microorganisms but are generally caused by those that infect or colonize the mucosal membranes of the lower tract and gain access to the upper tract by retrograde invasion or are transported by instrumentation.[44] Many cases of PID (salpingitis) are caused by *N. gonorrhoeae* and *C. trachomatis.*[45] *Streptococcus agalactiae* and *G. vaginalis* are frequently isolated from endometrial aspirates.[46] *Mycoplasma hominis* has also been associated with cases of PID. Abscesses frequently yield a mixture of strict and facultative anaerobes such as *Bacteroides* spp., *Prevotella* spp., *Fusobacterium* spp., and *Escherichia coli.* Isolation of *Actinomyces* spp. has been associated with intrauterine de-

COLLECTION AND TRANSPORT OF SPECIMENS FROM THE FEMALE GENITAL TRACT

Clinical Condition	Probable Organism(s)	Optimal Collection Site	Lab Test Method	Appropriate Collection Method	Transport
External genital lesions	HSV	Vesicle/lesion base	Culture/DFA	Syringe/Dacron swab	On ice
	HPV	Condyloma	DNA hybridization	Biopsy (not usually necessary)	
	T. pallidum	Chancre (soft)	Dark field/DFA	Aspiration/scraping	Saline at RT
	H. ducreyi	Chancre (hard)	Gram stain/culture	Swab of lesion base	Aerobic transport
	LGV	Inguinal node	Culture/DFA	Aspiration of node	Sucrose phosphate medium
					On ice
	Granuloma inguinale	Lesion	Fixed tissue stains	Biopsy	In formalin
	Molluscum contagiosum	Lesion	Fixed tissue stains or viral culture	Biopsy (not usually necessary)	In formalin Viral transport medium
Bartholinitis	N. gonorrhoeae C. trachomatis Mixed aerobes/ anaerobes	Drainage from duct or abscessed gland	Culture w/Gram Culture/DFA Aerobic culture Anaerobic culture	Collection of exudate with Dacron swab	Aerobic transport at RT Sucrose phosphate medium/kit slide Anaerobic Transport at RT
Vaginitis/vaginosis	Mixed aerobes/ anaerobes (BV)	Vaginal exudate/ discharge	Slide wet mount/ Gram stain	Collection of vaginal exudate	Microscopic examination at point of care 10% KOH pretreatment
	Yeast Vaginal exudate/ discharge				
	Trichomonas Vaginal exudate/ discharge		Wet mount/culture	Saline washings	Maintain washings at RT
Toxic shock syndrome	S. aureus	Vagina	Culture/toxin test	Swab of exudate	Aerobic transport
Prenatal screening for Group B Strep	Group B Strep	Vagina and perianum	Culture	Swab of vagina and perirectal area	Send swab in selective Todd-Hewett broth or aerobic transport
Cervicitis	N. gonorrhoeae C. trachomatis	Endocervix Endocervix	Culture/DNA probe/EIA/N.A. amplification	Collect: exudate endocervical cells/urine	Sucrose phosphate medium/kit transport devices
Upper genital tract infection	N. gonorrhoeae C. trachomatis Mixed aerobes/ anaerobes	Collection of tissue &/or fluids from site of infection	Culture/N.A. amplification	Tissue and/or fluids from site of infection, or Dacron swab	See above.
	Mycoplasma/ Ureaplasma				Mycoplasma/ ureaplasma: Send swab in balanced salt with albumin (e.g., M-4 medium)

Key: DFA = Direct fluorescent antibody
EIA = Enzyme immunoassay
N.A. = Nucleic acid
RT = room temperature
BV = bacterial vaginosis

vices.[47,48] *Clostridium perfringens* or *Streptococcus pyogenes* may be isolated from postoperative or postabortion cases with myometrial necrosis.

Tissues and fluids collected via laparotomy or laparoscopy are usually not contaminated with resident flora. These specimens should be placed in an anaerobic transport device, maintained at room temperature (cold storage may inhibit the subsequent growth of certain anaerobes and *N. gonorrhoeae*), and delivered to the laboratory within 2 h for Gram-stain examination as well as aerobic and anaerobic culture. In most clinical microbiology laboratories, cultures for the mycoplasmas or *C. trachomatis* require separate requests but can be performed from these same specimens as long as the transport time is within 1 to 2 h. If transport is to be delayed, the special transport containers mentioned above for recovery of these organisms should be used.

Specimens collected via the vaginal vault—e.g., cul-de-sac fluid—are vulnerable to extensive contamination, which can make interpretation of results difficult. To minimize contamination, effective decontamination of mucous membranes must occur prior to specimen collection. Specimens of the upper tract obtained via the endocervical canal should be collected using a catheter device such as the Pipelle, which should be advanced through the endocervix into the uterine cavity while trying to avoid touching the vaginal walls.[49,50] The entire catheter should be transported to the microbiology laboratory without delay for processing. Alternatively, the collected specimen can be expelled into an anaerobic transport tube and submitted.

Specimens collected by swab are suboptimal for recovery of anaerobes; however, they are occasionally used to sample placental membranes or the endometrial mucosal surface. Swabs should be placed into an anaerobic transport medium and sent at room temperature.

SUMMARY

Infections of both the upper and lower urogenital tract can be caused by a broad spectrum of microorganisms; they can frequently be polymicrobial infections involving aerobic, anaerobic, and obligate intracellular organisms, each with their own requirements for appropriate collection and transport to the diagnostic laboratory. Specimens should be collected in such a way as to minimize contamination by normal resident flora, which makes interpretation difficult, since many of the organisms causing upper tract infection are organisms that constitute the normal vaginal flora. There are numerous specimen collection and transport kits and devices available. The person collecting the specimens must be aware of the methods being used in the diagnostic laboratory to which the specimens are to be sent so that collection, transport, and detection methods are compatible. Culture methods that were considered state of the art are rapidly changing in favor of more rapid, non-growth-dependent techniques that require the use of special collection and transport kits. It is an obligation of the laboratory to communicate such changes to the clinical users of these services.

References

1. Sewell DH, Horn AS: Evaluation of a commercial enzyme-linked immunosorbent assay for the detection of herpes simplex virus. *J Clin Microbiol* 21:457, 1985.
2. Lafferty WE, Krofft SK, Remington M, et al: Diagnosis of herpes simplex virus by direct immunofluorescence and viral isolation from samples of external genital lesions in a high-prevalence population. *J Clin Microbiol* 25:323, 1987.
3. Nahass GT, Goldstein BA, Zhu WY, et al: Comparison of the Tzanck smear, viral culture, and DNA diagnostic methods in detection of herpes simplex and varicella zoster infection. *JAMA* 268:2541, 1992.
4. Soloman AR, Rasmussen JE, Varaini J, Pierson CL: The Tzanck smear in the diagnosis of cutaneous herpes simplex. *JAMA* 251:633, 1984.
5. Ashley R, Cent A, Maggs V, et al: Inability of enzyme immunoassays to discriminate between infections with herpes simplex virus types 1 and 2. *Ann Intern Med* 115:520, 1991.
6. Bauer HM, Ting Y, Greer CE, et al: Genital human papillomavirus infections in female university students as determined by a PCR-based method. *JAMA* 265:472, 1991.
7. Karlsen F, Kalantari M, Jenkins A, et al: Use of multiple PCR primer sets for optimal detection of human papillomavirus. *J Clin Microbiol* 34:2095, 1996.
8. Wilber DC, Reichman RC, Stoler MH: Detection of infection by human papillomavirus in genital condylomata: A comparison study using immunocytochemistry and in situ nucleic acid hybridization. *Am J Clin Pathol* 89:505, 1988.
9. Bergeron C, Ferenczy A, Shah KV, Naghashfar Z: Multicentric human papillomavirus infections of the female genital tract: Correlation of viral types with abnormal mitotic figures, colposcopic presentation and localization. *Obstet Gynecol* 69:736, 1987.
10. Larson SA, Steiner BM, Rudolph AH: Laboratory diagnosis and interpretation of tests for syphilis. *Clin Microbiol Rev* 8:1, 1995.
11. Hannah P, Greenwood JR: Isolation and rapid identification of *Haemophilus ducreyi*. *J Clin Microbiol* 16:861, 1982.
12. Hammond GW, Lian CJ, Wilt JC, Ronald AR: Comparison of specimen collection and laboratory techniques for isolation of *Haemophilus ducreyi*. *J Clin Microbiol* 7:39, 1978.

13. Sottnek FO, Biddle JW, Krause SJ, et al: Isolation and identification of *Haemophilus ducreyi* in a clinical study. *J Clin Microbiol* 12:170, 1980.

14. Dennis J, Oshiro LS, Bunter JW: Molluscum contagiosum, another sexually transmitted disease: Its impact on the clinical virology laboratory. *J Infect Dis* 151:376, 1985.

15. Eschenbach DA: Bacterial vaginosis and anaerobes in obstetric-gynecologic infection. *Clin Infect Dis* 16(suppl 4):S282, 1993.

16. Eschenbach DA, Hillier SL, Critchlow C, et al: Diagnosis and clinical manifestations of bacterial vaginosis. *Am J Obstet Gynecol* 158:819, 1988.

17. Spiegel CA, Amsel R, Holmes KK: Diagnosis of bacterial vaginosis by direct Gram stain of vaginal fluid. *J Clin Microbiol* 18:170, 1983.

18. Marquez-Davila G, Martinez-Barreda CE: Predictive value of the "clue cells" investigation and the amine votilization test in vaginal infections caused by *Gardnerella vaginalis* from clinical specimens. *J Clin Microbiol* 22:865, 1985.

19. Nugent RP, Krohn MA, Hillier SL: Reliability of diagnosing bacterial vaginosis is improved by a standardized method of Gram stain interpretation. *J Clin Microbiol* 29:297, 1991.

20. Joesoef MR, Hillier SL, Josodiwondo S, Linnan M: Reproducibility of a scoring system for Gram stain diagnosis of bacterial vaginosis. *J Clin Microbiol* 29:1730, 1991.

21. Redondo-Lopez V, Cook RL, Sobel JD: Emerging role of lactobacilli in the control and maintenance of the vaginal bacterial microflora. *Rev Infect Dis* 12:856, 1990.

22. Reed BD, Huck W, Zazove P: Differentiation of *Gardnerella vaginalis, Candida albicans* and *Trichomonas vaginalis* infections of the vagina. *J Fam Pract* 28:673, 1989.

23. Levett PN: A comparison of five methods for the detection of *Trichomonas vaginalis* in clinical specimens. *Med Lab Sci* 37:85, 1980.

24. Gelbart SM, Thomasen JL, Osypowski PJ, et al: Growth of *Trichomonas vaginalis* in commercial culture media. *J Clin Microbiol* 28:962, 1990.

25. Briselden AM, Hillier SL: Evaluation of Affirm VP microbial identification test for *Gardnerella vaginalis* and *Trichomonas vaginalis*. *J Clin Microbiol* 32:148, 1994.

26. Shands KN, Schmid GP, Dan BB, et al: Toxic shock syndrome in menstruating women: Association with tampon use and *Staphylococcus aureus* and clinical features in 52 cases. *N Engl J Med* 303:1436, 1980.

27. Musser JM: Clinical relevance of streptococcal pyrogenic exotoxins in streptococcal toxic shock-like syndrome and other severe invasive infections. *Pediatr Ann* 21:821, 1992.

28. Yancey MK, Armer T, Clark P, Duff P: Assessment of rapid identification tests for genital carriage of group B streptococci. *Obstet Gynecol* 80:1038, 1992.

29. Morales WJ, Lim D: Reduction of group B streptococcal maternal and neonatal infections in preterm pregnancies with premature rupture of membranes through a rapid identification test. *Am J Obstet Gynecol* 157:13, 1987.

30. Wanger AR: Cervical screening tests for group B streptococci. *Clin Microbiol Newsl* 14:149, 1992.

31. Wust J, Hebisch G, Peters K: Evaluation of two enzyme immunoassays for rapid detection of group B streptococci in pregnant women. *Eur J Clin Microbiol Infect Dis* 12:124, 1993.

32. Greenspoon JS, Fishman A, Wilcox JG, et al: Comparison of culture for group B streptococcus versus enzyme immunoassay and latex agglutination rapid tests: Results in 250 patients during labor. *Obstet Gynecol* 77:97, 1991.

33. Skoll MA, Mercer BM, Baselski V, et al: Evaluation of two rapid group B streptococcal antigen tests in labor and delivery patients. *Obstet Gynecol* 77:322, 1991.

34. Taylor-Robinson D, Munday PE: Mycoplasmal infection of the female genital tract and its complications, in Hare MJ (ed): *Genital Tract Infection in Women.* New York: Churchill Livingstone, 1988, pp 228–247.

35. Mahoney JB, Phernesky MA: Effect of swab type and storage temperature in the isolation of *Chlamydia trachomatis* from clinical specimens. *J Clin Microbiol* 22:865, 1985.

36. Aarnaes SL, Peterson EM, de la Maza LM: The effect of media and temperature on the storage of *Chlamydia trachomatis. Am J Clin Pathol* 81:237, 1984.

37. Forbes BA, Bartholoma N, McMillan J, et al: Evaluation of a monoclonal antibody test to detect *Chlamydia trachomatis* in cervical and urethral specimens. *J Clin Microbiol* 23:1127, 1986.

38. Cheresky MA, Mahoney JB, Castriciano S, et al: Detection of *Chlamydia trachomatis* antigens by enzyme immunoassay and immunofluorescence in genital specimens from symptomatic and asymptomatic men and women. *J Infect Dis* 154:141, 1986.

39. Krepel J, Laur I, Sposton A, et al: PCR and direct fluorescent-antibody staining confirm *Chlamydia trachomatis* antigens in swabs and urine below the detection threshold of Chlamydiazyme Enzyme Immunoassay. *J Clin Microbiol* 33:2847, 1995.

40. Kluytmans JAJW, Niesters HGM, Moulton JW, et al: Performance of a non-isotopic DNA probe for the detection of *Chlamydia trachomatis* in urogenital specimens. *J Clin Microbiol* 29:2685, 1991.

41. Limberger RJ, Biega R, Evancoe A, et al: Evaluation of culture and Gen-Probe Pace 2 assay for the detection of *Neisseria gonorrhoeae* and *Chlamydia trachomatis* in endocervical specimens transported to a state health laboratory. *J Clin Microbiol* 30:1161, 1992.

42. Schachter J, Moncada J, Whidden R, et al: Noninvasive tests for diagnosis of *Chlamydia trachomatis* infection: Application of ligase chain reaction to first-catch urine

specimens of women. *J Infect Dis* 172:1411, 1995.

43. Spence MR, Guzik DS, Katta LR: The isolation of *Neisseria gonorrhoeae*—A comparison of three culture transport systems. *Sex Transm Dis* 10:138, 1983.

44. Faro S: Vaginal flora and pelvic inflammatory disease. *Am J Obstet Gynecol* 169:470, 1993.

45. Patton DL, Askienazy-Elbhar M, Henry-Suchet J, et al: Detection of *Chlamydia trachomatis* in fallopian tube tissue in women with postinfection tubal infertility. *Am J Obstet Gynecol* 171:95, 1994.

46. Gibbs RS, Blanco JD, St Clair PJ, et al: Quantitative bacteriology of amniotic fluid from women with clinical intramnionic infection at term. *J Infect Dis* 145:1, 1982.

47. Pearlman M: Abdominal wall *Actinomyces* abscess associated with an intrauterine device. *J Reprod Med* 36:398, 1991.

48. Jones MC, Buschmann BO, Dowling EA, Pollock HM: The prevalence of *Actinomyces*-like organisms found in cervicovaginal smears of 300 IUD wearers. *Acta Cytol* 23:282, 1979.

49. Eschenbach DA, Rosene K, Tompkins LS, et al: Endometrial cultures obtained by a triple-lumen method from afebrile and febrile postpartum women. *J Infect Dis* 153:1038, 1986.

50. Martens MG, Faro S, Hammill HA, et al: Transcervical uterine cultures with a new endometrial suction curette: A comparison of three sampling methods in postpartum endometritis. *Obstet Gynecol* 74:273, 1989.

INDEX

Page numbers followed by *f* or *t* refer to figures or tables.

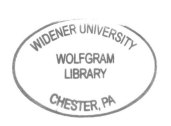

ISBN 0-07-049127-5

90000>

9 780070 491274